PA PASSifier

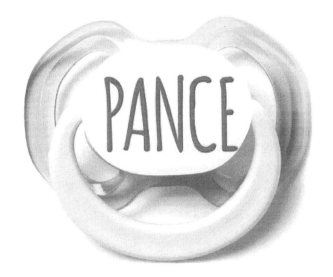

Matthew Bach PA-C

Shelby Bach PA-C

ISBN: 9798857948347

Acknowledgement

Special recognition goes out to the dedicated students or practitioners who are utilizing this study resource. Your commitment to reach this stage is commendable. We understand that there was a time when opening a study resource to learn medicine was just a distant dream. Today, that dream is your reality – a testament to your hard work.

We acknowledge the journey you've undertaken, marked by nights of uncertainty about your educational path to the days of excitement leading up to starting your PA program. This path of peaks and valleys will undoubtedly continue throughout your training and lead you to be a great practitioner.

In the midst of it all, please remember; every step you've taken and every challenge you've faced has brought you where you are today. You've earned every opportunity and achievement that lies before you. Embrace your accomplishments and let them fuel your drive as you continue to make a meaningful impact in the field of medicine. Your journey is a testament to your hard work.

You truly deserve this.

TABLE OF CONTENTS

Chapter 1
Cardiovascular

Dilated Cardiomyopathy

Etiology & Risk Factors	• Progressive dilation or enlargement of the ventricles resulting in a decreased left ventricular ejection fraction (less than 40%)
	• <u>Etiologies</u>: **idiopathic**; multiple genetic and environmental factors, **prolonged ischemia**
	   • <u>Infectious</u>: **post-viral myocarditis (most common identifiable cause)**; enterovirus, coxsackievirus B, Lyme's disease, parvovirus, HIV
	   • <u>Metabolic</u>: **obesity**, diabetes, thyroid dysfunction, vitamin B1 (thiamine) deficiency (alcohol abuse)
	• <u>Risk Factors</u>: **male**, advanced age, **alcohol and substance abuse, hypertension**, family history, autoimmune disorders, certain infectious disorders, certain metabolic disorders, certain ethnicities (African American descent are at 3x greater risk), pregnancy

Patho-physiology	• Myocardial remodeling causes left ventricle dilation resulting in systolic dysfunction secondary to poor contractility and weakness of cardiac myocytes, thus reducing the ejection fraction; progressive dilation can lead to significant mitral and tricuspid valve regurgitation • Renin-angiotensin aldosterone system activation causes increased heart rate and peripheral vascular system tone as compensatory mechanism that eventually fails

Signs & Symptoms	• <u>Left Sided Heart Failure</u>: **dyspnea is most common symptom**, fatigue, paroxysmal nocturnal dyspnea, orthopnea
	• <u>Right Sided Heart Failure</u>: **lower extremity edema**, hepatomegaly, **jugular venous distention**
	• May present with longstanding hypertension, thromboembolic events, arrhythmias, conduction changes
	• <u>Physical Exam</u>:
	   • <u>S3 Gallop</u>: caused by deceleration of inflow during diastole
	   • <u>Pulmonary Crackles/Rales</u>: due to fluid overload on lungs, particularly at lower lung fields
	   • <u>Cheyne-Stokes Respirations</u>: cyclical apneic and hyperventilating breathing patterns
	   • <u>Pulsus Alternans</u>: alternating strong and weak arterial beats
	   • <u>Tricuspid/Mitral Regurgitation Murmurs</u>: due to dilated ventricles/annular dilation

Diagnosis	• <u>**Echocardiogram**</u>: **preferred diagnostic test** to determine any valvular disorders, size and functional capacity; **demonstrates LV dilation/dysfunction, hypokinesis & LVEF <40%**
	• <u>Chest X-Ray (CXR)</u>: **cardiomegaly**, pulmonary effusions and venous congestion, and pleural effusions (**right more common** than left)
	• <u>Electrocardiogram (ECG)</u>: sinus tachycardia, left bundle branch block (LBBB), nonspecific ST-T wave changes, **left ventricular hypertrophy**, conduction abnormalities (ectopy)
	• <u>**Cardiac Markers**</u>:
	   • <u>**Brain Natriuretic Peptide (BNP)**</u>: **or N-terminal pro-BNP** aids in diagnosis and prognosis
	   • <u>**Troponin I or T**</u>: determines acute ischemic involvement
	• <u>Coronary Angiogram</u>: performed in patients with no known CAD history to rule out ischemic disease

Treatment	• <u>Lifestyle Modifications</u>: **alcohol cessation**; treat underlying condition, proper nutrition and exercise, cardiac rehabilitation, sleep hygiene, smoking cessation • <u>**Congestive Heart Failure Treatment**</u>: **ACE inhibitors** (decreases overall mortality), ARBs, beta blockers, **diuretics** (manages hypervolemia symptoms (dyspnea/edema); digoxin • **CCBs are contraindicated** • <u>Anticoagulation</u>: indicated in patients with history of atrial fibrillation, artificial heart valves, or identified mural thrombus • <u>Device Therapy</u>: cardioverter-defibrillators (ICDs) or cardiac resynchronization therapy (CRT) devices may be implanted to help regulate heart rhythm and improve pumping efficiency; considered if LVEF<35 • <u>Heart transplant</u>: indicated in severe cases with heart failure that does not respond to other treatments; may be considered as a last resort

Dilated left ventricle

Takotsubo Cardiomyopathy

Etiology & Risk Factors	• **Stress induced cardiomyopathy** ("broken-heart syndrome") • <u>Etiology</u>: not fully understood; **acute surge in catecholamines (stress hormones) due to emotional or physical stress** • <u>Risk Factors</u>: **emotional or physical stress (death, fear, medical diagnosis/illness, argument, financial loss, domestic abuse), female (most common in postmenopausal women)**, age (>50 years old most common), history of neurologic or psychiatric disorders, pre-existing cardiovascular risk factors (hypertension, atherosclerosis)
Patho-physiology	• **Acutely stressful or traumatizing events results in a major catecholamine discharge** leading to cardiac dysfunction • Catecholamines cause microvascular spasm/dysfunction or myocardial injury resulting in the characteristic ballooning or apical ballooning of the left ventricle • Estrogen has a protective element to the cardiovascular system through vasodilation and protection against endothelial dysfunction/atherosclerosis which may explain why post-menopausal women experience exaggerated vasoconstriction and sympathetic activation as a result of trauma or stress

Signs & Symptoms	• <u>**Chest Pain**</u>: **acute retrosternal chest pain, pressure, discomfort**; indistinguishable from acute myocardial infarction
	• <u>**Congestive Heart Failure (CHF)**</u>: dyspnea (due impaired contractility of the heart), fatigue, acute lower extremity edema, dizziness, syncope
	   • *May develop late systolic murmur due to left outflow obstruction*
	   • Cardiogenic shock & sudden congestive heart failure signs (approximately 10% of patients will develop cardiogenic shock)
	• <u>**Arrhythmias**</u>: supraventricular tachycardias, ventricular tachycardia/fibrillation due to the sudden and transient impairment of cardiac function

Diagnosis	• <u>Electrocardiogram (ECG)</u>: **ST segment elevation that can mimic STEMI** in anterior distribution; staging can mimic pericarditis • <u>Troponin</u>: may be elevated or normal but not as elevated as a traditional STEMI; • <u>Brain Natriuretic Peptide (BNP)</u>: may be elevated • <u>Echocardiogram</u>: systolic dysfunction (EF<25-35%); **left ventricle systolic apical ballooning** and reduced contractility • <u>Coronary Angiogram</u>: invasive procedure utilized only with ST segment elevation and/or troponin elevation • Will demonstrate **no evidence of significant coronary artery blockage**, no plaque rupture, and **patent coronary arteries**

Treatment	• <u>**Treat as Acute Coronary Syndrome**</u>: STEMI treatment until ACS can be ruled out
	   • **Aspirin** (antiplatelet); **nitroglycerin** (vasodilation); **beta-blocker** (rate/rhythm control); **heparin** (anticoagulant); *consider lipid-lowering agent*
	   • *Discontinue QTc prolonging drugs; consider repleting magnesium*
	• <u>Monitoring</u>: serial ECGs to monitor QTc intervals & arrhythmias; serial echocardiograms to detect wall motion abnormalities and ventricular ejection fraction
	• <u>Prevention</u>: cardio-selective beta-blockers & ACEI may be supportive in preventing recurrence

Key Words & Most Common	• Postmenopausal woman experiencing stressful event • Caused by catecholamine discharge; possible vasospasm • Symptoms comparable to acute MI • ECG mimics anterior STEMI; angiogram shows patent coronary arteries • Treat as STEMI until ACS ruled out

Apical ballooning on echocardiogram

Restrictive Cardiomyopathy

Etiology & Risk Factors	• Restrictive myocardial condition secondary to non-compliant or stiff ventricles as a result of infiltrative or fibrotic systemic disease
	• Etiologies:
	  • <u>Infiltrative Diseases</u>: **amyloidosis is most common cause**; sarcoidosis, hemochromatosis
	  • <u>Fibrosis and Scarring</u>: endomyocardial fibrosis, Löeffler endocarditis, and systemic sclerosis (scleroderma), postoperative changes
	  • <u>Other</u>: idiopathic, certain genetic disorders, radiation therapy, certain medications (ergotamine or serotonin containing drugs)

Patho-physiology	• Infiltrative diseases can lead to the accumulation of abnormal substances (amyloid fibrils, iron, or inflammatory cells) within the heart muscle, causing it to become stiff and less compliant resulting in diastolic dysfunction as stiff ventricles impede filling that may lead to mitral/tricuspid regurgitation and venous pulmonary hypertension • Ventricle wall thickening leads to high diastolic filling pressures and impaired filling; may cause AV blocks or arrhythmias if nodal/conduction tissue is affected

Signs & Symptoms	• <u>Left Sided Heart Failure</u>: **exertional dyspnea, orthopnea**, paroxysmal nocturnal dyspnea, and **peripheral edema**
	  • **Fatigue** (result of fixed cardiac output); angina or syncope
	  • **Diastolic heart failure**; pulmonary hypertension often present
	• <u>Physical Exam</u>:
	  • <u>Vascular Congestion</u>: low-volume and rapid carotid pulse, pulmonary crackles, pronounced jugular venous distention
	  • <u>Kussmaul's Sign</u>: paradoxical rise in jugular venous pressure occurring with inspiration

Diagnosis	• <u>Echocardiogram</u>: **preferred diagnostic test**; aids in differentiating from constrictive pericarditis
	  • **Diastolic dysfunction with preserved left ventricle (LV) ejection fraction; elevated left ventricle filling pressures**
	  • May show **atrial dilation**; myocardial hypertrophy with non-dilated ventricles (LV is small)
	• <u>Electrocardiogram (ECG)</u>: **low voltage QRS complex**; arrhythmias; AV blocks; pathologic Q waves
	• <u>Chest X-Ray (CXR)</u>: heart typically normal sized, atria may be enlarged, pulmonary congestion pattern
	• <u>Endomyocardial biopsy</u>: **definitive diagnosis**; differentiates restrictive disease from other forms of myopathies
	  • Biopsy for amyloidosis associated with immunoglobulins green birefringence with congo-red staining on biopsy

Treatment	• <u>Diuretics</u>: **indicated for peripheral edema and pulmonary vascular congestion to reduce fluid overload**
	  • *Caution with diuretics as cardiac output is dependent on preload*
	  • *Caution with afterload reduction to avoid abrupt hypotension*
	• <u>Beta blockers or Calcium Channel Blockers</u>: may be used to decrease heart rate and increase filling time
	• <u>Treat Underlying Disorder</u>: chelation or phlebotomy therapy for hemochromatosis; steroids for sarcoidosis

Key Words & Most Common	• Diastolic dysfunction caused by stiff ventricular walls that restricts filling; amyloidosis is most common cause • Dyspnea, orthopnea, peripheral edema • Echocardiogram shows dilation of atrium, diastolic dysfunction & elevated LV filling pressure; biopsy is definitive • Treat based on symptoms or underlying disorder

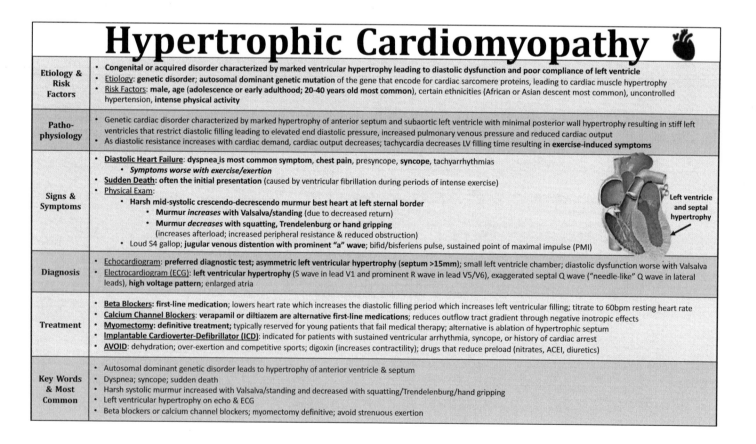

Stiff, non-compliant ventricles

Hypertrophic Cardiomyopathy

Etiology & Risk Factors	• **Congenital or acquired disorder characterized by marked ventricular hypertrophy leading to diastolic dysfunction and poor compliance of left ventricle** • <u>Etiology</u>: **genetic disorder; autosomal dominant genetic mutation** of the gene that encode for cardiac sarcomere proteins, leading to cardiac muscle hypertrophy • <u>Risk Factors</u>: **male, age (adolescence or early adulthood; 20-40 years old most common)**, certain ethnicities (African or Asian descent most common), uncontrolled hypertension, **intense physical activity**
Patho-physiology	• Genetic cardiac disorder characterized by marked hypertrophy of anterior septum and subaortic left ventricle with minimal posterior wall hypertrophy resulting in stiff left ventricles that restrict diastolic filling leading to elevated end diastolic pressure, increased pulmonary venous pressure and reduced cardiac output • As diastolic resistance increases with cardiac demand, cardiac output decreases; tachycardia decreases LV filling time resulting in **exercise-induced symptoms**

Signs & Symptoms	• <u>Diastolic Heart Failure</u>: **dyspnea is most common symptom, chest pain**, presyncope, **syncope**, tachyarrhythmias
	  • *Symptoms worse with exercise/exertion*
	• <u>Sudden Death</u>: **often the initial presentation** (caused by ventricular fibrillation during periods of intense exercise)
	• <u>Physical Exam</u>:
	  • **Harsh mid-systolic crescendo-decrescendo murmur best heart at left sternal border**
	    • Murmur *increases* with Valsalva/standing (due to decreased return)
	    • Murmur *decreases* with squatting, Trendelenburg or hand gripping
	      (increases afterload; increased peripheral resistance & reduced obstruction)
	  • Loud S4 gallop; **jugular venous distention with prominent "a" wave**; bifid/bisferiens pulse, sustained point of maximal impulse (PMI)

Diagnosis	• <u>Echocardiogram</u>: **preferred diagnostic test; asymmetric left ventricular hypertrophy (septum >15mm)**; small left ventricle chamber; diastolic dysfunction worse with Valsalva • <u>Electrocardiogram (ECG)</u>: **left ventricular hypertrophy** (S wave in lead V1 and prominent R wave in lead V5/V6), exaggerated septal Q wave ("needle-like" Q wave in lateral leads), **high voltage pattern**; enlarged atria
Treatment	• <u>Beta Blockers</u>: **first-line medication**; lowers heart rate which increases the diastolic filling period which increases left ventricular filling; titrate to 60bpm resting heart rate • <u>Calcium Channel Blockers</u>: **verapamil or diltiazem are alternative first-line medications**; reduces outflow tract gradient through negative inotropic effects • <u>Myomectomy</u>: **definitive treatment**; typically reserved for young patients that fail medical therapy; alternative is ablation of hypertrophic septum • <u>Implantable Cardioverter-Defibrillator (ICD)</u>: indicated for patients with sustained ventricular arrhythmia, syncope, or history of cardiac arrest • <u>AVOID</u>: dehydration; over-exertion and competitive sports; digoxin (increases contractility); drugs that reduce preload (nitrates, ACEI, diuretics)
Key Words & Most Common	• Autosomal dominant genetic disorder leads to hypertrophy of anterior ventricle & septum • Dyspnea; syncope; sudden death • Harsh systolic murmur increased with Valsalva/standing and decreased with squatting/Trendelenburg/hand gripping • Left ventricular hypertrophy on echo & ECG • Beta blockers or calcium channel blockers; myomectomy definitive; avoid strenuous exertion

Left ventricle and septal hypertrophy

Myocarditis

Etiology & Risk Factors	• Inflammation of the myocardium with necrosis of cardiac myocytes
	• Etiology:
	  • Viral: **enterovirus (Coxsackievirus B), parvovirus B19 and human herpes virus 6 most common**; adenovirus, influenza A&B; **COVID-19**;
	  • Bacterial: beta-hemolytic Streptococcus; Mycoplasma; Toxoplasma; Histoplasmosis; Lyme disease
	  • Drugs/Medications: **clozapine**, antibiotics, Indomethacin, sulfonamides, doxorubicin, cocaine
	  • Inflammatory Conditions: systemic lupus erythematosus, rheumatoid arthritis, sarcoidosis, Chagas disease (most common cause worldwide)
	• Risk Factors: **male, age (most common in young patients, 20-50 years old)**, recent viral illness, history of autoimmune disorder, radiation or chemotherapy

Patho-physiology	• The immune system's response to various triggers including viral infections, bacteria, parasites, or autoimmune processes which activates the immune cells to attack the myocardium, leading to inflammation, tissue damage, disruption of normal heart function and eventual necrosis of cardiac myocyte cells
Signs & Symptoms	• **Flu-Like Symptoms**: cardiac symptoms may be preceded by **fever**, myalgias, fatigue, URI symptoms, nausea and vomiting that progress to new onset heart failure symptoms • **Heart Failure Symptoms**: chest pain, dyspnea, fatigue, **tachycardia out of proportion to fever** • Chest pain worse with thoracic motion, cough, breathing, or swallowing food; relieved by sitting up and leaning forward • Physical Exam: **S3 gallop; pericardial friction rub** (pericarditis) • *Consider in septic appearing patient that decompensates after receiving IVF or in healthy patient with new onset heart failure/arrhythmias*
Diagnosis	• Chest X-Ray (CXR): cardiomegaly; pulmonary edema • Electrocardiogram (ECG): **sinus tachycardia**, low voltage pattern, prolonged QTc, **nonspecific diffuse ST elevations** and PR depressions in precordial leads (pericarditis) • Cardiac Enzymes: elevated cardiac troponin and creatine kinase muscle band isoenzyme (CK-MB) due to cardiac myocyte necrosis; **increased erythrocyte sedimentation rate** • Echocardiogram: decreased left ventricle ejection fraction (systolic dysfunction), wall motion abnormalities and hypokinesis • **Endomyocardial Biopsy**: **gold standard** but rarely used; demonstrates inflammatory infiltrate of myocardium and necrosis of myocytes
Treatment	• Treat Underlying Etiology: consider **antiviral agents** (nirmatrelvir, ritonavir, oseltamivir) as indicated; limited evidence of efficacy with IVIG/steroids in COVID-19 • **Treatment of Heart Failure**: ACEI, beta blockers, diuretics, nitrates to treat systolic heart failure symptoms
Key Words & Most Common	• Young patients with few risk factors with new onset systolic heart failure • Viral etiology is most common • Flu-like illness progresses to heart failure symptoms • Biopsy is gold standard • Supportive cardiac treatment; treat underlying cause **Myocyte necrosis seen on histopathology**

Sinus Arrhythmia

Etiology & Risk Factors	• Common rhythm variation often seen in **young patients or children;** considered indicator of good cardiovascular health • Etiology: changes in the normal electrical activity of the heart's sinus node • Risk Factors: **age (most common in young adults or children)**, more common in physically active patients or during certain physiological states (deep breathing or sleep)
Patho-physiology	• Respiratory drive leads to vagal nerve stimulation and changes in cardiac filling pressure during inspiration leading to an irregular R-R interval variation
Signs & Symptoms	• **Asymptomatic** • Normal finding (not considered pathologic unless new onset accompanied with hearth failure symptoms • Rhythm *increases* during periods of inspiration; rhythm *decreases* during periods of expiration

Diagnosis	• **Electrocardiogram (ECG)**: no acute abnormalities
	  • **Bradycardia**
	  • Normal monoformic P waves
	  • **R-R interval >0.12 seconds** with irregular rate
	  • **Decreased P-P intervals (faster rate) during inspiration; increased P-P intervals (slower rate) during expiration**
	• Auscultation: increased heart rate during periods of inhalation that slows during exhalation

Treatment	• **No Treatment Required**: considered indicator of good cardiovascular health • Atropine: consider if symptomatic bradycardia
Key Words & Most Common	• Young, healthy patient with few/no risk factors • Stimulation of vagus nerve • Increased rate with inspiration; decreased rate with expiration • ECG shows R-R interval >0.12s • No treatment required – indicator of good health

Sinus Tachycardia

Etiology & Risk Factors	• **Heart rate greater than 100 beats per minute**
	• Etiology: physiologic or pathologic; **considered first sign of serious pathology**
	  • Physiologic: **exercise**, stress, anxiety, pain; normal in young children or infants
	  • Pathologic:
	    • Cardiac: myocarditis, tamponade, ACS
	    • Respiratory: **pulmonary embolism**, hypoxia
	    • GI/Renal/Electrolyte: hypoglycemia, **hypovolemia/dehydration**, hyperkalemia, hypocalcemia, hypomagnesemia
	    • Infectious: acute infection or sepsis, fever
	    • Vascular: shock (cardiogenic, hypovolemic, obstructive, distributive)
	    • Hematologic: anemia, **hemorrhage**
	    • Endocrine: pregnancy, hyperthyroidism
	    • Medications: albuterol, amphetamines, antihistamines/decongestants, epinephrine, scopolamine
	    • Toxicology: cocaine, caffeine, carbon monoxide; withdrawal (alcohol, benzo, opioid, sedative hypnotics)

Patho-physiology	• **Increased impulse from the sinoatrial node** due to physiologic, pathologic, medication, or toxicology cause
Signs & Symptoms	• **Asymptomatic**: most common • Symptomatic: may have dizziness, dyspnea, chest pain, palpitations, presyncope/syncope
Diagnosis	• Evaluate Hemodynamic Status: hypoxia, altered mental status, hypotension or hypertension, volume status, shock • **Electrocardiogram (ECG): regular sinus rhythm greater than 100 beats per minute** • P wave followed by QRS complex & T wave; upright P wave in leads I, II, & aVL, negative in aVR • **Testing to Identify Underlying Etiology**: CXR, labs, toxicology screen, ABG, d-dimer • 24-hour Holter Monitor: may be utilized to determine arrhythmia
Treatment	• **Treat Underlying Etiology**: if pathologic; remove offending medication • **Beta Blockers**: may be used in management of acute myocardial ischemia for rate control
Key Words & Most Common	• Heart rate greater than 100 beats per minute • May be physiologic, pathologic, caused by medication or toxicologic cause • Often asymptomatic • ECG shows rhythm > 100 bpm • Treat underlying cause

Sinus Bradycardia

Etiology & Risk Factors	• **Heart rate less than 60 beats per minute**
	• Etiology: physiologic, pathologic, intrinsic or extrinsic
	  • Physiologic: young athletes, sleep, vasovagal response
	  • Pathologic: **ischemia**, carotid sinus sensitivity (carotid massage), hypoxia, sleep apnea, intracranial hypertension, anorexia nervosa/bulimia (vomiting), trauma, Lyme disease, rheumatic conditions, neuromuscular disorder, hypothyroidism, hypothermia
	  • Medications: beta blockers, calcium channel blockers, antiarrhythmics, digoxin, adenosine,
	  • Toxicology: cannabinoids, opioids
	• Risk Factors: **common in athletes** or adults over age of 65

Patho-physiology	• Cardiac rhythm with cardiac depolarization from the sinus node at less than 60 beats per minute • Increased vagal tone in healthy patient
Signs & Symptoms	• **Asymptomatic**: most common • **Symptomatic**: may have fatigue, dizziness, syncope or presyncope, exercise intolerance
Diagnosis	• Evaluate Hemodynamic Status: hypoxia, altered mental status, hypotension • **Electrocardiogram (ECG): regular rhythm less than 60 beats per minute** • P wave followed by QRS complex & T wave; upright P wave in leads I, II, & aVL, negative in aVR • **Testing to Identify Underlying Etiology**: blood glucose level, labs, toxicology screen, cardiac enzymes • 24-hour Holter Monitor: may be utilized to determine arrhythmia
Treatment	• **Observation**: no treatment required if asymptomatic • **Treat Underlying Etiology**: if pathologic; remove offending medication • **Atropine**: first-line medication in symptomatic patient • Atropine vs epinephrine vs transcutaneous pacing in setting of hemodynamically unstable patient
Key Words & Most Common	• Heart rate less than 60 beats per minute • May be physiologic, pathologic, caused by medication or toxicologic cause • Often asymptomatic • ECG shows rhythm <60 bpm • Treat underlying cause; evaluate hemodynamic status; atropine if symptomatic

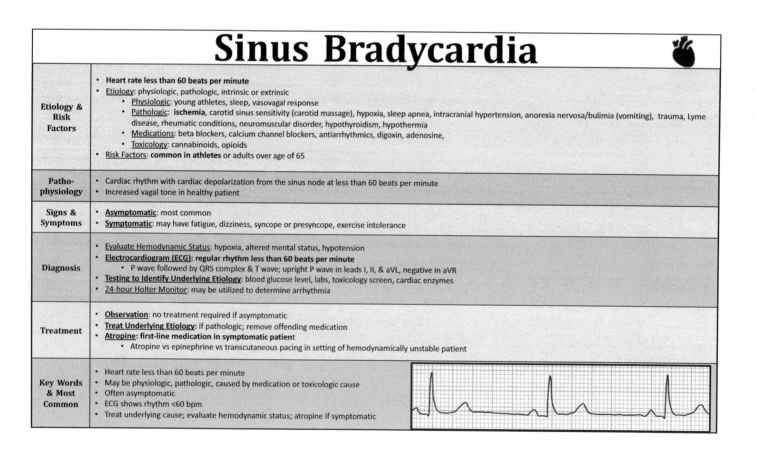

Sick Sinus Syndrome

Etiology & Risk Factors	• Sinus node dysfunction in which the sinoatrial node has impaired pacemaker function
	• Etiology: caused by intrinsic or extrinsic factors
	  • Intrinsic: **fibrosis is most common, age**, congenital disorder, surgery (specifically valve replacement surgery as damage to SA node possible)
	  • Extrinsic: carotid sinus hypersensitivity (carotid massage), vasovagal syncope
	  • Conditions: hypoxia, hypothermia, hypothyroidism, hyper or hypokalemia, sleep apnea
	  • Medications: class I-IV antiarrhythmics, lithium, digoxin

Patho-physiology	• Age-related fibrosis and degeneration of the sinoatrial node leads to impaired electrical conduction and rhythm disturbances in the heart
	• Disorder of the sinoatrial node
	  • Pacemaker "P cells" fail to generate action potential
	  • Transitional "T cells" fail to transmit impulse to right atrium

Signs & Symptoms	• **Asymptomatic**: most common in early stages
	• **Symptomatic**: exercise intolerance, lightheadedness
	  • **Alternating tachycardia & bradycardia symptoms**
	  • Hypoperfusion Symptoms: during instances of bradycardia
	    • Central Nervous System: **syncope or presyncope**
	    • Gastrointestinal: abdominal pain
	    • Renal: oliguria (decreased urine output)

Diagnosis	• Testing to Identify Underlying Etiology: electrolyte imbalance (CMP), sleep apnea, metabolic dysfunction • Evaluate Hemodynamic Status: hypoxia, altered mental status, hypotension, volume status • Electrocardiogram (ECG): **often does not capture due to episodic nature of condition** • **24-hour Holter Monitor or Telemetry**: periods of bradycardia alternating with atrial tachyarrhythmias; utilized due to episodic nature of condition
Treatment	• Treat Underlying Etiology: if pathologic; remove offending medication • **Atropine**: consider in hemodynamically unstable symptomatic patient • **Permanent Pacemaker**: indicated in symptomatic patients caused by bradycardia • **Anticoagulation**: in atrial tachyarrhythmias due to increased risk of stroke
Key Words & Most Common	• Sinus node dysfunction with alternating bradycardia & tachyarrhythmias • Fibrosis & age are most common causes • Symptoms as result of hypoperfusion • 24-hour Holter monitor or telemetry to capture rhythm • Atropine if unstable, pacemaker for symptomatic patients

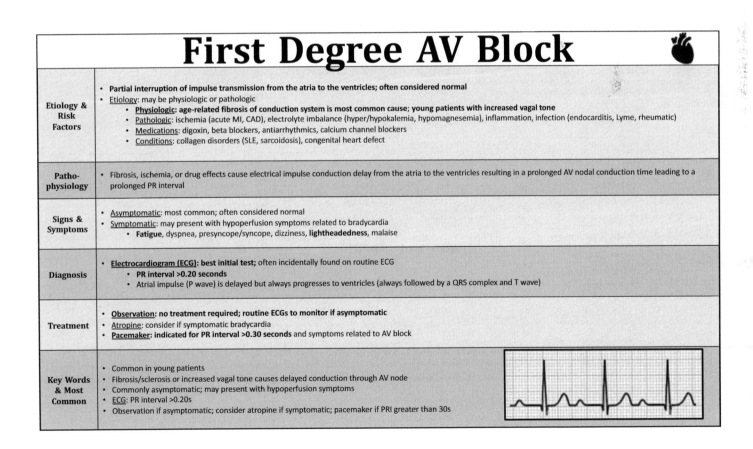

First Degree AV Block

Etiology & Risk Factors	• **Partial interruption of impulse transmission from the atria to the ventricles; often considered normal**
	• Etiology: may be physiologic or pathologic
	  • **Physiologic: age-related fibrosis of conduction system is most common cause; young patients with increased vagal tone**
	  • Pathologic: ischemia (acute MI, CAD), electrolyte imbalance (hyper/hypokalemia, hypomagnesemia), inflammation, infection (endocarditis, Lyme, rheumatic)
	  • Medications: digoxin, beta blockers, antiarrhythmics, calcium channel blockers
	  • Conditions: collagen disorders (SLE, sarcoidosis), congenital heart defect

Patho-physiology	• Fibrosis, ischemia, or drug effects cause electrical impulse conduction delay from the atria to the ventricles resulting in a prolonged AV nodal conduction time leading to a prolonged PR interval
Signs & Symptoms	• Asymptomatic: most common; often considered normal • Symptomatic: may present with hypoperfusion symptoms related to bradycardia • **Fatigue**, dyspnea, presyncope/syncope, dizziness, **lightheadedness**, malaise

Diagnosis	• Electrocardiogram (ECG): **best initial test;** often incidentally found on routine ECG
	  • **PR interval >0.20 seconds**
	  • Atrial impulse (P wave) is delayed but always progresses to ventricles (always followed by a QRS complex and T wave)

Treatment	• **Observation: no treatment required; routine ECGs to monitor if asymptomatic** • Atropine: consider if symptomatic bradycardia • **Pacemaker: indicated for PR interval >0.30 seconds** and symptoms related to AV block
Key Words & Most Common	• Common in young patients • Fibrosis/sclerosis or increased vagal tone causes delayed conduction through AV node • Commonly asymptomatic; may present with hypoperfusion symptoms • ECG: PR interval >0.20s • Observation if asymptomatic; consider atropine if symptomatic; pacemaker if PRI greater than 30s

Mobitz I Wenckebach	# Second Degree AV Block

Etiology & Risk Factors	• **Partial interruption atrial impulse to the ventricles;** often considered normal in patients with increased vagal tone in absence of structural heart disease
	• Etiology: may be physiologic or pathologic
	   • **Physiologic: age-related fibrosis of conduction system is most common cause; young patients with increased vagal tone**
	   • Pathologic: ischemia (acute MI, CAD), electrolyte imbalance (hyper/hypokalemia, hypomagnesemia), inflammation, infection (endocarditis, Lyme, rheumatic)
	   • Medications: digoxin, beta blockers, antiarrhythmics, calcium channel blockers
	   • Conditions: collagen disorders (SLE, sarcoidosis), congenital heart defect

Patho-physiology	• Dysfunction within the AV node results in progressive prolongation of AV node conduction until an atrial impulse is blocked and fails to conduct to the ventricles • Atrial impulse is transmitted during the relative refractory period resulting in a progressively slower conduction through the AV node until the impulse is transmitted during the absolute refractory period resulting in a blocked conduction • When an atrial impulse is blocked, there will be a **P wave without a corresponding QRS complex (dropped beat)**

Signs & Symptoms	• <u>Asymptomatic</u>: most common
	• <u>Symptomatic</u>: palpitations or sensation of "skipped beats"
	   • **Hypoperfusion Symptoms: symptoms related to bradycardia** fatigue, dyspnea, syncope/presyncope, dizziness, lightheadedness, malaise
	     • *Severe cases may present with angina, syncope, altered mental status, diaphoresis, pallor, or hypotension*

Diagnosis	• <u>Electrocardiogram (ECG)</u>: progressive increase of PR interval until atrial impulse is blocked leading to a P wave without a corresponding QRS complex • *After dropped QRS complex, PR interval progression resets* • <u>Labs</u>: cardiac enzymes (if ischemia is suspected cause); magnesium, serum electrolytes
Treatment	• <u>**Observation: no treatment required;**</u> routine ECGs to monitor if asymptomatic • <u>**Treat Underlying Etiology:**</u> remove or titrate dosing of offending medication • <u>**Atropine**</u>: indicated in setting of hypotension or symptomatic bradycardia • <u>**Transcutaneous or Transvenous Pacing: indicated if patients fails atropine therapy**</u>
Key Words & Most Common	• Often benign; may result from inferior myocardial ischemia (AV node ischemia) • May be asymptomatic; hypoperfusion symptoms if symptomatic • ECG: progressive prolongation of PR interval until dropped QRS complex • Atropine if hypotensive or symptomatic bradycardia

Mobitz II Wenckebach	# Second Degree AV Block

Etiology & Risk Factors	• **Partial interruption atrial impulse to the ventricles** • **Rarely seen in patients without structural heart disease;** often pathologic and associated with **myocardial ischemia, fibrosis or sclerosis** • Etiology: **blockage or damage to the His-Purkinje system** • Risk Factors: **age (>65 years old most common), structural heart abnormalities** (myocardial infarction, myocarditis, cardiomyopathies, congenital heart disorders, cardiac tumors), **certain medications** (beta blockers, antiarrhythmics, calcium channel blockers, digoxin), previous heart surgery or ablation, family history
Patho-physiology	• Dysfunction of the infra-nodal (blow the AV node)conduction system results in intermittent failure of electrical conduction from the atria to the ventricles due to blockage or damage to the His-Purkinje system resulting in occasional skipped ventricular beats and a fixed PR interval on the ECG before the blocked beat. • Regular conduction through the AV node (**regular PR interval**) until a P wave is **not** followed by a QRS complex • Often progresses to complete block

Signs & Symptoms	• <u>Asymptomatic</u>: most common
	• <u>Symptomatic</u>: palpitations or sensation of "skipped beats"
	   • <u>**Hypoperfusion Symptoms: symptoms related to bradycardia**</u> fatigue, dyspnea, syncope/presyncope, dizziness, lightheadedness, malaise
	     • *Severe cases may present with **angina, syncope**, altered mental status, diaphoresis, pallor, hypotension, or **sudden cardiac arrest***

Diagnosis	• <u>Electrocardiogram (ECG)</u>: **fixed PR interval with conducted QRS complex**
	   • Regular AV node conduction (**regular PR interval**) until intermittent non-conducted QRS complex (P wave is **not** followed by a QRS complex [dropped beat])
	   • *Be weary of P waves hidden inside T waves*
	• <u>Labs</u>: cardiac enzymes (if ischemia is suspected cause); magnesium, serum electrolytes

Treatment	• <u>**Treat Underlying Etiology**</u>: remove or titrate dosing of offending medication • <u>**Atropine**</u>: indicated in setting of hypotension or symptomatic bradycardia; most do not respond to atropine therapy • <u>**Cardiac Monitoring**</u>: admit to inpatient for monitoring & pacing (transcutaneous followed by transvenous) • <u>**Permanent Pacemaker**</u>: indicated due to chance of progression to complete AV block and poor prognosis
Key Words & Most Common	• Often pathologic; seen in patients with ischemia or iatrogenic causation with medications or cardiac surgery • Hypoperfusion symptoms that can progress to severe symptoms including sudden cardiac arrest • ECG: fixed PR interval with intermittent dropped beat; P wave may be hidden inside T wave • Often fail atropine • Admit for pacing → permanent pacemaker definitive

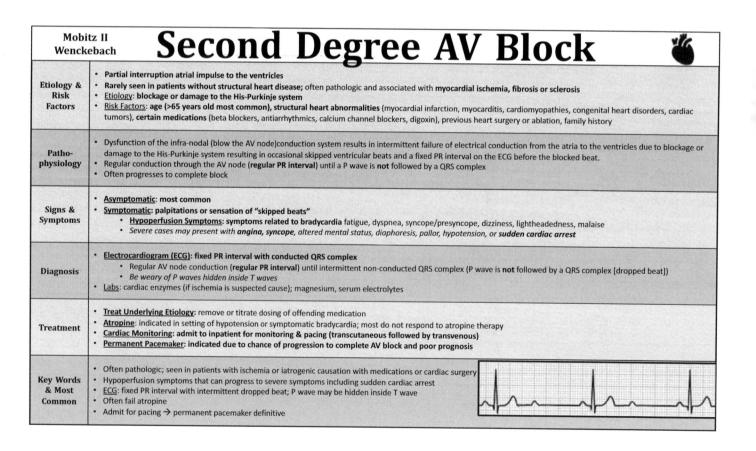

Third Degree AV Block

Etiology & Risk Factors	• **Complete interruption atrial impulse to the ventricles**; also known as **complete heart block** • <u>Etiology</u>: complete blockage of electrical impulses between the atria and the ventricles • <u>Risk Factors</u>: **age (>65 years old most common), structural heart abnormalities** (**inferior wall myocardial infarction**, myocarditis, cardiomyopathies, congenital heart disorders, cardiac tumors), **certain medications** (beta blockers, antiarrhythmics, calcium channel blockers, digoxin), previous heart surgery or ablation, family history
Patho-physiology	• Complete atrioventricular dissociation; electrical signals originating from the sinoatrial node are completely blocked from reaching the ventricles through the AV node, resulting in the two chambers beating independently • Ventricles are activated by an escape rhythm (junctional, fascicular or ventricular) while the SA node continues to send impulses to the atria independently in a regular rhythm therefore atrial rate will be slightly faster than the ventricular rate
Signs & Symptoms	• <u>Bradycardia</u>: **most common symptom**; typically less than 45-50 beats per minute • <u>**Hypoperfusion Symptoms**</u>: **symptoms related to bradycardia** fatigue, dyspnea, syncope/presyncope, dizziness, lightheadedness, malaise • *Severe cases may present with* **angina, syncope**, altered mental status, diaphoresis, pallor, or hypotension or **sudden cardiac arrest**

Diagnosis	• <u>Electrocardiogram (ECG)</u>: evaluate for rate, rhythm and signs of ischemia
	    • **Bradycardia is most common finding**
	    • **Fixed, regular P-P intervals unrelated to regular, slightly slower, R-R intervals**
	    • If block occurs *above* bundle of His, may have *narrow* QRS complex; if block occurs *below* bundle of His may have *wide* QRS complex
	• <u>Labs</u>: cardiac enzymes (if ischemia is suspected cause); magnesium, serum electrolytes, blood glucose

Treatment	• <u>Stabilize Patient</u>: patient will often be hemodynamically unstable • <u>Atropine</u>: indicated in setting of hypotension or symptomatic bradycardia; most do not respond to atropine therapy • <u>Transcutaneous or Transvenous Pacing</u>: **indicated if patients fails atropine therapy** • <u>Permanent Pacemaker</u>: **definitive treatment; indicated for most patients for long term management**
Key Words & Most Common	• Complete atrioventricular disassociation – P-P intervals are regular & unrelated to R-R intervals • Atrial rate>ventricular rate • Severe bradycardia with symptoms • ECG: regular P-P intervals with slightly slower R-R intervals • Often fails atropine; requires pacing

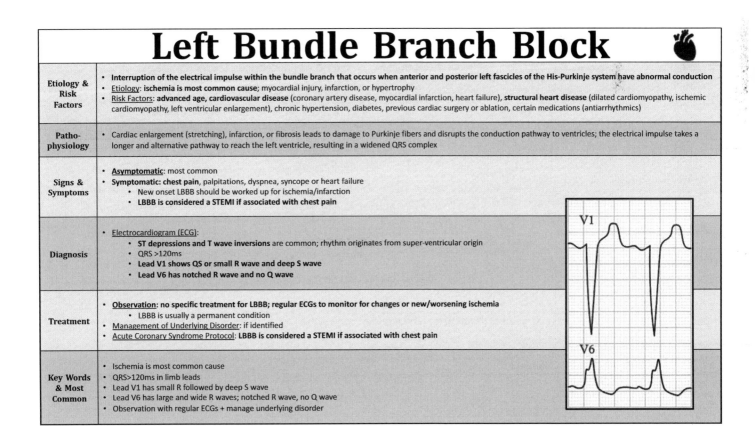

Left Bundle Branch Block

Etiology & Risk Factors	• **Interruption of the electrical impulse within the bundle branch that occurs when anterior and posterior left fascicles of the His-Purkinje system have abnormal conduction** • <u>Etiology</u>: **ischemia is most common cause**; myocardial injury, infarction, or hypertrophy • <u>Risk Factors</u>: **advanced age, cardiovascular disease** (coronary artery disease, myocardial infarction, heart failure), **structural heart disease** (dilated cardiomyopathy, ischemic cardiomyopathy, left ventricular enlargement), chronic hypertension, diabetes, previous cardiac surgery or ablation, certain medications (antiarrhythmics)
Patho-physiology	• Cardiac enlargement (stretching), infarction, or fibrosis leads to damage to Purkinje fibers and disrupts the conduction pathway to ventricles; the electrical impulse takes a longer and alternative pathway to reach the left ventricle, resulting in a widened QRS complex

Signs & Symptoms	• <u>Asymptomatic</u>: most common
	• **Symptomatic**: **chest pain**, palpitations, dyspnea, syncope or heart failure
	    • New onset LBBB should be worked up for ischemia/infarction
	    • **LBBB is considered a STEMI if associated with chest pain**

Diagnosis	• <u>Electrocardiogram (ECG)</u>:
	    • **ST depressions and T wave inversions** are common; rhythm originates from super-ventricular origin
	    • QRS >120ms
	    • **Lead V1 shows QS or small R wave and deep S wave**
	    • **Lead V6 has notched R wave and no Q wave**

Treatment	• <u>Observation</u>: no specific treatment for LBBB; regular ECGs to monitor for changes or new/worsening ischemia • LBBB is usually a permanent condition • <u>Management of Underlying Disorder</u>: if identified • <u>Acute Coronary Syndrome Protocol</u>: LBBB is considered a STEMI if associated with chest pain
Key Words & Most Common	• Ischemia is most common cause • QRS>120ms in limb leads • Lead V1 has small R followed by deep S wave • Lead V6 has large and wide R waves; notched R wave, no Q wave • Observation with regular ECGs + manage underlying disorder

Right Bundle Branch Block

Etiology & Risk Factors	• Abnormal conduction through the right bundle fascicles of the His-Purkinje system • <u>Etiology</u>: structural heart disease (coronary artery disease, myocardial infarction, cardiomyopathy) is most common cause • More commonly seen in patients with myocardial injury, infarction, or hypertrophy; can be caused by infiltrative, trauma, or iatrogenic (right heart catheterization) • <u>Risk Factors</u>: advanced age, dilated cardiomyopathy, ischemic cardiomyopathy, left ventricular enlargement • <u>Risk Factors</u>: **advanced age, cardiovascular disease** (coronary artery disease, myocardial infarction, heart failure), **structural heart disease** (dilated cardiomyopathy, ischemic cardiomyopathy, **right ventricular hypertrophy**), **pulmonary embolism**, chronic hypertension, diabetes, previous cardiac surgery or ablation (right heart catherization), certain medications (antiarrhythmics)
Patho-physiology	• Delay or blockage in the electrical signals that originates from the AV node conducts to the bundle of His and through the right bundle branch of the heart's conduction system. This results in the ventricles not contracting in a coordinated manner, leading to a delay in the right ventricle's activation • The left ventricle depolarizes initially while the right is delayed
Signs & Symptoms	• <u>**Asymptomatic**</u>: **most common**; may be found incidentally on routine ECG • <u>**Symptomatic**</u>: fatigue, weakness, palpitations, dyspnea

Diagnosis	• <u>Electrocardiogram (ECG)</u>:
	  • ST depressions and T wave inversions are common
	  • QRS > 120ms
	  • **rSR' wave in V1 & V2**
	    • First R wave in V1 is always **smaller** than the second
	  • **Slurred S wave in leads I and V6**

Treatment	• <u>**Observation**</u>: no specific treatment for RBBB; regular ECGs to monitor for changes or new/worsening ischemia • LBBB is usually a permanent condition • <u>Management of Underlying Disorder</u>: if identified
Key Words & Most Common	• Asymptomatic; may be found incidentally • rSR' wave in V1 & V2; slurred S wave in leads I and V6 • No specific treatment; treat underlying disorder

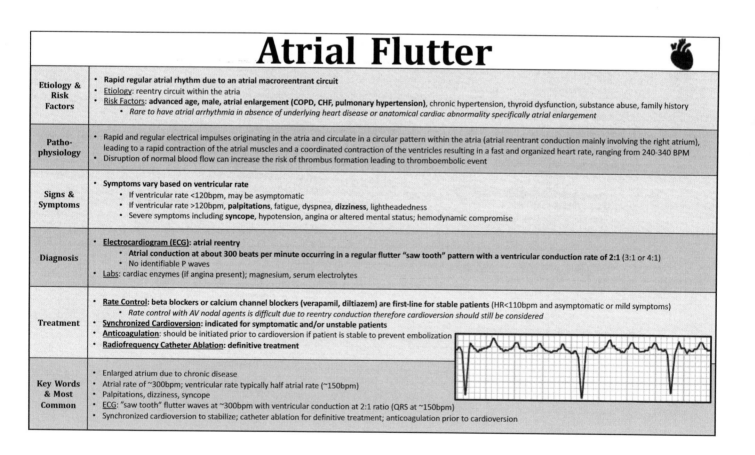

Atrial Flutter

Etiology & Risk Factors	• **Rapid regular atrial rhythm due to an atrial macroreentrant circuit** • <u>Etiology</u>: reentry circuit within the atria • <u>Risk Factors</u>: **advanced age, male, atrial enlargement (COPD, CHF, pulmonary hypertension)**, chronic hypertension, thyroid dysfunction, substance abuse, family history • *Rare to have atrial arrhythmia in absence of underlying heart disease or anatomical cardiac abnormality specifically atrial enlargement*
Patho-physiology	• Rapid and regular electrical impulses originating in the atria and circulate in a circular pattern within the atria (atrial reentrant conduction mainly involving the right atrium), leading to a rapid contraction of the atrial muscles and a coordinated contraction of the ventricles resulting in a fast and organized heart rate, ranging from 240-340 BPM • Disruption of normal blood flow can increase the risk of thrombus formation leading to thromboembolic event

Signs & Symptoms	• **Symptoms vary based on ventricular rate**
	  • If ventricular rate <120bpm, may be asymptomatic
	  • If ventricular rate >120bpm, **palpitations**, fatigue, dyspnea, **dizziness**, lightheadedness
	  • Severe symptoms including **syncope**, hypotension, angina or altered mental status; hemodynamic compromise

Diagnosis	• <u>Electrocardiogram (ECG)</u>: atrial reentry
	  • **Atrial conduction at about 300 beats per minute occurring in a regular flutter "saw tooth" pattern with a ventricular conduction rate of 2:1** (3:1 or 4:1)
	  • No identifiable P waves
	• <u>Labs</u>: cardiac enzymes (if angina present); magnesium, serum electrolytes

Treatment	• <u>Rate Control</u>: beta blockers or calcium channel blockers (verapamil, diltiazem) are first-line for stable patients (HR<110bpm and asymptomatic or mild symptoms) • *Rate control with AV nodal agents is difficult due to reentry conduction therefore cardioversion should still be considered* • <u>Synchronized Cardioversion</u>: indicated for symptomatic and/or unstable patients • <u>Anticoagulation</u>: should be initiated prior to cardioversion if patient is stable to prevent embolization • <u>Radiofrequency Catheter Ablation</u>: **definitive treatment**
Key Words & Most Common	• Enlarged atrium due to chronic disease • Atrial rate of ~300bpm; ventricular rate typically half atrial rate (~150bpm) • Palpitations, dizziness, syncope • ECG: "saw tooth" flutter waves at ~300bpm with ventricular conduction at 2:1 ratio (QRS at ~150bpm) • Synchronized cardioversion to stabilize; catheter ablation for definitive treatment; anticoagulation prior to cardioversion

Atrial Fibrillation

Etiology & Risk Factors	• **Rapid, irregularly irregular rhythm**; most common cardia arrhythmia • <u>Etiology</u>: multiple wavelets with chaotic reentry within the atria • <u>Risk Factors</u>: **advanced age**, cardiac disease (valvular, structural, or ischemia), pulmonary disease, electrolyte imbalance, hypertension, sleep apnea, genetics, medications, **alcohol** or drug use ("**holiday heart**"), sedentary lifestyle, previous heart surgery, certain genetic components • *Any disease or condition that attributes to physiologic stress, inflammation, ischemia, or disrupts the normal cardiac anatomy*
Patho-physiology	• Cardiac remodeling (enlargement) causes structural and electrical changes particularly of the atria which leads to **chaotic reentry**; atria never fully contract as the atrioventricular node is overwhelmed by continuous electrical impulse leading to inconsistent transmission of impulse and an **irregularly irregular ventricular rate** • Quivering of atria leads to turbulent blood flow which can **increase risk of thromboembolism** (commonly originates from **left atrial appendage**) • <u>Paroxysmal</u>: afib reverts to sinus rhythm spontaneously in **less than 7 days** (typically less than 24 hours) • <u>Persistent</u>: afib lasting for **greater than 7 days**; requires pharmacologic or electrical cardioversion • <u>Long-Standing Persistent</u>: Persistent afib for greater than 1 year; turns to Permanent Afib when unresponsive for pharmacologic or electrical cardioversion
Signs & Symptoms	• *Symptoms range from asymptomatic to devastating outcomes from thromboembolism* • **Palpitations is most common symptom,** angina, **fatigue**, dyspnea, lower extremity edema • Severe symptoms include **syncope**, hypotension, angina or altered mental status; hemodynamic compromise or stroke/organ failure from thromboembolism • <u>Physical Exam</u>: **pulse is irregularly irregular**; auscultation may reveal heart rate faster than peripheral pulse (decreased left ventricular stroke volume)
Diagnosis	• <u>Electrocardiogram (ECG)</u>: **irregularly irregular R-R intervals with fibrillating waves**, no discernable P wave; atrial rate often >300bpm best seen in V1; QRS often >140bpm • <u>Labs</u>: CBC; CMP; TSH; BNP; cardiac enzymes if ischemia suspected • <u>Echocardiogram</u>: **required prior to cardioversion** to rule out atrial thrombus (**transesophageal echo preferred**); assesses for structural or valvular cause • <u>Imaging</u>: consider risk for pulmonary embolism with PERC or WELLS score follow-up spiral CT imaging; consider CXR if heart failure suspected

Treatment	• <u>Rate Control</u>: **beta blocker (metoprolol) or calcium channel blocker (diltiazem)**; digoxin in hypotension or heart failure
	• <u>Rhythm Control</u>: **synchronized cardioversion** (immediate if unstable; must rule out atrial thrombus with TTE/TEE first if stable); chemical cardioversion with **Amiodarone**
	• <u>Anticoagulation</u>: recommended if afib <48hrs or **3 weeks prior to and 4 weeks after cardioversion if afib>48hrs**
	   • <u>Warfarin</u>: indicated with valve replacement & chronic kidney disease; requires heparin bridge & monitored with INR (2-3)
	   • <u>Non-Vitamin K Antagonist (NVKA)</u>: (cabigatran; **apixaban; rivaroxaban**) preferred over warfarin due to decreased risk of ischemic stroke and ease of use (no need to check INR); *not approved for use in patients with valve replacement*
	   • <u>Dual Antiplatelet</u>: (aspirin + clopidogrel) only indicated in patients in which anticoagulation is contraindicated
	• **Radiofrequency Catheter Ablation:** reserved for refractory cases to electrical or pharmacologic cardioversion

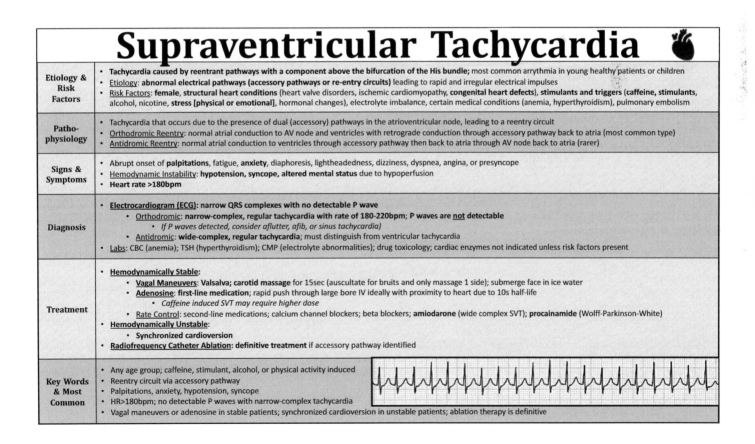

Supraventricular Tachycardia

Etiology & Risk Factors	• **Tachycardia caused by reentrant pathways with a component above the bifurcation of the His bundle**; most common arrythmia in young healthy patients or children • <u>Etiology</u>: **abnormal electrical pathways (accessory pathways or re-entry circuits)** leading to rapid and irregular electrical impulses • <u>Risk Factors</u>: **female**, **structural heart conditions** (heart valve disorders, ischemic cardiomyopathy, **congenital heart defects**), **stimulants and triggers (caffeine, stimulants,** alcohol, nicotine, **stress [physical or emotional]**, hormonal changes), electrolyte imbalance, certain medical conditions (anemia, hyperthyroidism), pulmonary embolism
Patho-physiology	• Tachycardia that occurs due to the presence of dual (accessory) pathways in the atrioventricular node, leading to a reentry circuit • <u>Orthodromic Reentry</u>: normal atrial conduction to AV node and ventricles with retrograde conduction through accessory pathway back to atria (most common type) • <u>Antidromic Reentry</u>: normal atrial conduction to ventricles through accessory pathway then back to atria through AV node back to atria (rarer)
Signs & Symptoms	• Abrupt onset of **palpitations**, fatigue, **anxiety**, diaphoresis, lightheadedness, dizziness, dyspnea, angina, or presyncope • <u>Hemodynamic Instability</u>: **hypotension, syncope, altered mental status** due to hypoperfusion • **Heart rate >180bpm**

Diagnosis	• **Electrocardiogram (ECG): narrow QRS complexes with no detectable P wave**
	   • <u>Orthodromic</u>: **narrow-complex, regular tachycardia with rate of 180-220bpm; P waves are <u>not</u> detectable**
	     • *If P waves detected, consider aflutter, afib, or sinus tachycardia)*
	   • <u>Antidromic</u>: **wide-complex, regular tachycardia**; must distinguish from ventricular tachycardia
	• <u>Labs</u>: CBC (anemia); TSH (hyperthyroidism); CMP (electrolyte abnormalities); drug toxicology; cardiac enzymes not indicated unless risk factors present

Treatment	• **Hemodynamically Stable:**
	   • **Vagal Maneuvers: Valsalva; carotid massage** for 15sec (auscultate for bruits and only massage 1 side); submerge face in ice water
	   • **Adenosine**: **first-line medication**; rapid push through large bore IV ideally with proximity to heart due to 10s half-life
	     • *Caffeine induced SVT may require higher dose*
	   • <u>Rate Control</u>: second-line medications; calcium channel blockers; beta blockers; **amiodarone** (wide complex SVT); **procainamide** (Wolff-Parkinson-White)
	• **Hemodynamically Unstable:**
	   • **Synchronized cardioversion**
	• **Radiofrequency Catheter Ablation: definitive treatment** if accessory pathway identified

Key Words & Most Common	• Any age group; caffeine, stimulant, alcohol, or physical activity induced • Reentry circuit via accessory pathway • Palpitations, anxiety, hypotension, syncope • HR>180bpm; no detectable P waves with narrow-complex tachycardia • Vagal maneuvers or adenosine in stable patients; synchronized cardioversion in unstable patients; ablation therapy is definitive

Wolff-Parkinson-White

Etiology & Risk Factors	• Tachycardia caused by antegrade conduction occurring over both the accessory pathway and the normal conducting system • <u>Etiology</u>: **ventricular preexcitation through accessory pathway** (outside the AV node) that combines with normal AV node conduction • <u>Risk Factors</u>: **male, age (young adults)**, family history, structural heart conditions (congenital heart defects **[Ebstein's anomaly]**, myocarditis, **hypertrophic cardiomyopathy**)
Patho-physiology	• **Conduction through accessory pathway (outside the AV node) combines with normal AV node conduction during sinus rhythm**; the accessory pathway (**Bundle of Kent**) is faster leading to the early ventricular depolarization (preexcitation) resulting in a **shorter P-R interval and a "slurred" upstroke of the QRS complex**
Signs & Symptoms	• May be asymptomatic • **Palpitations**, fatigue, **anxiety**, diaphoresis, lightheadedness, dizziness, dyspnea, angina, or presyncope • *More at risk for developing tachyarrhythmias* • <u>Hemodynamic Instability</u>: **hypotension, syncope, altered mental status** due to hypoperfusion

Diagnosis	• <u>Electrocardiogram (ECG)</u>: several ECG criteria
	   • <u>**Short PR Interval**</u>: less than 0.12 seconds; due to AV node conduction delay
	   • <u>**Wide QRS Complex**</u>: QRS greater than 0.12 seconds; due to fusion impulse from accessory pathway & normal AV node
	   • <u>**"Slurred" Upstroke QRS**</u>: **"delta wave"** due to early ventricular activation
	• <u>Labs</u>: CBC; CMP; TSH; BNP; cardiac enzymes if ischemia suspected

Treatment	• <u>**Hemodynamically Stable**</u>:
	   • <u>**Procainamide**</u>: **first-line medication**; safest due to preserving AV node conduction (delays but does not block)
	   • <u>**Avoid AV Nodal Blocking Medications**</u>: amiodarone, beta blockers, calcium channel blockers, digoxin generally contraindicated
	      • Will lead to increased conduction through accessory pathway (**Bundle of Kent**) due to normal AV node conduction blockade
	• <u>**Hemodynamically Unstable**</u>:
	   • **Synchronized Cardioversion**
	• <u>**Radiofrequency Catheter Ablation**</u>: **definitive treatment** if accessory pathway identified

Key Words & Most Common	• Conduction through Bundle of Kent (accessory pathway) combines with normal AV conduction • Palpitations, fatigue, anxiety; often asymptomatic • <u>ECG</u>: short PR interval; wide QRS; "slurred" upstroke of QRS (Delta wave) • Procainamide; Avoid ABCD AV nodal blocking medications if stable • Synchronized cardiovert if unstable; Ablation is definitive

Delta Wave

Premature Ventricular Contraction

Etiology & Risk Factors	• Type of abnormal heart rhythm originating from the ventricles • <u>Etiology</u>: **single ventricular impulses due to reentry within the ventricle or abnormal automaticity of ventricular cells** • <u>Risk Factors</u>: **advanced age, structural heart disease** (cardiomyopathies, myocardial ischemia or infarction, chronic hypertension), **electrolyte abnormalities** (hypokalemia, hypomagnesemia, hypercalcemia), stimulants or substances (caffeine, tobacco, alcohol, elicit drugs, ADD medication), sleep deprivation, anxiety, stress
Patho-physiology	• **Premature electrical impulse initiated from the Purkinje fibers in the ventricle** (rather than the SA node) leading to an early ectopic beat • Could be caused by a subthreshold potential within certain pacemaker cells being met with normal cardiac electrical activity leading to a premature beat • Electrolyte abnormalities may lead to spontaneous depolarization
Signs & Symptoms	• **Often asymptomatic** • **Intermittent palpitations are most common symptom**; may be described as flutters or pounding of chest • Prolonged run of PVC's may result in hypotension, dizziness

Diagnosis	• <u>Electrocardiogram (ECG)</u>:
	   • **Wide abnormally shaped QRS complex without a preceding P wave** followed by a compensatory pause
	   • Subsequent T wave is often opposite of the QRS complex
	   • *ECG often does not capture unless PVC occurs during ECG*
	• <u>Labs</u>: CBC, BMP, magnesium, thyroid stimulating hormone, Ionized calcium, consider drug toxicology
	• <u>**24-hour Holter Monitor**</u>: often be required for diagnosis

Treatment	• <u>**Observation**</u>: **no treatment required if asymptomatic**; routine ECGs to monitor if asymptomatic
	• <u>**Identify and Correct Underlying Etiology**</u>:
	   • Correct electrolyte imbalance particularly calcium, potassium, magnesium
	   • Discontinue offending medication, drug, or substance

Key Words & Most Common	• Common; may be due to caffeine, stimulants, or electrolyte abnormality • Premature impulse from ventricle rather than SA node leads to early beat • Often asymptomatic; may experience palpitations • <u>ECG</u>: wide abnormal QRS with subsequent inverted T wave • Treat underlying etiology

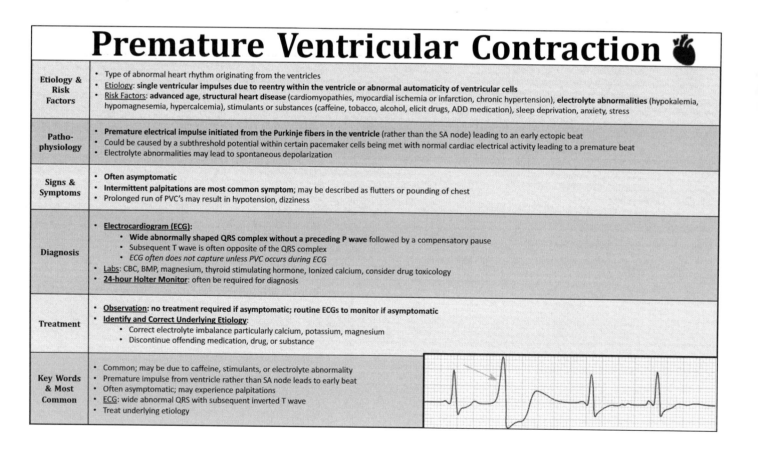

Ventricular Tachycardia

Etiology & Risk Factors	• **Abnormal electrical signals generate multiple rapid impulses, leading to a sustained ventricular heart rate above 100 beats per minute** • Etiology: **ischemic heart disease (myocardia infarction) is most common cause** • Risk Factors: **structural heart disease (cardiomyopathies, myocardial ischemia or infarction, chronic hypertension), electrolyte abnormalities (hypomagnesemia, hypokalemia, hypocalcemia)**, stimulant drug use **(cocaine** or amphetamines), sleep apnea, myocarditis, cardiomyopathies, long QT syndrome, hypertension, COPD
Patho-physiology	• Myocardial scarring as a result of ischemia or structural change leads to spontaneous reentry of electrical activity or slowed impulse through scarred tissue results in abnormal automaticity and early/late after-depolarizations and reentry of impulse • In myocardial infarction, ischemia leads to increased extracellular potassium
Signs & Symptoms	• **Palpitations**, syncope, altered mental status, **angina, diaphoresis**, pallor • Hemodynamic Instability: **hypotension, syncope, altered mental status** due to hypoperfusion • **Sudden cardiac arrest**

Diagnosis	• Electrocardiogram (ECG):
	    • **Multiple/sustained wide QRS complexes (>0.12s) with no preceding P waves**; HR>100bpm
	        • Non-sustained VTach: lasts *less* than 30 seconds
	        • Sustained VTach: lasts *more* than 30 seconds or less than 30 seconds accompanied with hemodynamic compromise
	        • Monomorphic: similar QRS morphology
	        • Polymorphic: changing QRS morphology
	• Labs: CBC, BMP, magnesium, ionized calcium, cardiac enzymes

Treatment	• **Antiarrhythmics**: indicated if stable
	    • Procainamide: **first-line medication**
	    • **Amiodarone** : indicated in acute MI; commonly used but does not usually work quickly
	    • *Failure of IV procainamide or IV amiodarone is an indication for cardioversion*
	• **Synchronized Cardioversion: indicated for unstable rhythm with pulse**
	• **Unsynchronized Cardioversion: indicated for unstable rhythm without pulse**; cardiopulmonary resuscitation (CPR) may be required
	• **Beta Blockers**: indicated for long term management
	• Implantable Cardioverter Defibrillator (ICD): utilized to prevent death in those with recurrent symptoms

Key Words & Most Common	• Most common cause is ischemic heart disease; MI; electrolyte abnormalities • Palpitations, syncope, sudden cardiac arrest • ECG: multiple wide QRS complexes with no preceding P wave • Procainamide or amiodarone • Synchronized vs unsynchronized cardioversion

Torsades de Pointes

Etiology & Risk Factors	• **Polymorphic ventricular tachycardia** variant with **oscillating QRS complex amplitudes;** French for "twisting of the points" • Etiology: **prolongation of QT interval** • Risk Factors: advanced age, structural heart disease, **electrolyte imbalance (hypomagnesemia, hypokalemia, hypocalcemia)**, medications (antipsychotics, antiemetics, **antiarrhythmics**, antifungals, antibiotics), diuretic use, bradycardia
Patho-physiology	• Inhibition of the delayed rectifier potassium current causes increased positively charged ions of the extracellular membrane (prolongs the repolarization phase) • If a PVC occurs during this repolarization phase (T wave) it is known as R on T phenomenon and may result in Torsades de Pointes • Heart rate of >200bpm or prolonged run of Torsades de Pointes can decompensate into ventricular fibrillation
Signs & Symptoms	• **Palpitations**, dizziness, lightheadedness, **syncope** • **Sudden cardiac arrest**

Diagnosis	• Electrocardiogram (ECG):
	    • Polymorphic ventricular tachycardia variant with **oscillating QRS complex around an isometric line**
	    • May be triggered as a **PVC occurring during a preceding T wave**
	• Labs: CBC, BMP, magnesium, ionized calcium, phosphorus
	    • **Hypomagnesemia, hypokalemia, hypocalcemia)**

Treatment	• Identify and Treat Underlying Etiology: **discontinue all QT prolonging medications; correct underlying electrolyte abnormalities** • **IV Magnesium Sulfate: first-line medication;** decreases calcium influx to suppress early after-depolarizations • Isoproterenol: may be necessary; increases heart rate & AV conduction • Overdrive Pacing: not utilized to convert Torsades de Pointes but effective to maintain sinus rhythm (target rate 90-120bpm) • *Avoid Amiodarone & Procainamide (can prolong QT interval)*
Key Words & Most Common	• QT prolonging medication or electrolyte abnormalities (low magnesium, low potassium, low calcium) • Palpitations, syncope • ECG: polymorphic VTach with oscillating QRS complex around isometric line • Magnesium Sulfate IV; discontinue QT prolonging medication • Treat underlying electrolyte abnormality

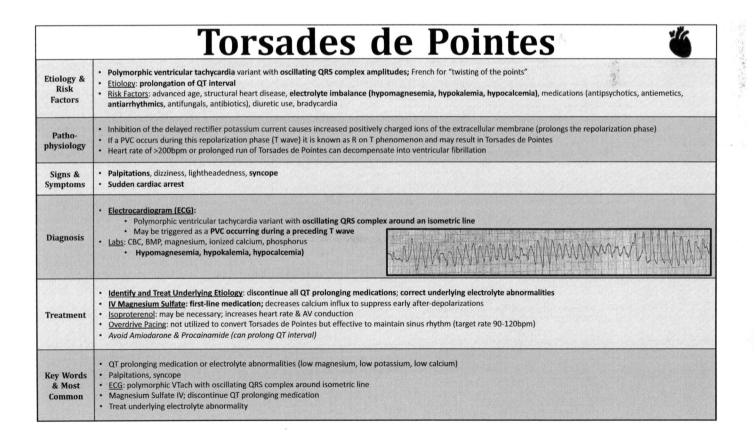

Ventricular Fibrillation

Etiology & Risk Factors	• **Dangerous uncoordinated quivering of the ventricle with no useful contractions; rate usually >300 beats per minute** • Etiology: ischemic heart disease (myocardial infarction) is most common cause • Risk Factors: **structural heart disease (cardiomyopathies, myocardial ischemia or infarction), electrolyte abnormalities (hypomagnesemia, hypokalemia, hypocalcemia),** stimulant drug use (**cocaine** or amphetamines), sleep apnea, myocarditis, cardiomyopathies, long QT syndrome, hypertension, COPD, hypothermia, hypoxia
Patho-physiology	• Inconsistent and uncoordinated depolarization of the ventricular myocardium leads to chaotic and irregular contractions, causing the heart to quiver rather than effectively pump blood which deprives the brain and other vital organs of oxygen • Functional or anatomic re-entry circuits caused by ischemia or structural change leads to abnormal impulse conduction
Signs & Symptoms	• Acute Coronary Syndrome Symptoms: **chest pain**, dyspnea, diaphoresis may precede arrhythmia symptoms • **Palpitations**, syncope, **loss of consciousness**, unresponsiveness, **pulseless** • **Sudden cardiac arrest**

Diagnosis	• Electrocardiogram (ECG):
	   • **Fibrillating waves of electrical impulses that vary in shape & amplitude**
	   • No identifiable P waves, QRS complexes, or T waves
	   • May have findings of acute MI
	• Labs: CMP, CBC, ABG, cardiac enzymes, BNP

Treatment	• **Acute Coronary Life Support (ACLS): protocol initiated immediately**
	   • **Unsynchronized Cardioversion (Defibrillation): indicated as soon as possible** and resume CPR
	   • **Epinephrine**: 1mg given after attempted defibrillation + resume CPR for 2 minutes if patient does not convert
	   • **Amiodarone**: 300mg after 2 attempted defibrillation + resume CPR for 2 minutes if patient does not convert
	• Implantable Cardioverter Defibrillator (ICD): indicated for most patients for long-term management/prevention
	• Antiarrhythmic Medications: often indicated to reduce the frequency of subsequent episodes of ventricular tachycardia/fibrillation

Key Words & Most Common	• Most common cause is MI or post-MI due to ischemia; electrolyte abnormalities (Mg or K) • Syncope, pulseless, sudden cardiac arrest • ECG: fibrillating waves with no identifiable P waves, QRS, or T waves • Initiate ACLS – unsynchronized cardioversion (defibrillation)

Patent Foramen Ovale

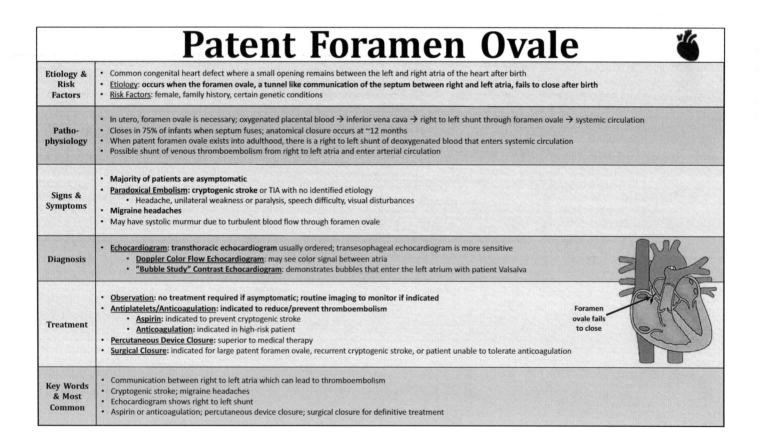

Foramen ovale fails to close

Etiology & Risk Factors	• Common congenital heart defect where a small opening remains between the left and right atria of the heart after birth • Etiology: **occurs when the foramen ovale, a tunnel like communication of the septum between right and left atria, fails to close after birth** • Risk Factors: female, family history, certain genetic conditions
Patho-physiology	• In utero, foramen ovale is necessary; oxygenated placental blood → inferior vena cava → right to left shunt through foramen ovale → systemic circulation • Closes in 75% of infants when septum fuses; anatomical closure occurs at ~12 months • When patent foramen ovale exists into adulthood, there is a right to left shunt of deoxygenated blood that enters systemic circulation • Possible shunt of venous thromboembolism from right to left atria and enter arterial circulation
Signs & Symptoms	• **Majority of patients are asymptomatic** • Paradoxical Embolism: **cryptogenic stroke** or TIA with no identified etiology • Headache, unilateral weakness or paralysis, speech difficulty, visual disturbances • **Migraine headaches** • May have systolic murmur due to turbulent blood flow through foramen ovale

Diagnosis	• Echocardiogram: **transthoracic echocardiogram** usually ordered; transesophageal echocardiogram is more sensitive
	   • **Doppler Color Flow Echocardiogram**: may see color signal between atria
	   • **"Bubble Study" Contrast Echocardiogram**: demonstrates bubbles that enter the left atrium with patient Valsalva

Treatment	• Observation: no treatment required if asymptomatic; routine imaging to monitor if indicated
	• Antiplatelets/Anticoagulation: indicated to reduce/prevent thromboembolism
	   • **Aspirin**: indicated to prevent cryptogenic stroke
	   • **Anticoagulation**: indicated in high-risk patient
	• Percutaneous Device Closure: superior to medical therapy
	• Surgical Closure: indicated for large patent foramen ovale, recurrent cryptogenic stroke, or patient unable to tolerate anticoagulation

Key Words & Most Common	• Communication between right to left atria which can lead to thromboembolism • Cryptogenic stroke; migraine headaches • Echocardiogram shows right to left shunt • Aspirin or anticoagulation; percutaneous device closure; surgical closure for definitive treatment

Atrial Septal Defect

Etiology & Risk Factors	• **Interatrial septum opening, causing a left-to-right shunt and volume overload of the right atrium and right ventricle; one of the most common congenital heart defects** • Etiology: not fully understood; combination of genetic and environmental factors • Risk Factors: certain genetic conditions (Down syndrome, Turner syndrome), maternal factors (exposure to cocaine or alcohol, gestational diabetes, advanced maternal age), family history, exposure to environmental toxins
Patho-physiology	• Pressure in right atrium is significantly less than pressure in left atrium leading to a **left to right shunt of blood and is considered noncyanotic** • Can become cyanotic if chronic volume overload causes remodeling of pulmonary vasculature and pulmonary hypertension (Eisenmenger syndrome) • Types: **ostium secundum most common** (75%), ostium primum (15-20%), sinus venous (5%), coronary sinus ASD is very rare

Signs & Symptoms	• **Asymptomatic: mostly asymptomatic in children**
	• **Symptomatic:** most patients will develop symptoms by 40 years old
	  • Young Children or Infants: may show decreased exercise tolerance, recurrent respiratory infections or failure to thrive
	  • Adults: may show decreased exercise tolerance, dyspnea, fatigue, palpitations, syncope, afib, pulmonary hypertension
	  • Stroke or TIA as result of paradoxical emboli
	• Physical Exam:
	  • Systolic ejection murmur at the left 2nd intercostal space (pulmonic area) with a **wide, fixed S2 split**
	  • Murmur does not change with respiration
	  • **Right ventricular heave**

Diagnosis	• **Echocardiogram: gold standard imaging modality;** evaluates size of defect, blood flow trajectory, cardiac anatomy, and estimate pulmonary artery pressure
	  • May show hypermobile atrial septum, right atrial enlargement, pulmonary artery dilation, high pulmonary artery pressure
	• **Electrocardiogram (ECG):**
	  • Incomplete right bundle branch block; **Crochetage pattern** (notch near apex of R wave in inferior limb leads); right axis deviation (pulmonary hypertension)
	• **Cardiac Catheterization: definitive diagnosis;** contraindicated in young patients/small defects

Treatment	• **Observation: indicated in ASD less than 5mm** as most will spontaneously close within first year of life • **Percutaneous Transcatheter vs Surgical Closure: indicated in ASD greater than 1cm** or symptomatic cases • Management of Complications: medical management of symptoms/complications (arrhythmia or pulmonary hypertension) • *Women with symptomatic ASD or pulmonary hypertension should avoid pregnancy*
Key Words & Most Common	• One of most common congenital heart defects; many spontaneous close • Left to right shunt & considered noncyanotic • Young are often asymptomatic; adults may be symptomatic by 40 years old; systolic murmur over pulmonic area • Echocardiogram is gold standard • Observe if <5mm; Intervention if >1cm or symptomatic

Ventricular Septal Defect

Etiology & Risk Factors	• **Defect in the interventricular septum between left and right ventricles;** typically associated with a **left-to-right shunt** • **Most common congenital cardiac abnormality in children;** can be isolated or in combination of other congenital cardiac anomalies (Tetralogy of Fallot) • Etiology: not fully understood; combination of genetic and environmental factors • Risks Factors: **certain genetic conditions** (Down syndrome), **maternal factors** (infection [**rubella**, influenza, or other febrile virus], gestational diabetes, **exposure to alcohol,** marijuana, cocaine or metronidazole, **advanced maternal age), fetal alcohol syndrome**
Patho-physiology	• Defect in the ventricular septum leads to a left-to-right shunt of blood through the opening; amount of shunted blood determines the clinical and hemodynamic significances of the VSD • 4 types: **perimembranous (most common),** trabecular muscular, inlet, and subpulmonary outlet
Signs & Symptoms	• **Symptoms increase as size of VSD increases** • **Poor feeding and inadequate weight gain** • Tachycardia and tachypnea worse during or after feedings, fatigue, diaphoresis • Frequent upper respiratory infections • Cyanotic Symptoms: cyanosis of fingers and lips; develop if large defect causing a right-to-left shunt of blood to occur (Eisenmenger syndrome) • Physical Exam: • **Harsh holosystolic murmur best heard at lower left sternal border;** smaller defects are associated with louder murmurs and palpable thrills
Diagnosis	• **Echocardiogram with Color Flow and Doppler: imaging test of choice;** determine important anatomic and hemodynamic information including size, location and blood flow • Electrocardiogram (ECG): mostly normal; may demonstrate biventricular hypertrophy (Katz-Wachtel phenomenon) in larger ASD • Chest X-Ray (CXR): normal or cardiomegaly with increased vascular markings
Treatment	• **Observation: no treatment required if small and asymptomatic; most will spontaneously close in early childhood** • **Surgical Repair:** percutaneous closure indicated in significantly symptomatic patients • Complications: unrepaired VSDs place patient at increased risk for pulmonary hypertension, endocarditis, arrhythmia, CHF
Key Words & Most Common	• Most common congenital cardiac abnormality; left to right shunt • Symptoms increase with size; poor feeding, tachypnea, frequent URI, fatigue • Echocardiogram is test of choice • Observation in small; surgical closure with significant symptoms

Defect in interventricular septum

Patent Ductus Arteriosus

Etiology & Risk Factors	• Persistence of the fetal connection (ductus arteriosus) between the aorta and pulmonary artery after birth; 2nd most common congenital heart defect • <u>Etiology</u>: not fully understood; combination of genetic and environmental factors • <u>Risk Factors</u>: **prematurity**, certain chromosomal abnormalities(trisomy 13/18/21), family history, maternal factors (infection [rubella], medication use [NSAIDs])
Patho-physiology	• Ductus arteriosus is a fetal vessel between the descending thoracic aorta and pulmonary artery that allows oxygenated blood from the placenta to bypass the lungs • Prostaglandins from the placenta keep vessel patent in utero; prostaglandin E1 production and low arterial oxygen after delivery may lead to patency of vessel • PDA results in blood being shunted from high pressure aorta to lower pressure pulmonary artery (left-to-right shunt) and may lead to pulmonary hypertension/edema • Shunting of blood during diastole results in increased cardiac output to compensate

Signs & Symptoms	• Often asymptomatic
	• **Symptoms worse with feeding/activity**
	   • **Dyspnea, tachycardia**, tachypnea, poor weight gain, irritability, poor feeding, recurrent respiratory infections, **diaphoresis**
	   • May develop **differential cyanosis** (cyanosis of lower extremities but not upper extremities)
	• <u>Physical Exam</u>:
	   • **Continuous machine-like murmur at left 2nd intercostal space (pulmonic area)**
	   • **Wide pulse pressures with bounding peripheral pulses**

Diagnosis	• <u>Echocardiogram</u>: imaging test of choice; demonstrates patent ductus arteriosus with left-to-right shunt; left atrial/ventricular enlargement • <u>Electrocardiogram (ECG)</u>: may demonstrate left atrial enlargement or left ventricular hypertrophy • <u>Chest X-Ray (CXR)</u>: normal or cardiomegaly; pulmonary edema or increased vascular markings

Treatment	• <u>Observation</u>: **no treatment required if small and asymptomatic; most will spontaneously close**
	   • Functional closure within hours; anatomical closure within weeks in healthy newborns
	• <u>Non-Steroidal Anti-Inflammatory Drugs (NSAIDs)</u>: **IV indomethacin** or ibuprofen **are first-line medications;** indicated with respiratory distress or cyanotic development
	   • Inhibit prostaglandin synthesis and blocks COX2 pathway
	• <u>Surgical Repair</u>: percutaneous catheter closure or surgical ligation indicated if failure to respond to medical therapy

Key Words & Most Common	• Prematurity is greatest risk factor; due to increased prostaglandin production keeps vessel patent • Continuous machine-like pulmonic murmur with wide pulse pressure • Dyspnea; respiratory distress; hypoxia; cyanotic lower extremities • Echocardiogram • NSAIDs (IV indomethacin) are first-line

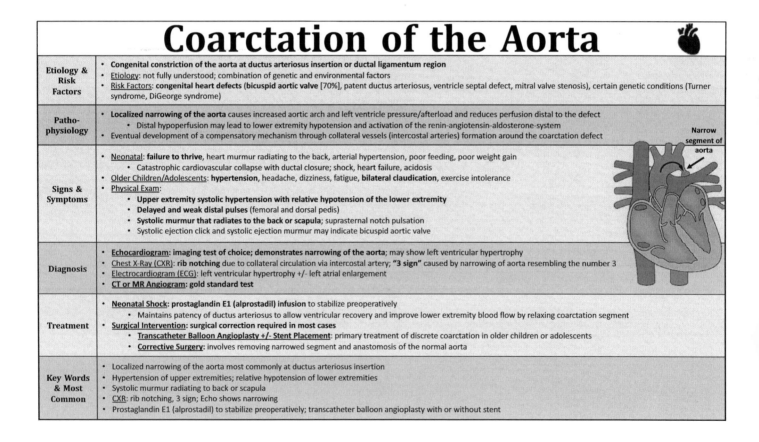

Coarctation of the Aorta

Etiology & Risk Factors	• **Congenital constriction of the aorta at ductus arteriosus insertion or ductal ligamentum region** • <u>Etiology</u>: not fully understood; combination of genetic and environmental factors • <u>Risk Factors</u>: **congenital heart defects (bicuspid aortic valve [70%]**, patent ductus arteriosus, ventricle septal defect, mitral valve stenosis), certain genetic conditions (Turner syndrome, DiGeorge syndrome)
Patho-physiology	• **Localized narrowing of the aorta** causes increased aortic arch and left ventricle pressure/afterload and reduces perfusion distal to the defect • Distal hypoperfusion may lead to lower extremity hypotension and activation of the renin-angiotensin-aldosterone-system • Eventual development of a compensatory mechanism through collateral vessels (intercostal arteries) formation around the coarctation defect

Signs & Symptoms	• <u>Neonatal</u>: **failure to thrive**, heart murmur radiating to the back, arterial hypertension, poor feeding, poor weight gain
	   • Catastrophic cardiovascular collapse with ductal closure; shock, heart failure, acidosis
	• <u>Older Children/Adolescents</u>: **hypertension**, headache, dizziness, fatigue, **bilateral claudication**, exercise intolerance
	• <u>Physical Exam</u>:
	   • **Upper extremity systolic hypertension with relative hypotension of the lower extremity**
	   • **Delayed and weak distal pulses** (femoral and dorsal pedis)
	   • **Systolic murmur that radiates to the back or scapula;** suprasternal notch pulsation
	   • Systolic ejection click and systolic ejection murmur may indicate bicuspid aortic valve

Diagnosis	• <u>Echocardiogram</u>: imaging test of choice; demonstrates narrowing of the aorta; may show left ventricular hypertrophy • <u>Chest X-Ray (CXR)</u>: **rib notching** due to collateral circulation via intercostal artery; **"3 sign"** caused by narrowing of aorta resembling the number 3 • <u>Electrocardiogram (ECG)</u>: left ventricular hypertrophy +/- left atrial enlargement • <u>CT or MR Angiogram</u>: **gold standard test**

Treatment	• <u>Neonatal Shock</u>: **prostaglandin E1 (alprostadil) infusion** to stabilize preoperatively
	   • Maintains patency of ductus arteriosus to allow ventricular recovery and improve lower extremity blood flow by relaxing coarctation segment
	• <u>Surgical Intervention</u>: surgical correction required in most cases
	   • <u>Transcatheter Balloon Angioplasty +/- Stent Placement</u>: primary treatment of discrete coarctation in older children or adolescents
	   • <u>Corrective Surgery</u>: involves removing narrowed segment and anastomosis of the normal aorta

Key Words & Most Common	• Localized narrowing of the aorta most commonly at ductus arteriosus insertion • Hypertension of upper extremities; relative hypotension of lower extremities • Systolic murmur radiating to back or scapula • <u>CXR</u>: rib notching, 3 sign; Echo shows narrowing • Prostaglandin E1 (alprostadil) to stabilize preoperatively; transcatheter balloon angioplasty with or without stent

Tetralogy of Fallot

Etiology & Risk Factors	• Congenital anomaly resulting in **4 distinct defects** • **(1) Right ventricle outflow obstruction (pulmonary stenosis) (2) Right ventricular hypertrophy (3) Ventricular septal defect (4) Overriding aorta** • <u>Etiology</u>: not fully understood; combination of genetic and environmental factors; most common cyanotic congenital heart disease • <u>Risk Factors</u>: **maternal factors (maternal diabetes, maternal retinoic acid intake, toxin exposures, rubella infection), certain chromosomal anomalies** (trisomy 13, 18, 21); gene 22q11.2; cleft palate/lip
Patho-physiology	• **Acute hypoxic episodes caused by a right to left shunt across the ventricular septal defect** • During cyanotic episodes there is increased pulmonary stenosis (RV obstruction) or decreased vascular resistance leading to the right-to-left shunt of blood flow • Pt may have history of squatting during episodes to increase systemic vascular resistance • Hypoxemia & hypercarbia results which further increases pulmonary vascular resistance and compounds on itself

Signs & Symptoms	• **Cyanosis during feeding & crying**
	• **"Tet spells": acute episode of hypoxia & cyanosis**
	    • **May be precipitated by increased activity, feeding or crying**
	    • **Child may squat**, or infants may bring knees to chest during episodes to increase systemic vascular resistance (increases afterload and decreases right-to-left shunt)
	• <u>Chronic Hypoxemia</u>: nailbed clubbing and elevated hematocrit
	• <u>Physical Exam</u>:
	    • **Early, harsh crescendo-decrescendo holosystolic murmur at left mid to upper sternal border** (ventricular septal defect/pulmonary stenosis)
	    • Murmur may radiate to back; right ventricular heave

Diagnosis	• <u>**Echocardiogram with Color Flow and Doppler Studies**</u>: **preferred imaging test** • <u>Chest X-Ray (CXR)</u>: **"boot-shaped heart"**; decreased vascular markings • <u>Electrocardiogram (ECG)</u>: right atrial/ventricular hypertrophy; right axis deviation
Treatment	• <u>Hypercyanotic Spells</u>: bring to knee-to-chest position, calming, supplemental oxygen, IV fluids • Try to avoid needle sticks during acute cyanotic event as crying worsens pulmonary vascular resistance • <u>**IV Prostaglandin E1**</u>: prostaglandin E1 indicated if infant does not respond to oxygen; maintains patent ductus arteriosus • <u>**Surgical Repair**</u>: cardiothoracic surgical repair performed ideally within first 3-11 months of life
Key Words & Most Common	• <u>4 Defects</u>: (1) Right ventricle outflow obstruction (pulmonary stenosis) (2) Right ventricular hypertrophy (3) Ventricular septal defect (4) Overriding aorta • "Tet spells" – cyanosis during feeding/crying; squatting or knees-to-chest position relieves cyanosis • Crescendo-decrescendo holosystolic murmur at left sternal border • Echo; CXR shows boot shaped heart • O$_2$→ prostaglandin E1

Labels on diagram: Overriding Aorta; Pulmonic Stenosis; Ventricular Septal Defect; Right Ventricular Hypertrophy

Transposition of the Great Arteries

Etiology & Risk Factors	• **Aorta originates from right ventricle while pulmonary artery from the left ventricle**; results in independent, parallel pulmonary and systemic circulations • <u>Etiology</u>: not fully understood; combination of genetic and environmental factors • <u>Risk Factors</u>: **maternal factors** (maternal diabetes, advanced maternal age, medication or toxin exposures), **certain genetic anomalies**

Patho-physiology	• **Two parallel circuits**
	    • **Deoxygenated systemic venous blood returns to right atrium and then back to systemic circulation via the right ventricle and aorta**
	    • **Oxygenated pulmonary venous blood returns to left atrium and then back to lungs via the left ventricle and pulmonary artery**
	• Survival is dependent on communication between the two circuits by either an ASD, VSD, PDA or patent foramen ovale

Signs & Symptoms	• **Cyanosis is most common sign**; determined by extent of communication between circuits; usually presents within first month of life • <u>Heart Failure</u>: tachypnea, dyspnea, tachycardia, diaphoresis, inability to gain weight • <u>Physical Exam</u>: • Pansystolic murmur at left lower sternal border (if VSD present)
Diagnosis	• <u>**Echocardiogram with Color Flow and Doppler Studies**</u>: **preferred imaging test** • <u>Electrocardiogram (ECG)</u>: initially normal; may show right axis deviation or right ventricular hypertrophy • <u>Chest X-Ray (CXR)</u>: "egg on a string"; great arteries form a narrow vascular pedicle when transposed; mild cardiomegaly; increased pulmonary vascular markings • <u>Cardiac Catheterization</u>: gold standard but rarely used
Treatment	• <u>**IV Prostaglandin E1**</u>: prostaglandin E1 indicated to maintain patent ductus arteriosus and supply intercirculatory mixing • <u>**Balloon Atrial Septostomy**</u>: indicated to stabilize severe hypoxemia due to inadequate mixing; indicated for severely hypoxemic neonates who do not respond to PGE1 • <u>**Arterial Switch Operation**</u>: **definitive repair**; typically performed within first 2 weeks of life • *Most patients (90%) will die within first year of life without treatment*
Key Words & Most Common	• Systemic venous blood returns to right atrium and reenters systemic circulation via right ventricle and aorta • Pulmonary venous blood returns to left atrium & reenters lungs via left ventricle and pulmonary artery • Cyanosis and tachypnea • Echo; CXR shows "egg on a string" • IV prostaglandins; arterial switch surgery

Labels on diagram: Pulmonary artery originates from left ventricle; Aorta originates from right ventricle

Angina Pectoris

Etiology & Risk Factors	• Clinical syndrome of precordial discomfort or pressure secondary to transient myocardial ischemia without infarction • <u>Etiology</u>: coronary artery stenosis (atherosclerosis) is most common cause of myocardial ischemia • <u>Risk Factors</u>: advanced age, **coronary artery disease, atherosclerosis, hyperlipidemia, diabetes mellitus, smoking**, obesity/metabolic syndrome, family history, hypertension, sedentary lifestyle, stress
Patho-physiology	• Cardiac function is dependent on oxygenation to support contractility; inadequate oxygen supply due to impaired perfusion leads to an increase in anaerobic glycolysis; the increased level of hydrogen, potassium, and lactate enters venous return to resupply heart; hydrogen ions compete with calcium causing hypokinesis

Signs & Symptoms	• **Chest Pain**: most common symptom
	  • Described as pressure, heavy, or tight
	  • Often substernal or poorly localized; may have radiation of symptoms to arm, jaw, shoulder, epigastric region
	  • <u>Stable</u>: exertional chest pain that **last less than 30 minutes & resolves within 5 minutes of rest or with nitroglycerine**
	  • <u>Unstable</u>: chest pain occurring for first time, **at rest**, or with increased severity/frequency
	• **Diaphoresis**, dyspnea, nausea/vomiting, fatigue out of proportion to activity level
	• *Women/elderly/obese may present atypically*

Diagnosis	• Clinical diagnosis for stable angina; physical exam typically benign (evaluate for pleuritic/palpated/positional chest pain to rule in/out other etiologies) • <u>Electrocardiogram (ECG)</u>: **initial test of choice**; may show **ST segment depression**, T wave inversions, or old infarct • <u>Chest X-Ray (CXR)</u>: utilized to rule out other causes of chest pain (infection, pneumothorax, trauma) • <u>Labs</u>: CBC, CMP, lipids, cardiac enzymes • <u>Stress Test</u>: **most important non-invasive test**; may use stress ECG, stress echocardiogram, or myocardial perfusion imaging • <u>Coronary angiography</u>: definitive test

Treatment	• <u>Lifestyle Modifications</u>: **tobacco cessation**, cholesterol reduction, blood pressure control, weight loss, aerobic exercise, diabetes control
	• <u>Medical Management</u>: prevention of ischemia
	  • <u>Antiplatelets</u>: aspirin, clopidogrel, prasugrel; inhibit platelet aggregation to reduce risk of ischemic events
	  • <u>Beta Blockers</u>: indicated in all patients; block sympathetic stimulation of the heart and reduce systolic BP, heart rate, contractility, and cardiac output
	  • <u>Nitrates</u>: nitroglycerin as needed; most effective medication during acute attack
	  • <u>Calcium Channel Blockers</u>: may be used if symptoms persist despite use of nitrates or if nitrates are not tolerated
	• <u>Revascularization Procedure</u>: **definitive treatment**
	  • <u>Percutaneous Coronary Interventions (PCI)</u>: **angioplasty vs stenting** indicated for <2 vessel stenosis not involving left main coronary artery
	  • <u>Coronary Artery Bypass Graft (CABG)</u>: indicated for **left main coronary artery stenosis, >2 vessel stenosis**, or left ventricle ejection fraction <40%

Prinzmetal Angina

Etiology & Risk Factors	• Secondary to epicardial coronary artery spasm; also known as **coronary artery vasospasm** or variant angina • <u>Etiology</u>: coronary artery vasospasm • <u>Risk Factors</u>: **female, age (most common <50 years old), history of vasospasm (migraines, Raynaud phenomenon)**, smoking, substance use (**cocaine**, amphetamines) • <u>Precipitating Factors</u>: alpha-agonist substances (**cocaine**, pseudoephedrine, oxymetazoline), cold weather, exercise, emotional stress, hyperventilation, or Valsalva
Patho-physiology	• **Exposure to vasoconstrictive stimuli causes coronary artery vasospasm** and temporary stenosis leads to ischemia and myocardial injury • Endothelial response may be inhibited due to imbalance of sympathetic and parasympathetic tone or impaired vasoconstriction/vasodilation regulatory mechanism
Signs & Symptoms	• **Chest Pain**: most commonly occurs at rest (non-exertional and persists through rest) • Chronic pattern occurring for 5-15minutes usually between midnight and early morning • Diaphoresis, nausea, palpitations; may be preceded by hyperventilation

Diagnosis	• <u>Electrocardiogram (ECG)</u>: **initial test of choice**
	  • **Transient ST elevations** during vasospasm; may have ST depressions or T-wave inversions
	  • **ECG changes resolve with nitroglycerin** or calcium channel blocker
	• <u>Labs</u>: **troponin often normal**; drug toxicology if cocaine suspected
	• <u>Coronary Angiography</u>: **confirms diagnosis**
	  • May show evidence of vasospasm spontaneously or with drug induction (ergonovine)

Treatment	• <u>Lifestyle Modification</u>: avoid potential triggers, avoid cold exposure, stress reduction, cessation of smoking or substance abuse
	• <u>Medical Management</u>:
	  • <u>Calcium Channel Blockers</u>: **first-line medication to prevent symptoms** and for chronic management; taken at night
	  • <u>Nitroglycerin</u>: may be used while symptomatic; promptly relieves variant angina
	  • *Avoid nonselective beta blockers as can worsen vasospasm (allows unopposed alpha-adrenergic vasoconstriction)*

Key Words & Most Common	• Relatively young, female patient with history of migraines or Raynaud phenomenon is classic patient; few risk factors for coronary artery disease • Coronary artery vasospasm caused by a trigger • Chest pain occurring at rest • ECG shows ST elevation • Nitroglycerin in acute phase; CCB for chronic management

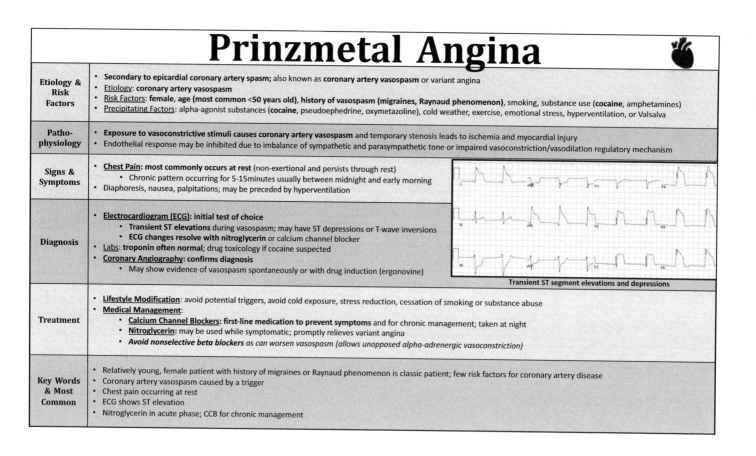

Transient ST segment elevations and depressions

Non-ST Elevation Myocardial Infarction ❤

Etiology & Risk Factors	• **Myocardial necrosis (as evident by positive cardiac biomarkers in blood)** *without* **acute ST-segment elevation; also known as NSTEMI** • <u>Etiology</u>: **coronary artery disease; atherosclerosis is most common** cause due to plaque formation • <u>Risk Factors</u>: **history of coronary artery disease is greatest risk factors**, male, advanced age, **diabetes mellitus, smoking, obesity**/metabolic syndrome, **hyperlipidemia**, family history, hypertension, age, sedentary lifestyle, poor diet, chronic kidney disease
Patho-physiology	• Partial occlusion of a coronary artery (usually due to the rupture of an atherosclerotic plaque) that exposes the underlying tissue, leading to platelet aggregation and the formation of a thrombus that partially obstructs cardiac perfusion • Inadequate oxygenation causes ischemia and necrosis of the cardiac myocytes, but without complete occlusion of the artery seen in STEMI

Signs & Symptoms	• <u>**Chest Pain**</u>: **described as pressure, heaviness or tightness**
	  • **Often substantial** or poorly localized; **may have radiation of symptoms to arm, jaw, shoulder, epigastric region**
	  • Not relieved with rest or with nitroglycerin
	• **Diaphoresis**, dyspnea, nausea/vomiting, dizziness, anxiety, tachycardia due to sympathetic stimulation
	• *Women/elderly/obese may present atypically*
	• <u>Physical Exam</u>:
	  • Often normal, may be tachycardic, anxious, diaphoretic

Diagnosis	• <u>**Electrocardiogram (ECG)**</u>: **initial test of choice; should be performed within first 10 minutes**
	  • Demonstrates no ST segment elevation; may show **ST depression**, T wave inversions, bradycardia or heart blocks
	• <u>**Cardiac Enzymes**</u>: serum markers of myocardial cell injury; elevated creatine kinase-MB isoenzyme (CK-MB) and cell contents (troponin I, troponin T, myoglobin)
	  • *Most patients with true ischemia will have elevated troponin within 6 hours*
	• <u>Coronary Angiography</u>: confirms diagnosis: within the first 24-48 hours in uncomplicated patient

Treatment	• <u>**Pre-Hospital Care**</u>: oxygen, aspirin, nitrates, triage to an appropriate medical center +/- morphine
	  • <u>**Aspirin (325mg)**</u>: indicated for antiplatelet, chewed for faster absorption
	  • <u>**Sublingual Nitroglycerin**</u>: potent vasodilator (increase coronary artery perfusion, decrease preload); *contraindicated if systolic BP<90 or use of PDE5 inhibitors*
	  • <u>Oxygen</u>: typically given at 2L/min nasal canula (4L/min if spO$_2$<90%)
	  • <u>Morphine</u>: consider judicious use of if nitroglycerin is contraindicated or if the patient has symptoms despite nitroglycerin therapy
	• <u>**Antithrombotics**</u>: unfractionated heparin or low-molecular weight heparin (LMWH) is routinely given if ST depression or T wave inversions unless contraindicated
	• <u>**Beta Blockers**</u>: decreases inotropic and chronotropic response to catecholamines; *contraindicated if <50bpm, systolic BP<90 or acute CHF*
	• <u>**Angiotensin-Converting Enzyme Inhibitors (ACEI)**</u>: decreases ventricular remodeling; indicated in CHF, hypertension, diabetes, or chronic kidney disease
	• <u>Observation</u>: serial ECGs and cardiac enzymes; medical management vs catheterization determined by level of risk for future cardiovascular events
	• <u>Fibrinolytics</u>: not indicated for any NSTEMI patients; risk outweighs potential benefit
	• <u>Coronary Angiography</u>: procedure within the first 24-48 hours of hospitalization to identify coronary lesions requiring PCI or CABG

ST Elevation Myocardial Infarction ❤

Etiology & Risk Factors	• **Myocardial necrosis (as evident by positive cardiac biomarkers in blood)** *with* **acute ST-segment elevation; also known as STEMI** • <u>Etiology</u>: **atherosclerotic plaque rupture in coronary arteries is most common cause; thrombus causes total occlusion and severe myocardial ischemia** • <u>Risk Factors</u>: **history of coronary artery disease is greatest risk factors**, male, advanced age, **diabetes mellitus, smoking, obesity**/metabolic syndrome, **hyperlipidemia**, family history, hypertension, age, sedentary lifestyle, poor diet, chronic kidney disease
Patho-physiology	• Atherosclerotic plaque rupture causes arterial thrombus leading to complete and persistent occlusion of myocardial perfusion; oxygen demand cannot be met

Signs & Symptoms	• <u>**Chest Pain**</u>: **described as pressure, heaviness or tightness**
	  • **Often substantial** or poorly localized; **may have radiation of symptoms to arm, jaw, shoulder, epigastric region**
	  • Not relieved with rest or with nitroglycerin
	• **Diaphoresis**, dyspnea, nausea/vomiting, dizziness, anxiety (**sense of impending doom**), tachycardia due to sympathetic stimulation
	• *Women/elderly/obese may present atypically*
	• <u>Physical Exam</u>:
	  • May be tachycardic, anxious, diaphoretic
	  • <u>**Levine's Sign**</u>: clenched fist held over the chest to describe ischemic chest pain
	  • <u>Triad for Right Ventricular Infarct</u>: hypotension + clear lung auscultation + increased JVP +/- Kussmaul's sign

Diagnosis	• <u>**Electrocardiogram (ECG)**</u>: **test of choice; should be performed within first 10 minutes**
	  • Demonstrates **ST segment elevation** >1mm in 2 or more contiguous leads with reciprocal changes
	    • ECG Progression: hyperacute T waves → ST segment elevation → Q waves
	• <u>**Cardiac Enzymes**</u>: serum markers of myocardial cell injury; elevated creatine kinase-MB isoenzyme (CK-MB) and cell contents (troponin I, troponin T, myoglobin)

Treatment	• <u>**Emergency Percutaneous Coronary Intervention (PCI)**</u>: **preferred treatment when readily available** (door to balloon-inflation time <90 minutes) • <u>**Fibrinolytics**</u>: most effective if utilized within first 30 minutes if PCI cannot commence within first 120 minutes (including hospital transfer); heparin is required after thrombolysis to prevent re-thrombus • <u>Adjunctive Therapy</u>: aspirin, antiplatelet (clopidogrel), oxygen, nitroglycerin, morphine, beta blockers, ACEI, statin
Key Words & Most Common	• Atherosclerosis is most common cause leading to plaque thrombus • Chest pain, diaphoresis, dyspnea • <u>ECG</u>: ST segment elevation >1mm in 2 contiguous leads; cardiac biomarkers elevated • Thrombolytics vs PCI; PCI preferred if can be started within 120 minutes

ST Elevation Myocardial Infarction
ECG and Cardiac Biomarker Interpretation

Locations	Ischemic Changes	Coronary Artery Involved
Anterior Wall	V1-V4	Left Anterior Descending
Anteroseptal	V1-V2	Proximal LAD
Lateral Wall	I, aVL, V5-V6	Circumflex
Anterolateral	I, aVL, V4-V6	Mid LAD or Circumflex
Inferior Wall	II, III, aVF	Right Coronary
Posterior Wall	ST depression V1-V2	Right Coronary (90%)

Type	Elevated Within	Peak Elevation	Return to Baseline
CK-MB	4-6 hours	12-24 hours	2-4 days
Troponin I & T	4-8 hours	10-24 hours	7-10 days
Myoglobin	1-4 hours	4-6 hours	1 day

I Lateral	aVR Aorta	V1 Septal	V4 Anterior
II Inferior	aVL Lateral	V2 Septal	V5 Lateral
III Inferior	aVF Inferior	V3 Anterior	V6 Lateral

Heart Failure

Etiology & Risk Factors	• Inability of the heart to supply sufficient perfusion to meet metabolic demands; abnormal retention of water and sodium result in venous congestion
	• Etiology: ventricular dysfunction
	  • **Left Side Heart Failure: coronary artery disease and hypertension are most common causes**
	  • **Right Side Heart Failure: left side heart failure is most common cause;** pulmonary disease (pulmonary hypertension, COPD)
	  • Systolic Heart Failure: decreased contractility (decreased ejection fraction); occurs secondary to myocardial infarction or dilated cardiomyopathy
	  • Diastolic Heart Failure: preserved contractility (normal ejection fraction); occurs secondary to hypertension, hypertrophy, hypertrophic or restrictive cardiomyopathy
	• Risk Factors: **coronary artery disease is greatest risk factor, advanced age,** smoking, hypertension, obesity, diabetes, valvular heart disease, uncontrolled arrhythmias, sedentary lifestyle, poor diet,

Patho-physiology	• Increased afterload and decreased myocardial contractility with impaired relaxation leads to increased myocardial oxygen demand; paradoxical need for increased cardiac output leads to myocardial cell death that then causes an overall decrease in cardiac output leading to heart failure • Decrease in cardiac output also leads to activation of RAAS causing increased sodium and fluid restriction and increased vasoconstriction; may lead to cardiac remodeling

	Left Side Heart Failure	Right Side Heart Failure

Signs & Symptoms	• **Pulmonary Vascular Congestion: dyspnea (most common symptom), cough with pink frothy sputum, fatigue, orthopnea, paroxysmal nocturnal dyspnea, nocturia**
	• Physical Exam:
	  • **Basilar rales** (fluid in alveoli), **wheezing, tachypnea, rhonchi,** cyanosis, **cool extremities, S3** (systolic), S4 (diastolic), **parasternal lift;** enlarged/displaced/hyperdynamic **apical impulse**
	  • **Cheyne-Stokes Breathing:** deep/fast breaths with gradual decrease/apnea)
		• **Systemic Vascular Congestion: dependent pitting edema;** decreased appetite/nausea (from GI tract edema) and
		• Physical Exam:
		  • **Jugular Venous Distension (JVD):** increased jugular venous pressure
		  • **Hepatomegaly: tender liver from hepatic congestion**
		  • **Peripheral Edema: lower extremity pitting edema;** may develop cyanosis

Diagnosis	• **Echocardiogram: most useful imaging to assess size/function of chamber, valves, pericardial effusion, shunts and ejection fraction** • Chest X-Ray (CXR): cardiomegaly, **pulmonary effusions/edema, perivascular or interstitial edema (Kerley B lines),** venous dilation, cephalization and alveolar fluid • Labs: CBC (rule out anemia), CMP, troponin/CK, **B-type natriuretic peptide (BNP),** thyroid panel in elderly patients, consider iron if hemochromatosis suspected • Electrocardiogram (ECG): **low voltage,** underlying arrhythmia (afib), conduction defect, **left ventricular hypertrophy,** evidence of new/old myocardial infarction
Treatment	• Lifestyle modifications: **sodium restriction** (<2g per day), exercise, smoking cessation, **fluid restriction** (<2L per day,) sleep upright, stress reduction • ACEI/ARB: **first-line medication;** most effective medication in mortality reduction by decreasing afterload and ventricular remodeling; improves other vasodilators • Beta Blockers: **improves ejection fraction by decreasing afterload,** reduces left ventricular dilation and reduces dysrhythmias • Diuretics: **most effective symptomatic treatment; added with fluid and sodium retention and edema;** Spironolactone may be used for potassium sparing • Hydralazine: decreases preload; may be combined with nitrates (preload and afterload reduction) • Digoxin: indicated for decompensated heart failure positive inotrope (↑ contractility), negative chronotrope (↓ heart rate) and negative dromotrope (↓conduction velocity)

Hypertension

Etiology & Risk Factors	• Defined as **systolic BP ≥130mmHg** and/or **diastolic BP ≥80mmHg**; Stage 2 HTN is systolic ≥140mmHg &/or diastolic ≥90mmHg
	• Etiology: may be primary or secondary
	   • **Primary (Essential): most common (95%) idiopathic**; multiple genetic and environmental factors that have compounding effects on cardiac and renal structure
	      • Family history, age >50, race or ethnicity (**African American**), alcohol, **smoking**, diabetes, dyslipidemia, anxiety, obesity, high sodium diet, sedentary lifestyle
	   • **Secondary**: due to underlying cause or agent that is often correctable
	      • Medications (OCP, NSAIDs, antidepressants, glucocorticoids, decongestants, stimulants); certain endocrine disorders (Cushing's, hyperaldosteronism, pheochromocytoma), obstructive sleep apnea, hyperthyroidism, kidney disease, substance abuse (cocaine, amphetamines)

Patho-physiology	• Increased sodium absorption and water retention leads to vascular volume expansion which impairs the renin-angiotensin-aldosterone system (RAAS) response and increases sympathetic nervous system activation to raise blood pressure; these changes lead to increased total peripheral resistance and afterload • Renovascular is most common cause of secondary HTN (renal artery stenosis); low blood flow to kidneys→renin secretion→water retention→fluid volume increase→HTN
Signs & Symptoms	• **Often asymptomatic** • **Nonspecific headache** is most common complaint is nonspecific headache • Moderate to Severe HTN: **hypertensive retinopathy**, retinal hemorrhages, exudates, **papilledema** • **HTN Urgency**: systolic BP >180mmHg or diastolic BP >110mmHg **with no symptoms** • **HTN Emergency**: systolic BP >180mmHg or diastolic BP >110mmHg **w/ end organ damage** (headache, dyspnea, chest pain, neurologic defects/stroke, signs of kidney failure, change in vision) Complications: • Cardiac: CAD, HF, MI, LVH, aortic aneurysm & dissection, ischemic heart disease • Neurologic: TIA, stroke, intracerebral hemorrhage (aneurysm rupture) • Nephropathy: CKD/renal disease, renal stenosis, MCC of renal disease • Ophthalmic: retinopathy, retinal hemorrhage
Diagnosis	• Labs: CBC (Hgb), CMP (creatinine/GFR, glucose), TSH, lipid panel; consider uric acid level, urine albumin to creatinine ratio, and urine pregnancy (preeclampsia) • Electrocardiogram: may show LVH • Fundoscopy: evaluate for **retinopathy**

Treatment	• Lifestyle changes: **low sodium diet**, smoking and alcohol cessation, exercise, weight loss
	• **Medical Management**: indicated for patients with DM/CKD and BP ≥140/90mmHg with BP target of <140/90mmHg; >60yo with BP ≥150/90mmHg to target BP <150/90mmHg
	   • **Diuretics: first-line medication without comorbidities**; reduces plasma volume to reduce peripheral resistance
	      • Thiazides: are most effects
	      • Loop: decrease lower extremity edema secondary to proteinuria (only diuretics in those w/ renal dysfunction when close electrolyte monitoring is assured)
	   • **ACEI/ARB: first-line with CKD or diabetes**; labs required prior to initiation to heck for hyperkalemia and kidney function (BUN/creatinine)
	   • **Beta Blockers**: used to decrease heart rate and cardiac output; reduces mortality post-MI (use with caution with pulmonary disease or diabetes)
	   • **Calcium Channel Blockers: preferred antihypertensive in African Americans and elderly**; causes peripheral vasodilation
	   • **Alpha Antagonists: consider as initial drug of choice in men with symptomatic prostatic hyperplasia**; lowers peripheral vascular resistance
	• Hypertensive Urgency: gradual reduction of BP no more than 25% over 24-48 hours with oral meds (**clonidine**, captopril, labetalol, nicardipine, or furosemide)
	• Hypertensive Emergency: gradual reduction 10-20% in first hour, then 5-15% over next 23 hours (no more than 25% reduction in first 24 hours); exceptions are aortic dissection or ischemic stroke (dissection requires rapid BP reduction to decrease shearing forces); IV formulary
	   • Preferred agents include sodium nitroprusside (NTG or BB if MI suspected); nitroprusside and BB (labetalol or esmolol) indicated for aortic dissection

Orthostatic Hypotension

Etiology & Risk Factors	• Defined as an excessive or sudden drop in blood pressure when an upright position is assumed
	• Etiology:
	   • Failure of Autonomic Reflex/Neurologic: diabetes, Parkinson disease, familial dysautonomia
	   • Intravascular Volume Depletion: **dehydration**, diuretic side effects, hemorrhage, vomiting
	   • Medication Side Effects: **antihypertensives**, diuretics, antipsychotic/antidepressants
	   • Cardiogenic: aortic stenosis, arrhythmia
	• Risk Factors: **advanced age (>65 years old most common); most common cause of falls in elderly, prolonged bed rest or immobility**, nervous system damage, anemia, pregnancy, alcohol consumption, antihypertensive medications

Patho-physiology	• Gravitational forces cause blood to accumulate in lower extremities when going from supine to standing resulting in decreased venous return contributing to decreased cardiac output which may lead to cerebral hypoperfusion • Normal compensation occurs with an increase in sympathetic and decrease in vagal tone (baroreceptor reflex) to increase peripheral vascular resistance which will raise venous return and cardiac output; *orthostatic hypotension is a result an impaired compensatory mechanism*
Signs & Symptoms	• **Hypoperfusion: sudden postural change leads to cerebral hypoperfusion** • **Dizziness, lightheadedness**, presyncope/syncope, blurred vision, palpitations, impaired cognition, nausea, headache • **Tachycardia**: suspect hypovolemia if accompanied by **rise in heart rate >15 bpm**
Diagnosis	• Orthostatic Vital Signs: patient lies supine while obtaining the blood pressure and heart rate. After five minutes, patient stands for 2-5 minutes and vital signs taken again • **Diagnosis confirmed with drop in systolic BP ≥20mmHg or diastolic BP ≥10mmHg from supine to standing** (within 3 minutes of position change) • **Tilt Table Test**: reduction of blood pressure with 60-degree incline of bed • Electrocardiogram (ECG): considered in those with no obvious cause to rule out cardiogenic etiology • Labs: CBC (**anemia**); BMP (BUN/Cr, electrolytes, glucose); findings of dehydration
Treatment	• **Address Underlying Etiology: first-line management; address volume status and medication** • **Medication Reconciliation**: diuretics, antihypertensives, vasodilators, antidepressants, dopaminergics • Supportive: **increase salt/fluid intake**, gradual position changes, compression stockings, fall prevention methods • **Aldosterone Analogues: fludrocortisone; first-line medication** for persistent symptoms; increases vascular tone • **Alpha-1 Agonists: midodrine**; may be used in refractory cases or if fludrocortisone is contraindicated; increases vascular tone
Key Words & Most Common	• Drop in systolic BP ≥20mmHg or diastolic BP ≥10mmHg from supine to standing • MCC is volume depletion; dizziness, lightheadedness, blurry vision most common symptom • Orthostatic vital signs or tilt table test • Treat underlying cause; fludrocortisone first line medication

Cardiogenic Shock

Etiology & Risk Factors	• Low output cardiac state resulting in circulatory failure resulting in organ hypoperfusion and tissue hypoxia • <u>Etiology</u>: **decreased circulating volume, decreased cardiac output and vasodilation** • **Myocardial infarction**, arrhythmias, heart failure, valvular/septal defects, hypertension, cardiomyopathies, medication overdose, electrolyte abnormalities • <u>Risk Factors</u>: **new or recent myocardial infarction is greatest risk factor,** advanced age, female, diabetes mellitus, history of left ventricular injury, hypertension, smoking, sedentary lifestyle, substance abuse
Patho-physiology	• Myocardial ischemia causes systolic and diastolic dysfunction which decreases myocardial contractility leading to **decreased cardiac output, hypotension and further cardiac ischemia**; myocardial injury → hypo-contractility → ↓cardiac output and ↓blood pressure → worsening hypoperfusion • Compensatory mechanisms such as tachycardia (increases myocardial oxygen demand and worsens ischemia and sympathetic activation) leads to **systemic vasoconstriction** and can increase afterload resulting in a self-perpetuating cycle causing global hypoperfusion and tissue death • <u>Metabolic Acidosis</u>: progressive tissue hypoxia → anaerobic metabolism → localized tissue death (lactic acid production)→ organ dysfunction
Signs & Symptoms	• **Usually acutely ill appearing** • <u>Organ Hypoperfusion</u>: altered mental status, **cool/mottled extremities, hypotension, oliguria,** diminished capillary refill and weak or absent peripheral pulses • <u>Congestive Heart Failure</u>: jugular venous distention (JVD), S3, pulmonary congestion/edema (rales), **peripheral edema, tachycardia/tachypnea**
Diagnosis	• <u>Clinical Criteria</u>: **systolic BP ≤90mmHg for greater ≥30 minutes or mechanical support to maintain systolic BP and urine output ≤30 mL/hr or cool extremities** • <u>Labs</u>: CBC, CMP, **blood type cross-match**, coagulation studies, lactate, **cultures** (investigate infection), cardiac biomarkers if suspecting MI, BNP • <u>CMP</u>: electrolytes, glucose, urinalysis, serum creatinine will help determine cause of shock; LFTs elevated with liver hypoperfusion • <u>Oxygen Saturation</u>: pulse oximetry or serial arterial blood gas (ABG) required to monitor tissue oxygenation • <u>Electrocardiogram (ECG)</u>: required to evaluate for myocardial ischemia or infarction • <u>Imaging</u>: chest x-ray (CXR) and transthoracic echocardiogram (TTE) should be considered

Treatment	• <u>Resuscitation</u>: true emergency requiring resuscitative therapy to preserve organ function; *early coronary blood flow restoration is most important intervention*
	   • **ABCDE's**: consider intubation (decreases O₂ demand but may worsen preload)
	   • Consider **small IV fluid challenge** (250-500cc normal saline) to avoid fluid overload dependent on patient's point on Starling curve; blood transfusion if Hgb<10
	• **Inotropic Support**: **dobutamine +/- norepinephrine** OR dopamine; consider milrinone or beta-blocker reversal if patient on beta-blocker; intra-aortic balloon pump
	• **Treat Underlying Etiology**: fibrinolytics vs angioplasty indicated for myocardial infarction

Key Words & Most Common	• Post MI • Low cardiac output state resulting in organ hypoperfusion and tissue hypoxia • <u>Organ Hypoperfusion</u>: AMS, cyanosis, hypotension, oliguria, tachypnea • Resuscitative therapy; only shock where large amounts of fluid are held; increase inotropy with dobutamine/norepinephrine

Distributive Shock

	Septic Shock	Anaphylactic Shock	Neurogenic Shock	Hypo-Adrenal Shock
Etiology & Risk Factors	• Systemic vasodilation and change in blood flow distribution results in tissue and organ hypoperfusion; decreased cardiac output and systemic vascular resistance (SVR) • Relative inadequacy of intravascular volume caused by arterial or venous vasodilation (circulating blood volume is normal)			
	• Bacterial infection with endotoxin release	• History of insect bite/sting, consumption of certain foods, medications, use of IV contrast	• Trauma or burns, spinal cord injury	• Addisonian crisis
Patho-physiology	• Infection leads to a dysregulated immune response producing systemic inflammation and cytokine release leading to vasodilation and decreased SVR	• IgE-mediated systemic hypersensitivity reaction causing a histamine release from mast cells and basophils leading to vasodilation and capillary fluid leak	• Sympathetic nervous system damage results in decreased adrenergic input causing vasodilation with resultant hypotension and paradoxical bradycardia	• Adrenal insufficiency leads to decreased alpha-1 receptor expression on arterioles secondary to decreased cortisol resulting in vasodilation
Signs & Symptoms	• **Infection symptoms** • Hypotension with wide pulse pressures, bounding peripheral pulses, tachycardia/tachypnea, **fever**, AMS • **Warm/flushed extremities (early)**	• **Urticaria, pruritus, angioedema** • Respiratory distress, hoarseness (laryngeal edema), throat swelling, tongue numbness	• Warm skin • **Bradycardia/hypotension**, wide pulse pressure, hypovolemia • **Evidence of trauma/burns**	• **Hypoglycemia** • **Hypotension that does not respond to fluid resuscitation**
Diagnosis	• <u>Electrocardiogram (ECG)</u>: identify arrhythmias • <u>Chest X-Ray (CXR)</u>: evaluate for pneumonia, pulmonary effusion/edema, pneumothorax • <u>Ultrasound</u>: bedside US to evaluate hemorrhage, pulmonary edema, pericardial tamponade • <u>Labs</u>: CBC, CMP, **blood type cross-match**, coagulation studies, **lactate, urine and blood cultures** (investigate infection), UA, lipase • <u>Consider for Workup</u>: procalcitonin (pneumonia), CT head or lumbar puncture, TSH (thyroid storm), pelvic exam (toxic shock syndrome), CT abdomen/pelvis (abdominal abscess, ruptured bowel or appendix)			
Treatment	• **Vasopressor Support: norepinephrine, dopamine**; fluid resuscitation • **Broad Spectrum IV Antibiotics:** • Piperacillin/tazobactam + Ceftriaxone; Vancomycin; Clindamycin + Metronidazole (for intra-abdominal infection); infection source control	• **Epinephrine**: indicated due to beta-2 stimulation for bronchodilation and mast cell stabilization) • **Antihistamines**: diphenhydramine • **Albuterol: bronchodilation** • **Corticosteroids**: may help prevent a late-phase reaction	• **Vasopressor Support**: norepinephrine, dopamine; fluid resuscitation • **Corticosteroids**: neuroprotective	• **Hydrocortisone**: 100mg if unresponsive to both fluids and vasopressors
	• **ABCDE's**: all patients with shock will benefit from IV fluid bolus (250-500cc's initially with normal saline or lactated ringers)			

Hypovolemic Shock

Etiology & Risk Factors	• Severe loss of fluid volume (blood) secondary to hemorrhage or extracellular fluid loss leading to hypoperfusion of the vital organs
	• Etiology:
	   • Hemorrhagic:
	      • <u>External</u>: hemoptysis (esophageal varices), ectopic pregnancy, trauma, GI bleed, **postpartum hemorrhage**
	      • <u>Internal</u>: **trauma is most common cause**
	        • <u>Thoracic</u>: thoracic aortic aneurysm rupture, trauma, fracture (clavicle, scapula, rib), cardiac tamponade
	        • <u>Peritoneal</u>: trauma (blunt force or penetrating), aortic aneurysm rupture
	        • <u>Retroperitoneal</u>: pelvic fracture
	   • <u>Fluid Loss</u>: severe **burns**, diabetic ketoacidosis (**osmotic diuresis**), vomiting/diarrhea, small bowel obstruction/pancreatitis (3rd space sequestration), diuretics

Patho-physiology	• Depletion of intravascular volume by hemorrhage or extracellular fluid loss causes increased sympathetic tone resulting in an increased HR and increased cardiac contractility but and an overall decrease in cardiac output due to impaired peripheral vasoconstriction • As oxygen delivery decreases, cells switch to anaerobic metabolism resulting in **lactic acidosis**
Signs & Symptoms	• <u>Early Volume Depletion</u>: **thirst**, muscle cramps and/or orthostatic hypotension • **Hypovolemia: hypotension, tachycardia, oliguria**/anuria; altered mental status • <u>Physical Exam</u>: • **Pale, cool, or cyanotic extremities**, >2s capillary refill time; dry mucous membranes
Diagnosis	• **Clinical Diagnosis** • <u>Labs</u>: **CBC** (increased Hgb/Hct due to **hemoconcentration**), CMP, **blood type cross-match**, coagulation studies, **lactate**, UA, urine osmolality, lipase, **ABG** • <u>**FAST (Focused Assessment with Sonography for Trauma) Exam**</u>: high specificity but low sensitivity for clinically significant hemorrhage; • <u>Decreased Central Venous Pressure</u>: initial increase in diastolic blood pressure with narrowed pulse pressure then drop in systolic blood pressure → broad hypotension
Treatment	• <u>**Address Hemodynamic Instability**</u>: **ABCDE's**; neurologic exam prior to intubation, assess C-Spine, identify and control source of hemorrhage or fluid loss • <u>**Aggressive Volume Resuscitation**</u>: normal saline or lactated ringers; monitor urine output to assess resuscitation progress • **Blood transfusion** if severe hemorrhage (packed RBC or O-/cross matched blood); treat coagulopathies • <u>Hypothermia Prevention</u>: warming blankets, warmed IV fluids if indicated
Key Words & Most Common	• Identify & treat source of fluid loss/hemorrhage • Tachycardia, hypotension, oliguria/anuria, cyanosis • FAST exam + fluid resuscitation

Dyslipidemia

Etiology & Risk Factors	• Genetic or acquired disorder describing elevated plasma cholesterol and/or triglyceride levels; >50% of American adults have elevated LDL levels while only <35% are managed
	• Etiology: be primary (familial) or secondary (acquired)
	   • <u>Primary (Familial)</u>: genetic disorder(s); familial hypercholesterolemia, familial combined hyperlipidemia
	   • <u>Secondary (Acquired)</u>: poor diet, obesity, sedentary lifestyle, medications (corticosteroids, amiodarone), diabetes, hypothyroidism, chronic kidney disease
	• **Hypercholesterolemia**: pregnancy, kidney failure, hypothyroidism, anorexia, obstructive liver disease, meds (amiodarone, diuretics, glucocorticoids), diet/obesity
	• **Hypertriglyceridemia**: uncontrolled diabetes, obesity, CKD, meds (**estrogen**, glucocorticoids), diet (**high carbohydrate diet; alcohol consumption**)

Patho-physiology	• Underlying endothelial damage, decreased nitric oxide, and focal inflammation, leading to lipid accumulation at the site and subsequent engulfment by macrophages, resulting in the formation of "foam cells."; the collection of cholesterol within these cells disrupts mitochondrial function and causes apoptosis of underlying tissue • Smooth muscle cells encapsulate the "foam cells" creating a fibrotic plaque and inhibits the underlying lipids (closest to endothelial wall) from being broken down

Signs & Symptoms	• <u>**Asymptomatic**</u>: most commonly asymptomatic until plaque stenosis reaches 70-80% obstruction of the vessel
	• <u>**Symptomatic**</u>: atherosclerotic cardiovascular disease (ASCVD); chest pain, shortness of breath, fatigue, leg pain/cramping (claudication), **pancreatitis (hypertriglyceridemia)**
	• <u>Physical Exam</u>:
	   • <u>**Xanthomas**</u>: waxy/yellow-ish fatty tissue collection under skin
	   • <u>**Xanthelasma**</u>: yellow-ish plaques on inner canthus of eyelid
	   • May have **carotid or femoral bruits**

Diagnosis	• <u>**Lipid Panel**</u>: total cholesterol, low density lipoprotein (LDL), high density lipoprotein (HDL), triglycerides; *patient should fast for 9-12 hours prior to test*
	   • **Men**: routine lipid panel starting at at 35 years old (with no other risk factors) or 25 years old (with risk factors or family history)
	   • **Women**: routine lipid panel starting at 45 years old (with no other risk factors) or 30-35 years old (with risk factors or family history)
	• <u>Labs</u>: **LFTs monitored when initiating statin**, Hgb A1C, TSH, amylase/lipase if symptomatic for pancreatitis

Treatment	• <u>**Lifestyle Modifications**</u>: **first-line**; alcohol cessation, treat underlying condition, weight reduction, proper nutrition, exercise, sleep hygiene, smoking cessation
	• <u>**Medication Management**</u>: determine overall cardiovascular risk (HTN, diabetes, age, race, gender, etc.) vs treating based solely on numbers
	   • <u>**Statins**</u>: atorvastatin, rosuvastatin; **lowers LDL** by inhibiting hepatic cholesterol synthesis (HMG-CoA reductase inhibition)
	      • Indicated in all patients with clinical ASCVD, LDL≥190 mg/dL, Age 40-75 years with diabetes and LDL 70-189 mg/dL, Age 40-75 years, with LDL-C 70-189 mg/dL and estimated 10-year risk of ASCVD ≥7.5%
	   • <u>**Fibrates**</u>: **lower triglycerides** by inhibiting synthesis & increases lipoprotein lipase (catabolizes triglyceride lipoproteins)
	   • <u>**Niacin**</u>: **increases HDL** & lowers triglycerides
	   • <u>**Bile Acid Sequestrants**</u>: **decreases LDL** by blocking enterohepatic reabsorption of bile

Key Words & Most Common	• Genetic vs acquired; hypercholesterolemia is elevated LDL; hypertriglyceridemia is elevated triglycerides • Xanthomas or xanthelasma may be present • Lipid panel drawn earlier if risk factors or family history • Statins are most effective drug to decrease LDL levels

Infective Endocarditis

Etiology & Risk Factors	• **Infection of the endocardium associated with bacteremia**; may affect native or prosthetic heart valves or internal cardiac devices
	• Etiology: endocardial injury followed by bacteremia
	  • *Staphylococcus aureus*: most common cause of **acute** bacterial endocarditis (more often with **native** valves); **most common organism in IV drug use**
	  • *Streptococcus viridans*: most common cause of **subacute** bacterial endocarditis (more often with **damaged** valves); associated with dental procedures/poor dentition
	  • *Staphylococcus epidermis*: *most* common cause of **prosthetic** valve endocarditis or affecting indwelling cardiac devices
	  • *Enterococcus spp.*: may be seen **after gastrointestinal or genitourinary surgery** (especially in men >50 years old)
	  • *HACEK (Haemophilus, Actinobacillus, Cardiobacterium hominis, Eikenella corrodens, Kingella kingae)*: gram negative bacteria that are difficult to culture
	• Risk Factors: **pre-existing heart valve abnormalities** (congenital heart defects, rheumatic valvular disease, bicuspid aortic valves, calcific aortic valves, mitral valve prolapse, hypertrophic cardiomyopathy), substance abuse (IVDU), immunocompromised, indwelling medical devices (central catheters, pacemaker), chronic kidney disease, dialysis

Pathophysiology	• Endocardial injury followed by bacteremia; turbulent blood flow around diseased leaflets or regurgitant cardiac defect allows vegetations to adhere to leaflets • Infection may result from direct intravascular contamination or bacteremia which is more common during dental, upper respiratory, urologic, and gastrointestinal procedures • **Mitral valve is most commonly affected valve overall; tricuspid valve most commonly affected in IV drug users**

Signs & Symptoms	• **Nonspecific Symptoms**: **fever, fatigue**, cough, dyspnea, arthralgias/myalgia, back/flank pain, malaise, unexplained weight loss
	• Physical Exam:
	  • **Murmur**: 85-90% will have a preexisting murmur (may be absent in right-sided infections); a **new or worsening murmur** is rare but diagnostically significant
	  • **Janeway Lesions**: small, non-tender erythematous/hemorrhagic macules on palms/soles (only few mm in diameter)
	  • **Splinter Hemorrhages**: red/brown linear hemorrhagic lesions of nail bed
	  • **Osler Nodes**: tender red/purple nodules on pads of distal fingers and toes or palms of hand (particularly at thenar/hypothenar eminence)
	  • **Roth Spots**: white centered (central clearing) retinal hemorrhage

Diagnosis	• **Duke Criteria**: **2 major** *OR* **1 major + 3 minor** *OR* **5 minor** accurately (80%) diagnose bacterial endocarditis
	  • **Major**: two positive blood cultures; evidence of endocardial involvement or valvular regurgitation on echocardiogram
	  • **Minor**: predisposing factors; fever >100.4; vascular phenomena' immunologic phenomena; one positive blood culture
	• **Blood Cultures**: 3 sets at least 1 hour apart should be obtained, ideally prior to antibiotics initiation (stable patient)
	• Electrocardiogram (ECG):: evaluate arrhythmias; **heart block** or ischemia
	• **Echocardiogram**: **presence of vegetations is diagnostic;** essential to diagnose and identify valve involvement (**TEE more sensitive** than TTE)
	• Labs: CBC (leukocytosis; normochromic normocytic anemia; thrombocytopenia); **marked elevation of ESR** and CRP

Treatment	• **Empiric Antibiotics:**
	• **Native Valve**: anti-staphylococcal penicillins (ampicillin/sulbactam; amoxicillin/clavulanate; oxacillin/nafcillin) + gentamicin
	  • **MRSA Coverage**: vancomycin + gentamicin + ciprofloxacin
	• **Prosthetic valve: vancomycin + gentamicin + rifampin**
	• **Prophylaxis**: indicated prior to invasive dental or respiratory procedures in setting of prosthetic valves, history of endocarditis, unrepaired congenital heart defect
	  • **Amoxicillin 2g (clindamycin 600mg if PCN allergic) given 1 hour prior to procedure**

Pericarditis

Etiology & Risk Factors	• Inflammation of the pericardium often accompanied by fluid within the pericardial space • Etiology: **idiopathic; inflammation secondary to viral infection** (*Coxsackievirus, Echovirus, Parvovirus B19,* **HIV**), bacterial infection (less common), inflammatory autoimmune conditions (SLE, RA), trauma, malignancy, radiation therapy • Risk Factors: males, age (<50 years old most common), infection, previous cardiac surgery, radiation therapy, certain medications (hydralazine, isoniazid), trauma
Pathophysiology	• Pericardium is the anchor within the thoracic cavity that surrounds the heart consisting of a visceral layer and richly innervated parietal layer • Inflammation may lead to fluid accumulation within pericardial sac leading to a pericardial effusion (may be serous, hemorrhagic or purulent based on etiology) resulting in restrictive pressure on the heart and eventually causing diastolic failure (pericardial tamponade)

Signs & Symptoms	• **Chest Pain**: sharp, pleuritic substernal chest pain
	  • **Worse while supine; improved when upright or leaning forward**
	  • Pain may radiate to back or **left trapezius ridge** (innervated by phrenic nerve which traverses pericardium)
	• **Pericardial Friction Rub**: **scratching, grating, high-pitched sound due to friction between pericardium and epicardium**
	  • Best heard wit diaphragm at LLSB with patient at end expiration while sitting and patient leaning forward
	• **Nonspecific Symptoms**: **fever**, dyspnea & hypotension may be present
	• **Dressler Syndrome**: post-myocardial infarction syndrome resulting in **pericarditis several weeks after incident**

Diagnosis	• Electrocardiogram (ECG): **initial test of choice;** must differentiate from STEMI
	  • Demonstrates *diffuse* **ST segment elevations** in V1-V6 (precordial leads) with concomitant **PR depressions** in those leads
	  • Should never produce ST depression unless V1 and aVR
	  • ST elevation in lead II>III favors pericarditis; ST elevation in lead III>II or Q waves favor STEMI
	• Labs: CBC, CMP, ESR, CRP, cardiac enzymes (may have **elevated CK levels but normal troponins**); consider TSH or ANA based on clinical suspicion
	• **Echocardiogram**: demonstrates extent of associated pericardial effusion or signs of cardiac tamponade (2/3rd of cases will have associated effusion)
	• Chest X-Ray (CXR): may show extent of effusion or pericardial calcification

Treatment	• **Non-Steroidal Anti-inflammatory Drugs (NSAIDs)**: **(ibuprofen** 600mg Q8h or **aspirin** 650mg Q6h) for 7-10d with tapering period of 3-4 weeks after • **Colchicine** or **Indomethacin** are second-line • **Corticosteroids**: prednisone; may be second-line in patients with contraindications to NSAIDs • **Pericardiocentesis**: **indicated with hemodynamic compromise to relieve fluid accumulation** if progresses to cardiac effusion/tamponade • Pericardial Window: surgical treatment indicated with recurrent effusions
Key Words & Most Common	• Inflammation of pericardial sac usually caused by viral infection • Sharp pleuritic chest pain worse supine improved when leaning/hunched forward and sitting upright; pericardial friction rub • ECG: diffuse ST segment elevations • Elevated CK levels with normal troponins • NSAIDs (ibuprofen, colchicine or indomethacin) first line treatment

Pericardial Effusion and Tamponade 🫀

Etiology & Risk Factors	• **Pericardial Effusion**: inflammation and fluid accumulation within the pericardial sac
	• **Pericardial Tamponade**: fluid accumulation within the pericardial sac **impedes cardiac filling due to pressure**
	• <u>Etiology</u>: accumulation of fluid within pericardial sac
	   • **Infection**: **viral infection** (*Coxsackievirus, Echovirus, Parvovirus B19,* **HIV**), bacterial infection (less common)
	   • **Inflammatory Disorders**: autoimmune conditions (SLE, RA, sarcoidosis), radiation therapy, certain medications
	   • **Malignancy**: **lung cancer most common malignant cause of pericardial effusion**; breast cancer is second most common cause; prostate, hematologic
	   • **Trauma**: blunt or penetrating trauma within cardiac box; *gunshot wound less likely as pericardial defect is larger*; cardiac surgery

Patho-physiology	• Inflammation or trauma leads to fluid accumulation within pericardial sac (may be serous, hemorrhagic or purulent based on etiology) • Rapidly accumulating or large volume of fluid may lead to restrictive pressure on the heart causing diastolic failure (pericardial tamponade) • Increased pericardial pressure from fluid → decreased right ventricle filling/diastolic failure → decreased cardiac output

Signs & Symptoms	• <u>Effusion</u>:
	   • **Chest Pain**: sharp, anterior, pleuritic substernal chest pain (if associated with pericarditis)
	   • **Muffled Heart Sounds**: due to fluid accumulation
	• <u>Tamponade</u>:
	   • **Beck's Triad**: distant/muffled heart sounds + hypotension + JVD
	   • **Pulsus Paradoxus**: decrease in systolic BP (>10mmHg) during inspiration
	   • <u>CHF Presentation</u>: dyspnea and peripheral edema, narrow pulse pressures, fatigue, tachycardia
	
	(ECG tracing labeled) Electrical Alternans

Diagnosis	• <u>**Echocardiogram**</u>: **test of choice**; demonstrates **fluid accumulation within pericardial space** (right sided **diastolic collapse with tamponade**) • <u>Electrocardiogram (ECG)</u>: electrical alternans, low QRS voltage, tachycardia • **Electrical Alternans**: beat-to-beat alternation of QRS amplitude; represents the swinging motion of the heart within the effusion • <u>Chest X-Ray (CXR)</u>: enlarged cardiac silhouette; "water bottle heart"
Treatment	• <u>**Treat Underlying Etiology**</u>: small effusions can be monitored with serial echocardiograms • <u>**Pericardiocentesis**</u>: indicated for large effusions or tamponade immediately to relieve pressure • <u>Hemodynamic Support</u>: IV fluid resuscitation indicated for tamponade to increase right ventricle volume and provide preload support; vasopressors if necessary
Key Words & Most Common	• Fluid accumulation within pericardial sac leads to pressure on heart & decreases cardiac filling & cardiac output • Beck's Triad: distant/muffled heart sounds + hypotension + JFD • Pulsus Paradoxus: decrease in systolic BP during inspiration • Echocardiogram demonstrates fluid accumulation in pericardial space +/- diastolic collapse; ECG may show electrical alternans • Pericardiocentesis for tamponade

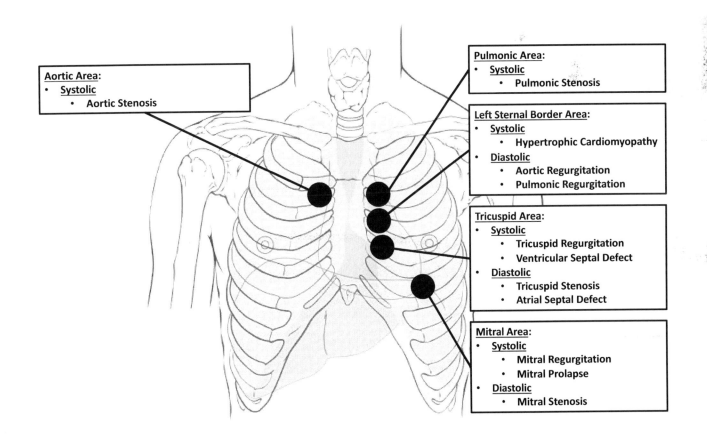

Aortic Area:
• <u>Systolic</u>
   • Aortic Stenosis

Pulmonic Area:
• <u>Systolic</u>
   • Pulmonic Stenosis

Left Sternal Border Area:
• <u>Systolic</u>
   • Hypertrophic Cardiomyopathy
• <u>Diastolic</u>
   • Aortic Regurgitation
   • Pulmonic Regurgitation

Tricuspid Area:
• <u>Systolic</u>
   • Tricuspid Regurgitation
   • Ventricular Septal Defect
• <u>Diastolic</u>
   • Tricuspid Stenosis
   • Atrial Septal Defect

Mitral Area:
• <u>Systolic</u>
   • Mitral Regurgitation
   • Mitral Prolapse
• <u>Diastolic</u>
   • Mitral Stenosis

Aortic Stenosis

Etiology & Risk Factors	• Narrowing of the aortic valve resulting in blood flow obstruction from the left ventricle to the ascending aorta during systole; most common valvular disorder
	• Etiology: may be degenerative, congenital or rheumatic
	   • **Degenerative/Calcific**: **most common cause**; aging and degeneration of the valve leads to calcium deposition and stiffening of the leaflets
	   • Congenital: **bicuspid aortic valve** (displaced blood flow; reduced valve opening, and jet angle causes damage, thickening and calcifications)
	   • Rheumatic: immune response toward untreated beta-hemolytic strep causing autoantibodies that attack and damage valve
	• Risk Factors: male, **age (>65 years old most common)**, congenital heart defects, chronic hypertension, dyslipidemia, family history

Patho-physiology	• Narrowed aortic orifice acts as a left ventricle (LV) outflow obstruction which creates a systolic pressure gradient increases the LV systolic pressure, ejection time and end-diastolic pressure; the increased afterload and volume overload causes LV chamber thickening (to fill appropriately) • Systolic function is preserved (fixed cardiac output) but diastolic function is lost

Signs & Symptoms	• **Chest Pain:** due to increased myocardial oxygen demand from increased LV pressure/muscle mass
	• **Syncope:** due to fixed cardiac output and arterial hypotension leading to **decreased cerebral perfusion**
	• Dyspnea: due to increased vascular congestion in lungs as end diastolic pressure increases
	• Physical Exam:
	   • **Narrow pulse pressure**
	   • **Crescendo-decrescendo harsh systolic "ejection" murmur best heard at the right upper sternal border & radiation to right carotid**
	      • **Increased murmur intensity while sitting and leaning forward, lying, squatting, or during expiration** (due to increased venous return)
	      • **Decreased murmur intensity with Valsalva or standing, isometric handgrip, or during inspiration** (due to decreased venous return)
	   • *Pulsus parvus et tardus:* slow-rising, delayed, weak carotid impulse

Diagnosis	• **Echocardiogram: test of choice**; may show **thickened/calcified aortic valve** with turbulent blood flow through aortic valve, LVH • Electrocardiogram (ECG): left ventricular hypertrophy; may show left atrial enlargement • Cardiac Catheterization: definitive diagnosis; only utilized prior to surgical procedure
Treatment	• **Aortic Valve Replacement (AVR): treatment of choice in symptomatic cases** or asymptomatic cases with EF <50% • Transcatheter Aortic Valve Replacement (TAVR): procedure utilized in high or intermediate risk patients • Percutaneous Aortic Valvuloplasty or Intra-Aortic Balloon Pump: may be utilized as bridge to aortic valve replacement in unstable patients • *Medical therapy does not significantly change disease progression* • Avoid negative inotropes (CCB & BB), venodilators (nitrates) and heavy exertional activity in severe aortic stenosis as cardiac output is highly dependent on preload
Key Words & Most Common	• Most common valvular disease in elderly; degenerative vs congenital causes narrowed aortic orifice and decreased compliance of valve leaflets • Angina, syncope, narrow pulse pressure; crescendo-decrescendo harsh systolic ejection murmur at right upper sternal border and radiates to right carotid • Echocardiogram shows thickened aortic valve • AVR vs TAVR is treatment of choice

Aortic Regurgitation

Etiology & Risk Factors	• **Incompetency of aortic valve leaflets cause reversal of blood flow through the aortic valve back into the left ventricle during diastole**
	• Etiologies: may be acute or chronic
	   • Acute: **aortic dissection**, infective endocarditis, acute myocardial infarction, blunt chest trauma
	   • Chronic: **Marfan syndrome**, aortic root dilation, congenital bicuspid aortic valve, rheumatologic conditions (SLE, RA, ankylosing spondylitis), syphilis
	• Risk Factors: **advanced age**, bicuspid aortic valve, chronic hypertension, family history

Patho-physiology	• Reversal of blood flow from the aorta back into the left ventricle leads a pressure gradient decrease within the left ventricle and subsequently causes fluid overload of fluid in the left ventricle; eccentric hypertrophy of the left ventricle occurs as a compensatory response which involves an enlargement and dilation of the chamber to accommodate the increased blood volume • Total stroke volume is equal to effect stroke volume + regurgitant volume (unlike aortic stenosis, aortic regurgitation is not dependent on preload) • Increased diastolic pressure and volume dilates the ventricle & thus decreases contractility; further dilation leads to decreased coronary perfusion & ischemia

Signs & Symptoms	• Asymptomatic: commonly asymptomatic until late in disease course
	• **Symptomatic: fatigue, dyspnea on exertion**, positional nocturnal dyspnea or orthopnea, **hypotension, lower extremity edema**, palpitations (arrhythmias)
	• Physical Exam:
	   • **Wide pulse pressure** (>40mmHg difference between systolic and diastolic BP); **bounding pulses**
	   • **Decrescendo diastolic "blowing" murmur best heard at the left upper sternal border worse when patient is sitting during expiration or isometric hand grip**

diagnosis			

Diagnosis			

Peripheral Sign	Description	Peripheral Sign	Description
Austin Flint Murmur	Low pitched rumbling mid diastolic at the apex (regurgitant blood flow through mitral valve)	Hills's Sign	Lower extremity blood pressure is greater than upper extremity blood pressure
Bisferians Pulse	Biphasic bounding pulse	Müller's sign	Pulsation of uvula during systole
Water Hammer Pulse	Forceful pulse with swift upstroke and descent of radial pulse	Quincke Sign	Capillary pulsation with light compression of fingernail
Corrigan's Pulse	Forceful pulse with swift upstroke and descent of carotid artery	De Musset's Sign	Head-bob with arterial pulsation

Diagnosis (row preceding table):
• **Doppler Echocardiogram**: best initial test; demonstrates **regurgitating jet** through aortic valve, left ventricular dilation; assesses aortic root/valve anatomy
• Cardiac Catheterization: definitive diagnosis; usually only utilized prior to surgical procedure

Treatment	• Medical Management: systemic hypertension management
	   • **Vasodilators**: dihydropyridine CCB, ACEI/ARB, hydralazine indicated to **reduce afterload**
	   • *Diuretics and nitrates are ineffective; avoid beta blockers as to not block compensatory tachycardia*
	• **Aortic Valve Replacement (AVR): treatment of choice in symptomatic cases** or asymptomatic cases with EF <50%
	   • Transcatheter Aortic Valve Replacement (TAVR): utilized in high or intermediate risk patients

Mitral Stenosis

Etiology & Risk Factors	• Narrowing or obstruction of the mitral valve orifice creating a dysfunction of normal forward blood flow from the left atrium to the left ventricle • Etiologies: **rheumatic fever is most common cause** (usually presents 30-40 years after episode) • Other: calcification or degeneration of mitral valve leaflets, **pregnancy**, congenital heart disease, endocarditis • Risk Factors: female, advanced age, **history of rheumatic fever**, limited access to medical care, certain autoimmune conditions, pulmonary hypertension, radiation
Patho-physiology	• Impediment of blood flow due to obstruction/narrowing of mitral valve orifice creates a pressure gradient (left atrial pressure>left ventricle pressure) leading to atrial dilation and pulmonary hypertension • Ventricular filling relies on the "atrial kick" during late diastole however atrial dilation can cause afib which disrupts the atrial kick leading to decreased cardiac output and CHF

Signs & Symptoms	• **Heart Failure Symptoms:** dyspnea is most common symptom, orthopnea/paroxysmal nocturnal dyspnea, hemoptysis, frequent URIs, pulmonary HTN, fatigue, weakness
	• **Palpitations:** atrial fibrillation secondary to atrial dilation
	• Physical Exam:
	   • **Mitral Facies: flushed cheeks** (cutaneous vasodilation) **with facial pallor** (chronic hypoxia)
	   • **Loud S1 due to increased force to close mitral valve, opening snap due to increased force to open mitral valve** (atrial>ventricular pressure)
	   • **Mid-diastolic, low-pitched, rumbling murmur best heard at apex accentuated with patient in left lateral decubitus position or isometric exercise**

Diagnosis	• **Doppler Echocardiogram: initial test of choice;** may show **thickened/calcified mitral valve leaflets** with turbulent blood flow, left atrial enlargement • Electrocardiogram (ECG): may show **atrial fibrillation**, left atrial enlargement (P wave changes; biphasic in V1/V2), right axis deviation or right ventricular hypertrophy secondary to pulmonary hypertension • Chest X-Ray (CXR): normal heart size with **straightening of left border of cardiac silhouette**, displacement of esophagus by enlarged atrium, prominent pulmonary vasculature • Cardiac Catheterization: definitive diagnosis; invasive test usually only performed prior to surgical procedure or if noninvasive tests are inconclusive

Treatment	• Medical Management:
	   • **Diuretics:** indicated to reduce fluid retention (pulmonary congestion/edema/hypertension)
	   • Beta Blockers or Calcium Channel Blockers: AV nodal blocking agents indicated for rate control
	   • **Anticoagulation: warfarin** indicated to prevent thromboembolism in patients with history atrial fibrillation, embolism, or a left atrial clot
	   • Antibiotics: primary prevention of rheumatic fever with penicillin antibiotics in setting of streptococcal pharyngitis
	• **Percutaneous Mitral Balloon Valvuloplasty:** invasive procedure to increase mitral valve diameter in young, symptomatic patients or asymptomatic with pulmonary HTN
	• **Mitral Valve Replacement:** indicated in patients with contraindication to percutaneous valvuloplasty due to mitral valve morphology or refractory symptoms
	   • Patient must be on warfarin after procedure with **target INR of 2.5-3.5** and pre-procedural antibiotics for endocarditis prophylaxis

Key Words & Most Common	• Rheumatic fever is most common cause • Dyspnea; afib; mitral facies (flushed cheeks with facial pallor); opening snap with a mid-diastolic rumbling murmur at apex worse with left lateral decubitus position • Echocardiogram shows thickened leaflets; ECG may show afib, biphasic P waves (atrial enlargement) • Diuretics for pulmonary congestion; Afib rate control; percutaneous mitral balloon valvuloplasty vs valve replacement

Mitral Regurgitation

Etiology & Risk Factors	• **Incompetency of mitral valve leaflets resulting in reversal of blood flow from left ventricle into left atrium through the mitral valve**
	• Etiology:
	   • **Primary (Degenerative or Organic): mitral valve prolapse is most common cause,** papillary muscle rupture, rheumatic heart disease, connective tissue disorders (Marfan/Ehlers-Danlos syndrome), endocarditis
	   • Secondary (Ischemic/Functional): **myocardial ischemia/infarct**, ischemic or dilated cardiomyopathy, annular dilatation due to chronic afib with left atrial enlargement
	• Risk Factors: **female, advanced age**, history of rheumatic fever or mitral valve prolapse, congenital heart defects, ischemic heart disease, connective tissue disorders

Patho-physiology	• Retrograde blood flow from left ventricle to left atrium leads to overload of the left ventricle volume from increase in stroke volume and preload during diastole • Left atrial and left ventricular dilation increases mitral valve annulus diameter leading to worsening regurgitation, hypocontractility, and decreased cardiac output

Signs & Symptoms	• **Heart Failure Symptoms: dyspnea,** peripheral edema, fatigue, weakness, hypertension
	• **Pulmonary Hypertension:** cough with clear or pink frothy sputum, orthopnea/paroxysmal nocturnal dyspnea, cyanosis, syncope, pleural effusions
	• **Palpitations: atrial fibrillation** secondary to atrial dilation
	• *Sudden dyspnea, tachycardia, hypotension, angina with new murmur suspect papillary muscle/chordae tendineae rupture secondary to acute myocardial infarct*
	• Physical Exam:
	   • **Blowing holosystolic murmur best heard at the apex with radiation to axilla accentuated with left lateral decubitus position and isometric handgrip**
	   • Diminished S1 & widely split S2 due to defective valve leaflets, **displaced apical impulse** and JVD

Diagnosis	• **Doppler Echocardiogram: initial test of choice;** demonstrates **regurgitating jet** through mitral valve; left atrial/ventricular dilation • Electrocardiogram (ECG): may show **atrial fibrillation**, left atrial enlargement (P wave changes), left ventricular hypertrophy, right axis deviation or right ventricular hypertrophy secondary to pulmonary hypertension • Chest X-Ray (CXR): may show cardiomegaly secondary to left atrial or right sided enlargement; pulmonary vascular congestion

Treatment	• Medical Management:
	   • **Diuretics:** indicated to reduce fluid retention (pulmonary congestion/edema/hypertension) and decrease regurgitant volume (afterload reduction)
	   • Beta Blockers or Calcium Channel Blockers: AV nodal blocking agents indicated for rate control
	   • **Anticoagulation: warfarin** indicated to prevent thromboembolism in patients with history atrial fibrillation, embolism, or a left atrial clot
	• Surgery: indicated in symptomatic patients with EF>30% or asymptomatic with EF 30-60% or cases refractory to medical management
	   • **Mitral Valve Repair: preferred over replacement** due to decreased recurrence
	   • **Mitral Valve Replacement:** indicated with extensive tissue damage (secondary to endocarditis)
	     • Mechanical preferred over bioprosthetic with replacement due to durability; **both require anticoagulation and pre-procedural prophylactic antibiotics**

Key Words & Most Common	• Mitral valve prolapse is most common cause • Dyspnea; blowing holosystolic murmur at apex with radiation to axilla • Echocardiogram shows regurgitating jet • Medical treatment with ACEI/ARB and diuretics for afterload reduction; surgical repair > replacement

Mitral Valve Prolapse

Etiology & Risk Factors	• Billowing (>2mm displacement) of anterior or posterior mitral valve leaflets beyond annulus into the left atrium during systole with or without mitral regurgitation • Etiology: **myxomatous degeneration of mitral valve is most common cause** 　• **Idiopathic, autosomal dominant inheritance,** connective tissue disorders (**Marfan**/Ehlers-Danlos/Loeys-Dietz syndrome, osteogenesis imperfecta) • Risk Factors: **female, age (15-30 most common)**, family history, connective tissue disorders, **psychological factors (anxiety or stress)**, impaired collagen production
Patho-physiology	• Prolapse of mitral valve leaflets secondary to myxomatous degeneration of mitral valve (causes weakening or elongation of chordae tendineae), mitral valve annular dilation or thickening of mitral valve tissue; mitral valve regurgitation occurs as mitral valve leaflets fail to approximate during systole
Signs & Symptoms	• Asymptomatic: most cases are benign and **asymptomatic** • **Autonomic Dysfunction: anxiety or panic attacks,** fatigue, exercise intolerance, atypical **chest pain, palpitations,** dizziness, presyncope/syncope, hypotension • Physical Exam: 　• **Mid-late systolic ejection click best heard at apex** 　　• **Increased intensity, earlier click with longer duration with Valsalva, standing, inspiration, isometric handgrip** due to **decreased** preload 　　• **Decreased intensity, delayed click with shorter duration with squatting, lying, expiration** due to **increased** preload 　　• Similar murmur to hypertrophic cardiomyopathy – **isometric handgrip ↑MVP murmur and ↓hypertrophic cardiomyopathy murmur** 　• **Evidence of connective tissue disorder** (narrow anterior-posterior diameter, pectus excavatum, low BMI, scoliosis, Marfanoid habitus)
Diagnosis	• **Doppler Echocardiogram: initial test of choice;** demonstrates >2mm displacement of anterior or posterior leaflet beyond mitral valve annulus into left atrium 　• Doppler may show regurgitating jet if associated with mitral regurgitation
Treatment	• **Observation:** asymptomatic cases generally require no treatment 　• Monitor with echocardiogram every year if associated mitral regurgitation; every 3-5 years without mitral regurgitation • **Beta Blockers:** propranolol; indicated for autonomic dysfunction symptoms • **Mitral Valve Repair vs Replacement:** indicated in mitral valve prolapse with severe mitral regurgitation to prevent congestive heart failure symptom development • Pre-Procedural Prophylactic Antibiotics: indicated if other cardiac conditions present, otherwise not routinely indicated
Key Words & Most Common	• Most common cause of mitral regurgitation in US; more common in younger women; Marfan syndrome is most common connective tissue disease cause • Mostly asymptomatic • Mid-late systolic ejection click best heard at apex that increases, earlier click and longer duration of murmur with isometric handgrip or Valsalva • No treatment in most cases; propranolol if associated with autonomic dysfunction

Pulmonic Stenosis

Etiology & Risk Factors	• **Narrowing or obstruction of pulmonic outflow tract causing obstruction of blood flow from the right ventricle to the pulmonary artery during systole** • Etiology: **congenital is most common;** may be associated with congenital heart conditions (**Tetralogy of Fallot or maternal rubella syndrome**) • Risk Factors: age (rare in adults), congenital heart defects, family history, rubella infection during pregnancy, advanced maternal age, myxoma
Patho-physiology	• Structural defects cause narrowing or obstruction of pulmonic valve creating an outflow obstruction at the right ventricle further which further reduces blood return to left ventricle and reduces overall cardiac output
Signs & Symptoms	• **Asymptomatic:** most cases are benign and asymptomatic • **Symptomatic: exertional dyspnea,** fatigue, right sided heart failure symptoms (peripheral edema, jugular venous distention [JVD]) • Physical Exam: 　• **Harsh, mid-systolic, crescendo-decrescendo ejection murmur best heard at left upper sternal border radiating to neck or back and intensifies with inspiration** 　• **Ejection click and wide split S2** from delay in pulmonic valve closure; S4 gallop
Diagnosis	• **Doppler Echocardiogram:** initial test of choice 　• Identifies extent of outflow obstruction; demonstrates increased doppler jet velocity through pulmonic valve • Electrocardiogram (ECG): may show right axis deviation
Treatment	• **Observation: indicated in asymptomatic cases** 　• Monitoring with echocardiogram based on extent of peak doppler gradient • **Percutaneous Pulmonic Balloon Valvuloplasty:** indicated in symptomatic patients or asymptomatic patients with increased peak doppler gradient (>60mmHg) • Surgical Replacement: reserved for dysplastic valvular annulus or severe stenosis with severe regurgitation
Key Words & Most Common	• Typically congenital and benign; may be associated with Tetralogy of Fallot • Mostly asymptomatic • Harsh, mid-systolic, crescendo-decrescendo ejection murmur at left upper sternal border radiating to neck or back accentuated with inspiration • Echocardiogram • Balloon valvuloplasty preferred in symptomatic patients

Pulmonic Regurgitation

Etiology & Risk Factors	• **Incompetency of the pulmonic valve causing retrograde blood flow from the pulmonary artery into the right ventricle during diastole** • Etiology: **pulmonary hypertension is most common secondary cause**; congenital heart disease, endocarditis, rheumatic heart disease, surgical repair of Tetralogy of Fallot
Patho-physiology	• Usually, the right ventricle pressure is greater than pulmonary artery pressure during systole which causes the pulmonic valve to remain open until late systole or early diastole • When the pulmonary artery pressure is greater than right ventricle pressure the pulmonic valve is forced closed; a defective valve will allow retrograde blood flow from the pulmonary artery to retrogradely flow back into right ventricle resulting in an increased right ventricle end diastolic volume causing a right sided overload

Signs & Symptoms	• **Asymptomatic**: most cases are benign and asymptomatic
	• **Symptomatic: exertional dyspnea**, fatigue, orthopnea, pulmonary hypertension, right ventricle dysfunction (peripheral edema, **jugular venous distention [JVD]**)
	• Physical Exam:
	  • **Graham-Steell Murmur**: **high-pitched "blowing" decrescendo early diastolic murmur best heart at left upper sternal border**
	    • **Increased intensity with full inspiration**; decreased intensity with Valsalva strain and expiration
	    • Caused when pulmonary artery pressure exceeds 55mmHg causing a high velocity regurgitant jet through a dilated pulmonic valve
	  • Hyperdynamic right ventricle on palpation

Diagnosis	• Doppler Echocardiogram: initial test of choice • Identifies extent of insufficiency by quantifying regurgitant jet; may show right atrial/ventricular enlargement • Electrocardiogram (ECG): may show right axis deviation; increased P wave amplitude in leads II, III, and aVF (right atrial enlargement) • Chest X-Ray (CXR): may show right ventricular enlargement
Treatment	• **Observation: indicated in asymptomatic cases** • Monitoring with echocardiogram based on extent of peak regurgitant jet • Treat Underlying Etiology: **treatment of pulmonary hypertension** • Transcatheter vs Surgical Pulmonary Valve Replacement: reserved for severely symptomatic patients refractory to medical management
Key Words & Most Common	• Pulmonary hypertension and congenital heart disease most common causes • Mostly asymptomatic; right sided heart failure symptoms if symptomatic • Graham-Steell Murmur: high-pitched blowing decrescendo early diastolic murmur at left upper sternal border with full inspiration • Echocardiogram • Asymptomatic requires no treatment → treat underlying pulmonary hypertension

Tricuspid Stenosis

Etiology & Risk Factors	• **Outflow obstruction caused by narrowing of the tricuspid valve orifice that obstructs blood flow from the right atrium to the right ventricle** • Etiology: **rheumatic fever is most common cause** (may coexist with mitral valve pathology); **large vegetations from infective endocarditis**; carcinoid syndrome • Risk Factors: female, **history of rheumatic fever** or endocarditis, congenital heart defects, radiation therapy, carcinoid syndrome, previous cardiac surgery
Patho-physiology	• Fibrous thickening and/or fusion of tricuspid leaflets in rheumatic heart disease leads to narrowing of tricuspid valve annulus • Right atrial pressure elevation leads to right atrial enlargement and right sided vascular congestion

Signs & Symptoms	• **Asymptomatic**: most cases are benign and asymptomatic
	• **Symptomatic: exertional dyspnea**, fatigue, orthopnea, pulmonary hypertension, right ventricle dysfunction (peripheral edema, **jugular venous distention [JVD]**)
	• Physical Exam:
	  • **Mid-diastolic rumbling murmur at left lower sternal border (4th intercostal space or xyphoid process) with soft opening snap**
	    • **Opening snap and murmur intensity increases with inspiration, leg raise, and squatting**
	    • Opening snap usually heard *after* opening snap of mitral stenosis

Diagnosis	• **Doppler Echocardiogram**: initial test of choice • Identifies extent of outflow obstruction; demonstrates increased doppler jet velocity through tricuspid valve • Electrocardiogram (ECG): may show right axis deviation or increased P wave amplitude in leads II, III, and aVF (right atrial enlargement)

Treatment	• **Observation: indicated in asymptomatic cases**
	  • Monitoring with echocardiogram based on extent of peak regurgitant jet
	• **Medical Management**: indicated with mild symptoms; **loop diuretics, ACEI, and sodium restriction** to decrease volume overload and vascular congestion
	• Tricuspid Valve Repair vs Replacement Surgery: indicated with right heart failure and decreased cardiac output
	  • **Tricuspid repair/replacement preferred over percutaneous balloon commissurotomy** as symptomatic tricuspid stenosis often present with tricuspid regurgitation; commissurotomy may produce or worsen regurgitation

Key Words & Most Common	• Rheumatic fever is most common cause; large vegetations from infective endocarditis • Mostly asymptomatic; may have right sided heart failure symptoms if progressed • Mid-diastolic murmur at left lower sternal border at Xyphoid process with opening snap accentuated with inspiration • Echocardiogram • Medical management with loop diuretics and sodium restriction; Tricuspid repair/replacement surgery preferred over commissurotomy

Tricuspid Regurgitation

Etiology & Risk Factors	• Incompetency of the tricuspid valve results in retrograde blood flow from the right ventricle to the right atrium during systole
	• <u>Etiology</u>: **dilation of right ventricle**; may be primary or secondary
	    • <u>**Primary**</u>: blunt chest trauma, carcinoid syndrome, congenital defects (**Ebstein anomaly**), idiopathic myxomatous, **rheumatic fever**
	    • <u>**Secondary**</u>: most common; leaflet tethering (annular dilation from chronic afib), papillary muscle displacement (RV dilation from chronic pulmonary hypertension)

Patho-physiology	• Increased annular diameters secondary to dilation of right ventricle leads to retrograde blood flow from right ventricle back to right atrium during systole • Tricuspid regurgitation increases with inspiration as right ventricle widens which further increases annulus diameter and regurgitant area • <u>Normal leaflet motion</u>: most commonly secondary to RV dilation from pulmonary HTN, mitral or pulmonic valve disease, left sided heart failure, or primary pulmonary disease • <u>Excessive leaflet motion</u>: myxomatous degeneration • <u>Restricted leaflet motion</u>: rheumatic fever, Ebstein anomaly (dysplasia of tricuspid valve)

Signs & Symptoms	• <u>Asymptomatic</u>: most cases are benign and asymptomatic
	• <u>Symptomatic</u>: symptoms secondary to right sided fluid overload resulting in right sided heart failure
	    • <u>**Right Ventricular Dysfunction**</u>: exertional dyspnea, fatigue, orthopnea, pulmonary hypertension, peripheral edema, **jugular venous distention (JVD)**
	    • <u>**Hepatic Congestion**</u>: ascites or pulsatile liver
	• <u>Physical Exam</u>:
	    • **High-pitched "blowing" holosystolic murmur best heart at left mid sternal border**
	        • **Increases in intensity during full inspiration;** decreases with Valsalva or during expiration
	    • <u>Carvallo's Sign</u>: accentuated murmur during full inspiration helps differentiate tricuspid regurgitation from mitral regurgitation

Diagnosis	• <u>**Doppler Echocardiogram**</u>: **initial test of choice** • Identifies extent of insufficiency by quantifying regurgitant jet; may show right atrial/ventricular enlargement • <u>Electrocardiogram (ECG)</u>: may show right axis deviation or increased P wave amplitude in leads II, III, and aVF (right atrial enlargement) • <u>Labs</u>: **elevated liver enzymes** or hyperbilirubinemia secondary to hepatic congestion

Treatment	• <u>**Observation**</u>: indicated in asymptomatic cases
	    • Monitoring with echocardiogram based on extent of peak regurgitant jet
	• <u>**Medical Management**</u>: indicated with mild symptoms; **loop diuretics, ACEI, and sodium restriction** to decrease volume overload and vascular congestion
	• <u>Tricuspid Valve Repair vs Replacement Surgery</u>: indicated with right heart failure and decreased cardiac output
	    • *Usually only performed when doing a left sided surgery as isolated tricuspid surgery is rare*

Key Words & Most Common	• Ebstein anomaly, rheumatic fever, RV dilation are most common causes • Mostly asymptomatic; may have right sided heart failure symptoms if progressed • High-pitched "blowing" holosystolic murmur at left mid sternal border accentuated with inspiration • Echocardiogram • Medical management with loop diuretics, ACEI and sodium restriction; tricuspid repair/replacement surgery

	Murmur	Description
Systolic Murmur	**Aortic Stenosis**	Crescendo-decrescendo harsh systolic "ejection" murmur best heard at the **right upper sternal border** & **radiation to right carotid**
	Pulmonic Stenosis	Harsh, mid-systolic, crescendo-decrescendo ejection murmur best heard at **left upper sternal border radiating to neck or back** and intensifies with inspiration; may have "ejection click"
	Mitral Regurgitation	Blowing holosystolic murmur best heard at the **apex** with **radiation to axilla** accentuated with left lateral decubitus position and isometric handgrip
	Tricuspid Regurgitation	High-pitched "blowing" holosystolic murmur best heart at **left mid sternal border** accentuated with full inspiration and decreases with expiration or Valsalva
Diastolic Murmur	**Aortic Regurgitation**	Decrescendo diastolic "blowing" murmur best heard at the **left upper sternal border** worse when patient is sitting during expiration or isometric hand grip
	Pulmonic Regurgitation	High-pitched "blowing" decrescendo early diastolic murmur best heart at **left upper sternal border** accentuated with full inspiration
	Mitral Stenosis	Mid-diastolic, low-pitched, rumbling murmur best heard at **apex** accentuated with patient in left lateral decubitus position or isometric exercise; may have "opening snap"
	Tricuspid Stenosis	Mid-diastolic murmur at **left lower sternal border**

Abdominal Aortic Aneurysm (AAA) ♥

Etiology & Risk Factors	• Potentially life-threatening focal dilation of the abdominal aorta • Etiology: weakening of the arterial wall most commonly secondary to atherosclerosis; trauma, postsurgical changes, vasculitis • Risk Factors: atherosclerosis and smoking are greatest risk factors, male, advanced age, Caucasian, chronic hypertension, family history, connective tissue disorders (Marfans, Loeys-Dietz, Ehlers-Danlos), certain medications (fluoroquinolones)
Patho-physiology	• Degeneration of the structural proteins (collagen lamellar units) causes gradual weakening of the aortic wall; chronic inflammation further weakens the lining of the aorta • There are less collagen lamellar units at the infrarenal portion of aorta as compared to thoracic; infrarenal aortic aneurysms are more common (85%) • Aneurysms increase in size at a rate proportional to the diameter; larger aneurysms (>5cm) are at a greater risk of rupture especially with concomitant hypertension

Signs & Symptoms	• Asymptomatic: most cases are asymptomatic; may be found incidentally on exam or imaging
	• Symptomatic:
	   • Unruptured: abdominal, flank, or back pain; compression of local viscera from enlarging aneurysm may manifest with GI or renal dysfunction
	   • Ruptured: diffuse abdominal pain and distension (described as sharp, sudden, or ripping sensation), shock (hypotension, AMS, syncope)
	• Physical Exam:
	   • Non-tender, pulsatile abdominal mass +/- abdominal bruit
	   • Flank Ecchymosis: indicates retroperitoneal hemorrhage (ruptured aneurysm)

Diagnosis	• Abdominal Ultrasound: initial screening study at bedside (may not reliably visualize rupture therefore should only be used as quick study in unstable patient)
	   • May be utilized for screening in asymptomatic patients
	• Computed Tomography (CT) with IV contrast: imaging test of choice; indicated in stable patient
	   • Determines location and size of aneurysm and identifies any involvement of other vessels
	• Labs: CBC, blood type and screen, coagulation studies, creatinine, urinalysis

Treatment	• Asymptomatic: routine screening based on size/extent of aneurysm;
	   • 3-4cm Diameter: every 12 months
	   • 4-5cm Diameter: every 6 months; vascular surgery evaluation
	   • 5-6cm Diameter: every month
	• Symptomatic or Ruptured: immediate endovascular vs open surgical repair (open repair is gold standard); endovascular may be used in high risk or elderly
	   • Do not waste time trying to stabilize in ER; antihypertensives vs pressors where applicable; resuscitate with blood products; pain control (avoid hypotension)
	• Beta Blockers: indicated in all patients to reduce risk of rupture

Key Words & Most Common	• Atherosclerosis and smoking are most common risk factors followed by Caucasian race and male gender • Non-tender, pulsatile abdominal mass +/- abdominal bruit on auscultation • Ruptured AAA: abdominal pain & distension, shock, flank ecchymosis • CT w/ IV contrast study of choice; US utilized if unstable or screening • Routine screening if asymptomatic; immediate surgical repair if symptomatic or ruptured

Aortic Dissection ♥

Etiology & Risk Factors	• Surge of blood through the aortic intima with separation of the intima and media • Etiology: tear in the intimal layer of the aorta allows blood to collect between intima and media creating a false lumen • Risk Factors: hypertension (especially abrupt/severe increase seen with weightlifting or sympathomimetic agents such as cocaine or ecstasy), advanced age, connective tissue disorder (Marfan, Loeys-Dietz, Ehlers-Danlos), male gender, family history, bicuspid aortic valve, preexisting aortic aneurysm, pregnancy and delivery, atherosclerosis
Patho-physiology	• Aortic wall consist of 3 layers: intima (inner), media (middle), and adventitia (outer); sheer stress and increased blood pressure lead to weakening and tearing of intima layer creating a false-lumen; as blood flows into the intima-media space aneurysm formation occurs which carries a potential for acute rupture • The most common site for aortic dissection is the ascending aorta particularly at the right lateral wall (where sheer forces are greatest) • DeBakey Classification: (I) involves ascending aorta to aortic arch (II) only involves ascending aorta (III) involves descending aorta and extends distally • Stanford Classification: (A) involves ascending aorta and/or aortic arch proximal to brachiocephalic artery (B) involves descending aorta distal to left subclavian artery

Signs & Symptoms	• Chest Pain: sudden, severe, tearing/ripping, chest pain that may radiate to the back
	• Malperfusion Symptoms: interruption of blood flow from dissection
	   • Stroke, myocardial infarction, intestinal infarction, renal insufficiency, paraparesis or paraplegia, limb weakness
	• Physical Exam:
	   • Blood pressures discrepancies on contralateral limbs (>20mmHg difference in systolic BP between arms); pulse deficits
	   • Wide pulse pressures and diastolic murmur at left upper sternal border (new onset aortic regurgitation)
	   • May have hypertension at presentation, hypotension is ominous sign indicative of a rupture

Diagnosis	• CT Angiogram (CTA): preferred imaging study; identifies false lumen, location of intimal dissection flap, areas of malperfusion, aortic dilation; assists in pre-surgical planning • Chest X-Ray (CXR): widened mediastinum (>8cm), possible left sided pleural effusion • Electrocardiogram (ECG): mandatory to rule out acute MI; may show LVH or nonspecific ST changes • Echocardiogram: may be performed at the bedside; TEE is more sensitive • MR Angiogram (MRA): gold standard imaging study; rarely utilized due to time constraints • Labs: CBC, CMP, D-dimer, cardiac enzymes

Treatment	• Immediate Surgical Consult: cardiothoracic and vascular surgery consult regardless of location of dissection
	• Medical Management: indicated to decrease arterial pressure, arterial shear stress, and ventricular contractility
	   • Beta Blockers: metoprolol, esmolol or labetalol; indicated for blood pressure and heart rate management
	   • Vasodilators: nicardipine or nitroprusside; indicated to further reduce blood pressure
	     • Nitroprusside must be given with BB or CCB (vasodilation causes reflex sympathetic activation, increasing ventricular inotropy and aortic shear stress)
	   • Goal to keep heart rate at 60bpm and systolic BP 100-120mmHg; SBP can be lowered rapidly to reduce sheer forces
	• Hemodynamic Support: aggressive fluid resuscitation and pressors if hypotension present
	• Immediate Surgical Repair: indicated for Stanford A/DeBakey I and II; aortic valve replacement may be required if aortic annulus involvement

False Lumen / True Lumen

True Lumen / False Lumen

Descending (Type B Stanford) Dissection

Peripheral Artery Disease

Etiology & Risk Factors	• Atherosclerotic plaques cause narrowing of the arteries that restrict blood flow to the lower extremities resulting in ischemia • Etiology: atherosclerotic plaques restrict blood flow • Risk Factors: **smoking is greatest risk factor (>70% of patients are past or current smokers)**, diabetes, obesity, hypertension, dyslipidemia, male, advanced age, family history, high homocysteine levels, sedentary lifestyle
Patho-physiology	• Atherosclerotic plaque builds up within the artery (particularly aorta, iliac, and femoral arteries) which react with compensatory dilation to continue to allow blood flow; eventually the blood vessel cannot dilate further and the flow lumen begins to narrow restricting blood flow to distal extremities • In severe cases, the atherosclerotic plaque may embolize and cause acute hemodynamic compromise of an extremity

Signs & Symptoms	• Asymptomatic: some patients may not sustain an exercise pace required to produce symptoms
	• Symptomatic: ambulation causes blood flow supply/demand mismatch and manifests as pain, cramping, or fatigue; nerve ischemia may cause burning of feet
	  • **Intermittent Claudication: pain in lower extremity worse with activity and relieved with rest is most common symptom;** may have leg pressure, fatigue, aching
	  • **Nerve Ischemia: burning pain on bottom of feet** most common at night relieved when foot dangled from side of bed (gravity)
	• Physical Exam: evidence of chronic ischemia
	  • **Shiny, hyperpigmented skin with hair loss**, muscle atrophy, cool extremities
	  • May have **decreased pulses** and **increased capillary refill (>3s)**
	  • May have **ulceration of the feet/toes** (lateral malleolus is most common location); more painful than venous ulcers

Diagnosis	• **Ankle-Brachial Index (ABI): quick, non-invasive, objective bedside screening**
	  • 0.91-1.3 is considered normal
	  • <0.90 considered peripheral artery disease
	• **CT Angiography/MR Angiography: gold standard imaging test;** indicated prior to revascularization procedure
	• Doppler Ultrasound: rule out DVT if clinically indicated
	• Labs: kidney function (BUN/creatinine) should be assessed

Treatment	• Lifestyle Modifications: daily exercise (fixed walking), **smoking cessation, alcohol cessation,** treat underlying condition (hypertension, diabetes, dyslipidemia management), proper nutrition and exercise, cardiac rehabilitation, sleep hygiene, smoking cessation
	• **Medication Management:**
	  • **Cilostazol:** indicated to relieve intermittent claudication; promotes vasodilation, enhance tissue oxygenation and suppresses vascular smooth muscle cell growth
	  • **Antiplatelets: aspirin, clopidogrel**, pentoxifylline; inhibit platelet aggregation to lessen symptoms and increase walking distance
	• Revascularization Procedures: **percutaneous balloon angioplasty** or stent placement; minimally invasive method for those that fail exercise or medication management

Key Words & Most Common	• Smoking is greatest risk factor • Intermittent claudication is most common symptom; burning pain on bottom of feet, decreased pulses, shiny & hyperpigmented skin • Ankle-Brachial Index is first line test • Lifestyle modifications (exercise & smoking cessation) → medication management with antiplatelets (Cilostazol, aspirin, or clopidogrel) → revascularization

Peripheral Artery Occlusion

Etiology & Risk Factors	• **Decrease in limb perfusion;** may be acute (embolism) or chronic (thrombosis)
	• Etiology: **thrombosis or embolism are most common causes;** aortic dissection and compartment syndrome
	  • Thrombosis (80%): formation of a blood clot that fully or partially blocks a blood vessel
	  • Embolism (20%): thrombus, blood clot or other foreign material that travels through a vessel until it reaches a vessel to small to allow passage and obstructs blood flow
	• Risk Factors: **smoking (>70% of patients are past or current smokers)**, diabetes, obesity, hypertension, hyperlipidemia, age, family history, high levels of homocysteine

Patho-physiology	• Atherosclerotic plaque builds up, narrowing the lumen of the blood vessel and creates a thrombosis; plaques may rupture and travel through vessel until it reaches a vessel to small to pass through and occludes the blood vessel (embolism) • Thrombosis occurs overtime so there is collateral vessels that form to preserve blood supply; embolism is an acute event and has little to no collateral blood supply
Signs & Symptoms	• **6 P's:** Pain, Paresthesia, Pallor, Paralysis, Pulselessness, Poikilothermic (limb cool to touch compared to contralateral side) • Symptoms are distal to the arterial obstruction; most common location is superficial femoral or popliteal artery • **Impaired Limb Perfusion: Decreased or absent pulses, delayed capillary refill (>2 seconds), limb weakness**
Diagnosis	• **Arterial Doppler Ultrasound:** utilized to assess pulses and location of occlusion; sensitivity decreases distally and is operator dependent • **CT Angiogram:** confirmatory test that is readily available • **Ankle-Brachial Index:** quick, non-invasive, objective bedside screening • Labs: CBC, CMP, coagulation studies (PT/PTT), CK; do not aid in diagnosis but to monitor concomitant condition and anticoagulation status

Treatment	• **Supportive:** indicated if non-limb threatening ischemia
	  • **Unfractionated heparin,** aspirin, pain control, dependent positioning
	• **Reperfusion Measures:** emergent vascular surgery and/or interventional radiology consult as ischemia can be limb threatening (amputation occurs in 10-15% of cases)
	  • **Embolism:** transcatheter or surgical embolectomy
	  • **Thrombosis:** intra-arterial thrombolysis (tPA), balloon angioplasty, stenting, surgical bypass

Key Words & Most Common	• Smoking is most common risk factor • Thrombosis occurs over time usually from atherosclerosis; Embolism is acute event and more associate with limb threatening emergencies • 6 P's: Pain, Paresthesia, Pallor, Paralysis, Pulselessness, Poikilothermic • CT angiogram vs arterial doppler • Reperfusion ASAP for limb threatening ischemia; supportive with heparin if non-limb threatening

Giant Cell Arteritis

Etiology & Risk Factors	• **Systemic inflammatory vasculitis of large and medium vessels particularly of the extracranial branches of the aorta** (carotid, **temporal**, occipital, ophthalmic artery) • Etiology: systemic inflammatory vasculitis • Risk Factors: **strongly associated with polymyalgia rheumatica** (40-60% of patients with giant cell arteritis have polymyalgia rheumatica symptoms), female, advanced age (>50 years old most common), certain ethnicities (Northern European [Scandinavian] most common), family history
Patho-physiology	• Not fully understood; innate or adaptive immune system dysregulation causes inflammation of medium to large arteries originating from the aortic arch Predominance of CD4+ T lymphocytes and macrophages on histopathology which undergo granulomatous organization and formation of giant cells

Signs & Symptoms	• **Nonspecific Symptoms**: fever, fatigue, weight loss, general malaise
	 • **Headache: unilateral temporal headache is most common**, scalp tenderness,
	   • Worse at night
	   • Usually does not respond to typical OTC analgesics
	 • Jaw Claudication: **jaw pain worse with mastication or talking**
	 • Temporal Artery Changes: **tender, pulseless, temporal artery**
	 • Myalgia: polymyalgia rheumatica and GCA share similar pathogenesis
	 • Unilateral Visual Loss: transient diplopia or amaurosis fugax if posterior ciliary artery affected

Diagnosis	• Labs: **elevated ESR and CRP** (CRP provides better sensitivity for inflammation due to less age-related increase) • **Temporal Biopsy**: gold standard definitive diagnosis; demonstrates transmural inflammation with intimal thickening • **American College of Rheumatology Criteria: diagnosis made with 3 or more of the following** • **(1)** Age ≥50 **(2)** New onset headache **(3)** ESR > 50mm/hr **(4)** Temporal artery abnormalities (tenderness or decreased pulsation) **(5)** Abnormal artery biopsy

Treatment	• **Corticosteroids: should be initiated immediately if GCA is suspected to prevent blindness and suppress disease activity**
	   • **IV Methylprednisolone**: 1,000mg for 3 days if **loss of vision** and/or neurological signs are present
	   • **Oral Prednisone: 50mg** daily for 2-4 weeks followed by taper if **no** loss of vision and neurological signs **are not** present
	 • Non-Steroidal Management: used if contraindications for steroid therapy
	   • Tocilizumab: IL-6 inhibitor that has gained importance in treatment in patients that are unable to tolerate corticosteroids
	   • Aspirin: adjuvant therapy that may reduce rate of vision loss

Key Words & Most Common	• Systemic inflammatory vasculitis MC affects temporal artery; may be associated with polymyalgia rheumatica • Unilateral temporal headache; jaw claudication • Elevated ESR & CRP • Corticosteroids: IV methylprednisolone with loss of vision; oral prednisone 50mg if no loss of vision • **Rule of 50's: affects patient >50yo with an ESR>50mm/hr and treated with 50mg of prednisone daily**

Superficial Thrombophlebitis

Etiology & Risk Factors	• Inflammatory condition of superficial veins with concomitant venous thrombosis; **most common in lower extremities (great saphenous vein is most common)** • Etiology: blood clot of a superficial vein secondary to inflammation • Risk Factors: IV infusion or catheterization is greatest risk factor, varicose veins, pregnancy, venous stasis, exogenous estrogens, obesity, autoimmune or infectious conditions, recent surgery • Types: **Sterile** (no infection), **Infectious** (prolonged IV use), **Traumatic** (blunt trauma, IV catheter, or chemical contact), **Migratory** (associated with malignancy) • **Trousseau Sign** – migratory thrombophlebitis associated with malignancy (**pancreatic** or visceral malignancy)
Patho-physiology	• Vessel wall injury, hypercoagulable state or venous stasis/turbulence causes microscopic thrombosis that can eventually lead to a larger thrombosis • Vascular injury causes an inflammatory reaction that results in platelet aggregation leading to further thrombus formation

Signs & Symptoms	• **Erythema or discoloration surrounding superficial vein**
	 • May have mild pruritus
	 • Physical Exam
	   • **Tender, indurated superficial vein; palpable cord** may be felt
	   • Minimal or no limb swelling

Diagnosis	• **Clinical Diagnosis** • **Compressive Ultrasound: confirms diagnosis**; used to rule out concomitant DVT and evaluate extent • May show noncompressible vein with vessel wall thickening • Malignancy Workup: patients >40yo with first case of thrombophlebitis; consider CEA, prostate specific antigen (PSA), CT scan, mammogram as clinically indicated • *D-Dimer and thrombophilia workup often not indicated*
Treatment	• **Supportive**: considered benign and self-limiting; **analgesia (NSAIDs), heat, compression**, elevation of extremity with follow-up in 7-10 days • Antibiotics: only indicated with infectious etiology, associated cellulitis, or clear evidence of infection • Anticoagulation: enoxaparin indicated if thrombosis >5cm • Thrombosis occurring within 5cm of sapheno-femoral junction should be treated as a DVT • Vein Ligation: indicated if varicose veins or recurrent superficial thrombophlebitis
Key Words & Most Common	• Most common at great saphenous vein in lower extremity • May occur as a result of IV catheterization or varicose veins • Erythematous, tender, induration, superficial vein +/- palpable cord • Clinical diagnosis • Supportive treatment

Deep Vein Thrombosis (DVT)

Etiology & Risk Factors	• Blood clot that forms within the deep venous system; DVT is the primary cause of pulmonary embolism
	• Etiology: clotting of blood in a deep vein of an extremity (usually calf or thigh) or the pelvis (can occur in upper extremity, mesenteric, or cerebral veins)
	• Risk Factors: Virchow's Triad
	   • **Venous Stasis:** **immobilization**, bed rest, prolonged sitting
	   • **Endothelial Injury:** trauma, **surgery**, IVDU, infection, indwelling catheter
	   • **Hypercoagulable State:** **malignancy, pregnancy, oral contraceptives**, thrombophilia, protein C or S deficiencies, antithrombin III deficiency, Factor V Leiden

Patho-physiology	• Virchow's Triad of venous stasis, endothelial wall injury, hypercoagulable state are three primary mechanisms leading to local cytokine production resulting in leukocyte adhesion to the endothelial wall, forming a thrombosis within a vessel • Most commonly occurs in areas of low-flow sites (especially in lower extremities)

Signs & Symptoms	• **Unilateral pain and swelling of lower extremity is most common**
	• Physical Exam:
	   • **Leg swelling >3cm** compared to contralateral side
	   • Unilateral discoloration if significant venous stasis
	   • Calf muscle tenderness
	   • **Homan's Sign:** deep pain while squeezing calf and simultaneously dorsiflexing foot

Diagnosis	• **Modified Well's Criteria** to determine testing modalities based on risk stratification (next slide) • Venous Duplex Ultrasound: **first-line imaging study** if high suspicion for DVT • D-Dimer: high-sensitivity, low-specificity test to rule out DVT in low-risk patients • Contrast Venography: gold standard test for definitive diagnostic; rarely performed due to difficult and invasive nature

Treatment	• **Anticoagulation: first-line therapy** for most DVT patients
	   • **Heparin: unfractionated or low molecular weight heparin** or fondaparinux given for 5 days followed by longer term oral treatment
	   • **Oral Vitamin K Analog:** warfarin; initiated within 24-48 hours after starting heparin; indicated for ≥3 months
	   • **Oral Factor Xa Inhibitor:** rivaroxaban, apixaban; does not require INR monitoring
	• Thrombolysis: alteplase; generally, not indicated but considered if symptomatic iliofemoral DVT
	• IVC Filter: indicated in recurrent DVT/PE despite anticoagulation; patients that cannot tolerate or contraindication to anticoagulation

Key Words & Most Common	• Risks include Virchow's Triad of venous stasis, hypercoagulable state, and endothelial injury; DVT carries significant risk for pulmonary embolism • Unilateral pain/swelling over lower extremity; + Homan's Sign • Well's Criteria utilized to determine D-Dimer vs Duplex Ultrasound studies. ultrasound first line if suspicious for DVT • Anticoagulation is first line therapy; heparin bridge to warfarin

Modified Well's Criteria (each 1 point)		
Active Cancer (<6mo)	Tenderness Along Deep Vein System	Unilateral Pitting Edema
Paralysis or Immobility of Extremity	Swelling of Leg	Collateral Superficial Veins
Bedrest >3 Days due to Procedure	Unilateral Calf Swelling >3cm	Previously Documented DVT
Alternative diagnosis as likely or more likely than DVT = −2 Points		

Well's Criteria Scoring		
-2 to 0 Points	**1 or 2 Points**	**3 or More Points**
Low Risk DVT prevalence <5%	**Moderate Risk** DVT prevalence 17%	**High Risk** DVT prevalence 17-53%
D-Dimer testing safe in this group and negative test decreases probability of DVT to <1%	D-Dimer test still effective and negative test decreases probability of DVT to <1% Consider US	Patient should receive Venous Duplex Ultrasound

Varicose Veins

Etiology & Risk Factors	• Dilated superficial veins and non-compliant venous valves causes retrograde venous blood flow contributing to the development of varicose veins and telangiectasias • Etiology: **primary venous valvular insufficiency or dilated venous walls** • Risk Factors: **female, advanced age, hormone changes (pregnancy, oral contraceptives)**, prolonged standing or sitting, obesity, sedentary lifestyle, history of DVT
Patho-physiology	• Intrinsic and extrinsic factors cause elevated venous pressures and/or defective venous valves which contribute to venous reflux; gravitational pull with non-compliant valves leads to increase pooling in lower extremities

Signs & Symptoms	• **Asymptomatic: mostly asymptomatic** but patient may seek treatment for aesthetic/cosmetic reasons
	• **Symptomatic:** may have swelling, **dull ache** and/or cramping of lower extremity, leg heaviness, exercise intolerance
	  • **Discomfort is worse with prolonged standing and relieved with rest and elevation of lower extremity**
	• Physical Exam:
	  • **Visibly distended veins** from thigh to ankle, discoloration, telangiectasias (spider veins)
	  • Severe cases may result in venous stasis ulcers

Diagnosis	• **Clinical Diagnosis** • Venous Duplex Ultrasound: assess anatomy and valve function; DVT should be ruled out as cause of clinical situation
Treatment	• **Supportive: mainstay of treatment; leg elevation, compression stockings** (20-30mmHg), and oral analgesia • Endovascular Treatment: catheter-based endovenous thermal ablation (EVTL) uses heat cautery where the catheter is located to direct blood flow to deep circulation • Surgical: surgical ligation and stripping of great saphenous vein • Liquid Sclerotherapy: treatment for superficial telangiectasias
Key Words & Most Common	• Retrograde venous blood flow and defective venous valves • Mostly asymptomatic; may have dull ache and discomfort with prolonged standing • Treatment with leg elevational and compression stockings

Chronic Venous Insufficiency

Etiology & Risk Factors	• **Prevalent disease process in which venous hypertension in lower extremities and impaired venous return leads to edema, skin changes, and discomfort** • Etiology: **incompetent venous valves is most common cause** • Risk Factors: **female, advanced age, prolonged sitting standing,** history of DVT or thrombophlebitis, smoking, obesity, sedentary lifestyle, hormonal changes (pregnancy, oral contraceptive pills)
Patho-physiology	• Weakened venous valves or dilated venous diameter leads to retrograde blood flow; gravitational pull with non-compliant valves leads to increase pooling in lower extremities • Chronically elevated venous pressure leads to symptoms; skin hyperpigmentation occurs as result of hemosiderin produced when RBCs leak into surrounding tissue

Signs & Symptoms	• **Pain, pruritus, burning,** cramping, aching or heaviness of lower extremity
	• **Symptoms worse with prolonged standing or seated with legs hanging and relieved with leg elevation and ambulation**
	  • Little to no correlation with exercise (differentiates from arterial claudication)
	  • Erythema improves with elevation (differentiates from cellulitis)
	• **Venous Stasis Dermatitis:** eczematous rash with **dark brown/purple hyperpigmented**, tight, dry, and hairless skin
	• Venous Stasis Ulcers: ulcer formation most commonly at the **medial malleolus**

Diagnosis	• **Clinical Diagnosis** • Must differentiate from other conditions including diabetic ulcers, cellulitis, PAD etc. • Venous Duplex Ultrasound: utilized to assess anatomy and valve function; DVT should be ruled out as cause of clinical situation • Ankle-Brachial Index: differentiates from peripheral artery disease

Treatment	• **Supportive: mainstay of treatment; leg elevation, compression stockings** (20-30mmHg), exercise, weight management
	• Ulcer Management: wound debridement of non-viable tissue, compression bandages with topical treatment
	  • Topical: antimicrobial (silver sulfadiazine), debriding agents (collagenase/hydrogels), antiseptic agents (cadexomer-iodine), moisturizors (hydrocolloids)
	  • Antibiotics: indicated for stasis ulcers or concomitant cellulitis; guidance based on wound culture results
	• Surgical: sclerotherapy, endovenous, or open vascular surgery reserved for cases that fail conservative management

Key Words & Most Common	• Weakened venous valves lead to venous stasis • Venous stasis dermatitis/ulcers; symptoms worse with standing and relieved with leg elevation; MC place for ulcer is at medial malleolus • Differentiate from cellulitis, PAD, diabetic ulcers; consider duplex US • Leg elevation, compression stockings, exercise and weight management

Works Cited

1. Major categories of cardiomyopathy.png. (2020, September 23). *Wikimedia Commons*. Retrieved 12:22, July 25, 2023 from https://commons.wikimedia.org/w/index.php?title=File:Major_categories_of_cardiomyopathy.png&oldid=468662590.
2. Takotsubo ultrasound.gif. (2021, June 6). *Wikimedia Commons*. Retrieved 12:25, July 25, 2023 from https://commons.wikimedia.org/w/index.php?title=File:Takotsubo_ultrasound.gif&oldid=567531869.
3. Respiratory sinus arrhythmia with RBBB (male, 21).jpg. (2022, May 28). *Wikimedia Commons*. Retrieved 15:28, July 24, 2023 from https://commons.wikimedia.org/w/index.php?title=File:Respiratory_sinus_arrhythmia_with_RBBB_(male,_21).jpg&oldid=659412765.
4. ECG Sinus Tachycardia 125 bpm.jpg. (2021, June 17). *Wikimedia Commons*. Retrieved 15:35, July 24, 2023 from https://commons.wikimedia.org/w/index.php?title=File:ECG_Sinus_Tachycardia_125_bpm.jpg&oldid=569531337.
5. Sinus bradycardia lead2.svg. (2023, January 7). *Wikimedia Commons*. Retrieved 15:56, July 24, 2023 from https://commons.wikimedia.org/w/index.php?title=File:Sinus_bradycardia_lead2.svg&oldid=723547176.
6. SSS ecg 001 (CardioNetworks ECGpedia).jpg. (2020, November 22). *Wikimedia Commons*. Retrieved 16:15, July 24, 2023 from https://commons.wikimedia.org/w/index.php?title=File:SSS_ecg_001_(CardioNetworks_ECGpedia).jpg&oldid=514248746.
7. Heart block.png. (2022, November 24). *Wikimedia Commons*. Retrieved 16:27, July 24, 2023 from https://commons.wikimedia.org/w/index.php?title=File:Heart_block.png&oldid=709177225.
8. Left Bundle Branch Block ECG Unlabeled.jpg. (2022, November 24). *Wikimedia Commons*. Retrieved 23:15, July 24, 2023 from https://commons.wikimedia.org/w/index.php?title=File:Left_Bundle_Branch_Block_ECG_Unlabeled.jpg&oldid=709168705.
9. Atrial flutter34.svg. (2023, January 8). *Wikimedia Commons*. Retrieved 23:47, July 24, 2023 from https://commons.wikimedia.org/w/index.php?title=File:Atrial_flutter34.svg&oldid=723814527.
10. ECG Atrial Fibrillation 98 bpm.jpg. (2021, June 17). *Wikimedia Commons*. Retrieved 13:18, July 25, 2023 from https://commons.wikimedia.org/w/index.php?title=File:ECG_Atrial_Fibrillation_98_bpm.jpg&oldid=569530625.
11. ECG AVNRT 181 bpm.jpg. (2022, February 18). *Wikimedia Commons*. Retrieved 14:29, July 25, 2023 from https://commons.wikimedia.org/w/index.php?title=File:ECG_AVNRT_181_bpm.jpg&oldid=630643262.
12. DeltaWave09.JPG. (2022, June 30). *Wikimedia Commons*. Retrieved 15:32, July 25, 2023 from https://commons.wikimedia.org/w/index.php?title=File:DeltaWave09.JPG&oldid=670154773.
13. De-Rhythm ventricular premature (CardioNetworks ECGpedia).png. (2023, April 28). *Wikimedia Commons*. Retrieved 16:11, July 25, 2023 from https://commons.wikimedia.org/w/index.php?title=File:De-Rhythm_ventricular_premature_(CardioNetworks_ECGpedia).png&oldid=755772216.
14. Vtach (CardioNetworks ECGpedia).jpg. (2022, August 3). *Wikimedia Commons*. Retrieved 16:31, July 25, 2023 from https://commons.wikimedia.org/w/index.php?title=File:Vtach_(CardioNetworks_ECGpedia).jpg&oldid=679983808.
15. Tosadesdepointes.jpg. (2023, February 13). *Wikimedia Commons*. Retrieved 17:05, July 25, 2023 from https://commons.wikimedia.org/w/index.php?title=File:Tosadesdepointes.jpg&oldid=732346834.
16. Ventricular fibrillation.png. (2023, January 7). *Wikimedia Commons*. Retrieved 17:43, July 25, 2023 from https://commons.wikimedia.org/w/index.php?title=File:Ventricular_fibrillation.png&oldid=723524313.
17. 2009 Congenital Heart Defects.jpg. (2023, April 15). *Wikimedia Commons*. Retrieved 18:34, July 25, 2023 from https://commons.wikimedia.org/w/index.php?title=File:2009_Congenital_Heart_Defects.jpg&oldid=750356056.
18. Thoracic landmarks anterior view.svg. (2022, March 3). *Wikimedia Commons*. Retrieved 18:37, August 21, 2023 from https://commons.wikimedia.org/w/index.php?title=File:Thoracic_landmarks_anterior_view.svg&oldid=634343099.
19. Ventricular septal defect.svg. (2022, July 25). *Wikimedia Commons*. Retrieved 19:43, July 25, 2023 from https://commons.wikimedia.org/w/index.php?title=File:Ventricular_septal_defect.svg&oldid=677657620.
20. Transposition of Great Arteries.png. (2023, March 1). *Wikimedia Commons*. Retrieved 21:09, July 25, 2023 from
21. from https://commons.wikimedia.org/w/index.php?title=File:Transposition_of_Great_Arteries.png&oldid=737145920.
22. Pericardial effusion with tamponade.png. (2020, October 2). *Wikimedia Commons*. Retrieved 21:16, August 17, 2023 from https://commons.wikimedia.org/w/index.php?title=File:Pericardial_effusion_with_tamponade.png&oldid=478437700.
23. Prinzmetal angina.png. (2020, October 13). *Wikimedia Commons*. Retrieved 22:03, July 25, 2023 from https://commons.wikimedia.org/w/index.php?title=File:Prinzmetal_angina.png&oldid=488402734.
24. AMI bloodtests engl.png. (2023, June 20). *Wikimedia Commons*. Retrieved 23:26, July 25, 2023 from https://commons.wikimedia.org/w/index.php?title=File:AMI_bloodtests_engl.png&oldid=775672557.
25. Contiguous leads.svg. (2020, October 1). *Wikimedia Commons*. Retrieved 23:33, July 25, 2023 from https://commons.wikimedia.org/w/index.php?title=File:Contiguous_leads.svg&oldid=477174609.
26. Contrast-enhanced CT scan demonstrating abdominal aortic aneurysm.jpg. (2023, January 3). *Wikimedia Commons*. Retrieved 21:20, August 17, 2023 from https://commons.wikimedia.org/w/index.php?title=File:Contrast-enhanced_CT_scan_demonstrating_abdominal_aortic_aneurysm.jpg&oldid=722464752.
27. Descending (Type B Stanford) Aortic Dissection.PNG. (2020, October 26). *Wikimedia Commons*. Retrieved 22:45, July 31, 2023 from https://commons.wikimedia.org/w/index.php?title=File:Descending_(Type_B_Stanford)_Aortic_Dissection.PNG&oldid=502783284.

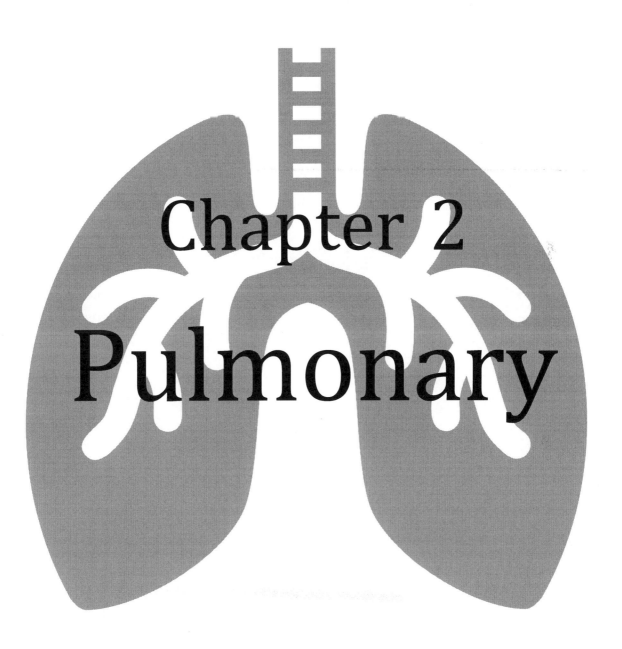

Chapter 2
Pulmonary

COPD	# Emphysema	🫁
Etiology & Risk Factors	• Steady, progressive, irreversible lung disease resulting in permanent enlargement of the terminal air space distal to the terminal bronchiole • Deterioration of lung parenchyma with associated loss of elasticity and no evidence of fibrosis • <u>Etiology</u>: **airflow limitation caused by an inflammatory response** • <u>Risk Factors</u>: **cigarette smoking/exposure is greatest risk factor, male, advanced age,** exposure to noxious gas, environmental pollutants or dust, recurrent lung infections, low birth weight, alpha-1-antitrypsin deficiency, coal mining exposure	
Patho-physiology	• Chronic inflammation and damage to airways distal to terminal bronchiole results in permanent dilation and destruction of airspace walls resulting in decreased capillary and alveolar surface area which impairs gas exchange • Elastase/anti-elastase imbalance leads to alveolar wall and capillary destruction and enlargement of airway; **loss of elastic recoil and airway collapse may lead to air trapping** • Cytotoxic T-cells release TNF-α which destroy alveolar wall epithelial cells	• <u>**Cetrilobar (Proximal Acinar):** **most common type and most associated with smoking history/exposure**</u> • <u>Panacinar</u>: most commonly associated with alpha-1 antitrypsin deficiency • <u>Paraseptal (Distal Acinar)</u>: may be alone or associated with other two types; most commonly seen with spontaneous pneumothorax if alone

Signs & Symptoms	• **Persistent dyspnea is most common symptom; chronic cough +/- sputum production,** hypoxemia, tachypnea
	• <u>Physical Exam</u>:
	  • Accessory respiratory muscle use, **"barrel chested" appearance (increased anteroposterior diameter)** due to **lung hyperinflation**
	  • Decreased breath sounds, **prolonged expiration,** wheezing, crackles in lower lung fields may be appreciated on auscultation
	  • <u>**"Pink Puffer"**</u>: cachectic and non-cyanotic (pink) appearance
	  • **Pursed lip expiration** prevents airway collapse by increasing airway pressure	

Diagnosis	• <u>**Pulmonary Function Test**</u>: **gold standard and most diagnostic; FEV1/FVC <0.7 is diagnostic;** air trapping confirmed with increased residual volume and total lung capacity • <u>Chest X-Ray (CXR)</u>: **hyperinflation of lungs, flattened diaphragm, increased AP diameter;** ordered to rule out pneumonia, CHF, pneumothorax effusions etc. • <u>Arterial Blood Gas (ABG)</u>: ordered if spO2 <92% and symptomatic hypercapnia (COPD exacerbation); may show respiratory acidosis	

Treatment	• <u>Supportive</u>: **smoking cessation,** exercise/pulmonary rehabilitation, **vaccination (pneumococcal and influenza),** avoid pollutants or irritants
	• <u>Oxygen</u>: indicated with paO2 ≤ 60mmHg or spO2< 88%; **goal spO2 88-92%** (>93% O2 associated with higher inpatient mortality due to Haldane effect)
	  • **Reduces mortality and improves quality of life** in advanced COPD
	• <u>Bronchodilators</u>: **albuterol (β2 agonist that relaxes smooth muscle in airway)** and **ipratropium (anticholinergic that inhibits acetylcholine induced bronchoconstriction)**
	• <u>Corticosteroids</u>: inhaled corticosteroids as add-on therapy to bronchodilators; IV (methylprednisolone) and oral steroids (prednisone) inhibit inflammatory cytokines
	• <u>Magnesium</u>: promotes bronchial smooth muscle relaxation in acute exacerbation
	• <u>Antibiotics</u>: indicated for patients with persistent purulent sputum or increased sputum production
	  • <u>Outpatient Healthy</u>: azithromycin, doxycycline, levofloxacin
	  • <u>Outpatient Unhealthy</u> (>65 years old, history of heart disease, >3 exacerbations per year): levofloxacin or amoxicillin/clavulanate
	  • <u>Inpatient</u>: levofloxacin OR cefepime OR piperacillin/tazobactam; indicated if concern for pseudomonas; *consider oseltamivir if during influenza season*
	• <u>Non-invasive Ventilation (CPAP or BiPaP)</u>: improves acidosis and relieves respiratory distress in acute exacerbation	

COPD	# Chronic Bronchitis	🫁
Etiology & Risk Factors	• Form of chronic obstructive pulmonary disease (COPD) characterized as a productive cough for more than 3 months out of the year for 2 consecutive years • <u>Risk Factors</u>: **cigarette smoking/exposure is greatest risk factor, male, advanced age,** exposure to noxious gas, environmental pollutants or dust, recurrent lung infections, low birth weight, alpha-1-antitrypsin deficiency, coal mining exposure, **history of asthma, bronchiectasis, or cystic fibrosis**	
Patho-physiology	• Chronic inflammation as a result of infectious or toxic stimuli causes mucous gland hyperplasia leading to **overproduction and hypersecretion of mucus by goblet cells** • Release of pro-inflammatory mediators (interleukin 8, colony stimulating factor, inflammatory cytokines) target alveolar epithelium • <u>Acute Exacerbation</u>: hyperemia (increased blood flow) and bronchial mucous membranes edema and decreased mucociliary function lead to obstruction and irritation of lungs	Opacity in inferior part of right upper lobe Hyperinflation of the lungs

Signs & Symptoms	• **Chronic cough with sputum production;** dyspnea
	  • Sputum color may be yellowish green, clear, or blood tinged (color may be dependent on infectious cause)
	• <u>Physical Exam</u>:
	  • **Wheezing** (due to airway inflammation); may lead to intermittent bronchospasm
	  • Crackles/rhonchi may be present
	  • <u>**"Blue Bloater"**</u>: obesity, peripheral edema and cyanosis	

Diagnosis	• <u>**Pulmonary Function Test**</u>: **gold standard and preferred test; FEV1/FVC <0.7 is diagnostic;** air trapping confirmed with increased residual volume and total lung capacity • <u>Chest X-Ray (CXR)</u>: **hyperinflation of lungs,** normal diaphragm, **increased AP diameter;** may show prominent vascular markings; **ordered to rule out pneumonia** • <u>Arterial Blood Gas (ABG)</u>: ordered if spO2 <92% and symptomatic hypercapnia (COPD exacerbation); may show respiratory acidosis • <u>Electrocardiogram (ECG)</u>: most common arrhythmias are **multifocal atrial tachycardia** or afib; cor pulmonale (RVH, right axis deviation, low voltage QRS) • <u>Labs</u>: CBC may show **increased hemoglobin and hematocrit** due to chronic hypoxia stimulating erythropoiesis; **sputum culture** if concern for infection	

Treatment	• <u>Supportive</u>: **smoking cessation,** exercise/pulmonary rehabilitation, **vaccination (pneumococcal and influenza),** avoid pollutants or irritants
	• <u>Oxygen</u>: indicated with paO2 ≤ 60mmHg or spO2< 88%; **goal spO2 88-92%** (>93% O2 associated with higher inpatient mortality due to Haldane effect)
	  • **Reduces mortality and improves quality of life** in advanced COPD
	• <u>Bronchodilators</u>: **albuterol (β2 agonist that relaxes smooth muscle in airway)** and **ipratropium (anticholinergic that inhibits acetylcholine induced bronchoconstriction)**
	• <u>Corticosteroids</u>: inhaled corticosteroids as add-on therapy to bronchodilators; IV (methylprednisolone) and oral steroids (prednisone) inhibit inflammatory cytokines
	• <u>Magnesium</u>: promotes bronchial smooth muscle relaxation in acute exacerbation
	• <u>Antibiotics</u>: indicated for patients with persistent purulent sputum or increased sputum production
	  • <u>Outpatient Healthy</u>: azithromycin, doxycycline, levofloxacin
	  • <u>Outpatient Unhealthy</u> (>65 years old, history of heart disease, >3 exacerbations per year): levofloxacin or amoxicillin/clavulanate
	  • <u>Inpatient</u>: levofloxacin OR cefepime OR piperacillin/tazobactam; indicated if concern for pseudomonas; *consider oseltamivir if during influenza season*
	• <u>Non-invasive Ventilation (CPAP or BiPaP)</u>: improves acidosis and relieves respiratory distress in acute exacerbation	

Cystic Fibrosis

Etiology & Risk Factors	• Autosomal recessive genetic disorder of exocrine glands that causes increasingly thick secretions • <u>Etiology</u>: mutations in the cystic fibrosis transmembrane conductance regulator (CFTR) gene • <u>Risk Factors</u>: male, certain ethnicities (Northern Europeans [Irish, Scottish, Ashkenazi Jewish ancestry] most common), family history, consanguinity (parents closely related [first-cousins]), age (median age of diagnosis is 6-8 months old; **predicted life expectancy <40 years old**)
Patho-physiology	• Mutation of the CTFR gene leads to defect in sodium/chloride exchange transport across exocrine glands • Defective chloride transport leads to thick, highly viscous secretions of lungs, liver, pancreas, reproductive and intestinal tract

Signs & Symptoms	• <u>Respiratory</u>: chronic bronchitis or **pneumonia colonized with *Pseudomonas aeruginosa***
	   • Chronic inflammation and infection leads to **bronchiectasis** (cystic fibrosis is most common cause of bronchiectasis in US)
	   • Increased risk of pneumothorax
	• <u>Gastrointestinal</u>:
	• **Malabsorption**: (especially fat-soluble vitamins [A, D, E, K]) leads to chronic diarrhea and malnutrition, distal intestinal obstruction, steatorrhea
	   • **Meconium Ileus**: failure to pass meconium within first 48 hours of life is earliest clinical indication of disease; infant may experience failure to thrive
	     • <u>Hepatobiliary</u>: pancreatic insufficiency and recurrent pancreatitis; biliary cirrhosis
	• <u>Reproductive</u>: infertility due to thickened cervical secretions in females and azoospermia in males
	• <u>Dermatologic</u>: "salty sweat", digital clubbing, cyanosis

Diagnosis	• <u>Sweat Chloride Test</u>: **most sensitive test**; chloride levels >60mmol/L on 2 separate instances • Pilocarpine (cholinergic drug that induces perspiration) is administered with electrode that draws pilocarpine into the skin and stimulates sweat glands • <u>Chest X-Ray (CXR)</u>: identifies pneumonia, bronchiectasis, hyperinflation, pneumothorax • **<u>Pulmonary Function Test</u>**: monitors disease progression; **demonstrates obstructive lung disease with air trapping** • <u>Sputum Cultures</u>: identify bacterial colonization (***Pseudomonas aeruginosa* most common**; *S. aureus* and *H. influenzae* common in first few months of life)
Treatment	• <u>Supportive</u>: **chest physiotherapy**; pancreatic enzyme and vitamin supplementation (A, D, E, K), optimizing nutrition (high fat diet), exercise, supplemental oxygen • <u>Antibiotics</u>: many patients placed on maintenance dose of azithromycin or other macrolide to prevent pneumonia • **Pseudomonas Coverage**: cefepime, imipenem, or **fluoroquinolone (levofloxacin)**; IV antibiotics if severe exacerbation • **<u>Bronchodilators</u>: albuterol (β2 agonist that relaxes smooth muscle in airway) and ipratropium (anticholinergic that inhibits acetylcholine induced bronchoconstriction)** • <u>Decongestants/Mucolytics</u>: reduce production of new mucous • **<u>Dornase Alfa</u>**: inhaled recombinant human deoxyribonuclease that hydrolyzes DNA in sputum to decrease viscosity and break down mucous plugs • <u>Nebulized Hypertonic Saline</u>: indicated to reduce sputum viscosity
Key Words & Most Common	• Autosomal recessive genetic disorder of exocrine glands leading to thick, highly viscous secretions of multiple organ systems • Pneumonia colonized with pseudomonas aeruginosa; meconium ileus; pancreatic insufficiency • Sweat chloride test is most accurate test; pulmonary function test to monitor disease • Antibiotics coverage pseudomonas (fluoroquinolones) + bronchodilators

Bronchiectasis

Etiology & Risk Factors	• **Chronic lung disease characterized by persistent dilation of bronchial airways and decreased mucociliary transport function caused by chronic inflammation/infection**
	• <u>Etiologies</u>: chronic inflammation or infection; **cystic fibrosis is most common cause in US**
	   • <u>Bacterial</u>: *Pseudomonas aeruginosa* (most common cause if related to cystic fibrosis), *H. influenzae*, *S. aureus*
	   • <u>Viral</u>: respiratory syncytial virus, measles
	   • <u>Pulmonary disease</u>: asthma, COPD, idiopathic pulmonary fibrosis, recurrent pneumonias
	   • <u>Congenital/Genetic</u>: cystic fibrosis, alpha-1 antitrypsin deficiency
	• <u>Risk Factors</u>: **cystic fibrosis is greatest risk factor**, frequent respiratory infections, immunosuppression, COPD, history of inhaled foreign body

Patho-physiology	• Chronic dilation of bronchial airways and decreased mucociliary transport function leads to airway bacterial colonization/infection, airway obstruction, cartilage destruction/fibrosis, mucous gland hyperplasia and inflammatory cell infiltration • Increased mucous build up leads to bacterial colonization which further causes airway damage/inflammation and eventually, dilated airways (harder to clear secretions)

Signs & Symptoms	• **Chronic, productive cough with thick sputum (may be purulent)**
	• Dyspnea; may have pleuritic chest pain; **hemoptysis due to airway neovascularization**
	• <u>Physical Exam</u>:
	   • **Crackles are most common finding**, wheezing on auscultation
	   • Hypoxia, digital clubbing, cyanosis may be present in advanced disease

Diagnosis	• **<u>High Resolution CT Scan</u>: most sensitive and specific test**; shows airway dilation and thickened bronchial walls with little tapering of airway
	   • **<u>Signet Ring Sign</u>**: thickened/dilated airway lie adjacent to smaller pulmonary artery branch
	   • **<u>Tram-Track Sign</u>: horizontal orientation of thickened, dilated airway**
	• <u>Chest X-Ray (CXR)</u>: nonspecific; may show airway wall thickening/dilation; tubular opacities secondary to mucous plug, linear atelectasis or perihilar densities
	• **<u>Pulmonary Function Test</u>**: airflow **obstructive** (↓FEV1) with air trapping (↑residual volume)
	• *Consider infectious workup if acute exacerbation*

Treatment	• <u>Supportive</u>: **chest physiotherapy**, regular exercise, supplemental oxygen, decongestants/mucolytics
	• <u>Antibiotics</u>: many patients on maintenance dose of a macrolide
	   • If no concern for *Pseudomonas*, may treat with amoxicillin/clavulanate, TMP-SMX, **azithromycin**
	   • If concern for Pseudomonas, cover with cefepime, imipenem, or **fluoroquinolone (levofloxacin)**; IV antibiotics if severe exacerbation
	• <u>Respiratory Adjuncts</u>: bronchodilators (albuterol/ipratropium)

Key Words & Most Common	• Chronic dilation of bronchial airways; most commonly caused by cystic fibrosis • Chronic productive cough with mucopurulent sputum; hemoptysis • High resolution CT shows tram-track sign (horizontal dilated/thickened airways); PFT shows obstructive pattern • Supportive with chest physiotherapy; antibiotics to cover for respiratory infection

Asthma

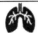

Etiology & Risk Factors	• **Chronic, intermittent, reversible, obstructive airways disease characterized by airway inflammation and narrowing**; may have acute exacerbations
	• <u>Etiology</u>: multiple genetic and environmental factors
	• <u>Risk Factors</u>: **atopic triad (allergic rhinitis, atopic dermatitis [eczema], asthma)**, **environmental exposures** (pollen, pet dander, dust mites, mold, smoke, air pollution)family history, childhood respiratory infections, obesity, smoking, formula fed during infancy
	   • <u>Intrinsic (Non-Allergic) Triggers</u>: emotional factors or stress, cold or dry air, viral URI, exercise, medications (aspirin or beta blockers), GERD, obesity
	   • <u>Extrinsic (Allergic) Triggers</u>: pollen/mold, animal dander, dust, cockroaches, tobacco smoke

Patho-physiology	• Inhalation of an irritant or allergen causes bronchoconstriction (smooth muscle contraction), airway inflammation, hypersensitivity and increased mucous production • Allergens bind to IgE receptors initiating mast cell activation and inflammatory cascade causing significant airway resistance
Signs & Symptoms	• **Dyspnea, wheezing, and cough**; may have chest tightness if acute exacerbation; *symptoms may be worse at night* • **Prolonged expiration with bilateral wheezes on auscultation** • <u>**Status Asthmaticus**</u>: life threatening form of asthma that rapidly progresses • <u>Ominous Signs</u>: **silent chest** (no air movement in or out), **altered mental status**, systemic hypoxia; patient in a **"tripod"** position (forward sitting to open airway), **paradoxical respirations** (chest deflation with abdominal protrusion during inspiration), peak expiratory flow <33% of personal best

Diagnosis	• <u>Clinical Diagnosis</u>; must monitor spO$_2$ (<90% indicative of respiratory distress and adverse outcome)
	• <u>**Pulmonary Function Test**</u>: gold standard diagnostic test; demonstrates airway obstruction (reduced FEV1 to FVC ratio) that is reversible with treatment
	   • Bronchial asthma diagnosed if there is a 12% or 200mL improvement of FEV1 from previous value after inhaled β2 agonist is administered
	   • <u>Bronchoprovocation Test</u>: methacholine/histamine challenge to determine airway hyperreactivity; rarely performed
	• <u>Peak Expiratory Flow Rate</u>: test to assess severity and response to treatment
	• <u>Chest X-Ray (CXR)</u>: may show hyperinflation consistent with bronchoconstriction; ABG not usually ordered (may show respiratory alkalosis secondary to tachypnea)

Treatment	• <u>Supportive</u>: allergen avoidance, environmental control, weight management if obese, smoking cessation, occupational change
	• <u>**Bronchodilators**</u>: first-line medication class
	   • <u>**Short Acting β2 agonist**</u>: **albuterol first-line treatment (inhaler or nebulizer)** to relax smooth muscle in airway
	   • <u>Anticholinergics</u>: **ipratropium** to inhibit acetylcholine induced bronchoconstriction
	   • <u>Long Acting β2 agonist</u>: salmeterol or formoterol
	• <u>**Corticosteroids**</u>: inhibit inflammatory cytokines
	   • <u>Inhaled corticosteroids</u>: budesonide or beclomethasone or fluticasone as add-on therapy to short acting bronchodilators for long term, persistent asthma
	   • <u>**IV (Methylprednisolone) and Oral Corticosteroids (Prednisone)**</u>: inhibit inflammatory cytokines in acute exacerbation; most exacerbations should be on short course
	• <u>Mast Cell Modifiers</u>: cromolyn, nedocromil; inhibit mast cell and leukotriene-mediated degranulation
	• <u>Magnesium</u>: promotes bronchial smooth muscle relaxation in acute exacerbation
	• <u>Leukotriene Modifiers</u>: **montelukast;** inhibits leukotriene mediated neutrophil migration and smooth muscle contraction

Clinical Classification of Asthma Severity

Severity	Symptom Frequency	SABA Use for Symptoms	Nighttime Symptoms	Limitation with Regular Activity	%FEV$_1$ of Predicted	FEV$_1$ Variability	Recommended Treatment
INTERMITTENT	≤2x per week	≤2 days per week	≤2x per month	None	≥80%	<20%	SABA inhaler as needed
MILD PERSISTENT	>2x per week	>2 days per week	3-4x per month	Minor Interference	≥80%	20-30%	SABA + Low Dose ICS
MODERATE PERSISTENT	Daily	Daily	>1x per week	Some Interference	60-80%	>30%	SABA + Low Dose ICS + LABA or Medium Dose ICS
SEVERE PERSISTENT	Continuously	>2x per day	Frequently, nightly	Extreme Interference	<60%	>30%	SABA + High Dose ICS + LABA +/- Omalizumab

ICS = inhaled corticosteroid
SABA = short acting β$_2$ agonist
LABA = long acting β$_2$ agonist

Severity of symptoms →

Step 1 – **SABA** (albuterol) as needed

Step 2 – **Low dose ICS** (beclomethasone, budesonide, fluticasone)

Step 3 – **Low dose ICS** (beclomethasone, budesonide, fluticasone) and **LABA** (salmeterol, formoterol)

Step 4 – **Medium dose ICS** (beclomethasone, budesonide, fluticasone) and **LABA** (salmeterol, formoterol)

Step 5 – **High dose ICS** (beclomethasone, budesonide, fluticasone) and **LABA** (salmeterol, formoterol) +/- **Omalizumab** for patients with allergies

Step 6 – **High dose ICS** (beclomethasone, budesonide, fluticasone) and **LABA** (salmeterol, formoterol) and oral corticosteroid (prednisone) +/- **Omalizumab** for patients with allergies

• Step up if needed.
• Step down if possible and asthma is well controlled for at least 3 months.
• Consult asthma specialist if step 3 and above

Sarcoidosis

Etiology & Risk Factors	• Chronic, multisystem inflammatory disease characterized by abnormal collection of noncaseating granulomas throughout multiple organ systems • Etiology: unknown, various associations possible with immune response to occupational/environmental exposures (beryllium, dust) or infection • Risk Factors: female, age (**20-40 years old most common**), **certain race or ethnicities (African Americans and Northern Europeans most common), female** (females more likely to have eye/skin involvement while males more likely to have cardiac involvement), immune system dysfunction, family history, environmental exposures
Patho-physiology	• Inflammatory response to environmental antigen in a genetically susceptible person • Antigen triggers a cell mediated immune response characterized by amplified T cell and macrophage accumulation, cytokine release, and granuloma formation • Granulomas accumulation deforms structure of affected organ can causes significant dysfunction • *Most common locations for granulomas are **lungs, skin, joints, and eyes**; less commonly affected is heart, kidney, exocrine glands and brain*
Signs & Symptoms	• Asymptomatic: about 50% of patients are asymptomatic and lesions found incidentally on routine imaging • Respiratory: **persistent dry cough**, dyspnea; **hilar or mediastinal lymphadenopathy** • Skin: **erythema nodosum** (red, indurated, painful nodules on anterior tibia, arms or trunk), **lupus pernio** (purplish plaque of nose, cheeks, lips, or ears) **is most specific** • Eyes: **uveitis** causing photophobia, blurred vision, and tearing • Cardiac: **restrictive cardiomyopathy**, arrhythmia or heart block secondary to conduction defects • Endocrine: hypercalcemia, hypothyroidism, adrenal insufficiency • Musculoskeletal: arthralgias (ankle, knee, wrist, elbow joint pain) • Neurologic: central diabetes insipidus, cranial neuropathy especially CNVII (facial nerve palsy) • Löfgren syndrome: triad of polyarthritis, erythema nodosum, and hilar adenopathy
Diagnosis	• Chest X-Ray (CXR): **best initial test; bilateral hilar lymphadenopathy is most common abnormality**; normal CXR does not exclude diagnosis • High Resolution CT: more sensitive test to detect hilar and mediastinal lymphadenopathy; may reveal ground glass opacities, interstitial infiltrates, fibrosis, cysts • Tissue Biopsy: **most accurate test** to confirm diagnosis; demonstrates noncaseating granulomas in absence of mycobacteria and fungi • Labs: hypercalcemia, **elevated serum ACE**, BUN; LFTs may be elevated with renal/hepatic involvement, consider 24-hour urine for hypercalciuria • Pulmonary Function Test: utilized to monitor progression and response to treatment; shows restrictive disease pattern • Electrocardiogram, echocardiogram, slit Lamp, PET Scan utilized to determine extrapulmonary involvement
Treatment	• Asymptomatic: requires no treatment, most patients often undergo spontaneous remission; monitoring with serial CXR and PFT at 3-6 month intervals • Symptomatic: **oral steroids (prednisone) are first-line** for symptomatic management • Immunosuppressants: methotrexate, azathioprine, or hydroxychloroquine in refractory cases or patients that cannot tolerate steroids
Key Words & Most Common	• Chronic multisystem inflammatory disease characterized by noncaseating granulomas; MC location is lungs and skin • ~50% of patients asymptomatic; persistent dry cough, erythema nodosum, lupus pernio, uveitis • CXR shows bilateral hilar lymphadenopathy; Tissue biopsy shows noncaseating granulomas • Oral steroids; observation if asymptomatic

Idiopathic Pulmonary Fibrosis

Etiology & Risk Factors	• Progressive lung disease characterized by scarring of the lungs; carries a poor prognosis (median survival time is 3 years from time of diagnosis) • Etiology: idiopathic; combination of genetic and environmental factors • Risk Factors: male, advanced age (most common >50 years old), **smoking**, metal/wood/dust exposure, chronic GERD, chronic aspiration
Patho-physiology	• Respiratory insult from environmental exposures leads to alveolar epithelial injury and activation of fibroblasts causing tissue destruction and fibrosis which prohibits adequate gas exchange leading to hypoxic respiratory failure

Signs & Symptoms	• **Progressive dyspnea**, dyspnea on exertion, **cough** (dry, nonproductive), fatigue
	• Physical Exam:
	  • **Fine, bibasilar "Velcro-like" crackles during inspiration**
	  • Digital clubbing (chronic hypoxia)
	  • Progressive hypoxia/respiratory failure; may co-exist with pulmonary hypertension and heart failure

Diagnosis	• Chest X-Ray (CXR): **diffuse reticular opacities and small cystic lesions (honeycombing)** in peripheral and lower lung fields; possible dilated airways • High Resolution CT: **preferred test**; diffuse/patchy reticular opacities in lower lobes; **bilateral subpleural honeycombing**; traction bronchiectasis • Ground glass opacities affecting >30% of lung suggest alternative diagnosis • Pulmonary Function Test: utilized to monitor progression and response to treatment every 3-6mo; shows restrictive disease pattern • Tissue Biopsy: **gold standard for definitive diagnosis** but not always necessary; demonstrates subpleural honeycombing & fibroblastic foci
Treatment	• Palliation: no effective medical management; treatments are controversial and carry questionable efficacy • Tyrosine Kinase Inhibitors: **pirfenidone and nintedanib are antifibrotic drugs that may slow disease progression** but do not improve mortality rate • Supportive: smoking cessation, **oxygen supplementation**, GERD medications, pneumococcal and influenza vaccination, pulmonary rehabilitation, support groups • **Lung transplant: shows survival benefit;** early referral recommended
Key Words & Most Common	• Progressive scarring/fibrotic lung disease from an unknown etiology with a poor prognosis • Dyspnea, dry/nonproductive cough • Fine, "Velcro" crackles during inspiration • HRCT is preferred test; shows reticular opacities in lower lobes and honeycombing • Pirfenidone and nintedanib may slow progression • Lung transplant only possible cure

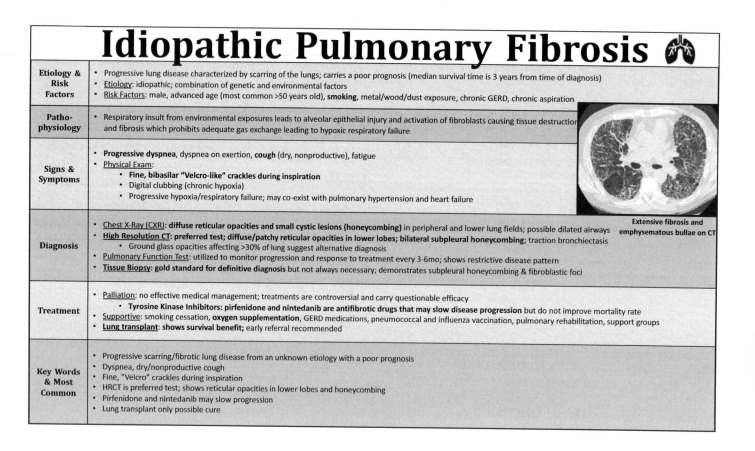

Extensive fibrosis and emphysematous bullae on CT

Silicosis

Etiology & Risk Factors	• Occupational pneumoconiosis characterized by nodular pulmonary fibrosis; **carries a 30x increased risk for developing tuberculosis** or mycobacterial disease
	• Etiology: **inhalation of silicon dioxide in form of crystalline silica dust**
	• Risk Factors: **occupational exposure (mining, construction, sandblasting, stone cutting)**, lack of personal protective measures, poor ventilation, smoking
	   • **Quarry workers/stonecutters/miners working with granite, slate, or quartz**
	   • **Sandblasting, ceramic pottery makers, glass or cement manufacturing**

Patho-physiology	• Alveolar macrophages engulf silica particles deposited in airways and subsequently release cytokines (TNF-α, IL-1) and growth factors which cause oxidative damage, stimulating inflammation and fibrosis • Silica released into surrounding tissue with macrophage death forms silicotic nodule which then turn into a fibrotic scar

Signs & Symptoms	• May initially be asymptomatic
	• **Progressive dyspnea and productive cough**
	• Weight loss and fatigue
	• Physical Exam:
	   • **Bilateral, diffuse crackles**
	   • Diminished breath sounds

Diagnosis	• Chest X-Ray: multiple small (<1cm) well-defined **nodular opacities located in upper lobes** • Chest CT Scan: **hilar and mediastinal lymph node calcification that may resemble eggshells**; pleural thickening • Biopsy: definitive diagnosis
Treatment	• **Supportive: removal from exposure source**; pulmonary rehabilitation, smoking cessation • No specific therapies; management with asthma medications (bronchodilators, inhaled/oral steroids) • Whole Lung Lavage: treatment of acute silicosis to remove or reduce the total mineral dust load in the lungs • Lung Transplant: last resort option; only effective long-term treatment • Monitoring: annual tuberculin skin test for TB surveillance
Key Words & Most Common	• Occupational history of silica exposure leading to nodular pulmonary fibrosis • Risk factors: quarry/stone/miner working with granite, slate, or quartz • Progressive dyspnea and symptomatic quote • CXR shows well defined upper lobe opacities • CT scan shows eggshell calcifications in hilar/mediastinal lymph nodes • Bronchodilators, inhaled corticosteroids

Coal Workers' Pneumoconiosis

Etiology & Risk Factors	• Also known as **black lung disease** • Occupational pneumoconiosis caused by inhalation and deposition of high-carbon coal dust particles usually over the course of 20 years • Etiology: **exposure to coal dust** • Risk Factors: coal mining/dust occupation exposures
Patho-physiology	• Alveolar macrophages engulf coal dust particles deposited in airways; macrophage release cytokines which stimulate inflammation and fibrosis • Macrophages collect in bronchiole and alveolar interstitium forming coal nodules that cause lung damage, airway obstruction, and impaired pulmonary function

Signs & Symptoms	• May initially be asymptomatic
	• **Progressive dyspnea and productive cough (may have black sputum as fibrotic lesions rupture into airway)**
	• Weight loss and fatigue
	• Physical Exam:
	   • Diffuse, fine crackles or diminished breath sounds on auscultation
	   • Massive fibrosis will eventually lead to respiratory failure
	   • **Caplan Syndrome: coal worker's pneumoconiosis with features of rheumatoid diathesis** (multiple rounded nodules appear in short timeframe)

Diagnosis	• **History of silica exposure** • Chest X-Ray (CXR): small, rounded, **nodular opacities located in upper lobes with lower lobe hyperinflation** • Chest CT Scan: more sensitive and specific for identifying coalescing nodules and fibrosis • Pulmonary Function Test: shows obstructive disease pattern • Biopsy: definitive diagnosis
Treatment	• **Supportive: removal from exposure source**; pulmonary rehabilitation, smoking cessation, supplemental oxygen • Monitoring: annual tuberculin skin test for TB surveillance
Key Words & Most Common	• Black lung disease characterized by chronic exposure to high-carbon coal dust • Progressive dyspnea and productive cough with black sputum • Small, rounded nodular opacities of upper lung with hyperinflation of lower lobes • Supportive treatment

Berylliosis

Etiology & Risk Factors	• Granulomatous pulmonary disease caused by occupational exposure to beryllium • Beryllium is an earth metal with low density & high thermal stability making it an ideal aerospace material; often alloyed with aluminum, copper, or nickel • <u>Etiology</u>: **exposure to beryllium** • <u>Risk Factors</u>: **beryllium mining, aerospace, electronics**, automotive/**aircraft manufacturing**, computer/electronic recycling, **metal alloy production**/machining, fluorescent light bulb manufacturing, jewelry making; *relatively rare now as industries have implemented production methods to limit exposure*
Patho-physiology	• Cell mediated hypersensitivity disease in which T-cells become sensitized to beryllium • Increased beryllium exposure leads to macrophage and CD4+ helper T-lymphocyte aggregation in the lungs forming noncaseating granulomas and pulmonary fibrosis

Signs & Symptoms	• **Progressive dyspnea** and dry cough
	• Fatigue, **weight loss and night sweats**
	• <u>Physical Exam</u>:
	  • Crackles or diminished breath sounds on auscultation
	  • Lymphadenopathy, joint pain, rash, and/or hepatosplenomegaly may be present

Diagnosis	• <u>Chest X-Ray (CXR)</u>: may be normal or **show diffuse infiltrates often with hilar lymphadenopathy** (resembles sarcoidosis) • <u>**Beryllium Lymphocyte Proliferation Test**</u>: **highly sensitive and specific**; lymphocyte culture with beryllium sulfate performed on blood, bronchoalveolar lavage fluid or both • <u>Chest CT Scan</u>: more sensitive and specific • <u>Pulmonary Function Test</u>: shows restrictive disease pattern *Diffuse infiltrates and hilar lymphadenopathy*
Treatment	• <u>Supportive</u>: removal from exposure source, **oxygen supplementation**, pulmonary rehabilitation, smoking cessation • <u>Corticosteroids</u>: decreases inflammation and symptoms and improves oxygenation; lifelong treatment usually required in chronic disease • **Prednisone** for 3-6 months with gradual taper • <u>Methotrexate</u>: indicated in refractory cases or when patients cannot tolerate corticosteroids • <u>Lung Transplant</u>: last resort open; only effective long-term treatment • <u>Mechanical Ventilation</u>: may be required in acute beryllium disease
Key Words & Most Common	• Occupational exposure to beryllium (aerospace/aircraft manufacturing, metal alloy production, computer/electronic manufacturing) • Progressive dyspnea, dry cough, weight loss, night sweats • CXR resembles sarcoidosis; diffuse infiltrates +/- hilar lymphadenopathy • Beryllium Lymphocyte Proliferation Test • Corticosteroids, supplemental oxygen

Byssinosis

Etiology & Risk Factors	• Occupational lung disease caused by inhalation of **cotton, flax, or hemp dust**; also known as cotton worker's lung or "Monday fever" • <u>Etiology</u>: **exposure to cotton, flax, or hemp dust** • <u>Risk Factors</u>: **textile industry employees; exposure to raw, unprocessed cotton** • Relatively rare in US now as industries have implemented production methods to limit exposure • Still prevalent in countries where textile manufacturing flourish (India, Sri Lanka, Pakistan, Indonesia, Bangladesh etc.)
Patho-physiology	• Gram negative bacteria that are contained within cotton dust produce an endotoxin which causes bronchoconstriction, bronchitis, and decreased pulmonary function
Signs & Symptoms	• **Dyspnea, cough, chest tightness that lessens with repeated exposure** • **Symptoms may be worse at beginning of workweek** hence "Monday fever" that improve towards end of shift or end of workweek • Differentiates from occupational asthma (which is worse at end of shift or end of workweek) • Productive cough if progresses to chronic byssinosis
Diagnosis	• **History of cotton/flax/hemp dust exposure** • **Clinical Diagnosis**; no known diagnostic test specific for byssinosis • <u>Chest X-Ray (CXR)</u>: ordered to rule out other pathology; may show flattened diaphragm, hyperlucency, or emphysema • <u>Pulmonary Function Test</u>: shows obstructive disease pattern
Treatment	• <u>Supportive</u>: **removal from exposure source**, smoking cessation, pulmonary rehabilitation, use of personal protection equipment • No specific therapies; management with asthma medications (bronchodilators, inhaled/oral steroids)
Key Words & Most Common	• Raw cotton exposure • Symptoms (dyspnea, cough, chest tightness) worse during beginning of week and improve toward end of week • No known diagnostic test • Supportive treatment; asthma medications

Asbestosis

Etiology & Risk Factors	• Form of progressive interstitial pulmonary fibrosis caused by asbestos fiber inhalation
	• Etiology: exposure to asbestos fibers
	• Risk Factors: **occupational exposure through demolition of old buildings, shipbuilders**, construction workers, welders, carpenters/plumbers/electricians, etc.
	  • Higher risk of disease associated with duration and intensity of exposure
	  • Asbestos has heat-resistant, electrical/thermal insulation, and structural properties making it useful in construction, insulation, ship building materials, automobile brakes, and fire-resistant products

Patho-physiology	• Alveolar macrophages engulf asbestos particles deposited in airways; macrophage release cytokines and fibroblast growth factors causing oxidative damage which stimulate inflammation and fibrosis • Asbestos fibers are toxic to lung tissue leading to inflammation

Signs & Symptoms	• May initially be asymptomatic
	• **Progressive dyspnea, nonproductive cough, fatigue**
	  • Productive cough and wheezing are unusual; may be associated with smoking
	• Physical Exam:
	  • Advanced disease may have digital clubbing, **bibasilar crackles**, restricted chest expansion, right sided heart failure

Diagnosis	• **History of asbestos fiber exposure**
	• Chest X-Ray (CXR): best initial test
	  • Bilateral linear reticular opacities (fibrosis) involving lower lobes
	  • **Pleural thickening and calcified pleural plaques (pathognomonic of disease)**
	  • "Shaggy heart" diffuse reticulonodular infiltrates at lung bases cause indistinct heart border
	• Chest CT Scan: more sensitive and specific for identifying above abnormalities
	• Pulmonary Function Test: shows restrictive disease pattern
	• Lung Biopsy: definitive diagnosis; shows interstitial fibrosis and distinct asbestos bodies

Treatment	• **Supportive: removal from exposure source**; pulmonary rehabilitation, smoking cessation, oxygen supplementation • No specific therapies; management with asthma medications (bronchodilators, inhaled/oral steroids) • Lung Transplant: last resort open; only effective long-term treatment
Key Words & Most Common	• Asbestos exposure – most common in construction, demolition, and ship building • Progressive dyspnea, nonproductive cough • CXR/CT: pleural plaques & thickening • Supportive treatment – no specific therapies; management with asthma medications

Pleural Plaques

Bilateral Reticular Opacities

Influenza

Etiology & Risk Factors	• Viral illness affecting the upper and lower respiratory tract • Etiology: **influenza viruses** (classified as type A or B) • Risk Factors: age (<2 or >65 years old), chronic medical comorbidities, immunocompromised, pregnancy, obesity, seasonal (fall/winter months in temperate climates) • Complications: primary viral pneumonia, secondary bacterial pneumonia, acute respiratory distress syndrome, meningitis, myocarditis, death • Transmission: droplet transmission occurs within 3-6ft radius; viral shedding lasts about 5days (24-48hr prior to symptom onset); *n95 or surgical mask reduces transmission*
Patho-physiology	• Acute viral illness targeting upper and lower respiratory tract; immune reaction and interferon response cause viral symptom syndrome as a result of viral infection • Influenza A can have multiple subtypes based on combination of hemagglutinin (H) and neuraminidase (N) protein expression on viral surface (i.e. H1N1, H3N2, etc.) • Hemagglutinin binds to respiratory tract epithelial cells allowing infection to progress; neuraminidase breaks bond holding virus together allowing transmission
Signs & Symptoms	• *Influenza A is associated with a more severe disease course* • **Sudden onset fever/chills, headache**, nonproductive cough, fatigue, pharyngitis • **Myalgias (particularly lower back and legs)** • Acute symptoms generally subside after 2-3 days; fever may persist for 5 days
Diagnosis	• **Clinical Diagnosis** • Rapid Influenza Nasal Swab or Viral Culture: specific but variable sensitivity • Reverse Transcriptase-Polymerase Chain Reaction (RT-PCR): sensitive and specific; used in hospital or ER setting • Chest X-Ray (CXR): may be ordered to rule out primary viral or secondary bacterial pneumonia

Treatment	• Supportive: symptomatic treatment with acetaminophen/NSAIDs as needed (avoid aspirin if <18 due to risk of Reye syndrome); adequate hydration; rest
	• Antivirals: recommended for hospitalized or high-risk patients; **all antivirals are most effective if initiated within 48 hours of symptoms**
	  • Neuraminidase Inhibitors: **oseltamivir (Tamiflu)** slow spread by interfering viral release from infected cells
	  • Endonuclease Inhibitor: **baloxavir (Xofluza)** block viral RNA transcription to interfere with viral replication
	  • Adamantanes: amantadine and rimantadine are no longer indicated due to 99% resistance
	• Prevention: **annual influenza vaccination**; pre/post-exposure prophylactic antivirals

Key Words & Most Common	• Seasonal virus characterized by abrupt onset of fever/chills, headache, myalgias of lower back and legs • Diagnosed clinically; rapid influenza may be used in office but lacks sensitivity; RT-PCR more sensitive but usually only used in inpatient/ER setting • Supportive symptomatic treatment is mainstay • Antivirals may be initiated if <48 hours since onset of symptoms • Prevention with annual vaccination

Acute Bronchitis

Etiology & Risk Factors	• Inflammation of the tracheobronchial tree commonly secondary to a viral upper respiratory infection; most common during fall and winter
	• Etiology: viral, bacterial or irritants/allergens
	   • **Viral**: influenza A & B, rhinovirus, parainfluenza, respiratory syncytial virus, coronavirus
	   • **Bacterial**: <10% of total cases
	   • **Irritants/Allergens**: smoke inhalation, air pollution, dust, animal dander, perfume exposure, cold weather exposure
	• Risk Factors: smoking, history of seasonal allergies, immunocompromised, chronic respiratory conditions (COPD, asthma), exposure to cold

Patho-physiology	• Triggers such as viral infection, irritants/allergies, etc. lead to inflammation of bronchial wall which triggers epithelial-wall flaking, increased mucous production, and decreased mucociliary function which further promotes bronchial irritation

Signs & Symptoms	• **Prodrome of URI**: rhinorrhea, sore throat, malaise, low-grade fever is common
	• **Cough +/- sputum production is most common symptom** (may be clear, yellow, or purulent); typically persists for 1-3 weeks but can last longer (avg is 18 days)
	   • Purulence does not always indicate bacterial infection
	   • **May have associated wheeze**
	• Physical Exam:
	   • **Expiratory wheeze on auscultation may be present**
	   • Rales/rhonchi/focal consolidation may indicate pneumonia

Diagnosis	• **Clinical diagnosis** • Chest X-Ray (CXR): often normal or nonspecific; used to rule out pneumonia • Indications for CXR: ill-appearing, hypoxia, tachycardia/tachypnea, fever, consolidations or egophony/fremitus on exam, age >65yo, night sweats
Treatment	• **Supportive: symptomatic treatment** with antitussives (codeine, dextromethorphan), analgesics, adequate hydration, rest • Antibiotics: not routinely necessary • Bronchodilators: albuterol; indicated if wheezing present
Key Words & Most Common	• Viral etiology in 95% of cases; often preceded by viral URI • Cough +/- sputum production is most common symptom; wheeze may be present • Clinical diagnosis; CXR only to rule out pneumonia if indicated • Supportive symptom-based treatment; antibiotics often not necessary

Pertussis (Whooping Cough)

Etiology & Risk Factors	• Highly communicable disease most commonly occurring in children and adolescents • Etiology: *Bordetella pertussis*; a gram-negative coccobacillus • Risk Factors: **age (<2 years old or adults with waning immunity most common)**, pregnancy, endemic exposure to illness, unvaccinated, close contact to illness • Endemic disease; 3-5 year infection cycles in the US; rarely seen due to widespread vaccination
Patho-physiology	• Gram-negative bacteria that adheres to ciliated respiratory epithelial cells and creates toxins damaging respiratory epithelium resulting in local inflammation • Aerosolized respiratory droplet transmission causing diseases in >80% of close contacts

Signs & Symptoms	• 7-14 day incubation period; three distinct phases
	• **Catarrhal Phase**: most contagious phase that lasts 1-2 weeks
	   • URI Symptoms: sneezing, coryza, dry cough
	• **Paroxysmal Phase**: lasts 2-4 weeks
	   • Increased severity/frequency of cough
	   • **Severe coughing fits during single inspiration followed by a hurried/deep inspiration ("whoop")**; **vomiting is common after coughing fits**; patient may appear well between coughing episodes
	• Convalescent Phase: lasts weeks to months
	   • Symptoms diminish but residual cough remains

Diagnosis	• **Clinical Diagnosis** • Nasopharyngeal Culture: more sensitive during first 2 weeks; requires special culture media so results may take 3-7 days • **Nasopharyngeal Polymerase Chain Reaction (PCR): most sensitive and specific test** • Chest X-Ray (CXR): nonspecific; may show peri bronchial thickening, atelectasis, and/or consolidation • Labs: may have **elevated WBC (leukocytosis)** specifically with large amounts of lymphocytes (**lymphocytosis**)

Treatment	• **Supportive**: mainstay of treatment; hydration, suction of secretions, oxygen, avoidance of respiratory irritants and disturbance (can precipitate coughing fit)
	• Antibiotics: initiated during catarrhal phase may reduce duration/severity of symptoms; Indicated for bacterial complications (otitis media, pneumonia, sinusitis)
	   • **Macrolides: azithromycin first line** (clarithromycin, erythromycin alternatives)
	   • Trimethoprim Sulfamethoxazole (TMP-SMX) is second line
	   • *Post-exposure antibiotic prophylaxis recommended for close contacts*
	• Prevention: **pertussis vaccination** (DTaP) at 2, 4, 6, 15-18 months and 4-6 years of age; one-time Tdap booster for adults to reduce transmission to children; Tdap for third-trimester pregnant women (no harm to fetus in third trimester); Strict isolation through catarrhal and paroxysmal phase

Key Words & Most Common	• Highly contagious illness that most commonly affects children <2 years old • Three phases: Catarrhal (URI symptoms); Paroxysmal (increased cough, coughing fits followed by a "whoop" inspiration, post-tussive vomiting); Convalescent • Nasopharyngeal PCR most sensitive/specific test; labs may show leukocytosis • Supportive treatment; Azithromycin indicated during catarrhal phase and for post-exposure prophylaxis

Bronchiolitis

Etiology & Risk Factors	• Common lower respiratory viral infection typically occurring in young patients • <u>Etiology</u>: **respiratory syncytial virus (RSV) is most common cause** (70% of cases), rhinovirus, parainfluenza virus, influenza, adenovirus • <u>Risk Factors</u>: **infants** (most common in infants <2 years old, **peak incidence 2-6 months old**), **premature infants** (<36weeks of gestation), parental smoking, crowded environment (day care) • Patients with congenital heart disease and chronic lung diseases, younger age (<3mo) and immunodeficiency are at risk for severe disease
Patho-physiology	• Virus infects airway epithelial cells which induce an inflammatory response and cause mucociliary dysfunction and accumulation of cellular debris • Cytokine release causes airway edema which progresses to decreased lung compliance and air trapping
Signs & Symptoms	• <u>**Upper Respiratory Infection Symptoms**</u>: **low grade fever, cough, rhinorrhea for 24–72 hours** • Progresses to symptoms of **respiratory distress** (apnea, wheezing, tachypnea, retractions, nasal flaring) • <u>**Dehydration**</u>: as a result of vomiting and decreased oral intake (tachypnea interferes with feeding) • Severe disease may have apnea/tachypnea, cyanosis/hypoxemia, respiratory failure, lethargy
Diagnosis	• **Clinical Diagnosis** • <u>Pulse Oximeter</u>: best predictor of disease course in children; further testing not required if normal spO$_2$ • <u>Chest X-Ray (CXR)</u>: not routinely necessary; nonspecific findings (hyperinflation, hilar markings, atelectasis); consider if diagnosis is unclear or severe symptoms • *Consider RSV testing (PCR or rapid antigen)*
Treatment	• <u>**Supportive**</u>: **mainstay of treatment; aggressive hydration (oral and/or IV), humidified oxygen**, nebulized saline, cool mist humidifier, suction of secretions • <u>Supplemental Oxygen</u>: goal spO$_2$>90% with high flow nasal canula • <u>Endotracheal Intubation</u>: reserved for severe cases with apnea, hypoxemia, or unable to clear secretions • <u>Bronchodilators</u>: generally not effective and may aggravate symptoms • Corticosteroids: dexamethasone; reserved for severe cases
Key Words & Most Common	• Acute, viral, lower respiratory infection typically occurring in young patients <2yo with peak incidence in 2–6-month-olds • URI symptoms for 24-72 hours that progress to respiratory distress; MC complication is dehydration • Clinical diagnosis, pulse oximeter should be monitored • Supportive treatment with aggressive hydration and supplemental oxygen with goal spO2 >90%

Epiglottitis

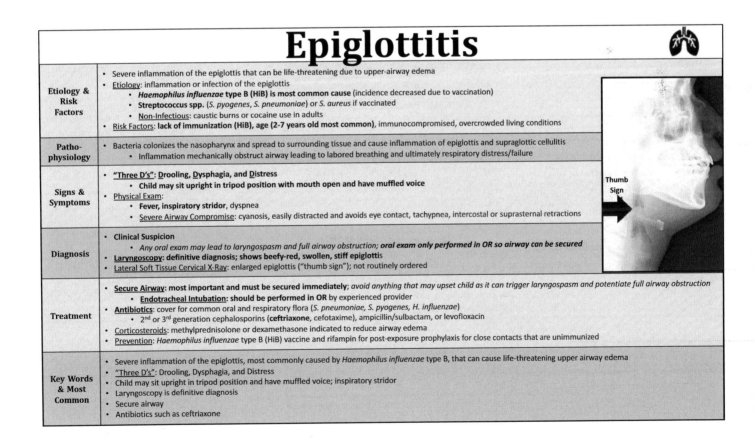

Thumb Sign

Etiology & Risk Factors	• Severe inflammation of the epiglottis that can be life-threatening due to upper-airway edema
	• <u>Etiology</u>: inflammation or infection of the epiglottis
	   • ***Haemophilus influenzae* type B (HiB) is most common cause** (incidence decreased due to vaccination)
	   • **Streptococcus spp.** (*S. pyogenes*, *S. pneumoniae*) or *S. aureus* if vaccinated
	   • <u>Non-Infectious</u>: caustic burns or cocaine use in adults
	• <u>Risk Factors</u>: **lack of immunization (HiB), age (2-7 years old most common)**, immunocompromised, overcrowded living conditions

Patho-physiology	• Bacteria colonizes the nasopharynx and spread to surrounding tissue and cause inflammation of epiglottis and supraglottic cellulitis • Inflammation mechanically obstruct airway leading to labored breathing and ultimately respiratory distress/failure

Signs & Symptoms	• **"Three D's"**: <u>Drooling, Dysphagia, and Distress</u>
	   • **Child may sit upright in tripod position with mouth open and have muffled voice**
	• <u>Physical Exam</u>:
	   • **Fever, inspiratory stridor**, dyspnea
	   • <u>Severe Airway Compromise</u>: cyanosis, easily distracted and avoids eye contact, tachypnea, intercostal or suprasternal retractions

Diagnosis	• **Clinical Suspicion** • *Any oral exam may lead to laryngospasm and full airway obstruction; **oral exam only performed in OR so airway can be secured*** • <u>Laryngoscopy</u>: **definitive diagnosis; shows beefy-red, swollen, stiff epiglottis** • <u>Lateral Soft Tissue Cervical X-Ray</u>: enlarged epiglottis ("thumb sign"); not routinely ordered

Treatment	• <u>**Secure Airway**</u>: **most important and must be secured immediately**; *avoid anything that may upset child as it can trigger laryngospasm and potentiate full airway obstruction*
	   • **Endotracheal Intubation: should be performed in OR** by experienced provider
	• <u>Antibiotics</u>: cover for common oral and respiratory flora (*S. pneumoniae, S. pyogenes, H. influenzae*)
	   • 2nd or 3rd generation cephalosporins (**ceftriaxone**, cefotaxime), ampicillin/sulbactam, or levofloxacin
	• <u>Corticosteroids</u>: methylprednisolone or dexamethasone indicated to reduce airway edema
	• <u>Prevention</u>: *Haemophilus influenzae* type B (HiB) vaccine and rifampin for post-exposure prophylaxis for close contacts that are unimmunized

Key Words & Most Common	• Severe inflammation of the epiglottis, most commonly caused by *Haemophilus influenzae* type B, that can cause life-threatening upper airway edema • "Three D's": Drooling, Dysphagia, and Distress • Child may sit upright in tripod position and have muffled voice; inspiratory stridor • Laryngoscopy is definitive diagnosis • Secure airway • Antibiotics such as ceftriaxone

Laryngotracheitis (Croup)

Etiology & Risk Factors	• Common respiratory illness that causes inflammation of the upper and lower airways particularly the larynx and subglottic airway • <u>Etiologies</u>: **parainfluenza virus is most common cause**; respiratory syncytial virus (RSV), adenovirus, rhinovirus, influenza A/B; may also be bacterial • <u>Risk Factors</u>: **age (6months-3 years old; peaks at 2 years old)**, seasonal (fall and early winter most common), parental smoking, crowded environment (day care)
Patho-physiology	• Infection causes white blood cell infiltration resulting in edema of the larynx, trachea, and bronchi to subglottic airway obstruction • Subglottic airway obstruction leads to labored breathing and the characteristic turbulent airflow (stridor)

Signs & Symptoms	• **Upper respiratory infection symptoms for 1-3 days followed by a harsh, spasmodic, "seal-like barking" cough and inspiratory stridor**
	   • **Most commonly occurring at night**
	   • Total duration of illness is 4-7 days; most severe on days 3-4
	• May have low grade fever, voice hoarseness, dyspnea
	• Child may awaken at night with tachypnea, retractions, and/or respiratory distress
	• **NO drooling or dysphagia**
	• Severe cases may have hypoxia and cyanosis
	
	R ← Steeple Sign

Diagnosis	• **Clinical Diagnosis** (obstructive conditions such as epiglottitis, bacterial tracheitis, and airway foreign body should be ruled out) • <u>AP Neck X-Ray</u>: may show subglottic airway stenosis (**steeple sign**) but is rarely performed
Treatment	• <u>Supportive</u>: **cool mist humidifier**, antipyretics, hydration • <u>**Corticosteroids**</u>: **firs- line treatment; dexamethasone PO/IM** provides significant relief and associated with faster resolution and decreased relapse • <u>**Nebulized Epinephrine**</u>: provides symptomatic relief through vasoconstriction; reserved for moderate to severe cases; patient should be observed for 3-4 hours after • <u>Intubation</u>: rarely required; ½ size smaller tube should be used due to airway edema • **Bronchodilators: contraindicated; do NOT give albuterol as may worsen airway edema (vasodilation)**
Key Words & Most Common	• Common respiratory illness most commonly caused by Parainfluenza virus resulting in upper/lower airway inflammation • Most common in 6mo-3yo (peaks at 2 years old) • URI symptoms for 1-3 days followed by harsh, "seal-like barking" cough and inspiratory stridor; worse at night • Clinical diagnosis; steeple sign on AP neck x-ray • Supportive with cool mist humidifier; dexamethasone is first-line for symptomatic relief

Bacterial Pneumonia

Etiology & Risk Factors	• <u>Community Acquired Pneumonia</u>: infection of the lung parenchyma caused by a pathogen acquired from outside the hospital or within 48hrs of hospital admission
	• <u>Hospital Acquired Pneumonia</u>: infection caused by pathogen acquired from within hospital or 48 hours after admission; often caused by Pseudomonas or MRSA
	• <u>Etiologies</u>:
	   • <u>Typical</u>: *Streptococcus pneumoniae* **(most common typical)**, *Haemophilus influenzae, Klebsiella pneumoniae, Staphylococcus aureus*
	   • <u>Atypical</u>: *Mycoplasma* **pneumonia (most common atypical)**, *Chlamydia, Legionella, Moraxella* spp.
	   • <u>Hospital Acquired</u>: MRSA and gram negatives most common; *Pseudomonas* **most common cause in ICUs (**carries the worst prognosis)
	• <u>Risk Factors</u>: altered level of consciousness, smoking, alcohol, malnutrition, Age>65, COPD/CF/Bronchiectasis, lung cancer, immunosuppressant drugs

Patho-physiology	• Microaspiration of contaminated oropharyngeal secretions enter lower respiratory tract and cause pneumonitis • Macrophages and neutrophils attempt to inactivate bacteria and cytokines are released leading to immune system activation; neutrophils, bacteria and fluid fill alveoli and may cause lung lobe consolidation

Signs & Symptoms	• <u>Typical</u>: **Sudden Fever, chills, rigor (severe chills with shaking)**, malaise, pleuritic chest pain, dyspnea, tachypnea/tachycardia
	   • **Cough with purulent sputum production**
	   • <u>Physical Exam</u>: **inspiratory crackles and/or decreased breath sounds**, dullness to percussion, **egophony or tactile fremitus**
	• <u>Atypical</u>: **Low-grade fever**, relatively mild pulmonary symptoms (nonproductive cough), extrapulmonary symptoms (myalgias, malaise, headache, N/V/D, sore throat)
	   • <u>Physical Exam</u>: **often normal**; may have inspiratory crackles and/or rhonchi, no evidence of consolidation

Diagnosis	• <u>**Chest X-Ray (CXR)**</u>: **best initial test; lobar consolidation** (typical) or **interstitial infiltrates** (atypical), peribronchial shadowing; may have negative imaging if early in course • <u>Procalcitonin</u>: levels rise in response to proinflammatory stimulus, especially bacterial infection. Elevated levels may support bacterial versus viral origin • <u>Pulse Oximetry</u>: monitor oxygenation status • <u>Sputum Testing</u>: gram stain and culture; may help identify causative organism; usually not performed prior to starting treatment • <u>Polymerase Chain Reaction (PCR)</u>: helpful to identify atypical or viral cause

Treatment	• <u>Supportive</u>: hydration, antipyretics, analgesics, rest, supplemental O_2; those that without significant risk factors or comorbidities may be managed outpatient
	• <u>**Antibiotics**</u>:
	   • <u>Community Acquired Outpatient</u>: **amoxicillin +/- macrolide (azithromycin/clarithromycin) OR doxycycline;** amoxicillin/clavulanate is alternative
	   • <u>Community Acquired Inpatient or risk factors/comorbidities</u>: **amoxicillin/clavulanate + macrolide** (azithromycin/clarithromycin) *OR* **doxycycline** *OR* **broad-spectrum fluoroquinolone** (levofloxacin, moxifloxacin)
	   • <u>Hospital Acquired</u>: **Anti-Pseudomonal β-lactam (cefepime or ceftazidime) + fluoroquinolone (levofloxacin, moxifloxacin) + Vancomycin**
	      • Consider Piperacillin/tazobactam + ciprofloxacin + vancomycin if multi-drug resistance suspected
	• <u>Hospital Admission</u>: neutropenia, involvement of more than 1 lobe, or bacterial resistance indicates need for hospitalization
	      • Consider admission for those >50yo w/ comorbidities, >65yo, altered mental status, uremia or hemodynamic instability

(Typical) Bacterial Pneumonia Comparison

Streptococcus pneumoniae	Haemophilus influenzae	Staphylococcus aureus
• Most common cause of CAP • Sudden onset fever/chills and rigors • Productive cough with blood-tinged sputum (rust color) • <u>Gram Stain</u>: gram positive diplococci	• 2nd most common cause of CAP • Increased risk in those of extreme age (>65yo or <5yo), immuno-compromised or chronic lung disease (CF, COPD, asthma) • <u>Gram Stain</u>: gram negative bacilli	• Implicated after viral infection (post-influenza pneumonia) or hospital-acquired pneumonia (MRSA) • Hematogenous spread possible (IV drug users) • <u>CXR</u>: Bilateral, multilobar infiltrates or cavitary lesions (abscess) • <u>Gram Stain</u>: gram positive cocci in clusters
Klebsiella pneumoniae	**Moraxella catarrhalis**	**Group A Streptococcus**
• Severe illness in alcoholics, chronic illness (diabetes), or aspiration risk patients • Cough with thick red/purple-colored sputum (currant jelly) • <u>CXR</u>: cavitary lesions • <u>Gram Stain</u>: gram negative bacilli	• Increased risk in chronic lung disease (COPD), malnourished, or immunocompromised patients • <u>Gram Stain</u>: gram negative diplococci	• <u>CXR</u>: Fulminant pneumonia with emphysema • <u>Gram Stain</u>: gram positive cocci in chains

Pneumococcal Vaccines

Pneumococcal Polysaccharide Vaccine (PPSV23)	Pneumococcal Conjugate Vaccine (PCV) 13
• **Pneumococcal polysaccharide vaccine (PPSV23)** is recommended for **children age 2-5, >65 yo, or anyone with chronic illness** (CP disease, sickle cell, tobacco abuse, splenectomy, liver) • All patients that were vaccinated before age 65 should get revaccinated at age 65 (unless <10 years)	• **Pneumococcal conjugate vaccine (PCV) 13** is 7-valent vaccine and protects against 13 serotypes that cause up to 85% of invasive infection • Recommended as series of **4 doses for children at 2, 4, 6, and 12-15 months of age** (booster shots every 6 years)

• If eligible for both: patient should receive PCV13 followed by PPSV23 8 weeks later
• If patient received PPSV23 in past, PCV13 should be given 1 year after the administration of PPSV23

Mycoplasma Pneumonia

Atypical Bacterial Pneumonia	
Etiology & Risk Factors	• Common cause of community acquired pneumonia and transmission occurs via respiratory droplets; also known as "walking" pneumonia • <u>Etiology</u>: *Mycoplasma pneumoniae*; **most common cause of atypical pneumonia** • <u>Risk Factors</u>: age (typically <40 years old, **young and otherwise healthy** [school-aged children, college students, military recruits]), crowded environments (**dormitories,** schools, hospitals, military barracks, nursing homes, long-term care facilities)
Patho-physiology	• *M. pneumoniae* has proteins that adhere to respiratory tract epithelium and produce hydrogen peroxide and superoxide causing ciliary and epithelial cell injury resulting in activation of inflammatory cytokines

Signs & Symptoms	• Long incubation period of 2-3 weeks
	• **Gradual onset** of low-grade fever, malaise, headaches, and **URI symptoms (pharyngitis, rhinorrhea, ear pain)**
	• **"Nagging", persistent, dry and nonproductive cough**
	• <u>Extrapulmonary Symptoms</u>: hemolysis, joint pain, gastrointestinal symptoms
	   • Hemolytic anemia occurs as IgM antibodies produce cold agglutin reaction
	• <u>Physical exam</u>: often normal; may have wheezing
	   • <u>Bullous Myringitis</u>: vesicles on tympanic membrane; rare and nonspecific

Diagnosis	• **Clinical Diagnosis** • **Chest X-Ray (CXR): reticulonodular pattern most common**; may have diffuse or patchy areas of consolidation more prominent in lower lobes • <u>Polymerase Chain Reaction (PCR)</u>: test of choice and rapid • <u>Cold Agglutinin Titers</u>: supports diagnosis; elevated in >50% of patients with mycoplasma disease but is nonspecific (also elevated in CMV or EBV) • *M. pneumoniae* lacks a cell wall and is fastidious so gram-stain and culture not useful

Treatment	• <u>Supportive care</u>: hydration, antipyretics, analgesics, rest
	• <u>Antibiotics</u>: empiric treatment for atypical pneumonia (**lacks a cell wall therefore resistant to beta-lactams**)
	   • <u>Macrolides</u>: **first-line treatment; azithromycin is most common** (or clarithromycin); macrolide resistance is emerging
	   • <u>Tetracyclines</u>: **doxycycline is second-line alternative**
	   • <u>Respiratory Fluoroquinolones</u>: **levofloxacin or moxifloxacin**

Key Words & Most Common	• M. pneumoniae is most common cause of atypical pneumonia and commonly affects young and otherwise healthy patients • Gradual onset of URI followed by a nagging dry cough; extrapulmonary symptoms (GI) • CXR has reticulonodular pattern; PCR and Cold Agglutinin Titers support diagnosis • Macrolides (azithromycin)

Legionella Pneumonia

Etiology & Risk Factors	• Pneumonia caused by *Legionella pneumophila*; also known as Legionnaire's disease • <u>Etiology</u>: *Legionella pneumophila* is a small, aerobic, gram-negative bacillus that is primarily spread through aerosolized water droplets • <u>Risk Factors</u>: exposure to contaminated water sources (air conditioners, ventilation/plumbing systems, cooling towers, medical equipment, hot tubs), smoking, elderly, immunocompromised, chronic lung disease, diabetes • Incubation 2-10 days
Patho-physiology	• Inhalation of aerosolized contaminated water leads to bacterial infection; bacterium adheres to respiratory epithelial cells and enter alveolar macrophages. Bacteria multiplies intracellularly in alveolar macrophages and recruited neutrophils, monocytes, and bacterial enzymes cause alveolar inflammation
Signs & Symptoms	• <u>Flu-Like Symptoms</u>: acute fever, myalgias, malaise, headache • <u>Extrapulmonary Symptoms</u>: **nausea/vomiting, diarrhea** (watery, non-bloody), abdominal pain, arthralgias, relative bradycardia compared to fever • <u>Respiratory Symptoms</u>: **cough +/- sputum production (1/3rd of patients have hemoptysis)**, dyspnea, pleuritic chest pain
Diagnosis	• <u>Chest X-Ray (CXR)</u>: consolidation at lung bases, patchy infiltrates • <u>Labs</u>: hypophosphatemia, hyponatremia, elevated LFTs (2-5x normal), elevated ESRCRP, elevated ferritin (>2x normal) • <u>Urine Antigen Testing</u>: **sensitive and highly specific; rapid**; only identifies most common serogroup • <u>Sputum Cultures</u>: **highly specific and can identify all serogroups**; takes 3-5 days to result

Treatment	• <u>Notify Health Department</u>: reportable disease
	• <u>Antibiotics</u>:
	    • <u>Macrolides</u>: **azithromycin is first-line for mild disease**
	    • <u>Doxycycline</u>: alternative for immunocompetent patients with mild disease
	    • <u>Respiratory Fluoroquinolones</u>: levofloxacin, moxifloxacin; indicated in severe cases or immunocompromised
	• <u>Prevention</u>: disinfection of contaminated water source

Key Words & Most Common	• Aerobic gram-negative bacteria spread through aerosolized water droplets • Outbreaks related to water sources including air conditions, medical equipment, plumbing • Flu like symptoms + cough + GI symptoms • Urine antigen testing vs sputum culture for diagnosis • Azithromycin first-line

Viral Pneumonia

Etiology & Risk Factors	• Viral infection affecting the upper or lower respiratory tract; **variable but often associated with seasonal epidemics and upper respiratory symptoms** • May be classified by the causative virus or clinically correlated according to the syndrome (common cold, bronchiolitis, croup, pneumonia) • <u>Etiologies</u>: influenza, coronavirus (COVID-19), respiratory syncytial virus (RSV), parainfluenza, adenovirus • <u>Risk Factors</u>: **age >65 or <2 years old**, altered mental status, smoking, alcohol, malnutrition, pregnancy, **other respiratory conditions** (COPD, CF, bronchiectasis, lung cancer), immunocompromised
Patho-physiology	• Contaminated airborne/droplet particles are inhaled and invade lung parenchyma; virus enters type 1 pneumocytes to multiply which become damaged and eventually die • Injured pneumocytes release signals to lymphocytes to destroy virus infected cells; stronger type 2 pneumocytes replace damaged/dead cells
Signs & Symptoms	• **Symptoms vary based on underlying causative virus or syndrome** • Generally gradual onset of fever (lower grade), myalgias, headache, cough, fatigue, pharyngitis • **Cough +/- sputum production (viral tends to be more watery sputum and are not purulent)** • Acute symptoms generally subside after 2-3 days; fever may persist for 5 days
Diagnosis	• <u>Chest X-Ray (CXR)</u>: **best initial test** if clinically suspicious • **Bilateral opacification (bacterial tends to be more focal) or** patchy distribution; may have negative imaging • <u>Labs</u>: procalcitonin (elevated levels may support bacterial origin); CBC (**minimal or no elevated WBC count**) • <u>Pulse Oximetry</u>: monitor oxygenation status • <u>Sputum Testing</u>: gram stain and culture; may help identify causative organism • <u>Polymerase Chain Reaction (PCR)</u>: helpful to identify causative organism to guide treatment Right lower lung opacification

Treatment	• <u>Supportive care</u>: hydration, antipyretics, analgesics, rest, **supplemental O₂**; those that without significant risk factors or comorbidities may be managed outpatient
	    • Patients may have continued cough for weeks after URI; symptom-based treatment with inhaled bronchodilator or corticosteroids
	• <u>Antivirals</u>:
	    • <u>Oseltamivir (Tamiflu) or baloxavir (Xofluza)</u>: initiated within first 48 hours for influenza
	    • <u>Ribavirin</u>: inhibits RNA and DNA viral replication; reserved for hospitalized infants or immunocompromised to treat RSV, COVID-19, parainfluenza, adenovirus
	• <u>Antibiotics</u>: **not routinely indicated for prophylaxis in most**; indicated for secondary bacterial infections or those with chronic lung disease
	    • Clinical correlation for superimposed bacterial infection
	• <u>Isolation</u>: to prevent spread; viral cause typically contagious for 4-10 days

Key Words & Most Common	• Viral cause of upper and lower respiratory symptoms; often associated with seasonal epidemics • +/- more gradual onset of fever, cough with or without sputum production • <u>CXR</u>: bilateral opacification; PCR to diagnose causative organism • Supportive care; antivirals as clinically indicated; antibiotics not routinely necessary for prophylaxis

Aspiration Pneumonia

Etiology & Risk Factors	• Abnormal entry of oropharyngeal secretions or gastric content into the lower respiratory tract that leads to infection
	• Etiology: aspiration of oropharyngeal sections or gastric contents
	  • Community Acquired (CAP): *Pneumococcus, Staphylococcus aureus, Haemophilus influenzae, Enterobacter* spp.
	  • Hospital Acquired (HAP): *Pseudomonas*, gram-negatives, MRSA
	• Risk Factors: advanced age, **impaired cognition or level of consciousness, GERD, esophageal dysmotility**, GI procedures, tube feedings, prolonged supine position

Patho-physiology	• Disruption of the normal mucociliary response and alveolar macrophage defense mechanisms that clear aspirated content allow secretions to enter the respiratory tract • Fluid entering the alveolar space triggers an inflammatory reaction; oxygen-free radicals are generated which further airway damage • Gastric contents are acidic and can cause chemical burn of airway/lungs which can lead to bronchoconstriction, edema, and alveolar hemorrhage
Signs & Symptoms	• **Sudden onset fever, dyspnea, productive cough with foul smelling sputum ("rotten egg" smell)** • Tachypnea, tachycardia, hypoxemia • Altered mental status • Physical Exam: • Crackles on auscultation

Diagnosis	• Chest X-Ray (CXR): unilateral focal/patchy consolidation in dependent lung segments
	  • Upper Lobe Infiltrate: aspiration in recumbent position
	  • Lower Lobe Infiltrate: aspiration in upright position
	  • **Right Lower Lobe: most common area; due to more vertical angle of right mainstem bronchus**
	  • Right Upper Lobe: more common when aspiration in prone position and those with alcohol use
	• Chest CT Scan: more sensitive and specific
	  • Utilized if clinical suspicion is high with negative chest x-ray; can detect cavitary lesions associated with abscess
	
	Right lower lobe consolidation

Treatment	• Supportive: **raise head of bed, suction of secretions**, supplemental oxygen
	• Antibiotics:
	  • CAP: **amoxicillin/clavulanate, clindamycin**, moxifloxacin
	  • HAP: coverage for gram negative or MRSA with Ceftriaxone + clindamycin *OR* piperacillin/tazobactam + clindamycin *OR* levofloxacin + clindamycin

Key Words & Most Common	• Abnormal inhalation of secretions/gastric content into lungs leading to infection • Sudden onset fever, dyspnea, cough with foul smelling sputum • CXR: unilateral consolidation; right lower lobe is most common • Supportive treatment + antibiotics (coverage for gram - & MRSA if hospital acquired)

Pneumocystis jirovecii Pneumonia

Etiology & Risk Factors	• Common cause of pneumonia in immunosuppressed patients • Etiology: ***Pneumocystis jirovecii*** (formerly known as *carinii*); an atypical yeast-like fungus • Risk Factors: **immunocompromised** (malignancy, cancer treatment, transplant recipients, HIV, immunosuppressive medication), malnutrition, chronic corticosteroid use • **Most common opportunistic infection associated with HIV, especially when CD4+ count < 200 cells/uL**
Patho-physiology	• Fungus is inhaled, attaches to alveolar epithelium and transitions from small trophic form to larger cystic form • Inflammation then leads to alveolar damage and further lung injury, impaired gas exchange, and possibly respiratory failure
Signs & Symptoms	• **Classic Triad: fever + nonproductive cough + progressive dyspnea** (starts with dyspnea on exertion and progresses to at-rest) • Hypoxemia, respiratory distress • Physical exam: • 50% will have normal breath sounds; may have crackles, rhonchi, tachypnea/tachycardia
Diagnosis	• Labs: ↑LDH, ↑beta-D-glucagon (contained in fungi cellular wall), ↓CD4+ count, ABG if respiratory distress • Chest X-Ray (CXR): **diffuse, bilateral, perihilar interstitial infiltrates**; normal CXR in 25% • Chest CT Scan: more sensitive and specific; shows ground glass infiltrative pattern • Sputum Histopathology: obtained through induced sputum or bronchoalveolar lavage • Methenamine silver stain, Wright-Giemsa stain, and modified monoclonal antibody stain may be used • Lung Biopsy: definitive diagnosis but rarely performed

Treatment	• **Antibiotics:**
	  • **Trimethoprim-sulfamethoxazole (TMP-SMX) is first line**; therapy for 21 days
	  • Sulfa Allergy: primaquine + clindamycin, atovaquone, trimethoprim + dapsone, or IV pentamidine
	• **Corticosteroids: prednisone indicated if HIV+ and severe respiratory compromise** (room air PaO_2<70mmHg *OR* A-a gradient>35mmHg *OR* hypoxic)
	• Prophylaxis: TMP-SMX once daily if CD4+ <200 cells/uL

Key Words & Most Common	• Most common in HIV+ patients with CD4+ <200 • Fever, nonproductive cough, progressive dyspnea • CXR: diffuse, bilateral, perihilar interstitial infiltrates • Trimethoprim-sulfamethoxazole (TMP-SMX) is first line; steroids if HIV+ and hypoxic

Histoplasmosis

Etiology & Risk Factors	• Pulmonary and hematogenous disease caused by *Histoplasma capsulatum*
	• Etiology: *Histoplasma capsulatum;* a dimorphic soil-based yeast
	   • Mold found in soil that contains bird or bat feces
	   • **Endemic to Ohio, Missouri, and Mississippi river valleys** and southeastern US
	• Risk Factors: **immunocompromised (AIDS with CD4+ ≤150 cells/uL)**; demolition of old buildings (inhabited by birds/bats), farmers, **cave explorers**, or cave excavators

Patho-physiology	• Disruption of soil containing the fungus causes spores to become airborne, inhaled by the host, and become lodged in the alveoli • Spore is engulfed by neutrophils and macrophages which then organize and form granulomas that fibrose and calcify

Signs & Symptoms	• <u>Asymptomatic</u>: **90% of cases**; usually self limited
	• <u>Symptomatic</u>: 1-4 weeks after exposure; **flu-like illness**
	   • Fever/chills, myalgias, headache, arthralgias, dyspnea, nonproductive cough (may have hemoptysis)
	• <u>Disseminated</u>: involves multiple organ systems & affects immunocompromised
	   • Hepatosplenomegaly, fever, weight loss, oropharyngeal mucosal or GI ulcers, bloody diarrhea, hematologic disturbance, pericarditis (mimics TB)

Diagnosis	• <u>Labs</u>: CBC (mild anemia); elevated alkaline phosphatase and elevated LDH in disseminated • <u>Chest X-Ray (CXR)</u>: may be normal in 40-70% of cases • Pneumonitis with **hilar/mediastinal lymphadenopathy**, focal pulmonary infiltrates (light exposure) or diffuse miliary pulmonary infiltrates (heavy exposure) • <u>Antigen Testing</u>: **serum or urine antigen testing is highly specific** • <u>Sputum Culture</u>: **most specific test**; poses serious risk to lab personnel (blood culture may be positive in disseminated)
Treatment	• <u>Asymptomatic</u>: **no treatment necessary**; resolves without treatment (pulmonary symptoms less than 1 month) • <u>Acute Primary</u>: **itraconazole is first line** if symptoms >1 month; treatment for 3 months • <u>Chronic Pulmonary</u>: **itraconazole** for 1 year • <u>Progressive Disseminated</u>: **amphotericin B** for 1 week followed by itraconazole for 1 year • *Untreated disseminated disease has >90% mortality rate*
Key Words & Most Common	• Soil-based fungus found in soil containing bird or bat feces • Endemic to Ohio and Mississippi river valleys • Asymptomatic and self limiting in 90% of cases; flu-like illness if symptomatic • Serum or urine antigen testing; CXR may show hilar/mediastinal lymphadenopathy • Asymptomatic requires no treatment; Itraconazole if symptoms >1mo

Diffuse pulmonary infiltrates with hilar lymphadenopathy

Cryptococcosis

Etiology & Risk Factors	• **Pulmonary or disseminated infection acquired by inhalation of soil contaminated with the encapsulated yeasts *Cryptococcus neoformans* or *C. gattii*** • Etiology: *Cryptococcus neoformans*; encapsulated, budding, round yeast • **Fungus found in soil contaminated with bird droppings (especially pigeons)** • Risk Factors: **immunocompromised (AIDS [CD4+ <100 cells/uL]**, lymphoma, sarcoidosis, organ transplant, long-term corticosteroid use, diabetes)
Patho-physiology	• Disruption of soil containing the fungus causes spores to become airborne and inhaled by the host. • Spread of the disease is through hematogenous dissemination in immunosuppressed patients (frequently to brain and meninges)

Signs & Symptoms	• <u>Central Nervous System</u>: symptoms as a result of cerebral edema
	   • **Meningoencephalitis is most common clinical manifestation**; CNS symptoms as a result of cerebral edema
	   • Low-grade fever, **headache**, general malaise, **neck stiffness**, **photophobia**, nausea/vomiting, blurred vision, depression, agitation, confusion, altered mental status
	• <u>Respiratory</u>: nonspecific; cough, dyspnea, **pneumonia**
	• <u>Skin</u>: pustular, papular, nodular, or **ulcerated lesions** may be seen if disseminated

Diagnosis	• <u>Lumbar Puncture and Cerebrospinal Fluid Analysis</u>: ↑ or normal WBC, ↓glucose, ↑protein
	   • <u>Cryptococcal Antigen via latex agglutination or ELISA</u>: highly sensitive and specific
	   • <u>Cryptococcal Culture</u>: 95-100% sensitive; takes 3-7 days
	   • <u>India Ink Stain</u>: **shows encapsulated yeast**
	• <u>CT Brain</u>: soap bubble lesions; may be normal
	• <u>Chest X-Ray (CXR)</u>: variable findings; may have infiltrates, mediastinal lymphadenopathy

Treatment	• **Pneumonia**:
	   • <u>AIDS-Associated</u>: **fluconazole for 6-12 months**
	   • <u>Not AIDS-Associated</u>: fluconazole or itraconazole for 6-12 months
	• **Meningoencephalitis**: **amphotericin B + flucytosine** for 4 weeks, **followed by oral fluconazole** for 8 weeks
	• *Therapy is discontinued when CD4+ count is >200 cells/uL and asymptomatic for 6 months*

Key Words & Most Common	• Pulmonary or disseminated infection caused by *Cryptococcus neoformans*; found in soil contaminated with pigeon droppings • Immunocompromised (AIDS patients with CD4+ count <100) • Meningoencephalitis is most common clinical manifestation • Diagnose with CSF analysis for antigen or identify encapsulated yeast on India ink stain • Pulmonary: Fluconazole • Meningitis: Amphotericin B + Flucytosine followed by oral fluconazole

Blastomycosis

Etiology & Risk Factors	• Pyogranulomatous fungal infection caused by inhaling spores of the dimorphic fungus *Blastomyces dermatitidis* • Etiology: ***Blastomyces dermatitidis***; a dimorphic fungus • **Fungus found in moist soil or decaying wood near Mississippi and Ohio River valleys and Great Lakes** (also Northern Midwest, Upstate NY, and southern Canada) • Risk Factors: **more common in immunocompetent males**, occupational and recreational exposure (**outdoor activities near water**); immunocompromised
Patho-physiology	• Fungal colony disturbed during outdoor activity causing spores to become airborne and inhaled which are then phagocytized by mononuclear cells & killed by macrophages and neutrophils; in the lungs, the inhaled spores convert to larger invasive yeasts, forming broad-based buds and may disseminate hematogenous
Signs & Symptoms	• Up to 50% of cases will be asymptomatic; 3-6 week incubation period • General: flu-like symptoms (fever/chills, cough, myalgias, arthralgias, malaise), weight loss, night sweats • Pulmonary: **most common site of involvement**; acute or chronic pneumonia, diffuse pneumonitis, ARDS • Cutaneous: **most common extrapulmonary site**; verrucous (wart-like) lesions with irregular border, **subcutaneous nodules, well-demarcated ulcers** that bleed easily • Disseminated: bone involvement (osteomyelitis, paravertebral abscess, **lytic bone lesions),** central nervous system (meningitis, brain/epidural abscess) and genitourinary system (prostatitis, epididymitis)
Diagnosis	• Chest X-Ray (CXR): **alveolar infiltrates, mass lesion**; lacks specificity • Vertebral X-Ray: well-circumscribed osteolytic lesion; may show lytic lesions at anterior vertebral body and destruction of disk space • Fungal Culture: sputum stained with fungal stain • Potassium Hydroxide (KOH) Wet Mount): sputum sample demonstrates **round yeast with thick double walls and broad-based budding**; may take 5-10 days • Antigen Testing: urine or serologic
Treatment	• Mild to Moderate: **itraconazole is first-line;** fluconazole for 6-12 months • Severe: **amphotericin B** if progressive, or CNS involvement
Key Words & Most Common	• Fungus found in moist soil/decaying wood near Mississippi & Ohio River valleys and Great Lakes • Immunocompetent male participating in outdoor activities near water • Flu-like symptoms; skin is most common extrapulmonary site • KOH shows round yeast with thick double walls and broad-based budding • Itraconazole if mild; Amphotericin B if severe

Aspergillosis

Etiology & Risk Factors	• **Opportunistic infection affecting the lower respiratory tract and is caused by inhaling spores of the filamentous fungus** *Aspergillus* • Etiology: *Aspergillus fumigatus;* a filamentous, monomorphic **fungus with septate hyphae that branch at 45° angles,** and affects the lungs, sinuses, and CNS • **Fungus is most commonly found in garden and houseplant soils, decaying vegetation and compost** • Risk Factors: **immunocompromised (AIDS, leukemia, organ transplant,** long-term corticosteroid use, diabetes), environmental or occupational exposure (**construction or farming industries),** smoking marijuana contaminated with fungus, chronic lung diseases (asthma, cystic fibrosis, COPD)		
Patho-physiology	• Aspergillus spores are inhaled and taken up by respiratory phagocytes that then germinate into hyphae due to increased body temperature within the lung • In immunocompetent patients, beta-D-glucan is secreted by phagocytes which activates neutrophils that kill the hyphae and prevent infection; inn immunocompromised patients, these defense mechanisms are impaired leading to infection		
	Allergic Bronchopulmonary Aspergillosis	**Aspergilloma**	**Acute Invasive Aspergillosis**
Signs & Symptoms	• **Type 1 hypersensitivity** to *A. fumigatus*; **most commonly affects patients with asthma or cystic fibrosis** • **Cough productive of brownish mucus plug** in sputum, hemoptysis, fever, malaise +/- allergic fungal sinusitis	• Affects those with preexisting pulmonary cavitary lung disease (TB, sarcoidosis); fungus colonizes the lesion (fungal ball) • May be asymptomatic and incidentally found on CXR; cough +/- hemoptysis if symptomatic	• Occurs in severely immunocompromised (leukemia, organ transplant, chemotherapy) • Fever, cough, dyspnea, **pleuritic chest pain, hemoptysis, invasive chronic sinusitis** (may develop necrotizing cutaneous lesions around sinus)
Diagnosis	• **Increased IgE** (2x increase from baseline), **eosinophilia**; positive skin test for *Aspergillus fumigatus* • CXR: central bronchiectasis, mucoid impaction, migratory pulmonary infiltrates (eosinophilic pneumonia)	• **Positive precipitin Ab test** • Biopsy: **septate hyphae that branch at 45° angles**; may be necrotic appearing • CXR/CT: **upper lobe "fungal ball" mass in preexisting cavity that changes position with patient; air crescent sign** (crescent of air outlining solid mass)	• Galactomannan level (cell wall component of Aspergillus release into blood); beta-D-glucan assay; sputum culture • CXR/CT: **halo sign** (nodules with surrounding ground glass opacities); cavitary lesions, wedge-shaped or pleural-based infiltrates
Treatment	• **Oral corticosteroids (3-6wks followed by taper) and chest physiotherapy is first-line**; add itraconazole if chronic	• **Oral itraconazole + surgical resection**; observation if asymptomatic	• **Voriconazole is drug of choice**; posaconazole or amphotericin B are alternatives
Key Words & Most Common	• Fungus found in gardens and decaying vegetation; affects immunocompromised • Allergic is type 1 hypersensitivity affecting asthma/cystic fibrosis; increased IgE and eosinophilia; treated with oral steroids • Aspergilloma affects preexisting pulmonary lung disease; "fungal ball" mass of upper lobe; air crescent sign; treated with itraconazole • Acute invasive: pleuritic chest pain & hemoptysis; halo sign (nodule with surrounding opacification); treated with voriconazole		

53

Coccidioidomycosis

Etiology & Risk Factors	• Pulmonary or hematogenous spread disseminated disease caused by the fungi *Coccidioides immitis* and *C. posadasii* • Etiology: *Coccidioides immitis* or *C. posadasii* a dimorphic fungus • Fungus most commonly found in soil of arid/desert regions; endemic to southwestern US (New Mexico, Arizona, West Texas, Southern California) • <u>Risk Factors</u>: **immunocompromised (HIV)** 2nd & 3rd trimester **pregnancy**, advanced age, **certain ethnicities** (Filipino, African American, Native American, Hispanics, Asians), environmental exposure (hiking, outdoor recreation, **farming, construction work**); *about 30-60% of people that live in endemic area have been exposed during lifetime*
Patho-physiology	• Disruption of soil containing the fungus causes spores to become airborne and inhaled by the host where they convert to large spherules which may rupture and release thousands of endospores; local release of endospores causes host response and acute inflammation leading to fibrosis

Signs & Symptoms	• <u>Primary Illness</u> : 1-4 weeks after exposure; 60% are asymptomatic
	  • Mild **flu-like symptoms** that may resemble bronchitis/pneumonia (fever, cough, pleuritic chest pain, chills, sputum production, sore throat, hemoptysis)
	• <u>Progressive Illness</u>: 1-3 weeks after primary pulmonary disease presentation
	  • **Fever, arthralgias** (especially knee and ankles), anorexia, weight loss, and weakness.
	  • <u>Erythema Nodosum</u>: erythematous, painful, subcutaneous nodules most common on the lower extremities
	• <u>Disseminated Illness</u>: more common in the immunosuppressed and pregnant women
	  • CNS involvement **(meningitis)** in 50%; vertebral osteomyelitis; skin lesions; **joint involvement (knees)**, dramatic sweats, weight loss

Diagnosis	• <u>Serologic Testing</u>: enzyme immunoassay detects IgM and IgG antibodies (usually first test ordered); elevated ESR, eosinophilia • <u>Fungal Culture</u>: most definitive test • <u>Microscopic Analysis</u>: **thick-walled spherule containing endospores seen within samples of** sputum, pleural fluid, cerebrospinal fluid (CSF), exudate, or biopsied specimens • <u>Polymerase Chain Reaction (PCR)</u>: highly sensitive and specific test; not widely available • <u>Chest X-Ray (CXR)</u>: unilateral infiltrates, miliary pneumonia, persistent cavitation • <u>CSF Analysis</u>: presence of complement-fixing antibodies is diagnostic; ↓glucose, lymphocytosis (ordered if meningitis suspected)
Treatment	• <u>Asymptomatic or Mild</u>: self-limited and requires no treatment • <u>Mild to Moderate Nonmeningeal Extrapulmonary Involvement</u>: **fluconazole or itraconazole** • <u>Severe</u>: **amphotericin B** • High dose fluconazole for meningitis
Key Words & Most Common	• Caused by fungus found in arid/desert regions of southwestern US • Primary Pulmonary (flu-like illness) followed by "Valley Fever" (triad of fever, arthralgias, and erythema nodosum); Dissemination may occur in immunocompromised • <u>Labs</u>: enzyme immunoassay to detect IgM & IgG; eosinophilia • Most cases self-limited; Fluconazole in moderate cases, Amphotericin B in severe cases

	Pneumocystis Jirovecii Pneumonia	Histoplasmosis	Cryptococcosis	Blastomycosis	Aspergillosis	Coccidioidomycosis
Etiology	• *Pneumocystis jirovecii:* atypical yeast-like fungus	• *Histoplasma capsulatum:* dimorphic soil-based yeast	• *Cryptococcus neoformans:* encapsulated yeast	• *Blastomyces dermatitidis:* dimorphic fungus	• *Aspergillus:* **fungus with septate hyphae that branch at 45° angles**	• *Coccidioides immitis:* dimorphic fungus
Risk Factors	• Most common opportunistic infection associated with HIV • **CD4+ count <200 cells/uL**	• Bird or **bat droppings** • OH, MO, and MS river valleys • **CD4+ ≤150 cells/uL**	• **Pigeon droppings** • CD4+ <100 cells/uL	• **Moist soil or decaying wood** • **MS & OH river valleys & Great Lakes**	• Garden soil/compost	• **Soil of arid/desert regions** • **Southwestern US**
Symptoms	• <u>Classic Triad</u>: **fever**, nonproductive **cough**, progressive **dyspnea**	• <u>Acute</u>: asymptomatic or flu-like illness • <u>Disseminated</u>: HSM, fever, oropharyngeal ulcers, bloody diarrhea	• Meningitis: MCC of fungal meningitis • <u>Pneumonia</u>: **cough, pleuritic pain, dyspnea**	• Flu-like symptoms • Skin is MC extrapulmonary site	• <u>Allergic</u>: hypersensitivity rxn in asthma and CF; cough with thick brown mucous plugs • <u>Aspergilloma</u>: colonizes preexisting cavitary lesion • <u>Invasive</u>: fever, cough, dyspnea, chest pain, hemoptysis	• <u>Primary</u>: flu-like illness • <u>Valley Fever</u>: fever, arthralgias, erythema nodosum • <u>Disseminated</u>: **meningitis**
Diagnosis	• <u>Labs</u>: ↑LDH, ↑beta-D-glucagon, ↓CD4+ count • <u>CXR</u>: diffuse, bilateral, perihilar interstitial infiltrates • <u>CT</u>: ground glass	• Sputum cultures/antigen • Urine antigen • Fungal blood cultures • CXR variable **(miliary infiltrates)**	• CSF: ↓glucose, ↑protein • **Cryptococcal Antigen** • **India Ink Stain** shows encapsulated yeast	• Sputum/CSF/urine cultures budding yeast with thick double walls	• <u>Allergic</u>: elevated IgE and eosinophilia • <u>Aspergilloma</u>: "fungal ball" with air crescent sign on CXR • <u>Invasive</u>: halo sign	• IgG and IgM antibodies • Histopathology with fungal culture
Treatment	• **Trimethoprim-sulfamethoxazole (TMP-SMX)** is first line • Steroids if HIV+ and hypoxic	• <u>Acute</u>: Itraconazole • <u>Disseminated</u>: Amphotericin B	• <u>Pneumonia</u>: Fluconazole • <u>Meningoencephalitis</u>: **Amphotericin B + Flucytosine**	• Itraconazole is first line • Amphotericin B if severe	• <u>Allergic</u>: corticosteroids • <u>Aspergilloma</u>: surgery + itraconazole • <u>Invasive</u>: voriconazole	• Mild: self limited • Moderate: Fluconazole • Severe: Amphotericin B

Tuberculosis

Etiology & Risk Factors	• Chronic, progressive multi-system disease caused by **Mycobacterium tuberculosis** and **spread through inhalation of airborne respiratory droplets** • Etiology: **Mycobacterium tuberculosis** • Risk Factors: close contact exposure to someone with TB, **crowded living conditions (homeless shelters, prisons)**, HIV (CD4+ <500 cell/uL, immunosuppression (steroid use, diabetes), **recent immigration from high-prevalence areas**, healthcare workers, malnutrition • Epidemiology: estimated that 1/4th of entire world population is infected; **most cases in Southeast Asia** (India, Indonesia), Africa, and the Western Pacific (China)
Patho-physiology	• *M. tuberculosis* is inhaled and deposit deep in lung (middle/lower lobe) and ingested by alveolar macrophages; infected macrophages can migrate to regional lymph nodes and enter the bloodstream; *M. tuberculosis* replicates inside which eventually kills host macrophage causing inflammatory mediators to go to area and creating a focal pneumonitis

Signs & Symptoms	• Primary: usually **asymptomatic**; may be rapidly progressive in immunocompromised
	• Reactivation: **fever, night sweats**, malaise, fatigue, **weight loss**
	  • **Pulmonary**: cough +/- mucous production, hemoptysis, dyspnea, pleuritic chest pain
	  • **Extrapulmonary**: painless lymphadenopathy (Scrofula), Pott's disease (TB osteomyelitis of vertebrae), pericarditis, adrenal insufficiency, meningitis, peritonitis
	• Latent: asymptomatic, positive purified protein derivative (PPD), no CXR findings of active infection
		• Primary: initial infection (often self-limiting), primary progressive may be present in children in endemic areas; **contagious**
		• Reactivation: **more common in immunocompromised patients**; cavitary lesions in upper lobe (secondary to ↑O_2 in lung apices); **contagious**
		• Latent: **caseating granuloma formation** leads to central necrotic, acidic and ↓O_2 environment decreases *M. tuberculosis* growth and inhibits symptomatic infection; **not contagious**

Diagnosis	• **Chest X-Ray (CXR): most common initial test**
	  • Primary: **middle or lower lobe consolidation**, hilar or mediastinal lymphadenopathy
	  • Reactivation: fibrocavitary lesions in **upper lobe**
	  • Latent: upper lobe/hilar nodules, fibrotic lesion, **Ghon's complex** (calcified caseating granuloma), **Ranke's complex** (healed Ghon's complex)
	  • Miliary TB: diffuse **millet-seed** (2-4mm) nodular lesions
	• Sputum Cytology: acid-fast bacilli, culture, nucleic acid amplification test	

Treatment	• Active: 4-drug therapy (RIPE) **Rifampin + Isoniazid + Pyrazinamide + Ethambutol for 2 months**, followed by **Isoniazid & Rifampin for 4 months** • Latent: **Isoniazid + Pyridoxine (vitamin B6) for 9 months;** Consider treatment for newly positive PPD, close contact exposure to active TB, immunocompromised	

Screening	• Purified Protein Derivative (PPD): transdermal administration & examined 48-72h after for transverse induration (erythema is not considered positive)
	  • Reaction considered POSITIVE in following situations
	    • ≥5mm: Immunosuppressed, HIV+, calcified granuloma or fibrotic changes on CXR, close contact exposure to active TB
	    • ≥10mm: Children <4yo, healthcare/prison employees, comorbid conditions (dialysis, diabetes, malignancy, IVDU), exposure to high prevalence area
	    • ≥15mm: No known risk factors
	• Interferon Gamma Release Assay (QuantiFERON Gold Assay): blood test with no reader bias, no false positive with BCG vaccine, and improved specificity	

Solitary Pulmonary Nodule

Etiology & Risk Factors	• **Single lung opacity measuring <3cm** that is well-circumscribed, discrete, and is surrounded by lung parenchyma (does not touch lung pleura, mediastinum or hilum)
	• Etiology: **generally benign; infectious granulomas are most common cause** (TB, fungal); primary/metastatic cancer, autoimmune (rheumatoid nodules), benign tumors (fibroma, lipoma), infection
	• Risk Factors: **smoking**, previous history of cancer, family history of cancer, current lung condition (COPD, interstitial lung disease)
	  • Risk of malignancy *increases* with larger nodule with **irregular border** or shape, **age >40yo**, upper lobe involvement, smoker
	  • Risk of malignancy *decreases* if small and well circumscribed, **dense calcifications**, age <30yo, no smoking history

Patho-physiology	• Not fully understood; inflammatory process causing alveolar epithelial injury has been implicated
Signs & Symptoms	• **95% are asymptomatic;** most often an incidental finding picked up during routine imaging or imaging for another reason • Symptoms may relate to underlying etiology
Diagnosis	• Chest X-Ray (CXR): **most common initial test** that identifies nodule; **commonly picked up on routine imaging or imaging for another reason** • Chest CT Scan: **most sensitive; test of choice to determine likelihood of malignancy;** may be used as follow-up imaging for incidental finding on CXR • PET Scan: used to differentiate benign and malignant nodules	**Radiographic Characteristics of Malignancy** • Growth Rate: no enlargement in >2 years suggests benign nature • Calcification: suggests benign nature • Margins: irregular or spiculated suggests malignancy • Diameter: **<1.5cm suggests benign nature; >5cm suggests malignancy** • Location: **upper lobe is more likely to be malignant**
Treatment	• Low Probability of Malignancy: **observation with routine imaging** to monitor for changes • Moderate Probability of Malignancy: close observation; diagnostic biopsy with transthoracic needle aspiration if peripheral lesion or bronchoscopy if central lesion • High Probability of Malignancy: surgical resection	
Key Words & Most Common	• Small <3cm lesion; often benign • Mostly asymptomatic • CXR: most common initial test; often picked up incidentally • CT: most sensitive; used to determine malignancy • Observation with routine imaging if stable; surgical resection if high risk	

Bronchial Carcinoid Tumor

Etiology & Risk Factors	• **Rare, slow-growing neuroendocrine** (enterochromaffin cell) **tumor with low metastatic potential**
	• Etiology: **tumor developed from neuroendocrine cells in the GI tract (most common)**, pancreas, pulmonary bronchi, and genitourinary tract
	  • May secrete biologically active chemical substances (serotonin, ACTH, ADH, somatostatin and bradykinin)
	• Risk Factors: **age (40-60 years old most common)**, female, family history, certain genetic syndromes (multiple endocrine neoplasia type 1and neurofibromatosis type 1)
	  • Not typically associated with smoking

Patho-physiology	• Develop from enterochromaffin cells within the bronchial mucosa or from the epithelium of the tracheobronchial tree cartilage • Neuroendocrine function through secretion of neuroamines and peptides such as serotonin, ACTH, ADH, somatostatin and bradykinin
Signs & Symptoms	• **Most are asymptomatic** • **Symptoms of Airway Obstruction**: nonproductive cough, dyspnea, wheezing (mimics asthma) • Recurrent pneumonia, **hemoptysis** (has vascular stroma and tends to bleed) • **Carcinoid Syndrome**: **flushing, tachycardia, and bronchospasm** (histamine release); **diarrhea** (serotonin release); **hypotension** (bradykinin release)
Diagnosis	• Chest X-Ray (CXR): hyperinflation due to air trapping; atelectasis; **mass in main, lobar, or segmental bronchi**; usually picked up incidentally • Chest CT Scan: helps identify location of lesion; reveals tumor calcification • **Bronchoscopy with Biopsy: definitive diagnosis**; pink/purple highly vascularized tumor that is centrally located • Biochemical Markers: urinary 5-hydroxyindoleacetic acid and serum chromogranin A support diagnosis
Treatment	• **Complete Surgical Resection: definitive management**; offers good prognosis • With or without chemotherapy and/or radiation therapy; often resistant to chemotherapy and radiation • Octreotide: may decrease secretion of active hormones and control symptoms
Key Words & Most Common	• Rare, slow-growing neuroendocrine tumor; may secrete chemical substances • Mostly asymptomatic • Carcinoid Syndrome: tachycardia and bronchospasm + diarrhea + hypotension • Bronchoscopy with Biopsy • Complete Surgical Resection

Bronchogenic Carcinoma

Etiology & Risk Factors	• **Most common cause of cancer-related deaths in the US**
	• Etiology: **lung tumor originating from the lung parenchyma or bronchi**
	• Risk Factors: **smoking is greatest risk factor; asbestos exposure**, radiation exposure for non-lung cancers, metal exposure (chromium, nickel, arsenic), radon exposure; other respiratory conditions (idiopathic pulmonary fibrosis, TB, and/or COPD), family history
	  • **Smoking and asbestos exposure combined compound to further increase risk**
	• **Two Main Types: small cell cancer and non-small cell cancer**
	  • **Small Cell:** highly aggressive and rapidly growing; roughly 80% of patients have metastatic disease at the time of diagnosis
	  • **Non-Small Cell:** variable behavior; 40% of patients will have metastatic disease at the time of diagnosis

Patho-physiology	• Repeated exposure to carcinogens leads to lung epithelium dysplasia and causes genetic mutations and affects protein synthesis; this leads to carcinogenesis as it disrupts the regular cell cycle
Signs & Symptoms	• Non-Specific Symptoms: **cough, dyspnea, hemoptysis, weight loss, chest pain** • Most patients have advanced disease at initial presentation
Diagnosis	• **Contrast Enhanced CT Chest**: assists with staging, location, and identifying metastatic lymph nodes or mediastinal invasion of the tumor • PET Scan: directed at sites of metastases, may identify recurrence vs. metabolic changes after radiation therapy • Biopsy: histologically differentiates cancer; performed through bronchoscopy or CT-guided
Treatment	*Treatment largely depends on cell type, location and extent of disease* • **Surgical Resection**: lobectomy or pneumonectomy with mediastinal lymph node sampling; likely with chemotherapy and radiation • **Adjuvant Chemotherapy**: etoposide, cisplatin, carboplatin **and radiation** • Screening: US Preventative Services Task Force recommends annual chest CT (low-dose) in patients 55-80 years old who currently smoke or have quit within 15 years
Key Words & Most Common	• Most common cause of cancer-related death in US • Smoking and asbestos biggest risk factors; synergistic • Two types: small cell and non-small cell cancer • Contrast Enhanced CT assists with staging and location of tumor • Chemotherapy and radiation vs Surgical Resection

Centrally located left lobar mass

	Non-Small Cell Lung Cancer			Small Cell Lung Cancer
	Lung Adenocarcinoma	**Squamous Cell Lung Carcinoma**	**Large Cell Carcinoma**	**Small Cell Carcinoma**
Etiology	• **Most common lung cancer subtype** • Arises from mucosal glands • Common in non-smokers and underlying lung disease • Peripheral nodules or masses	• 2nd most common lung CA subtype • **Arises in central/proximal bronchi**	• Heterogenous group of poorly differentiated tumors • Typically, peripheral mass	• Highly aggressive • Often presents with lymph node involvement or early metastases at time of presentation • Typically, hilar mass
Risk Factors	• **Smoking greatest risk factor;** asbestos, silica, heavy metal exposure	• **Strongest association with smoking**	• Smoking greatest risk factor	• Smoking greatest risk factor • Male gender

Symptoms	• **Typically, asymptomatic in early disease**
	• Peripheral lesions
	  • Cough, dyspnea, pain due to pleural or chest wall invasion
		• **Centrally located lesions**
		  • Cough, hemoptysis, wheeze, stridor, dyspnea, post-obstructive pneumonia
		• **Pancoast syndrome**
			• Peripheral lesions
			  • Cough, dyspnea, pain due to pleural or chest wall invasion
				• **Centrally located lesions**
				  • Cough, hemoptysis, wheeze, stridor, dyspnea, post-obstructive pneumonia
				• **Paraneoplastic Syndrome**

Diagnosis	• Histology: **neoplastic gland formation and mucin production**	• CXR: widened mediastinum, cavitary lesions • Hypercalcemia • Histology: **presence of keratin or intracellular desmosomes**	• Histology: **lack cytologic features;** diagnosis of exclusion	• CXR: centrally located mass • Histology: **round, oval, or angulated cells;** about 2x size of lymphocytes; no distinct nucleoli
Treatment	• Surgical Resection +/- chemo & radiation	• Surgical Resection +/- chemo & radiation	• Chemotherapy +/- radiation	• Chemotherapy +/- radiation • Often metastatic at time of presentation

Superior Vena Cava Syndrome 🫁

Etiology & Risk Factors	• Type of paraneoplastic syndrome characterized by **partial or complete obstruction of blood flow** through the superior vena cava (SVC) • Etiology: **extrinsic malignant mass most common;** thrombus from indwelling catheter or pacemaker • Risk Factors: **lung cancer (small cell bronchogenic carcinoma),** thrombophilia, Non-Hodgkins lymphoma, indwelling catheter/pacemaker, goiter, radiation treatment
Patho-physiology	• Compression and obstruction of the superior vena cava by a mass (usually malignancy) results in increased vascular resistance and SVC pressure while venous return decreases • SVC with significant stenosis leads to formation of collateral blood vessels to compensate and bypass the obstruction and return normal venous flow
Signs & Symptoms	• **Facial swelling (worse in morning and improves throughout the day)** • Cough, dyspnea, cyanosis • **Distended neck and chest veins** • Headache
Diagnosis	• Chest X-Ray (CXR): may show **mediastinal or parenchymal lung mass** • Contrast Enhanced CT: greater sensitivity to determine degree of obstruction and evaluates etiology (mass vs thrombus)
Treatment	• Supportive: elevate head of bed, treat underlying etiology • Malignancy: mediastinal radiation • Thrombus: anticoagulation, removal of indwelling catheter, consider thrombolytics
Key Words & Most Common	• Obstruction of blood flow through SVC caused by malignant mass (lung cancer) or thrombus • Facial swelling, distended neck/chest veins • CXR/CT shows lung mass • Supportive: elevate head of bed; treat underlying cause

Distended chest veins

Superior Sulcus (Pancoast) Tumor

Etiology & Risk Factors	• Tumor originating near the apex of the lung and involves surrounding structures • <u>Etiology</u>: **non-small cell lung carcinoma (squamous cell carcinoma most common)** make up 80-85% of cases, thyroid carcinoma, metastasis from primary carcinoma • <u>Risk Factors</u>: **smoking**, exposure to carcinogens, age (>50 years old most common), male, family history, history of other pulmonary disease (COPD, IPF)
Patho-physiology	• Tumor invades surrounding structures, putting compression on the brachial plexus leading to arm/shoulder pain • Structures affected include the brachial plexus, cervical paravertebral sympathetic nervous system, and stellate ganglion leading to distinct signs and symptoms described as **Pancoast Syndrome** • Tumor may involve sympathetic nervous system causing ipsilateral facial flushing and sweating
Signs & Symptoms	• <u>Shoulder and Arm Pain</u>: **most common initial symptom** • Medial half of $4^{th}/5^{th}$ finger, medial side of forearm and hand due to C8, T1 radiculopathy; may lead to weakness and atrophy • <u>Horner Syndrome</u>: ipsilateral ptosis (eyelid drooping), miosis (constriction of pupil), anhidrosis (lack of perspiration) • <u>Respiratory Symptoms</u>: cough, dyspnea do not develop until advanced disease as tumors are apically located
Diagnosis	• <u>**Chest X-Ray (CXR)**</u>: **initial test**; may show **apical mass** • <u>Magnetic Resonance Imaging (MRI)</u>: neck, chest, and abdomen to stratify extent of brachial plexus and vascular involvement; more sensitive • <u>**CT Guided Core Biopsy**</u>: **diagnostic test of choice**
Treatment	• **Chemotherapy followed by Surgical Resection: standard of care**
Key Words & Most Common	• Apical tumor that may involve surrounding structures including brachial plexus • Non-small cell lung carcinoma; squamous cell carcinoma are most common cause • Shoulder and arm pain with ulnar neuropathy • CXR initial test; CT guided core biopsy is test of choice • Chemotherapy followed by surgical resection

Right Apical Mass

Foreign Body Aspiration

Etiology & Risk Factors	• Aerodigestive foreign body causing varying amount of airway obstruction leading to difficulty with ventilation and oxygenation • **Main cause of death is associated with hypoxic-ischemic brain injury** • <u>Etiology</u>: **peanuts are most common**, toys, balloons, coins, food • <u>Risk Factors</u>: **age (<3 years old most common), play habits (playing with small items)**, dentures, substance abuse, neurologic conditions (stroke affecting swallowing reflex), intellectual disabilities, dental procedures
Patho-physiology	• **Mean age of 2 years old** due to dental development; **children can bite food with incisors but unable to grind food due to absence of molar teeth** • Young children are more likely to stick objects into their mouth and become distracted/playful while eating and have narrower tracheobronchial tree • **Most common site is right mains bronchus due to a wider and more vertical airway**
Signs & Symptoms	• May be asymptomatic if small • **Sudden onset of cough, dyspnea, choking, stridor** • Physical Exam: • Unilateral wheeze or absent/asymmetric breath sounds on auscultation

Diagnosis	• <u>**Chest X-Ray (CXR)**</u>: **best initial test**; may show atelectasis, pneumothorax, or **air trapping (most common)**
	   • **May show foreign body if radiopaque**
	   • Normal CXR does not rule out foreign body aspiration
	   • Additional neck x-ray may be indicated
	• <u>Chest CT Scan</u>: ordered if negative x-ray on symptomatic patient with suggestive history
	• <u>**Rigid Bronchoscopy**</u>: **definitive diagnostic test**; therapeutic as object can be removed during procedure

Treatment	• <u>**Bronchoscopy**</u>: **diagnostic and therapeutic to remove foreign body**
	   • **Rigid preferred to flexible**
	   • Rigid allows ventilation, improved visualization, and allows greater versatility of instruments

Key Words & Most Common	• Peanuts are most common object • Most common among ~2 year olds • Sudden onset cough, dyspnea, choking • CXR best initial test; shows air trapping • Rigid bronchoscopy is diagnostic and therapeutic

Coin in esophagus of child

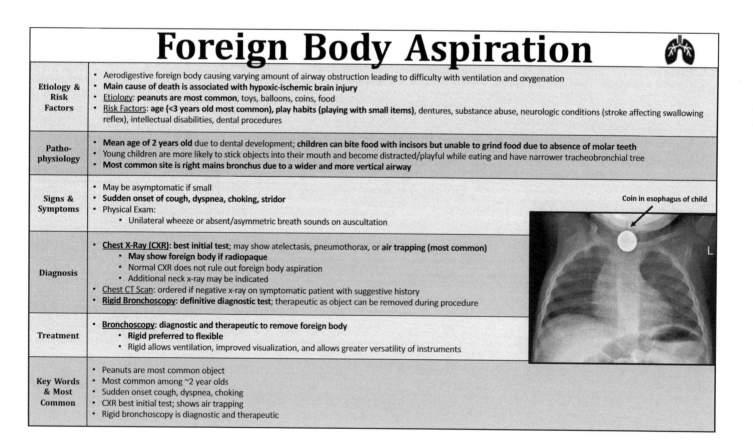

Costochondritis

Etiology & Risk Factors	• Chest wall pain caused by inflammation of the costal cartilage (the cartilage connecting ribs to the sternum) • Etiology: **inflammation of costal cartilage** • Risk Factors: **trauma** (impact/contusion, **physical exertion**, heavy breathing, heavy lifting) or **post-viral** (**excessive coughing**, sneezing), arthritis, joint hypermobility, certain medical conditions (fibromyalgia, ankylosing spondylitis)
Patho-physiology	• Inflammation of cartilage caused by trauma or excessive coughing, sneezing as a result of recent viral illness
Signs & Symptoms	• **Chest pain worse with certain positions or body movements, deep inspiration, coughing/sneezing** • May be sharp or dull in nature; **pleuritic** • **Reproducible point tenderness to chest wall at costosternal or costochondral joints** • Tietze Syndrome: palpable edema
Diagnosis	• **Diagnosis of Exclusion**: must rule out ACS, pneumonia, pulmonary embolism etc. as clinically correlated • Additional testing not required to diagnose costochondritis; rules out other causes of chest pain • Labs: used to rule out other causes • Chest X-Ray (CXR): consider for trauma etiology; rule out pneumonia, pneumothorax, lung mass • Electrocardiogram (ECG): to rule out ischemia
Treatment	• **Analgesia: non-steroidal anti-inflammatory drugs (NSAIDs) are mainstay** • Supportive: heat, gentle stretching, slow deep breathing exercises • Physical Therapy: if refractory or persistent
Key Words & Most Common	• Inflammation of costal cartilage from trauma or coughing • Chest pain worse with coughing or deep inspiration • Diagnosis of exclusion • NSAIDs

Pleural Effusion

Etiology & Risk Factors	• Accumulation of fluid between the parietal and visceral pleura that may result from infectious, inflammatory, or malignant cause
	• Etiology: classified as transudate or exudate based on Light's criteria
	  • Transudate: **CHF is most common cause, nephrotic syndrome, liver cirrhosis**, hypoalbuminemia, (conditions that ↑hydrostatic pressure or ↓oncotic pressure)
	  • Exudate: **infection (pneumonia, TB), inflammatory disorders** (malignancy, pancreatitis, lupus, rheumatoid arthritis, **pulmonary embolism**)

Patho-physiology	• Pleural cavity contains a small amount of pleural fluid that acts as lubrication for two pleural surfaces • Increased hydrostatic pressure from parietal pleura vessels drives interstitial fluid into pleural space;
Signs & Symptoms	• May be asymptomatic • **Dyspnea, pleuritic chest pain, cough** • Physical Exam: • Fullness at intercostal spaces, **dullness to percussion, decreased breath sounds, decreased tactile and vocal fremitus**

Diagnosis	• **Chest X-Ray (CXR): best initial test; shows blunting of costophrenic angles (meniscus sign)**
	  • Minimum 200mL effusion required to view on **upright PA view**
	  • Minimum 50mL effusion required to view on **lateral decubitus view; can detect smaller effusions**
	• Chest CT/US: more sensitive; may be useful to plan thoracentesis
	• **Thoracentesis: gold standard;** can be diagnostic and therapeutic; differentiates between exudate and transudate
	  • **Light's Criteria**: effusion is exudative if any of the following 3 are present
	    • Pleural fluid/serum protein ration >0.5
	    • Pleural fluid/serum LDH ratio >0.6
	    • Pleural fluid LDH > 2/3 of upper limit of normal LDH

Treatment	• **Treat Underlying Condition**: evaluate and treat underlying disorder • Therapeutic Thoracentesis: may aid in diagnosis as well; not always necessary unless underlying infection present • Do not drain >1500mL during one procedure as can lead to re-expansion pulmonary edema • **Chest Tube Drainage + Antibiotics: indicated for empyema** (pleural fluid **pH <7.2, glucose <40 mg/dL** or **presence of organisms** on gram stain)
Key Words & Most Common	• Transudate (CHF is MCC) vs Exudate (infection/inflammation) • Dyspnea, pleuritic chest pain, cough • CXR shows blunting of costophrenic angles • Thoracentesis is gold standard; diagnostic and therapeutic • Treat underlying cause; chest tube & antibiotics if empyema

Left sided pleural effusion

Pneumothorax

Etiology & Risk Factors	• Collection of air outside the lung but within the pleural cavity which adds positive intrapleural air pressure and leads to lung collapse • Etiology: • **Primary Spontaneous**: due to bleb rupture; occurs in those with **no underlying lung disease; classically tall, thin, male 20-40 years old with history of smoking** • **Secondary Spontaneous**: occurs in those with **underlying lung disease** (COPD, CF, Asthma) • Traumatic: result of penetrating or blunt chest injuries • **Tension: positive air pressure pushing mediastinum to contralateral side**; ventilation mismatch, barotrauma, penetrating/blunt trauma; **considered emergent**
Patho-physiology	• Intrapleural pressure is usually negative due to inward lung and outward chest wall recoil • Communication between alveoli and pleural space causes air to accumulate in intrapleural space, changing the pressure gradient (↑intrapleural pressure, ↓lung volume) causing the lung to collapse to restore equilibrium
Signs & Symptoms	• **Chest Pain**: unilateral, pleuritic, sharp/severe • May be sudden and radiate to ipsilateral shoulder • Physical Exam: • **Hyperresonance to percussion**, asymmetrical lung expansion, **decreased breath sounds** and fremitus • Tension: hypotension, tachycardia, **JVD**
Diagnosis	• Chest X-Ray (CXR): **initial test of choice** • Radiolucent air and/or absence of lung markings between collapsed lobe and parietal pleura • **Tracheal deviation or mediastinal shift towards the opposite side** may occur with large pneumothoraxes • Ultrasound: **more sensitive**; no lung sliding seen, no comet-tail artifact, lung point presence
Treatment	• Supportive: indicated for small primary spontaneous pneumothorax (<20% diameter of hemithorax or depth <2cm) • **Supplemental oxygen** and observation if asymptomatic, and stable vital signs • Decompression: indicated for large primary spontaneous pneumothorax (depth >3cm) • Needle aspiration vs. chest tube thoracostomy • **Needle Aspiration followed by Chest Tube Thoracostomy: indicated in tension pneumothorax; considered emergent** • Video Assisted Thoracoscopic Surgery (VATS): if recurrent, continuous air leak >1week, high-risk professional patient (diver, pilot, etc.) • *Patient should avoid high pressure changes for minimum 2 weeks after (airplane travel, high altitude, smoking, scuba diving)*
Key Words & Most Common	• Primary Spontaneous: most common in tall, thin, male age 20-40 with no underlying lung disease or smokers. • Secondary Spontaneous: most common in those with underlying lung disease • Tension: emergent • Unilateral pleuritic chest pain; hyperresonance to percussion, decreased breath sounds, may have wheezing • CXR: initial test of choice; if tension pneumothorax, should be treated based on symptoms and exam • Needle aspiration followed by chest tube thoracostomy

Absent Lung Markings
Mediastinal Shift to the Right
Collapsed Left Lung

Pulmonary Hypertension

Etiology & Risk Factors	• Elevated pulmonary artery pressure ≥20 mmHg • Etiology: **increased pressure in the pulmonary circulation** • Primary: **idiopathic (most common in middle-aged women with metabolic syndrome and HTN)**, toxin-induced, connective tissue disorders • Secondary: left-sided heart failure, COPD, chronic pulmonary thromboembolism, **sleep apnea**, autoimmune disorders, **pregnancy** • Risk Factors: female, age (middle-aged adults most common), family history, connective tissue disorders, congenital heart disease, left heart disease, certain medications (stimulant appetite suppressants; fenfluramine and dexfenfluramine), living at high altitudes (due to the lower oxygen levels and the body's adaptive responses to altitude)
Patho-physiology	• Increased arterial vascular resistance and vessel narrowing leads to right ventricular hypertrophy and increased pressure ultimately causing right-sided heart failure
Signs & Symptoms	• **Exertional dyspnea is most common symptom** • Fatigue, weakness, chest pain, palpitations, lower extremity edema; dizziness, presyncope/syncope if severe • Physical Exam: • Accentuated S2, tachycardia, pulmonary or tricuspid regurgitation murmurs; right-sided heart failure signs (increased JVP, peripheral edema, ascites)
Diagnosis	• Chest X-Ray (CXR): right atrial enlargement, prominent pulmonary vasculature (congestion), pulmonary artery dilation • Electrocardiogram (ECG): **cor pulmonale (right ventricular hypertrophy, right axis deviation, right atrial enlargement, right bundle branch block)**; S1Q3T3, PAC's • Echocardiogram: **pulmonary artery systolic pressure >40 mmHg or mean pulmonary artery pressure >25 mmHg**; right ventricle hypertrophy, tricuspid valve regurgitation, dilated right ventricle • Labs: CBC may show polycythemia with elevated hematocrit; elevated BNP • Pulmonary Artery Catheterization: invasive but definitive test; can test pulmonary artery pressure(PAP) and pulmonary capillary wedge pressure (PCWP) • Mean PAP >25 mmHg with associated PCWP <15 mmHg is diagnostic of PAH • Elevated mean PAP and PCWP >15 mmHg is typical in patients with pulmonary hypertension as a result of left sided heart disease
Treatment	• Address/Correct Underlying Etiology: smoking, pregnancy, high-altitude, use of sympathomimetics • **Calcium Channel Blockers**: nifedipine, diltiazem, amlodipine; **first-line with positive vasoreactivity trial** • **Prostacyclin Analogs**: epoprostenol, iloprost; activate prostacyclin receptor causing pulmonary vasodilation • **Phosphodiesterase-5 Inhibitors**: sildenafil, tadalafil; inhibit enzymatic process which increases c-GMP causing systemic vasodilation • Endothelin Receptor Antagonists: bosentan, ambrisentan; antagonize endothelin receptors and inhibit vasoconstriction • Adjunctive Therapy: **supplemental oxygen**, diuretics, long-term anticoagulation • Heart-Lung Transplant: definitive treatment; last-resort treatment
Key Words & Most Common	• Elevated pulmonary artery pressure ≥20 mmHg; most common in middle-aged women with metabolic syndrome and HTN; sleep apnea, pregnancy; COPD • Exertional dyspnea • ECG: cor pulmonale; echo shows increased pulmonary artery pressures; pulmonary artery catheterization is definitive but invasive test • Treatment relies of pulmonary vasodilation and inhibiting vasoconstriction; CCBs first line if vasoreactivity

Pulmonary Embolism (PE)

Etiology & Risk Factors	• Occlusion of the pulmonary arteries secondary to a blood clot (thromboembolism from lower extremity DVT)
	• Etiology: occlusion of pulmonary arteries
	  • **Thromboembolism: venous thromboembolism originating from deep vein in legs or pelvis is most common cause**
	  • **Non-Thrombotic Sources:** air embolism, fat embolism, infected material, foreign body, tumor, central venous catheters
	• Risk Factors: **Virchow's Triad (endothelial damage** [trauma, inflammation, infection] + **venous stasis** [**surgery**, prolonged sitting, immobilization] + **hypercoagulability** [OCP use, **malignancy**, pregnancy, smoking, genetic risk factors])

Patho-physiology	• Clot breaks off from a lower extremity thrombus and embolizes into pulmonary vascular circulation and eventually obstructs pulmonary blood flow • Larger emboli may lead to reflexive increase in ventilation, hypoxemia (as a result of ventilation/perfusion [V/Q] mismatch) and low venous oxygenation content (secondary to low cardiac output), atelectasis (due to alveolar hypocapnia) • Increased pulmonary vascular resistance from mechanical obstruction and vasoconstriction may cause tachycardia and hypotension

Signs & Symptoms	• **Sudden onset dyspnea (most common symptom), pleuritic chest pain, hemoptysis**, cough, palpitations, calf/thigh pain
	• Physical Exam:
	  • **Tachypnea (most common sign), tachycardia, hypoxia**, arrythmias
	  • **Evidence of DVT:** calf/thigh swelling, palpable cord, discoloration, + Homan sign)
	  • **Homan's Sign:** pain behind the knee upon forced dorsiflexion of the foot

Diagnosis	• Assess Pre-Test Probability: **Modified Well's Criteria**; assess for lower extremity DVT (lower extremity doppler US)
	• Labs: **D-Dimer** (elevated due to acute thrombotic process, high negative predictive value); ABG (may show respiratory alkalosis and hypoxemia)
	• Electrocardiogram (ECG): sinus tachycardia is most common finding; nonspecific ST segment and T wave changes; **S1Q3T3 is most specific for PE** (deep S wave lead I, Q wave and inverted T wave in lead III); right bundle branch block, right ventricular strain
	• Chest X-Ray: often normal, may show atelectasis
	  • **Westermark's Sign:** focal loss of vascular markings distal to PE
	  • **Hampton's Hump:** wedge shaped density due to infarction
	• **CT Pulmonary Angiography: best initial test to confirm pulmonary embolism**, >95% sensitivity and specificity
	• Ventilation Perfusion (V/Q) Scan: utilized when CT scan contraindicated (**pregnancy**, renal disease)
	• Pulmonary Angiography: **gold standard definitive test** but not commonly ordered

Treatment	• Supportive: supplemental oxygen, hemodynamic support (pressors, IV fluids) • **Anticoagulation: first-line therapy; low-molecular weight heparin**, fondaparinux or heparin bridge with warfarin or newer oral anticoagulants (apixaban, rivaroxaban, dabigatran) • IVC Filter: indicated in patients that cannot tolerate anticoagulation (bleeding disorder, bleed risk), **recurrent PE**; unsuccessful anticoagulation • Thrombolysis: indicated for hemodynamically unstable patients or massive PE • Surgical Embolectomy: indicated for massive PE and thrombolysis is contraindicated or fails

Acute Respiratory Distress Syndrome (ARDS)

Etiology & Risk Factors	• Acute, diffuse inflammatory lung injury; can be **life threatening**
	  • Characterized by bilateral pulmonary infiltrates, progressive hypoxemia, rapid onset, and absence of cardiogenic pulmonary edema
	• Etiology: airspace filling
	  • **Elevated alveolar capillary hydrostatic pressure** (left ventricular failure [pulmonary edema] or hypervolemia)
	  • **Increased alveolar capillary permeability**
	  • **Blood** (diffuse alveolar hemorrhage) **or inflammatory exudates** (pneumonia, inflammatory lung conditions)
	• Risk Factors: **critically ill patients (gram negative sepsis is most common)**, trauma, pancreatitis, aspiration, drowning, drug overdose, burns, advanced age, female, smokers, alcohol use, recent cardiac or vascular surgery

Patho-physiology	• Diffuse alveolar-capillary damage characterized by inflammation, apoptosis, necrosis, and increased alveolar-capillary permeability • Increased permeability leads to the development of noncardiogenic alveolar edema which reduces gas exchange and causes **hypoxemia without hypercarbia**

Signs & Symptoms	• **Acute dyspnea and hypoxemia**, altered mental status
	• Physical Exam:
	  • Tachypnea, labored breathing
	  • Diffuse crackles on auscultation

Diagnosis	• Pulse Oximetry/ABG: **hypoxemia** • **Chest X-Ray (CXR): bilateral diffuse pulmonary infiltrates that do not affect costophrenic angles** (non cardiogenic origin)

Treatment	• Treat Underlying Etiology: cover for sepsis (broad spectrum antibiotics)
	• Supplemental Oxygen: non-rebreather, full-mask CPAP, BiPAP, high-flow nasal cannula
	• Mechanical Ventilation: secure airway
	  • Low Tidal Volume: decreases non-pulmonary organ failure, prevents volutrauma
	  • Positive End-Expiration Pressure: reduces hypoxemia by preventing alveolar collapse, improves ventilation/perfusion mismatch
	• Extracorporeal Membrane Oxygenation (ECMO): salvage therapy for refractory ARDS patients

Bilateral diffuse pulmonary infiltrates; sparing of costophrenic angles

Key Words & Most Common	• Life threatening inflammatory lung injury most common in critically ill (septic) patients • Acute dyspnea and hypoxemia • Hypoxemia on pulse ox and ABG • CXR shows bilateral diffuse pulmonary infiltrates • Oxygen support +/- Mechanical ventilation

Hypoxemia	PaO_2/FiO_2 Ratio (mmHg)
Severe	100 or less
Moderate	101-200
Mild	201-300

Obstructive Sleep Apnea

Etiology & Risk Factors	• Characterized by periodic episodes of complete (apnea) or partial (hypopnea) cessation of normal respiration during sleep; often associated with decline in oxygen saturation • <u>Etiology</u>: **partial or complete closure of the upper airway occurring during sleep** • <u>Risk Factors</u>: **obesity (most common risk factor)**, high BMI, advanced age, males, pregnancy, central fat distribution, large neck circumference • **Anatomical Predisposition**: prominent tongue base, thick pharyngeal walls, "crowded" oropharynx
Patho-physiology	• Upper airway obstruction as a result of anatomical reduction of upper airway size or soft tissue collapse • Decreased transmural pressure of oropharynx causes airway reduction and pharyngeal closure leading to hypercapnia, hypoxia, and/or apnea leading to heightened arousal (waking) to maintain respiratory effort and maintain an open airway
Signs & Symptoms	• **Excessive, chronic, daytime sleepiness** (insidious in onset) • Snoring, gasping, breathing cessation (most commonly noticed by partner) • Headaches (worse in morning, bifrontal)
Diagnosis	• <u>Nighttime In-Laboratory Polysomnography</u>: **gold-standard diagnostic test** • Patient is monitored with EEG leads, pulse ox, temperature and nasal/oral airway pressure sensors • <u>Home Sleep Testing</u>: good for patients with high pre-test probability • <u>Labs</u>: CBC to check for polycythemia secondary to chronic hypoxemia • <u>Epworth Sleepiness Scale or STOP-Bang Questionnaire</u>: helps quantify severity
Treatment	• <u>Lifestyle Modifications</u>: **weight loss**, positional change while sleeping (elevating head of bed), exercise, abstaining from alcohol or sedative medications • **Continuous Positive Airway Pressure (CPAP): most effective treatment** • <u>Oral Appliance Therapy</u>: bite guard pulls lower jaw forward to open airway; used as adjunct if CPAP is unsuccessful • <u>Surgery</u>: surgical resection of obstructing lesion; nasal septoplasty or uvulopalatopharyngoplasty • *Evaluate for other causes including allergic rhinitis, deviated septum, thyroid lesion*
Key Words & Most Common	• Periods of apnea or hypopnea episodes during sleep • Obesity and large neck circumference is most common risk factor • Excessive daytime sleepiness; snoring/gasping • Polysomnography is gold standard • Weight loss + CPAP Partial obstruction of upper airway Prominent tongue base

Cor Pulmonale

Etiology & Risk Factors	• **Hypertrophy or dilation of the right ventricle primarily caused by respiratory system disorder and/or pulmonary hypertension** • *Right-sided heart failure that occurs as a result of left-sided heart failure or congenital heart disease is not considered cor pulmonale* • <u>Etiology</u>: **COPD is most common cause**; pulmonary hypertension, interstitial lung disease, obstructive sleep apnea, autoimmune or cystic fibrosis, pulmonary embolism • <u>Risk Factors</u>: advanced age, male, family history, smoking, high-altitude living, chronic lung disease, sleep-disordered breathing
Patho-physiology	• Chronic vasoconstriction (secondary to chronic hypoxemia) causes endothelial remodeling leading to increased pulmonary vascular resistance, pulmonary arterial pressure, right ventricular workload that eventually causes right ventricular failure • Right ventricular remodeling occurs (hypertrophy, dilation, or both)

Signs & Symptoms	• **Dyspnea on exertion (most common symptom)**, fatigue, lethargy, cough, hemoptysis
	• Physical Exam:
	   • <u>Heart Failure Signs</u>: **jugular venous distension (JVD)**, tachypnea, lower extremity edema, hepatomegaly, ascites
	   • Loud S2, tricuspid or pulmonic insufficiency murmurs

Diagnosis	• <u>Chest X-Ray (CXR)</u>: **prominent pulmonary vasculature**, cardiomegaly • <u>Electrocardiogram (ECG)</u>: **right ventricular hypertrophy**, right axis deviation, right bundle branch block • <u>Echocardiogram</u>: **right ventricular enlargement/dilation**, increased right sided pressure, tricuspid/pulmonic insufficiency • <u>CT Angiography vs V/Q Scan</u>: rules out PE as possible etiology
Treatment	• <u>Treat Underlying Etiology</u>: manage COPD or underlying lung disease, smoking cessation • <u>Supplemental Oxygen</u>: decreases pulmonary vasoconstriction to increase cardiac output • <u>Diuretics</u>: decreases right ventricular filling volume • <u>Calcium Channel Blockers</u>: causes vasodilation of pulmonary arteries to reduce vascular resistance Right ventricular hypertrophy and dilation RV LV
Key Words & Most Common	• Hypertrophy or dilation of right ventricle as a result of respiratory disorder and/or pulmonary hypertension • COPD is most common cause • Dyspnea on exertion; jugular venous distension • CXR shows prominent pulmonary vasculature; ECG shows right side strain • Treat underlying etiology

Hyaline Membrane Disease

Etiology & Risk Factors	• Also known as neonatal respiratory distress syndrome; common cause of respiratory distress in newborn presents immediately or within minutes to hours after birth • <u>Etiology</u>: **surfactant deficiency from immature lung formation** or inadequate surfactant production; may be genetic • <u>Risk Factor</u>: **small for gestational age, prematurity**, monozygotic twins, Cesarean section or rapid delivery, maternal diabetes
Patho-physiology	• Surfactant deficiency in setting of immature lungs increases surface tension within alveoli and small airways and decreases overall lung compliance • Balance of air-fluid pressure is necessary to prevent alveolar collapse or filling with fluid

Signs & Symptoms	• <u>Respiratory Distress</u>: usually immediately after birth
	  • **Tachypnea** (>60 respirations per minute), tachycardia, **chest wall retractions with use of accessory muscles**, nasal flaring, cyanosis, expiratory grunting
	  • **Presents at birth or within minutes to hours after birth**

Diagnosis	• <u>Chest X-Ray (CXR)</u>: **best initial test**
	  • **Ground-glass reticulo-granular opacities with air bronchograms is pathognomonic**
	  • Bell-shaped thorax (decreased lung volume), peri-hilar streaking (lymph system engorgement)
	• <u>Arterial Blood Gas (ABG)</u>: **hypoxemia** (may or may not be responsive to supplemental oxygen), may show respiratory and metabolic acidosis

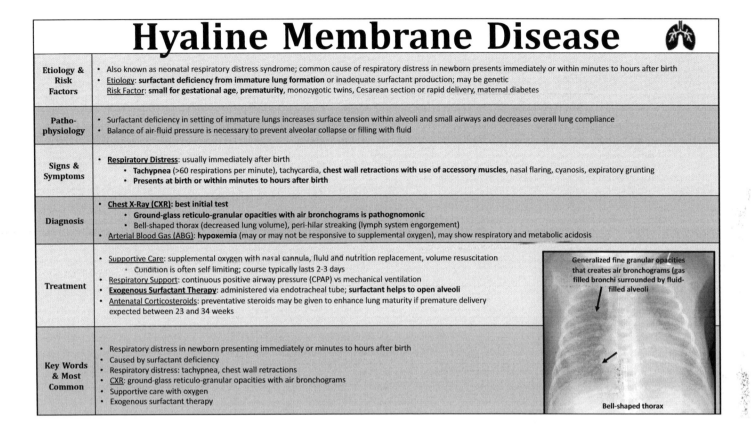

Generalized fine granular opacities that creates air bronchograms (gas filled bronchi surrounded by fluid-filled alveoli

Bell-shaped thorax

Treatment	• <u>Supportive Care</u>: supplemental oxygen with nasal cannula, fluid and nutrition replacement, volume resuscitation • Condition is often self limiting; course typically lasts 2-3 days • <u>Respiratory Support</u>: continuous positive airway pressure (CPAP) vs mechanical ventilation • <u>Exogenous Surfactant Therapy</u>: administered via endotracheal tube; **surfactant helps to open alveoli** • <u>Antenatal Corticosteroids</u>: preventative steroids may be given to enhance lung maturity if premature delivery expected between 23 and 34 weeks
Key Words & Most Common	• Respiratory distress in newborn presenting immediately or minutes to hours after birth • Caused by surfactant deficiency • Respiratory distress: tachypnea, chest wall retractions • CXR: ground-glass reticulo-granular opacities with air bronchograms • Supportive care with oxygen • Exogenous surfactant therapy

References

1. Article river a52123f05cfb11e9afb233c9de065d31-fig-3.png. (2022, January 22). *Wikimedia Commons*. Retrieved 15:41, August 3, 2023 from https://commons.wikimedia.org/w/index.php?title=File:Article_river_a52123f05cfb11e9afb233c9de065d31-fig-3.png&oldid=623540517.
2. Pulmon fibrosis.PNG. (2020, September 15). *Wikimedia Commons*. Retrieved 15:32, August 3, 2023 from https://commons.wikimedia.org/w/index.php?title=File:Pulmon_fibrosis.PNG&oldid=459680530.
3. Chronic beryllioisis - Case 293 (15528999565).jpg. (2023, April 10). *Wikimedia Commons*. Retrieved 15:20, August 3, 2023 from https://commons.wikimedia.org/w/index.php?title=File:Chronic_beryllioisis_-_Case_293_(15528999565).jpg&oldid=748894942.
4. Asbestosis 2.jpg. (2023, January 3). *Wikimedia Commons*. Retrieved 15:15, August 3, 2023 from https://commons.wikimedia.org/w/index.php?title=File:Asbestosis_2.jpg&oldid=722403848.
5. Epiglottitis.jpg. (2020, October 28). *Wikimedia Commons*. Retrieved 17:37, August 3, 2023 from https://commons.wikimedia.org/w/index.php?title=File:Epiglottitis.jpg&oldid=504879377.
6. Croup steeple sign.jpg. (2022, dicembre 21). *Wikimedia Commons*. Retrieved 17:34, agosto 3, 2023 from https://commons.wikimedia.org/w/index.php?title=File:Croup_steeple_sign.jpg&oldid=718568196.
7. Chest X-ray in influenza and Haemophilus influenzae - annotated.jpg. (2020, September 30). *Wikimedia Commons*. Retrieved 18:14, August 6, 2023 from https://commons.wikimedia.org/w/index.php?title=File:Chest_X-ray_in_influenza_and_Haemophilus_influenzae_-_annotated.jpg&oldid=476158629.
8. Wikipedia contributors. (2023, August 3). Aspiration pneumonia. In *Wikipedia, The Free Encyclopedia*. Retrieved 18:15, August 6, 2023, from https://en.wikipedia.org/w/index.php?title=Aspiration_pneumonia&oldid=1168509090
9. Chest X-ray acute pulmonary histoplasmosis PHIL 3954.jpg. (2022, February 11). *Wikimedia Commons*. Retrieved 18:30, August 6, 2023 from https://commons.wikimedia.org/w/index.php?title=File:Chest_X-ray_acute_pulmonary_histoplasmosis_PHIL_3954.jpg&oldid=629119845.
10. Solitary pulmonary nodule CT arrow.jpg. (2020, October 29). *Wikimedia Commons*. Retrieved 19:58, August 6, 2023 from https://commons.wikimedia.org/w/index.php?title=File:Solitary_pulmonary_nodule_CT_arrow.jpg&oldid=505964824.
11. LungCACXR.PNG. (2023, July 5). *Wikimedia Commons*. Retrieved 20:55, August 6, 2023 from https://commons.wikimedia.org/w/index.php?title=File:LungCACXR.PNG&oldid=780632283.
12. Superior.vena.cava.syndrome.aak.jpg. (2023, January 7). *Wikimedia Commons*. Retrieved 21:04, August 6, 2023 from https://commons.wikimedia.org/w/index.php?title=File:Superior.vena.cava.syndrome.aak.jpg&oldid=723539625.
13. Pancoast Tumor 1.jpg. (2020, September 30). *Wikimedia Commons*. Retrieved 21:23, August 6, 2023 from https://commons.wikimedia.org/w/index.php?title=File:Pancoast_Tumor_1.jpg&oldid=476533134.
14. Foreign body aspiration.jpg. (2020, October 21). *Wikimedia Commons*. Retrieved 21:40, August 6, 2023 from https://commons.wikimedia.org/w/index.php?title=File:Foreign_body_aspiration.jpg&oldid=496741551.
15. Costal Cartilage.png. (2020, October 24). *Wikimedia Commons*. Retrieved 21:46, August 6, 2023 from https://commons.wikimedia.org/w/index.php?title=File:Costal_Cartilage.png&oldid=498968734.
16. Left-sided Pleural Effusion.jpg. (2022, September 29). *Wikimedia Commons*. Retrieved 21:51, August 6, 2023 from https://commons.wikimedia.org/w/index.php?title=File:Left-sided_Pleural_Effusion.jpg&oldid=692841363.
17. 05-Spontanpneumothorax.jpg. (2023, February 28). *Wikimedia Commons*. Retrieved 13:08, August 7, 2023 from https://commons.wikimedia.org/w/index.php?title=File:05-Spontanpneumothorax.jpg&oldid=736717144.
18. ARDSSevere.png. (2023, June 20). *Wikimedia Commons*. Retrieved 14:34, August 7, 2023 from https://commons.wikimedia.org/w/index.php?title=File:ARDSSevere.png&oldid=775791009.
19. Obstruction ventilation apnée sommeil.svg. (2022, December 11). *Wikimedia Commons*. Retrieved 15:32, August 7, 2023 from https://commons.wikimedia.org/w/index.php?title=File:Obstruction_ventilation_apn%C3%A9e_sommeil.svg&oldid=714114092.
20. 525-cor-pulmonale-echocardiogram-s118-springer-high ru.jpg. (2023, May 31). *Wikimedia Commons*. Retrieved 17:34, August 7, 2023 from https://commons.wikimedia.org/w/index.php?title=File:525-cor-pulmonale-echocardiogram-s118-springer-high_ru.jpg&oldid=768904718.
21. X-ray of infant respiratory distress syndrome (IRDS).png. (2020, September 17). *Wikimedia Commons*. Retrieved 18:27, August 7, 2023 from https://commons.wikimedia.org/w/index.php?title=File:X-ray_of_infant_respiratory_distress_syndrome_(IRDS).png&oldid=462195611.

Chapter 3
Gastrointestinal

Cholelithiasis

Etiology & Risk Factors	• Hardened deposits of digestive fluid (gallstones) that form in the gallbladder; may develop complications including cholecystitis, choledocholithiasis, pancreatitis, or cholangitis
	• <u>Etiology</u>: biliary sludge often evolves into gallstones
	• <u>Risk Factors</u>: obesity, age, female gender, cirrhosis, pregnancy, infection, rapid weight loss, hypertriglyceridemia, oral contraceptive use
	   • <u>5 F's</u>: **Fat, Forty, Fair, Fertile, Female**
	• <u>Types</u>:
	   • <u>**Cholesterol**</u>: **most common type (90%)**
	   • <u>Black</u>: hemolysis, cirrhosis, sickle cell anemia, cystic fibrosis
	   • <u>Brown</u>: southeast Asian population; chronic bacterial or parasitic infection

Patho-physiology	• <u>Cholesterol Saturation</u>: liver produces more cholesterol than bile can dissolve; cholesterol may precipitate crystals and form stones • <u>Excess Bilirubin</u>: certain hematologic conditions may lead to excess bilirubin production which can cause gallstone formation • <u>Gallbladder Hypomotility</u>: gallbladder does not effectively empty bile; bile becomes concentrated and stagnant and forms gallstones
Signs & Symptoms	• **Mostly asymptomatic** • Symptoms occur when gallstone enters cystic duct opening • <u>Biliary Colic</u>: intermittent episodes of **right upper quadrant pain that slowly resolve over 30-90 minutes** • **Often triggered by fatty/greasy or large meal**
Diagnosis	• <u>Abdominal Ultrasound</u>: **first-line and most sensitive initial test** • <u>Abdominal CT Scan</u>: may be utilized to determine other causes of abdominal pain; does not increase sensitivity to cholelithiasis diagnosis

Treatment	• <u>Asymptomatic</u>: **observation**, dietary modifications (avoid greasy/fatty/spicy foods); educate on signs and symptoms of biliary colic and when to seek medical attention
	• <u>Symptomatic</u>:
	   • <u>Medical Management</u>: ursodeoxycholic acid; takes 9-12 months to reach therapeutic levels and only effective on stones <1cm, cholesterol, only effective in 50%
	   • <u>**Elective Cholecystectomy**</u>: **definitive treatment**

Key Words & Most Common	• 5 F's = Fat, Forty, Fair, Fertile, Female • Cholesterol is most common type • Asymptomatic; biliary colic (RUQ pain that is triggered by high fat/greasy/spicy meal) • US is first line test • Asymptomatic = observation; symptomatic = elective cholecystectomy

Acute Cholecystitis

Etiology & Risk Factors	• Inflammation of the gallbladder secondary to obstruction of the cystic duct • <u>Etiology</u>: gallstones are **most commonly cause; biliary sludge** • <u>Risk Factors</u>: **recent spicy or greasy meal** (stimulates emptying of bile from the gallbladder, cholelithiasis blocks cystic duct); history of cholelithiasis, female, obesity, oral contraceptive pills, high-fat diet
Patho-physiology	• Gallbladder is stimulated to empty bile through cystic duct to duodenum after a high-fat meal; obstruction of cystic duct leads to acute inflammation • Inflammation can eventually lead to ischemia of the gallbladder wall which increases risk of infection

Signs & Symptoms	• **Right upper quadrant pain**
	   • Pain may radiate to back or shoulder
	• Inability to tolerate certain foods (especially **high fat/greasy** or spicy foods; large meals) leading to bloating, gas, nausea/vomiting
	   • May be a specific dietary etiology "I had cheeseburger and chili cheese fries"
	• <u>Physical Exam</u>: fever (low grade); enlarged gallbladder
	   • <u>**Murphy's Sign**</u>: RUQ pain with inspiratory arrest with deep palpation of the gallbladder
	   • <u>Boas Sign</u>: referred pain to right shoulder (phrenic nerve pain)

Diagnosis	• <u>**Abdominal Ultrasound**</u>: **best initial test**; may show thickened walls (>3mm) and pericholecystic fluid (indicates infection), gallstones, sonographic Murphy's sign • <u>Abdominal CT Scan</u>: if lack of evidence to support diagnosis with just US; evaluates for other complications including pancreatitis or gallbladder perforation • <u>Labs</u>: CBC shows ↑WBCs (leukocytosis with left shift), ↑LFTs (obstructive), ↑bilirubin; *consider amylase/lipase to evaluate pancreatitis* • <u>HIDA Scan</u>: **gold standard test**; ordered when other tests are equivocal
Treatment	• <u>Supportive</u>: nothing by mouth (**NPO**), **IV fluid hydration**, analgesia (NSAIDs [ketorolac] if tolerated) • <u>Nasogastric Suction</u>: indicated if vomiting or ileus present for gastric decompression • <u>Antibiotics</u>: metronidazole + ceftriaxone *OR* metronidazole + ciprofloxacin; piperacillin/tazobactam • <u>**Surgery**</u>: **laparoscopic cholecystectomy is preferred and definitive treatment** • <u>Percutaneous Cholecystostomy</u>: reserved for high-risk surgical patients
Key Words & Most Common	• Inflammation of gallbladder secondary to gallstone obstruction of cystic duct • Most commonly follows high fat, greasy, or spicy meal • RUQ pain, + Murphy's sign • US is best initial test; HIDA scan gold standard • NPO, IV fluids, IV antibiotics, followed by cholecystectomy

Gallbladder wall thickness

Stones within gallbladder

Acute Ascending Cholangitis

Etiology & Risk Factors	• **Life-threatening ascending bacterial infection of the common bile duct** • <u>Etiology</u>: **choledocholithiasis** (stones in common bile duct) **is most common cause**; biliary tract strictures, malignancy, pancreatic cancer, parasites, biliary sludge deposits • <u>Risk Factors</u>: high triglycerides, sedentary lifestyle, high BMI (>30), rapid weight loss • <u>Causative Pathogens</u>: ***E. coli* is most common cause**, *Klebsiella, Enterobacter, Pseudomonas, B. fragilis*
Patho-physiology	• Acute infection and inflammation of the common bile duct caused by obstruction of biliary flow • Bacteria and endotoxins released lead to infection and may cause biliary septicemia or hepatic abscess
Signs & Symptoms	• <u>**Charcot's Triad**</u>: **fever + right upper quadrant pain + jaundice** • <u>**Reynold's Pentad**</u>: fever + right upper quadrant pain + jaundice + altered mental status + sepsis/hypotension
Diagnosis	• <u>Labs</u>: CBC (**leukocytosis** with neutrophil predominance); LFTs (↑**Alkaline phosphatase, ↑GGT and ↑conjugated bilirubin**); consider blood cultures • <u>**Abdominal Ultrasound**</u>: **first-line imaging test**; shows dilated common bile duct and choledocholithiasis • <u>Abdominal CT Scan</u>: helps to identify pathologies such as tumors, metastases or abscess • <u>Magnetic Resonance Cholangiopancreatography (MRCP)</u>: most sensitive imaging test • <u>**Endoscopic Retrograde Cholangiopancreatography (ERCP)**</u>: **gold standard** to establish diagnosis and may be used for intervention
Treatment	• <u>Sepsis Resuscitation</u>: IV fluids, electrolyte replacement, antipyretics, ABCs, hemodynamic support • <u>**IV Antibiotics**</u>: metronidazole + ceftriaxone *OR* metronidazole + ciprofloxacin; piperacillin/tazobactam, ampicillin/sulbactam • <u>**Endoscopic Retrograde Cholangiopancreatography (ERCP)**</u>: **gold standard treatment for biliary decompression**; performed once patient is stable and afebrile for ~48 hours • <u>Percutaneous Transhepatic Cholangiogram (PTC)</u>: biliary decompression method if unable to do ERCP
Key Words & Most Common	• Ascending bacterial infection of common bile duct most commonly caused by choledocholithiasis • E. coli is most commonly implicated bacteria • <u>Charcot's Triad</u>: fever + right upper quadrant pain + jaundice • <u>Reynold's Pentad</u>: fever + right upper quadrant pain + jaundice + altered mental status + sepsis/hypotension • US is first line imaging test but CT scan utilized to determine source of obstruction • ERCP is diagnostic and therapeutic

Neonatal Jaundice

Etiology & Risk Factors	• Neonatal hyperbilirubinemia is caused by elevated serum bilirubin and presents as **yellow discoloration of skin, sclera, mucosal membranes and conjunctiva** • **60% of full-term and 90% of pre-term neonates develop jaundice within 1 week after birth** • <u>Etiology</u>: biliary stasis • <u>Risk Factors</u>: **prematurity, maternal diabetes**, poor oral intake, congenital hypothyroidism, intestinal obstruction, gestational exposure to sulfa or cephalosporins

Patho-physiology	• <u>Physiologic Jaundice</u>: presents about 24 hours after delivery and peaks at 2-4 days; usually resolves within 2-3 weeks
	  • Inadequate uridine diphosphate glucuronosyltransferase (UGT) – the enzyme needed for bilirubin conjugation
	  • Inadequate number of bowel movements (bilirubin excreted through feces)
	  • Poor metabolization of lipid processing by immature liver
	• <u>Pathologic Jaundice</u>: if presents on first day of life and lasts more than 2 weeks; bilirubin levels continue to rise
	  • Crigler-Najjar syndrome, Gilbert syndrome, hemolytic anemia affect bilirubin clearance

Signs & Symptoms	• <u>Jaundice</u>: yellowish discoloration of skin, sclera, mucosal membranes and conjunctiva
	  • **Bilirubin level > 5 mg/dL**
	• Weight loss, evidence of dehydration, few bowel movements
	• <u>**Kernicterus**</u>: encephalopathy secondary to bilirubin deposits in brain tissue
	  • Poor feeding, lethargy, seizures, developmental delays, altered sleep, abnormal tone
	  • **Bilirubin level > 20mg/dL**

Diagnosis	• <u>**Total and Direct Bilirubin Levels**</u>: should trend levels over day(s) • <u>Complete Blood Count (CBC)</u>: evaluates for hemolytic anemia or polycythemia • <u>Coombs Test</u>: distinguishes immune vs non-immune hemolytic disorder
Treatment	• <u>**Observation**</u>: indicated for physiologic jaundice; daily monitoring of bilirubin levels • <u>**Phytotherapy**</u>: **first-line treatment of choice**; initiate based on total bilirubin level (see chart) • <u>Exchange Transfusion</u>: consider for bilirubin encephalopathy
Key Words & Most Common	• Elevated serum bilirubin; more common in pre-term infants • Jaundice: yellow discoloration of skin, sclera, and mucosal membranes/conjunctiva • Kernicterus: bilirubin encephalopathy • Monitor total and direct bilirubin levels • Phytotherapy is first line treatment of choice

Phytotherapy Guidelines
Total Bilirubin Cutoff by Risk Group

Age	Low Risk	Medium Risk	High Risk
Birth	7.0	5.0	4.0
24 hrs	11.5	9.0	8.0
48 hrs	15.0	14.0	10.0
72 hrs	17.5	15.0	14.0
96 hrs	20	17.5	14.5
5+ days	21	17.5	15

• Low risk = born full-term with no risk factors
• Medium Risk = born full-term with risk factors or born 35-57 weeks without risk factors
• High Risk = born <38 weeks with risk factors

Constipation

Etiology & Risk Factors	• Decreased frequency of bowel movements (less than 2 per week) with associated straining or pain, hard stool, or sensation of incomplete void
	• Etiology: multiple
	   • Functional: withholding behaviors; other causes ruled out
	   • Anatomical: anal/intestinal stricture or stenosis; malignancy (mass causing partial obstruction)
	   • Muscular: Down syndrome, muscular dystrophy
	   • Neurologic Abnormality/Outlet Delay: Hirschsprung's disease, spinal cord defect, dementia, cerebral palsy
	   • Medication: anticholinergics, opioids, vitamin D intoxication
	   • Metabolic: hypokalemia, hypercalcemia, diabetes
	   • Other: cystic fibrosis, allergies, inflammatory bowel disease, celiac disease, irritable bowel syndrome
	• Risk Factors: **poor diet, dehydration**, low fiber, caffeine intake, psychologic condition, hypothyroidism

Patho-physiology	• Slow motility of intestine leads to increased water absorption which causes firmer stool making it harder to pass
Signs & Symptoms	• **2 or fewer bowel movements per week** • **Hard or painful stool**; large fecal mass • Physical Exam: • Assess for "alarm" signs/symptoms such as fever, abdominal distention/pain, weight loss, nausea, vomiting
Diagnosis	• **Clinical Diagnosis** • Digital Rectal Exam: stool in rectal vault • Abdominal X-Ray: may show stool particularly in descending or sigmoid colon • Abdominal CT Scan: if concern for obstruction
Treatment	• Supportive: adequate fluid intake, fibrous foods, exercise, sorbitol containing juices (apple juice, prune juice) • Emollient: docusate sodium is a stool softener that facilitates stool fat and water combination • Osmotic Laxatives: polyethylene glycol, lactulose, saline laxative (milk of magnesia); causes stool water retention through osmotic effect • Bulk Forming Laxative: psyllium, methylcellulose, wheat dextran helps stool absorb water and increase mass • Stimulant Laxative: senna, bisacodyl increases peristalsis and stimulates colonic motility to pass stool
Key Words & Most Common	• Decreased frequency of bowel movements most commonly as a result of poor diet or dehydration • <2 bowel movements per week; hard or painful stool • Clinical diagnosis; digital rectal exam v CT/Xray if concerned for obstruction • Supportive with fluid intake, fiber, and exercise is mainstay

Significant stool in colon

Fecal Impaction

Etiology & Risk Factors	• Impaction occurs when hardened, bulky fecal matter is retained in the rectum and cannot be evacuated with normal peristalsis
	• Etiology: large, hardened mass of stool
	   • Medications: anticholinergics, **opioids**, antipsychotics
	   • Anatomic: malignancy, anorectal disorder, Hirschsprung's disease
	   • Neurologic: dementia, cerebral palsy, spinal cord injury, pelvic floor dysfunction, psychiatric or cognitive disorders
	• Risk Factors: **advanced age (most common among elderly especially in hospital or institutional care)**, chronic constipation, low fiber diet, **dehydration**, lack of physical activity, neurologic disorders, malignancy

Patho-physiology	• Slow motility of intestine leads to increased water absorption which causes firmer stool making it harder to pass • Fecal impaction then puts intraluminal pressure on sigmoid colon (narrowest section) which may decrease perfusion to colonic wall
Signs & Symptoms	• **Rectal pain or fullness** • **Inability to evacuate stool** or feeling of incomplete evacuation • **Progressive abdominal pain, discomfort, distension** and bloating • Nausea and vomiting, loss of appetite
Diagnosis	• Digital Rectal Exam (DRE): palpable firm stool at rectal vault • Abdominal X-Ray: if DRE is not conclusive; evaluate for free air (perforation) • Abdominal CT Scan: if severe presentation
Treatment	• Distal Impaction: **digital disimpaction** followed by rectal suppository or enema (warm-water enema with mineral oil) • Proximal Impaction: respond better to oral laxatives; **polyethylene glycol** • Surgery: indicated for severe cases and/or signs of perforation, colitis, or peritonitis • Prevention: address risk factors or underlying etiology and maintain bowel regimen
Key Words & Most Common	• Hard bulky fecal matter retained in rectum • Most common in elderly or opioid use • Diagnose with digital rectal exam • Manual digital disimpaction first line followed by rectal suppository • Polytheylene glycol if proximal impaction

Anorectal Abscess and Fistula ⟆

Etiology & Risk Factors	• Bacterial infection of glandular crypts of the rectum/anus
	• Etiology: bacterial infection
	   • Anorectal Abscess: **localized collection of pus forming around the anus or rectum**
	   • Anorectal Fistula: **tubelike tract between anal canal and perianal skin**; seen with deep abscesses
	      • Perianal is most common type of anorectal abscess; **posterior rectal wall most common site**
	   • Pathogens: ***S. aureus* most common**, *E. coli, Proteus, Streptococcus*
	• Risk Factors: **inflammatory bowel disease, Crohn's disease**, chronic constipation, trauma, diabetes mellitus, chronic steroid use, diverticulitis, STIs, poor hygiene, obesity, anal intercourse

Patho-physiology	• Anal glands empty to ducts that drain into the anal crypts; if no adequate drainage, infection can occur and form an abscess that expands and enters perianal or perirectal area • Fluid collection expands and follows "path of least resistance" which may form a fistula to the intersphincter space of anal canal

Signs & Symptoms	• **Rectal pain**; may be described as sharp, dull, or throbbing
	   • **Pain worse with prolonged sitting, defecating, Valsalva**
	• May have spontaneous purulent or bloody drainage especially if fistula present
	• Physical Exam:
	   • **Focal erythema, edema induration of surrounding tissue** (cellulitis), and **fluctuance of abscess**

Diagnosis	• **Clinical Diagnosis** • CT/MRI: may be utilized to establish fistula diagnosis and extent; pre-procedural planning
Treatment	• Incision and Drainage (I&D): **first line and preferred treatment**; commonly performed in outpatient or ER setting • Antibiotics: not always required unless surrounding cellulitis or risk factors (diabetic, elderly, systemic signs, valvular condition) • Anorectal abscesses rarely respond to antibiotics without proper I&D • Surgery: **fistulotomy is gold standard treatment** for acute fistula
Key Words & Most Common	• Bacterial infection of rectum/anus; Perianal most common type • Crohn's disease or inflammatory bowel disease most common causes • Rectal pain +/- spontaneous drainage, surrounding cellulitis • Clinical diagnosis • I&D is mainstay of treatment

Anal Fissure ⟆

Etiology & Risk Factors	• Superficial linear tear/crack of the skin distal to the dentate line of the anus • Etiology: **constipation**, passing of large/hard stool, anal trauma, anal sexual intercourse • Risk Factors: **chronic diarrhea or constipation**, dehydration, low-fiber diet, inflammatory bowel disease
Patho-physiology	• Epithelium of anoderm inferior to dentate line is very sensitive and susceptible to microtrauma. This skin may tear when exposed to trauma or pressure to area. • Skin tear may expose underlying sphincter muscle causing severe pain
Signs & Symptoms	• **Severe sharp rectal pain worse during or immediately after bowel movements** • **Bright red rectal bleeding** (typically small amounts) • Physical Exam: • **Superficial longitudinal tear that extends proximally; most common site is posterior midline**
Diagnosis	• **Clinical Diagnosis** • Valsalva maneuver may help expose fissure to aid in diagnosis • *If atypical location or ulcerating, Crohn's disease should be ruled out*

Treatment	• Supportive: **first-line**; warm Sitz baths (especially after bowel movement), analgesics, stool softeners, increased hydration, high-fiber diet
	   • Most (80%+) resolve spontaneously
	• Topical Treatments: usually used in combination
	   • **Topical Lidocaine:** pain control
	   • **Topical Corticosteroids:** hydrocortisone ointment; anti-inflammatory
	   • **Topical Nitroglycerin:** vasodilator to increase blood flow and aid healing
	   • **Topical Nifedipine:** reduces anal sphincter tone
	• Surgery: lateral internal sphincterotomy for chronic cases that do not respond to conservative measures

Key Words & Most Common	• Linear tear/crack of skin most common at posterior midline • Severe sharp rectal pain with or after a bowel movement • Clinical Diagnosis Warm Sitz baths, topical lidocaine, stool softeners, high-fiber diet

Hemorrhoids

Etiology & Risk Factors	• Vascular tissue of the anal canal submucosa comprised of connective tissue, smooth muscle and blood vessels; **can be internal or external** • Risk Factors: family history, **age, pregnancy**, chronic diarrhea or constipation, sedentary lifestyle, obesity, anal sexual intercourse, inflammatory bowel disease	
	INTERNAL	**EXTERNAL**
	• Originate from superior hemorrhoid vein and **proximal to the dentate line** • Covered with **anorectal mucosa** • Naturally occurring in most individuals; not always pathologic • **More likely to bleed** and usually **painless**	• Originate from inferior hemorrhoid vein and **distal to dentate line** • Covered with **squamous epithelium** • More likely to be pathologic (engorged, prolapsed, or thrombosed) • **Less likely to bleed** and more **painful**
Patho-physiology	• **Raised intraabdominal pressure** leads to decreased venous return from hemorrhoidal veins causing a pathologic engorgement of venous plexuses • Firm stool leads to increased strain which further raises intra-abdominal pressure; as engorgement continues, circulation slows and may become thrombosed	
	INTERNAL	**EXTERNAL**
Signs & Symptoms	• **Intermittent rectal bleeding; bright red blood** coating stool or on toilet paper • **Painless** • May have rectal fullness	• **Perianal pain worse with bowel movement** • **Painful** • May have palpable mass or skin tags • Dark blue/purple and firm if thrombosed
Diagnosis	• Clinical Diagnosis with visual inspection +/- Valsalva • Anoscopy: may be used for direct visualization • Proctosigmoidoscopy or Colonoscopy: indicated in patients with red flag symptoms • Weight loss, continued bleeding, anemia, change in bowel habits	• **Clinical Diagnosis with direct visualization** • Digital rectal exam
Treatment	• Supportive: **high-fiber diet, hydration, warm Sitz baths**, physical activity, witch hazel wipes/pads, avoid hot/spicy/greasy foods • **Topical Medications**: topical steroid ointment (hydrocortisone), topical analgesics (lidocaine) • Procedures: **rubber band ligation (most common)**, injectable sclerotherapy, infrared photocoagulation, excision of thrombosed • Hemorrhoidectomy: surgical procedure indicated for stage IV or failed conservative management	
Key Words & Most Common	• Pregnancy, chronic diarrhea/constipation • Internal more likely to bleed and painless • External less likely to bleed and painful • High fiber diet, hydration, Sitz baths vs rubber band ligation or hemorrhoidectomy if refractory	

External anal sphincter — Internal anal sphincter — Anoderm — External Hemorrhoid — Perianal Vessels — Prolapsing Internal Hemorrhoid — Internal Hemorrhoid Pectinate Line

Diverticulitis

Etiology & Risk Factors	• Inflammation of the diverticulum; can be complicated (perforation, abscess, obstruction, fistula formation) or uncomplicated • Etiology: **inflammation or infection of diverticulum (outpouching herniation of mucosa into wall of colon) due to micro-perforation** • Risk Factors: **low fiber diet, age (>40 years old most common)**, obesity, constipation, **inflammatory diet, medications (NSAIDs**, steroids, opioids), bacterial overgrowth, family history, sedentary lifestyle
Patho-physiology	• Increased intraluminal pressures leads to erosion of the diverticular wall thickened/dehydrated fecal matter which causes micro-perforation leading to inflammation and necrosis of area • Most common pathogens are gram negative rods and anaerobes

Signs & Symptoms	• **Left lower quadrant abdominal pain (most common symptom)**
	     • **Sigmoid colon is most common site** (secondary to high intraluminal pressure)
	 • **Fever**, nausea/vomiting, bloating, increased flatulence
	 • **Change in bowel habits (constipation most common**; diarrhea, painless hematochezia)
	 • Physical Exam:
	     • LLQ tenderness to palpation, tender mass if abscess present
	     • Peritoneal signs (rigidity, guarding, or rebound tenderness) indicates perforation

Diagnosis	• **Clinical Diagnosis** • Labs: may show leukocytosis; elevated inflammatory markers (ESR and CRP) • **CT Scan with IV and PO Contrast: imaging test of choice for diagnosis; indicated for initial presentation** • Shows bowel wall thickening, pericolic fat stranding • Endoscopy/Colonoscopy: should be avoided in acute phase due to risk of perforation

Treatment	• Uncomplicated: mild disease with minimal systemic signs
	     • **Supportive: bowel rest (clear liquid diet** with slow progression/low fiber foods); managed as outpatient
	     • Antibiotics: **metronidazole + ciprofloxacin** OR Metronidazole + trimethoprim/sulfamethoxazole OR amoxicillin/clavulanate
	 • Complicated: perforation, abscess, obstruction, fistula formation, excessive vomiting, immunocompromised, advanced age, high fever
	     • Admission with **IV antibiotics, IV fluids, and pain management**
	     • Large abscesses (>3cm) may be drained percutaneously with CT-guidance
	 • Surgery: frequent recurrence, perforation, or refractory to medical therapy

Key Words & Most Common	• Inflammation of diverticulum due to micro-perforation • Sigmoid colon is most common site • Left lower quadrant abdominal pain; fever • CT scan with IV and PO contrast • Bowel rest + Antibiotics (metronidazole and ciprofloxacin)

Outpouching of the colonic wall, wall thickening, and surrounding fat stranding

Toxic Megacolon

Etiology & Risk Factors	• **Nonobstructive dilation of colon (≥6cm in diameter)** with systemic toxicity as a result of colonic inflammation
	• <u>Etiology</u>: **colonic inflammation**
	   • <u>**Inflammatory**</u>: **ulcerative colitis is most common cause**, Crohn's disease
	   • <u>Infectious</u>: **C. difficile**, Shigella, Campylobacter colitis, **Cytomegalovirus**, E. coli O157
	   <u>Ischemia</u>: volvulus, diverticulitis, obstructive malignancy
	   • <u>Other</u>: medications (antimotility, opioids, anticholinergics); hypokalemia; colonoscopy

Patho-physiology	• Mucosal inflammation leads to release of bacterial byproducts and inflammatory mediators which prompt nitric oxide release can causes colonic dilation • Dilation leads to further smooth muscle inflammation resulting in colonic paralysis and worsening dilation

Signs & Symptoms	• **Abdominal pain +/- distension**
	• **Diarrhea (may or may not be bloody)**; nausea, vomiting
	• <u>**Toxicity Signs**</u>: fever, tachycardia, may have hypotension or altered mental status
	• <u>Physical Exam</u>:
	   • Abdominal tenderness, decreased bowel sounds
	   • Peritoneal signs (fever, rigidity, guarding, rebound tenderness) may indicate perforation

Diagnosis	• **Abdominal X-Ray: best initial imaging test; shows >6cm of colonic dilation**; loss of haustra, air-fluid levels, bowel edema
	   • <u>Dilation of colon AND at least 3 of following</u>: fever, heart rate >120bpm, neutrophilic leukocytosis >10,500/microliter, anemia
	   • <u>AND at least 1 of following</u>: dehydration, altered mental status, electrolyte disturbance, hypotension
	• <u>Labs</u>: leukocytosis, hypokalemia, hypomagnesemia, ↑inflammatory markers (ESR/CRP), anemia, hypoalbuminemia
	• <u>Abdominal CT Scan</u>: may be used to assess for perforation

Treatment	• <u>**Supportive**</u>: bowel rest, nasogastric tube decompression, IV fluid and electrolyte replacement (address hypokalemia/hypomagnesemia)
	• <u>Treat Underlying Etiology</u>:
	   • <u>**Corticosteroids**</u>:: hydrocortisone or methylprednisolone if inflammatory bowel disease
	   • <u>Antiviral</u>: ganciclovir if CMV
	   • <u>Guided Antibiotic Therapy</u>: ceftriaxone + metronidazole; consider **oral vancomycin if known C. diff**; triple therapy with ampicillin + metronidazole + gentamicin

Key Words & Most Common	• Nonobstructive dilation of colon >6cm in diameter • Ulcerative colitis is most common cause; C. difficile • Abdominal pain +/- distension +/- bloody diarrhea • Abdominal x-ray is best initial test • Supportive treatment + treat underlying etiology

Dilation of colon

Crohn's Disease

Etiology & Risk Factors	• Idiopathic immunologically mediated inflammatory bowel disease
	• <u>Etiology</u>: **transmural inflammation**; affects any part of GI tract and inflammation extends through full thickness of bowel wall (mucosa to serosa)
	   • **Terminal ileum is most commonly affected bowel segment**
	   • 30% have small bowel involvement, 20% only colon involvement, 50% have both small bowel and colon involvement; **rectum is often unaffected**
	• <u>Risk Factors</u>: family history, immune system dysfunction (autoimmune), environmental factors (smoking, poor diet, GI infections), altered gut microbiome (frequent use of antibiotics), stress and psychological factors

Patho-physiology	• Multifactorial involving immunologic, infectious, genetic predisposition, dietary, and environmental causes that lead to inflammation of the bowel • Infiltrate forms in intestine which ulcerates to involve deeper layer of mucosa. Inflammation may cause non-caseating granuloma formation.
Signs & Symptoms	• <u>Gastrointestinal Symptoms</u>: **crampy abdominal pain (right lower quadrant), diarrhea** (may contain mucous or blood), **weight loss**, perianal fissures or fistulas, malabsorption • <u>Extraintestinal Symptoms</u>: • **Aphthous mouth ulcers** • <u>Peripheral Arthritis</u>: polyarticular or monoarticular, low back pain with morning stiffness, sacroiliitis • <u>Ocular</u>: uveitis (blurring of vision, photophobia, scleral injection); episcleritis (burning/itching without pain, hyperemia of sclera/conjunctiva) • <u>Dermatologic</u>: erythema nodosum (red, painful nodules or extensor surfaces); pyoderma gangrenosum (ulcerative necrotic lesions at pretibial/trunk region) • <u>Hepatobiliary</u>: cholelithiasis, fatty liver, autoimmune hepatitis
Diagnosis	• <u>Abdominal X-Ray</u>: rule out small bowel obstruction, perforation, or toxic megacolon) • <u>**Upper GI Series**</u>: fluoroscopic x-ray; **initial test of choice**; **"string sign" (barium flowing through stricture formation or spasm) is classic finding** • <u>Endoscopy</u>: shows **segmental "skip areas"** (unaffected area of mucosa among affected area); **cobblestone of mucosa**, aphthous ulcer formation • <u>Labs</u>: anemia (iron or **B12 deficiency** due to malabsorption), elevated inflammatory markers (ESR/CRP) • **Normal anti-neutrophil cytoplasmic antibodies (ANCA)** and **positive anti-saccharomyces cerevisiae antibodies (ASCA)** can distinguish Crohn disease from ulcerative colitis

Treatment	**Acute Treatment**
	• <u>Supportive</u>: bowel rest, IV fluids, electrolyte replacement, analgesia
	• <u>Glucocorticoids</u>: IV methylprednisolone and/or oral prednisone
	   • Anti-inflammatory properties
	• <u>Antidiarrheals</u>: contraindicated
		Chronic Treatment
		• <u>**Aminosalicylates**</u>: 5-ASA, **mesalamine, sulfasalazine** with probiotics
		• <u>**Immunomodulators**</u>: 6-mercatopurine, methotrexate, azathioprine
		   • Steroid-sparing agents used in fistulas or surgical contraindication; slower onset of action
		• <u>Anti-TNF</u>: adalimumab, infliximab; indicated in medically resistant moderate/severe disease

Key Words & Most Common	• Idiopathic autoimmune inflammatory bowel disease causing transmural inflammation affecting any part of GI tract • Most commonly affects terminal ileum • Crampy abdominal pain + weight loss + diarrhea; extraintestinal symptoms include aphthous mouth ulcers, arthritis, uveitis • Upper GI Series – string sign • Acute treatment = steroids; chronic = aminosalicylates vs immunomodulators vs anti-TNF

Ulcerative Colitis

Etiology & Risk Factors	• Idiopathic autoimmune inflammatory bowel disease causing diffuse friability and superficial erosions of colonic mucosa; most common form of inflammatory bowel disease • **Inflammation restricted to colonic mucosa and submucosa; starts at rectum and extends proximally** • <u>Etiology</u>: not fully understood; combination of genetic, environmental, and immune system factors • <u>Risk Factors</u>: genetic component/family history, immune system dysfunction (autoimmune), environmental factors (toxin exposure, diet, infections), altered gut microbiome (frequent use of antibiotics), stress and psychological factors • Some evidence shows smoking may be protective
Patho-physiology	• **Ulcerative colitis begins at rectum and may extend proximally**; inflammation affects mucosa and submucosa with sharp border between normal and affected tissue • Defect of epithelial barrier leads to increased permeability (defective regulation of tight junctions); loss of barrier enables increased uptake of luminal antigens • Breakdown of the colonic homoeostatic microbiotic balance between mucosal immunity and enteric microflora results in autoimmune response against non-pathogenic commensal flora
Signs & Symptoms	• **Bloody diarrhea with or without mucous** • **Crampy abdominal pain (left lower quadrant); tenesmus** (frequent urge to go to the bathroom without being able to go) • <u>Mild</u>: <4 bowel movements per day, no systemic symptoms, few extraintestinal symptoms, episodic constipation and rectal bleeding <u>Moderate</u>: >4 bowel movements per day, abdominal pain • <u>Severe</u>: >6 bowel movements per day, anemia (bloody stool), signs of systemic toxicity (fever, weight loss, extraintestinal symptoms)
Diagnosis	• <u>Flexible Sigmoidoscopy</u>: allows visual confirmation; **uniform erythema and ulceration that involves rectum and extends proximally** • <u>Double Contrast Barium Enema</u>: "stovepipe sign" (cylindrical bowel with loss of haustra markings) <u>Labs</u>: elevated inflammatory markers (ESR/CRP) +/- leukocytosis; anemia • **Positive perinuclear anti-neutrophil cytoplasmic antibodies (P-ANCA)** and normal or elevated **anti-saccharomyces cerevisiae antibodies (ASCA)**
Treatment	• <u>**Topical Aminosalicylates (5-ASA)**</u>: **first-line**; **mesalamine or sulfasalazine** by suppository; oral 5-ASA may be added • <u>**Corticosteroids**</u>: IV methylprednisolone and/or prednisone; topical steroids • <u>**Probiotics**</u>: supplementation or consumption of fermented foods or dairy products (yogurt, kefir, sauerkraut, kimchi etc.) to restore gut microbiome • <u>**Immunomodulators**</u>: 6-mercaptopurine, methotrexate, azathioprine; steroid-sparing agents indicated if fistula formation or surgical contraindication; slower onset of action • <u>Anti-TNF</u>: adalimumab, infliximab; indicated for medically resistant, moderate/severe disease
Key Words & Most Common	• Idiopathic autoimmune inflammatory bowel disease; begins at rectum and extends proximally • Bloody diarrhea with or without mucous; crampy abdominal pain; tenesmus • Flexible sigmoidoscopy visualizes erythema and ulceration • + P-ANCA and normal or + ASCA • Topical 5-ASA is first line followed by steroids

	Ulcerative Colitis	Crohn Disease
Site of Origin	• Rectum	• Terminal Ileum
Distribution	• **Begins at rectum** and limited to colon	• Any segment of GI tract from **mouth to anus**
Spread	• Proximally Contiguous	• Discontinuous/regular = "skip lesions"
Thickness of Inflammation	• Mucosa and submucosa	• Transmural
Symptoms	• **LLQ abdominal pain** • **Bloody Diarrhea** • **Tenesmus/urgency**	• **Crampy RLQ abdominal pain** • Weight loss • Diarrhea w/o blood
Complications	• Hemorrhage, **toxic megacolon**, cholangitis	• Perianal disease: fistula, abscess • Obstruction • Malabsorption: iron and B12 deficiency
Radiographic Findings (Barium Study)	• "Stovepipe sign" = loss of haustra	• **"String Sign" = barium flows through narrow area due to stricture formation or spasm**
Colonoscopy	• Uniform inflammation with ulceration • Affects rectum and extends proximally	• Segmental **"Skip Areas"** = unaffected area of mucosa among affected area • **Cobblestone of mucosa**, aphthous ulcer formation
Risk of Colon Cancer	• Marked Increase	• Slight Increase
Labs	• + perinuclear anti-neutrophil cytoplasmic antibodies (P-ANCA)	• Normal or + **anti-saccharomyces cerevisiae antibodies** (ASCA)
Surgery	• Curative	• Non-curative; reserved for complications (stricture)

Acute Mesenteric Ischemia

Etiology & Risk Factors	<ul><li>Sudden onset of small bowel and colon hypoperfusion</li><li>**Superior mesenteric artery (SMA) is most commonly affected (involves small bowel and right colon)**</li><li>Etiology: hypoperfusion secondary to thrombosis or embolism<ul><li>Mesenteric Arterial Embolism: **embolism from atrial fibrillation is most common**; cardiomyopathy, valve disease, endocarditis</li><li>Mesenteric Artery Thrombosis: atherosclerosis or vasculopathy Nonocclusive Arterial Ischemia: hypovolemia/hypoperfusion secondary to shock, diuretics, vasopressors, toxin (cocaine induced vasospasm)</li><li>Mesenteric Venous Thrombosis: hypercoagulable state (pregnancy, cancer, clotting disorder) causes venous outflow obstruction</li></ul></li></ul>
Patho-physiology	<ul><li>Intestinal mucosa has high metabolic rate and respective blood flow therefore is sensitive to hypoperfusion; ischemia alters the mucosal barrier which allows release of toxins, vasoactive mediators and even bacteria leading to a systemic inflammatory response syndrome and ultimately organ failure</li></ul>
Signs & Symptoms	<ul><li>**Abdominal Pain:** diffuse severe tenderness to palpation that generalized and colicky<ul><li>**Pain out of proportion to exam**</li><li>Pain may be worse on left side at SMA watershed areas (splenic flexure and rectosigmoid junction)</li></ul></li><li>May have nausea, vomiting, diarrhea (bloody)</li><li>Severe Ischemia/Necrosis: peritonitis (rigidity, guarding, rebound tenderness), hypotension, altered mental status, severe/worsening pain</li></ul>
Diagnosis	<ul><li>**CT Angiography: preferred imaging test to evaluate ischemia; demonstrates bowel wall edema (thickened bowel wall)**</li><li>Mesenteric Arteriography: gold standard but rarely used as patient is often critically ill</li><li>Labs: **leukocytosis, metabolic acidosis, elevated lactate and LDH**</li></ul>
Treatment	<ul><li>Supportive: aggressive IV fluid resuscitation, correct electrolyte abnormalities, broad-spectrum antibiotics (prevent sepsis if necrotic)</li><li>**Surgical Revascularization:** surgical embolectomy *OR* mesenteric bypass *OR* retrograde angioplasty with stenting</li><li>Bowel Resection: necrotic bowel may be resected after revascularization procedure if bowel is avascular/necrotic</li><li>Anticoagulation: heparin with warfarin bridge</li><li>Thrombolysis: tPA intra-arterial thrombolysis</li></ul> 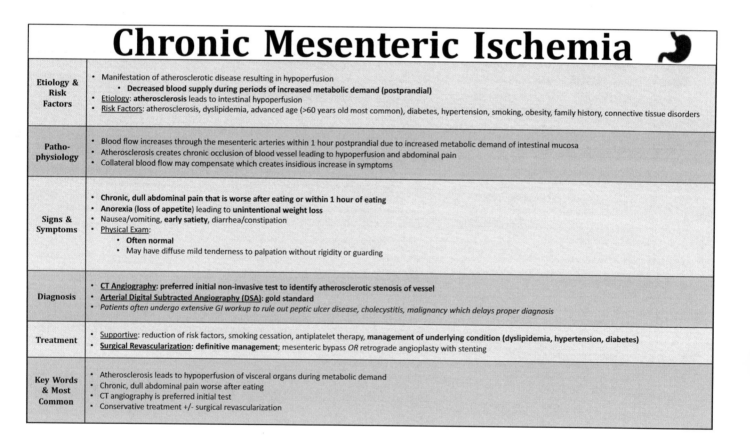 Dilated bowel with thickened bowel wall
Key Words & Most Common	<ul><li>Sudden onset of small bowel/colon hypoperfusion most commonly by embolism</li><li>Superior mesenteric artery most commonly affected</li><li>Abdominal pain out of proportion to exam</li><li>CT angiography preferred imaging study</li><li>IVF resuscitation, correct electrolytes, antibiotics + surgical revascularization +/- bowel resection if necrotic</li></ul>

Chronic Mesenteric Ischemia

Etiology & Risk Factors	<ul><li>Manifestation of atherosclerotic disease resulting in hypoperfusion<ul><li>**Decreased blood supply during periods of increased metabolic demand (postprandial)**</li></ul></li><li>Etiology: **atherosclerosis** leads to intestinal hypoperfusion</li><li>Risk Factors: atherosclerosis, dyslipidemia, advanced age (>60 years old most common), diabetes, hypertension, smoking, obesity, family history, connective tissue disorders</li></ul>
Patho-physiology	<ul><li>Blood flow increases through the mesenteric arteries within 1 hour postprandial due to increased metabolic demand of intestinal mucosa</li><li>Atherosclerosis creates chronic occlusion of blood vessel leading to hypoperfusion and abdominal pain</li><li>Collateral blood flow may compensate which creates insidious increase in symptoms</li></ul>
Signs & Symptoms	<ul><li>**Chronic, dull abdominal pain that is worse after eating or within 1 hour of eating**</li><li>**Anorexia (loss of appetite)** leading to **unintentional weight loss**</li><li>Nausea/vomiting, **early satiety**, diarrhea/constipation</li><li>Physical Exam:<ul><li>**Often normal**</li><li>May have diffuse mild tenderness to palpation without rigidity or guarding</li></ul></li></ul>
Diagnosis	<ul><li>**CT Angiography: preferred initial non-invasive test to identify atherosclerotic stenosis of vessel**</li><li>**Arterial Digital Subtracted Angiography (DSA): gold standard**</li><li>*Patients often undergo extensive GI workup to rule out peptic ulcer disease, cholecystitis, malignancy which delays proper diagnosis*</li></ul>
Treatment	<ul><li>Supportive: reduction of risk factors, smoking cessation, antiplatelet therapy, **management of underlying condition (dyslipidemia, hypertension, diabetes)**</li><li>**Surgical Revascularization: definitive management**; mesenteric bypass *OR* retrograde angioplasty with stenting</li></ul>
Key Words & Most Common	<ul><li>Atherosclerosis leads to hypoperfusion of visceral organs during metabolic demand</li><li>Chronic, dull abdominal pain worse after eating</li><li>CT angiography is preferred initial test</li><li>Conservative treatment +/- surgical revascularization</li></ul>

Colon Polyps

Etiology & Risk Factors	• Protrusion of tissue from bowel wall into colon lumen; **most commonly arise from mucosal layer** and may be adenomatous, serrated, or non-neoplastic • Etiology: **sporadic (most common)**; syndromes • Risk Factors: advanced age, **male gender**, **poor diet** (high-fat/low-fiber), **smoking**, excessive alcohol intake, **family history**

Patho-physiology	• **Hyperplastic Polyps: most common non-neoplastic polyp** with low malignant potential
	• Pseudopolyps: secondary to inflammatory bowel disease; not considered malignant
	• **Adenomatous Polyps: most common neoplastic polyp; 95% of colon adenocarcinomas originate from polyps**
	  • **Villous Adenoma: highest cancer risk**
	  • Tubular Adenoma: most common type of adenomatous polyp; nonpedunculated; least risk of cancer among adenomatous group
	  • Tubuvillous: moderate cancer risk

Signs & Symptoms	• **Mostly asymptomatic** and found during routine colonoscopy • Painless rectal bleeding, mucous stool, diarrhea/constipation • Symptoms of iron deficiency anemia (chronic bleeding); fatigue, weakness, pallor
Diagnosis	• Labs: CBC to evaluate anemia, CMP to evaluate electrolyte abnormalities • Fecal Occult Blood Test (FOBT): evaluate for blood in GI tract • **Colonoscopy: gold-standard for diagnosis and polypectomy; direct visualization of polyps**
Treatment	• **Colonic Polypectomy: gold-standard for diagnostic and therapeutic purposes; performed during colonoscopy** • Prophylactic Colectomy: for Familial Adenomatous Polyposis (FAP) and MUTYH-associated polyposis (MAP) or polyps with high-risk features of malignancy • *Address underlying anemia*
Key Words & Most Common	• Protrusion of mucosal tissue into colon lumen • Family history, male gender, and smoking are greatest risk factors • Mostly asymptomatic; may cause painless rectal bleeding or stool changes • Colonoscopy with polypectomy is gold standard to diagnosis and treatment

Colorectal Cancer

Etiology & Risk Factors	• Colorectal cancer most commonly arises from adenomatous polyps; third most common diagnosed and second most common cause of death related to malignancy
	• Risk Factors: **age >50** (peaks at age 65), obesity, smoking, alcohol use, African Americans, family history, **inflammatory bowel disease, diet** (low-fiber, processed foods)
	• Genetic Component:
	  • Familial Adenomatous Polyposis: colonic adenoma begin in childhood and develops to cancer by age 45; treated with prophylactic colectomy
	  • Lynch Syndrome (Hereditary Non-polyposis Colorectal Cancer): autosomal dominant; develops cancer between age 20-50
	• Protective Factors: physical activity, diet (fiber, resistant starches, fish, fruits/vegetables), vitamin supplements (folate, Ca, Mg, vitamin D and B6), aspirin/NSAID use

Patho-physiology	• Transformation of normal colonic epithelium to precancerous adenoma to invasive carcinoma • Dysplastic change arises from chronic inflammation of bowel resulting chromosomal instability, mismatch repair, and hypermethylation causing alteration in oncogene and tumor suppressors equilibrium
Signs & Symptoms	• **Mostly asymptomatic** and found during routine colonoscopy • **Painless rectal bleeding**, mucous stool, diarrhea/constipation, symptoms of iron deficiency anemia (chronic bleeding) • Large lesions may cause bowel obstruction (most common in left sided lesion)
Diagnosis	• **Colonoscopy: diagnostic test of choice for diagnosis and tissue biopsy; polypectomy may be performed** • CT Colonography: may aid with staging; screening test for those unwilling to undergo colonoscopy • Labs: **iron deficiency anemia**, electrolyte abnormalities, ↑**serum carcinoembryonic antigen (CEA) (nonspecific tumor marker)**,
Treatment	• **Surgical Resection**: via radical vs endoscopic • Attempt to cure with **wide resection of bowel segment**, regional lymphatic system and tumor +/- chemotherapy or radiation to destroy residual cells • Adjuvant Therapy: chemotherapy improves survival rates by 10-30%; preoperative chemotherapy/radiation may reduce metastasis risk
Key Words & Most Common	• Age, inflammatory bowel disease, smoking and genetic component are major risk factors • Mostly asymptomatic, may have rectal bleeding • Colonoscopy is diagnostic test of choice with tissue biopsy • Surgical resection +/- chemotherapy/radiation

Esophagitis

Etiology & Risk Factors	• Inflammation or injury to the esophageal mucosa
	• Etiologies:
	  • **Erosive/Inflammatory**: gastroesophageal reflux disease (GERD) is most common cause
	  • Infectious: fungal (candida), cytomegalovirus, herpes simplex virus; most common in immunocompromised patients
	  • Eosinophilic: allergic; chronic immune-antigen related esophageal inflammation from eosinophil infiltration
	  • Pill-Induced: bisphosphonates, antibiotics (tetracycline, doxycycline, clindamycin), NSAIDs, aspirin, ferrous sulfate, potassium chloride, ascorbic acid
	  • Radiation-Induced: radiotherapy related toxicity

Patho-physiology	• Erosive/Inflammatory: gastric content refluxes into esophagus causing mucosal injury • Infectious: Impairment of host mechanisms (immunocompromised) lead to colonization of organisms • Eosinophilic: allergic disorder caused by antigen sensitivity through food or airborne allergens • Pill-Induced: direct irritant effect disrupting mucosal protective factors; caustic injury from doxycycline, tetracycline or ferrous sulfate (pH of 3 when dissolved) • Radiation-Induced: DNA damage from radiation creates volatile oxygen-free radicals which destroys epithelial cells
Signs & Symptoms	• **Retrosternal chest pain** • **Odynophagia** (painful swallowing); **dysphagia** (trouble swallowing) • Globus sensation, reflux, dyspepsia, wheezing/chronic cough
Diagnosis	• Clinical Diagnosis • **Upper Endoscopy**: allows for direct visualization of esophageal mucosa +/- biopsy • *Consider HIV workup if infectious etiology*
Treatment	• Treat Underlying Etiology: management of risk factors, remove offending agent, treat infection/condition • Erosive/Inflammatory: **PPI/H2 blockers for acid suppression**, lifestyle modification, elevate head of bed, elimination/modified diet • Infectious: **oral fluconazole for candida; ganciclovir for CMV; acyclovir for HSV** • Eosinophilic: PPI/H2 blockers for acid suppression, topical/systemic steroids (topical budesonide or fluticasone), dietary modification if a food allergy is suspected • Pill-Induced: discontinue/switch offending medication; take pills with 4+ oz of water and remain upright for >30 minutes after
Key Words & Most Common	• Inflammation or injury to esophageal mucosa • Most common cause is GERD • Retrosternal chest pain + odynophagia + dysphagia • Clinical with upper endoscopy to confirm • Treat underlying etiology

Irritable Bowel Syndrome (IBS)

Etiology & Risk Factors	• **Chronic, idiopathic gastrointestinal disease with no organic cause** • Etiology: not fully understood • Risk Factors: **age (most common 13-30 years old)**, **female**, abnormal GI motility, alterations in gut microbiome, intestinal inflammation, family history, food sensitivities, **stress and psychologic factors**
Patho-physiology	• **Visceral Hyperalgesia**: hypersensitivity to normal amounts of intestinal distention, heightened perception of GI related pain; may result from gut-brain axis neural pathway remodeling • **Altered Gut Motility**: serotonin and acetylcholine imbalances within the intestine leads to abnormal motility (constipation if slow colonic transit; diarrhea if fast colonic transit) and abdominal pain • **Psychosocial Factors**: concomitant depression, anxiety, or somatization disorder may lead to altered CNS processing; underlying past abuse; sleep disturbances • Other: hormone fluctuations may lead to increased rectal sensitivity during menses; altered gut microbiome; food intolerances (FODMAPs)
Signs & Symptoms	• **Abdominal discomfort/pain related to defecation/bowel habits** • **Discomfort associated with alteration of stool frequency (diarrhea and/or constipation) and consistency (loose vs hard)** • **Pain often relieved with defecation** • Symptoms may be triggered by stress or foods • RED FLAGS: age >45, weight loss, rectal bleeding, anorexia or weight loss, iron deficiency anemia, family history of GI cancer, IBD or celiac disease, nocturnal diarrhea

Diagnosis	• Diagnosis of Exclusion: normal GI workup with imaging (colonoscopy/abdominal CT), stool studies/culture, and labs to rule out other etiologies
	• Rome IV Criteria: requires at least 3 days per month for last 3 months to be associated with at least 2 or more of following:
	  • **Abdominal pain/discomfort related to defecation**
	  • Onset associated with **change in frequency of stool**
	  • Onset associated with **change in form or appearance of stool**

Treatment	• Lifestyle Modifications: dietary modifications are first-line
	  • Diet: whole foods with no processed foods; elimination diet
	    • Avoidance of: wheat products, onions, fructose/sorbitol (apples/raisins) or gas producing foods (beans, cruciferous vegetables) and some dairy which contain short-chain, poorly absorbed, highly fermentable carbohydrates (FODMAPs) which are related to increased GI symptoms in the IBS patient
	  • Probiotics: supplementation or consumption of fermented foods or dairy products (yogurt, kefir, sauerkraut, kimchi etc.) to restore gut microbiome
	• Constipation: fiber supplements, psyllium or laxatives
	  • Lubiprostone (chloride channel activator) or linaclotide (guanylate cyclase G agonist) if no relief from conservative treatment
	• Diarrhea: **loperamide** (antidiarrheal), **rifaximin** (antibiotic that helps with bloating/loose stool), **dicyclomine** (antispasmodic)
	  • Tricyclic Antidepressants: nortriptyline/amitriptyline; downregulate cortical afferent pathways from the gut

Hiatal Hernia

Etiology & Risk Factors	• Condition in which the upper portion of the stomach or other abdominal structures bulge through the esophageal hiatus opening of the diaphragm • <u>Etiology</u>: stretching of the fascial attachments between the esophagus and diaphragm at the hiatus • <u>Risk Factors</u>: advanced age, **conditions with elevated intraabdominal pressure** (COPD, **obesity**, pregnancy, chronic constipation), abdominal trauma, sedentary lifestyle

Patho-physiology	• <u>4 Classifications</u>:
	  • **<u>Type I (sliding)</u>: most common type (95%); occurs when the gastroesophageal junction (GEJ) "slides" upward toward the hiatus**
	  • <u>Type II (rolling)</u>: paraesophageal hernia in which fundus of stomach bulges through diaphragm parallel to esophagus; GEJ remains in anatomical location.
	  • <u>Type III</u>: paraesophageal and sliding hernia; both GEJ and part of stomach migrate into mediastinum
	  • <u>Type IV</u>: stomach and any abdominal structures herniate into mediastinum

Signs & Symptoms	• **Mostly asymptomatic** • Epigastric/substernal Pain • **Gastric reflux symptoms**, postprandial fullness, nausea, chronic cough
Diagnosis	• <u>Chest X-Ray (CXR)</u>: large hiatal hernias may be found incidentally on CXR • <u>Barium Swallow</u>: evaluates size and contour of hernia; may detect small hernias • <u>Upper Endoscopy</u>: definitive diagnosis; allows for direct visualization of esophagus
Treatment	• <u>Asymptomatic</u>: no specific therapy; observation • <u>Supportive</u>: **weight loss, exercise** (strengthens diaphragm), dietary modifications, elevate head of bed, alcohol and smoking cessation • <u>Type I Sliding</u>: GERD management with **PPI/H2 blockers for gastric acid suppression**, lifestyle modification, elevate head of bed, elimination/modified diet • <u>Type II-IV Paraesophageal</u>: surgical repair considered to prevent complications (strangulation, volvulus, obstruction)
Key Words & Most Common	• Condition in which upper portion of stomach or other abdominal structures bulge through opening of diaphragm • Type I sliding hiatal hernia is most common type • Mostly asymptomatic; may have gastric reflux symptoms • May be found incidentally on CXR; confirmed with upper endoscopy • Conservative with weight loss, exercise, diet modification is first line • GERD management (PPI) for sliding

Retrocardiac mass with air-fluid level

Gastroesophageal Reflux Disease (GERD)

Etiology & Risk Factors	• Incompetence of lower esophageal sphincter allowing reflux of gastric contents into esophagus
	  • *One of most commonly diagnosed GI condition in United States; affects upwards of 20% of population*
	• <u>Etiology</u>: **reflux of gastric contents into esophagus**
	  • <u>3 Classifications</u>: non-erosive reflux disease (NERD), erosive esophagitis (EE), and Barrett esophagus (BE)
	• <u>Risk Factors</u>: **lying down after meals, carbonated beverages, caffeine, obesity**, age (>50 years old most common), low socioeconomic status, **alcohol/tobacco use, pregnancy**, postprandial supination, **poor diet** (spicy, acidic, fatty foods), medications (NSAIDs, aspirin, muscle relaxers, CCBs), delayed gastric emptying (gastroparesis)

Patho-physiology	• Incompetency of the lower esophageal sphincter and transient relaxation allows retrograde passing of gastric contents into esophagus • Hiatal hernia presence may hinder function of the lower esophageal sphincter • Delayed gastric emptying or inadequate esophageal peristalsis causes decreased clearance of gastric content, gastric distention and leads to reflux into the esophagus

Signs & Symptoms	• <u>Pyrosis</u>: **heartburn is most common symptoms; pain described as retrosternal**
	  • Symptoms **worse postprandial and while supine**
	  • May have nausea, cough, dyspepsia
	• <u>Gastric Regurgitation</u>: sour/foul taste in mouth, cough, sore throat, chronic clearing of the throat, **halitosis** (bad breath), dental erosions (if chronic)
	• <u>Atypical symptoms</u>: wheezing/asthma, chest pain, laryngitis, dysphonia, dental erosions, globus sensation

Diagnosis	• **Clinical Diagnosis**; *cardiac causes of chest pain may need to be ruled out* • <u>Proton Pump Inhibitor (PPI) Trial</u>: may aid in presumptive diagnosis if symptoms improve or resolve with PPI use • <u>Ambulatory Esophageal Reflux Monitoring</u>: pH monitoring using telemetry or transnasal catheter; used to assess correlation of symptoms with acid exposure • <u>Esophagogastroduodenoscopy (EGD)</u>: utilized if symptoms persistent/fail treatment, or associated atypical symptoms

Treatment	• <u>Lifestyle Modifications</u>: **exercise/weight loss, dietary modifications (avoid foods that delay gastric emptying** such as caffeine, fatty/spicy foods, chocolate, citrus, carbonated drinks), smoking and alcohol cessation, elevate head of bead, avoid lying supine for 3 hours after eating
	• <u>Medical Management</u>:
	  • **<u>Histamine Receptor Antagonists (H2 blockers)</u>: famotidine**; blocks action of histamine on parietal cells to decrease acid secretion to stomach
	  • **<u>Proton Pump Inhibitors (PPI)</u>: omeprazole**; most effective treatment; inhibits secretion of gastric acid by blocking the hydrogen/potassium ATP enzyme system
	• <u>Laparoscopic Nissen Fundoplication</u>: gold-standard surgical procedure in the management of GERD patients refractory to medical and conservative therapy

Complications	• **<u>Barrett's Esophagus</u>**: normal squamous epithelium of the distal esophagus is replaced with metaplastic columnar epithelium during healing phase of acute esophagitis
Key Words & Most Common	• Incompetents of lower esophageal sphincter allows reflux of gastric contents into esophagus • Heartburn, dyspepsia, cough, gastric regurgitation (foul taste, clearing throat) are most common symptoms • Mostly clinical diagnosis; EGD if atypical symptoms • Lifestyle modifications first line; H2 blockers (famotidine); PPI (omeprazole)

Esophageal Cancer

	Adenocarcinoma	Squamous Cell Carcinoma

Etiology & Risk Factors	• Most common cause of esophageal cancer in **US**
	• Location: most common at distal esophagus and esophagogastric junction
	• Risk Factors: **Barrett's esophagus (GERD), obesity, smoking** (alcohol is not important risk factor)
	   • **4x more common in Caucasians than African-Americans**
	   • Age (can be seen in young patients)
		• Most common cause of esophageal cancer **worldwide**
		• Location: most common at mid to upper 1/3rd of esophagus
		• Risk Factors: **alcohol and tobacco use** (any form), poor diet, achalasia, **human papilloma virus (HPV) infection**, sclerotherapy, thermal injury from hot food/drinks
		   • **4-5x more common in African Americans than Caucasians**
		   • Age (peaks at 50-70 years old)

Patho-physiology	• **Barrett's Esophagus**: normal squamous epithelium of the distal esophagus is replaced with metaplastic columnar epithelium during healing phase of acute esophagitis	• The alcohol metabolite aldehyde is a recognized carcinogen which causes mutations and increased risk of developing SCC.
Signs & Symptoms	• Asymptomatic in early stages • **Progressive Dysphagia: most common presenting symptom;** difficulty swallowing solid food, then soft food, then liquids, then saliva); odynophagia • **Weight loss**, loss of appetite, iron deficiency anemia (chronic blood loss), chest pain, cough, hematemesis, regurgitation • Compression of laryngeal nerve may lead to **hoarse voice**	
Diagnosis	• *No routine screening tests available* • **Upper Endoscopy with Biopsy: diagnostic test of choice;** may demonstrate plaques, nodules or ulceration of tissue • **Endoscopic Ultrasound: standard therapy for locoregional staging;** allows for fine needle biopsy of surrounding lymph nodes • CT Scan: imaging of neck/abdomen/thorax to evaluate extent of primary tumor and potential metastases • PET/CT Scan: pretreatment study aids in establishment of potential metastases	
Treatment	• Endoscopic Esophageal Resection: utilized for superficial limited mucosal disease +/- chemotherapy • Systemic Treatment: radiation/chemotherapy (cisplatin/5-fluorouracil) • Palliation: manual dilation or orally inserted stents utilized to improve dysphagia by reducing esophageal obstruction	
Key Words & Most Common	• Adenocarcinoma: 4x more common in whites than blacks; most common at distal esophagus; Barrett's esophagus and smoking most common risk factor • Squamous Cell: 4x more common in blacks than whites; most common at mid to upper 1/3rd of esophagus; alcohol/tobacco, HPV, and poor nutrition most common risk factor • Progressive dysphagia and weight loss • Upper endoscopy with biopsy diagnostic test of choice • Endoscopic Esophageal Resection +/- chemotherapy	

Achalasia

Etiology & Risk Factors	• **Esophageal smooth muscle motility disorder causing loss of peristalsis and failure to relax lower esophageal sphincter (LES)** • Etiology: **mostly idiopathic**; may have genetic predisposition, autoimmune or viral infection component • Risk Factors: **age (30-60 years old most common)**, family history, autoimmune disorders, viral infections (HSV), certain environmental factors, nerve degeneration, esophageal infections
Patho-physiology	• May be caused by degeneration of myenteric plexus and vagus nerve fibers leading to increased lower esophageal sphincter pressure resulting in disruption of normal lower esophageal sphincter relaxation • Degeneration leads to functional obstruction causing esophageal dilation, disrupting normal peristalsis
Signs & Symptoms	• **Dysphagia: most common presenting symptom;** difficulty swallowing foods and liquids • Regurgitation of undigested food, chest pain, nocturnal cough • Anorexia, weight loss, dehydration

Diagnosis	• **Esophageal Manometry: most accurate and preferred test**
	   • Demonstrates incomplete relaxation of lower esophageal sphincter and lack of peristalsis
	• **Barium Esophogram: complementary initial test**
	   • Demonstrates classic "bird's beak" appearance at level of lower esophageal sphincter
	   • Narrowing of LES with proximal esophageal dilation, loss of peristalsis distal to LES
	• Upper Endoscopy: recommended to rule out malignant lesions prior to initiating treatment

Treatment	• No treatment will fully restore peristalsis; **treatment guided to reduce LES pressure**
	• Non-Surgical:
	   • **Calcium Channel Blockers**: block smooth muscle contraction to reduce LES pressure
	   • **Vasodilators**: nitrates and **5-phosphodiesterase** promote smooth muscle relaxation
	   • Endoscopic Botulinum Toxin Injection: blocks acetylcholine release at level of LES
	   • Endoscopic Pneumatic Dilatation of the Esophagus: most cost-effective non-surgical therapy for achalasia
	• Surgical:
	   • Laparoscopic or Endoscopic Myotomy: more definitive treatment; incises circular muscle fibers of LES to promote relaxation

Key Words & Most Common	• Esophageal smooth muscle motility disorder • Dysphagia of foods and liquids • Esophageal Manometry is most accurate and preferred test • Treatment guided to reduce LES pressure • Non-Surgical: CCBs/Nitrates/5-PDE to promote smooth muscle relaxation; endoscopic botulinum toxin injection, pneumatic dilation • Surgical: definitive; myotomy

Dilated esophagus with retained column of barium and "bird's beak"

Zenker's Diverticulum

Etiology & Risk Factors	• Type of diverticulum involving the hypopharynx forming a pharyngoesophageal pouch 　• **"False" diverticulum only involves mucosa and submucosa** (does not involve muscle layer) • Etiology: not fully understood; acquired mucosal herniation • Risk Factors: **male, age (>60 years old most common), weakening of the muscles in the throat and upper esophagus,** impaired swallowing, chronic inflammation, family history, alcohol consumption and smoking
Patho-physiology	• Fibrotic changes cause impaired cricopharyngeal compliance leading to increased hypopharyngeal pressure resulting in **outpouching of mucosa and submucosa at weak points** just above the cricopharyngeal muscle and lower inferior pharyngeal constrictor muscle (Killian's triangle) • False diverticulum retains food particles and leads to symptoms and halitosis
Signs & Symptoms	• **Dysphagia with globus sensation (sensation of food caught in throat)** • **Regurgitation of *undigested* food** • **Halitosis** (bad breath due to retained food in pouch) • Cough, neck mass, choking sensation
Diagnosis	• **Barium Esophagram with Video Fluoroscopy: test of choice** to evaluate size, location, and characteristics of mucosal lining • Upper Endoscopy: confirmatory test; performed during presurgical evaluation; may reveal pooling of food at diverticulum
Treatment	• Observation: indicated if asymptomatic or lesion is small (<2cm) • Surgery: cricopharyngeal myotomy for large or symptomatic lesions; high recurrent rate
Key Words & Most Common	• "False" diverticulum involving mucosa and submucosa causing outpouch at cricopharyngeal level • Dysphagia with choking sensation • Regurgitation of undigested food • Halitosis • Barium Esophagram with video fluoroscopy is test of choice • Observation vs Surgery if large or symptomatic

Inferior pharyngeal constrictor muscle

Zenker's diverticulum

Cricopharyngeal muscle

Barium Esophagram

Diffuse Esophageal Spasm

Etiology & Risk Factors	• **Esophageal motility disorder characterized by rapid, simultaneous, uncoordinated, non-peristaltic esophageal contractions** • Etiology: uncoordinated esophageal contractions • Risk Factors: chronic GERD, hyperglycemia, high cholesterol, **elevated BMI**, female gender, Caucasian
Patho-physiology	• Imbalance of inhibitory and excitatory postganglionic pathway innervation leading to premature and rapid esophageal contractions • Acetylcholine release may be contributing factor
Signs & Symptoms	• **Substernal chest pain worse with hot or cold liquids** 　• Angina-like symptoms without exertional pain • **Dysphagia of solids and liquids** • Globus sensation (sensation of food caught in throat)
Diagnosis	• **Barium Esophagram:** severe disordered contractions with poor progression of bolus (poor peristalsis); may show **"corkscrew" esophagus** • **Esophageal Manometry: definitive, most specific test;** shows aperistalsis, simultaneous or premature contractions at distal esophagus • *ACS must be ruled out as clinically indicated*
Treatment	• Medication Management: **calcium channel blockers and nitrates are first-line;** tricyclic antidepressants 　• **Calcium Channel Blockers:** block smooth muscle contraction to reduce lower esophageal sphincter (LES) pressure 　• **Nitrates:** promote smooth muscle relaxation • Endoscopic Botulinum Toxin Injection: second-line; blocks acetylcholine release at level of LES • Endoscopic Myotomy: more definitive treatment; cuts circular muscle fibers of LES to cause relaxation
Key Words & Most Common	• Esophageal motility disorder with uncoordinated non-peristaltic esophageal contractions • Substernal chest pain worse with hot/cold liquids • Dysphagia of solids and liquids • Esophageal manometry is definitive and most specific • Barium esophogram may show "corkscrew" esophagus • CCBs vs Nitrates first line

Corkscrew appearance of the esophagus on upper GI series (esophagram)

Hypercontractile Esophagus

Etiology & Risk Factors	• Esophageal motility disorder characterized by increased pressure and sequential smooth muscle contractions of esophagus during peristalsis • Also known as the "jackhammer" or "nutcracker" esophagus • <u>Etiology</u>: **idiopathic, gastric junction outflow obstruction** • <u>Risk Factors</u>: **age (>60 years old most common)**, female, family history, **history of GERD**, certain neurological disorders (Parkinson's disease or multiple sclerosis), psychological factors (stress, anxiety)
Patho-physiology	• Excess acetylcholine release and asynchrony of longitudinal and circular muscle contractions • Inflammation of myositis by eosinophilic infiltration may lead to increased esophageal muscle thickness
Signs & Symptoms	• **Substernal chest pain** • Angina-like symptoms without exertional pain • **Dysphagia of solids and liquids** • Globus sensation (sensation of food caught in throat)

Diagnosis	• <u>**Esophageal Manometry**</u>: **definitive, most specific test**
	   • **Shows increased pressure during peristalsis (this differentiates from esophageal spasm)**
	   • **Multi-peaked contractions** (resembles jackhammer)
	• <u>Upper Endoscopy and Barium Esophagram</u>: usually normal
	• *ACS must be ruled out as clinically indicated*

Treatment	• <u>Medication Management</u>: **calcium channel blockers and nitrates are first-line**; tricyclic antidepressants
	   • <u>**Calcium Channel Blockers**</u>: block smooth muscle contraction to reduce lower esophageal sphincter (LES) pressure
	   • <u>**Nitrates**</u>: promote smooth muscle relaxation
	• <u>Endoscopic Botulinum Toxin Injection</u>: second-line; inhibits acetylcholine release at level of LES

Key Words & Most Common	• "Jackhammer" esophagus • Motility disorder with increased pressure and sequential smooth muscle contractions of esophagus during peristalsis • Substernal chest pain; dysphagia of solids and liquids • Esophageal Manometry is definitive; shows increased pressure and multi-peaked contractions during peristalsis • CCBs vs nitrates are first line; endoscopic Botox injections as second line

Diagram of esophageal motility study for nutcracker esophagus (left is a schematic of esophagus as it relates to each peaked contraction)

Mallory-Weiss Syndrome

Etiology & Risk Factors	• Longitudinal superficial lacerations through mucosa and submucosa occurring primarily at the gastroesophageal junction
	   • May extend proximally to lower esophagus
	   • May extend distally to gastric cardia
	• <u>Etiology</u>: **sudden rise of intraabdominal pressure (forceful vomiting/retching, straining, coughing, blunt abdominal trauma)**
	• <u>Risk Factors</u>: **alcoholism**, hiatal hernia, forceful vomiting (bulimia nervosa, hyperemesis gravidarum, cannabinoid hyperemesis syndrome), chronic gastroesophageal reflux disease (GERD), chronic cough, trauma

Patho-physiology	• Sudden increase in intraabdominal pressure causes rush of gastric contents or gastric prolapse into esophagus • Increased excessive pressure causes longitudinal tears to mucosa and submucosa • **Excessive pressure often from retching or vomiting after alcohol binge**

Signs & Symptoms	• <u>**Symptoms of Upper GI Bleed**</u>:
	   • **Hematemesis following retching or vomiting**
	      • **"Coffee ground" emesis**
	   • **Melena**
	• May develop abdominal or back pain
	• <u>Severe Bleeding</u>: hypotension, dizziness, syncope

Diagnosis	• <u>Labs</u>: bleeding workup with CBC, CMP, coagulation studies, type and screen, stool guaiac
	• <u>**Upper Endoscopy**</u>: **gold standard test**
	   • **Demonstrates longitudinal superficial mucosal lacerations**
	   • May show active bleeding, clot, or fibrin crust over erosions

Treatment	• <u>**Supportive**</u>: **most cases are self-limiting** and recurrence rates are low
	• <u>**Medication Management**</u>:
	   • <u>**PPI/H2 Blockers**</u>: decrease gastric acidity and promote healing
	   • <u>**Antiemetics**</u>: ondansetron or promethazine used to control nausea/vomiting
	• <u>Severe Bleed</u>: resuscitation efforts (ABCs, IV access, fluid replacement)
	   • Endoscopic band ligation, local epinephrine injection (vasoconstriction), multipolar electrocoagulation (MPEC), argon plasma coagulation
	   • Sengstaken-Blakemore tube compression is last resort for balloon tamponade

Key Words & Most Common	• Longitudinal superficial mucosal lacerations at gastroesophageal junction • Excessive pressure from retching/vomiting after alcohol binge • Hematemesis following repeated retching or vomiting, "coffee ground" emesis, melena • Upper endoscopy is gold standard • Most self-limiting; supportive treatment with PPI/H2 blockers and anti-emetics

Boerhaave Syndrome

Etiology & Risk Factors	• Spontaneous full-thickness esophageal rupture secondary to forceful retching or vomiting or sudden rise in intraesophageal pressure • Most common site of rupture is left posterolateral wall of distal esophagus • <u>Etiology</u>: **iatrogenic (endoscopy), forceful vomiting/retching**, thoracic trauma, caustic ingestion, foreign body • <u>Risk Factors</u>: vomiting (**alcoholism**, bulimia nervosa, hyperemesis gravidarum, cannabinoid hyperemesis syndrome), chronic gastroesophageal reflux disease (GERD), **weightlifting**, childbirth, constipation/defecation, seizure
Patho-physiology	• Full transmural esophageal rupture secondary to sudden rise in intraesophageal pressure • Intrathoracic esophageal perforations lead to mediastinal inflammation, emphysema and necrosis secondary to gastric contents entering the area

Signs & Symptoms	• <u>**Mackler's Triad:**</u>
	    • <u>**Chest Pain:**</u> often worse with inspiration, neck flexion and swallowing; often occurs after forceful vomiting
	    • <u>**Vomiting**</u>: may have hematemesis
	    • <u>**Subcutaneous Emphysema:**</u> may have crepitus on auscultation
	• Pain may occur at the retrosternal, neck, or epigastric area depending on level of rupture
	• <u>Physical Exam:</u>
	    • **Crepitus on auscultation** from subcutaneous emphysema
	    • <u>**Hamman's Sign:**</u> mediastinal "crackle" with every heartbeat in left lateral decubitus position
	
	Pneumomediastinum adjacent to the thoracic aorta

Diagnosis	• <u>Chest X-Ray (CXR)</u>: pneumomediastinum, mediastinal widening, pleural effusion • <u>Contrast Esophogram</u>: **diagnostic test of choice**; uses a water-soluble contrast such as Gastrografin; shows extravasation of contrast at perforation site • <u>Chest CT Scan</u>: more sensitive to diagnose pneumomediastinum but does not localize perforation well
Treatment	• <u>Supportive</u>: IV fluid resuscitation, broad-spectrum IV antibiotics (Gentamicin + metronidazole; piperacillin/tazobactam) • <u>Surgical Repair</u>: primary esophageal repair through open thoracotomy vs. **video assisted thoracoscopic surgery (VATS) with fundic reinforcement (gold standard)**
Key Words & Most Common	• Sudden rise in intraesophageal pressure causes full-thickness esophageal rupture • Forceful vomiting secondary to alcohol is most common cause • <u>Mackler's Triad of Symptoms</u>: chest pain, vomiting, subcutaneous emphysema • Contrast esophogram is test of choice • Supportive with surgical consult

Esophageal Web and Ring

	Esophageal Web	Esophageal Ring (Shatzki)

Etiology & Risk Factors	• Noncircumferential membrane that may partially occlude esophageal lumen
	• **Most common at mid to upper esophagus**
	• <u>Etiology</u>:
	    • <u>Plummer-Vinson Syndrome</u>: triad of dysphagia, iron deficiency anemia, esophageal webs
	    • Zenker's diverticulum, pemphigus vulgaris, bullous pemphigoid
		• Circumferential diaphragm of tissue that indents into esophageal lumen
		• **Most common at lower esophagus** (squamocolumnar junction)
		• <u>Etiology</u>:
		    • **Almost always associated with hiatal hernia**
		    • Eosinophilic esophagitis

Patho-physiology	• Chronic inflammation may irritate esophageal mucosa and cause webs and rings to form • If webs/rings are large enough, may partially occlude esophageal lumen leading to dysphagia and possible food impaction	
Signs & Symptoms	• Many cases are asymptomatic • **Dysphagia to solid foods (especially meats and bread)**	

Diagnosis	• <u>**Barium Esophagram**</u>: **diagnostic test of choice**
	• <u>Upper Endoscopy</u>: may be necessary for confirmation of diagnosis
	    • <u>Esophageal Webs</u>: thin membranes that ***do not*** span the entire circumference of the esophagus
	    • <u>Esophageal Rings</u>: thin membranes, that ***do*** span the entire circumference of the esophagus.
		Esophageal Web

Treatment	• <u>**Endoscopic Esophageal Dilation**</u>: safe and low risk procedure to relieve dysphagia • Biopsy may be required for esophageal rings to rule out eosinophilic esophagitis • <u>Proton Pump Inhibitor (PPI) Therapy</u>: long term acid suppression to prevent recurrence (rings may be close to gastroesophageal junction)	
Key Words & Most Common	• <u>Webs</u>: noncircumferential membrane most common in mid/upper esophagus • <u>Rings</u>: circumferential membrane most common at lower esophagus • Asymptomatic; dysphagia to solid foods • Barium esophagram • Endoscopic esophageal dilation + PPI	**Esophageal Ring**

Esophageal Varices

Etiology & Risk Factors	• Dilated collateral submucosal veins located at distal esophagus secondary to portal vein hypertension • <u>Etiology</u>: **elevated pressure in the portal venous system** • <u>Risk Factors</u>: **cirrhosis is most common cause**, alcoholism, portal vein obstruction, portal vein thrombosis, splenomegaly, right sided heart failure, pericarditis
Patho-physiology	• Portal venous system has no valves therefore vascular resistance leads to retrograde blood flow and elevated pressure • Collateral submucosal veins eventually enlarge and will connect portal venous system to systemic circulation • Congested veins become dilated and tortuous until rupture occurs *Prominent varices*

Signs & Symptoms	• **Sudden, painless, upper GI bleed**
	  • **Hematemesis, "coffee ground" emesis**
	  • **Melena**
	• Jaundice, anorexia, weight loss
	• <u>Physical Exam</u>:
	  • **Jaundice**
	  • Evidence of liver disease (spider angiomata of chest/back, palmar erythema, jaundice, gynecomastia, testicular atrophy), **ascites**
	  • <u>Severe</u>: shock symptoms; hypotension, tachycardia, altered mental status

Diagnosis	• <u>**Upper Endoscopy**</u>: **test of choice**; identifies site, size, and extend of bleed; may be used for treatment (band ligation) • <u>Labs</u>: CBC (serial hemoglobin), CMP, coagulation profile, fibrinogen, type and screen, guaiac

Treatment	• <u>Resuscitation</u>: 2 large bore IV lines, IV fluids, treat coagulopathy (packed red blood cells; fresh frozen plasma may increase rebleeding risk)
	• <u>**Endoscopic Variceal Ligation**</u>: **initial treatment of choice**; less risk of rebleed and fewer complications than sclerotherapy
	• <u>Medical Management</u>:
	  • <u>**Vasoconstrictors**</u>: **octreotide is first-line medication** (somatostatin analog that lowers portal venous pressure and causes portal venous vasoconstriction)
	    • Vasopressin is second-line (decreases portal venous pressure)
	  • <u>Proton Pump Inhibitor (PPI)</u>: pantoprazole reduces rate of rebleeding
	  • <u>Antibiotics</u>: ceftriaxone or ciprofloxacin to prevent infectious complications
	• <u>Balloon Tamponade</u>: used for life-threatening hemorrhage if endoscopy not available
	• <u>Surgical Decompression</u>: transjugular intrahepatic portosystemic shunt (TIPS) procure indicated as a salvage procedure for continuous bleed despite other procedures

Key Words & Most Common	• Dilated collateral veins at distal esophagus that form secondary to portal vein hypertension • Sudden, painless, upper GI bleed • Hematemesis • Upper endoscopy is test of choice • Endoscopic variceal ligation is initial treatment of choice • Octreotide is a first line vasoconstrictor that lowers portal venous pressure

Celiac Disease

Etiology & Risk Factors	• **Autoimmune-mediated small bowel inflammation secondary to gluten exposure in the diet (wheat, rye, barley)** • Also known as gluten sensitivity enteropathy or celiac sprue • <u>Etiology</u>: sensitivity to the gliadin fraction of gluten (protein found in wheat) • <u>Risk Factors</u>: **family history, female**, type 1 diabetes, other autoimmune disorders (Hashimoto's thyroiditis), genetic (HLA dominant DQ2 or DQ8 genes), trisomy 21
Patho-physiology	• Autoimmune disorder caused by a reaction to gliadin (peptide protein found in wheat/rye/barley) producing a T-cell activation response and inflammation • Inflammatory response leads to mucosal villous atrophy and subsequent malabsorption; hindered nutrient absorption can have systemic effects
Signs & Symptoms	• May be asymptomatic or only have nutritional deficiency symptoms • <u>**Malabsorption**</u>: **intermittent diarrhea, abdominal pain/distention, steatorrhea** (pale, bulky, greasy, foul-smelling stool), **bloating** • Weight loss, iron deficiency anemia, aphthous ulcers of mouth, chronic fatigue, chronic headaches • <u>**Dermatitis Herpetiformis**</u>: atypical; intensely pruritic papulovesicular rash that is symmetric and most commonly affects extensor areas, neck, trunk and scalp
Diagnosis	• *Diagnosis may be clinical if symptoms improve with avoidance of gluten in diet* • <u>Serology</u>: **transglutaminase IgA antibodies is initial test of choice**; anti-endomysial antibody • <u>**Duodenal Mucosa (Small Bowel) Biopsy**</u>: **gold standard for diagnosis; shows villous atrophy**
Treatment	• <u>**Gluten-Free Diet**</u>: strict avoidance all wheat, rye, barley; oats may be cross contaminated so should assess tolerance • May require dietician/nutritionist consult • <u>Nutritional Supplementation</u>: vitamin D, ferrous sulfate, folate, calcium
Key Words & Most Common	• More common in females and those with family history • Autoimmune disorder causes Inflammation which leads to mucosal villous atrophy and malabsorption • Malabsorption symptoms: diarrhea, abdominal distention/bloating, steatorrhea • Dermatitis herpetiformis is intensely pruritic papulovesicular symmetric rash • Transglutaminase IgA antibodies serologic test of choice • Duodenal (small bowel) biopsy is gold standard; shows villous atrophy • Gluten-free diet *Dermatitis Herpetiformis*

Lactose Intolerance

Etiology & Risk Factors	• **Deficiency of the lactase digestive enzyme results in failure to hydrolyze lactose into absorbable glucose and galactose** • Etiology: lack of lactase digestive enzyme • Risk Factors: age (lactase enzyme production naturally declines with age), certain ethnicities (South American, Asian, African descent); secondary lactase deficiency from GI injury (gastroenteritis, inflammatory bowel disease, Celiac disease, antibiotic use)
Patho-physiology	• Lactase enzyme is located in brush border of small intestine • Lactase deficiency causes increased amount of unabsorbed lactose to be present; undigested lactose causes influx of fluid to bowel and lead to osmotic diarrhea • Bacterial fermentation of carbohydrate in bowel leads to increased gas production that causes flatulence and bloating
Signs & Symptoms	• **Symptoms appear 30 minutes to 2 hours after consuming dairy or milk-containing products**; *severity usually determined by amount consumed* • **Diarrhea**, abdominal pain/**bloating, flatulence**, nausea/vomiting, **borborygmi (gurgling noises** within bowel caused by movement of fluid/gas)
Diagnosis	• Elimination Diet: clinical diagnosis; symptoms improve with avoidance of dairy in diet and exacerbated by consuming dairy • Hydrogen Breath Test: test of choice; hydrogen is produced from bacterial fermentation of carbohydrate/undigested lactose in the bowel • Lactose Tolerance Test: serum glucose is measured 0, 30, 60 minutes after consuming lactose; diagnosis made if glucose rises by <20g

Treatment	• Dietary Modification: avoid lactose containing products (cheese, cream, milk, ice cream, sour cream, yogurt, pancakes/waffles, butter)
	   • Yogurt has varying amounts of lactose; Greek yogurt has lowest
	• Nutritional Supplementation: vitamin D and calcium supplements; probiotics (*Lactobacillus acidophilus*)
	   • **Lactase supplements** help breakdown lactose

Key Words & Most Common	• Lactase enzyme deficiency results in inability to properly digest lactose • Diarrhea, bloating, flatulence appearing 30-120 minutes after consuming dairy • Hydrogen breath test is test of choice • Dietary modifications first line + nutritional supplementation

Nut Allergy

Etiology & Risk Factors	• Lifelong allergy to peanuts or tree nuts that may cause a fatal reaction if ingested • Etiology: **type 1 IgE mediated reaction** due to exposure to nuts • Risk Factors: history of atopy, family history of nut allergy, maternal consumption of peanuts/tree nuts during pregnancy, use of peanut oils to fry foods • **Delayed, minimal, or no exposure to nuts/nut butters prior to age 3 increases risk**
Patho-physiology	• Initial sensitization to nuts stimulates IgE antibodies; ingestion can trigger antibody cross-linking to IgE receptors on effector cells (basophils/mast) which causes a histamine, cytokine, chemokine release which propagates the inflammatory/allergic response
Signs & Symptoms	• Common Symptoms: skin flushing, **pruritus, urticaria**, local erythema/edema, sneezing, congestion • Serious Symptoms: **angioedema, tingling of mouth/throat/lips, wheezing, dyspnea**, cough • Symptoms frequently progress to **anaphylaxis**
Diagnosis	• **Clinical Diagnosis** • Skin Testing: drop of nut extract applied to skin; wheal/flare response after 10-20 minutes indicates positive sensitivity • Serum IgE: peanut specific IgE antibodies tested in serum • Oral Food Challenge: most reliable test performed under provider supervision to determine severity of reaction; performed if skin test/serum IgE test is positive
Treatment	• **Dietary Modifications: complete avoidance of allergen is crucial** • **Epinephrine**: prevent or treat anaphylaxis in setting of accidental exposure/consumption • Adjuvant Therapy: antihistamines, steroids, bronchodilators • Peanut Immunotherapy: newer strategy to desensitize/prevent food allergy
Key Words & Most Common	• Type 1 IgE mediated reaction that can be fatal if nut consumed • History of atopy/family history of nut allergy biggest risk factors • Skin reactions: pruritus, urticaria, skin flushing • Serious: angioedema, wheezing/dyspnea, anaphylaxis • Skin testing vs serum IgE test • Avoidance of allergen; Epinephrine if accidental exposure

Peptic Ulcer Disease

Etiology & Risk Factors	• Erosion of inner lining of gastrointestinal tract secondary to gastric acid secretion or pepsin; most common site is at proximal duodenum followed by stomach
	• Etiology:
	  • Common: *Helicobacter pylori* is most common cause, NSAIDs/Aspirin is second most common cause (inhibit prostaglandin synthesis)
	  • Rare: Zollinger-Ellison Syndrome (gastrin producing tumor), alcohol, stress (acute illness, trauma, burns), radiation, Crohn disease

Patho-physiology	• Imbalance between gastric mucosal protective factors (mucous/bicarbonate production, prostaglandin synthesis) and destructive factors (HCl, *H. pylori*) • Defect in protective superficial mucosal layer leads to acidic damage extending to muscularis mucosa • *H. pylori* colonizes and inflames gastric mucosa, secretes urease which neutralizes stomach acid leading to hypochlorhydria, inflammation, and tissue ulceration • NSAIDs inhibit prostaglandin synthesis which leads to decreased gastric mucous and decreased bicarbonate production (mucosal protective factors)
Signs & Symptoms	• <u>Abdominal Pain</u>: epigastric abdominal pain (gnawing/burning) is most common symptom, **dyspepsia**, nausea/vomiting, weight loss • <u>Upper GI Bleed</u>: PUD is most common cause of upper GI bleed; hematemesis, melena, iron deficiency anemia • <u>Perforated Ulcer</u>: sudden onset severe abdominal pain +/- radiation to back or shoulder, rebound tenderness, guarding • <u>Duodenal Ulcer</u>: **nocturnal symptoms**, symptoms *relieved* with food but returns 2-3 hours after meal, • <u>Gastric Ulcer</u>: no consistent pattern; symptoms *worse* with food; weight loss

Diagnosis	• <u>Upper Endoscopy with Biopsy</u>: gold standard and most sensitive test; repeat EGD should be performed to assess treatment success
	• <u>H. Pylori Testing</u>:
	  • <u>Upper Endoscopy with Biopsy</u>: gold standard test
	  • <u>Urea Breath Test</u>: high sensitivity/specificity; noninvasive; urease (*H. pylori* enzyme) is a radiolabeled CO_2 produced by the stomach and exhaled by the lungs
	  • <u>Stool Antigen</u>: highly specific; may be used to determine treatment success
	  • <u>Serologic Antibodies</u>
	• <u>Abdominal X-Ray vs CT</u>: if suspected perforated ulcer or gastric outflow obstruction

Treatment	• <u>Antisecretory Medications</u>: **PPIs** (block acid production), H_2 blockers (reduces pepsin secretion), misoprostol (prostaglandin analog), antacids, bismuth, sucralfate
	• *H. pylori* Eradication:
	  • <u>Triple Therapy</u>: PPI + Clarithromycin + Metronidazole OR Amoxicillin; use quadruple therapy if patient has recent macrolide use or PCN allergy
	  • **<u>Quadruple Therapy</u>: first-line; PPI + Tetracycline + Metronidazole + Bismuth subsalicylate**
	• <u>Surgery</u>: parietal cell vagotomy vs partial gastrectomy

Key Words & Most Common	• *H. pylori* is most common cause; PUD is most common cause of upper GI bleed • Gnawing epigastric pain, hematemesis, melena; Upper endoscopy with biopsy is gold standard; Urea Breath Test to diagnose *H. pylori* • Triple Therapy: PPI + Clarithromycin + Amoxicillin OR Metronidazole

Gastritis

Etiology & Risk Factors	• Inflammation of stomach mucosa caused by infection, drugs, stress, or autoimmune • <u>Acute Gastritis</u>: polymorphonuclear leukocyte infiltration of stomach antrum and body mucosa • <u>Chronic Gastritis</u>: atrophy or metaplasia of antrum ($\downarrow$gastrin secretion) or corpus ($\downarrow$acid and pepsin secretion) • Etiology: ***H. pylori*** infection is most common cause, **NSAIDs/Aspirin is second most common cause**, alcohol, stress (acute illness, trauma, burns), medications, radiation, bile acid reflux, autoimmune
Patho-physiology	• Imbalance between gastric mucosal protective factors (mucous/bicarbonate production, prostaglandin synthesis) and destructive factors (HCl, *H. pylori*) • *H. pylori* colonizes and inflames gastric mucosa, secretes urease which neutralizes stomach acid leading to hypochlorhydria, inflammation, and tissue ulceration • NSAIDs inhibit prostaglandin synthesis which leads to decreased gastric mucous and decreased bicarbonate production (mucosal protective factors)
Signs & Symptoms	• May be asymptomatic • Sudden onset **epigastric pain, dyspepsia, heartburn**, nausea, vomiting • Early satiety, **bloating**

Diagnosis	• <u>Upper Endoscopy with Biopsy</u>: gold standard and most sensitive test
	• <u>H. Pylori Testing</u>:
	  • <u>Upper Endoscopy with Biopsy</u>: gold standard test; thick erosions
	  • <u>Urea Breath Test</u>: high sensitivity/specificity; noninvasive; urease (*H. pylori* enzyme) is a radiolabeled CO_2 produced by the stomach and exhaled by the lungs

Treatment	• <u>Antisecretory Medications</u>: **PPIs** (block acid production), H_2 blockers (reduces pepsin secretion), misoprostol (prostaglandin analog), antacids, bismuth, Sucralfate
	• *H. pylori* Eradication:
	  • **<u>Triple Therapy</u>: PPI + Clarithromycin + Metronidazole OR Amoxicillin**
	  • <u>Quadruple Therapy</u>: **PPI + Tetracycline + Metronidazole + Bismuth subsalicylate** if patient had recent macrolide use or PCN allergy

Key Words & Most Common	• Inflammation of stomach mucosa most commonly caused by *H. pylori* infection or chronic NSAID use • May be asymptomatic • Epigastric pain, dyspepsia, heartburn, N/V • Upper endoscopy with biopsy is gold standard • Urea breath test for *H. pylori* testing • PPIs, H_2 blockers • Triple Therapy: PPI + Clarithromycin + Amoxicillin OR Metronidazole if *H. pylori*

Zollinger-Ellison Syndrome

Etiology & Risk Factors	• Gastrinoma is a gastric neuroendocrine malignancy (gastrin-secreting tumor) leading to hypersecretion of hydrochloric acid by parietal cells • **Most common site is duodenum**, followed by pancreas, and lymph nodes • <u>Etiology</u>: **sporadic cause; multiple endocrine neoplasia type 1 (MEN1)** (approximately 50% of patients with MEN1 also have ZES)
Patho-physiology	• Ectopic gastrin-secreting tumor stimulates hypersecretion of hydrochloric acid by parietal cells of the stomach • Gastrin leads to gastrointestinal mucosal ulceration
Signs & Symptoms	• **Abdominal pain, heartburn, diarrhea** • **Multiple refractory ulcers** • Malabsorption (pancreatic enzymes inactivated by hyperchlorhydria) leading to weight loss, chronic diarrhea, anorexia
Diagnosis	• <u>**Fasting Serum Gastrin Level**</u>: **best initial test**; (pH<2 or gastrin level > 1,000pg/mL); patient should avoid PPI for 1 week and H2 blockers for 48 hours prior to test • <u>**Secretin Stimulation Test**</u>: **confirmatory test**; measures fasting serum gastrin level at 2 to 15 minutes after intravenous secretin administration (positive if >200pg/mL) • <u>**Somatostatin Receptor Scintigraphy (SRS)**</u>: more sensitive than conventional imaging (CT/MRI) and more specific for extrahepatic gastrinoma; detects primary and secondary lesions • <u>MEN1 Screening</u>: serum calcium, parathyroid hormone level, prolactin, and pancreatic polypeptide

Treatment	• <u>**Acid Suppression Medication**</u>:
	   • <u>**Proton Pump Inhibitor (PPI)**</u>: **omeprazole is drug of choice;** blocks acid production
	   • <u>H$_2$ blockers</u>: famotidine; reduces pepsin secretion
	   • <u>Octreotide</u>: decreases acid production
	• <u>Surgical Resection</u>: local tumor resection; surgical resection of metastases (liver, abdominal lymph nodes)
	• <u>Chemotherapy</u>: indicated for metastatic disease (streptozocin + 5-fluorouracil or doxorubicin is the preferred chemotherapy for islet cell tumors)

Key Words & Most Common	• Gastrin-secreting neuroendocrine tumor leading to ↑HCl secretion • Most common site is duodenum • Associated with MEN1 • Abdominal pain, heartburn, diarrhea, refractory ulcers • Fasting Serum Gastrin Level is best initial test • Secretin Stimulation Test to confirm • Acid Suppression with PPI is initial treatment of choice

Carcinoid Tumor

Etiology & Risk Factors	• **Slow-growing well-differentiated tumor arising from neuroendocrine enterochromaffin cells capable of secreting peptides and neuroamines** • **Most common site is GI system, particularly the small intestine**; lungs second most common site • <u>Etiology</u>: tumor arising from neuroendocrine cells • <u>Risk Factors</u>: **age (50-70 years old most common)**, female, certain genetic syndromes (MEN1, NF1), family history, chronic inflammatory bowel disease, smoking

Patho-physiology	• Tumor arising from neuroendocrine enterochromaffin cells of the GI tract
	• Tumor may secrete peptides and neuroamines that can disrupt many processes
	   • Paracrine agents and growth factors increase cell proliferation and potentiate mutations in oncogenes and tumor suppressor genes
	   • Secretion of vasoactive substances such as serotonin, prostaglandins, histamine, and hormones

Signs & Symptoms	• Many are asymptomatic
	• <u>**Carcinoid Syndrome**</u>:
	   • <u>**Histamine and Kinin Production**</u>: **vasodilation, episodic flushing,** hypotension, **tachycardia and bronchoconstriction**
	   • <u>**Serotonin Release**</u>: **watery diarrhea;** may be present with fasting

Diagnosis	• <u>Biochemical Screening</u>:
	   • <u>Chromogranin A</u>: nonspecific neuroendocrine marker that may aid in prognostics
	   • <u>Pancreastatin</u>: negative prognostic indicator
	   • <u>**24-hour Urine for 5-hydroxyindoleacetic acid (5-HIAA)**</u>: **serotonin degradation product**
	• <u>Imaging</u>: CT/MRI; Upper Endoscopy to visualize accessible lesions; Somatostatin Receptor Scintigraphy (SRS) is more sensitive than conventional imaging (CT/MRI)

Treatment	• <u>Surgical Resection</u>: local tumor resection if possible depending on site • <u>**Somatostatin Analogues**</u>: **mainstay of medical therapy** • <u>**Octreotide**</u>: binds to somatostatin receptors to reduce diarrhea and flushing; may control growth of tumor
Key Words & Most Common	• Tumor arising from neuroendocrine enterochromaffin cells • Most common site is small intestine • Carcinoid Syndrome: flushing, diarrhea, tachycardia, bronchoconstriction • Screening: 24-hour urine 5-HIAA • Somatostatin Analogues: octreotide

Gastric Cancer

Etiology & Risk Factors	• **Most common is adenocarcinoma**
	• <u>Etiology</u>: multifactorial; **most common type is adenocarcinoma (95%)**
	  • <u>Two Types of Gastric Adenocarcinomas</u>: intestinal (well-differentiated) and diffuse (undifferentiated)
	• <u>Risk Factors</u>: males, age (>40 years old most common)
	  • <u>**Infection**</u>: ***H. pylori* infection (biggest risk factor)**
	  • <u>Dietary</u>: **high-salt diet**, preserved foods containing nitrites/nitrates, smoked/cured meats, smoking, contaminated drinking water, obesity, poor diet
	  • <u>Medications</u>: aspirin and NSAID use associated with decreased risk
	  • <u>Conditions</u>: non-Hodgkin lymphoma (most common extra-nodal site), **pernicious anemia**, chronic gastritis

Patho-physiology	• Chronic inflammation caused by *H. pylori*, pernicious anemia, or high-salt diets cause loss of parietal cells and reduction of acid production leading to chronic gastritis • This chronic inflammation then leads to intestinal metaplasia, dysplasia, and culminates to adenocarcinoma.

Signs & Symptoms	• Most patients are at advanced stage by time of presentation
	• <u>**Non-Specific Symptoms**</u>: **weight loss, persistent abdominal pain,**
	• <u>**Gastrointestinal Symptoms**</u>: hematemesis, **early satiety**, anorexia, dysphagia, dyspepsia, nausea/vomiting (especially post-prandial)
	• <u>Physical Exam</u>:
	  • Palpable abdominal mass is most common finding
	  • Metastatic signs (see chart below)

Diagnosis	• <u>**Upper Endoscopy with Biopsy**</u>: **initial test of choice; direct visualization** • <u>Abdominal CT Scan</u>: evaluate metastatic disease
Treatment	• <u>Endoscopic Resection vs Surgical Resection</u>: for local gastric cancer offers best chance of survival with surgery alone • <u>Chemotherapy/Radiation</u>: for advanced stages and/or when resection unable to be performed • <u>Palliative Care</u>: most patients present with advanced disease and offer **poor prognosis**

Key Words & Most Common	• Most common is adenocarcinoma • Most common risk factor is H. pylori infection causing chronic inflammation • Weight loss, abdominal pain, early satiety, post-prandial vomiting • Metastatic Signs (see chart) • Upper Endoscopy with Biopsy is test of choice • Poor prognosis; resection +/- chemotherapy and radiation	**Metastatic Signs**	
		<u>Virchow's Node</u>: Left Supraclavicular Lymphadenopathy	<u>Krukenburg Tumor</u>: Ovarian Mass
		<u>Sister Mary Joseph's Node</u>: Peri-Umbilical Nodule	<u>Blumer's Shelf</u>: Rectal Mass
		<u>Irish Node</u>: Left Axillary Nodule	Ascites or Hepatomegaly

Pyloric Stenosis

Etiology & Risk Factors	• Infantile hypertrophy and hyperplasia of the pylorus muscles leading to gastric outlet obstruction • <u>Etiology</u>: hypertrophy/hyperplasia of pylorus muscle • <u>Risk Factors</u>: **males (4x greater risk), Caucasian, first-born infant, post-natal exposure to erythromycin**, preterm birth, cesarean section delivery, smoking during pregnancy
Patho-physiology	• Hypertrophy and hyperplasia of circular and longitudinal muscle layers of the pylorus leading to narrowing of the gastric antrum lumen • This causes a gastric outlet obstruction which prevents gastric emptying into the duodenum and stomach becomes dilated • Obstruction leads to immediate postprandial, nonbilious, projectile emesis

Signs & Symptoms	• **Symptoms most common in first 3-6 weeks of life**
	• **Nonbilious, projectile emesis most common; immediately post-prandial**
	• <u>Severe</u>: **dehydration** (depressed fontanelles, dry mucous membranes, decreased skin tearing, fatigue/lethargy, minimal tearing), weight loss, anorexia
	• <u>Physical Exam</u>:
	  • **Palpable, non-tender, firm pylorus muscle about 1-2cm in diameter ("olive shaped") at the right epigastrium**
	  • May see reverse peristaltic wave

Diagnosis	• <u>**Abdominal Ultrasound**</u>: **primary test of choice**
	  • **Demonstrates thickened (>3mm) and elongated (>15mm) pylorus**
	• <u>Labs</u>: classic finding is **hyperchloremic, hypokalemic, metabolic alkalosis**
	• <u>Barium Upper GI Series</u>: rarely required; utilized if abdominal US inconclusive
	  • May show elongated pylorus, delayed gastric emptying
	  • <u>String Sign</u>: thin "string" of barium through a narrowed pylorus
	  • <u>Railroad Track Sign</u>: excess mucosa in the pylorus resulting in 2 channels of barium

Treatment	• <u>Medical Management</u>: supportive
	  • Rehydration (**IV fluids**) and **correction of electrolyte abnormalities** (potassium, sodium, chloride)
	  • Correction of bicarbonate (may post hypoventilation risk)
	  • Consider nasogastric (NG) tube placement
	• <u>Surgery</u>: **pyloromyotomy is curative**

Key Words & Most Common	• Most common in first 3-6 weeks of life, males, white, first-born infant • Nonbilious, projectile vomiting immediately after eating • Palpable, non-tender, firm pylorus muscle at right epigastrium ("olive shaped") • Abdominal Ultrasound is primary test of choice • IV rehydration + electrolyte replacement • Pyloromyotomy is curative

Thickened and elongated pylorus muscle

Autoimmune Hepatitis

Etiology & Risk Factors	• Idiopathic hepatocellular inflammation caused by autoimmune pathology
	• 2 Types:
	   • <u>Type 1</u>: presence of anti-smooth muscle antibodies (ASMA) +/- anti-nuclear antibodies (ANA)
	   • <u>Type 2</u>: positive anti-liver/anti-kidney microsome (anti-LMK) type 1 antibodies or anti-liver cytosol (anti-LC) type 1 antibodies
	• <u>Etiology</u>: **idiopathic**
	• <u>Risk Factors</u>: **age (15-40 years old most common)**, **female**, genetic predisposition, environmental factors, immune dysregulation (Grave's, rheumatoid arthritis, celiac, T1DM, ulcerative colitis)

Patho-physiology	• Immune tolerance failure in susceptible patient causes T-cell mediated inflammatory response to a trigger • This leads to chronic inflammation of hepatocytes and hepatic fibrosis
Signs & Symptoms	• May be asymptomatic • <u>Nonspecific Symptoms</u>: **Fatigue, malaise, abdominal pain** (epigastric/RUQ), nausea, **arthralgias**, **jaundice**, cirrhosis • <u>Physical Exam</u>: hepatomegaly, jaundice, and ascites seen in severe severe disease

Diagnosis	• <u>Labs</u>:
	   • <u>Autoantibodies</u>: **elevated antinuclear antibody (ANA)**, **smooth muscle antibodies (SMA)**, and antibodies to liver kidney microsome type 1 (anti-LKM1)
	   • <u>Liver Function Tests (LFT)</u>: **marked elevation of ALT/AST (1.5 50x normal) and gamma-globulin**; mild to moderate elevation of alkaline phosphatase
	   • <u>CBC</u>: may show leukopenia, hemolytic anemia, thrombocytopenia
	• **<u>Liver Biopsy</u>: definitive diagnosis**; may show bridging or multilobular necrosis

Treatment	• <u>Monotherapy</u>: **corticosteroids** (prednisone taper) • <u>Combination Therapy</u>: **corticosteroids + azathioprine** (immunosuppressant) • <u>Liver Transplant</u>: may be necessary in cases with severe cirrhosis or liver failure
Key Words & Most Common	• Idiopathic hepatocellular inflammation • Most common in young women • Nonspecific Symptoms: fatigue, malaise, abdominal pain, arthralgias, jaundice • Labs: elevated ANA and SMA; marked ALT/AST elevation • Liver biopsy is required for definitive diagnosis • Steroids + azathioprine

Acute Liver Failure

Etiology & Risk Factors	• Fulminant hepatitis resulting in severe liver dysfunction in a patient with no preexisting liver disease • <u>Etiology</u>: **drug-induced (acetaminophen toxicity) is most common cause**; hepatitis (A and E); Reye Syndrome (child given aspirin after viral infection); viral • <u>Risk Factors</u>: hepatitis (A and E), **drug toxicity (acetaminophen)**, toxin exposure (poisonous mushrooms, industrial chemicals), hepatic ischemia, metabolic disorder, pregnancy (HELLP syndrome)
Patho-physiology	• Hepatocyte necrosis/apoptosis occurs when oxidative stress causes ATP to become depleted leading to cellular edema and cell membrane interference • Ammonia able to cross blood brain barrier causing cerebral edema
Signs & Symptoms	• <u>General</u>: **abdominal pain, nausea**/vomiting, fatigue, edema, **changes in urine or stool** (dark-colored urine due to the presence of bilirubin and pale-colored stools due to lack of bile secretion), **generalized pruritus (bile salt accumulation)**, myalgia • <u>Encephalopathy</u>: **altered mental status**, vomiting, hyperreflexia, **asterixis** (hand tremor with wrist extension), cerebral edema • <u>Coagulopathy</u>: easy bruising, bleeding gums, nosebleeds • <u>Reye Syndrome</u>: rash of palms of hands and feet, vomiting, altered mental status, confusion, hyperventilation, fever, dilated pupils • <u>Physical Exam</u>: • Tender hepatomegaly, jaundice, right upper quadrant pain

Diagnosis	• <u>Liver Function Tests (LFT)</u>: **alanine transaminase (ALT), aspartate transaminase (AST), alkaline phosphatase (ALP), bilirubin**
	   • <u>Alanine Transaminase</u>: ALT is more specific to liver
	   • **<u>Aspartate Transaminase</u>: extreme elevation indicates acetaminophen toxicity**; moderate elevation indicates viral hepatitis; mild elevation indicates alcoholic hepatitis
	   • <u>Alkaline Phosphatase and Bilirubin</u>: elevated in cholestasis disease
	• <u>Coagulation Studies</u>: reflects liver's ability to produce coagulation factors; INR>1.5, increased PT and eventual increase in PTT
	• <u>Other</u>: elevated ammonia (encephalopathy), low serum albumin, thrombocytopenia, hypoglycemia (hepatic gluconeogenesis)
	   • Acetaminophen level, viral hepatitis serologies

Treatment	• <u>Supportive</u>: IV hydration, electrolyte replacement, monitor hypoglycemia, blood products (platelets, fresh frozen plasma for coagulopathy) • <u>Medical Management</u>: **N-acetyl cysteine if acetaminophen toxicity suspected**, mannitol (cerebral edema with elevated ICP) • <u>Liver Transplant</u>: definitive; high risk of graft complication
Key Words & Most Common	• Acute liver dysfunction in patient with no preexisting liver disease • Most common cause is acetaminophen toxicity • Hepatomegaly, jaundice, nausea, RUQ pain • Encephalopathy: AMS, vomiting, asterixis • Elevated AST/ALT, Alkaline phosphatase, bilirubin, INR/PT/PTT, ammonia, albumin • Supportive therapy and treat underlying cause

Hepatitis A

Etiology & Risk Factors	• Acute viral illness transmitted by fecal-oral route affecting the liver • <u>Etiology</u>: hepatitis A virus (HAV); a single-stranded RNA picornavirus • <u>Risk Factors</u>: **IV drug users, men who have sex with men**, isolated communities, homelessness, **occupational exposure** (healthcare, day care), institutionalization, oyster consumption, international travel to endemic area • <u>Transmission</u>: **fecal-oral**; contaminated food, water, or close contact to infectious person • Most common transmission from asymptomatic child to adult
Patho-physiology	• <u>Incubation Period</u>: 15-50 days • Single-stranded RNA virus that replicates within hepatocytes • Virus is taken up by GI system after ingestion; T-cell mediated release of cytotoxic interferon-gamma leads to inflammation of liver. Resulting hepatocellular apoptosis and inflammation from the innate immune reaction
Signs & Symptoms	• Most patients are **asymptomatic** • Prodrome of nausea/vomiting, right upper quadrant pain, fatigue/malaise, **fever**, myalgia, anorexia • May develop dark urine, clay-colored stool; jaundice, scleral icterus, pruritus
Diagnosis	• <u>Liver Function Tests (LFT)</u>: elevated ALT, AST, and bilirubin • <u>**Acute Phase**</u>: **elevated anti-hepatitis A virus IgM** • <u>Past Exposure</u>: elevated anti-hepatitis A virus IgG
Treatment	• <u>Supportive</u>: no specific treatment required; **virus is self limiting** (not associated with chronic state or liver failure) • Antiemetics, IV fluids, avoiding hepatotoxic medications • <u>Prevention</u>: improving sanitation and handwashing, food safety, immunization

	Pre-Exposure	Post-Exposure
Prophylaxis	• Indicated in children 12 months or older, international travel to endemic area, homosexuals, intravenous drug users, occupational risk exposure • <u>Standard Adult Dosing</u>: two doses of the vaccine 6-12 months apart	• <u>Healthy 1-40yo</u>: hepatitis A virus vaccine within 2 weeks of exposure • <u>Healthy >40yo</u>: hepatitis A virus (+/- immunoglobulin) within 2 weeks of exposure • <u>Immunocompromised</u>: hepatitis A vaccine + immunoglobulin

Key Words & Most Common	• Acute viral illness transmitted fecal-oral route • IV drug users, homosexuals and occupational exposure are greatest risk factors • Mostly asymptomatic, may have nausea/vomiting, fever, RUQ pain progressing to dark urine, pale stool, jaundice • Elevated anti-HAV IgM test • Supportive treatment; virus is self limiting

Hepatitis E

Etiology & Risk Factors	• Acute, self-limiting viral infection of the liver due to hepatitis E virus; **most common cause of acute viral hepatitis worldwide** • <u>Etiology</u>: hepatitis E virus (HEV); a non-enveloped RNA virus • <u>Risk Factors</u>: living in **developing countries**, travel to endemic area, **consumption of contaminated food/water or undercooked meat (pork)** • <u>Transmission</u>: **fecal-oral**
Patho-physiology	• <u>Incubation Period</u>: 2-10 weeks (usually 4-6 weeks) • Non-enveloped RNA virus spread fecal-oral route • After ingestion, hepatitis E is infiltrated through GI system mucosa and reaches liver through portal circulation • High infantile mortality and fetal loss as HEV can be transmitted vertically from mother to infant during gestation
Signs & Symptoms	• Most patients are **asymptomatic** • Prodrome of nausea/vomiting, right upper quadrant pain, fatigue/malaise, **fever**, myalgia, anorexia • **Pregnant women tend to have more severe disease**, increased risk for liver failure and fetal loss
Diagnosis	• <u>Liver Function Tests (LFTs)</u>: elevated ALT, AST, and bilirubin • <u>**Immunoglobulin Tests**</u>: **elevated anti-hepatitis E virus IgM** • <u>Polymerase Chain Reaction (PCR) Test</u>: hepatitis E virus detected in stool
Treatment	• <u>Supportive</u>: no specific treatment required; **virus is self limiting** (not associated with chronic state or liver failure) • Antiemetics, IV fluids, avoiding hepatotoxic medications • **Highest mortality rate secondary to liver failure during pregnancy** (mortality rate goes up to 10-25% during third trimester pregnancy)
Key Words & Most Common	• Acute viral illness transmitted fecal-oral route • Living in developing country or consumption of contaminated food/water greatest risk factors • Mostly asymptomatic, may have nausea/vomiting, fever, RUQ pain • Pregnant women have more severe disease • Elevated AST/ALT, elevated anti-HEV IgM • Supportive treatment; virus is self limiting

Hepatitis C

Etiology & Risk Factors	• Viral infection of the liver due to hepatitis C virus; most common infectious cause of chronic liver disease, cirrhosis, and liver transplant • Etiology: hepatitis c virus (HCV); a single-stranded RNA flavivirus • Risk Factors: **IV drug use is most common cause**, needlestick injury, blood transfusion recipient prior to 1992 • Transmission: **bloodborne**; not commonly transmitted sexual, perinatal or breastfeeding
Patho-physiology	• Single-stranded RNA flavivirus • Hepatitis C virus enters hepatocyte through endocytosis; chronic infection may be secondary to weak CD4+ and CD8+ T-cell response, failing to control viral replication • Liver fibrosis correlates with increased risk of hepatocellular carcinoma
Signs & Symptoms	• Most patients are **asymptomatic; >75% of cases progress to chronic infection** • Nausea/vomiting, **right upper quadrant pain**, **fatigue/malaise** (from electrolyte disruption), myalgia, anorexia, **general unwell feeling** • May develop dark urine, **clay-colored stool**, pruritus • Physical Exam: • **Jaundice, scleral icterus**, gynecomastia, small testes, temporal wasting, hepatomegaly, caput medusae, paraumbilical hernia

	Acute HCV	Chronic HCV	Prior HCV
HCV Antibodies	+/-	+	+
HCV RNA	+	+	-

Diagnosis	• Liver Function Tests (LFT): elevated ALT, AST, and bilirubin • Screening: **hepatitis C virus antibodies** (turns positive within 6 weeks) • Confirmation: **hepatitis C virus RNA**; more sensitive; determines active from past infection • Liver Biopsy: gold standard; may help with staging

Treatment	• Supportive: alcohol cessation, avoidance of hepatotoxic medication (acetaminophen)
	• **Antiviral Therapy:**
	  • **Direct-Acting Antiviral Drugs (DAAs): sofosbuvir-ledipasvir combination or grazoprevir-elbasvir combination; cure rate is 90-97%**
	• Previous Regimen: injected pegylated interferon alpha + ribavirin
	  • Low cure rate (40-60%) and many side effects (thrombocytopenia, flu like illness, leukopenia, arthralgias, severe anemia, and psychosis

Key Words & Most Common	• Most common infectious cause of chronic liver disease and cirrhosis; 75% of cases progress to chronic HCV • Bloodborne transmission; IV drug use is most common cause • Mostly asymptomatic; may develop general unwell feeling/malaise, RUQ pain, jaundice, scleral icterus, clay colored stool • HCV antibodies for screening; HCV RNA for confirmation • Antiviral therapy with DAAs

Hepatitis B

Etiology & Risk Factors	• Potentially life-threatening viral liver infection caused by the hepatitis B virus
	• Etiology: hepatitis B virus (HBV); a DNA virus
	• Risk Factors: **IV drug users**, homosexual males, hemodialysis patients, healthcare workers, primary contact exposure
	• Transmission: horizontal or vertical transmission
	  • Horizontal Transmission: sexual (oral, vaginal, anal) or mucosal surface contact (saliva, vaginal secretion, semen, blood)
	  • Vertical Transmission: mother to newborn perinatal transmission during delivery

Patho-physiology	• Incubation Period: 4-25 weeks • HBsAg is transmitted through blood or body secretion contact. HBsAg and other nucleocapsid proteins then promote T cells to induce lysis of infected cells • Cytotoxicity T-cell immune response to hepatitis B virus causes hepatocyte injury

Signs & Symptoms	• Most patients are **asymptomatic**
	• Anicteric Phase: fever, skin rash, nausea/vomiting, arthralgia, **RUQ pain, fatigue/malaise**/myalgia, anorexia, **decrease smoking desire**
	• Icteric Phase: **jaundice**
	  • May develop dark urine, **clay-colored stool**, pruritus, that progresses into liver failure
	• Physical Exam:
	  • **Jaundice, scleral icterus**, ascites, gynecomastia, small testes, temporal wasting, hepatomegaly, caput medusae, paraumbilical hernia

Diagnosis	• Liver Function Tests (LFT): elevated ALT, AST, and bilirubin (jaundice); **AST/ALT in thousands in acute phase**, hundreds in chronic phase • **Hepatitis B Serologies: hepatitis B surface antigen, surface antibody, core antibody** (see chart on next slide) • Confirmation: **hepatitis B virus DNA**; more sensitive; determines viral load • Liver Biopsy: gold standard and may help with staging

Treatment	• Supportive Care: indicated for acute phase; most will not progress to chronic
	  • Alcohol cessation, avoid hepatotoxic medication (acetaminophen)
	• **Antiviral Therapy:** indicated if persistent, jaundice (bilirubin >10mg/dL), liver biopsy inflammation, severe symptoms
	  • Interferons (peginterferon alfa-2a, interferon alfa-2b), nucleoside analogs (**entecavir**, lamivudine, telbivudine), and nucleotide analogs (adefovir, **tenofovir**)
	• Liver Transplant: definitive; high risk of graft complication

Vaccination	• **Schedule: birth, 1 month, 6 months** • Adults at high risk of HBV infection should be screened and vaccinated if they are not immune or infected
Key Words & Most Common	• Transmitted through sexual or mucosal surface contact • Most patients are asymptomatic; may have constitutional symptoms (fever, rash, N/V, arthralgia) that progresses to jaundice +/- liver failure • ALT/AST, bilirubin elevation, Hepatitis B serologies • Supportive Care + antiviral therapy as indicated

Hepatitis B Serology Chart

Marker	Meaning	Acute Infection	Window Period	Recovered Infection	Immunization	Inactive Chronic Carrier
HBcAb	Exposure	IgM	IgM	IgG	–	IgG
HBsAg	Infection	+	–	–	–	–
HBsAb	Immunity	–	–	+	+	–

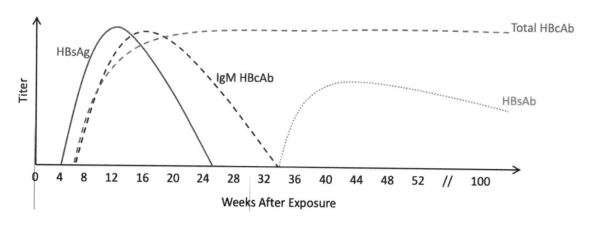

Hepatocellular Carcinoma

Etiology & Risk Factors	• Primary tumor of the liver; **will affect 85% of patients with cirrhosis** • Etiology: **complication of cirrhosis is most common cause** • Risk Factors: **viral hepatitis (hepatitis B and C), alcoholic liver disease, cirrhosis**, non-alcoholic liver disease, aflatoxin B1 exposure (*Aspergillus* spp), iron overload, glycogen storage disease, Wilson disease, alpha-1-antitrypsin disease
Patho-physiology	• Genetic alteration and mutations of hepatocytes leads to oncogenesis • Chronic inflammation leads to hepatic fibrosis, necrosis, and cellular regeneration which increases likelihood of hepatocellular carcinoma

Signs & Symptoms	• Many are asymptomatic in early stages of disease
	• **Malaise, weight loss, jaundice, abdominal pain**
	• May have fever, hypoglycemia, hyperlipidemia
	• Physical Exam:
	    • **Right upper quadrant mass** may be palpable,
	    • Hepatic friction rub/bruit, jaundice

Diagnosis	• Liver Function Tests (LFT): elevated ALT, AST, and bilirubin • **Elevated Alpha-Fetoprotein (AFP)**: signifies dedifferentiation of hepatocytes • **Abdominal Ultrasound**: non-invasive test to screen or for surveillance • **US primary surveillance modality every 6 months +/- alpha-fetoprotein in high-risk patients** • Contrast-Enhanced Abdominal CT Scan: characterizes lesions and greater sensitivity/specificity • Liver Biopsy: not routinely performed due to risk of seeding and bleeding
Treatment	• **Surgical Resection**: indicated if early stage and confined to a lob without cirrhosis • **Liver Transplant**: indicated to remove tumors; offers a better prognosis • **Systemic Chemotherapy: first-line for advanced stage**, macrovascular infiltration, or extrahepatic spread
Key Words & Most Common	• Primary tumor of liver that will affect 85% of patients with cirrhosis • Cirrhosis and hepatitis are biggest risk factors • Asymptomatic in early stages; progress to malaise, abdominal pain, weight loss, jaundice • Elevated liver enzymes and alpha-fetoprotein • US for surveillance and screening; Contrasted CT to characterize lesion and is more sensitive/specific • Surgical Resection vs Liver Transplant vs Chemo

Budd-Chiari Syndrome

Etiology & Risk Factors	• **Hepatic vein outflow obstruction** leading to impaired liver drainage and resultant portal hypertension and cirrhosis
	• Etiology: obstruction of hepatic vein
	  • **Primary: caused by thrombosis or phlebitis** (75%)
	  • Secondary: caused by compression of hepatic vein or inferior vena cava due to a mass, pregnancy
	• Risk Factors: **myeloproliferative disorders** (essential thrombocythemia, **polycythemia vera**), presence liver lesions (**malignancy,** cysts, adenoma, aneurysm) causing compression, increased estrogen level (pregnancy or oral contraception pill use), coagulation disorders

Patho-physiology	• Occlusion of hepatic vein causes venous congestion and subsequent expansion of the liver capsule; interstitial fluid filtration worsens liver congestion • Filtered interstitial fluid may exceed lymphatic drainage ability leading to ascites • Thrombosis and venous occlusion leads to portal hypertension and decreased liver perfusion causing hepatocyte hypoxia and injury
Signs & Symptoms	• **Classic Triad: right upper quadrant abdominal pain + hepatomegaly + ascites** • Acute Obstruction: classic triad + fatigue, nausea/vomiting, mild jaundice (**most commonly caused by pregnancy**) • Chronic Obstruction: may range from **asymptomatic to liver failure; cirrhosis, lower extremity edema**, progressive ascites, splenomegaly, **jaundice**
Diagnosis	• **Clinical Diagnosis:** no definitive test to diagnose; clinical suspicion in patients with hepatomegaly, liver failure, ascites, or cirrhosis with no easily identifiable cause • Liver Function Tests (LFT): elevated ALT, AST, and bilirubin • **Doppler Abdominal Ultrasound: initial screening imaging test; shows direction of blood flow and level of thrombi or obstruction** • Abdominal CT/MRI: performed if ultrasound is non-diagnostic; consider if mechanical obstruction from mass is suspected cause • Venography: gold standard test; more invasive so rarely performed • Liver Biopsy: rarely performed due to invasive nature of test; helps determine if cirrhosis has developed; may show necrosis/hemorrhage
Treatment	• Supportive: aimed to treat complications (liver failure, varices, ascites) with **diuretics, sodium restriction, therapeutic paracentesis to remove fluid excess** • **Anticoagulation: mainstay of treatment; low-molecular-weight heparin bridge to warfarin** • Thrombolysis and Stenting: placement of Transjugular intrahepatic portosystemic shunt (TIPS procedure) • Surgical Decompression: removal of mass effect • Liver Transplant: if failed therapy and has cirrhosis or liver failure
Key Words & Most Common	• Hepatic vein outflow obstruction most commonly caused by thrombosis; may also be caused by pregnancy/malignancy • Classic Triad of RUQ abdominal pain, hepatomegaly, ascites • Doppler Ultrasound is initial screening test of choice • Supportive therapy with diuretics, sodium restriction, paracentesis • Anticoagulation

Cirrhosis

Etiology & Risk Factors	• Chronic injury of the liver leads to fibrosis and nodular formation of the liver parenchyma leading to liver failure • Etiology: **chronic hepatitis C is most common cause, alcoholic liver disease**, nonalcoholic fatty liver disease (diabetes, hypertriglyceridemia, obesity), autoimmune hepatitis, primary biliary cirrhosis, primary sclerosing cholangitis, drug induced (acetaminophen, amiodarone), hemochromatosis, alpha-1-antitrypsin deficiency

Patho-physiology	• Hepatocyte hyperplasia (nodule regeneration) and angiogenesis results from chronic inflammation and injury to liver leading to hepatic insufficiency
	  • Angiogenesis connect hepatic artery and portal vein to hepatic venules, leading to low-volume, high-pressure venous drainage
	  • Portal vein pressure then increases contributing to portal hypertension

Signs & Symptoms	• Abdominal distension/pain, fatigue, weakness and muscle cramping (electrolyte abnormalities), anorexia, weight loss, **generalized pruritus** (bile salt accumulation) • Hepatic Encephalopathy: **altered mental status**, confusion, lethargy (secondary to toxic levels of ammonia), **asterixis** (hand tremor with wrist extension) • Physical Exam: • Ascites, hepatosplenomegaly, **caput medusa, muscle wasting**, gynecomastia, **jaundice**, telangiectasias, spider nevi, Dupuytren's contractures, nail clubbing
Diagnosis	• **Liver Function Tests (LFT):** normal or modestly **elevated ALT, AST, bilirubin; elevated or normal gamma-glutamyl transpeptidase (GGT) and alkaline phosphatase (ALP)** • Coagulation Studies: INR>1.5, increased PT; reflects liver's ability to produce coagulation factors • Other Labs: **elevated ammonia** (encephalopathy), **low serum albumin**, thrombocytopenia, normocytic anemia (macrocytic if secondary to alcohol) • **Abdominal Ultrasound:** may show small, nodular liver; used to screen for hepatocellular carcinoma every 6 months +/- alpha-fetoprotein • Abdominal CT/MRI with and without Contrast: detects nodular texture, esophageal varices, portal/splenic venous thrombosis; delineates suspected malignancy • **Liver Biopsy: gold standard** but rarely performed due to invasive nature; may show necrosis/hemorrhage

Treatment	• Supportive: liver damage is permanent; treatment is aimed to slow progression
	  • **Lifestyle Modifications: alcohol cessation,** HBV/HCV vaccination, maintain **proper nutrition** and balanced diet, weight reduction, avoid hepatotoxic medications
	  • **Symptomatic Treatment: diuretics, sodium restriction, therapeutic paracentesis to remove fluid excess**
	• Treat Underlying Etiologies: if possible; antiviral medications for HBV/HCV, steroids/immunosuppressant medications for autoimmune hepatitis, ursodeoxycholic acid for primary biliary cholangitis, copper chelation therapy for Wilson disease, and iron chelation/phlebotomy in hemochromatosis
	• Medication Management:
	  • **Lactulose: indicated for encephalopathy;** GI flora converts to lactic acid which neutralizes ammonia
	  • **Cholestyramine:** indicated for pruritus; reduces bile salt accumulation in skin
	• Thrombolysis and Stenting: placement of transjugular intrahepatic portosystemic shunt (TIPS procedure) if portal hypertension develops
	• Liver Transplant: indicated if liver failure or hepatocellular carcinoma develops

Key Words & Most Common	• Chronic fibrosis and nodular regeneration of liver; most commonly caused by chronic hepatitis C or alcoholic liver disease • General symptoms of abdominal distension, fatigue, muscle cramping/weakness, weight loss • Ascites, hepatomegaly, caput medusa, jaundice • Elevated liver enzymes, GGT, ALP, ammonia, low serum albumin • Avoid alcohol, proper nutrition; lactulose for hepatic encephalopathy

Ascites secondary to portal hypertension

Spontaneous Bacterial Peritonitis

Etiology & Risk Factors	• Acute infection of ascites fluid without a district source of infection (no bowel perforation); common complication of cirrhosis • <u>Etiology</u>: **most commonly caused by gram-negative aerobic organisms (*Escherichia coli* and *Klebsiella pneumoniae*)**; gram-positive *Streptococcus pneumoniae*
Patho-physiology	• Bacterial overgrowth in the GI tract (secondary to prolonged intestinal transit time) is common in cirrhosis patients • Reduced protein production (low complement levels in serum and ascites) results in a decreased immune system capability to clear microorganisms which contributes to bacterial overgrowth within the ascites fluid
Signs & Symptoms	• **Abdominal pain, fever/chills**, malaise, diarrhea, paralytic ileus, altered mental status • <u>Physical Exam</u>: • **Ascites** (fluid wave, shifting dullness), abdominal tenderness to palpation (guarding, rebound tenderness), increased abdominal girth

Diagnosis	• <u>Paracentesis</u>: **test of choice**; peritoneal fluid analysis with cell count, differential, culture, lactate level, pH
	   • <u>**Polymorphonuclear Leukocyte (PMN)**</u>: **PMN count of > 250 cells/mcL**
	   • <u>Serum Ascites Albumin Gradient (SAAG)</u>: >1.1 indicates portal hypertension diagnosis
	   • <u>Protein</u>: <1 g/dL
	   • <u>Glucose</u>: >50mg/dL
	   • <u>Gram Stain</u>: identifies class of organism; often negative
	   • <u>Culture</u>: most accurate; identifies gram-negative aerobic organism or gram-positive (anaerobes are very rare)
	• <u>Abdominal CT Scan</u>: if bowel perforation is suspected source

Treatment	• <u>**Empiric Antibiotics**</u>: **third-generation cephalosporin (cefotaxime or ceftriaxone)**; ciprofloxacin if beta-lactam allergic • <u>IV Albumin</u>: reduces renal failure from hepatorenal syndrome
Key Words & Most Common	• Acute infection of ascites fluid without bowel perforation • E. coli is most common organism • Abdominal pain + fever in patient with ascites • Paracentesis is test of choice; PMN>250, SAAG>1.1 • Culture is most accurate • Empiric antibiotics with cefotaxime or ceftriaxone; IV albumin to reduce renal failure

Primary Biliary Cholangitis

Etiology & Risk Factors	• Autoimmune disorder leading to gradual destruction of intrahepatic small bile ducts leading to cirrhosis, portal hypertension, decreased bile salt excretion, and liver failure • <u>Etiology</u>: **autoimmune destruction of intrahepatic small bile ducts** • <u>Risk Factors</u>: **female, age (middle age; 35-70 years old most common), genetic predisposition (X chromosome), autoimmune mechanism** (systemic sclerosis, Sjogren syndrome, scleroderma, autoimmune thyroiditis), **environmental triggers** (UTI, nail polish, hormone replacement, cigarette smoking, toxic waste exposure)
Patho-physiology	• Instigating event/trigger leads to autoimmune response with T cell destruction of intrahepatic small bile ducts • Destruction of bile ducts leads to inability to form and excrete bile (cholestasis) causing retention of toxic materials causing further hepatocytes inflammation • Hepatocyte inflammation decreases as fibrosis progresses to cirrhosis
Signs & Symptoms	• Most are asymptomatic • **Fatigue (most common initial symptom), pruritus**, right upper quadrant abdominal pain, dry mouth, dry eyes • Fat malabsorption may lead to vitamin deficiency and osteoporosis • <u>Physical Exam</u>: • **Hepatomegaly, jaundice, xanthelasmas**, hyperpigmentation, osteoporosis, cirrhosis (if progressive disease)
Diagnosis	• <u>Liver Function Tests (LFT)</u>: • <u>Cholestatic Liver Disease Pattern</u>: **elevated gamma-glutamyl transpeptidase (GGT) and alkaline phosphatase (ALP);** minimally abnormal ALT/AST; bilirubin normal • <u>**Antimitochondrial antibody (AMA)**</u>: **hallmark of disease**; elevated titer (1:40+); differentiates from primary sclerosing cholangitis • <u>Dyslipidemia</u>: HDL decreases, LDL increases • <u>Abdominal Ultrasound</u>: initial imaging test to screen for extrahepatic obstruction; MRCP/ERCP may be required • <u>Liver Biopsy</u>: definitive diagnosis; shows nonsuppurative cholangitis and interlobular bile ducts destruction or lesion
Treatment	• <u>**Ursodeoxycholic Acid**</u>: **first-line medication**; hydrophilic bile salt stabilizes hepatocyte membranes to inhibit apoptosis and fibrosis • <u>**Cholestyramine**</u>: indicated to treat pruritus (reduces bile salts in skin) • <u>**Vitamin Supplementation**</u>: fat soluble vitamin malabsorption leads to deficiencies in vitamins A, D, E, K; may lead to osteoporosis • <u>Statin Therapy</u>: treat hyperlipidemia
Key Words & Most Common	• Autoimmune disorder leading to intrahepatic small bile duct destruction • Clinical suspicion in middle-aged female patient with classic symptoms (pruritus, fatigue, right upper quadrant discomfort, jaundice) • Elevated gamma-glutamyl transpeptidase (GGT) and alkaline phosphatase (ALP) • Positive antimitochondrial antibody (AMA) differentiates from primary sclerosing cholangitis • Ursodeoxycholic acid is first line • Supportive treatment with vitamin supplementation, cholestyramine, statins

Primary Sclerosing Cholangitis 🫃

Etiology & Risk Factors	• Chronic, progressive, autoimmune cholestatic liver disorder leading to **inflammation, fibrosis, and stricture of intrahepatic and extrahepatic biliary ducts** • <u>Etiology</u>: not fully understood • <u>Risk Factors</u>: **inflammatory bowel disease (UC)**, male, age 20-40 years old most common), family history, certain genetic conditions (**HLA B8, HLA DR3 genes have higher risk**) • **Most commonly associated with inflammatory bowel disease particularly ulcerative colitis (60-80% of cases)**
Patho-physiology	• Genetically susceptible individual (HLA) with exposure a possible environmental source leads to persistent chronic injury of the cholangiocytes • Inflammation and fibrosis leads to cholestasis and furthers parenchymal injury eventually causing permanent scarring
Signs & Symptoms	• Most are asymptomatic • **Fatigue (most common initial symptom), pruritus**, right upper quadrant abdominal pain, weight loss, fever • <u>Physical Exam</u>: **hepatomegaly, jaundice, xanthelasmas**, excoriations from pruritus, cirrhosis (if progressive disease)
Diagnosis	• <u>Liver Function Tests (LFT)</u>: • <u>Cholestatic Liver Disease Pattern</u>: **elevated gamma-glutamyl transpeptidase (GGT) and alkaline phosphatase (ALP)**; minimally abnormal ALT/AST; bilirubin normal • **Positive P-ANCA: hallmark of disease; differentiations from primary biliary cholangitis** • <u>Ultrasound</u>: initial imaging test to screen for extrahepatic obstruction • <u>MRCP/ERCP</u>: **most accurate test**; shows narrowing/strictures/beading of intrahepatic or extrahepatic biliary ducts
Treatment	• <u>Ursodeoxycholic Acid</u>: **first-line medication**; hydrophilic bile salt stabilizes hepatocyte membranes to inhibit apoptosis and fibrosis • <u>Cholestyramine</u>: Indicated to treat pruritus (reduces bile salts in skin) • <u>ERCP Dilation of Strictures</u>: provides symptomatic relief • <u>Liver Transplant</u>: definitive treatment that is curative and improves life expectancy
Key Words & Most Common	• Chronic autoimmune cholestatic liver disorder affecting intrahepatic and extrahepatic biliary ducts • Commonly associated with inflammatory bowel disease (ulcerative colitis) • Most asymptomatic • Fatigue, pruritus, RUQ abdominal pain, weight loss • Hepatomegaly, jaundice, excoriations from pruritus • Elevated GGT and ALP • Positive P-ANCA differentiates from primary biliary cholangitis • Ursodeoxycholic acid first line; cholestyramine for pruritus • Liver transplant definitive

Wilson's Disease 🫃

Etiology & Risk Factors	• Autosomal recessive disorder resulting in **excess copper accumulation in the body** (liver, basal ganglia of brain, kidney, joints, cornea) • <u>Etiology</u>: **copper metabolism disorder; genetic mutation on chromosome 13** • <u>Risk Factors</u>: family history, age (often initially presents in first decade of life with neuropsychiatric symptoms seen in 30s-40s)
Patho-physiology	• Mutation of ATP7B gene on chromosome 13 which controls protein transporter responsible for regulating copper excretion into bile and out of body • Copper begins to accumulate in liver and other tissues (brain, kidney, joints, cornea) causing fibrosis and ultimately cirrhosis of liver
Signs & Symptoms	• <u>General</u>: fatigue, **weakness**, insomnia, arthralgias (copper deposition in joints), amenorrhea, miscarriage • <u>Hepatic</u>: abdominal pain, jaundice, **hepatosplenomegaly**, cirrhosis, liver failure • <u>Neurologic</u>: **dysarthria (most common)**, gait abnormalities, dystonia, Parkinsonism (bradykinesia, rigidity, tremors), migraines • <u>Psychiatric</u>: **depression**, personality/behavioral change, **psychosis, delusions** • <u>Ophthalmic</u>: **Kayser-Fleischer Rings** are gold or greenish/gold pigmented rings due to copper deposition in the cornea seen under slit-lamp examination

Diagnosis	• <u>Labs</u>:
	   • <u>LFT</u>: elevated AST/ALT
	   • <u>CBC</u>: **hemolytic anemia** (Coombs negative)
	   • **Low serum ceruloplasmin**
	   • **Elevated 24-hour urinary copper excretion**
	   • <u>Serum Copper Concentration</u>: low sensitivity; may be elevated, normal, or low
	   • <u>Genetic Testing</u>: testing to detect mutation of ATP7B gene
	• <u>Slit-Lamp Examination</u>: evaluate for Kayser-Fleischer Rings
	• **Liver Biopsy: gold standard, definitive diagnosis** to measure hepatic copper concentration
	
	Kayser-Fleischer Ring: golden, or greenish gold ring at corneal lumbus (copper deposition)

Treatment	• <u>Supportive</u>: low copper diet (avoiding liver, cashews, black-eyed peas, shellfish, mushrooms, cocoa), avoid copper containing vitamins, assess drinking water for copper
	• **Copper-Chelation Therapy:**
	   • **Penicillamine: is most common first-line chelation drug**
	   • **Trientine**: second line; less side effects
	• <u>Zinc Supplementation</u>: prevents copper accumulation and reduces intestinal copper absorption; do not supplement if taking penicillamine or trientine

Key Words & Most Common	• Autosomal recessive disorder causing excess copper accumulation in the body • Hepatosplenomegaly, dysarthria, cirrhosis, Parkinsonism, Kayser-Fleischer Rings • Low serum ceruloplasmin, elevated 24-hour urinary copper excretion; Liver biopsy is gold standard • Copper-chelation therapy with penicillamine vs trientine • Zinc supplementation

Inguinal Hernia

	INDIRECT HERNIA	DIRECT HERNIA
Etiology & Risk Factors	• Bowel protrusion at the internal inguinal ring traversing into the inguinal canal • Origin is *lateral* to inferior epigastric artery • **Most common type of hernia**, more common in men	• Bowel protrusion extending directly forward through transversalis fascia and not passing through the inguinal canal • Origin is *medial* to the inferior epigastric artery
Patho-physiology	• Often congenital secondary to a persistent **patent process vaginalis** which allows bowel protrusion through internal inguinal ring into the inguinal canal and possibly into scrotum as a result of increased intraabdominal pressure	• Occurs secondary to weakness in floor of inguinal canal • May have higher proportions of type III collagen compared to type I; type I typically has higher tensile strength
Signs & Symptoms	• Many have vague discomfort or are asymptomatic • <u>Reducible</u>: **soft hernia sac** that is **easily reducible** through defect; swelling/fullness at hernia site that **enlarges with increased intraabdominal pressure** • Indirect hernia may lead to scrotal swelling • <u>Incarceration</u>: **enlarged, firm, and painful hernia sac** that is unable to be reduced; nausea/vomiting present in case of bowel obstruction • <u>Strangulated</u>: **severely painful, firm, ischemic hernia that is irreducible**; hypoperfusion leads to systemic toxicity; erythema of overlying skin	
Diagnosis	• **Clinical Diagnosis** with history and physical exam • Patient should be examined standing with Valsalva maneuver or coughing (increases intraabdominal pressure) • <u>Groin Ultrasound</u>: **initial imaging of choice** if physical exam is equivocal • <u>CT Scan</u>: if concern for incarceration of strangulation	
Treatment	• <u>Surgery</u>: **elective surgery indicated** due to risk of incarceration/strangulation • <u>Strangulated Hernia</u>: surgical emergency	

Key Words & Most Common	• Protrusion at internal inguinal ring into inguinal canal
	• Lateral to inferior epigastric artery
	• Reducible is soft hernia sac easily reducible
	• Incarceration is enlarged, firm, painful
	  Strangulated is severely painful and irreducible with signs of ischemia
	• Clinical diagnosis vs US if equivocal
	• Surgery
		• Protrusion extending through transversalis fasia NOT passing through inguinal canal
		• Medial to inferior epigastric artery
		• Reducible is soft hernia sac easily reducible
		• Incarceration is enlarged, firm, painful
		  Strangulated is severely painful and irreducible with signs of ischemia
		• Clinical diagnosis vs US if equivocal
		• Surgery

Indirect Inguinal Hernia	Direct Inguinal Hernia	Femoral Hernia
• Bowel protrusion at the internal inguinal ring traversing into the inguinal canal • Origin is **lateral** to inferior epigastric artery	• Bowel protrusion extending directly forward through transversalis fascia and not passing through the inguinal canal • Origin is **medial** to the inferior epigastric artery	• Bowel protrusion into **femoral canal *below*** inguinal ligament
• More common in men	• More common on right side	• More common in women

Umbilical Hernia	Incisional (Ventral) Hernia	Obturator Hernia
• Herniation through **umbilical fibromuscular ring** • Congenital from umbilical ring closure failure • Increased abdominal pressure from ascites, pregnancy, or obesity	• Herniation through weak point of abdominal wall • May be spontaneous or acquired • Due to **excess abdominal wall tension or poor wound healing or surgical incision infection**	• Rare herniation of abdominal/pelvic contents through pelvic floor and obturator foramen • Almost always presents as partial or complete bowel obstruction
• More common in **premature neonates** (often resolve by age 2 with observation; surgery indicated if persistent at age 5+)	• Most common in **obese patients** after vertical abdominal wall incision (surgery)	• Most common in **multiparous women** or **women with significant weight loss**

Type	Description	Relationship to Inferior Epigastric Vessels	Internal Spermatic Fascia Coverage	Onset
Direct	Protrusion through weak point in abdominal wall fascia	Medial	No Coverage	Adulthood
Indirect	Protrusion through inguinal ring; failure of processus vaginalis to close	Lateral	Coverage	Congenital or Adulthood

Norovirus Gastroenteritis

Etiology & Risk Factors	• Most common cause of viral gastroenteritis in US • <u>Etiology</u>: norovirus; a nonenveloped, positive-sense, single-stranded virus • <u>Risk Factors</u>: **crowded living spaces** (common outbreaks seen on **cruise ships**, schools, military barracks, **restaurants, healthcare facilities), seasonal** (peak incidence in **winter**; may occur at any time of year), consumption of high-risk foods (**raw foods**, particularly fruits and vegetables, oysters, fish/sushi) • <u>Transmission</u>: **fecal-oral route from contaminated food/water or surface fomite contamination** • Very low inoculum to cause infection (highly contagious)
Patho-physiology	• Norovirus invades, infects and replicates in immune cells including macrophages, dendritic cells, and B cells; may directly invade enterocytes lining the gut lumen • Virus may interact with host's gut flora to enhance infection and replication

Signs & Symptoms	• Onset 12-72 hours after exposure (24 hours average); may be abrupt onset
	• <u>General Symptoms</u>: fever, malaise, headache, anorexia
	• <u>Gastrointestinal Symptoms</u>:
	   • **Intense nausea and recurrent vomiting are predominant symptoms**
	   • Non-bloody diarrhea without mucous
	   • Abdominal cramping

Diagnosis	• **Clinical Diagnosis** • <u>Enzyme Immunoassays and Reverse Transcription Polymerase Chain Reaction (RT-PCR)</u>: may aid in detection but rarely used • <u>Labs</u>: CBC/CMP to evaluate hypovolemia/electrolyte abnormalities if profuse vomiting

Treatment	• **Fluid Replacement**:
	   • **Oral Hydration**: **preferred** method of rehydration; oral glucose-electrolyte solution, bouillon, broths
	   • **IV Hydration**: reserved for intractable vomiting, hypovolemia, severe dehydration
	• **Antiemetics**: **ondansetron** alleviates nausea to allow for proper oral rehydration
	• <u>Prevention</u>: proper hygiene; wash hands with warm soap and water; disinfect bathroom (*virus may aerosolize with vomiting, defecation, or when flushing toilet*)

Key Words & Most Common	• Fecal-oral transmission from contaminated food/water (raw fruits/vegetables, fish) • Abrupt onset of vomiting • Clinical diagnosis • Oral hydration vs IV hydration • Ondansetron for symptomatic relief

Rotavirus Gastroenteritis

Etiology & Risk Factors	• Most common cause of viral gastroenteritis in worldwide; most common in unimmunized kids • <u>Etiology</u>: **rotavirus**; a double-stranded virus • <u>Transmission</u>: **fecal-oral route from contaminated hands or surface fomite contamination** (food/water contaminations less likely), seasonal (peak incidence in **later winter to early spring**; may occur at any time of year) • Common outbreaks seen in day dare facilities or elementary schools
Patho-physiology	• Viral replication occurs in mature enterocytes throughout small intestine lumen causing alteration in epithelial cells. This causes an osmotically active food bolus to rapidly transmit through large intestine and impairing water absorption thus causing the typical watery diarrhea
Signs & Symptoms	• Onset 24-72 hours after exposure • **Copious, watery diarrhea is predominant symptom, vomiting, fever** • May have general symptoms like fever, abdominal cramping, fatigue, malaise, headache, dehydration (tachycardia, dry mucous membranes, decreased urine output) • *Symptoms are more severe in infants and children*
Diagnosis	• **Clinical Diagnosis** • <u>Enzyme Immunoassays and Reverse Transcription Polymerase Chain Reaction (RT-PCR)</u>: may aid in detection but rarely used • <u>Labs</u>: CBC/CMP to evaluate hypovolemia/electrolyte abnormalities if profuse diarrhea

Treatment	• **Fluid Replacement**:
	   • **Oral Hydration**: **preferred** method of rehydration; oral glucose-electrolyte solution, bouillon, broths
	   • **IV Hydration**: reserved for intractable vomiting, hypovolemia, severe dehydration
	• **Antiemetics**: **ondansetron** alleviates nausea to allow for proper oral hydration; avoid in children
	• <u>Antidiarrheals</u>: loperamide may offer symptomatic relief; avoid in children
	• <u>Prevention</u>: proper hygiene; wash hands with warm soap and water; oral immunization given to infants

Key Words & Most Common	• Fecal-oral transmission from contaminated hands or surface fomites • Copious, watery diarrhea, vomiting, fever • Clinical diagnosis • Oral hydration vs IV hydration • Ondansetron/loperamide for symptomatic relief; avoid in children

Staphylococcus aureus Gastroenteritis

Non-Invasive Infectious

Etiology & Risk Factors	• Gastroenteritis resulting from consumption of foods containing preformed enterotoxin from *S. aureus* • Etiology: ***Staphylococcus aureus*** • Risk Factors: **improper food handling, prepared foods, foods with high protein content**, cross contamination during food preparation, warm/humid environment, inadequate storage, poor personal hygiene • Transmission: **contaminated food source (dairy products, mayonnaise, meats, eggs, salads),** food may be room temperature and may not look/smell spoiled
Patho-physiology	• *S. aureus* is commonly present on skin or within nose and can be transferred to food if improper hand washing prior to handling food. • Bacteria can multiply and produce toxin if left at permissive temperature (room temperature)
Signs & Symptoms	• Rapid onset following ingestion of contaminated food (usually 1–6 hours) • **Abrupt onset of hypersalivation, vomiting and nausea** • May have fever, headache, diarrhea • Symptoms typically resolve within 24 hours
Diagnosis	• **Clinical Diagnosis** • Enzyme Immunoassays and Reverse Transcription Polymerase Chain Reaction (RT-PCR): may aid in detection but rarely used • Evaluate hypovolemia/electrolyte abnormalities (CBC, CMP) if profuse diarrhea/vomiting

Treatment	• Fluid Replacement: mainstay of therapy
	  • **Oral hydration preferred** (oral glucose-electrolyte solution, bouillon, broths)
	  • **IV Hydration** reserved for intractable vomiting, hypovolemia, severe dehydration
	• Antiemetics: ondansetron alleviates nausea to allow for proper oral hydration; avoid in children
	• Proper Hygiene: wash hands with warm soap and water

Key Words & Most Common	• Contaminated food source (dairy, mayo, meat, eggs, salad) • Rapid onset (within 1-6 hours after consumption) • Vomiting, nausea, hypersalivation • Clinical diagnosis • Oral hydration vs IV hydration • Ondansetron for symptomatic relief; avoid in children

Bacillus cereus Gastroenteritis

Non-Invasive Infectious

Etiology & Risk Factors	• Etiology: Bacillus cereus; a gram-positive, beta-hemolytic, rod-shaped, toxin-producing, facultatively anaerobic bacterium
	  • Commonly found in environment and can contaminate food
	  • Enterotoxin that can survive reheating
	• Risk Factors: improper food handling, starchy foods (rice, pasta, potatoes), reheating of food, inadequate storage, cross contamination during preparation, large batches of food (slow cooling), foods held at buffets
	• Transmission: **contaminated food source (fried rice most common**, potato, pasta, cheese)

Patho-physiology	• Occurs through endospore survival when food (rice) is improperly cooked where temperature is not great enough to kill bacterial spores. • Bacterial growth results in production of heat-stable enterotoxins causing gastroenteritis
Signs & Symptoms	• Rapid onset following ingestion of contaminated food (usually 1–6 hours) • Diarrheal-Type Illness: **profuse watery diarrhea, abdominal cramping; nausea/vomiting rarely seen;** onset 6-15 hours after exposure • Emetic-Type Illness: **abrupt onset vomiting and nausea**; +/- diarrhea; onset within 30 minutes to 6 hours after exposure • May have fever, headache, diarrhea • Symptoms typically resolve within 24 hours
Diagnosis	• **Clinical Diagnosis** • Bodily Fluid Analysis: detect enterotoxin through serology or biological tests; may aid in detection but rarely used • Evaluate hypovolemia/electrolyte abnormalities (CBC, CMP) if profuse diarrhea/vomiting

Treatment	• Fluid Replacement: mainstay of treatment
	  • **Oral Hydration: preferred method of rehydration** (oral glucose-electrolyte solution, bouillon, broths)
	  • **IV Hydration:** reserved for intractable vomiting, hypovolemia, severe dehydration
	• Antiemetics: ondansetron alleviates nausea to allow for proper oral hydration; avoid in children
	• Antidiarrheals: loperamide may offer symptomatic relief; avoid in children
	• Proper Hygiene: wash hands with warm soap and water

Key Words & Most Common	• Contaminated food source (fried rice) • Rapid onset (within 1-6 hours after consumption) • Vomiting, nausea, hypersalivation • Clinical diagnosis • Oral hydration vs IV hydration • Ondansetron for symptomatic relief; avoid in children

Enterotoxigenic *E. Coli*

Non-Invasive Infectious	
Etiology & Risk Factors	• **Most common cause of traveler's diarrhea**; affects 40-60% of those that travel (location dependent) • Etiology: *Escherichia coli*; a gram-negative bacilli that produces heat-stable toxins and heat-labile toxins • Risk Factors: **poor hygiene** in resource-limited areas with regards to food handling and preparation, lack of refrigeration and poor food storage practice, certain geographical locations (most common in sub-Saharan Africa, Latin America, Middle East, South Asia) • Transmission: fecal-oral route through contaminated food and water; **water most common source** (brushing teeth, ice from local water, food washed with local water)
Patho-physiology	• Cytotoxin release and mucosal invasion from *E. coli* bacterium leads to destruction of the intestinal mucosa resulting in loss of surface mucosa which decreases water absorption and causes diarrhea
Signs & Symptoms	• Onset 12-72 hours after exposure • **Abrupt onset of copious, watery diarrhea (non-bloody), vomiting**, abdominal cramping, +/- fever • May have general symptoms like fatigue, myalgias, dehydration (tachycardia, dry mucous membranes, decreased urine output) • Symptoms are more severe in patients taking medications to decrease stomach acidity (antacids, H2 blockers, PPIs)
Diagnosis	• **Clinical Diagnosis** • Stool Culture and Gram Stain: confirms diagnosis; rarely used • Evaluate hypovolemia/electrolyte abnormalities (CBC, CMP) if profuse diarrhea/vomiting

Treatment	• **Fluid Replacement: mainstay of therapy**
	  • **Oral Hydration: preferred method of rehydration** (oral glucose-electrolyte solution, bouillon, broths)
	  • **IV Hydration**: reserved for intractable vomiting, hypovolemia, severe dehydration
	• **Antiemetics: ondansetron**; alleviates nausea to allow for proper oral hydration
	• Antidiarrheals: **bismuth subsalicylate; prophylaxis can reduce incidence by 50%;** loperamide may offer symptomatic relief
	• Antibiotics: **ciprofloxacin is first-line**; azithromycin second-line; indicated if fever, profuse vomiting, abdominal cramping, and/or bloody diarrhea present
	• Proper Hygiene: wash hands with warm soap and water, avoiding contaminated foods/water, **using clean filtered or bottled water**

Key Words & Most Common	• Contaminated water source (brushing teeth, ice, raw fruits/vegetables washed) • Abrupt onset of watery diarrhea and vomiting • Clinical diagnosis • Oral hydration vs IV hydration • Ondansetron and/or loperamide for symptomatic relief • Bismuth subsalicylate may reduce incidence by 50% if used as prophylaxis • Ciprofloxacin is first line antibiotic if severe

Cholera

Non-Invasive Infectious	
Etiology & Risk Factors	• Gastrointestinal infection due to *Vibrio cholerae* • Etiology: *Vibrio cholerae*; a gram-negative, enterotoxin-producing bacteria • Risk Factors: patients with blood type O are more likely to have severe disease, residing in or travel to endemic areas (Asia, Africa, and Central/South America); poor sanitary conditions, regions afflicted by natural disasters and/or humanitarian crises • Transmission: **fecal-oral route** through contaminated food/water **(seafood/shellfish)**; humans are only known host; can live freely in fresh/salt water
Patho-physiology	• Small intestine is colonized by bacterium that produces enterotoxins causing increase in cell cAMP leading to hypersecretion of isotonic electrolytes by the mucosa into the gut lumen causing intense secretory diarrhea
Signs & Symptoms	• Onset 24-72 hours after exposure • **Abrupt onset of copious, watery diarrhea (white/gray stool with flecks of mucous "rice water stool"**; may have "fishy odor"), **vomiting**, abdominal cramping • May develop **severe dehydration** (tachycardia, dry mucous membranes, decreased urine output, weakness, muscle cramps) **from fluid and electrolyte loss** • Fluid loss can be as high as 1L/hr • *Fatality rate as high as 70% without treatment due to dehydration, arrythmia (electrolyte abnormalities), paralytic ileus*
Diagnosis	• **Clinical Diagnosis** • Stool Culture: on TCBS medium; confirms diagnosis • Polymerase Chain Reaction (PCR): detects specific antigens or genetic material in stool sample • Labs: indicated to evaluate hypovolemia/electrolyte abnormalities (CBC, CMP); may show hyponatremia, hypokalemia, hypoglycemia, hemoconcentration

Treatment	• Fluid Replacement: mainstay of therapy
	  • **Oral Hydration: preferred method of rehydration** (oral glucose-electrolyte solution, bouillon, broths)
	  • **IV Hydration**: reserved for intractable vomiting, hypovolemia, severe dehydration
	• Antibiotics: antibiotics have been shown to decrease the severity and duration of disease
	  • **Doxycycline is first-line**; azithromycin or ciprofloxacin are alternatives
	• Proper Hygiene: wash hands with warm soap and water, avoiding contaminated foods/water, using clean filtered or bottled water
	• *Antiemetics and antidiarrheals are found to have little benefit*

Key Words & Most Common	• Contaminated food/water source (seafood/shellfish) • Abrupt onset of watery diarrhea; white/gray flecks of mucous "rice water" stool • Severe dehydration • Clinical diagnosis • Oral hydration vs IV hydration • Doxycycline is first line antibiotic

Invasive Infectious	# *Clostridioides difficile*
Etiology & Risk Factors	• Most common cause of antibiotic-associated colitis and infectious diarrhea in hospitalized patients • <u>Etiology</u>: ***Clostridioides difficile*** (formerly *Clostridium*); a spore-forming, toxin-producing, gram-positive anaerobic bacterium • <u>Risk Factors</u>: **recent antibiotic use (clindamycin,** cephalosporins, penicillin, fluoroquinolones), **advanced age**, recent hospitalization, resident at nursing home, use of PPI/H2 blockers, chemotherapy
Patho-physiology	• *C. diff* colonizes in large intestine; use of antibiotics then alter the microbial flora increasing susceptibility of infection and overgrowth of C. diff bacteria • Diarrhea and colitis secondary to clostridial glycosylation exotoxins and enterotoxins which leads to hypersecretion of fluid into intestinal lumen and develops characteristic pseudomembranes (yellow-white plaques), and watery, foul-smelling diarrhea
Signs & Symptoms	• Onset typically 5-10 days after starting antibiotic • <u>Diarrhea</u>: **foul-smelling, watery** diarrhea (may have mucous and occult blood), **abdominal cramping**, low-grade fever, nausea, vomiting, anorexia • <u>Fulminant Colitis</u>: severe diarrhea, diffuse abdominal pain/distension, hypovolemia that may lead to sepsis, toxic megacolon, or perforated bowel
Diagnosis	• *Consider testing patients with >3 loose stools within 24 hours + risk factors* • <u>Stool Assay</u>: tests for ***C. difficile*** toxin (initial test of choice); **glutamate dehydrogenase (GDH) antigen** and polymerase chain reaction (PCR) for toxin gene • <u>Labs</u>: leukocytosis and elevated WBC count • <u>Sigmoidoscopy</u>: confirms pseudomembrane presence; used for patients with high suspicion and negative toxin assay

Treatment	• **<u>Discontinue Offending Antibiotic</u>: first step in management if possible**
	• **<u>Fluid Replacement</u>:**
	    • **<u>Oral Hydration</u>: preferred method of rehydration;** oral glucose-electrolyte solution, bouillon, broths
	    • **<u>IV Hydration</u>:** reserved for hypovolemia or severe dehydration
	• **<u>Antibiotics</u>:**
	    • **Oral vancomycin or oral fidaxomicin are first-line**
	    • Metronidazole is an alternative
	• <u>Fecal Transplant</u>: transplantation of microbiota using colonoscopy indicated for severe (3+) recurrence
	• <u>Prevention</u>: **proper hygiene, contact precautions**; hand washing with warm soap and water (spores resistant to alcohol-based hand sanitizer)
	• <u>Recurrence</u>: consider pulse-taper with oral vancomycin/fidaxomicin +/- metronidazole

Key Words & Most Common	• Recent antibiotic use (clindamycin); common cause of infectious diarrhea in hospitalized patients • Foul-smelling, watery diarrhea • Stool Assay test for *C. diff* toxin • Discontinue antibiotic • Oral Vancomycin or oral Fidaxomicin • Contact precautions

Invasive Infectious	# *Yersinia enterocolitica*
Etiology & Risk Factors	• <u>Etiology</u>: *Yersinia enterocolitica*; a gram-negative coccobacillus with bipolar stain • <u>Risk Factors</u>: **consumption of raw or undercooked pork**, untreated water source, unpasteurized milk consumption, blood transfusion, immunocompromised, iron-overloaded • <u>Transmission</u>: **fecal-oral route**
Patho-physiology	• Pathogen is ingested and traverses through stomach and gut wall and localizes in lymphoid tissue and mesenteric lymph nodes • Bacteria can produce ureases that can form ammonia to protect itself from gastric acidity • Bacteria cannot chelate iron; iron overload can increase severity of infection
Signs & Symptoms	• Symptom duration 12-22 days • **Diarrhea (can become bloody), fever, abdominal pain, nausea, vomiting** • **Right lower quadrant pain that can mimic appendicitis** • **Mesenteric lymphadenitis** can lead to abdominal tenderness and guarding
Diagnosis	• <u>Stool Culture</u>: **best way to detect**; gram-stain may reveal "safety-pin like organism" • Culture of mesenteric lymph nodes, pharyngeal exudates, peritoneal fluid, or blood may also be obtained • <u>Serology</u>: enzyme-linked immunosorbent assays (ELISA); not commonly used • <u>Abdominal Ultrasound or CT</u>: utilized to rule out acute appendicitis

Treatment	• *Must rule out appendicitis*
	• **<u>Fluid Replacement</u>:**
	    • **<u>Oral Hydration</u>: preferred method of rehydration;** oral glucose-electrolyte solution, bouillon, broths
	    • **<u>IV Hydration</u>:** reserved for hypovolemia or severe dehydration
	• <u>Antibiotics</u>: indicated for severe cases, elderly, immunocompromised, or diabetics
	    • **Ciprofloxacin or Trimethoprim-Sulfamethoxazole**
	• <u>Prevention</u>: proper hygiene habits, safe food processing, treated water consumption, avoiding raw or undercooked pork

Key Words & Most Common	• Most common source is raw or undercooked pork consumption • RLQ pain that mimics appendicitis; mesenteric lymphadenitis • Stool culture • US/CT to rule out appendicitis • Oral rehydration • Ciprofloxacin or Trimethoprim-Sulfamethoxazole for severe cases

Campylobacter jejuni Enteritis

Invasive Infectious	
Etiology & Risk Factors	• Most common cause of bacterial enteritis in the US; commonly affects children and young adults • Etiology: *Campylobacter jejuni*; a motile, gram-negative, non-spore-forming bacteria • Risk Factors: consumption of **raw/unpasteurized milk, undercooked poultry, and contaminated water**; contact with animal feces (puppies) • Transmission: **fecal-oral route**
Patho-physiology	• **C. jejuni is strongly associated with subsequent development of Guillain-Barré syndrome (GBS)** secondary to a cross-reaction between *C. jejuni* antibodies and human gangliosides; autoantibodies may react with peripheral nerves causing demyelination and ascending paralysis • Bacterial invasion of intestinal epithelium causes inflammatory lesions and mucosal damage leading to bloody and mucous-like diarrhea
Signs & Symptoms	• Onset is 1-3 days after exposure with symptoms lasting 5-7 days • Prodrome phase of fever, rigors, body aches, dizziness • **Diarrhea (initially watery progressing to bloody or mucous-like), fever, abdominal pain, nausea, vomiting** • **Periumbilical pain (may mimic appendicitis)**
Diagnosis	• **Stool Culture: confirms diagnosis**; gram-stain may reveal "S or comma shaped organism" • Rapid Molecular or Antigen Test: detects specific antigens in stool sample • Enzyme-linked Immunosorbent Assays (ELISA) or Polymerase Chain Reaction (PCR): detects the genetic material in stool samples; not commonly used • Ultrasound or CT: utilized to rule out acute appendicitis if warranted

Treatment	• Fluid Replacement:
	  • **Oral Hydration: preferred method of rehydration**(oral glucose-electrolyte solution, bouillon, broths)
	  • **IV Hydration:** reserved for intractable vomiting, hypovolemia, severe dehydration
	• Antibiotics: indicated for severe cases, elderly, immunocompromised, or diabetics
	  • **Azithromycin is first-line;** ciprofloxacin may be used but growing resistance
	• Antidiarrheals: avoided in invasive diarrheas
	• Prevention: proper hygiene habits, safe food processing, treated water consumption

Key Words & Most Common	• Most common source is raw milk or undercooked poultry • Watery diarrhea that may become bloody or mucous-like • Stool culture • Oral rehydration • Azithromycin for severe cases

Enterohemorrhagic *E. coli* 0157:H7

Invasive Infectious	
Etiology & Risk Factors	• Etiology: *Escherichia coli 0157:H7*; a shiga-like toxin producing gram-negative bacteria • Transmission: **fecal-oral route** • Risk Factors: consumption of **raw/unpasteurized milk or apple cider, undercooked ground beef, and contaminated water or unwashed fruits/vegetables**; day care centers, petting zoos, age (most commonly affects children and elderly adults)
Patho-physiology	• Bacteria produce shiga-like verotoxins that cause direct damage to vascular endothelial cells and mucosal cells of the large intestinal wall • Intestinal mucosal cells may slough off causing bloody diarrhea • Shiga-like toxin can have systemic effects causing vasculitis which manifests as hemolytic uremic syndrome
Signs & Symptoms	• Onset is 4-9 days after exposure • **Acute onset of watery diarrhea progressing to grossly bloody diarrhea within 24 hours** • Abdominal pain, nausea, vomiting • Typically low-grade or no fever • Hemolytic-Uremic Syndrome: may have hypertension and evidence of fluid overload
Diagnosis	• Labs: most patients will have leukocytosis • Hemolytic-uremic syndrome may have sharp decrease in hematocrit and platelets, elevated creatinine • **Stool Culture: best way to detect** • Stool Assay: antigen stool test, enzyme-linked immunosorbent assays (ELISA) or polymerase chain reaction (PCR); not commonly used • *Evaluate for other causes of bloody diarrhea*

Treatment	• **Fluid Replacement:**
	  • **Oral Hydration: preferred method of rehydration**(oral glucose-electrolyte solution, bouillon, broths)
	  • **IV Hydration:** reserved for intractable vomiting, hypovolemia, severe dehydration
	• Antibiotics: **should be avoided due to increase release of shiga-like toxins leading to hemolytic uremic syndrome**
	• Antidiarrheals: avoided in invasive diarrheas
	• Prevention: proper hygiene; wash hands with warm soap and water, safe food processing, treated water consumption

Key Words & Most Common	• Most common source is unpasteurized milk or apple cider, undercooked ground beef, contaminated water • Watery diarrhea that may become bloody • Stool culture • Oral rehydration • Avoid antibiotics due to increased chance of developing hemolytic uremic syndrome

Typhoid Fever

Invasive Infectious	
Etiology & Risk Factors	• <u>Etiology</u>: *Salmonella typhi* and *Salmonella paratyphi*; gram-negative bacilli • <u>Risk Factors</u>: consumption of **contaminated water,** undercooked foods; travel to overcrowded and unhygienic areas (South-Central Asia, Mexico, Peru, India), age (most commonly affects children and young adults) • Major sources are eggs, poultry • <u>Transmission</u>: **fecal-oral route**
Patho-physiology	• Bacteria is ingested and invades epithelium wall of intestine through transferring of bacterial proteins or M cells (epithelial cells serving as antigen-present cells in gut mucosa or lymphoid tissue) or direct penetration of gut mucosa • Pathogen may become systemic through lymphatic and bloodstream infiltration; may colonize in gallbladder of chronic carriers
Signs & Symptoms	• Onset is 8-14 days after exposure • <u>Initial Symptoms</u>: may be gradual; **abdominal pain, fever, constipation and headache** • <u>Subsequent Symptoms</u>: **diarrhea** (may be "pea soup" green or bloody), "step-ladder" fever (rises one day, falls the next), cough, anorexia, malaise • Constipation may be predominant over diarrhea in some cases due to Payer patch hypertrophy • <u>Physical Exam</u>: • **Bradycardia relative to fever** • **Rose spots** (pink/salmon-colored macular rash of trunk and extremities) • **Hepatosplenomegaly**, dehydration, delirium
Diagnosis	• <u>**Blood, Urine and Stool Cultures**</u>: **best way to detect**; antibiotic susceptibility indicated due to increasing drug resistance • <u>Bone Marrow Culture</u>: gold standard; highly invasive and expensive so rarely ordered • <u>Enzyme-Linked Immunosorbent Assays (ELISA) or Polymerase Chain Reaction (PCR)</u>: expensive and not commonly used
Treatment	• <u>**Fluid Replacement**</u>: • <u>**Oral Hydration**</u>: **preferred method of rehydration**(oral glucose-electrolyte solution, bouillon, broths) • <u>**IV Hydration**</u>: reserved for intractable vomiting, hypovolemia, severe dehydration • <u>Antibiotics</u>: **ciprofloxacin is first-line; azithromycin or ceftriaxone are alternatives**; guided treatment based on culture susceptibility • <u>Prevention</u>: proper hygiene habits, safe food processing, treated water consumption
Key Words & Most Common	• Most common source is contaminated water; contact with contaminated eggs, poultry; travel to endemic area • Abdominal pain, fever, constipation, headache progressing to diarrhea, cough, general symptoms • Bradycardia relative to fever, Rose spots, hepatosplenomegaly • Blood, urine and stool cultures; bone marrow culture is gold standard • Fluid replacement • Ciprofloxacin is first-line; azithromycin or ceftriaxone

Non-Typhoidal Salmonella

Invasive Infectious	
Etiology & Risk Factors	• Food borne disease caused by *Salmonella enteriditis*; most common cause of foodborne illness in US • <u>Etiology</u>: *Salmonella enteriditis*; a gram-negative bacilli • <u>Transmission</u>: fecal-oral route • <u>Risk Factors</u>: **consumption of contaminated water or foods** (poultry, eggs, peanut butter, unwashed produce), contact with reptiles (**turtles**)
Patho-physiology	• Bacteria is ingested and invades epithelium wall of intestine through transferring of bacterial proteins or M cells (epithelial cells serving as antigen-present cells in gut mucosa or lymphoid tissue) or direct penetration of gut mucosa • Pathogen may become systemic through lymphatic and bloodstream infiltration; may colonize in gallbladder of chronic carriers
Signs & Symptoms	• Onset is 8-72 hours after exposure • <u>Initial Symptoms</u>: may be gradual; **abdominal pain, fever, constipation and headache** • <u>Subsequent Symptoms</u>: **diarrhea** (may be "pea soup" green or bloody), **"step-ladder" fever** (rises one day, falls the next), cough, anorexia, malaise • *Constipation may be predominant over diarrhea in some cases due to Payer patch hypertrophy* • <u>Physical Exam</u>: **bradycardia relative to fever; Rose spots** (pink/salmon-colored macular rash of trunk and extremities), **hepatosplenomegaly**, dehydration, delirium
Diagnosis	• <u>**Blood, Urine and Stool Cultures**</u>: **best way to detect**; order with antibiotic susceptibility due to increasing drug resistance • <u>Bone Marrow Culture</u>: gold standard; highly invasive and expensive so rarely ordered • <u>Enzyme-Linked Immunosorbent Assays (ELISA) or Polymerase Chain Reaction (PCR)</u>: expensive and not commonly used
Treatment	• <u>Fluid Replacement</u>: mainstay of therapy • <u>**Oral Hydration**</u>: **preferred method of rehydration**(oral glucose-electrolyte solution, bouillon, broths) • <u>**IV Hydration**</u>: reserved for intractable vomiting, hypovolemia, severe dehydration • <u>Antibiotics</u>: guided treatment based on culture susceptibility • **Ciprofloxacin is first-line** • **Azithromycin or ceftriaxone are alternatives** • <u>Prevention</u>: proper hygiene habits, safe food processing, treated water consumption
Key Words & Most Common	• Most common source is contaminated water; contact with contaminated eggs, poultry, turtles; travel to endemic area • Abdominal pain, fever, constipation, headache progressing to diarrhea, cough, general symptoms • Bradycardia relative to fever, Rose spots, hepatosplenomegaly • Blood, urine and stool cultures; bone marrow culture is gold standard • Fluid replacement • Ciprofloxacin is first-line; azithromycin or ceftriaxone

Shigellosis

Etiology & Risk Factors	• Bacterial diarrhea caused by the anaerobic gram-negative bacilli *Shigella* spp. • Etiology: ***Shigella sonnei* (most common in US),** *flexneri, boydii,* and *dysenteriae* (produces most toxin) • Risk Factors: consumption of **contaminated water/food**, immunocompromised, age (elderly, children <5yo), overcrowded areas with inadequate sanitization (**daycare**) • Transmission: **fecal-oral route**; humans are only natural reservoirs; can be spready by flies; *requires very small inoculum to cause disease*
Patho-physiology	• Bacteria is ingested and then multiplies in the small intestine before entering colon. Shigella bacterium invades colonic mucosa and produces a "Shiga" enterotoxin which is cytotoxic, neurotoxic and enterotoxic; intestinal mucosal cells may slough off causing bloody diarrhea • Shiga toxin can have systemic effects causing vasculitis which manifests as hemolytic uremic syndrome
Signs & Symptoms	• Onset is 1-4 days after exposure • **Generalized crampy abdominal pain, fever, tenesmus** (urgency to defecate) • **Explosive watery diarrhea (progresses to bloody or mucous-like)** • Severe Symptoms: delirium, anuria, encephalopathy, seizures (febrile seizures may be more common in young children) • Physical Exam: fever, tachycardia, hypotension, evidence of dehydration, distended abdomen, hyperactive bowel sounds, lower abdominal tenderness
Diagnosis	• Labs: shows **marked leukocytosis** • Stool Culture: confirms diagnosis; stool analysis may show fecal leukocytes and blood • Polymerase Chain Reaction (PCR): detects specific antigens or genetic material in stool sample • Sigmoidoscopy: diffuse erythema with small punctate ulcerations

Treatment	• Fluid Replacement: mainstay of therapy
	  • **Oral Hydration: preferred method of rehydration**(oral glucose-electrolyte solution, bouillon, broths)
	  • **IV Hydration:** reserved for intractable vomiting, hypovolemia, severe dehydration
	• Antibiotics: guided treatment based on culture susceptibility
	  • **Ciprofloxacin is first-line**
	  • **Azithromycin (first-line for pediatrics) or ceftriaxone are alternatives**
	• Antidiarrheals: should be avoided as retained toxins can worsen or prolong illness
	• Prevention: proper hygiene habits, safe food processing, treated water consumption

Key Words & Most Common	• Most common source is contaminated water; contact with contaminated eggs, poultry, turtles; travel to endemic area • Crampy abdominal pain, fever, tenesmus • Explosive watery diarrhea (bloody or mucous-like) • Stool cultures; CBC shows marked leukocytosis • Fluid replacement • Ciprofloxacin is first-line; azithromycin or ceftriaxone

Giardiasis

Etiology & Risk Factors	• Small intestine infection; most common cause of parasitic diarrhea worldwide • Etiology: ***Giardia lamblia (duodenalis)***; a flagellated intestinal protozoan parasite • Risk Factors: **consumption of contaminated water from remote streams or wells; wilderness travelers, international travelers, daycare workers,** poor sanitation • "Backpacker's diarrhea" or "beaver fever" • Transmission: fecal-oral; **contaminated water most common;** most common during summer months
Patho-physiology	• Infected animals excrete cysts into water; ingestion of cysts through consumption of contaminated water leads to infection • Cysts undergo excystation within the intestines which then release trophozoites that adhere to the intestinal epithelium. This disrupts the epithelial cell wall junctions and brush border enzymes leading to altered intestinal motility and permeability
Signs & Symptoms	• Onset is 1-14 days after exposure • **Most are asymptomatic**; *asymptomatic patients can still excrete infective cysts in stool* • **Watery, foul-smelling, pale diarrhea (no blood or mucous)** • **Abdominal cramping and distension, flatulence,** malaise, low-grade fever • Fat and sugar malabsorption can occur with chronic diarrhea
Diagnosis	• Stool Antigen Assay: uses enzyme-linked immunosorbent assays (ELISA); more sensitive than microscopy • Stool Microscopy: evaluation for ova and parasites; demonstrates motile trophozoites and cysts • Labs: normal WBCs, no eosinophilia

Treatment	• Fluid Replacement:
	  • **Oral Hydration: preferred method** for rehydration; oral glucose-electrolyte solution, bouillon, broths
	  • **IV Hydration:** reserved for hypovolemia or severe dehydration
	• Antiparasitics: **Metronidazole is first-line**; Tinidazole, Albendazole, Quinacrine are alternatives
	• Prevention: proper hygiene habits, safe food processing, treated water consumption

Key Words & Most Common	• Most common source is contaminated water from remote streams, lakes, or wells Most common among wilderness travelers, hikers or daycare workers • Watery, foul-smelling, pale diarrhea (no blood/mucous) • Stool antigen test • Fluid replacement • Metronidazole is first-line; albendazole, tinidazole are alternatives

Protozoan Infection	# Amebiasis

Etiology & Risk Factors	• Parasitic protozoan infection transmitted by ingestion of cysts from fecal contaminated food/water • <u>Etiology</u>: ***Entamoeba histolytica***; a motile protozoan • <u>Risk Factors</u>: **inadequate sanitation practices, contaminated food or water**, poor personal hygiene, **migrants from or travelers to endemic areas** (Central America, western South America, western and southern Africa, India), immunocompromised, living in crowded or institutional settings (refugee camps)
Patho-physiology	• Upon ingestion of contaminated food or water, the cysts of the parasite survive the acidic environment of the stomach and transform into trophozoites in the intestines where they feed on bacteria and tissue, reproduce and colonize the lumen and the mucosa of the large intestine. • The trophozoites can invade the intestinal lining, leading to inflammation, tissue damage, ulcer formation; trophozoites can spread to other organs, such as the liver

Signs & Symptoms	• **Mostly asymptomatic**
	• <u>Gastrointestinal Symptoms</u>: develop 1 to 3 weeks after ingestion of cysts
	  • **Intermittent diarrhea and constipation, flatulence, cramping abdominal pain**
	• <u>Amebic Dysentery</u>:
	  • Frequent semiliquid stools that often contain blood and mucous
	  • Abdominal pain, fever, weight loss
	• <u>Liver Abscess</u>: significantly more common in men
	  • **Fever**, chills, diaphoresis, nausea, vomiting, weakness, weight loss
	  • **RUQ pain (may radiate to right shoulder)**

Diagnosis	• <u>Stool Microscopy</u>: evaluation of ova and parasites; diagnosis supported by finding amebic trophozoites, cysts, or both in stool or tissues • <u>Enzyme Immunoassay (EIA)</u>: most widely used antigen test; sensitive and rapidly performed • <u>Stool Polymerase Chain Reaction (PCR)</u>: **diagnostic gold standard**; detects parasitic DNA in the stool • <u>Abdominal Imaging</u>: ultrasonography, CT, or MRI indicated to diagnose liver abscess; may require CT guided aspiration

Treatment	• <u>Fluid Replacement</u>:
	  • **Oral Hydration: preferred method of rehydration** (oral glucose-electrolyte solution, bouillon, broths)
	  • **IV Hydration:** reserved for intractable vomiting, hypovolemia, severe dehydration
	• <u>Amebicides</u>:
	  • **Metronidazole or tinidazole followed by paromomycin**, iodoquinol, or diloxanide furoate to eradicate residual cysts in the intestine
	  • *Asymptomatic cases should be treated with paromomycin, iodoquinol, or diloxanide furoate alone*

Key Words & Most Common	• Parasitic protozoan infection caused by Entamoeba histolytica contracted from contaminated food/water • Mostly asymptomatic → GI symptoms that range from mild to dysentery • Liver abscess (fever + RUQ pain) • Stool microscopy, EIA, PCR + abdominal imaging if concern for liver abscess • Metronidazole followed by paromomycin (to eradicate cysts)

Protozoan Infection	# Whipple's Disease

Etiology & Risk Factors	• <u>Etiology</u>: ***Tropheryma whipplei***; a gram-positive bacilli that causes a systemic disorder • <u>Risk Factors</u>: **male, age (30-60 years old most common), most commonly seen in farmers**, genetic factors (associated with HLA B27 haplotype) • <u>Transmission</u>: fecal-oral; **contaminated soil**
Patho-physiology	• Bacteria shares antigenic similarity to Streptococcal B and G • Organism is ingested by macrophages which can be absorbed through periodic acid-Schiff-positive • Malabsorption occurs due to disrupted villi function

Signs & Symptoms	• <u>**Four Main Symptoms: arthralgias + diarrhea + abdominal pain + weight loss**</u>
	  • First symptoms are often fever and arthralgia progressing to intestinal symptoms (diarrhea, abdominal pain, etc.)
	• <u>Malabsorption</u>: chronic diarrhea, **steatorrhea**, nutritional deficiency
	• <u>CNS Involvement</u>: seizures, delirium, impaired memory, abnormal body movements
	• <u>Physical Exam</u>:
	  • Peripheral lymphadenopathy seen in >50%

Diagnosis	• <u>**Duodenal Biopsy: periodic acid-Schiff-positive macrophages**</u>; villus atrophy • <u>Polymerase Chain Reaction (PCR)</u>: detection of *T. whipplei* or detection of the specific bacteria RNA • <u>Immunohistochemical Staining</u>: with *T. whipplei* antibodies • <u>Labs</u>: malabsorption (iron deficiency anemia, vitamin B12 and folate deficiency)
Treatment	• <u>**Antibiotics: ceftriaxone or penicillin for 2 weeks followed by trimethoprim-sulfamethoxazole for 12 months (maintenance therapy)**</u> • Doxycycline + hydroxychloroquine is alternative therapy • *Evaluate treatment with test for cure (PCR of bodily fluids)*
Key Words & Most Common	• Most commonly seen in farmers (males) aged 30-60 years old • Four main symptoms: arthralgia, diarrhea, abdominal pain, weight loss • Malabsorption: steatorrhea • Duodenal biopsy shows period acid-Schiff-positive macrophages • Antibiotics treatment with ceftriaxone or penicillin followed by TMP-SMX

Glucose-6-Phosphate Dehydrogenase (G6PD) Deficiency

Etiology & Risk Factors	• X-linked recessive enzyme disorder that may allow increased cellular damage from reactive oxygen species leading to acute hemolytic anemia • Etiology: **X-linked enzymatic defect** • Risk Factors: **male** (x-linked recessive), certain ethnicities (**African descent** [10-15% of men of African descent are positive], Mediterranean, or southeast Asian descent) • Precipitating Factors: **infection**, fava beans, medications (**nitrofurantoin, dapsone, sulfonamides**, methylene blue, phenazopyridine, **ciprofloxacin, antimalarials**)
Patho-physiology	• G6PD is an enzyme that plays role in preventing RBC damage from reactive oxygen species by catalyzing NADP to its reduced form, NADPH. • NADPH serves as substrate to glutathione reductase (a potent antioxidant) which can convert hydrogen peroxide to water, protecting against RBC membrane and destruction (hemolysis) • Deficiency of the G6PD enzyme leads to oxidative form of methemoglobin (denatured hemoglobin precipitates as Heinz bodies)
Signs & Symptoms	• Most patients asymptomatic until periods of oxidative stress • **Hemolytic Anemia: pallor, jaundice (dark urine), splenomegaly, back or abdominal pain, fatigue, dark urine** • Profound Hemolysis: hemoglobinuria, **acute kidney injury** • **Neonatal Jaundice**

Diagnosis	• Peripheral Blood Smear: may be normal if not in acute phase or crisis; nonpersistent in patients with intact spleen
	  • **Schistocytes: "bite cells"**; 1 micron "bite" taken from cell periphery
	  • **Heinz Bodies:** denatured hemoglobin particles
	• Labs: increased reticulocytes, increased indirect bilirubin; normocytic hemolytic anemia only during acute phase or crisis
	• G6PD Enzyme Assay: performed immediately after acute phase; fluorescent spot or DNA testing

Treatment	• Supportive Care: **self-limiting; identify and discontinue precipitating agent** (avoid foods/medications, treat underlying infection) • Supplementation: iron and folic acid supplementation if severe anemia present • Blood Transfusion: indicated for severe anemia (Hgb <7 • Phototherapy: first-line treatment for neonatal jaundice
Key Words & Most Common	• X-linked recessive enzyme disorder than may cause hemolytic anemia • Most common in males of African descent • Can be precipitated by infection (most common) or medications Hemolytic anemia: pallor, jaundice, splenomegaly, back/abdominal pain, dark urine Peripheral blood smear shows schistocytes ("bite cells"); Heinz Bodies • Supportive care; avoid/treat precipitating agent

Paget Disease

Etiology & Risk Factors	• Skeletal growth disorder resulting in abnormal bone remodeling occurs in multifactorial ways leading to larger and weaker bones • Condition presents with increase in osteoclastic resorption with compensatory increase in osteoblastic bone formation • Risk Factors: certain ethnicities (**most common in Caucasians of Northern and Western European descent**), family history, **age (>50 years old most common)**
Patho-physiology	• Increased osteoclastic resorption with subsequent increase in osteoblastic bone formation leads to bone turnover acceleration at involved sites • Active osteoclasts are large with many nuclei while osteoblastic repair is hyperactive and with thickened lamellae and trabeculae leading to weakness within the bone secondary to abnormal structure despite being larger and sclerotic
Signs & Symptoms	• Most are asymptomatic (>70%); often found incidentally on x-ray or due to high alkaline phosphatase • **Bone Pain: bone pain at affected sites (pelvis, femur, spine and skull most common) is most common symptom** • Usually worse at night • Bone Remodeling: pathologic fractures, osteoarthritis, bowing of long bones • Skull Enlargement: bitemporally and frontal enlargement, **deafness** (secondary to CN VIII compression), headache, "increase in hat size", dilated scalp veins

Diagnosis	• Labs:
	  • **Marked alkaline phosphatase elevation**
	  • **Normal calcium and phosphate levels;** normal parathyroid levels, normal GGT levels
	  • Urine levels of hydroxyproline, C-telopeptide, and N telopeptide
	  • **Hyperuricemia** seen due to high bone turnover
	• Plain X-Ray: of affected sites
	  • Initial lesion may be destructive and radiolucent (especially skull)
	  • Involved bones may have sclerosis with increased trabecular markings; expanded and dense
	  • Stress fissure microfractures in long bones
	  • **Skull has "cotton wool" appearance;** poorly defined/fluffy appearance with disorganized trabeculae and sclerosis
	• Radionucleotide Bone Scan: evaluates baseline extent of disease and follow treatment
	
	Paget disease of right pelvis

Treatment	• **Observation: asymptomatic patients do not require treatment;** NSAIDs or acetaminophen for pain • **Bisphosphonates: first-line treatment option;** influences bone remodeling • Vitamin D and Calcium Supplementation: prevents hypocalcemia during bisphosphonate treatment; may provide symptomatic relief • Calcitonin: second-line treatment; assists with bone resorption
Key Words & Most Common	• Most common in Caucasians of European descent • Bone pain at affected site (pelvis, femur, spine, skull most common) • Skull enlargement may lead to deafness • Marked alkaline phosphatase elevation; X-ray will show sclerosis or radiolucency; skull has "cotton wool" appearance • Bisphosphonates are first line

Phenylketonuria (PKU)

Etiology & Risk Factors	• **Autosomal recessive disorder** caused by an inborn error of amino-acid metabolism leading to toxic accumulation of phenylalanine in urine and blood • <u>Etiology</u>: **deficiency of the enzyme phenylalanine hydroxylase (PAH)** • <u>Risk Factors</u>: certain ethnicities (Caucasian, Turkish and Native Americans most common), genetic inheritance, history of consanguinity (marriage between close blood relatives) within family, advanced maternal age
Patho-physiology	• Excess dietary phenylalanine is normally converted by the hepatic enzyme phenylalanine hydroxylase to tyrosine • Genetic mutation leads to absence or deficiency of phenylalanine hydroxylase leading to excess accumulation of phenylalanine metabolized to phenylketones • Phenylketones are neurotoxic; neurotoxicity irreversible if not detected by age 3.

Signs & Symptoms	• **Most children are asymptomatic at birth**
	   • Children tend to be lighter complexion (blond, blue-eyed, fair skin)
	• Symptoms present over course of months as phenylalanine accumulates
	   • **Intellectual and mental disability**, irritability, **hyperactivity**, gait disturbances, eczema-like rash, convulsions, **increased deep tendon reflexes**
	   • **Mousy body odor (phenylacetic acid) of urine and sweat**

Diagnosis	• <u>Labs</u>: **increased serum phenylalanine** • <u>Urine</u>: musty/mousy odor from phenylacetic acid • In US, neonates are routinely screened at 24-48 hours after birth

Treatment	• <u>Dietary Modifications</u>: **lifelong restriction of phenylalanines (milk, cheese, meats, eggs, nuts, fish, chicken, legumes, aspartame in diet pop)**
	   • Consumption of low-protein natural foods encouraged (fruits, vegetables, certain cereals)
	   • Nutritional deficiencies may develop (especially selenium, copper, magnesium, and zinc)
	• <u>Tyrosine Supplementation</u>: tyrosine is an essential amino acid
	• Women of childbearing age with PKU should be counseled on appropriate diet to avoid fetal complications

Key Words & Most Common	• Autosomal recessive disorder leading to toxic accumulation of neurotoxic Phenylketones in body • Intellectual and mental disability most common symptom Hyperactivity, irritability, increased deep tendon reflexes • Mousy (musty) body odor and urine secondary to phenylacetic acid • Increased serum phenylalanine • Dietary restriction of phenylalanines (low-protein foods) + tyrosine supplementation

Vitamin A Deficiency

Etiology & Risk Factors	• Vitamin A is a fat-soluble vitamin that is essential for cellular and embryo development, metabolism, immune and reproductive function, and vision • **Most common cause of blindness in developing world** • <u>Risk Factors</u>: **dietary restriction or deprivation**; liver disease (vitamin A stored in liver), alcoholics, **low-fat or vegan diets**, fat malabsorption conditions (CF, celiac disease, pancreatic insufficiency, duodenal bypass surgery), premature infants • <u>Sources</u>: **organ meats (liver, kidney), egg yolks**, fish, **milk products, butter**, green leafy vegetables, orange-colored vegetables
Patho-physiology	• Vitamin A is essential for rhodopsin (photoreceptor pigment within retina) formation; if deficiency persists, retinal rods will degenerate leading to xeropthalmia (eye dryness) and then true blindness • Vitamin A maintains epithelial tissues and immune function; Deficiency leads to mucosal membrane and immune dysfunction and chronic infections

Signs & Symptoms	• <u>Night Blindness</u>: **earliest manifestation**
	• <u>Xeropthalmia</u>: **drying and thickening of cornea and conjunctiva of eye is pathognomonic**
	• <u>Immune Dysfunction</u>: **frequent GI, respiratory, and urinary tract infections; poor wound healing**
	• <u>Toxicity</u>: blurry vision, nausea/vomiting, idiopathic intracranial HTN, vertigo, teratogenicity, alopecia, hepatotoxicity
	• Physical Exam:
	   • **Bitot Spots**: small white "foamy" patches on corneal conjunctiva
	   • Skin drying, flaking, and follicular thickening

Diagnosis	• **Clinical Diagnosis** • <u>Serum Retinol Level</u>: levels may only be decreased in advanced disease as liver has large store of vitamin A • <u>Liver Biopsy</u>: gold standard to quantify retinal concentration; rarely performed
Treatment	• <u>Nutritious Diet</u>: consumption of foods high in vitamin A; organ meats (liver, kidney), **egg yolks**, fish, **milk products, butter**, green leafy and orange-colored vegetables • <u>Vitamin A Supplementation</u>: dosing based on severity of deficiency; pregnant women get lower dose due to risk of fetotoxicity
Key Words & Most Common	• Fat soluble vitamin essential for cellular, embryonic, metabolic, immune and visual function • Night blindness, xeropthalmia, frequent infection, poor wound healing • Bitot spots (white "foamy" patches on corneal conjunctiva • Clinical diagnosis; serum retinol level to confirm • Nutritious Diet + Vitamin A Supplementation

Vitamin B1 (Thiamine) Deficiency

Etiology & Risk Factors	• Vitamin B1 is a water-soluble vitamin that supports carbohydrate, fat, amino acid metabolism, alcohol metabolism, and aids in nerve cell function • <u>Risk Factors</u>: **chronic alcoholism (most common)**, inadequate dietary intake, gastric bypass surgery, diarrhea, diuretic use, pregnancy/lactation • <u>Sources</u>: **meat** (beef, pork, liver), whole grains, legumes, nuts, potatoes, fortified cereal products
Patho-physiology	• Thiamine acts as energy catalyst through decarboxylation of branched chain amino acids (BCAAs) • Thiamine aids in propagating nerve impulses and maintaining myelin sheath integrity • Deficiency leads to degeneration of peripheral nerves, cerebellum, and muscle fibers
Signs & Symptoms	• <u>"Dry" Beriberi</u>: **symmetric peripheral neuropathy** occurring in "stocking-glove" distribution (paresthesia starts in toes/feet), impaired reflexes/coordination, muscle cramps • <u>"Wet" Beriberi</u>: vasodilation, wide pulse pressure, diaphoresis, tachycardia leading to **high output heart failure** causing orthopnea, edema • <u>Wernicke Encephalopathy</u>: neurologic emergency; most common in alcoholics; **ataxia** (gait and balance difficulty), **mental impairment/confusion, ocular nerve palsy** • <u>Korsakoff Psychosis</u>: **amnesia** (especially short term), time disorientation, **confabulation**, emotional changes
Diagnosis	• **Clinical Diagnosis** • Diagnosis can be made with therapeutic trial of vitamin supplementation • 24-Hour Urinary Thiamine Excretion • Erythrocyte Transketolase Activity
Treatment	• <u>**Nutritious Diet**</u>: **consumption of foods high in thiamine**; meat (beef, pork, liver), whole grains, legumes, nuts, potatoes, fortified cereal products • <u>**Thiamine Supplementation**</u>: dosing based on severity of deficiency; take with food to aid in absorption • IV thiamine followed by oral thiamine in acute crisis with cardiovascular and/or neurological symptoms

Key Words & Most Common	• Water-soluble vitamin found in red meats,
	• Chronic alcoholism is most common risk factor
	  Dry Beriberi: symmetric peripheral neuropathy
	• Wet Beriberi: high output heart failure
	• Wernicke Encephalopathy: ataxia, confusion, ocular nerve palsy
	  Korsakoff Psychosis: amnesia, confabulation
	• Clinical Diagnosis
	• Nutritious Diet + Thiamine Supplementation

Vitamin B2 (Riboflavin) Deficiency

Etiology & Risk Factors	• Vitamin B2 is a heat-stable, water-soluble vitamin that aids in carbohydrate, fat, and protein metabolism into glucose for ready-energy; antioxidant of immune system • <u>Risk Factors</u>: **inadequate dietary intake, veganism**, chronic diarrhea, malabsorption, liver disorders, dialysis, alcoholism, **women taking birth control pills** • <u>Sources</u>: eggs, milk, cheese, liver, fortified cereal product
Patho-physiology	• Riboflavin is involved in RBC production, migraine prevention, collagen synthesis, iron absorption and oxygen transport (supports hemoglobin) • Riboflavin is precursor of flavin cofactors of electron transport chain; supports mitochondrial function • Deficiency impairs above functions

Signs & Symptoms	• **Fatigue**
	• <u>**Angular Stomatitis/Cheilitis**</u>: **most common symptom** (pallor and maceration of mucosa at corners of mouth)
	   • May develop candida albicans infection
	   • May progresses to form painful fissures
	• **Magenta colored tongue**
	• <u>**Seborrheic Dermatitis**</u>: of nasolabial folds, ears, eyelids, labia majora or scrotum

Diagnosis	• **Clinical Diagnosis** • Diagnosis can be made with therapeutic trial of vitamin supplementation • <u>Urinary Excretion of Riboflavin</u>: <40mcg/day
Treatment	• <u>**Nutritious Diet**</u>: **consumption of foods high in riboflavin**; eggs, milk, cheese, liver, fortified cereal product • <u>**Riboflavin Supplementation**</u>: dosing based on severity of deficiency; take with food to aid in absorption • *Riboflavin has a green/yellow fluorescent pigment which may turn urine a bright yellow*
Key Words & Most Common	• Water-soluble vitamin found in eggs, milk, cheese, liver • Risks include inadequate diet, veganism, OCP pills, malabsorption/diarrhea, alcoholism Angular stomatitis is most common symptom; cheilitis • Magenta colored tongue • Clinical Diagnosis • Nutritious Diet + Riboflavin Supplementation

Angular Cheilosis

Vitamin B3 (Niacin/Nicotinic Acid) Deficiency

Etiology & Risk Factors	• Deficiency also known as **pellagra** • Vitamin B3 also known as niacin, nicotinic acid, or nicotinamide • <u>Risk Factors</u>: **inadequate dietary intake, veganism, diets high in untreated corn** (lacks niacin and tryptophan) chronic diarrhea, malabsorption, liver disorders, dialysis, **alcoholism**, carcinoid syndrome (increased tryptophan metabolism to form serotonin) • <u>Sources</u>: **red meat** (beef, pork, liver), fish, poultry, whole grains, legumes, nuts, potatoes, fortified cereal products
Patho-physiology	• Niacin is important cofactor in production of NAD+ and NADH/NADPH which are vital for redox reactions; aids in metabolism of carbohydrates, fat, and protein • Deficiency leads to altered metabolism • Altered metabolism of tryptophan which cannot be converted to niacin

Signs & Symptoms	• <u>Three D's</u>: **D**ermatitis, **D**iarrhea, **D**ementia
	   • **Dermatitis**: rash and skin photosensitivity; may be erythematous and scaly especially on sun-exposed areas, often mistaken for sunburn
	   • **Diarrhea**: due to impaired cell turnover
	   • **Dementia**: disorientation, **delusions**, depression, anxiety

Diagnosis	• **Clinical Diagnosis** • Diagnosis can be made with therapeutic trial of vitamin supplementation • Urinary Excretion of N1-methylnicotinamide
Treatment	• <u>**Nutritious Diet**</u>: **consumption of foods high in vitamin B3;** red meat (beef, pork, liver), fish, poultry, whole grains, legumes, nuts, potatoes, fortified cereal products • <u>**Nicotinamide Supplementation**</u>: dosing based on severity of deficiency; nicotinamide preferred over niacin which can cause flushing, itching/burning of skin
Key Words & Most Common	• Vitamin found in red meat, fish, poultry, whole grains, legumes • Risks include inadequate diet, veganism, diets high in untreated corn, alcoholism • Dermatitis: rash and skin photosensitivity • Diarrhea • Dementia: disorientation, delusion • Clinical diagnosis • Nutritious Diet + Nicotinamide Supplementation

Vitamin B6 (Pyridoxine) Deficiency

Etiology & Risk Factors	• Vitamin B6 includes compounds pyridoxine, pyridoxal, and pyridoxamine • Cofactor for enzymatic reactions involved with carbohydrate, lipid and amino acid metabolism, gluconeogenesis, and cellular function • <u>Risk Factors</u>: **inadequate dietary intake, veganism or vegetarian diet**, obesity, isoniazid use, chronic diarrhea, malabsorption GI conditions, liver disorders, dialysis, alcoholism, **women taking oral contraceptive pills**, dialysis • <u>Sources</u>: **red meat (beef**, pork, liver), fish, poultry, whole grains, legumes, nuts, potatoes, fortified cereal products
Patho-physiology	• Vitamin B6 includes compounds pyridoxine, pyridoxal, and pyridoxamine which metabolize to pyridoxal phosphate, a coenzyme important in CNS, blood, and skin metabolic functions; absorbed within small intestine and metabolized in mitochondria and cytosol to active form • Plays a role in cognitive development via neurotransmitter synthesis, immune function through IL-2 production, and formation of hemoglobin.
Signs & Symptoms	• **Peripheral neuropathy**, headaches, depression, mood changes • <u>Pellagra-Like Syndrome</u>: seborrheic dermatitis, glossitis, angular cheilitis, anemia, flaky skin
Diagnosis	• **Clinical Diagnosis** • Diagnosis can be made with therapeutic trial of vitamin supplementation • <u>Serum Pyridoxal 5'-Phosphate</u>: not commonly available
Treatment	• <u>**Nutritious Diet**</u>: **consumption of foods high in vitamin B6;** red meat (beef, pork, liver), fish, poultry, whole grains, legumes, nuts, potatoes, fortified cereal products • <u>**Pyridoxine Supplementation**</u>: dosing based on severity of deficiency
Key Words & Most Common	• Water-soluble vitamin found in meat, whole grains, fortified cereal • Risks include inadequate diet, veganism, OCP pills, isoniazid use, malabsorption/diarrhea, alcoholism • Peripheral neuropathy, mood changes • Glossitis, cheilosis • Clinical Diagnosis • Nutritious Diet + Riboflavin Supplementation

Vitamin B12 (Cobalamin) Deficiency

Etiology & Risk Factors	• Water-soluble vitamin that is a cofactor for synthesis of DNA, fatty acids, and myelin
	• Sources: **animal products**; red meat, eggs, dairy products, seafood/shellfish
	• Etiology: **decreased absorption is most common cause**; decreased intake
	   • **Decreased Absorption: pernicious anemia is most common cause** (lack of intrinsic factors due to parietal cell antibodies leading to malabsorption and gastric atrophy), **Crohn disease** (affects terminal ileum), pancreatic insufficiency, gastric bypass surgery, gastritis, Celiac disease, alcoholism, certain medications (**oral contraceptive pills**, H2 blockers/PPIs [decreased acidity decreases absorption], metformin, anticonvulsants), parasites
	   • Decreased Intake: **vegetarian or vegan diet**
	• Risk Factors: **inadequate dietary intake, vegetarian or vegan diet**, gastrointestinal disorders resulting in chronic diarrhea, advanced age, liver disorders, dialysis, alcoholism, **gastric bypass surgery**

Patho-physiology	• Vitamin B12 is involved with nucleic acid metabolism, methyl transfer, and myelin synthesis; necessary for multiple metabolic pathways, neurologic and hematologic function • Vitamin B12 is bound to intrinsic factor (protein secreted by gastric parietal cells); B12 intrinsic factor complex is absorbed by the terminal ileum and stored in liver
Signs & Symptoms	• Hematologic: **anemia symptoms; fatigue, pallor**, exercise intolerance • Gastrointestinal: **diarrhea, malabsorption**, hepatomegaly/splenomegaly, weight loss Neurologic: **symmetrical peripheral neuropathy is most common initial symptom**; ataxia, weakness • Dorsal Column Demyelination: impaired vibratory and proprioception senses, hypotonia
Diagnosis	• **CBC with Peripheral Smear: macrocytic anemia (increased MCV)** • **Megaloblastic Anemia**: hyper segmented neutrophils, high RDW, low reticulocyte count; leukopenia/thrombocytopenia if severe • **Serum B12 Level: decreased levels** • **Methylmalonic Acid: elevated methylmalonic acid distinguishes B12 from folate deficiency** (MMA is normal in folate deficiency) • Other: LDH and bilirubin may be elevated; **elevated homocysteine**

Treatment	• **Nutritious Diet: consumption of foods high in riboflavin**; eggs, milk, cheese, liver, fortified cereal product
	• **Vitamin B12 Supplementation**: dosing based on severity of deficiency
	   • **Intramuscular Injection**: weekly cyanocobalamin injection then tapered; indicated for symptomatic anemia or neurologic symptoms
	   • *Pernicious anemia patients need lifelong IM B12 injections*

Key Words & Most Common	• Water-soluble vitamin found in animal products; red meat, eggs, dairy • Risks include pernicious anemia, inadequate diet, veganism, OCP pills, malabsorption/diarrhea, alcoholism • Anemia symptoms (fatigue, pallor); malabsorption, diarrhea • Symmetrical peripheral neuropathy is most common initial symptom • CBC with peripheral smear: macrocytic anemia • Nutritious Diet + Vitamin B12 Supplementation (IM injections if symptomatic or pernicious anemia patient)

Vitamin C Deficiency

Etiology & Risk Factors	• **Also known as scurvy** • Etiology: inadequate oral intake or decreased absorption • Risk Factors: **diets low in fruits and vegetables, alcoholism**, infants only consuming pasteurized milk, smokers, malnourished (eating disorders), elderly, drug use, hyperthyroidism, burns • Sources: **fresh fruits and vegetables**; citrus fruits, potatoes, spinach, tomatoes, berries, broccoli, red peppers • **Vitamin C is heat sensitive** (pasteurization, boiling, or cooking denatures vitamin and removes nutritional value)
Patho-physiology	• Vitamin C plays vital role in collagen, carnitine, hormone, and amino acid formation; important cofactor for hydroxylation of proline and lysine into collagen • Forms main components of bone, skin (basement membrane), and blood vessels; potent antioxidant that supports immune system function; aids in iron absorption • When deficient, basement membrane and intercellular substances of connective tissue becomes weak leading to weakened capillaries (hemorrhage), poor bone and dentin formation, poor wound healing
Signs & Symptoms	• Symptoms appear 8-12 weeks of inadequate intake • **Hyperkeratosis: hyperkeratotic follicular papules, petechiae**, corkscrew coiled hair • **Hemorrhage**: weakened capillaries from poor collagen synthesis; **perifollicular hemorrhage, gingival bleeding, easy bruising, impaired wound healing** • **Hematologic**: anemia (Vit C promotes iron absorption), malaise, weakness, glossitis, bleeding into joint with minimal trauma • Mood disturbance, delusions, depression, cognitive impairments
Diagnosis	• **Clinical Diagnosis** • **Serum Ascorbic Acid Level**: levels <0.2mg/dL
Treatment	• **Nutritious Diet: fresh fruits and vegetables**; citrus fruits, potatoes, spinach, tomatoes, berries, broccoli, red peppers • **Ascorbic Acid Supplementation**: oral 100-500mg TID for 1-2 weeks until symptoms resolve
Key Words & Most Common	• Vitamin C plays role in collagen and amino acid formation; supports immune system • Risks include diets low in fresh fruits and vegetables; alcoholism • Hyperkeratosis: hyperkeratotic follicular papules, petechia • Hemorrhage: gingival bleeding, easy bruising, poor wound healing • Hematologic: anemia • Clinical diagnosis; serum ascorbic acid level • Nutritious diet + ascorbic acid supplementation

Vitamin D Deficiency

Etiology & Risk Factors	• Vitamin D is a fat-soluble vitamin used for bone development and maintenance by amplifying calcium, magnesium, and phosphate absorption • Deficiency can lead to osteomalacia and rickets in children and osteomalacia in adults • <u>Etiology</u>: inadequate oral intake or decreased absorption • <u>Risk Factors</u>: **inadequate sunlight exposure (dark skin, sunscreen use, living in colder climate)**, inadequate dietary intake, veganism, impaired absorption (Crohn's, CF, pancreatic insufficiency), renal/hepatic failure • <u>Sources</u>: **direct sunlight**, fortified milk, egg yolks, fish liver oils, saltwater fish
Patho-physiology	• Hydroxylated in liver to 25-hydroxyvitamin D which is then hydroxylated in kidney enzymes to 1,25-dihydroxyvitamin D (active form) • Vitamin D stimulates calcium absorption and phosphorus level maintenance for bone development; modulates immune function and inflammation reduction • Hypocalcemia can lead to secondary hyperparathyroidism leading to accelerated demineralization
Signs & Symptoms	• **Muscle aches and pain, muscle weakness** (proximal), muscle fasciculations (spasming/twitching) • **Bone pain**; hip pain may lead to antalgic gait • **Bowing of long bones** • <u>Rickets</u>: **delayed fontanel closure**, bossing of skull, and costochondral thickening; **genu varum** (lateral bowing of lower extremities)
Diagnosis	• <u>Serum 25-hydroxyvitamin D Level</u>: normal 75-250 nmol/L; insufficiency 25-75 nmol/L • <u>Labs</u>: **decreased calcium, decreased phosphate**, increased alkaline phosphatase and PTH • <u>X-Ray</u>: **bone demineralization** of spine, pelvis, lower extremities; pseudo-fracture lines (narrow, incomplete lines of demineralized bone) • <u>Rickets</u>: **widening of epiphyseal plate**, enlargement of costochondral junction; less distinct cortex most evident at distal radius/ulna
Treatment	• <u>Nutritious Diet</u>: fortified milk, egg yolks, fish liver oils, saltwater fish • <u>Sunlight Exposure</u>: **short durations during morning and evening hours** lowers risk of overexposure • <u>Vitamin D Supplementation</u>: vitamin D3 (cholecalciferol) more efficacious; dosing based on severity of deficiency • Supplementation should be initiated for those with risk factors
Key Words & Most Common	• Fat-soluble vitamin used for bone development and maintenance • Sources include direct sunlight, fortified milk, egg yolks, fish liver oil • Risks include inadequate sunlight or dietary intake, veganism • Muscle aches/pain/weakness; bone pain • Rickets: delayed fontanel closure, genu varum • Serum 25-hydroxyvitamin D level; decreased calcium and phosphate • X-ray shows bone demineralization • Nutritious Diet + Adequate Sunlight + Vitamin D Supplementation

Acute Pancreatitis

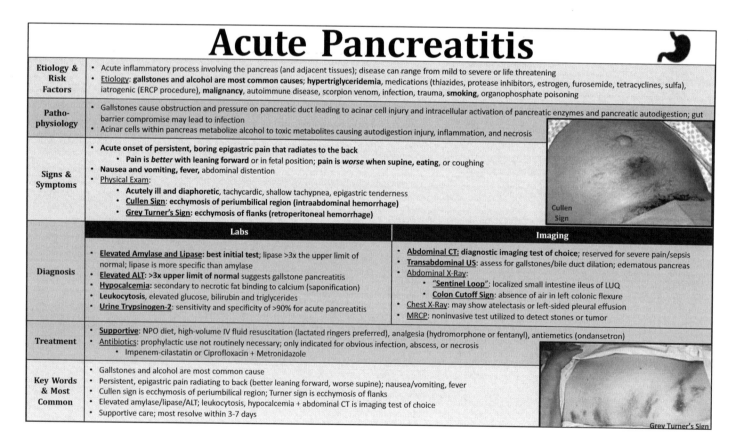

Etiology & Risk Factors	• Acute inflammatory process involving the pancreas (and adjacent tissues); disease can range from mild to severe or life threatening • <u>Etiology</u>: **gallstones and alcohol are most common causes; hypertriglyceridemia**, medications (thiazides, protease inhibitors, estrogen, furosemide, tetracyclines, sulfa), iatrogenic (ERCP procedure), **malignancy**, autoimmune disease, scorpion venom, infection, trauma, **smoking**, organophosphate poisoning		
Patho-physiology	• Gallstones cause obstruction and pressure on pancreatic duct leading to acinar cell injury and intracellular activation of pancreatic enzymes and pancreatic autodigestion; gut barrier compromise may lead to infection • Acinar cells within pancreas metabolize alcohol to toxic metabolites causing autodigestion injury, inflammation, and necrosis		

Signs & Symptoms	• **Acute onset of persistent, boring epigastric pain that radiates to the back**
	  • Pain is *better* with leaning forward or in fetal position; pain is *worse* when supine, eating, or coughing
	• **Nausea and vomiting, fever,** abdominal distention
	• <u>Physical Exam</u>:
	  • **Acutely ill and diaphoretic,** tachycardic, shallow tachypnea, epigastric tenderness
	  • <u>Cullen Sign</u>: ecchymosis of periumbilical region **(intraabdominal hemorrhage)**
	  • <u>Grey Turner's Sign</u>: ecchymosis of flanks **(retroperitoneal hemorrhage)**
			Cullen Sign

	Labs	Imaging

Diagnosis	• <u>Elevated Amylase and Lipase</u>: **best initial test**; lipase >3x the upper limit of normal; lipase is more specific than amylase
	• <u>Elevated ALT</u>: >3x upper limit of normal suggests gallstone pancreatitis
	• <u>Hypocalcemia</u>: secondary to necrotic fat binding to calcium (saponification)
	• <u>Leukocytosis</u>, elevated glucose, bilirubin and triglycerides
	• <u>Urine Trypsinogen-2</u>: sensitivity and specificity of >90% for acute pancreatitis
		• <u>Abdominal CT</u>: **diagnostic imaging test of choice**; reserved for severe pain/sepsis
		• <u>Transabdominal US</u>: assess for gallstones/bile duct dilation; edematous pancreas
		• <u>Abdominal X-Ray</u>:
		  • **"Sentinel Loop"**: localized small intestine ileus of LUQ
		  • **Colon Cutoff Sign**: absence of air in left colonic flexure
		• <u>Chest X-Ray</u>: may show atelectasis or left-sided pleural effusion
		• <u>MRCP</u>: noninvasive test utilized to detect stones or tumor

Treatment	• <u>Supportive</u>: NPO diet, high-volume IV fluid resuscitation (lactated ringers preferred), analgesia (hydromorphone or fentanyl), antiemetics (ondansetron) • <u>Antibiotics</u>: prophylactic use not routinely necessary; only indicated for obvious infection, abscess, or necrosis • Impenem-cilastatin or Ciprofloxacin + Metronidazole
Key Words & Most Common	• Gallstones and alcohol are most common cause • Persistent, epigastric pain radiating to back (better leaning forward, worse supine); nausea/vomiting, fever • Cullen sign is ecchymosis of periumbilical region; Turner sign is ecchymosis of flanks • Elevated amylase/lipase/ALT; leukocytosis, hypocalcemia + abdominal CT is imaging test of choice • Supportive care; most resolve within 3-7 days

Grey Turner's Sign

Chronic Pancreatitis

Etiology & Risk Factors	• Chronic, progressive, inflammatory disorder causing permanent changes to the pancreatic parenchyma resulting in loss of pancreatic endocrine and exocrine function • Etiology: **alcohol abuse is most common cause**, idiopathic, ductal obstruction (malignancy, trauma), genetics (CF, familial pancreatitis), chemotherapy, autoimmune conditions, hypercalcemia, hyperlipidemia
Patho-physiology	• Alcohol consumption or other factors causes increased acinar cell protein secretion resulting in viscous pancreatic fluid which plugs ducts and lobules • Ductal obstruction, fibrosis, and calcification results in loss of endocrine/exocrine function • Complications include diabetes mellitus, malabsorption of fat-soluble vitamins, and adenocarcinoma

Signs & Symptoms	• **Prolonged abdominal pain (epigastric pain or abdominal pain that radiates to the back)**
	   • May be intermittent
	   • May be relieved with sitting or leaning forward
	• **Weight loss**; fatigue
	• Nausea/vomiting
	• **Steatorrhea (greasy, foul-smelling, pale stool) or diarrhea**

Multiple calcifications in the pancreas

	Labs	Imaging
Diagnosis	• **Amylase and Lipase: usually normal or minimally elevated** • LFTs: may show elevated bilirubin and alkaline phosphatase • **Fecal Elastase-1 Level: most sensitive and specific test**	• Abdominal X-Ray: demonstrates pancreatic calcifications • Abdominal CT Scan: **shows intraductal calcifications of pancreas**; may help exclude other pathology (malignant obstruction) • MRCP: noninvasive test utilized to detect stones or tumor

Treatment	• Supportive: alcohol cessation, pain control (NSAIDs, TCAs, pregabalin), diet modifications (small, frequent, low-fat meals), vitamin supplementation (Vit A,D,E,K) • Pancreatic Enzymes: taken with meals; may alleviate pain • Acid Suppression Therapy: H2 blockers, PPIs • Surgery: indicated if pain refractory to medical therapy; required for pancreatic abscess/fistula, mechanical obstruction of common bile duct
Key Words & Most Common	• Chronic inflammatory disorder of pancreas most commonly secondary to alcohol abuse • Prolonged, epigastric abdominal pain; weight loss, N/V, fatigue • Steatorrhea (greasy, pale stool) • Amylase/Lipase usually normal • Fecal Elastase-1 Level is most sensitive and specific • Abdominal x-ray/CT shows pancreatic calcifications • Supportive measures +/- pancreatic enzyme supplementation

Pancreatic Cancer

Etiology & Risk Factors	• Exocrine tumors arising from ductal and acinar cells within the pancreas; 4th leading cause of cancer-related death in the US • Risk Factors: age (>65 years old most common), **smoking, diabetes mellitus**, family history, male, obesity, poor diet, history of chronic pancreatitis, cirrhosis, *H. pylori* infection, occupational exposures
Patho-physiology	• Chronic inflammation leads to activation of oncogenes through point mutation and amplification • 80% of carcinoma located at head of pancreas • Adenocarcinoma (ductal) is most common (90%+); islet cell carcinoma (5-10%) • Serous, seromucinous, or mucinous

Signs & Symptoms	• Often asymptomatic in early disease course; most patients present late in course (after metastases)
	• **Painless jaundice (obstruction of common bile duct) and weight loss most common symptoms**
	• **Abdominal pain** radiating to back
	• Weakness, **skin pruritus (bile salt accumulation in the skin)**, anorexia, **acholic (light colored) stool**, dark urine
	• Physical Exam
	   • Trousseau's Malignancy Sign: migratory phlebitis; nonspecific
	   • **Courvoisier's Sign: palpable, nontender, distended gallbladder**

Diagnosis	• **Abdominal CT Scan: initial imaging test of choice**; uses pancreatic technique • MRI/MRCP: for preoperative evaluation • **Pancreas-Associated Antigen CA 19-9**: utilized to monitor after treatment or screen for high risk • Amylase/Lipase: usually normal

Adenocarcinoma tumor at the head of the pancreas

Treatment	• **Neoadjuvant Treatment**: chemotherapy and/or radiation is preferred for locally advanced, non-resectable adenocarcinoma • **Whipple Procedure: pancreaticoduodenectomy; procedure of choice for adenocarcinoma involving head of pancreas** • Postoperative chemotherapy with 5-FU, Gemcitabine, radiotherapy • Prognosis: poor prognosis; only ~20% are resectable; 5-year survival rate <20%
Key Words & Most Common	• Risks: smoking, age, obesity, diabetes • Painless jaundice, weight loss most common symptoms • Abdominal pain radiation to back, skin pruritus, pale stool • CT Scan initial imaging test of choice • Pancreas associated antigen CA 19-9 to monitor or screen for high-risk • Neoadjuvant treatment • Whipple procedure if involves head of pancreas

Meckel's Diverticulum

Etiology & Risk Factors	• Congenital abnormality of the small intestine involving an incomplete involution of the embryonic vitelline duct (omphalomesenteric duct) • Involution usually occurs by 7th week of gestation • Most common congenital abnormality of the GI tract • **Rule of 2's:** • Affects 2% of infants; • Affects males 2x as often • 2% become symptomatic • Children most often 2 years old at time of presentation • Located 2 feet proximal to ileocecal valve • 2 inches in length or less • May have 2 types of mucosal lining (gastric or pancreatic)
Patho-physiology	• The vitelline or omphalomesenteric duct connects the midgut to the yolk sac; if obliteration does not occur by 7th week of gestation, then Meckel's diverticulum develops • Meckel diverticulum contains heterotopic gastric or pancreatic tissue which may secrete hydrochloric acid or other digestive hormones which may lead to ulceration of adjacent tissue
Signs & Symptoms	• **Usually asymptomatic** and incidental finding on imaging studies • **Painless rectal bleeding is most common symptom** (most often presents by age 5) • Commonly described as "currant jelly" or "brick colored" stool (stool composed of blood and mucous) • Abdominal pain (often periumbilical and may mimic appendicitis) • May lead to intussusception, volvulus, or obstruction in children (diverticulitis in adults)
Diagnosis	• **Technetium-99m Pertechnetate Scan (Meckel scan):** may identify **ectopic gastric mucosa** in the ileal area • Abdominal CT Scan: may show inflammation or obstruction at level of diverticulum • Mesenteric Angiogram: definitive diagnosis; only indicated if nuclear (Meckel) scan is negative w/ high suspicion
Treatment	• **Surgical Excision:** laparoscopic vs open technique if symptomatic • Asymptomatic diverticulum do not always need to be excised • Assess volume status (blood loss)
Key Words & Most Common	• Rule of 2's • Usually asymptomatic • Painless rectal bleeding most common symptom; abdominal pain • Currant jelly or brick colored stool • Meckel scan identifies ectopic gastric tissue • Surgical Excision

Duodenal Atresia

Etiology & Risk Factors	• Congenital closure of duodenum resulting in gastric outlet obstruction • Etiology: complete or partial obstruction of the duodenum • Risk Factors: **polyhydramnios (increased amniotic fluid)**, **Down syndrome** (25-40% of cases), disruption of blood flow during fetal development, maternal diabetes
Patho-physiology	• During week 6-7 of embryologic development, GI tract becomes occluded then recanalizes at week 8-10; error of recanalization leads to duodenal atresia • Associated with other congenital defects of cardiac, renal, or vascular systems • **VACTERL:** **V**ertebral anomalies, **A**nal atresia, **C**ardiac malformations, **T**racheoesophageal fistula, **E**sophageal atresia, **R**enal anomalies and **R**adial aplasia, and **L**imb anomalies
Signs & Symptoms	• **Neonatal intestinal obstruction** usually occurring within first 24-38 hours of life after first feeding • **Bilious vomiting** • **Abdominal distention** (with or without visible/palpable loops of bowel) • May have signs of dehydration
Diagnosis	• Abdominal X-Ray: double-bubble sign • **Double-Bubble Sign:** distended air-filled stomach and proximal duodenum with pyloric valve separation; absence of distal gas) • Prenatal US: used to screen those with risk factors (polyhydramnios, Down syndrome) • Upper GI Series: may be used preoperatively to identify GI anatomy Pyloric valve separation
Treatment	• Supportive: decompressing of GI tract with nasogastric suction, NPO, fluid/electrolyte replacement • **Surgery: duodenoduodenostomy is definitive management**
Key Words & Most Common	• Risks: polyhydramnios, Down syndrome • Neonatal intestinal obstruction • Bilious vomiting, distended abdomen • Abdominal X-ray shows double-bubble sign (distended stomach and duodenum separated by pyloric valve) • Supportive care • Surgery (Duodenoduodenostomy) is definitive Double-Bubble Sign

Volvulus

Etiology & Risk Factors	• Occurs when loop of bowel twists on itself at the mesenteric attachment site leading to bowel obstruction • **Sigmoid colon and cecum most commonly** implicated in older adults; midgut and ileum most common in children • <u>Risk Factors</u>: intestinal malrotation, Hirschsprung's disease, pregnancy, dilated colon, **abdominal adhesions, high-fiber diet, chronic constipation**, chronic laxative use
Patho-physiology	• Dilated bowel fills with stool leading to torsion; loop of bowel twists at mesenteric attachment site leading to obstruction and strangulation of vascular supply • Adhesions may develop leading to fixed twisted position
Signs & Symptoms	• <u>Classic Triad</u>: **abdominal pain + abdominal distention + constipation** • **Bilious vomiting**, tympanitic abdomen • <u>Strangulation of Vascular Supply</u>: **fever**, tachycardia, peritonitis (guarding, rebound tenderness) • <u>Newborns</u>: **sudden onset bilious vomiting**, hematochezia, abdominal distention, inconsolable cry

Diagnosis	• <u>Abdominal X-Ray</u>: **best initial imaging test**
	   • <u>Sigmoid</u>: "bent inner tube" or "coffee bean" sign (U-shaped, air-filled, closed loop of distended bowel with lack of haustral markings)
	   • <u>Cecal</u>: air-fluid level, paucity of gas, distended small and large bowel
	• <u>Contrast Enema</u>: "bird's beak" appearance at point of proximal and distal bowel rotate to form volvulus; contraindicated if peritonitis present
	• <u>Abdominal CT Scan</u>: highly sensitive and specific; definitive diagnosis
	
	Sigmoid volvulus

Treatment	• <u>Supportive</u>: decompressing of GI tract with nasogastric suction, NPO, fluid/electrolyte replacement, antibiotics (if gangrenous bowel suspected) • **<u>Endoscopic Decompression (proctosigmoidoscopy)</u>: initial treatment of choice**; may use air insufflation at site of torsion to decompress looped bowel • <u>Bowel Resection</u>: often performed after decompression due to high rate of recurrence (especially cecal volvulus)
Key Words & Most Common	• <u>Risks</u>: high-fiber diet, chronic constipation; most common in "elderly constipated male" • Classic triad of abdominal pain, distention, constipation +/- bilious vomiting • Newborns may present with sudden onset bilious vomiting • Abdominal X-ray is best initial test; shows loop of distended bowel with lack of haustral markings • Contrast Enema shows "bird beak" narrowing at point of proximal/distal bowel rotation • Endoscopic decompression +/- bowel resection

Small Bowel Obstruction

Etiology & Risk Factors	• Partial or full mechanical blockage of small bowel • <u>Etiology</u>: **post-surgical intraabdominal adhesions (most common cause), incarcerated hernias**, malignancy, Crohn disease, intussusception, stool impaction, foreign bodies, volvulus
Patho-physiology	• Intraabdominal adhesions, malignancy etc. leads to mechanical obstruction of bowel causing ingested food, digestive secretions, and gas to accumulate proximal to the obstruction. Proximal bowel distention occurs causing the distal bowel to collapse which depresses the normal secretory and peristaltic function of the bowel • Strangulation occurs as result of volvulus, intussusception, or hernia; may progress to full incarceration leading to infarction and gangrene

Signs & Symptoms	• **Crampy abdominal pain, distention, nausea/vomiting and obstipation** (not passing gas)
	• Constipation; may have thin, loose bowel movements
	• <u>Physical Exam</u>:
	   • **Abdominal distention**, diffuse tenderness to palpation, signs of dehydration
	   • **High-pitched "tinkling" bowel sounds**
	   • Peritonitis signs (guarding, rebound tenderness) if late in course
	
	Small bowel obstruction with multiple air fluid levels

Diagnosis	• <u>Abdominal X-Ray</u>: **best initial test**
	   • Air-fluid levels and "ladder-like" appearance of dilated bowel loops
	   • <u>String of Pearls Sign</u>: small gas pockets along small bowel trapped between thin, circular loops of mucosa is diagnostic
	• <u>Abdominal CT Scan w/ Contrast</u>: **gold-standard**; consider if abdominal x-ray nondiagnostic
	   • Shows transition zone from dilated loops of bowel with contrast to area without contrast (ischemia)
	• <u>Abdominal Ultrasound</u>: sensitive and specific; no radiation exposure

Treatment	• **<u>Supportive</u>: decompression of GI tract with nasogastric (NG) suction, NPO, fluid/electrolyte replacement, antibiotics** (if bowel ischemia/infarct suspected) • <u>Surgical Consult</u>: early laparotomy indicated; resection or palliative gastrojejunostomy • Ileus and partial obstructions can be treated conservatively
Key Words & Most Common	• Partial or complete blockage of small bowel • Most common cause is post-surgical adhesions; incarcerated hernias, malignancy • Crampy/colicky abdominal pain, distention, N/V, obstipation • High-pitched "tinkling" bowel sounds • <u>Abdominal X-Ray</u>: best initial test; dilated bowel loops trapped between circular loops of bowel • <u>Abdominal CT Scan w/ Contrast</u>: gold standard • Supportive care (NG suction) + Surgical consult

Splenic Rupture

Etiology & Risk Factors	• Spleen is encapsulated organ at the posterior aspect of the left upper quadrant of the abdomen within the peritoneal cavity near 9th, 10th, and 11th ribs
	• **Spleen is most common organ injured secondary to trauma**
	• Etiology: traumatic and nontraumatic mechanisms
	    • <u>Trauma (most common cause)</u>: **motor vehicle accidents**, direct blows, falls, sports related injuries; associated with rib fractures
	    • <u>Nontraumatic</u>: idiopathic, infectious mononucleosis due to Ebstein-Barr Virus infection (predisposes to rupture with minimal trauma)

Patho-physiology	• Splenic rupture leads to hemorrhage into the peritoneal cavity; may be minimal or massive depending on extent of rupture and mechanism • Blood loss may lead to hemorrhagic shock
Signs & Symptoms	• **Abdominal pain (LUQ)**, abdominal distention, rib pain • Signs of hemorrhagic shock; tachycardia, hypotension, altered mental status • <u>Kehr Sign</u>: referred pain to tip of left shoulder secondary to compression of diaphragm and phrenic nerve from peritoneal bleed
Diagnosis	• <u>Splenic Ultrasound</u>: indicated for unstable patients to search for free fluid; FAST (focused assessment with sonography for trauma) • <u>Abdominal CT Scan</u>: for stable patients to determine extent of injury
Treatment	• <u>Observation</u>: goal is to preserve spleen; indicated for hemodynamically stable patients; monitor with serial abdominal exams, hematocrit level, vital signs • <u>Splenectomy</u>: indicated for uncontrollable bleed • <u>Endovascular Embolization</u>: may be indicated for stable patient that fails conservative management
Key Words & Most Common	• Most common organ injured due to trauma • Motor vehicle accidents, direct impacts, falls, rib fractures • Splenic enlargement secondary to Ebstein-Barr Virus predisposes to rupture with minimal trauma • Abdominal pain, distention; signs of hemorrhagic shock • <u>Kehr Sign</u>: left shoulder referred pain • Ultrasound if unstable, CT scan if stable • Observation if stable, Splenectomy if unstable

Ileus

Etiology & Risk Factors	• Decreased or absence of peristalsis without mechanical/structural obstruction
	• Also known as "sleepy bowel"
	• Etiology:
	    • <u>Surgery</u>: **abdominal or pelvic surgery is most common cause**
	    • <u>Inflammation</u>: appendicitis, diverticulitis, peptic ulcer, colitis, gallstone ileus, pancreatitis
	    • <u>Hematomas</u>: ruptured AAA, trauma
	    • <u>Metabolic</u>: hypokalemia, hypercalcemia
	    • <u>Medications</u>: opioids

Patho-physiology	• Neuroimmune interaction in which autonomic nervous system and immune system leads to inflammation which inhibits afferent/efferent communication • Bowel manipulation (surgery or other) leads to immune macrophages to release anti-peristaltic cytokines that activate pro-inflammatory cells • Bowel stress then leads to further inflammation and inhibition of sympathetic activity within the bowel

Signs & Symptoms	• **Abdominal distention and bloating**, nausea/vomiting, obstipation, inability to tolerate PO intake
	• Physical Exam:
	    • **Decreased/absent bowel sounds** (SBO has high-pitched bowel sounds)
	    • Diffuse tenderness to palpation, tympany, no peritoneal signs

Diagnosis	• <u>Abdominal X-Ray</u>: **dilated bowel loops with *no* transition zone**; shows air in colon and rectum • <u>Abdominal CT Scan</u>: helps delineate transition point; rules out other abdominal pathology • <u>Labs</u>: CBC, CMP (electrolytes + LFTs), amylase, lipase (look for reversible causes of ileus
Treatment	• <u>Treat Underlying Etiology</u>: if possible • <u>Supportive</u>: **NPO with slow progression of diet (clear liquids to full liquid etc.), fluid/electrolyte replacement** (avoid excessive as bowel edema can worsen ileus) • Chewing gum can stimulate cephalocaudal reflex and improve bowel function • <u>Nasogastric Decompression</u>: if persistent nausea/vomiting
Key Words & Most Common	• Decreased/absent peristalsis most commonly after abdominal/pelvic surgery • Abdominal distention/bloating, N/V, obstipation • Decreased/absent bowel sounds (differentiates from SBO) • Abdominal X-Ray: dilated bowel loops with NO transition zone; air in colon/rectum • Supportive treatment

Intussusception

Etiology & Risk Factors	• Telescoping of portion of the intestine into an adjacent segment of intestinal lumen leading to bowel obstruction • Most common site is ileocolic junction • Etiology: **idiopathic most common**, Meckel diverticulum, hyperplasia of Peyer's patches, anatomical factors, polyps, altered motility, submucosal hematoma • Risk Factors: **children (6-18 months old most common)**, males, post-viral, post-vaccination (rotavirus vaccine), recent gastroenteritis
Patho-physiology	• Peristaltic activity of intestine pulls proximal segment of bowel into lumen of distal segment of bowel • Trapped segment of bowel can become ischemic if blood supply is impacted • Mucosal is sensitive to ischemia leading to sloughing of mucus, blood, and mucosa into gut causing "currant jelly" stool

Signs & Symptoms	• **Sudden, colicky abdominal pain**, nausea, **vomiting**
	• **"Currant Jelly" Stool**: stool mixed with mucus, blood and sloughed gut mucosa
	• Physical Exam:
	  • **Child may pull legs to chest**
	  • **Palpable sausage-shaped mass** at right upper quadrant
	  • Dance Sign: retraction of right iliac fossa due to bowel telescoping

Diagnosis	• **Abdominal Ultrasound: best initial imaging test**
	  • **Target or Donut Sign**: central core of hyperechoic bowel surrounded by hypoechoic edematous outer bowel, confirms diagnosis
	• Abdominal X-Ray: lack of air within bowel
	  • **Barium, water-soluble, or air enema confirms diagnosis** and successfully reduces it; air enema more commonly used; water-soluble preferred over barium
	• Abdominal CT Scan: consider if high susception with equivocal imaging

Treatment	• **Supportive: decompression of GI tract with nasogastric (NG) suction, NPO, fluid/electrolyte replacement** • Reduction: pneumatic or hydrostatic (saline/contrast) decompression of intussuscepted segment; pneumatic (air) is preferred especially if peritonitis present • Surgery: manual reduction may be attempted; bowel resection if unable to be reduced
Key Words & Most Common	• Telescoping of intestine on itself • Most common in children age 6-18 months • Sudden, colicky abdominal pain, vomiting • "Currant jelly" stool: stool mixed with mucus, blood and sloughed gut mucosa • Ultrasound is best initial test; target/donut sign • Water soluble/air enema can be diagnostic and therapeutic • Supportive treatment with reduction through pneumatic/hydrostatic decompression

Intussusception of the Bowel

Hirschsprung Disease

Etiology & Risk Factors	• Congenital megacolon due to absence of ganglion cells at the Meissner (submucosa) and Auerbach (muscularis) autonomic plexus in the intestinal wall leading to obstruction • **Most common site is distal colon and terminal rectum**; may extend proximally • Etiology: absence of nerve cells (ganglion cells) in the lower part of the large intestine (colon) • Risk Factors: **male (4:1), Down syndrome**, family history, prematurity at birth, maternal diabetes, consanguineous marriages (marriages between close blood relatives)
Patho-physiology	• Disruption of the complete neural crest migration leads to absence of enteric ganglion cells at the Meissner and Auerbach plexus in intestinal wall • This leads to failure persistent release of acetylcholine causing intestinal overactivity (contraction) of the affected segment and subsequent relaxion of the aganglionic segment leading to functional obstruction
Signs & Symptoms	• Neonatal Intestinal Obstruction: **delayed passage of meconium after birth (>48 hours); bilious vomiting, abdominal distention**, obstipation • Children: **constipation**, anorexia, no urge to defecate, **absence of stool in rectal vault** (may palpate stool proximally in colon and explosive passage of stool when withdrawing finger "blast sign")
Diagnosis	• **Barium Contrast Enema: shows narrowed colon and dilated proximal bowel with transition zone** • Abdominal X-Ray: distended colon with absence of air in rectum • Anorectal Manometry: demonstrates increased sphincter pressure with impaired internal sphincter relaxation • **Rectal Suction Biopsy: definitive diagnosis**; shows absence of ganglionic cells
Treatment	• **Supportive: while waiting on surgical consult;** decompression of GI tract with nasogastric suction, NPO, fluid/electrolyte replacement • Surgery: resection of affected segment; brings normal bowel segment to anus while preserving sphincters
Key Words & Most Common	• Absence of ganglion cells leads to functional obstruction in neonate • Males most commonly affected • Most common site distal colon and terminal rectum • Neonate: delayed passage of meconium (meconium ileus), vomiting, abdominal distention • Barium contrast enema shows narrowed colon and dilated proximal bowel • Rectal suction biopsy required for definitive diagnosis • Surgery

113

Appendicitis

Etiology & Risk Factors	• Acute inflammation of the vermiform appendix, a hollow organ located at the cecum • **Most common cause of acute abdomen in children (12-18 years old)** • <u>Etiology</u>: fecalith obstruction, lymphoid hyperplasia (secondary to infection), malignancy, foreign body, parasite, benign or malignant tumors • <u>Risk Factors</u>: **age (10-30 years old most common)**, female, family history, poor diet (low-fiber), smoking
Patho-physiology	• Obstruction of vermiform appendix lumen leads to increase in intraluminal and intramural pressure causing small blood vessel occlusion and lymphatic stasis • Inflammation, distention, bacterial overgrowth and ischemia increases as appendix fills which can all lead to increased pressure and eventual perforation

Signs & Symptoms	• **Epigastric or periumbilical abdominal pain** followed by anorexia, nausea/vomiting (usually occurs after pain)
	   • After several hours (usually 12-18), **pain localizes to right lower quadrant**
	• May have **fever**
	• ***Sudden improvement suggests perforation***
	• <u>Physical Exam</u>:
	   • Epigastric or right lower quadrant tenderness; rebound tenderness, guarding, rigidity
	   • **McBurney's Point**: maximal tenderness to palpation 2/3 of way from umbilicus to right anterior superior iliac spine
	   • **Rovsing Sign**: RLQ pain with LLQ palpation
	   • **Obturator Sign**: RLQ pain with internal and external hip rotation
	   • **Psoas Sign**: RLQ pain with extension of right leg at hip while patient lies on left side
	
	Enlarged appendix with increased wall thickness

Diagnosis	• <u>**Abdominal Ultrasound**</u>: initial imaging choice for children and pregnant women
	   • Demonstrates noncompressible enlarged appendix with increased wall thickness
	• <u>**Abdominal CT Scan**</u>: imaging test of choice for men and non-pregnant women; more sensitive and specific
	   • Demonstrates enlarged appendix with increased wall thickness; can identify perforation

Treatment	• <u>**Supportive**</u>: NPO, fluid/electrolyte replacement, analgesics, antiemetics • <u>**Antibiotics**</u>: initiated prior to surgery with coordination from surgeon; 3rd generation cephalosporins preferred • <u>**Surgery**</u>: open vs laparoscopic appendectomy
Key Words & Most Common	• Acute inflammation of appendix • Most commonly due to fecalith obstruction or lymphoid hyperplasia • Epigastric/periumbilical abdominal pain that localizes to RLQ • Nausea/vomiting +/- fever • McBurney's Point; Rovsing Sign; Obturator Sign; Psoas Sign • Ultrasound for children and pregnant women; CT scan for men and non-pregnant women • Supportive care + antibiotics • Appendectomy

References

1. Acute cholecystitis as seen on ultrasound axial view.jpg. (2023, July 9). *Wikimedia Commons.* Retrieved 19:06, August 7, 2023 from https://commons.wikimedia.org/w/index.php?title=File:Acute_cholecystitis_as_seen_on_ultrasound_axial_view.jpg&oldid=781841923.
2. Constipation(lots).png. (2020, October 13). *Wikimedia Commons.* Retrieved 20:28, August 7, 2023 from https://commons.wikimedia.org/w/index.php?title=File:Constipation(lots).png&oldid=488959365.
3. Internal and external hemorrhoids.png. (2023, May 19). *Wikimedia Commons.* Retrieved 20:54, August 7, 2023 from https://commons.wikimedia.org/w/index.php?title=File:Internal_and_external_hemorrhoids.png&oldid=764940668.
4. Diverticulitis.png. (2022, March 27). *Wikimedia Commons.* Retrieved 21:07, August 7, 2023 from https://commons.wikimedia.org/w/index.php?title=File:Diverticulitis.png&oldid=644400039.
5. Toxic Megacolon in Ulcerative Colitis.jpg. (2020, October 23). *Wikimedia Commons.* Retrieved 21:35, August 7, 2023 from https://commons.wikimedia.org/w/index.php?title=File:Toxic_Megacolon_in_Ulcerative_Colitis.jpg&oldid=498131737.
6. Ischemicbowel.PNG. (2020, September 17). *Wikimedia Commons.* Retrieved 22:16, August 7, 2023 from https://commons.wikimedia.org/w/index.php?title=File:Ischemicbowel.PNG&oldid=462562416.
7. X-ray of hiatal hernia.jpg. (2022, September 28). *Wikimedia Commons.* Retrieved 22:52, August 7, 2023 from https://commons.wikimedia.org/w/index.php?title=File:X-ray_of_hiatal_hernia.jpg&oldid=692525907.
8. Acha.JPG. (2023, July 7). *Wikimedia Commons.* Retrieved 23:22, August 7, 2023 from https://commons.wikimedia.org/w/index.php?title=File:Acha.JPG&oldid=781175678.
9. Zenker2.jpg. (2022, March 30). *Wikimedia Commons.* Retrieved 23:43, August 7, 2023 from https://commons.wikimedia.org/w/index.php?title=File:Zenker2.jpg&oldid=645326436.
10. Radiology 0012 Nevit.jpg. (2023, January 8). *Wikimedia Commons.* Retrieved 14:25, August 8, 2023 from https://commons.wikimedia.org/w/index.php?title=File:Radiology_0012_Nevit.jpg&oldid=723908881.
11. Nutcracker manometry.jpg. (2023, May 15). *Wikimedia Commons.* Retrieved 14:45, August 8, 2023 from https://commons.wikimedia.org/w/index.php?title=File:Nutcracker_manometry.jpg&oldid=763498699.
12. CXR Pneumomediastinum.jpg. (2021, May 1). *Wikimedia Commons.* Retrieved 16:40, August 8, 2023 from https://commons.wikimedia.org/w/index.php?title=File:CXR_Pneumomediastinum.jpg&oldid=556825590.
13. Esophageal web.jpg. (2020, October 18). *Wikimedia Commons.* Retrieved 16:45, August 8, 2023 from https://commons.wikimedia.org/w/index.php?title=File:Esophageal_web.jpg&oldid=493041383.
14. Schatzki ring 2.jpg. (2022, April 26). *Wikimedia Commons.* Retrieved 16:45, August 8, 2023 from https://commons.wikimedia.org/w/index.php?title=File:Schatzki_ring_2.jpg&oldid=651968739.
15. Gastric Varices.jpg. (2020, September 27). *Wikimedia Commons.* Retrieved 16:54, August 8, 2023 from https://commons.wikimedia.org/w/index.php?title=File:Gastric_Varices.jpg&oldid=472818159.
16. Dermatitis-herpetiformis.jpg. (2020, October 28). *Wikimedia Commons.* Retrieved 17:02, August 8, 2023 from https://commons.wikimedia.org/w/index.php?title=File:Dermatitis-herpetiformis.jpg&oldid=505273148.
17. Pyloric-stenosis.jpg. (2022, December 18). *Wikimedia Commons.* Retrieved 18:11, August 8, 2023 from https://commons.wikimedia.org/w/index.php?title=File:Pyloric-stenosis.jpg&oldid=715968256.
18. Hepaticfailure.jpg. (2020, September 22). *Wikimedia Commons.* Retrieved 19:46, August 8, 2023 from https://commons.wikimedia.org/w/index.php?title=File:Hepaticfailure.jpg&oldid=467921195.
19. Kayser-Fleischer ring.jpg. (2022, April 26). *Wikimedia Commons.* Retrieved 20:37, August 8, 2023 from https://commons.wikimedia.org/w/index.php?title=File:Kayser-Fleischer_ring.jpg&oldid=652054012.
20. Blausen 0560 InguinalHernia.png. (2021, May 14). *Wikimedia Commons.* Retrieved 21:22, August 8, 2023 from https://commons.wikimedia.org/w/index.php?title=File:Blausen_0560_InguinalHernia.png&oldid=560318918.
21. Paget's disease of Right Hip Bone.jpg. (2023, April 5). *Wikimedia Commons.* Retrieved 22:58, August 8, 2023 from https://commons.wikimedia.org/w/index.php?title=File:Paget%27s_disease_of_Right_Hip_Bone.jpg&oldid=747138201.
22. Angular Cheilitis.JPG. (2020, September 2). *Wikimedia Commons.* Retrieved 23:13, August 8, 2023 from https://commons.wikimedia.org/w/index.php?title=File:Angular_Cheilitis.JPG&oldid=467530714.
23. Hemorrhagic pancreatitis - Grey Turner's sign.jpg. (2022, September 4). *Wikimedia Commons.* Retrieved 17:41, August 10, 2023 from https://commons.wikimedia.org/w/index.php?title=File:Hemorrhagic_pancreatitis_-_Grey_Turner%27s_sign.jpg&oldid=686634096.
24. Cullen's sign.jpg. (2022, September 4). *Wikimedia Commons.* Retrieved 18:01, August 10, 2023 from https://commons.wikimedia.org/w/index.php?title=File:Cullen%27s_sign.jpg&oldid=686661705.
25. Chronische Pankreatitis mit Verkalkungen - CT axial.jpg. (2022, March 31). *Wikimedia Commons.* Retrieved 18:05, August 10, 2023 from https://commons.wikimedia.org/w/index.php?title=File:Chronische_Pankreatitis_mit_Verkalkungen_-_CT_axial.jpg&oldid=645461880.
26. MBq cystic-carcinoma-pancreas.jpg. (2021, August 30). *Wikimedia Commons.* Retrieved 18:26, August 10, 2023 from https://commons.wikimedia.org/w/index.php?title=File:MBq_cystic-carcinoma-pancreas.jpg&oldid=587515703.
27. DuodAtres.png. (2022, April 2). *Wikimedia Commons.* Retrieved 19:34, August 10, 2023 from https://commons.wikimedia.org/w/index.php?title=File:DuodAtres.png&oldid=646082078.
28. Sigmoidvolvulus.jpg. (2022, July 13). *Wikimedia Commons.* Retrieved 20:13, August 10, 2023 from https://commons.wikimedia.org/w/index.php?title=File:Sigmoidvolvulus.jpg&oldid=674032849.
29. Upright abdominal X-ray demonstrating a bowel obstruction.jpg. (2020, September 25). *Wikimedia Commons.* Retrieved 21:01, August 10, 2023 from https://commons.wikimedia.org/w/index.php?title=File:Upright_abdominal_X-ray_demonstrating_a_bowel_obstruction.jpg&oldid=471394385.
30. Intussusception.png. (2020, September 20). *Wikimedia Commons.* Retrieved 21:25, August 10, 2023 from https://commons.wikimedia.org/w/index.php?title=File:Intussusception.png&oldid=465711547.
31. AppendicitisMark.png. (2022, October 22). *Wikimedia Commons.* Retrieved 22:10, August 10, 2023 from https://commons.wikimedia.org/w/index.php?title=File:AppendicitisMark.png&oldid=698241144.

Chapter 4

Musculoskeletal

Compartment Syndrome

Etiology & Risk Factors	• Increased pressure within a closed osteofascial compartment resulting in impaired tissue perfusion and muscle/nerve ischemia • Anterior compartment of leg following tibia fracture is most common location • <u>Etiology</u>: **trauma; fracture of long bones is most common cause; crush injuries**, immobilization, constriction (casts, splints, burns), snake bites, prolonged tourniquet application, drug overdose
Patho-physiology	• Increased intra-compartmental fluid (bleeding) secondary to trauma leads to increased compartment pressure as fascia is non-compliant • As compartment pressure increases, venous outflow is reduced causing increased venous pressure. If venous pressure is greater than arterial pressure, then arterial inflow is reduced leading to decreased perfusion and tissue ischemia.

Signs & Symptoms	• **Pain out of proportion to severity of injury is most specific**
	• **5 P's: Pain, Paresthesia, Paralysis, Pallor, Pulselessness**
	• <u>Physical exam</u>:
	    • Edematous, tender, **tense compartment**; may be described as "wood-like"
	    • **Pain with passive stretching of affected muscles**

Diagnosis	• <u>X-Ray</u>: obtain if fracture is suspected • **<u>Compartment Pressure Measurement</u>: increased intra-compartmental pressure >30 mmHg or Δ pressure <30 mmHg indicates need for fasciotomy** • Δ Pressure = [Diastolic Pressure] − [Compartment Pressure] • <u>Labs</u>: **elevated creatine kinase** (rhabdomyolysis); CMP may show hyperkalemia
Treatment	• **<u>Emergency Fasciotomy</u>: decompresses compartmental pressure through large skin incision** • <u>Supportive</u>: removal of constrictive dressing (cast/splint), analgesia, supplemental oxygen, fluid/electrolyte replacement • <u>Amputation</u>: indicated if extensive necrosis or prolonged ischemia
Key Words & Most Common	• Most common at anterior compartment of leg following tibia fracture • Trauma and fracture of long bones most common etiology • Pain out of proportion to injury • Pain, Paresthesia, Paralysis, Pallor, Pulselessness • Tense compartment; pain with stretching of affected muscle • Compartment pressure measurement • Emergency fasciotomy

Osteomyelitis

Etiology & Risk Factors	• Acute or chronic inflammation of bone secondary to infection • <u>Children</u>: femur and tibia most commonly affected • <u>**Adults**</u>: **spinal vertebrae most commonly affected** • <u>Etiology</u>: **contiguous spread from infected tissue** (infected prosthetic joint, infected diabetic ulcer); **bloodborne organisms** (IV drug user, sickle cell disease); **open wounds** (open fractures, surgery) • <u>Risk Factors</u>: diabetes mellitus, prosthetic joint, IV drug user, sickle cell disease, open fracture
Patho-physiology	• Infection of bone via direct inoculation, hematogenous or contiguous spread results in vascular insufficiency and occlusion of surrounding vasculature leading to necrosis and local spread of infection • Infection may expand through bone cortex and under periosteum	**Organisms** • ***Staphylococcus aureus*: most common organism overall** • *Staphylococcus epidermis*: most commonly affects prosthetic joints • *Salmonella*: sickle cell disease • Group B *Streptococcus*: neonate osteomyelitis • *Pseudomonas aeruginosa*: calcaneal osteomyelitis s/p puncture injury through shoe
Signs & Symptoms	• <u>Peripheral Bones</u>: **fever**, weight loss, fatigue; **localized warmth, tenderness, swelling, erythema and/or bone pain**, decreased ROM and functional strength • <u>Vertebral</u>: **localized back pain and tenderness, paravertebral muscle spasms**, radiculopathy, weakness; often afebrile
Diagnosis	• <u>Labs</u>: **elevated ESR and CRP, leukocytosis**, blood cultures • <u>X-Ray</u>: **initial imaging test**; may be normal early in course (infection not apparent until 2+ weeks after symptoms) • **Periosteal reaction** with soft tissue edema → **bone demineralization**, lytic lesions, periosteal destruction • **<u>Magnetic Resonance Imaging (MRI)</u>: imaging test of choice; highest sensitivity and specificity especially early** • <u>Technetium-99 Bone Scintigraphy</u>: sensitive but lacks specificity

Treatment	• <u>Antibiotics</u>: empiric treatment followed by guided therapy based on culture results; requires 2-6 weeks of treatment
	    • <u>Acute</u>: **Vancomycin (preferred)** or Nafcillin or Oxacillin *PLUS* **3rd generation cephalosporin** (cefepime or ceftazidime or **cefotaxime**)
	    • <u>Chronic</u>: Vancomycin + piperacillin/tazobactam
	• <u>Surgical Debridement</u>: may be required for persistent or extensive infection

Key Words & Most Common	• Infection of bone; femur/tibia in children, spinal vertebrae in adults • Staphylococcus aureus is most common organism overall • Fever, localized warmth/swelling/pain • Elevated ESR/CRP, leukocytosis • MRI imaging test of choice • Broad spectrum antibiotics

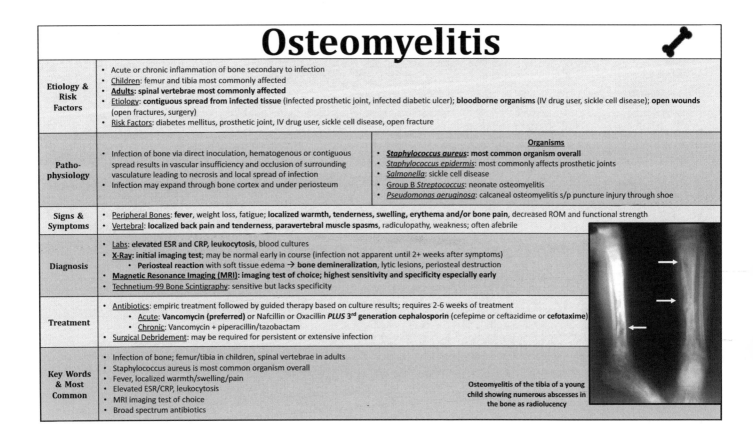

Osteomyelitis of the tibia of a young child showing numerous abscesses in the bone as radiolucency

Osteoarthritis

Etiology & Risk Factors	• Chronic arthropathy characterized by joint cartilage, bone degeneration, and bone hypertrophy (osteophyte) • Symptoms may range from mild intermittent to physically debilitating; **weight bearing joints most affected**. If hands, **DIPJ** > PIPJ/MCP • <u>Risk Factors</u>: **advanced age, female gender, obesity, family history**, trauma/injury, heavy labor, poor muscle tone
Patho-physiology	• Tissue damage leads to pro-inflammatory mediators to be released leading to cartilage matrix damage and bone remodeling. This triggers inflammatory cycle leading to chondrocyte apoptosis • Attempts at bone repair leads to subchondral sclerosis and osteophyte formation and margins of the joint (meant to attempt to stabilize joint)

Signs & Symptoms	• <u>Joint Pain</u>: gradual increase in **joint pain, stiffness, and restricted range of motion**
	  • Symptoms **worse in afternoon/evening** and correlated with activity or weather changes
	  • Pain may resolve with rest
	• <u>Mechanical Symptoms</u>: instability, "buckling" or "giving away" (sign of muscle weakness)
	• <u>Physical Exam</u>:
	  • **Hard/bony joint, joint effusion, crepitus** (grating sound due to friction within joint), **limited ROM**
	  • **Heberden nodes** (posterolateral swelling of DIPJ) and **Bouchard nodes** (posterolateral swelling PIPJ)

Diagnosis	• **Clinical Diagnosis** • <u>X-Ray</u>: **demonstrates joint space narrowing, subchondral sclerosis/cysts, marginal osteophytes** • <u>Labs</u>: normal CBC, ESR, rheumatoid factor, and ANA; may be ordered to rule out inflammatory arthritis • <u>Ultrasound</u>: may show synovial inflammation, effusion, and osteophytes • <u>MRI</u>: not typically ordered unless other pathology suspected

Treatment	• <u>Lifestyle Modifications</u>: **weight loss**, moderate exercise to **improve muscle strength**, activity modifications, use of assistive devices (braces/splints, canes, walkers)
	• <u>Medication Management</u>:
	  • **Acetaminophen**: indicated for mild to moderate OA
	  • **NSAIDs**: ibuprofen, naproxen sodium; more effective but have more side effects (especially in elderly); topical NSAIDs (diclofenac) have safer profile
	  • **Duloxetine**: serotonin norephinephrine reuptake inhibitor may provide modest pain relief if NSAIDs contraindicated
	• **Intraarticular Corticosteroid Injection**: methylprednisolone or triamcinolone preparations; usually mixed with lidocaine; provides temporary relief
	• <u>Hyaluronic Acid Injections</u>: may provide some relief; studies show strong placebo effect
	• <u>Joint Replacement</u>: if conservative measures fail and significantly compromised function

Key Words & Most Common	• Gradual joint pain/stiffness in weight bearing joints; worse in afternoon/evening and after activity +/- mechanical symptoms • Physical exam shows hard/bony joint, effusion, crepitus • X-Ray: joint space narrowing, osteophytes • Lifestyle modifications → acetaminophen/NSAIDs → Intraarticular injections → joint replacement

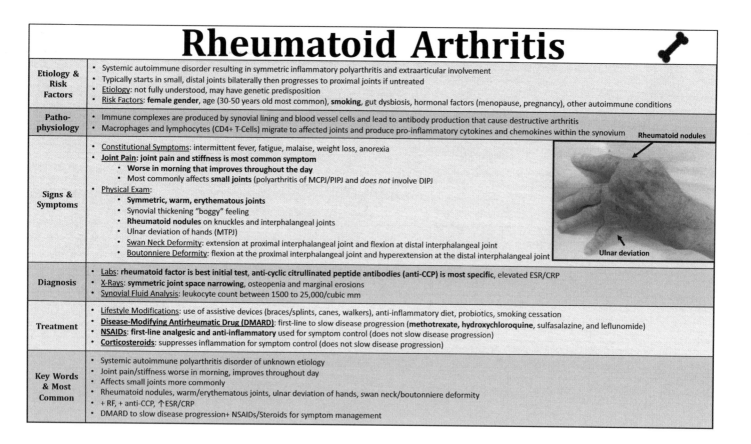

Osteophytes
Joint space narrowing
Increased subchondral bone density

Rheumatoid Arthritis

Etiology & Risk Factors	• Systemic autoimmune disorder resulting in symmetric inflammatory polyarthritis and extraarticular involvement • Typically starts in small, distal joints bilaterally then progresses to proximal joints if untreated • <u>Etiology</u>: not fully understood, may have genetic predisposition • <u>Risk Factors</u>: **female gender**, age (30-50 years old most common), **smoking**, gut dysbiosis, hormonal factors (menopause, pregnancy), other autoimmune conditions
Patho-physiology	• Immune complexes are produced by synovial lining and blood vessel cells and lead to antibody production that cause destructive arthritis • Macrophages and lymphocytes (CD4+ T-Cells) migrate to affected joints and produce pro-inflammatory cytokines and chemokines within the synovium

Signs & Symptoms	• <u>Constitutional Symptoms</u>: intermittent fever, fatigue, malaise, weight loss, anorexia
	• <u>Joint Pain</u>: **joint pain and stiffness is most common symptom**
	  • **Worse in morning that improves throughout the day**
	  • Most commonly affects **small joints** (polyarthritis of MCPJ/PIPJ and *does not* involve DIPJ)
	• <u>Physical Exam</u>:
	  • **Symmetric, warm, erythematous joints**
	  • Synovial thickening "boggy" feeling
	  • **Rheumatoid nodules** on knuckles and interphalangeal joints
	  • Ulnar deviation of hands (MTPJ)
	  • <u>Swan Neck Deformity</u>: extension at proximal interphalangeal joint and flexion at distal interphalangeal joint
	  • <u>Boutonniere Deformity</u>: flexion at the proximal interphalangeal joint and hyperextension at the distal interphalangeal joint

Diagnosis	• <u>Labs</u>: **rheumatoid factor is best initial test, anti-cyclic citrullinated peptide antibodies (anti-CCP) is most specific**, elevated ESR/CRP • <u>X-Rays</u>: **symmetric joint space narrowing**, osteopenia and marginal erosions • <u>Synovial Fluid Analysis</u>: leukocyte count between 1500 to 25,000/cubic mm
Treatment	• <u>Lifestyle Modifications</u>: use of assistive devices (braces/splints, canes, walkers), anti-inflammatory diet, probiotics, smoking cessation • **Disease-Modifying Antirheumatic Drug (DMARD)**: first-line to slow disease progression (**methotrexate, hydroxychloroquine**, sulfasalazine, and leflunomide) • **NSAIDs**: first-line analgesic and anti-inflammatory used for symptom control (does not slow disease progression) • <u>Corticosteroids</u>: suppresses inflammation for symptom control (does not slow disease progression)
Key Words & Most Common	• Systemic autoimmune polyarthritis disorder of unknown etiology • Joint pain/stiffness worse in morning, improves throughout day • Affects small joints more commonly • Rheumatoid nodules, warm/erythematous joints, ulnar deviation of hands, swan neck/boutonniere deformity • + RF, + anti-CCP, ↑ESR/CRP • DMARD to slow disease progression+ NSAIDs/Steroids for symptom management

Rheumatoid nodules
Ulnar deviation

Septic Arthritis

Etiology & Risk Factors	• **Inflammation of a joint secondary to infectious etiology** (bacteria most common); constitutes an orthopedic emergency • **Knee is most common joint affected in adults and older children** • **Hip is most common joint affected in younger children** • Sternoclavicular and sacroiliac joint in IVDU • <u>Etiology</u>: **direct penetration** (surgery, trauma, bites), infection extension (osteomyelitis, adjacent abscess), hematogenous spread • <u>Risk Factors</u>: **advanced age, immunosuppression, prosthetic joint implant, trauma**, chronic arthropathy (gout, RA, OA), **diabetes**, sickle cell disease		
Patho-physiology	• Bacterial inoculation of the synovium lead to joint destruction mediated by inflammatory cytokines and proteases • Neutrophiles then migrate to joint, phagocytose the organism resulting in lysosomal enzyme release which damages the cartilage, synovium, and ligaments	**Organisms** • <u>*Staphylococcus aureus*</u>: most common organism overall; MRSA seen with IVDU • <u>*Staphylococcus epidermis*</u>: prosthetic joint implant • <u>*Streptococcal spp.*</u>: 2nd most common organism; more common in young kids/neonates • <u>*Neisseria gonorrhoeae*</u>: sexually active young adults • <u>*Pseudomonas spp.*</u>: immunocompromised; trauma/puncture wounds; IVDU • <u>*Salmonella*</u>: sickle cell disease		
Signs & Symptoms	• <u>Constitutional Symptoms</u>: **fever**, chills, malaise/fatigue, diaphoresis, myalgias, tachycardia • <u>Local Symptoms</u>: **swollen, warm, erythematous, painful joint; limited ROM** with active and passive movement,		
Diagnosis	• <u>**Arthrocentesis with Synovial Fluid Analysis**</u>: most useful and accurate test; culture, Gram stain, crystals analysis, white blood cell count with differential • **WBC >50,000** (90% neutrophil predominance), WBC>1,100 considered positive in prosthetic joints • <u>Labs</u>: elevated ESR and CRP (nonspecific); blood cultures (if Neisseria suspected, cultures obtained from the cervix, rectum, and/or throat) • <u>X-Ray</u>: nonspecific; joint space widening, soft tissue bulging, or subchondral bony change		

Treatment	• <u>Antibiotics</u>: empiric treatment followed by guided therapy based on culture results
	   • **Vancomycin is preferred antibiotic**
	   • **Nafcillin** *or* **Oxacillin** *PLUS* 3rd **generation cephalosporin** (cefepime or ceftazidime or **cefotaxime; ceftriaxone**) is alternative
	• <u>Procedures</u>: joint aspiration vs open surgical debridement vs arthroscopic irrigation		

Key Words & Most Common	• Knee most common in adults/older children; hip most common in young children • *S. aureus* most common organism; S. epidermis most common with prosthetic joint • Fever + warm/swollen/erythematous joint • Synovial fluid analysis (WBC>50k); elevated ESR/CRP • Antibiotics (Vanco + cephalosporin) +/- surgical drainage or irrigation		

Developmental Dysplasia of the Hip

Etiology & Risk Factors	• Disorder that results due to abnormal development of the femoral head and acetabulum leading to instability of the joint • <u>Risk Factors</u>: **female gender**, first-born infant, **breech position in 3rd trimester**, family history, postmaturity (prematurity not associated with increased risk), swaddling
Patho-physiology	• Interference with proper contact between femoral head and acetabulum in utero or during infancy can lead to DDH • Swaddling in extreme positions (adducted, extended hip), or positioning in utero leads to malalignment and impaired contact causing hypertrophy of capsule, ligament teres, and acetabular edge which impedes proper hip development

Signs & Symptoms	• **Limited hip abduction** in infant, **asymmetrical gait** in toddler
	• <u>Physical Exam</u>: examinations occur at birth and during well visits until infant is walking
	   • **Ortolani Maneuver**: detects the hip sliding back *into* the acetabulum
	      • Infant is supine with hip flexed 90°; gentle abduction of hip while anterior force is applied to the thigh. If hip is dislocated, a "jerk or clunk" will be felt as hip is reduced back into acetabulum
	   • **Barlow Maneuver**: detects the hip sliding *out of* the acetabulum
	      • Infant is supine with hip flexed 90°, gentle adduction of hip while posterior force is applied to the thigh. A "jerk or clunk" indicates the hip slid out of the acetabulum
	   • <u>Galeazzi Sign</u>: difference in knee height with hip/knee flexion while feet flat on the table
	   • Asymmetry of skin folds/femur length; limited hip abduction

Diagnosis	• **Clinical diagnosis**; imaging used to confirm • **Hip Ultrasound: used in children <4 months of age** • **Hip X-Ray: used in children >4 months of age** (bones have started to ossify) • Disruption of Shenton's Line (arc that connects the femoral neck to the superior margin of the obturator foramen)
Treatment	• **Referral to Pediatric Orthopedic Specialist** • <u>0-6 Months</u>: **Pavlik harness** (hold the affected hips abducted and externally rotated) • <u>>6 Months</u>: closed reduction with hip spica cast
Key Words & Most Common	• Breech position in 3rd trimester greatest risk factor • Limited hip abduction, asymmetry of skin folds • <u>Ortolani</u>: detects hip sliding into acetabulum (anterior force in abduction) • <u>Barlow</u>: detects hip sliding out of acetabulum (posterior force in adduction) • US vs Hip X-Ray • <6 months = Pavlik harness; >6 months = closed reduction with hip spica cast **Dislocated right hip in child**

Pelvic Fractures

Etiology & Risk Factors	• Fracture involving hip bones, sacrum, coccyx, or bones that form the pelvic ring • <u>Mechanism</u>: **high-impact injuries (motor vehicle accident**, blunt force trauma, fall from height), hip dislocations, falls in the elderly, athletic injuries in adolescent • <u>3 Mechanisms of Injury</u>: anteroposterior compression injuries (APC), lateral compression injuries (LC), and vertical shear injuries (VS)
Patho-physiology	• The pelvis is a highly stable structure due to inherent ring anatomy; the amount of force required to fracture increases likelihood there is vascular or neurologic injury • Significant vascular and neurologic anatomic structures traverse the pelvis; vascular injuries (iliac vein injuries) may occur leading to significant hemorrhage • Hemorrhage may be external (open fracture)

Signs & Symptoms	• **Pelvic/hip pain following traumatic injury**
	  • May have **groin/lower back pain**
	• Inability to ambulate
	• <u>Physical Exam</u>:
	  • May have findings of further vascular or neurologic injury: **blood at urethral meatus**, hematuria, abdominal pain, rectal bleeding, **perineal ecchymosis, weakness/loss of sensation of lower extremities, incontinence vs urinary retention**

Diagnosis	• <u>Pelvic X-Ray</u>: initial test to determine fracture and extent • <u>CT Scan</u>: **gold standard imaging test, more sensitive**; obtain in all stable patients with fracture on x-ray (except avulsion) • <u>Retrograde Cystourethrogram</u>: **obtain (before foley) if blood at urethral meatus,** high riding prostate or hematuria • <u>Labs</u>: CBC to monitor blood loss, type and screen
Treatment	• <u>Stable Fractures</u>: symptomatic treatment, pain control • <u>Unstable Fractures</u>: external fixation or open reduction internal fixation (ORIF) • <u>Significant Hemorrhage</u>: pelvic binder + IV fluid resuscitation + angiographic embolization • Treat associated injuries
Key Words & Most Common	• High-impact injury (MVA, fall from height) • Pelvic/hip pain following traumatic injury; groin/lower back pain • Pelvic X-ray • CT Scan gold standard • Unstable Fractures require external fixation vs ORIF • Pelvic binder + IVF + embolization for significant hemorrhage

Acetabular fracture

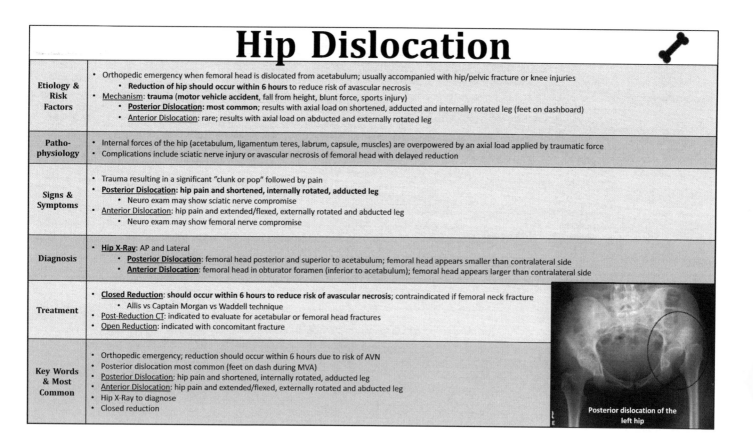

Posterior dislocation of the left hip

Hip Dislocation

Etiology & Risk Factors	• Orthopedic emergency when femoral head is dislocated from acetabulum; usually accompanied with hip/pelvic fracture or knee injuries
	  • **Reduction of hip should occur within 6 hours** to reduce risk of avascular necrosis
	• <u>Mechanism</u>: **trauma (motor vehicle accident**, fall from height, blunt force, sports injury)
	  • <u>Posterior Dislocation</u>: most common; results with axial load on shortened, adducted and internally rotated leg (feet on dashboard)
	  • <u>Anterior Dislocation</u>: rare; results with axial load on abducted and externally rotated leg

Patho-physiology	• Internal forces of the hip (acetabulum, ligamentum teres, labrum, capsule, muscles) are overpowered by an axial load applied by traumatic force • Complications include sciatic nerve injury or avascular necrosis of femoral head with delayed reduction

Signs & Symptoms	• Trauma resulting in a significant "clunk or pop" followed by pain
	• <u>Posterior Dislocation</u>: **hip pain and shortened, internally rotated, adducted leg**
	  • Neuro exam may show sciatic nerve compromise
	• <u>Anterior Dislocation</u>: hip pain and extended/flexed, externally rotated and abducted leg
	  • Neuro exam may show femoral nerve compromise

Diagnosis	• <u>Hip X-Ray</u>: AP and Lateral
	  • <u>Posterior Dislocation</u>: femoral head posterior and superior to acetabulum; femoral head appears smaller than contralateral side
	  • <u>Anterior Dislocation</u>: femoral head in obturator foramen (inferior to acetabulum); femoral head appears larger than contralateral side

Treatment	• <u>Closed Reduction</u>: **should occur within 6 hours to reduce risk of avascular necrosis**; contraindicated if femoral neck fracture • Allis vs Captain Morgan vs Waddell technique • <u>Post-Reduction CT</u>: indicated to evaluate for acetabular or femoral head fractures • <u>Open Reduction</u>: indicated with concomitant fracture
Key Words & Most Common	• Orthopedic emergency; reduction should occur within 6 hours due to risk of AVN • Posterior dislocation most common (feet on dash during MVA) • <u>Posterior Dislocation</u>: hip pain and shortened, internally rotated, adducted leg • <u>Anterior Dislocation</u>: hip pain and extended/flexed, externally rotated and abducted leg • Hip X-Ray to diagnose • Closed reduction

Hip Fractures

Etiology & Risk Factors	• Fracture of the proximal femur that may occur in the head, neck, or below the trochanters • Mechanism: **falls in elderly is most common cause**, high energy trauma, indirect trauma • Risk Factors: **osteoporosis, advanced age, female gender**, malignancy, use of walking aids, history of falls, gait abnormalities, vertigo, neurologic conditions (Parkinson disease) • Types: Intracapsular (femoral head, femoral neck); Extracapsular (intertrochanteric, subtrochanteric)
Patho-physiology	• Osteoblasts (bone matrix cells that mineralize bone) and osteoclasts (cells that resorb bone) are regulated by parathyroid hormone, calcitonin, estrogen, vitamin D, various cytokines, and other local factors (prostaglandins) • Menopause leads to decreased cortical thickness and trabeculae size resulting in an increased porosity which weakens bone structure (osteopenia/osteoporosis) • Trauma (even minimal such as rolling over in bed, getting up from a chair, walking) can lead to fracture

Signs & Symptoms	• **Groin/hip/thigh pain**
	• Inability to ambulate
	• Physical Exam:
	   • **Shortened, abducted, externally rotated leg**
	   • Should also assess head trauma

Diagnosis	• Hip/Femur X-Ray: AP and lateral • MRI: most sensitive imaging study; ordered if x-ray is negative with high suspicion

Treatment	• Analgesia: pain control (consider nerve block); NSAIDs, opioids as tolerated/indicated
	• Surgery:
	   • **Open Reduction Internal Fixation (ORIF)**: Nondisplaced/impacted femoral neck fractures in elderly and femoral neck fractures in younger patients
	   • Joint Arthroplasty: if displaced femoral neck fracture in elderly
	• Physical Therapy: initiated as soon as possible

Key Words & Most Common	• Falls in elderly most common cause • Risks include osteoporosis, advance age, female • Groin/hip/thigh pain after injury; inability to ambulate • Shortened, abducted, externally rotated leg • X-ray • ORIF

Intertrochanteric hip fracture

Legg-Calvé-Perthes Disease

Etiology & Risk Factors	• Idiopathic avascular osteonecrosis of the capital femoral epiphysis of the femoral head • Epiphysis fails to grow due to ischemia; usually unilateral • Risk Factors: **age (3-12; 5-7 years old most common), male gender**, family history, coagulopathies, secondhand smoke exposure, short stature, low birth weight
Patho-physiology	• Disruption of blood flow leads to capital femoral epiphysis ischemia and growth retardation; bone infarcts leading to necrosis • Bone reabsorbs necrotic bone; osteoblastic activity takes over resulting in femoral head remodeling

Signs & Symptoms	• **Painless gait disturbance (limp)**
	• **Gradual hip pain and limp** may develop; pain may radiate to groin, thigh, or knee
	   • **Pain worse with activity and relieved with rest** (pain worse at end of day)
	• Physical Exam:
	   • **Restricted range of motion (decreased hip abduction and internal rotation)**
	   • Thigh muscle atrophy

Diagnosis	• Hip X-Ray: AP and frog-leg lateral
	   • Early: may be normal; widening of joint space (epiphyseal cartilage hypertrophy), minimal flattening of femoral head
	   • Late: **flattening of femoral head, "Crescent Sign"** (subchondral fracture with bony collapse)

Treatment	• Supportive: good outcomes in most cases; revascularization within 2-3 years
	   • **Activity modifications (protective weight bearing), physical therapy, orthotics**
	• Surgical: indicated in children >8 years old or advance disease
	   • **Femoral or pelvic osteotomy**

Key Words & Most Common	• Avascular necrosis of capital femoral epiphysis • Most common in males aged 5-7 years old • Painless gait → gradual increase in hip pain with limp; worse with activity • Restricted ROM ↓hip abduction and internal rotation • Hip X-Ray shows flattening of femoral head and "crescent sign" (subchondral fracture) • Supportive vs surgical

Legg-Calvé-Perthes Disease

Slipped Capital Femoral Epiphysis

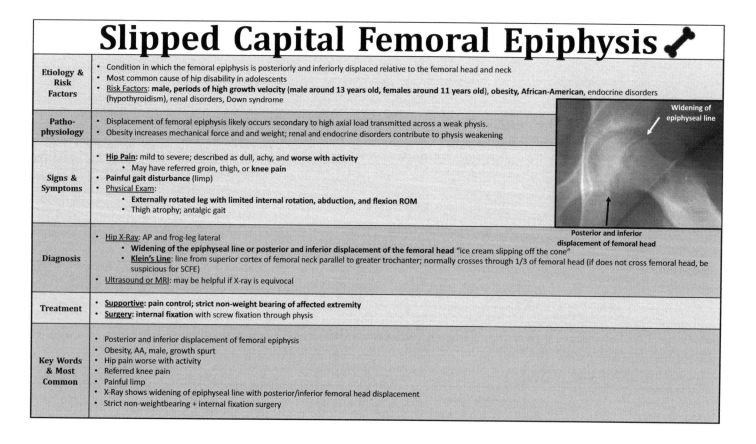

Etiology & Risk Factors	• Condition in which the femoral epiphysis is posteriorly and inferiorly displaced relative to the femoral head and neck • Most common cause of hip disability in adolescents • <u>Risk Factors</u>: **male, periods of high growth velocity (male around 13 years old, females around 11 years old)**, **obesity, African-American,** endocrine disorders (hypothyroidism), renal disorders, Down syndrome
Patho-physiology	• Displacement of femoral epiphysis likely occurs secondary to high axial load transmitted across a weak physis. • Obesity increases mechanical force and and weight; renal and endocrine disorders contribute to physis weakening

Signs & Symptoms	• <u>Hip Pain</u>: mild to severe; described as dull, achy, and **worse with activity**
	   • May have referred groin, thigh, or **knee pain**
	• **Painful gait disturbance** (limp)
	• <u>Physical Exam</u>:
	   • **Externally rotated leg with limited internal rotation, abduction, and flexion ROM**
	   • Thigh atrophy; antalgic gait

Diagnosis	• <u>Hip X-Ray</u>: AP and frog-leg lateral
	   • **Widening of the epiphyseal line or posterior and inferior displacement of the femoral head** "ice cream slipping off the cone"
	   • <u>Klein's Line</u>: line from superior cortex of femoral neck parallel to greater trochanter; normally crosses through 1/3 of femoral head (if does not cross femoral head, be suspicious for SCFE)
	• <u>Ultrasound or MRI</u>: may be helpful if X-ray is equivocal

Treatment	• <u>**Supportive**</u>: pain control; **strict non-weight bearing of affected extremity** • <u>**Surgery**</u>: **internal fixation** with screw fixation through physis
Key Words & Most Common	• Posterior and inferior displacement of femoral epiphysis • Obesity, AA, male, growth spurt • Hip pain worse with activity • Referred knee pain • Painful limp • X-Ray shows widening of epiphyseal line with posterior/inferior femoral head displacement • Strict non-weightbearing + internal fixation surgery

Avascular Necrosis of the Hip

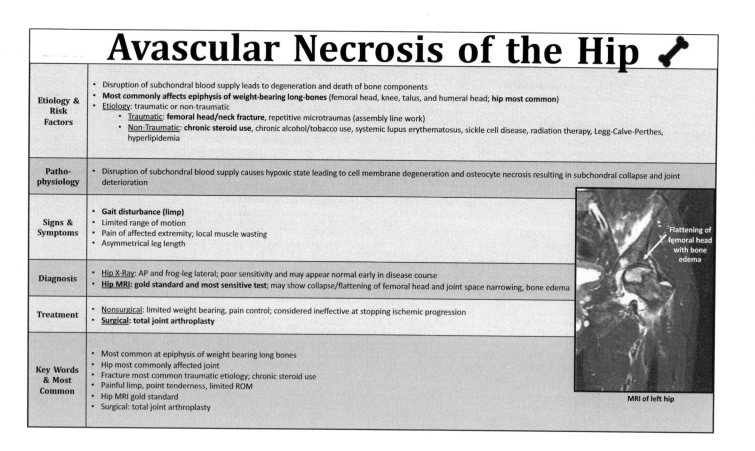

Etiology & Risk Factors	• Disruption of subchondral blood supply leads to degeneration and death of bone components
	• **Most commonly affects epiphysis of weight-bearing long-bones** (femoral head, knee, talus, and humeral head; **hip most common**)
	• <u>Etiology</u>: traumatic or non-traumatic
	   • <u>Traumatic</u>: **femoral head/neck fracture**, repetitive microtraumas (assembly line work)
	   • <u>Non-Traumatic</u>: **chronic steroid use**, chronic alcohol/tobacco use, systemic lupus erythematosus, sickle cell disease, radiation therapy, Legg-Calve-Perthes, hyperlipidemia

Patho-physiology	• Disruption of subchondral blood supply causes hypoxic state leading to cell membrane degeneration and osteocyte necrosis resulting in subchondral collapse and joint deterioration
Signs & Symptoms	• **Gait disturbance (limp)** • Limited range of motion • Pain of affected extremity; local muscle wasting • Asymmetrical leg length
Diagnosis	• <u>Hip X-Ray</u>: AP and frog-leg lateral; poor sensitivity and may appear normal early in disease course • **Hip MRI: gold standard and most sensitive test**; may show collapse/flattening of femoral head and joint space narrowing, bone edema
Treatment	• <u>Nonsurgical</u>: limited weight bearing, pain control; considered ineffective at stopping ischemic progression • <u>**Surgical**</u>: **total joint arthroplasty**
Key Words & Most Common	• Most common at epiphysis of weight bearing long bones • Hip most commonly affected joint • Fracture most common traumatic etiology; chronic steroid use • Painful limp, point tenderness, limited ROM • Hip MRI gold standard • Surgical: total joint arthroplasty

Medial and Lateral Collateral Ligament Injury

	Medial Collateral Ligament (MCL)	Lateral Collateral Ligament (LCL)
Etiology & Risk Factors	• MCL originates at medial femoral epicondyle and inserts at the medial condyle of tibia • Functions to provide **valgus stability to knee** (lateral impacted trauma) • Etiology: **sports injury (skiing)**, fall	• LCL originates at lateral femoral epicondyle and inserts at the fibular head • Functions to provided **varus stability to knee** (medial impacted trauma) and prevent posterior-lateral rotation of the knee • Etiology: **sports injury** (tennis/gymnastics), trauma, motor vehicle accidents, falls
Patho-physiology	• **Direct blow to the lateral knee causing valgus stress** • More common to injure than LCL	• **Direct blow to the anteromedial knee causing varus stress and hyperextension** • Can also be from non-contact varus stress or hyperextension injury

Signs & Symptoms	• **Localized medial-sided knee pain**, swelling, stiffness +/- ecchymosis
	• Physical Exam:
	  • Tenderness to MCL
	  • **Pain and laxity with valgus stress**
		• **Localized lateral-sided knee pain**, swelling, stiffness +/- ecchymosis
		• Physical Exam:
		• Tenderness to MCL
		• **Pain and laxity with varus stress**

Diagnosis	• **Clinical Diagnosis**
	• Physical Exam: **valgus stress test (MCL); varus stress test (LCL)**
	  • Grade I: sprain; pain along ligament with little/no joint opening
	  • Grade II: incomplete tear; some opening of joint but with firm endpoint
	  • Grade III: complete tear; significant joint opening with no firm endpoint
	• Knee X-Ray: should be performed to rule out fracture
	• MRI: **gold standard imaging test**	

Treatment	• **Conservative**: pain control (NSAIDs), rest, activity modification, compression, physical therapy • Grade I and II: conservative treatment + **non-weightbearing with crutches for 1 week** • **Hinged knee brace for 1 month during functional rehab** • Grade III: **surgical reconstruction**	
Key Words & Most Common	• MCL provides valgus stability to knee; LCL provides varus stability • Common sports related injury • MCL has pain/laxity with valgus stress; LCL has pain/laxity with varus stress • Physical exam + X-ray (r/o fx) +/- MRI • Grade I and II Sprain: conservative + non-weightbearing + brace • Grade III Tear: surgical reconstruction	

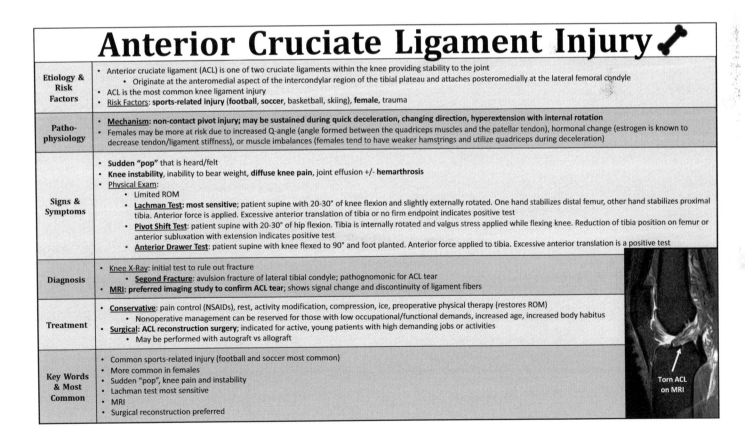

Anterior Cruciate Ligament Injury

Etiology & Risk Factors	• Anterior cruciate ligament (ACL) is one of two cruciate ligaments within the knee providing stability to the joint • Originate at the anteromedial aspect of the intercondylar region of the tibial plateau and attaches posteromedially at the lateral femoral condyle • ACL is the most common knee ligament injury • Risk Factors: **sports-related injury (football, soccer, basketball, skiing), female**, trauma
Patho-physiology	• **Mechanism: non-contact pivot injury; may be sustained during quick deceleration, changing direction, hyperextension with internal rotation** • Females may be more at risk due to increased Q-angle (angle formed between the quadriceps muscles and the patellar tendon), hormonal change (estrogen is known to decrease tendon/ligament stiffness), or muscle imbalances (females tend to have weaker hamstrings and utilize quadriceps during deceleration)

Signs & Symptoms	• **Sudden "pop"** that is heard/felt
	• **Knee instability**, inability to bear weight, **diffuse knee pain**, joint effusion +/- **hemarthrosis**
	• Physical Exam:
	  • Limited ROM
	  • **Lachman Test: most sensitive**; patient supine with 20-30° of knee flexion and slightly externally rotated. One hand stabilizes distal femur, other hand stabilizes proximal tibia. Anterior force is applied. Excessive anterior translation of tibia or no firm endpoint indicates positive test
	  • **Pivot Shift Test**: patient supine with 20-30° of hip flexion. Tibia is internally rotated and valgus stress applied while flexing knee. Reduction of tibia position on femur or anterior subluxation with extension indicates positive test
	  • **Anterior Drawer Test**: patient supine with knee flexed to 90° and foot planted. Anterior force applied to tibia. Excessive anterior translation is a positive test

Diagnosis	• Knee X-Ray: initial test to rule out fracture • **Segond Fracture**: avulsion fracture of lateral tibial condyle; pathognomonic for ACL tear • **MRI: preferred imaging study to confirm ACL tear**; shows signal change and discontinuity of ligament fibers

Treatment	• **Conservative**: pain control (NSAIDs), rest, activity modification, compression, ice, preoperative physical therapy (restores ROM)
	  • Nonoperative management can be reserved for those with low occupational/functional demands, increased age, increased body habitus
	• **Surgical: ACL reconstruction surgery**; indicated for active, young patients with high demanding jobs or activities
	  • May be performed with autograft vs allograft

Key Words & Most Common	• Common sports-related injury (football and soccer most common) • More common in females • Sudden "pop", knee pain and instability • Lachman test most sensitive • MRI • Surgical reconstruction preferred

Torn ACL on MRI

Posterior Cruciate Ligament Injury

Etiology & Risk Factors	• Posterior Cruciate Ligament (PCL) is one of two cruciate ligaments within the knee providing stability to the joint • Originates at the anterolateral aspect of the medial femoral condyle in the intercondylar notch and inserts at the posterior tibial plateau • About 1.5-2x as thick and 2x as strong as the ACL • <u>Mechanism</u>: **motor vehicle accident (dashboard injury)**, sports-related injury (football, soccer, basketball, skiing), **trauma (fall onto flexed knee)**
Patho-physiology	• Anterior force applied to proximal tibia with knee flexed to 90° puts posterior translative force on the PCL leading to sprain or rupture

Signs & Symptoms	• **Knee instability**, inability to bear weight
	• **Posterior knee pain**, joint effusion
	• <u>Physical Exam</u>:
	   • Limited ROM
	   • **<u>Posterior Drawer Test</u>: most sensitive**; patient supine with hip flexed to 45° and knee flexed to 90°. Posterior force applied to tibia. Excessive posterior translation of tibia or no firm endpoint indicates positive test

Diagnosis	• <u>Knee X-Ray</u>: initial test to rule out fracture • 45° flexion view may show **positive sag** compared to contralateral side • **<u>MRI</u>: preferred imaging study to confirm PCL tear**; shows signal change and discontinuity of ligament fibers
Treatment	• **<u>Conservative</u>**: pain control (NSAIDs), rest, activity modification, compression, ice, physical therapy (restores ROM and strength) • Nonoperative management can be reserved for those with low occupational/functional demands or minimal symptoms (PCL can scar down and may heal) • **<u>Surgical</u>: PCL reconstruction surgery**; may be performed with autograft vs allograft
Key Words & Most Common	• Most common as result of dashboard injury during MVA or fall onto flexed knee • Posterior knee pain/instability • Posterior drawer test to diagnose • MRI • Conservative if minimal symptoms or low occupational/functional demands • PCL reconstruction surgery definitive

Meniscal Tears

Etiology & Risk Factors	• Medial and lateral menisci are crescent-shaped fibrocartilage structures that function as load bearing transmission and shock absorption within the knee joint • Menisci are wedge shaped within joint with thicker edge at periphery of articular surface which improves joint congruency and stability • **Medial meniscus tears more common** than lateral • <u>Risk Factors</u>: **sports-related injury (football, soccer, basketball, skiing), trauma, male, age (>40 years old most common), occupations requiring frequent squatting/kneeling**
Patho-physiology	• <u>Mechanism</u>: axial loading with rotation or shearing force (kneeling/squatting, deceleration, quick direction change, lifting/carrying heavy objects) • Inner 2/3 of meniscus is avascular and does not have propensity to heal

Signs & Symptoms	• May or may not have inciting event
	• **Pain along joint line with joint effusion**
	• **Mechanical symptoms** (popping, locking, catching)
	• Instability during walking or ascending/descending stairs
	• <u>Physical Exam</u>:
	   • Joint effusion, restricted ROM
	   • <u>McMurray Test</u>: patient supine with knee in fully flexed position. Knee is extended with internal rotation of the tibia and varus stress, then returned to starting position. Knee is then extended with external rotation of the tibia and a valgus stress. Test is positive with pain, snapping, clicking, or locking of joint
	      • Internal rotation of tibia + varus stress = lateral meniscus
	      • External rotation of tibia + valgus stress = medial meniscus
	   • <u>Apley Grind Test</u>: patient prone with knee flexed to 90° and tibia is internally/externally rotated to induce pain

Diagnosis	• <u>Knee X-Ray</u>: initial test to rule out fracture • **<u>MRI</u>: preferred imaging study to confirm meniscus tear** • Demonstrates signal change or disruption of normal meniscal morphology
Treatment	• **<u>Conservative</u>**: pain control (NSAIDs), rest, activity modification, compression, ice, physical therapy (restores ROM and strength) • **<u>Surgical</u>: arthroscopic meniscus repair vs partial meniscectomy surgery**
Key Words & Most Common	• Medial meniscus more common • Occupational injury requiring squatting/kneeling, sports-related injury • Pain along joint line + effusion +/- mechanical symptoms • McMurray Test • MRI • Conservative vs arthroscopic surgery

Signal change at medial meniscus

Patellar Fracture

Etiology & Risk Factors	• Patella serves as insertion of quadriceps tendon and acts as fulcrum to maximize extensor mechanism; provides protection to anterior knee • <u>Risk Factors</u>: osteopenia/osteoporosis, arthritis, inadequate bone stock, male, history of falls, increased activity level
Patho-physiology	• <u>Mechanism</u>: **direct impact injury to anterior knee most common** (falling on flexed knee, forceful quadricep contraction, dashboard injury), **hyperflexion injury** • Rapid knee flexion occurs during active contraction of the quadriceps, the 3-force bending forces may cause the patella to fail in compression

Signs & Symptoms	• **Pain and swelling at anterior knee**
	• Inability to bear weight
	• <u>Physical Exam</u>:
	  • Limited or no range of motion
	  • **Patellar crepitus,**
	  • **Lack of extensor mechanism with straight leg raise**
	  • May have visible deformity if displaced fracture
	  • Loss of extensor mechanism if displaced fracture

Diagnosis	• <u>Knee X-Ray</u>: **best initial test**; AP, lateral and sunrise • Identify fracture and assess displacement • <u>Knee CT Scan</u>: may be ordered prior to surgery
Treatment	• <u>Nondisplaced</u>: **knee immobilizer in extension and strict non-weightbearing** with crutches; pain control, ice • <u>Displaced</u>: above treatment + early referral for **open reduction internal fixation (ORIF)** • Surgery indicated if displacement >3mm, open fractures, or loss of extensor mechanism
Key Words & Most Common	• Most common as result of direct impact to anterior knee (fall, dashboard injury), hyperflexion injury • Pain/swelling of anterior knee • Patellar crepitus, loss of extensor mechanism • Knee X-ray (lateral + sunrise) • Nondisplaced: immobilize + non-weightbearing • Displaced: ORIF

Patellar Instability

Etiology & Risk Factors	• Condition in which the patella subluxates (incomplete dislocation) or dislocates from articulation point (trochlear groove of femur) • Most commonly dislocates laterally • <u>Risk Factors</u>: **age (adolescence most common), female,** sports (soccer, basketball), history of patellar instability, muscular imbalances, connective tissue disorders, anatomical predisposition
Patho-physiology	• <u>Mechanism</u>: **externally rotated tibia with foot planted on ground,** medial impact to knee (forces patella laterally) • Patella dislocates laterally due to shallower trochlear groove and quadricep pull is lateral to mechanical axis; increased Q-angle in females • Medial patellofemoral ligament (MPFL) is check rein to lateral displacement of patella; almost always torn in setting of acute dislocation

Signs & Symptoms	• **Acute anterior knee pain with effusion**
	• **Laterally displaced patella** (deformity) if active dislocation
	• <u>Physical Exam</u>:
	  • Joint effusion with restricted ROM
	  • **J Sign**: "J" tracking of patella; lateral patellar deviation from flexion to extension
	  • **Apprehension Sign**: knee is placed at 20-30° of flexion and lateral force applied to patella
	    • Patient will have apprehension or guarding if positive

Diagnosis	• **Clinical Diagnosis** • <u>Knee X-Ray</u>: used to rule out fracture or establish anatomical etiology of recurrent instability • <u>Knee MRI</u>: assesses soft tissue integrity (**MPFL tear**, ligamentous injury)
Treatment	• <u>Closed Reduction</u>: place hip in mid flexion, gently extend knee while pushing patella anteromedially to reduce • Post reduction films to rule out fracture • <u>Conservative</u>: **pain control** (NSAIDs), rest, **knee immobilizer** in extension and non-weightbearing with crutches, ice, physical therapy (restores ROM and strength) • <u>Surgery</u>: **Medial patellofemoral ligament reconstruction** surgery if recurrent instability or MPFL tear
Key Words & Most Common	• Most common in adolescent female • Externally rotated tibia with foot planted • Anterior knee pain with effusion +/- laterally displaced patella • J sign; apprehension sign • Clinical diagnosis; MRI to assess MPFL integrity • Closed reduction if acutely dislocated • MPFL reconstruction if recurrent

Laterally dislocated patella

Osgood-Schlatter Disease

Etiology & Risk Factors	• Osteochondrosis or traction apophysitis of the tibial tubercle • Inflammation of distal patellar tendon at tibial tubercle insertion point • Risk Factors: **overuse** (repetitive stress), **high intensity sports** (basketball, volleyball, gymnastics, football, sprinting) **periods of high growth velocity** (male around 13 years old, females around 11 years old), **male**, poor flexibility
Patho-physiology	• Increased patellar tendon tension across apophysis when bone growth exceeds flexibility of tendon • Microavulsion fracture as a result of repetitive excessive traction of patellar tendon on an immature epiphyseal insertion point

Signs & Symptoms	• **Anterior knee pain and swelling over tibial tubercle**
	  • Often **worse during activity** (jumping, sprinting, kneeling) and relieved with rest
	• Physical Exam:
	  • **Prominence at anterior tibial tubercle**
	  • Tenderness and swelling, may have poor flexibility of quadriceps and hamstrings

Diagnosis	• **Clinical Diagnosis** • Knee X-Ray: may show elevated tibial tubercle, apophyseal fragmentation, distal patellar tendon calcification
Treatment	• <u>Conservative</u>: **mainstay of treatment**; pain control (NSAIDs), rest, activity modification, compression, ice, physical therapy (restores ROM and strength), stretching of quadriceps/hamstrings, **patellar tendon strap**, immobilization • <u>Surgery</u>: only indicated in skeletally mature patient with refractory symptoms
Key Words & Most Common	• Overuse injury often seen in athletes playing jumping/running sports • Most common in males during growth spurts • Anterior knee pain/swelling over tibial tubercle • Clinical diagnosis • Conservative treatment

Fragmentation of the tibial tubercle with overlying soft tissue swelling

Quadriceps/Patella Tendon Rupture

Etiology & Risk Factors	• Rupture of extensor mechanism of lower leg resulting in loss of extension and severe tendon damage • **Quadricep rupture more common than patellar tendon rupture** • Quadricep rupture typically >40 years old; patellar tendon rupture typically <40 years old • Risk Factors: **medications (fluoroquinolones**, corticosteroids, anabolic steroids), **diabetes**, **obesity**, **sedentary lifestyle**, **chronic kidney disease**, hyperparathyroidism, hypercholesterolemia, hyperuricemia, autoimmune
Patho-physiology	• <u>Mechanism</u>: **forceful/sudden contraction of quadricep muscle** (jump/land mechanism, fall on flexed knee, hyperflexion of knee) • Majority of quadricep tendon rupture occurs at myotendinous junction as a result of degeneration of tissue from chronic health conditions or lack of activity

Signs & Symptoms	• **Audible "pop" or tearing sensation** following traumatic mechanism
	• **Knee pain, significant effusion, ecchymosis**
	• Inability to ambulate
	• Physical Exam:
	  • **Complete loss of extensor mechanism** (inability to perform straight leg raise)
	  • <u>Quadricep Tendon Rupture</u>: palpable defect above patella
	  • <u>Patellar Tendon Rupture</u>: palpable defect below patella

Diagnosis	• Knee X-Ray: initial test to rule out patella fracture
	  • <u>Quadricep Tendon Rupture</u>: **patella baja** (low-riding patella)
	  • <u>Patellar Tendon Rupture</u>: **patella alta** (high-riding patella)
	• Knee Ultrasound: may be used to detect tendon defect and assess gap at rupture point
	• Knee MRI: usually more sensitive and specific; often ordered preoperatively

Treatment	• <u>Supportive</u>: **knee immobilizer in extension and strict non-weightbearing** with crutches; pain control, ice • <u>Surgery</u>: quadriceps/patellar tendon repair within 48-72 hours (delayed intervention leads to retraction of tendon)
Key Words & Most Common	• Quad rupture >40; patellar rupture <40 • Medications (fluoroquinolone, steroids), diabetes, CKD, obesity/sedentary • Audible pop + knee pain + ecchymosis • Loss of extensor mechanism • Knee X-Ray patella baja (quad rupture), patella alta (patellar rupture) • Knee immobilizer in extension + non-weightbearing • Surgical

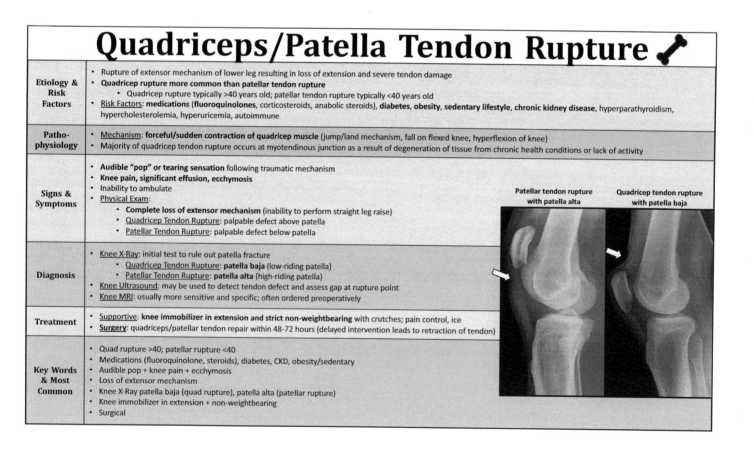

Patellar tendon rupture with patella alta   Quadricep tendon rupture with patella baja

Knee (Tibiofemoral) Dislocation

Etiology & Risk Factors	• Devastating limb-threatening emergency in which tibiofemoral joint is dislocated • Anterior/posterior most common and may have associated popliteal artery injury • <u>Mechanism</u>: **high velocity trauma (car accident, fall from height)**, sports related injury
Patho-physiology	• Anterior cruciate ligament, posterior cruciate ligament, medial collateral ligament, lateral collateral ligament are 4 ligamentous stabilizers within the knee • High energy trauma may rupture several or all of these supporting ligaments opening knee to dislocation • Popliteal artery lies posterior to knee joint and is most at risk for injury due to location

Signs & Symptoms	• **Severe knee pain following injury**
	• May have obvious deformity, effusion, ecchymosis
	• <u>Physical Exam</u>:
	   • Multidirectional instability
	   • Must assess neurovascular status distal to injury

Diagnosis	• <u>Knee X-Ray</u>: order to rule out fracture
	• <u>**Neurovascular Assessment**</u>:
	   • <u>**Peripheral Pulses**</u>: popliteal and distal pulses
	   • <u>**Peroneal Nerve**</u>: foot drop or reduced sensation to dorsal side of foot
	   • <u>**Ankle Brachial Index (ABI)**</u>: if <0.9 should order arterial duplex or CT angiogram
	• <u>Arterial Duplex vs CT Angiography</u>: asymmetric pulses, ABI<0.9, or ischemia/expanding hematoma

Treatment	• <u>**Immediate Reduction**</u>: orthopedic consult for closed reduction and neurovascular assessment followed by post-reduction x-ray • <u>**Surgery**</u>: orthopedics for surgical reduction and/or ligament reconstruction; vascular surgery needed for vascular injury
Key Words & Most Common	• Dislocation of knee joint with associated multiligament and popliteal artery injury • Severe knee pain following high velocity trauma • X-Ray + vascular assessment → arterial duplex if compromised • Immediate reduction with orthopedic consult • Surgery necessary for ligament reconstruction or vascular repair

Posterior knee dislocation

Femoral Condyle Fracture

Etiology & Risk Factors	• Fracture of the supracondylar or intercondylar region of the distal femur • Bimodal distribution affecting young athletes or elderly • <u>Risk Factors</u>: **advanced age, osteopenia/osteoporosis, obesity**, history of joint replacement, history of falls
Patho-physiology	• <u>Mechanism</u>: **axial loading** (fall from height), **high-energy impact** (motor vehicle accident, pedestrian hit by car), **sports related** (direct blow to femur) • Muscle attachments then cause fractured segments to displace which may lead to vascular injury

Signs & Symptoms	• **Severe pain and swelling**
	• **Inability to bear weight**
	• <u>Physical Exam</u>:
	   • Noticeable deformity may be present
	   • Must assess neurovascular status distal to injury

Diagnosis	• <u>Knee X-Ray</u>: order evaluate fracture
	• <u>**Neurovascular Assessment**</u>:
	   • <u>**Peripheral Pulses**</u>: popliteal and distal pulses
	   • <u>**Peroneal Nerve**</u>: foot drop or reduced sensation to dorsal side of foot
	   • <u>**Ankle Brachial Index (ABI)**</u>: if <0.9 should order arterial duplex or CT angiogram
	• <u>Arterial Duplex vs CT Angiography</u>: asymmetric pulses, ABI<0.9, or ischemia/expanding hematoma

Treatment	• <u>Conservative</u>: if minimal displacement; **knee immobilizer in extension and strict non-weightbearing** with crutches; pain control, ice • <u>**Surgery**</u>: if displaced; open reduction internal fixation vs intramedullary nailing
Key Words & Most Common	• Distal femur fracture affecting young athletes or elderly • Advanced age, osteopenia/osteoporosis, obesity • High-energy trauma • Severe pain/swelling and inability to bear weight • X-ray to assess fracture, neurovascular assessment • Minimally displaced can be treated conservatively • Many require surgery due to displacement

Tibial Plateau Fracture

Etiology & Risk Factors	• Fracture of the tibial plateau and may involve soft tissue injuries to nearby vasculature, nerves, ligaments, or menisci • Bimodal distribution affecting young athletes or elderly • Risk Factors: **advanced age, osteopenia/osteoporosis, obesity**, athlete
Patho-physiology	• Mechanism: **varus/valgus load +/- axial loading** (fall from height), **high-energy impact** (motor vehicle accident), **sports related** (direct blow to planted foot) • May involve meniscal or ligament tears (lateral meniscus most common) due to mechanism and anatomical location • Lateral tibial plateau is most common site Lateral tibial plateau fracture with depression

Signs & Symptoms	• **Severe pain/swelling and hemarthrosis**
	• **Inability to bear weight**
	• Physical Exam:
	  • Joint line tenderness
	  • Must assess neurovascular status distal to injury

Diagnosis	• Knee X-Ray: order evaluate fracture; may show sclerotic area indicating compression, malalignment, or articular surface depression
	• Neurovascular Assessment:
	  • Peripheral Pulses: **popliteal and distal pulses**
	  • Peroneal Nerve: foot drop or reduced sensation to dorsal side of foot
	• Knee CT Scan: faster/easier to obtain in acute setting to assess articular surface for depression, size, and extent of fracture; may be ordered preoperatively
	• Knee MRI: more sensitive to evaluate soft tissue, ligament, or meniscus pathology

Treatment	• Conservative: if minimal displacement; **hinged knee brace with partial weightbearing** with crutches; passive range of motion, pain control, ice, orthopedic follow-up • Surgery: if displaced; open reduction internal fixation
Key Words & Most Common	• Fracture of tibial plateau and accompanied soft tissue/ligament injury • Sports injury, fall from heigh, MVA • Severe pain/swelling +/- hemarthrosis • Knee X-ray to assess fracture + NV assessment • CT Scan vs MRI • Conservative if no displacement with hinged knee brace + crutches • Surgery indicated if displaced

Patellofemoral Chondromalacia

Etiology & Risk Factors	• Softening of the patellar articular cartilage that may lead to subsequent fissuring or erosion of the patellofemoral hyaline cartilage • Also known as patellofemoral syndrome or **runner's knee** • Etiology: **iatrogenic injections to knee** (corticosteroid injections may soften cartilage), abnormal microtrauma from **repetitive use** • Risk Factors: **overuse** (runners/cyclists, occupational), **female (increased Q angle), pes planus (flat feet),** high-heel shoe wear, obesity, abnormal patellar tracking
Patho-physiology	• Destruction of hyaline cartilage may result from chondrotoxic agents injected within the joint or from repetitive microtraumas (overuse) that place increased load and compressive stress on patellofemoral joint

Signs & Symptoms	• **Anterior knee pain behind or adjacent to patella**
	• Pain exacerbated with **knee flexion** (prolonged sitting, climbing stairs, jumping, running, cycling)
	• Physical Exam:
	  • **Patellar crepitus**
	  • Patellar Grind Test: pain or crepitus with compression of patella during knee extension

Diagnosis	• **Clinical Diagnosis** • Knee X-ray: may be performed to determine joint space narrowing or patellar tilt (sunrise view) • Knee MRI: definitive diagnosis; demonstrates signal change of affected cartilage; helps rule out other pathology
Treatment	• Conservative: **mainstay of treatment**; pain control (NSAIDs), rest, activity modification, compression, ice, physical therapy (restores ROM and strength), quadricep strengthening, **patellar stabilizing brace** • Surgery: arthroscopic chondroplasty if refractory symptoms to conservative management
Key Words & Most Common	• Softening of patellar cartilage from overuse • Runner/cyclist; female wearing high-heels • Anterior knee pain behind patella; worse with knee flexion • Clinical diagnosis • Conservative treatment

Ankle Sprain

Etiology & Risk Factors	• Ankle sprains can range in severity depending on mechanism of injury (high vs low energy injury), position of foot during injury, and rotational force • <u>Lateral Ankle Sprain</u>: **most common**; involves injury to **anterior talofibular ligament (ATFL)** or calcaneofibular (CFL) during inversion injury of foot • **ATFL is most common stabilizing ligament that is injured with foot inversion** • <u>Medial Ankle Sprain</u>: involves injury to deltoid ligament during eversion injury of foot
Patho-physiology	• Ankle is stabilized by three ligamentous systems: lateral ligament complex, medial deltoid ligament, and syndesmotic ligaments • Lateral complex include the anterior talofibular (ATFL), the calcaneofibular (CFL), and posterior talofibular (PTFL) ligament which may be injured during inversion injury • Medial deltoid ligament the strongest of the stabilizing ligaments and may be injured during eversion injury • Syndesmotic ligament stabilizes distal tibia and fibula and may be injured during ankle dorsiflexion and/or externally rotation

Signs & Symptoms	• **Ankle pain, swelling, and inability to bear weight after an injury**
	• May have audible "pop" at time of injury
	• <u>Physical Exam</u>:
	   • Tenderness to palpation over ligament; bony tenderness suggests fracture over sprain (should palpate proximal fibula for Maisonneuve fracture)
	   • <u>Anterior Drawer Test</u>: differentiates between 2nd and 3rd degree tear of ATFL; one hand stabilizes anterior distal tibia while other hand cups heel and pulled anteriorly. Forward movement of foot indicates 3rd degree tear.

Diagnosis	• **Clinical Diagnosis**
	• <u>Ankle/Foot X-Ray</u>: ordered to rule out fracture
	   • <u>Ottawa Ankle Rules</u>: X-ray should be ordered if (1) pain along lateral/medial malleolus (2) midfoot (navicular) pain (3) 5th metatarsal pain (4) inability to walk more than 4 steps at time of injury
	   • <u>Maisonneuve Fracture</u>: **(1)** spiral fracture of proximal fibula **(2)** Tibiofibular syndesmosis disruption **(3)** Deltoid ligament rupture **(4)** Medial malleolus fracture
		Degree of Injury	**Symptoms**	**Time to Heal**	

		1st Degree	Minimal pain/swelling. Weak ankle.	Hours to days
		2nd Degree	Pain + swelling + bruising Pain with ambulation and weight bearing	Days to weeks
		3rd Degree	Significant pain + swelling + bruising Inability to bear weight; joint instability	6-8 weeks

Treatment	• <u>Conservative</u>: **mainstay of treatment**; pain control (NSAIDs), rest, ice, compression, elevation, activity modification, physical therapy (restores ROM and strength)
	   • **Protected weight bearing with crutches**
	   • ACE wrap vs boot (depends on severity of sprain), lace-up ankle brace with return to activity
	• <u>Surgery</u>: reconstructive surgery reserved for recurrent ankle instability

Key Words & Most Common	• Lateral ankle sprain inversion injuring the ATFL most common • Ankle pain, swelling, inability to weight bear + TTP over ligament; anterior drawer test • Clinical Diagnosis +/- X-ray • Conservative treatment with NSAIDs, RICE, PT, protected weight bearing, orthotic support

Achilles Tendon Rupture

Etiology & Risk Factors	• Most common tendon rupture of lower extremity • **Most common ages 30-50 years old** • <u>Risk Factors</u>: **prior tendinopathy, fluoroquinolone use**, prolonged steroid use, **poor conditioning prior to exercise ("weekend warriors")**, overexertion during exercise • Chronic medical conditions (gout, **diabetes**, chronic kidney disease, thyroid disorders)
Patho-physiology	• <u>Mechanism</u>: **sudden forceful plantar flexion**, direct trauma, and/or mechanical overload with eccentric contraction • Long-standing tendinopathy or degenerative conditions increase likelihood of rupture • Most common site of rupture is 2-6cm proximal to calcaneal insertion point where blood supply is the weakest

Signs & Symptoms	• **Sudden, severe pain at posterior calf/ankle** (typically with sudden acceleration or pivoting)
	• **May have audible "pop" or tearing sensation**
	   • **Patient may describe sensation of being kicked or hit with ball in lower leg**
	• Inability to bear weight
	• <u>Physical Exam</u>:
	   • Unable to stand on toes; weak plantar flexion of ankle
	   • **Palpable defect in calcaneal tendon** 2-6cm proximal to calcaneal insertion point
	   • <u>Thompson Test</u>: patient prone with knee flexed to 90°; positive test if absent plantar flexion with squeezing of gastrocnemius muscle

Diagnosis	• **Clinical Diagnosis** • <u>Ankle X-Ray</u>: ordered to rule out fracture • <u>Ankle Ultrasound</u>: used to confirm diagnosis • <u>Ankle MRI</u>: **most accurate test to confirm diagnosis**; typically ordered prior to surgery
Treatment	• <u>Conservative</u>: pain control (NSAIDs), rest, elevation and functional bracing, **protected weight bearing with crutches** • **Short leg posterior splint vs cast with slight ankle plantar flexion** • <u>Surgery</u>: Achilles tendon repair; allows for earlier range of motion and quicker return to activity
Key Words & Most Common	• Most common in 30-50 year old "weekend warriors" • Prior tendinopathy or fluoroquinolone use • Sudden, severe pain with sudden acceleration or push-off +/- pop/tearing sensation • Clinical diagnosis with palpable defect of tendon + positive Thompson Test (absent plantar flexion with squeezing of calf muscle) • MRI used to confirm diagnosis • Conservative: short leg posterior splint/cast with slight ankle plantar flexion • Surgery provides quicker return to activity

Visible defect of left calcaneal tendon

Stress Fracture

Etiology & Risk Factors	• "March fractures" are stress fractures caused by repetitive weight bearing stress • Risk Factors: **overuse**, female, **high-impact or weight bearing exercise** (college athletes, **military training**), long distance runners, history of prior stress fracture, vitamin D or calcium deficiency, improper footwear
Patho-physiology	• **Most commonly affects metatarsal bones (2nd and 3rd most common)**; can also affects tibia, fibula, navicular • Repetitive stress to metatarsal bones during weight-bearing activity leads to microtrauma and bone fatigue which eventually consolidates to stress fracture

Signs & Symptoms	• **Gradual onset of localized bone pain** +/- swelling
	  • **Pain is worse with activity** and improves with rest
	  • May be described as dull/achy
	• Physical Exam:
	  • Focal bony tenderness
	  • Antalgic gait (limp)
	
	Stress fracture of 2nd metatarsal

Diagnosis	• X-Ray: **initial imaging test of choice**; high false-negative rate as fracture may not be visible until 2-4 weeks after pain onset • May show frank fracture, subtle periosteal reaction, cortex blurring; callus formation evident of more mature fracture • MRI: **sensitive and specific**; performed if x-ray is negative for suspected stress fracture in high-risk area or persistent symptoms • Labs: BMP, vitamin D level may be ordered for suspected nutritional deficiency
Treatment	• Conservative: **mainstay of treatment**; pain control (NSAIDs), rest, activity modification, compression, ice, gait training, physical therapy, orthotic inserts • **Immobilization + controlled weight bearing**; may gradually bear weight over 6-12 weeks (if asymptomatic); strict non-weightbearing if 5th metatarsal • Surgery: orthopedic referral for surgical fixation (risk of nonunion) • Supplementation: consider vitamin D or calcium supplements, or nutritional counseling if suspected etiology
Key Words & Most Common	• Repetitive weight bearing stress from high-impact exercise (athletes, military training) • 2nd and 3rd metatarsal most commonly affected • Gradual onset of dull/achy pain worse with activity • X-ray may be negative early → MRI • Immobilization with gradual return to weight bearing activity • Surgery if risk of nonunion (5th metatarsal)

Plantar Fasciitis

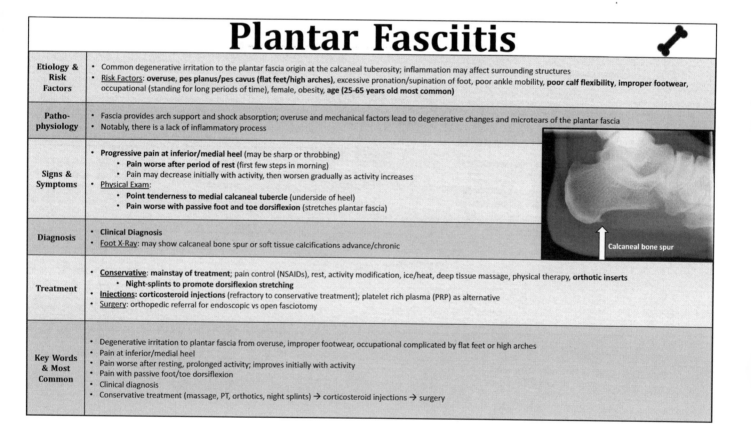

Etiology & Risk Factors	• Common degenerative irritation to the plantar fascia origin at the calcaneal tuberosity; inflammation may affect surrounding structures • Risk Factors: **overuse**, pes planus/pes cavus (flat feet/high arches), excessive pronation/supination of foot, poor ankle mobility, **poor calf flexibility, improper footwear**, occupational (standing for long periods of time), female, obesity, **age (25-65 years old most common)**
Patho-physiology	• Fascia provides arch support and shock absorption; overuse and mechanical factors lead to degenerative changes and microtears of the plantar fascia • Notably, there is a lack of inflammatory process

Signs & Symptoms	• **Progressive pain at inferior/medial heel** (may be sharp or throbbing)
	  • **Pain worse after period of rest** (first few steps in morning)
	  • Pain may decrease initially with activity, then worsen gradually as activity increases
	• Physical Exam:
	  • **Point tenderness to medial calcaneal tubercle** (underside of heel)
	  • **Pain worse with passive foot and toe dorsiflexion** (stretches plantar fascia)
	
	Calcaneal bone spur

Diagnosis	• **Clinical Diagnosis** • Foot X-Ray: may show calcaneal bone spur or soft tissue calcifications advance/chronic
Treatment	• Conservative: **mainstay of treatment**; pain control (NSAIDs), rest, activity modification, ice/heat, deep tissue massage, physical therapy, **orthotic inserts** • Night-splints to promote dorsiflexion stretching • Injections: corticosteroid injections (refractory to conservative treatment); platelet rich plasma (PRP) as alternative • Surgery: orthopedic referral for endoscopic vs open fasciotomy
Key Words & Most Common	• Degenerative irritation to plantar fascia from overuse, improper footwear, occupational complicated by flat feet or high arches • Pain at inferior/medial heel • Pain worse after resting, prolonged activity; improves initially with activity • Pain with passive foot/toe dorsiflexion • Clinical diagnosis • Conservative treatment (massage, PT, orthotics, night splints) → corticosteroid injections → surgery

Tarsal Tunnel Syndrome

Etiology & Risk Factors	• Entrapment neuropathy secondary to compression of structures within tarsal tunnel (similar to carpal tunnel of the lower extremity) • Tarsal tunnel contains posterior tibialis tendon, flexor digitorum longus, and flexor hallucis longus tendon; posterior tibial artery and vein, posterior tibial nerve • Etiology: compression of structures within tarsal tunnel • Risk Factors: **poorly fitting or restrictive footwear, overuse, trauma**, post-surgical scarring, overuse, **lower extremity edema**, tendinopathy, tenosynovitis, mass lesions, diabetes, hypothyroidism, gout
Patho-physiology	• Compression of posterior tibial nerve by above etiology as it travels through the tarsal tunnel

Signs & Symptoms	• **Retromalleolar pain** (burning/tingling); may extend along plantar medial heel
	  • **Pain worse with standing/walking** and increases throughout the day
	    • **Pain typically *does not* improve with rest**
	• Physical Exam:
	  • **Focal tenderness to area posterior/inferior to medial malleolus**
	  • **Tinel Sign**: tapping on tarsal tunnel causes distal tingling sensation

Diagnosis	• **Clinical Diagnosis** • Electromyography: used to confirm diagnosis
Treatment	• **Conservative**: **mainstay of treatment**; pain control (NSAIDs), rest, activity modification, ice, **properly fitting shoes**, physical therapy, **orthotic inserts** • Injections: corticosteroid injections (refractory to conservative treatment) • Surgery: orthopedic referral for tunnel release if severe
Key Words & Most Common	• Entrapment neuropathy of posterior tibial nerve by poorly fitting/restrictive footwear, overuse, trauma, edema • Retromalleolar pain/burning/tingling • Worse with standing/walking and does not improve with rest • + Tinel Sign • Clinical diagnosis + electromyography to confirm • Conservative treatment

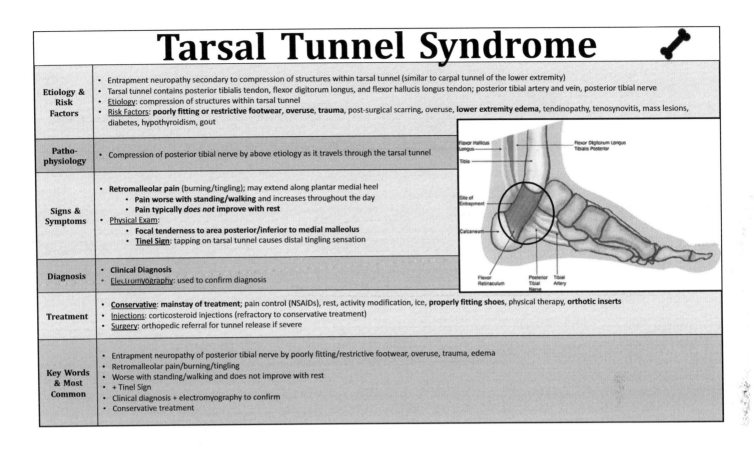

Hallux Valgus (Bunion)

Etiology & Risk Factors	• Prominence/deformity at the first metatarsophalangeal (MTP) joint with lateral deviation of the proximal phalanx • Risk Factors: **female, poorly fitting/tight/pointed footwear**, pes planus, history of rheumatoid arthritis, anatomical predisposition (short or dorsiflexed 1st metatarsal)
Patho-physiology	• Increased pressure at the head of the of the first metatarsal causes medial angulation and thus increasing the hallux angle and forcing the hallux laterally to accommodate the muscle stabilization • Medial collateral ligaments become strained resulting in worsening deformity • Synovitis and bursitis occurs and causes pain/deformity
Signs & Symptoms	• **Joint pain and prominence at MTP joint with lateral deformity** • Physical Exam: • **Adventitial bursitis** (painful, warm, cystic, fluctuant/mobile, inflammation at MTP)
Diagnosis	• **Clinical Diagnosis** • Foot X-Rays: may help to establish diagnosis of osteoarthritis or gout (periarticular erosions)
Treatment	• **Conservative**: **mainstay of treatment** • Pain control (NSAIDs), rest, activity modification, ice, **properly fitting shoes (wide toe box)**, orthotic inserts, bunion pads • Injections: corticosteroid injections (refractory to conservative treatment) • Surgery: orthopedic referral for surgical release or realignment if severe
Key Words & Most Common	• Prominence/deformity at first MTP caused by poorly fitting/tight/pointed footwear • Joint pain + prominence at MTP with lateral deformity • Warm/painful/inflamed MTP bursa • Clinical Diagnosis • Conservative treatment (wide toe box shoes, orthotics, bunion pads) → steroid injection → surgery

Bony prominence at MTP joint with lateral deformity

Hammer Toe

Etiology & Risk Factors	• Most common deformity of forefoot caused by misalignment and flexion of the proximal interphalangeal joint (IPJ) and hyperextension of MTP and DIP joint • **2nd digit is most commonly affected** • Risk Factors: **poorly fitting/tight/pointed footwear, diabetes**, history of rheumatoid arthritis, anatomical predisposition (short 1st metatarsal), hallux valgus, pes planus
Patho-physiology	• Weak intrinsic muscles and strong extrinsic muscles of the metatarsophalangeal joint create imbalance • Excessive pronation leads to hyperpronation of subtalar joint resulting in flexor stabilization resulting in hammering of digit to increase stability
Signs & Symptoms	• **Pain of proximal interphalangeal joint** of affected digit especially while wearing narrow toe box shoes • Physical Exam: • Flexion of PIP joint and hyperextension of MTP and DIP joint
Diagnosis	• **Clinical Diagnosis** • Foot X-Ray: may be used to evaluate arthritis or fracture of foot *Hammer toe of 3rd digit*
Treatment	• <u>Conservative</u>: **mainstay of treatment**; pain control (NSAIDs), rest, activity modification, **properly fitting shoes (wide toe box), orthotic inserts, metatarsal pads** • Surgery: orthopedic referral for arthroplasty/arthrodesis if severe
Key Words & Most Common	• Misalignment of toe (flexed PIP joint and hyperextension of MTP and DIP joint • Caused by tight/poorly fitting footwear • Pain of proximal interphalangeal joint • Clinical Diagnosis • Conservative treatment with wide toe box shoes, orthotic inserts with metatarsal pads

Neuropathic (Charcot) Arthropathy

Etiology & Risk Factors	• Destructive joint disorder resulting from peripheral neuropathy initiated by trauma to an affected extremity • Can lead to fracture or dislocations of the foot • Risk Factors: **diabetes (diabetic neuropathy is most common cause)**, neuropathy, trauma, metabolic abnormalities, peripheral vascular disease
Patho-physiology	• Repeated microtrauma, autonomic dysfunction and impaired sensation leads to resorption and weakening of bone
Signs & Symptoms	• Acute: **joint pain, minimally tender, prominent effusion** (may be hemorrhagic), warmth, erythema • Chronic: **deformity**/alteration of joint, **audible crepitus**, massive synovial effusion, subluxation and instability of the joint

Diagnosis	• X-ray: similar to osteoarthritis
	  • **Joint space narrowing/obliteration, bone fragmentation/destruction**, joint disorganization
	  • New bone growth or increased bone density
	• MRI: may be used to rule out other etiologies (osteomyelitis)
	
	Diffuse joint space obliteration with bone fragmentation/destruction

Treatment	• <u>Conservative</u>: mainstay of treatment; rest, **accommodating footwear, diabetes management,** smoking cessation • **Protected weight-bearing** (Total contact casts (TCC) with a controlled ankle motion (CAM) walker) • Medication: Bisphosphonates and Calcitonin help prevent osteoclastic resorption • Surgery: orthopedic referral for severe deformity
Key Words & Most Common	• Destructive joint disorder most commonly as a result of diabetic neuropathy initiated by trauma • Joint pain, effusion, deformity, audible crepitus • X-Ray shows joint space obliteration, bone fragmentation • Treatment with accommodating footwear, protected weight bearing; bisphosphonates/calcitonin • Management of underlying condition

Interdigital (Morton's) Neuroma

Etiology & Risk Factors	• Compressive neuropathy of the forefoot interdigital nerve • Neuropathy secondary to compressive irritation to the plantar aspect of the transverse intermetatarsal ligament • Most common location for Morton neuroma is between 3rd and 4th metatarsals • <u>Risk Factors</u>: **females, age (25-50 years old most common), improper footwear (narrow toe-box), high-heeled shoes (cause toe hyperextension and toe deviation), pes planus (flat feet)**, intermetatarsal bursitis, transverse metatarsal ligament thickening, forefoot trauma, high-impact activity, lipoma
Patho-physiology	• Repetitive compression and trauma to the common digital nerve of the forefoot leads to vascular changes, edema, and bursal thickening resulting in perineural fibrosis

Signs & Symptoms	• **Plantar foot pain at forefoot**
	  • **Most common between 3rd and 4th metatarsals**
	  • Described as as **burning**, stabbing, or tingling
	  • Pain worse with specific footwear (narrow toe box)
	• May have **numbness/paresthesia** of toe or plantar aspect of foot
	• <u>Physical Exam</u>:
	  • **Tenderness to palpation of plantar aspect of forefoot**
	  • Pain reproducible by squeezing interdigital space
	  • <u>**Mulder's Sign**</u>: squeezing the two metatarsal heads together with one hand, while applying pressure on the interdigital space with the other
	    • Pain or clicking indicates positive test

Diagnosis	• **Clinical Diagnosis** • <u>Ultrasound/MRI</u>: may be used to confirm diagnosis or ordered prior to surgery
Treatment	• <u>**Conservative**</u>: **mainstay of treatment** • **Properly fitting shoes (wide toe box), orthotic inserts, metatarsal pads,** pain control (NSAIDs), rest, activity modification, ice • <u>Injections</u>: corticosteroid injections (refractory to conservative treatment) • <u>Surgery</u>: orthopedic referral for surgical resection if severe
Key Words & Most Common	• Neuropathy of forefoot most commonly between 3rd and 4th metatarsals • Female age 25-50 wearing high-heeled/narrow shoes is most common • Burning plantar forefoot pain between 3rd and 4th metatarsals +/- paresthesia • Clinical Diagnosis • Properly fitting shoes, orthotic inserts with metatarsal pads → cortisone injections → surgery

Representation of plantar nerve anatomy

Fifth Metatarsal Fracture

	<u>Jones Fracture</u>	<u>Pseudo-Jones Fracture</u>	<u>Stress Fracture</u>
Etiology & Risk Factors	• **Transverse fracture through diaphysis at metaphyseal-diaphyseal junction** • **Involves the 4th and 5th metatarsal articulation** • High risk (15-30%) of nonunion or malunion	• **Fracture through the tuberosity of fifth metatarsal** • **Most common of 5th metatarsal fractures** • *Does not* involve 4th-5th intertarsal junction	• **Fracture through diaphyseal area** • Increased risk of nonunion or malunion
Patho-physiology	• Occurs with significant adduction force to the foot with a lifted heel • Athlete suddenly changes direction	• Occurs when hindfoot is inverted during plantar flexion • Athlete lands awkwardly after a jump	• Occurs as chronic injury with repetitive microtraumas
Signs & Symptoms	• **Lateral foot pain** • May have **ecchymosis and edema** • <u>Physical Exam</u>: • Point tenderness to 5th metatarsal, inability to bear weight, pain with resisted eversion		

Diagnosis	• <u>**Foot X-Ray**</u>: initial imaging test of choice; AP, lateral, oblique views
	  • <u>Jones</u>: **Transverse fracture through diaphysis at metaphyseal-diaphyseal junction**
	  • <u>Pseudo-Jones</u>: **Fracture through the tuberosity of fifth metatarsal**
	  • <u>Stress</u>: **Fracture through diaphyseal area**
	• <u>Foot CT/MRI</u>: may be ordered in setting of delayed healing		

Treatment	• <u>**General Fracture Management**</u>: pain control (NSAIDs), rest, activity modification, ice, orthopedic referral
	  • <u>Jones</u>: strict non-weightbearing
	  • <u>Pseudo-Jones</u>: walking boot or hard shoe; weight-bearing as tolerated
	  • <u>Stress</u>: strict non-weightbearing
	• <u>Surgery</u>: **Jones or displaced fracture frequently requires ORIF/pinning due to risk of nonunion**		

Key Words & Most Common	• <u>Jones</u>: Transverse diaphyseal fracture at metaphyseal-diaphyseal junction • <u>Pseudo-Jones</u>: tuberosity fracture • <u>Stress</u>: diaphyseal fracture • Lateral foot pain + bruising + swelling • X-ray • General fracture management; non-weightbearing, ortho referral • Jones/displaced fracture often requires surgery (nonunion)		

Proximal fractures of the 5th metatarsal

Location	Associated with
Proximal diaphysis	Stress fracture
Metaphysis	Jones fracture
Tuberosity	Pseudo-Jones
Apophysis	Normal at 10 - 16 years

Os vesalianum Present in 0.1–1%

Lisfranc Injury

Etiology & Risk Factors	• Fracture and/or dislocation of the midfoot disrupting one or more tarsometatarsal joints • **Lisfranc joint is articulation point of first, second, third metatarsal heads and respective cuneiform bones** • <u>Risk Factors</u>: **high-risk activity** (football, motorcyclist, horseback riders), male, **age (30-40 years old most common)**
Patho-physiology	• <u>Mechanism</u>: direct blow to foot or indirect **force/axial load applied to foot in plantar flexion (fall onto foot while in plantar flexion)** • Lisfranc ligament attaches 2nd metatarsal head to medial cuneiform; injury to 2nd metatarsal often results in dislocation of other metatarsals as articulation is disrupted
Signs & Symptoms	• **Severe midfoot pain** • Pain worse with "push off" during ambulation • Inability to bear weight (especially on tiptoe) • <u>Physical Exam</u>: • **Midfoot ecchymosis**, edema, point tenderness of tarsometatarsal joint • Pain with pronation and abduction of foot
Diagnosis	• <u>Foot X-Ray</u>: AP, lateral, oblique views (weight bearing views should be attempted) • **Fracture of base of 2nd metatarsal is pathognomonic** • May show chip fracture of cuneiform • Disruption of tarsometatarsal joint • <u>Foot CT Scan</u>: may be used to confirm diagnosis; more sensitive
Treatment	• <u>General Fracture Management</u>: pain control (NSAIDs), **strict non-weightbearing**, orthopedic referral • <u>Surgery</u>: **ORIF or fusion is definitive**
Key Words & Most Common	• Fracture/dislocation of midfoot • Mechanism involves fall onto foot while in plantar flexion • Severe midfoot pain/ecchymosis • Foot X-Ray shows fracture of base of 2nd metatarsal • ORIF + non-weightbearing

L

Fracture of base of 2nd metatarsal

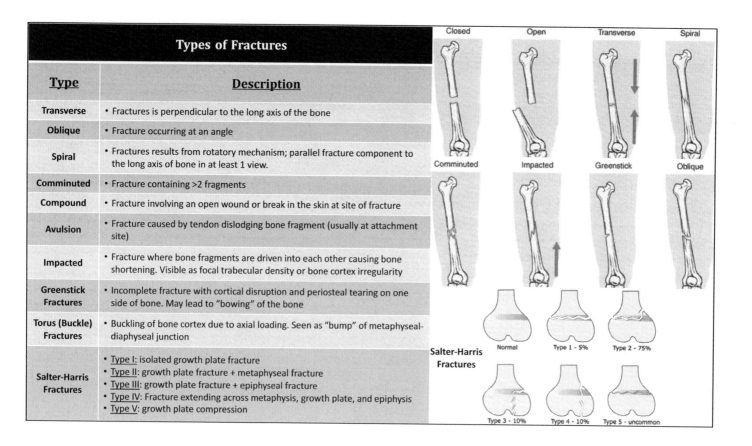

Types of Fractures	
Type	**Description**
Transverse	• Fractures is perpendicular to the long axis of the bone
Oblique	• Fracture occurring at an angle
Spiral	• Fractures results from rotatory mechanism; parallel fracture component to the long axis of bone in at least 1 view.
Comminuted	• Fracture containing >2 fragments
Compound	• Fracture involving an open wound or break in the skin at site of fracture
Avulsion	• Fracture caused by tendon dislodging bone fragment (usually at attachment site)
Impacted	• Fracture where bone fragments are driven into each other causing bone shortening. Visible as focal trabecular density or bone cortex irregularity
Greenstick Fractures	• Incomplete fracture with cortical disruption and periosteal tearing on one side of bone. May lead to "bowing" of the bone
Torus (Buckle) Fractures	• Buckling of bone cortex due to axial loading. Seen as "bump" of metaphyseal-diaphyseal junction
Salter-Harris Fractures	• <u>Type I</u>: isolated growth plate fracture • <u>Type II</u>: growth plate fracture + metaphyseal fracture • <u>Type III</u>: growth plate fracture + epiphyseal fracture • <u>Type IV</u>: Fracture extending across metaphysis, growth plate, and epiphysis • <u>Type V</u>: growth plate compression

Closed   Open   Transverse   Spiral

Comminuted   Impacted   Greenstick   Oblique

Salter-Harris Fractures

Normal   Type 1 - 5%   Type 2 - 75%

Type 3 - 10%   Type 4 - 10%   Type 5 - uncommon

Osteosarcoma

Etiology & Risk Factors	• Malignant osseous neoplasm of osteoblastic proliferation • **Most common primary bone cancer of childhood** • Bimodal distribution **most common in adolescents** 10-14 years old and second peak at 50-60 years old • <u>Risk Factors</u>: **Paget disease**, electrical burns, trauma, exposures (beryllium, alkylating agents, **ionizing radiation**), orthopedic prosthetics, previous bone infection
Patho-physiology	• **Most commonly occurs in metaphysis of long bones** (**distal femur most common site**, proximal tibia, proximal humerus, skull, mandible, pelvis) • Most common METS site is lungs • Caused by overproduction of osteoid and immature bone by malignant osteoblasts; osteoblastic proliferation

Signs & Symptoms	• **Bone pain worse with activity** (parents may think it's a sprain, growing pains etc.)
	  • **Nocturnal bone pain**
	• Absence of constitutional symptoms
	• <u>Physical Exam</u>:
	  • Joint effusion
	  • **Palpable mass** (may be tender)
	  • Limited ROM of affected joint, may have antalgic gait
	  • Respiratory findings with metastatic forms

Diagnosis	• <u>X-Ray</u>:
	  • "Sunburst" Appearance – lytic lesion with metaphyseal periosteal reaction and cortical disruption
	  • Codman's Triangle – subperiosteal bone formation when the periosteum is raised
	• <u>MRI</u>: further characterizes lesion
	• **Biopsy: definitive diagnosis**; malignant osteoid cells
	• *Consider CXR + CT of chest to evaluate metastatic disease*

Treatment	• <u>**Neoadjuvant Chemotherapy + Surgical Removal**</u>: **indicated for most cases**
	  • <u>Limb Sparing Surgery</u>: if not neovascular
	  • <u>Amputation</u>: if neovascular

Key Words & Most Common	• Most common primary bone cancer of childhood; peaks age 10-14 and 50-60 • Distal femur most common site • Bone pain worse with activity and at night +/- painful mass • X-Ray: lytic lesion with periosteal reaction • Biopsy for definitive diagnosis • Chemotherapy + surgical removal

Chondrosarcoma

Etiology & Risk Factors	• Malignant cartilaginous neoplasm • Malignant transformation occurs in 5% of osteochondromas • <u>Risk Factors</u>: age (40+ years old most common), males, chromosomal abnormalities • <u>Location</u>: **most common on flat bones** (scapula, pelvis, sternum, ribs); can occur on long bones (proximal femur, proximal humerus)
Patho-physiology	• Cytogenetic analyzation shows chromosomal structural abnormalities and genetic instability increase likelihood of chondrosarcoma • Overproduction of chondroid matrix in the medullary cavity
Signs & Symptoms	• **Localized pain and swelling** • Long duration of symptoms (months to years) • Initial presentation may be **pathologic fracture**
Diagnosis	• <u>X-Ray</u>: punctate calcifications (popcorn calcification or rings and arcs calcification) and cortical bone destruction • <u>CT/MRI</u>: used to assess extent of bone involvement • Osteolytic lesion with ill-defined margins and with calcifications • <u>**Biopsy: definitive diagnosis**</u>
Treatment	• <u>**Surgical Excision**</u>: **definitive treatment** • Chemotherapy is generally not effective; may be used in select advanced disease cases
Key Words & Most Common	• Malignant cartilaginous neoplasm • Most common on flat bones (pelvis, scapula) • Localized pain and swelling; insidious onset • X-ray shows punctate calcifications, cortical bone destruction • Biopsy • Surgical Excision

Periosteal reaction of the pelvis

Osteolytic lesion with ill-defined margins and calcifications seen on CT scan

Ewing Sarcoma

Etiology & Risk Factors	• **Highly aggressive osseous neoplasm arising from neuroectoderm cells** • Second most common primary bone neoplasm in children/young adults (peaks 10-15 years old) • **25% of patients will be metastatic at time of presentation** (spin and lungs most common metastasis site) • <u>Location</u>: **most common sites are pelvis, axial skeleton, and femur** • <u>Risk Factors</u>: no established association with environmental or drug exposure, radiation history, or familial cancer history
Patho-physiology	• Chromosome t(11;22)(q24;q12) translocation is associated with 85% of tumors • Underlying etiology not well established
Signs & Symptoms	• **Localized bone pain and swelling worse with activity** • **Nocturnal pain** • May have constitutional symptoms; fever, fatigue, weight loss, night sweats • <u>Physical Exam</u>: **palpable mass**, localized pain, joint effusion
Diagnosis	• <u>X-Ray</u>: **layered periosteal reaction with periosteal bone formation (described as "onion peel") and osseous destruction (described as "moth eaten")** • <u>Labs</u>: **LDH is prognostic factor**; may have increased ESR or leukocytosis • **Biopsy: definitive diagnosis** • <u>CT/MRI/PET</u>: may be used to evaluate metastases
Treatment	• **Neoadjuvant Chemotherapy + Surgical Resection: indicated in most cases** • Limb sparing surgery if possible • <u>Radiation Therapy</u>: utilized when complete surgical excision is not possible
Key Words & Most Common	• Highly aggressive osseous neoplasm that is commonly metastatic at time of presentation • Most common site is pelvis, axial skeleton, femur • Localized bone pain/swelling worse with activity and at night • X-Ray shows layered periosteal reaction and bone formation (onion peel) and osseous destruction (moth eaten) • LDH prognostic factor • Biopsy is for definitive diagnosis • Chemotherapy; surgical resection; radiation therapy

Osteochondroma

Etiology & Risk Factors	• Benign cartilage-capped osseous surface lesion arising from external metaphysis surface of a bone or areas of tendon insertion • Most common benign osseous tumor; grows until skeletal maturity • **Femur is most common bone affected**; tibia, humerus • <u>Risk Factors</u>: **age (10-20 years old most common), male**, radiation exposure, trauma (surgery or Salter-Harris fractures)
Patho-physiology	• May be a developmental lesion as a result of cell separation at the epiphyseal growth plate occurring after trauma or irradiation • Fragment of growth plate herniates at periosteum level (which continues to grow) resulting in sessile or pedunculated lesion at the metaphysis
Signs & Symptoms	• **Asymptomatic** (found incidentally on x-ray) • **Painless, palpable mass** • May cause neurovascular compression
Diagnosis	• <u>X-Ray</u>: **pedunculated (narrow stalk) growth that grows adjacent and away from the joint with medullary and cortical continuity** • <u>Biopsy</u>: definitive diagnosis • <u>MRI</u>: compressive symptom evaluation
Treatment	• **Observation: if asymptomatic**; may grow until patient reaches skeletal maturity • <u>Surgery</u>: **surgical resection indicated for large, symptomatic lesions** or lesions with concerning imaging factors (growth in skeletally mature patient, irregular margins, focal radiolucency, osseous erosions)
Key Words & Most Common	• Benign osseous tumor that grows until skeletal maturity • Femur most commonly affected • Asymptomatic vs painless palpable mass • X-Ray shows pedunculated growth growing away from joint with medullary/cortical continuity • Observation if asymptomatic • Surgical resection if symptomatic

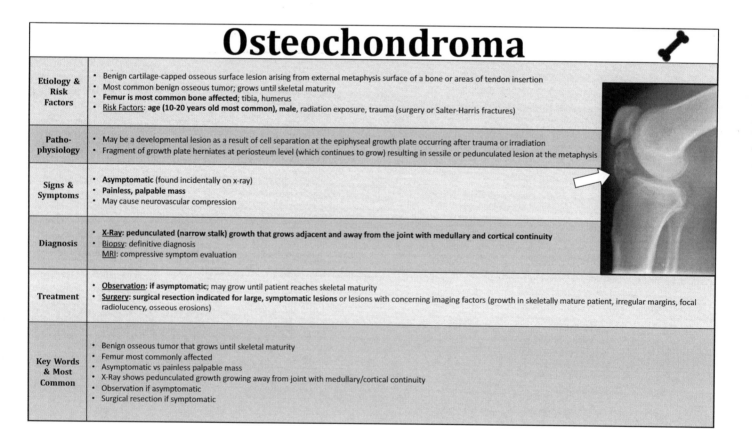

Osteoid Osteoma

Etiology & Risk Factors	• Benign osseous tumor frequently affecting long bones (femur, tibia) • <u>Location</u>: **proximal femur most common** site; tibia, spine • <u>Etiology</u>: not fully understood; benign neoplasm vs trauma/inflammatory process • <u>Risk Factors</u>: age (5-25 years old most common), male (3x greater risk)
Patho-physiology	• Tumor may be a result of neoplasia or trauma to area • Nerve fibers receive stimulation from increased blood flow as a result of **prostaglandin release from the nidus** (well vascularized "core" of the tumor) • Prostaglandin release shown to be 100-1000x greater at osteoid osteoma site than normal bone

Signs & Symptoms	• **Progressive bone pain**
	   • **Not related to activity level**
	   • **Nocturnal pain**
	   • **Pain relieved with NSAIDs** (prostaglandin inhibition)
	• <u>Physical Exam</u>:
	   • Localized swelling, tenderness, limited range of motion
	   • Antalgic gait; may lead to limb length discrepancy
	
	Marked sclerosis around the nidus of the lesser trochanter

Diagnosis	• <u>X-Ray</u>: **small, round, radiolucent nidus with surrounding sclerotic margin**; nidus may contain calcifications • <u>CT/MRI</u>: more sensitive imaging test (CT preferred)
Treatment	• <u>**Conservative**</u>: NSAIDs with serial x-rays to monitor changes **(6 months)**; long-term NSAID use side effects prevent it from being definitive treatment • <u>Surgery</u>: surgical resection if symptomatic refractory to conservative treatment
Key Words & Most Common	• Benign osseous tumor most common at proximal femur • Adolescent male most common • Progressive bone pain, NOT related to activity, worse at night • Pain relieved with NSAIDs • X-Ray shows small, round, radiolucent nidus with sclerotic margin • NSAIDs + monitoring → surgical resection

Fibromyalgia

Etiology & Risk Factors	• Condition characterized by chronic musculoskeletal pain perception of unknown etiology • <u>Etiology</u>: no specific etiology; may be triggered by physical and/or emotional stressors, or infection (Lyme disease, COVID-19) • <u>Risk Factors</u>: **age (20-55 years old most common), female**, history of rheumatic disease
Patho-physiology	• Patient becomes hypersensitive to pain possibly due to elevated levels of glutamate and substance P neurotransmitters, diminished levels of dopamine and norepinephrine, prolonged pain sensation, and dopamine dysregulation
Signs & Symptoms	• **Chronic, widespread, musculoskeletal pain and stiffness** (most common in neck/shoulders) • **Fatigue** • <u>Cognitive Disturbances</u>: "fibro fog", difficulty with attention or completing tasks • May have associated anxiety/depression **18 Tender Points**
Diagnosis	• **Clinical diagnosis**; normal findings in imaging and laboratory tests • Fibromyalgia Classification Criteria: • **Tenderness in at least 11 of 18 defined trigger points + chronic pain for greater than 3 months**

Treatment	• <u>**Conservative**</u>: reassurance and education, proper sleep hygiene, stretching, local heat, massage, stress management
	• <u>**Exercise**</u>: low-impact aerobic exercise (swimming, biking, walking)
	• <u>**Medications**</u>: tricyclic antidepressants **(amitriptyline) is first-line medication**; SSRI/SNRI (duloxetine, milnacipran) are alternatives
	   • **Cyclobenzaprine** for mild/moderate symptoms; may promote deeper sleep and decrease muscle pain
	   • Gabapentin/**pregabalin** may be used as adjuncts (pregabalin is FDA approved for fibromyalgia)
	   • Opioids should be avoided

Key Words & Most Common	• Chronic muscle pain with no known etiology • Most common in females age 20-55yo • Chronic musculoskeletal pain/stiffness + fatigue • May have cognitive disturbances, anxiety/depression • Clinical diagnosis • Conservative + exercise • TCAs (amitriptyline) first line; cyclobenzaprine; pregabalin

Polymyalgia Rheumatica

Etiology & Risk Factors	• Rheumatic condition characterized by pain/stiffness of neck/shoulder/hip area • <u>Etiology</u>: unknown etiology; idiopathic inflammation of joints, tendons, and bursa • <u>Risk Factors</u>: **age (>55 years old most common), female, Caucasian, history of giant cell arteritis, history of EBV**
Patho-physiology	• Immune-mediated disorder with elevated inflammatory markers secondary to decreased number of circulating B cells resulting in increased IL-6 response

Signs & Symptoms	• **Pain and stiffness of proximal muscles and joints** (especially **shoulder**, neck, **hips**, pelvis)
	  • **Shoulders and hips most common**
	  • **Pain/stiffness worse in morning and after prolonged rest**
	  • May be abrupt in onset
	• May have constitutional symptoms (fatigue/malaise, low-grade fever, anorexia, weight loss)
	• <u>Physical Exam</u>:
	  • Decreased range of motion (especially hip/shoulder); **normal muscle strength**

Diagnosis	• **Clinical Diagnosis** • <u>Labs</u>: **increased ESR/CRP**; may have normocytic anemia • Antinuclear antibody (ANA), rheumatoid factor (RF), creatine kinase (CK) and anti-citrullinated protein antibodies (Anti-CCP AB) are negative
Treatment	• <u>**Low-Dose Corticosteroids**</u>: **initial treatment of choice**; dosing may need to be titrated to prevent relapse • Consider vitamin D and calcium supplements for patients with long-term steroid use • <u>Methotrexate</u>: alternative medication if steroids are not tolerated or contraindicated
Key Words & Most Common	• Idiopathic inflammation of joints/tendons/bursa • Most common in Caucasian females >55yo • Pain/stiffness of proximal muscles and joints • Worse in morning and after rest • Increased ESR/CRP; negative ANA/RF/CK/Anti-CCP AB • Steroids first-line

Shoulders and hips most common

Rhabdomyolysis

Etiology & Risk Factors	• Acute breakdown and necrosis of muscle leading to release of intracellular constituents (myoglobin, sarcoplasmic proteins, electrolytes) into bloodstream • <u>Etiology</u>: **breakdown and necrosis of muscle** • <u>Risk Factors</u>: **trauma, extreme exertion, prolonged immobility** (opioid or alcohol intoxication), sepsis, crush injury, **seizures**, muscle hypoxia, infection, drugs (**cocaine**), toxins, **statin therapy**, metabolic or electrolyte disorders, snake bites, electric shock
Patho-physiology	• Skeletal muscle electrolyte exchange, adenosine triphosphate (ATP) metabolism, and myocyte membrane is disrupted resulting in cell breakdown. • Myoglobin and creatine kinase is then released to circulation which is toxic to renal tubular cells resulting in acute tubular necrosis (acute kidney injury)
Signs & Symptoms	• **Triad: muscle pain + muscle weakness + myoglobinuria (reddish-brown "tea colored" urine)** • May have fever or altered mental status; signs of dehydration

Diagnosis	• <u>**Electrocardiogram (ECG)**</u>: **most important initial test**; evaluate for changes secondary to electrolyte abnormalities (hyperkalemia – peaked T waves, prolonged PR interval)
	• <u>Urine Tests</u>:
	  • <u>**Urine Dipstick/Urinalysis**</u>: **first lab test; positive for blood but negative for RBCs** (indicates myoglobin is spilling into urine)
	  • <u>**Urine Myoglobin**</u>: **most specific test**
	• <u>Labs</u>:
	  • <u>Electrolytes</u>: **hyperkalemia, hyperuricemia, hypocalcemia**, hypophosphatemia, **elevated creatinine** (acute kidney injury)
	  • <u>Muscle Enzymes</u>: **elevated creatinine kinase (CK)** elevated LDH, ALT/AST

Treatment	• <u>**IV Fluids**</u>: **first-line treatment**; liberal amounts (10L) with target urine output goal of 200-300 ml/hr
	• <u>Electrolyte Abnormalities</u>:
	  • **Hyperkalemia: D50 + insulin** (shifts K+ intracellularly), **IV sodium bicarbonate, calcium gluconate** (stabilizes cardiac membranes; use with caution)
	  • <u>Hypocalcemia</u>: IV calcium gluconate
	  • <u>Hyperuricemia</u>: allopurinol
	  • *Peritoneal dialysis may be required*
	• **Osmotic diuretics (mannitol) or alkalinization of urine (sodium bicarbonate drip)** may be used in severe rhabdomyolysis (crush injuries)

Key Words & Most Common	• Acute muscle breakdown leading to release of myoglobin into blood stream • Trauma, exertion, immobility, crush injuries, seizures, cocaine are most common causes • Triad of muscle pain + weakness + tea/Coke colored urine • ECG may show hyperkalemia signs • Urine shows blood but no RBCs; urine myoglobin most specific test • Elevated CK • IV Fluids; electrolyte correction

Polymyositis

Etiology & Risk Factors	• Idiopathic autoimmune condition leading to inflammatory myopathy; primarily affects proximal muscles, neck, and pharynx • <u>Risk Factors</u>: **age (30-50 years old most common), female, African American**, history of viral infection/malignancy/autoimmune disorder, medication use (hydralazine, statins, ACEI)
Patho-physiology	• Direct myocyte damage secondary to cellular immune responses from abnormal cytotoxic T cell (CD8) and macrophage activation against muscular antigens

Signs & Symptoms	• **Progressive, symmetrical, proximal muscle weakness**
	  • Most commonly affects shoulders/pelvic muscles
	  • May have difficulty brushing/washing hair, rising from chair, kneeling climbing chairs, raising hands above head
	• **Generally painless**
	• **May develop arthralgias**, dysphagia
	• <u>Constitutional</u>: low-grade fever, anorexia, arthralgia, and weight loss
	• <u>Physical Exam</u>:
	  • **Decreased muscle strength** especially proximal muscles; may have muscle atrophy

Diagnosis	• <u>Labs</u>:
	  • **Muscle Enzymes: elevated creatine kinase (CK) and aldolase; best initial tests**
	  • <u>Inflammatory Markers</u>: elevated C-Reactive Protein (CRP), erythrocyte sedimentation rate (ESR), and rheumatoid factor (RF), antinuclear antibody (ANA)
	  • Complete Blood Count (CBC): may have lymphocytosis and thrombocytosis
	  • **Autoantibodies: anti-signal recognition particle (SRP) is most specific for polymyositis**; Anti-Jo-1 is a marker for fibrosing alveolitis
	• <u>**Abnormal Electromyography (EMG)**</u>: may show varying amplitude/velocity of membranous action potential or fibrillations with membrane irritability
	• <u>**Muscle Biopsy: definitive diagnosis**</u>; shows endomysial inflammation

Treatment	• <u>**High-Dose Corticosteroids: first-line; followed by steroid taper**</u> • <u>Immune-Modulators</u>: methotrexate, azathioprine, cyclosporine second-line; used for those that do not respond to steroids or have adverse side effects to steroids
Key Words & Most Common	• Idiopathic autoimmune inflammatory myopathy • Most commonly affects females age 30-50 • Progressive, symmetrical, proximal muscle weakness; painless • Decreased muscle strength (differentiates from polymyalgia rheumatica) • Elevated CK/aldolase; anti-signal recognition particle is most specific • High-dose corticosteroids + taper is first-line

Dermatomyositis

Etiology & Risk Factors	• Idiopathic autoimmune muscle disease characterized by muscle inflammation and dermatologic manifestations (rash) • <u>Etiology</u>: **unknown**; several genetic, immunologic, infectious (Coxsackie B, parvovirus, enterovirus), drugs (anti-neoplastic, antibiotics, NSAIDs, vaccines) and environmental factors (UV radiation, pollution) are implicated in dermatomyositis • <u>Risk Factors</u>: **age (40-50 years old most common), female, history of cancer** (lung, ovarian, GI)
Patho-physiology	• Inflammatory myopathy secondary to immune complex deposition within the vessels (complement-mediated vasculopathy) • Hypoxic injury leads to atrophy, degeneration, and necrosis

Signs & Symptoms	• **Progressive, symmetrical, proximal muscle weakness**
	• **Generally painless; may develop arthralgias**, dysphagia
	• <u>Constitutional</u>: low-grade fever, anorexia, arthralgia, and weight loss
	• <u>Physical Exam</u>:
	  • <u>**Decreased Muscle Strength**</u>: especially proximal muscles; may have muscle atrophy
	  • <u>**Gottron's Papules**</u>: erythematous/violaceous papules and raised scaly patches of the dorsal metacarpophalangeal/interphalangeal joints +/- ulceration
	  • <u>**Heliotrope Rash**</u>: purple/blue erythematous rash of the upper eyelids +/- periorbital edema
	  • <u>**Shawl Sign**</u>: erythema of posterior neck, upper back, and shoulders
	  • <u>V Sign</u>: erythematous macules of anterior neck and upper chest
	  • May have malar rash, photosensitivity, nail changes

Diagnosis	• <u>Labs</u>: underlying malignancy workup should be considered
	  • **Muscle Enzymes: elevated creatine kinase (CK) and aldolase; best initial tests**
	  • Elevated C-Reactive Protein (CRP), erythrocyte sedimentation rate (ESR), and rheumatoid factor (RF), antinuclear antibody (ANA)
	  • May have normocytic normochromic anemia
	  • <u>**Autoantibodies: Anti-Mi2 is most specific for dermatomyositis**</u>; Anti-Jo-1 is a marker for fibrosing alveolitis
	• <u>**Abnormal Electromyography (EMG)**</u>: may show varying amplitude/velocity of membranous action potential or fibrillations with membrane irritability
	• <u>**Muscle Biopsy: definitive diagnosis**</u>; shows endomysial inflammation

Treatment	• <u>**High-Dose Corticosteroids: first-line; followed by steroid taper**</u> • <u>**Hydroxychloroquine: utilized for skin rashes**</u> • <u>Immune-Modulators</u>: methotrexate, azathioprine second-line; indicated for those that do not respond to steroids or have adverse side effects to steroids
Key Words & Most Common	• Idiopathic autoimmune inflammatory myopathy • Most commonly affects females age 40-50 • Progressive, symmetrical, proximal muscle weakness; painless; decreased muscle strength; rash of hands, upper eyelids • Elevated CK/aldolase; Anti-Mi2 is most specific • High-dose corticosteroids + taper is first-line; hydroxychloroquine for rash

Gottron's Papules

Systemic Lupus Erythematosus (SLE) 🦴

Etiology & Risk Factors	• Chronic systemic autoimmune condition with multi-organ systemic involvement • <u>Risk Factors</u>: **age (20-30yo), female, African America or Asian**, genetic, environmental factors, **sun exposure**, infection (Epstein-Barr Virus), **estrogen (oral contraceptive pills)**, drugs (procainamide, hydralazine, sulfa drugs), vitamin D deficiency
Patho-physiology	• Activation of autoimmunity by an infectious, environmental, or exposure results in cellular dysfunction causing the immune system to be exposed to self-antigens • This leads to T and B cell activation and eventually a chronic immune response

Signs & Symptoms	• <u>Triad</u>: **joint pain + fever + malar "butterfly" rash**
	• <u>Constitutional Symptoms</u>: fever, fatigue, malaise, anorexia, weight loss, night sweats, arthralgias
	• <u>Mucocutaneous Symptoms</u>: variety of erythematous, firm, maculopapular lesions occurring on exposed face/neck, upper chest, elbows; alopecia; photosensitivity
	  • **Malar "Butterfly" Rash**: fixed erythematous rash of the bilateral cheeks and/or bridge of nose that spares nasolabial folds
	  • **Discoid Lupus**: annular erythematous plaques that progress to atrophic scars; cluster at light-exposed areas (face, scalp, ears)
	  • **Raynaud Syndrome**: distal extremity vasospasm leads to blanching and cyanosis of fingers/toes
	• <u>Systemic Symptoms</u>:
	  • **Central Nervous System (CNS)**: mild cognitive impairment, headache, personality changes, psychosis, seizures
	  • **Cardiopulmonary**: recurrent pleurisy, pericarditis, PE, pulmonary hypertension
	  • **Other**: **glomerulonephritis**, general lymphadenopathy, recurrent miscarriages, retinitis *Malar "Butterfly" Rash*

Diagnosis	• <u>**Anti-Nuclear Antibodies (ANA)**</u>: **initial screening test of choice; most sensitive test** (lacks specificity) • <u>**Anti-Double-Stranded DNA (anti-dsDNA) or Anti-Smith (anti-Sm)**</u>: **positive test is pathognomonic; highly specific test** (lacks sensitivity) • <u>Antiphospholipid Antibodies</u>: associated with thrombotic events and adverse pregnancy-related outcomes • <u>**Complement C3 and C4**</u>: decreased complement levels; correlates with disease activity • <u>Other</u>: leukopenia (lymphopenia), thrombocytopenia, hemolytic anemia, anemia of chronic disease, elevated ESR/CRP, urinalysis may show RBC/WBC casts
Treatment	• <u>**Supportive**</u>: education, emotional support, exercise, sleep hygiene, sun protection (skin coverings, sunscreen), smoking cessation, topical corticosteroids for rash • <u>**Mild**</u>: (joint, skin, mucosal involvement); **hydroxychloroquine +/- NSAIDs**; alternatives include chloroquine or low-dose corticosteroids • <u>**Moderate**</u>: (multiple organ involvement, but not organ threatening); **hydroxychloroquine + short term corticosteroids** • <u>**Severe**</u>: (life or organ threatening); **high-dose corticosteroids (IV methylprednisolone) + immunosuppressants** (cyclophosphamide, mycophenolate, azathioprine) • Rituximab for recurrent or refractory cases
Key Words & Most Common	• Female, age 20-30 • Triad of joint pain + fever + malar rash (cheeks and bridge of nose, spares nasolabial folds); multi-organ involvement • ANA screening (most sensitive); anti-dsDNA or anti-Sm to diagnose (most specific); decreased complement C3/C4 • Treatment based on severity of condition • Hydroxychloroquine +/- NSAIDs +/- steroids • High-dose steroids + immunosuppressants if severe

Drug-Induced Lupus 🦴

Etiology & Risk Factors	• Autoimmune condition similar to systemic lupus erythematosus caused by use of certain medications • <u>Etiology</u>: **hydralazine, procainamide, isoniazid, quinidine**, antihypertensives (diuretics, CCBs, BB), proton pump inhibitors (omeprazole, pantoprazole), anti-TNF drugs (adalimumab), and antifungals (terbinafine)
Patho-physiology	• Demethylation of DNA and alteration of self-antigens by medication leading to lupus-like phenomenon
Signs & Symptoms	• <u>Lupus-Like Symptoms</u>: fever, rash, arthralgias, serositis (pleurisy, pericarditis) • *Less systemic involvement than SLE*
Diagnosis	• <u>**Anti-Nuclear Antibodies (ANA)**</u>: **elevated** • <u>**Anti-Histone Antibodies**</u>: **hallmark of condition** • *Decreased complement levels or anti-dsDNA are not typically seen*
Treatment	• <u>**Discontinuation of Offending Medication**</u>: **mainstay of management** • <u>Analgesia</u>: NSAIDs +/- topical or oral corticosteroids for symptomatic management
Key Words & Most Common	• Lupus-like phenomenon caused by certain medications • Hydralazine and procainamide most commonly implicated • Fever, rash, arthralgias • ANA + Anti-Histone Antibodies • D/C offending medication • Symptom management (NSAIDs/steroids)

Anti-Phospholipid Syndrome

Etiology & Risk Factors	• Idiopathic autoimmune disorder characterized by arterial/venous thrombosis due to autoantibodies that are directed against phospholipid-binding proteins • **Hallmark is presence of antiphospholipid antibodies (APLA) in setting of arterial/venous thrombus and/or loss of pregnancy** • May occur as primary condition or in setting of other conditions including systemic lupus erythematosus • <u>Risk Factors</u>: **systemic lupus erythematosus**, smoking, immobilization, **increased estrogen (OCPs, pregnancy, hormone replacement therapy)**, malignancy, nephrotic syndrome, hypertension, hyperlipidemia
Patho-physiology	• Antiphospholipid antibodies are pathogenic antibodies that lead to complement-mediated thrombosis by interacting with protein C, annexin V, platelets, proteases, tissue factor, and by impairing fibrinolysis
Signs & Symptoms	• <u>Vascular Thrombosis</u>: deep vein thrombosis (DVT), pulmonary embolism (PE), arterial thrombus (manifests as transient ischemic attack or stroke) • <u>Pregnancy Morbidity</u>: pregnancy loss in 2nd or 3rd trimester; multiple/recurrent miscarriages; may develop HELLP syndrome, preeclampsia, premature birth • <u>Cutaneous Involvement</u>: livedo reticularis (mottled reticulated vascular pattern appearing as lace-like purple/blue discoloration of the skin) • <u>Valvular Involvement</u>: mitral and aortic valves most commonly involved; manifests as thickening, nodules, or vegetations leading to stenosis/insufficiency
Diagnosis	• <u>**Lupus Anticoagulant Test**</u>: **prolonged partial thromboplastin time (PTT) with associated thrombosis**; strongest predictor for adverse pregnancy-related events • <u>**Anticardiolipin and Anti-Beta-2-Glycoprotein I Antibodies**</u>: antiphospholipid antibodies in plasma are measured by immunoassays of IgG/IgM antibodies that bind to phospholipid/beta-2 glycoprotein 1 complexes • <u>Mixing Studies</u>: prolonged PTT that does not correct when mixed with normal plasma due to presence of inhibitor • Returns to normal after adding quantity of phospholipids • <u>Other</u>: thrombocytopenia, anemia, elevated ESR, renal involvement

Treatment	• <u>Anticoagulation</u>: unfractionated heparin, low molecular weight heparin (LMWH) or warfarin (**warfarin contraindicated in pregnancy**)
	    • **LMWH may be used in pregnancy to prevent fetal loss**
	    • Recurrent thrombosis may require lifelong anticoagulation; aspirin has been used for prophylaxis
	• <u>Hydroxychloroquine</u>: indicated if patient has systemic lupus erythematosus

Key Words & Most Common	• Presence of antiphospholipid antibodies in setting of arterial/venous thrombus and/or loss of pregnancy • SLE, estrogen exposure are risk factors • Vascular thrombosis (DVT/PE/TIA) + pregnancy morbidity (recurrent miscarriages) • Lupus anticoagulant test; anticardiolipin/anti-beta-2-glycoprotein I antibody test • Anticoagulation with heparin; LMWH in pregnancy to prevent fetal loss; warfarin contraindicated in pregnancy

Sjögren Syndrome

Etiology & Risk Factors	• Systemic autoimmune condition due to lymphocytic infiltration of exocrine glands (lacrimal and salivary glands) • May present alone (primary) with other autoimmune disorders (secondary) including rheumatoid arthritis (RA) and systemic lupus erythematosus (SLE), Hashimotos • <u>Risk Factors</u>: **age (45-55 years old), female (90%)**, history of autoimmune condition, genetic predisposition (HLA-DR3)
Patho-physiology	• Infiltration of CD4+ T cells (and some B cells) of lacrimal, salivary, and other exocrine glands; inflammatory cytokines are produced which damage the secretory ducts

Signs & Symptoms	• <u>Glandular Manifestations</u>: **parotid gland enlargement**
	    • **Dry Eyes (keratoconjunctivitis sicca)**: sandy, gritty sensation, corneal damage
	    • **Dry Mouth (xerostomia)**: difficulty chewing/swallowing, secondary *Candida* infection, tooth decay
	    • <u>Vaginal Dryness</u>: presents as painful intercourse (dyspareunia)
	    • <u>Upper Respiratory Dryness</u>: cough, nosebleeds
	• <u>Extra-glandular Manifestations</u>: **arthralgias**, lymphadenopathy, Raynaud syndrome, interstitial lung disease, vasculitis, peripheral neuropathy

Diagnosis	• <u>**Anti-Nuclear Antibodies**</u>: sensitive screening test • <u>**AntiSS-A (Ro) and AntiSS-B (La) Autoantibodies**</u>: best initial test; antiSS-A Ro is most sensitive/specific autoantibody test but not diagnostic • <u>**Schirmer Test**</u>: positive if decreased tear production using filter paper strip on lower eyelid (<5mm of filter paper moistened is positive; normal is 15mm moistened) • <u>**Lip or Parotid Gland Biopsy**</u>: **definitive diagnosis**; shows focal lymphocytic sialadenitis • <u>Other</u>: elevated ESR, positive rheumatoid factor, anemia, leukopenia

Treatment	• <u>Supportive</u>:
	    • <u>Dry Eyes</u>: **artificial tears, topical ocular cyclosporine**
	    • <u>Dry Mouth</u>: **increased fluids, chewing gum**, saliva substitutes, closed mouth breathing habits
	    • <u>Dry Mucosa</u>: humidifiers, nasal saline
	• <u>Hydroxychloroquine</u>: recommended for inflammatory polyarthritis and slow progression of disease
	• <u>Corticosteroids</u>: recommended for extra-glandular (systemic) treatment
	• <u>Cholinergic Medications</u>: **Pilocarpine or Cevimeline** to stimulate secretion production
	• <u>Immune Modulators</u>: DMARDs (methotrexate, azathioprine) may be used as steroid-sparing agents

Key Words & Most Common	• Autoimmune condition resulting in exocrine gland (lacrimal/salivary) dysfunction; most common among females age 45-55yo • Dry eyes, dry mouth, dry mucous membranes • ANA screening, antiSS-A (Ro) and antiSS-B (la) autoantibodies are more sensitive/specific; Schirmer test • Supportive care + hydroxychloroquine for arthralgias; steroids for systemic treatment • Pilocarpine or Cevimeline (cholinergic) to stimulate glandular secretions

Dry Mouth

Dry Eyes

Parotid gland enlargement

Scleroderma

Etiology & Risk Factors	• Chronic autoimmune connective tissue condition characterized by collagen deposition leading to skin, soft tissue, and organ fibrosis; also known as systemic sclerosis • <u>Etiology</u>: no known specific etiology; multiple genetic and environmental factors may contribute • <u>Risk Factors</u>: **age (30-50 years old most common), female**
Patho-physiology	• Endothelial cells produce large quantities of endothelin I leading to vasoconstriction, vascular damage and fibroblast activation which also produces activated oxygen species leading to further vascular remodeling. • Vascular remodeling leads to collagen and extracellular protein overproduction and accumulation
Signs & Symptoms	• <u>Localized</u>: limited to skin and underlying tissue affecting face/neck and distal to elbows/knees; <u>Diffuse</u>: involves proximal extremities/trunk/organs • <u>CREST Syndrome</u>: **C**alcinosis cutis (calcium deposits in soft tissue), **R**aynaud's phenomenon (white, purple/blue, red vasospastic discoloration of digits), **E**sophageal motility disorder, **S**clerodactyly (taut skin of hand causing claw-like deformity), **T**elangiectasias • <u>Skin/Nail Manifestations</u>: **taut, shiny, hypo/hyperpigmented, thickened skin,** telangiectasias, digital ulcers, abnormal microvasculature of nails, **sclerodactyly** • <u>Joint Manifestations</u>: polyarthralgia, flexion contractures of fingers, wrist, elbows • <u>GI Manifestations</u>: esophageal dysfunction, dysphagia, GERD, malabsorption • <u>Cardiopulmonary Manifestations</u>: lung fibrosis, interstitial lung disease can lead to exertional dyspnea and restrictive disease pattern, pulmonary hypertension
Diagnosis	• <u>**Anti-Nuclear Antibodies**</u>: sensitive screening test; nonspecific • <u>**Anti-Centromere Antibodies**</u>: specific to diagnosing CREST syndrome (limited) • <u>**Anti-SCL-70 (Topoisomerase I) Antibodies**</u>: specific to diagnosing diffuse disease
Treatment	• **Treatment is specific to symptoms or organ involvement** • <u>GERD</u>: proton pump inhibitors (PPIs), elevate head of bed, smaller meals • <u>Raynaud's Phenomenon</u>: vasodilators; calcium channel blockers (CCB), bosentan, sildenafil; protection from cold, smoking cessation • <u>Immune Modulators</u>: DMARDs (methotrexate, azathioprine) may be used in severe disease • <u>Hypertension/Renal Crisis</u>: ACE inhibitors • <u>Pain/Inflammation</u>: corticosteroids • <u>Pulmonary Fibrosis</u>: cyclophosphamide • <u>Localized Scleroderma</u>: topical corticosteroids
Key Words & Most Common	• Chronic autoimmune conditions leading to skin, soft tissue, organ fibrosis; more common in females age 30-50 • CREST Syndrome: Calcinosis, Raynaud's, Esophageal dysfunction, Sclerodactyly, Telangiectasias • Skin is taut, shiny, hypo/hyperpigmented and thickened • ANA sensitive screening; anti-centromere antibodies for limited disease, anti-SCL-70 antibodies for diffuse disease • Treatment specific to symptoms/organ involvement

Kawasaki Disease

Etiology & Risk Factors	• Acute, self-limited, small/medium vessel vasculitis that may involve the coronary arteries; also known as mucocutaneous lymph node syndrome • <u>Etiology</u>: unknown, may be unidentified respiratory/viral agent • <u>Risk Factors</u>: **age (<5 years old most common), male, Asian (specifically children of Japanese descent)**
Patho-physiology	• Infectious agent enters body through respiratory tract and activates lymphocytes, cytokines, and proteinases, (tumor necrosis factor alpha (TNF-a), Interleukin 1, 4 and 6) leading to myocarditis and vasculitis
Signs & Symptoms	• <u>**Fever:**</u> **abrupt onset of fever** (usually lasting >5 days) • Associated fatigue, malaise, lethargy, colicky abdominal pain • <u>**Rash:**</u> **described as polymorphous, erythematous macular rash on trunk and accentuated on perineum** • <u>Mucositis</u>: Injected pharynx; conjunctivitis; erythematous, swollen or fissured lips; **erythematous tongue with prominent papillation (strawberry tongue)** • <u>Other</u>: tender cervical lymphadenopathy, extremity changes (erythema, variable edema of palms/soles), desquamation of superficial skin layer, arthralgias

Diagnosis	• <u>**Clinical Criteria**</u>: **fever > 5 days + 4 of the following 5 (CREAM mnemonic)**
	  1. **C**onjunctivitis: bilateral, nonexudative
	  2. **R**ash: polymorphous truncal exanthem
	  3. **E**xtremity Changes: edema, erythema, desquamation
	  4. **A**denopathy: cervical lymphadenopathy
	  5. **M**ucositis: injection, fissuring, strawberry tongue
	• <u>Labs</u>: leukocytosis, normocytic anemia, thrombocytosis, elevated ESR/CRP, WBCs in urine (with negative urine culture), hypoalbuminemia
	• <u>ECG and Echocardiogram</u>: performed to rule out complications (coronary vessel arteritis/aneurysm, valvular abnormalities, MI, myocarditis, pericarditis)

Treatment	• <u>**High Dose IV Immunoglobulin + Aspirin**</u>: indicated to decrease inflammation of coronary arteries and for symptomatic relief

Key Words & Most Common	• Acute vasculitis that may involve coronary arteries; most common in young Asian males
	• Fever + 4/5 of following
	  • Conjunctivitis
	  • Rash
	  • Extremity edema/erythema
	  • Cervical lymphadenopathy
	  • Oral Mucositis (strawberry tongue)
	• IV immunoglobulin + aspirin

Polyarteritis Nodosa

Etiology & Risk Factors	• Systemic necrotizing vasculitis primarily involving medium-sized vessels • **Most commonly affects renal, peripheral nerve, skin, muscle and GI vessels; pulmonary vessels are *not* involved** • **Most common at arterial bifurcation/branch sites** • <u>Etiology</u>: **idiopathic**; secondary PAN results from hepatitis B, hepatitis C, or malignancy (hairy cell leukemia) • <u>Risk Factors</u>: **middle age** (peaks at 50 years old), male
Patho-physiology	• Transmural necrotizing vasculitis and intimal proliferation leads to vessel thickening and inflammation • Vessel narrowing, inflammation and reduction of blood flow occurs and may result in thrombosis or aneurysm
Signs & Symptoms	• <u>Constitutional</u>: fever, fatigue, malaise, anorexia, night sweats, weight loss, myalgias, arthralgias and generalized weakness • <u>Nervous System</u>: **multiple peripheral neuropathies** (peroneal nerve most common, ulnar, median), headache, mononeuritis multiplex, stroke, seizures • <u>Renal</u>: **hypertension** (renal artery stenosis), oliguria, uremia, renal infarct/ischemia can lead to renal failure • <u>Gastrointestinal</u>: **postprandial abdominal pain** (mesenteric artery vasculitis), nausea, vomiting • <u>Cardiac</u>: coronary artery disease (may be asymptomatic) • <u>Cutaneous</u>: **livedo reticularis** (mottled reticulated vascular pattern appearing as lace-like purple/blue discoloration of the skin), skin ulcers, bullous/vesicular eruptions, palpable purpura (fingers, ankles, malleoli, pretibial), Raynaud phenomenon • <u>Genital</u>: orchitis may occur

Diagnosis	• <u>Labs</u>: **non-specific**
	    • <u>CBC</u>: leukocytosis, thrombocytosis
	    • <u>Urinalysis</u>: proteinuria, microscopic hematuria
	    • Elevated ESR; hepatitis B and C serologies to rule out secondary etiology
	    • ANCA negative (P-ANCA positive in <20%)
	• **Arteriography: renal or mesenteric; shows microaneurysms or stenosis of medium-sized vessels**
	• **Biopsy: definitive diagnosis**; shows necrotizing vessel vasculitis with no granuloma inflammation

Treatment	• **Corticosteroids: initial treatment** if mild symptoms; often requires months of treatment • **Cyclophosphamide:** if severe cases or refractory; used in combination with steroids • **Immune Modulators:** DMARDs (methotrexate, azathioprine) may be if unable to tolerate or refractory to steroids • Hypertension management (ACEI); Hepatitis B treatment if applicable
Key Words & Most Common	• Systemic necrotizing vasculitis most commonly affecting renal, peripheral nerve, skin/muscle, and GI medium-sized vessels • New onset HTN in adult; multiple peripheral neuropathy, postprandial abdominal pain, livedo reticularis • Non-specific lab testing, hepatitis B/C serologies; arteriography shows microaneurysms; biopsy for definitive diagnosis • Corticosteroids +/- cyclophosphamide; immune modulators

Eosinophilic Granulomatosis with Polyangiitis

Etiology & Risk Factors	• Systemic necrotizing granulomatous vasculitis of small and medium sized vessels • Also known as Churg Straus Syndrome • Characterized by extravascular necrotizing granulomas, eosinophilia, and eosinophilic tissue infiltration • <u>Etiology</u>: unknown; allergies, infections, medications considered; may be associated with leukotriene inhibitor use (montelukast and zafirlukast)
Patho-physiology	• Possible allergic mechanism with eosinophil/neutrophil degranulation products leading to tissue injury and activation of T lymphocytes leading to inflammation
Signs & Symptoms	• **Triad: Asthma + Eosinophilia + Chronic Sinusitis** • <u>Prodrome</u>: allergic rhinitis, nasal polyposis, asthma, or a combination • <u>Eosinophilic Phase</u>: multiorgan involvement (particularly skin, lungs, and GI tract) caused by eosinophilic infiltration; subcutaneous nodules, eosinophilic pneumonia, abdominal pain, eosinophilic gastroenteritis • <u>Vasculitis Phase</u>: potentially life-threatening vasculitis vascular and extravascular granulomatosis; presents as constitutional symptoms (fever, weight loss, malaise)
Diagnosis	• Clinical Diagnosis • <u>Labs</u>: **eosinophilia; positive P-ANCA**, elevated ESR/CRP, positive rheumatoid factor (RF) • <u>Chest X-Ray (CXR)</u>: may show transient, patchy pulmonary infiltrates • <u>Biopsy</u>: most sensitive/specific test; shows granulomatous necrotizing vasculitis
Treatment	• **Corticosteroids: mainstay of treatment**; inhibits eosinophilic survival in extravascular tissue • **Cyclophosphamide**: if severe or refractory to steroids • <u>Immune Modulators</u>: DMARDs (methotrexate, azathioprine) may be if unable to tolerate or refractory to steroids
Key Words & Most Common	• Systemic necrotizing granulomatous vasculitis of unknown etiology (may be associated with montelukast) • Triad of asthma + eosinophilic + chronic sinusitis • Labs show eosinophilia, positive P-ANCA, elevated ESR/CRP • Biopsy is most sensitive/specific test • Corticosteroids +/- cyclophosphamide

Granulomatosis with Polyangiitis 🦴

Etiology & Risk Factors	• Systemic necrotizing condition characterized by granulomatous inflammation, small/medium sized vasculitis, and focal necrotizing glomerulonephritis • Also known as Wegener's Granulomatosis • **Most commonly affects upper respiratory tract, lungs, and kidneys** • <u>Etiology</u>: not fully understood; genetic link, medications or microbial infection etiology may be implicated
Patho-physiology	• Neutrophilic microabscesses progress to macronecrosis; granuloma inflammation ultimately result in partial or total occlusion of blood vessels • Central area of necrosis is surrounded by lymphocytes, plasma cells, macrophages, and giant cells further damaging the submucosa

Signs & Symptoms	• **Triad: upper respiratory + lower respiratory tract + kidney involvement**
	   • <u>Upper Respiratory Tract</u>: **sinusitis**, rhinitis, **saddle nose deformity, otitis media**, mastoiditis, hearing loss, refractory sinusitis, epistaxis
	   • <u>Lower Respiratory Tract</u>: **cough, dyspnea**, hemoptysis, wheezing, pulmonary nodules/infiltrates, alveolar hemorrhage (does not respond to antibiotics)
	   • <u>Kidney Involvement</u>: **glomerulonephritis**; rapidly progressive, hematuria, RBC casts

Diagnosis	• <u>Labs</u>: leukocytosis, anemia, thrombocytosis, elevated ESR/CRP; kidney function may be affected
	   • <u>**Cytoplasmic Anti-Nuclear Cytoplasmic Antibodies (C-ANCA)**</u>: **positive; best initial lab test**
	• <u>Urinalysis</u>: hematuria, proteinuria
	• <u>Chest X-Ray/CT</u>: nonspecific abnormalities; evaluate for pulmonary lesions or hemorrhage
	• <u>Biopsy</u>: **definitive diagnosis**; lung more accurate than kidney biopsy
	   • Lung shows necrotizing granulomas
	   • Renal shows necrotizing focal crescentic or noncrescentic **glomerulonephritis**

Treatment	• <u>**Corticosteroids + Cyclophosphamide**</u>: indicated in moderate to severe disease • <u>Corticosteroids + Methotrexate</u>: indicated in mild disease (no glomerulonephritis or organ-threatening disease)
Key Words & Most Common	• Systemic necrotizing condition affecting upper respiratory tract, lungs, kidneys • <u>Upper</u>: Sinusitis, saddle nose deformity, otitis media • <u>Lower</u>: Cough/dyspnea, wheezing • <u>Kidney</u>: glomerulonephritis • C-ANCA positive • Biopsy is definitive diagnosis • Corticosteroids + Cyclophosphamide

Microscopic Polyangiitis 🦴

Etiology & Risk Factors	• Systemic necrotizing vasculitis without immune globulin deposition affecting small and medium vessels • **Not associated with upper respiratory symptoms** or granulomatous inflammation • Primarily affects small vessels (capillaries and postcapillary venules) • <u>Etiology</u>: not fully understood; genetic causes, infections, medications have been implicated
Patho-physiology	• Unknown pathogenesis; may stem from activation of neutrophils and MPO-ANCA with receptors present on the endothelial surface leading to small vessel vasculitis
Signs & Symptoms	• <u>Prodromal Illness</u>: fever, arthralgia, malaise, weight loss • <u>Renal</u>: hematuria, **acute glomerulonephritis** • <u>Cutaneous</u>: **palpable purpura**; may have nailbed infarcts/splinter hemorrhages • **Respiratory**: cough, dyspnea, hemoptysis; **does not affect upper respiratory tract**
Diagnosis	• <u>Labs</u>: leukocytosis, anemia, thrombocytosis, elevated ESR/CRP; elevated BUN/Creatinine • <u>**Perinuclear Anti-Nuclear Cytoplasmic Antibodies (P-ANCA)**</u>: **positive; best initial lab test** • <u>Chest X-Ray (CXR)</u>: nonspecific findings; may show bilateral patchy infiltrates • **Biopsy**: **definitive diagnosis**; shows non-granulomatous inflammation and/or focal segmental necrotizing glomerulonephritis (renal biopsy)
Treatment	• **Corticosteroids + Cyclophosphamide** in moderate to severe disease • Corticosteroids + Methotrexate in mild disease (no glomerulonephritis or organ-threatening disease)
Key Words & Most Common	• Systemic necrotizing vasculitis affecting small/medium vessels • Does not affect upper respiratory tract • Constitutional symptoms • Acute glomerulonephritis • Palpable purpura • Lower Respiratory symptoms • P-ANCA positive • Biopsy is definitive • Corticosteroids + Cyclophosphamide

Henoch-Schönlein-Purpura

Etiology & Risk Factors	• Acute systemic immunoglobulin A (IgA) mediated small-vessel vasculitis • **Most common vasculitis in children** (90% occur in children) • Etiology: small-vessel vasculitis • Risk Factors: **age (3-15 years old most common; most cases occur by 10 years old); often preceded by upper respiratory infection (Group A Streptococcus,** Coxsackievirus, parvovirus B19, adenovirus); other environmental or genetic factors
Patho-physiology	• Antigenic exposure from infection leads to IgA-antibody immune complexes to deposit in the small vessels of the skin, joints, kidneys, and gastrointestinal tract • Influx of pro-inflammatory mediators to specific site leads to clinical manifestations
Signs & Symptoms	• Symptoms may develop over days to weeks • Rash: palpable purpura; begins as erythematous/macular/urticarial wheals that progress into ecchymosis and petechiae • **Most common in lower extremities/buttocks** • Abdominal Pain: acute pain described as diffuse and colicky; may have GI bleeding • Arthritis: migratory arthralgia; typically affects knees and ankles • Glomerulonephritis: azotemia (elevated BUN/creatinine), hematuria, proteinuria
Diagnosis	• **Clinical Diagnosis** • Labs: may have elevated BUN/creatinine; normal PT/PTT and platelets (purpura secondary to vasculitis rather than coagulopathy) • Urinalysis: hematuria, proteinuria, RBC casts • Kidney Biopsy: definitive diagnosis; shows mesangial IgA deposits and leukoclastic vasculitis; unnecessary if clinical diagnosis is clear
Treatment	• **Supportive: self-limiting disease**; hydration, NSAIDs for pain (if no renal involvement) • **Corticosteroids:** for severe arthralgias, abdominal pain, or renal insufficiency
Key Words & Most Common	• Acute IgA mediated vasculitis most commonly seen in children • Preceded by URI (GAS most common) • Rash (palpable purpura) + Abdominal pain + Arthritis + Glomerulonephritis • Clinical Diagnosis • Kidney biopsy for definitive diagnosis, rarely performed • Supportive care +/- steroids

Diffuse palpable purpura of buttocks/lower extremities

Psoriatic Arthritis

Etiology & Risk Factors	• Spondyloarthropathy and chronic inflammatory arthritis associated with psoriasis • About 20% of patients with psoriasis develop psoriatic arthritis • Risk Factors: **HLA-B27 genotype positive,** family history of psoriasis, age (30-40 years old most common)
Patho-physiology	• IL-23 is a central cytokine produced when an environmental trigger (infection or mechanical stress) initiates a chronic inflammatory process involving the skin/joints
Signs & Symptoms	• Arthritis: joint pain/stiffness • **Distal interphalangeal (DIP) joints of fingers/toes especially affected** • Dactylitis: **sausage-shaped deformity of digits** of hands/feet due to inflammation • Enthesopathy: tendinous insertion point inflammation (Achilles tendinitis, patellar tendinitis, elbow epicondylitis) • Sacroiliitis: manifests usually as unilateral low back pain • Psoriasis: **erythematous plaques with thick silvery-white scales** and nail pitting commonly affecting the back of the forearms, shins, navel area, and scalp.

Diagnosis	• **Clinical Diagnosis**
	• Labs: no specific diagnostic lab test; **rheumatoid factor (RF) may be positive;** elevated ESR/CRP; will have negative anti-CCP (highly specific for rheumatoid arthritis)
	• X-Ray: **best initial test**
	  • **"Pencil in Cup" Deformity of DIPJ:** periarticular bony erosions and bone resorption; thin bone inserts into thickened part of adjacent bone
	  • Erosive changes, gross joint destruction, joint space narrowing

Treatment	• **NSAIDs: first-line initial medication** for pain control • Immune-Modulators: **methotrexate is preferred medication** for severe disease • TNF-α Antagonists: adalimumab, infliximab; if refractory to methotrexate • Interleukin Antagonists: ustekinumab, secukinumab; indicated if refractory to TNF-α antagonists

Key Words & Most Common	• Chronic inflammatory arthritis in patient with psoriasis
	  Arthritis (especially DIPJ)
	  Dactylitis (sausage fingers)
	• Psoriasis (erythematous plaques with silver scale)
	• Clinical diagnosis
	• RF +; anti-CCP -
	• X-Ray shows pencil in cup deformity
	• NSAIDs → methotrexate

Pencil-In-Cup

Periarticular erosions and bone resorption

Thin bone inserts into thickened part of adjacent bone

Ankylosing Spondylitis

Etiology & Risk Factors	• Chronic inflammatory arthropathy of the axial skeleton affecting the spine and sacroiliac joints • <u>Etiology</u>: not fully understood • <u>Risk Factors</u>: **age (20-30 years old most common) males, HLA-B27 genotype positive**, history of autoimmune condition, family history of ankylosing spondylitis
Patho-physiology	• Idiopathic etiology causes a cytokine (TNF-α and TGF-b) mediated inflammatory process leading to inflammation, fibrosis and ossification points of enthesitis

Signs & Symptoms	• **Progressive back pain/stiffness**
	  • **Worse in morning**
	  • **Improves with activity/exercise**
	  • **No improvement with rest**
	  • **Sacroiliitis**
	• Decreased trunk range of motion
	• **Kyphosis** (loss of lumbar lordosis with a fixed "bent-forward" posture)
	• <u>Systemic Manifestations</u>: Achilles and patellar tendinitis, dactylitis, **uveitis**, aortic insufficiency, cardiac conduction abnormalities, dyspnea/cough (pulmonary fibrosis)

Diagnosis	• <u>Labs</u>: **elevated ESR/CRP**; negative RF and ANA; HLA-B27 positivity (90%)
	• <u>Spinal X-Ray</u>: subchondral erosions, sclerosis, and joint fusion of sacroiliac (SI) joint (**sacroiliitis**)
	  • **"Squaring" of vertebral bodies**
	  • **Bamboo Spine:** thoracolumbar or lumbosacral fusion by syndesmophytes; **loss of lumbar curvature**
	• <u>Spinal MRI</u>: most accurate imaging test

Treatment	• <u>Supportive</u>: exercise, physical therapy, posture training, ROM exercises • <u>**NSAIDs**</u>: **first-line for pain control and suppress joint inflammation** • <u>Sulfasalazine</u>: reduces peripheral joint symptoms • <u>**TNF-α Antagonists**</u>: etanercept, adalimumab, infliximab; effective treatment for inflammatory back pain especially if refractory to NSAIDs
Key Words & Most Common	• Chronic inflammatory spinal/SI arthropathy • Young male with +HLA-B27 genotype • Progressive back pain/stiffness; worse in morning; improves with rest • Kyphosis; uveitis • Elevated ESR • X-Ray shows squaring of vertebral bodies; Bamboo Spine • NSAIDs +/- TNF-α Antagonists

Squaring of vertebral bodies

Loss of lordosis

Reactive Arthritis

Etiology & Risk Factors	• Inflammatory arthritis that presents days/weeks after a GI/GU infection or inflammation to another anatomical site • Also known as Reiter Syndrome • <u>Etiology</u>: triggered by a bacterial infection of the genitourinary tract (***Chlamydia trachomatis,*** *Neisseria gonorrhea*) or **gastrointestinal tract** (*Salmonella, Shigella, Campylobacter, Yersinia*) • <u>Risk Factors</u>: **age (20-30 years old most common), male**, HLA-B27 genotype positive, history of sexual intercourse (often with new partner) or high-risk sexual behavior
Patho-physiology	• Cytotoxic T lymphocytes are induced by fragments of bacteria when they reach systemic circulation which then attack the synovium; unknown why the localization to synovium of joints occurs
Signs & Symptoms	• <u>**Triad**</u>: **arthritis + ocular involvement (conjunctivitis, uveitis) + genital involvement (urethritis, cervicitis)** • <u>Preceding Infection</u>: gastroenteritis, **urethritis** • <u>Musculoskeletal</u>: **arthritis** (large joints of lower extremity), **enthesitis** (pain at tendonous insertion point), dactylitis (sausage shaped digits), low back pain • <u>Extra-Articular</u>: **conjunctivitis**, uveitis, dysuria, oral lesions • **Keratoderma Blennorhagicum**: yellowish-brown vesicles/pustules occurring on palms and soles that become hyperkeratotic and form crusts
Diagnosis	• **Clinical diagnosis** • <u>Urine STD Screen</u>: **Nucleic acid amplification test (NAAT) for gonorrhea/chlamydia** • <u>Synovial Fluid Analysis</u>: rule out septic arthritis; may test for gonorrhea/chlamydia • <u>Labs</u>: elevated ESR/CRP; negative RF and ANA; HLA-B27 positivity

Treatment	• First-Line:
	  • **NSAIDs: pain management**
	• Second-Line:
	  • <u>Sulfasalazine</u>: reduces peripheral joint symptoms
	  • <u>Methotrexate</u>: second-line treatment if refractory to NSAIDs
	  • <u>Intraarticular Corticosteroid Injection</u>: local steroid injection to reduce inflammation
	• <u>Antibiotics</u>: **treatment of underlying infectious etiology**
	  • **Ceftriaxone + doxycycline for Gonorrhea + Chlamydia infection**; treatment often for 3-6 months

Key Words & Most Common	• Inflammatory arthritis that may occur as result of GI/GU infection (chlamydia/gonorrhea most common) • Arthritis +/- conjunctivitis +/- urethritis • <u>Keratoderma Blennorhagicum</u>: yellow/brown vesicles of palms/soles that become hyperkeratotic • Clinical Diagnosis; test for gonorrhea/chlamydia • NSAIDs first line for pain; treat underlying infection

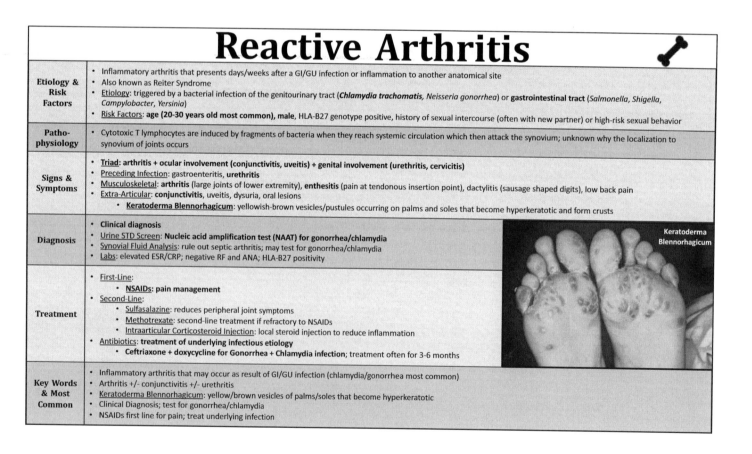

Keratoderma Blennorhagicum

Gout

Negatively birefringent, needle-shaped urate crystals

Etiology & Risk Factors	• Inflammatory arthritis characterized by monosodium urate monohydrate crystal(uric acid) deposition in the tissues
	• <u>Etiology</u>: **hyperuricemia** secondary to renal hypo-excretion of uric acid or overproduction of uric acid
	• <u>Risk Factors</u>: **male (90%)**, **metabolic disorder (diabetes, obesity)**, diet, medications, renal disorder, trauma to area, dehydration
	   • <u>Purine-Rich Diet</u>: **alcohol**, **seafood** (shellfish), organs (liver, kidney), **red meat** (beef, pork), sweetened drinks (soda pop), high-fructose corn syrup
	   • <u>Medication</u>: **diuretics**, ACEI/ARBs (except Losartan) pyrazinamide, ethambutol, aspirin
	   • <u>Comorbid Conditions</u>: **diabetes, obesity**, heart disease, renal insufficiency, hypertension

Patho-physiology	• Monosodium urate crystals (product of purine metabolism) deposited into bone/joint/tissue resulting in inflammatory arthritis

Signs & Symptoms	• **Sudden onset of focal joint pain**; can be excruciating and is progressive over hours/days
	   • Often **nocturnal**
	   • **Metatarsophalangeal (MTP) joint of a great toe is most commonly affected joint** (podagra); can also occur in knee, ankle, wrist, elbow
	• **Erythema, effusion, warmth, tenderness** of affected joint; may have fever
	• <u>Tophi</u>: firm, yellow/white subcutaneous nodules under transparent skin; occur from granuloma formation around crystal deposits

Diagnosis	• **Clinical Diagnosis** • <u>**Synovial Fluid Analysis**</u>: diagnostic test of choice; **negatively birefringent, needle-shaped monosodium urate crystals** • <u>X-Ray</u>: unnecessary for diagnosis; may show punched-out bony erosions with sclerotic margins (mouse/rate bite lesions); gouty tophi • <u>Labs</u>: elevated ESR/CRP, elevated serum uric acid level

Treatment	• <u>Supportive</u>: alcohol cessation (especially beer), low-purine diet, weight loss, discontinue diuretics
	• <u>Acute</u>:
	   • **NSAIDs; initial treatment of choice for pain control**
	   • <u>Corticosteroids</u>: if refractory to or unable to tolerate NSAIDs; oral vs. intraarticular injection
	   • <u>Colchicine</u>: alternative to NSAIDs
	• <u>Chronic</u>:
	   • **Allopurinol**: first-line for chronic management (Febuxostat alternative); xanthine oxidase inhibitor to block urate production and prevent acute flares
	   • <u>Probenecid</u>: uricosuric drug (promotes urate excretion); contraindicated in renal insufficiency

Key Words & Most Common	• Inflammatory arthritis most common in males; precipitated by diet high in purines, medications or comorbid conditions • Sudden onset of pain; most common at first MTP joint; erythema, effusion, warmth • Synovial fluid analysis shows negatively birefringent, needle-shaped monosodium urate crystals • <u>Acute</u>: NSAIDs vs steroids vs colchicine • <u>Chronic</u>: allopurinol

Calcium Pyrophosphate Dihydrate Crystal Deposition Disease

Positively birefringent, rhomboid-shaped calcium pyrophosphate crystals

Etiology & Risk Factors	• Crystal deposition arthropathy resulting from **calcium pyrophosphate dihydrate deposition** to the synovial and periarticular tissue leading to inflammation • Also known as **pseudogout** • <u>Risk Factors</u>: **hyperparathyroidism**, osteoarthritis, rheumatoid arthritis, and **hemochromatosis**; osteoporosis, **hypomagnesemia**, renal insufficiency, calcium supplementation • **Knee is most commonly affected joint**; other joints include elbow, wrist, MCP joint
Patho-physiology	• Pyrophosphate production and pyrophosphatase level in diseased cartilage imbalance leads to further pyrophosphate deposits in the synovium and adjacent tissue • These deposits then combines with calcium to form calcium pyrophosphate crystals causing inflammation and bone destruction
Signs & Symptoms	• **Asymptomatic**; may be incidental finding on x-ray • <u>**Pseudogout**</u>: similar to gout; **acute arthritis with pain, erythema, warmth, effusion, tenderness of the joint** • May resemble RA or OA
Diagnosis	• <u>**Synovial Fluid Analysis**</u>: diagnostic test of choice; **positively birefringent, rhomboid-shaped calcium pyrophosphate crystals** • <u>X-Ray</u>: unnecessary for diagnosis; may show linear cartilage calcifications (chondrocalcinosis)
Treatment	• <u>Supportive</u>: ice, restricted weight-bearing • <u>**NSAIDs**</u>; initial treatment of choice for pain control • <u>Corticosteroids</u>: if refractory to or unable to tolerate NSAIDs; oral vs. intraarticular injection • <u>Colchicine</u>: alternative to NSAIDs; may be used as first-line therapy
Key Words & Most Common	• Calcium pyrophosphate dihydrate crystal deposits to synovium and soft tissue • AKA Pseudogout • Risk factors: Hyperparathyroidism, hemochromatosis, hypomagnesaemia, renal insufficiency • Symptoms similar to gout; pain, erythema, warmth, effusion, tenderness • <u>Synovial fluid analysis</u>: positively birefringent, rhomboid-shaped calcium pyrophosphate crystals • NSAIDs vs steroids vs colchicine

Juvenile Rheumatoid Arthritis 🦴

Etiology & Risk Factors	• Idiopathic inflammatory arthropathy affecting children less than 16 years old for greater than 6 weeks • <u>Etiology</u>: autoimmune response triggered by environmental factors in genetically susceptible patient • <u>Risk Factors</u>: antibiotic exposure, C-section delivery
Patho-physiology	• Imbalance of regulatory T cells of adaptive immunity lead to release of proinflammatory cytokines such as IL-1 beta, IL-6, and IL-18 leading to systemic arthritis
Signs & Symptoms	• <u>Systemic</u>: **fever**, splenomegaly, generalized lymphadenopathy, pericardial effusion, pleuritis • <u>Rash</u>: **faint, erythematous (salmon-colored) macular coalescing rash on the trunk, palms, soles** • <u>Arthritis</u>: often polyarticular • <u>Enthesitis</u>: tendon insertion pain of iliac crest and spine, greater trochanter of femur, patella, tibial tuberosity, Achilles or plantar fascia insertions • <u>Iridocyclitis</u>: inflammation of the anterior chamber and anterior vitreous • <u>Growth Complications</u>: epiphyseal growth disturbances, premature physeal fusion, limb length discrepancy
Diagnosis	• **Clinical diagnosis** • <u>Labs</u>: no specific lab test; may have elevated ESR/CRP, elevated ferritin, leukocytosis, anemia, thrombocytosis • <u>Slit-Lamp Exam</u>: used to diagnose iridocyclitis
Treatment	• <u>Supportive</u>: ice, physical therapy • **NSAIDs; initial treatment of choice for pain control** • **Corticosteroids**: if refractory to or unable to tolerate NSAIDs • <u>Disease-Modifying Antirheumatic Drugs (DMARDs)</u>: particularly **methotrexate** as second-line therapy or for severe disease • <u>Biologic Agents</u>: **anakinra** or etanercept as second-line therapy or for severe disease
Key Words & Most Common	• Idiopathic inflammatory arthropathy in kids less than 16 years old for >6wks • Fever; salmon-colored rash on trunks/palms/soles; arthritis • Iridocyclitis (anterior uveitis) • Clinical diagnosis • NSAIDs → steroids → DMARDs (methotrexate) or biologics (anakinra)

Osteoporosis 🦴

Etiology & Risk Factors	• Progressive loss of bone mineral density by altered bone matrix secondary to bone resorption and bone formation imbalance that predisposes patient to fractures
	• Osteopenia is precursor to osteoporosis
	• Etiology: primary or secondary
	  • <u>Primary</u>: postmenopausal women
	  • <u>Secondary</u>: high cortisol state (**chronic corticosteroid** use, Cushing's syndrome), **hyperparathyroidism**, diabetes, low estrogen, hypogonadism, low body weight
	    • <u>Medications</u>: glucocorticoids, anti-epileptics, chemotherapy agents, PPIs, thiazolidines, levothyroxine
	• <u>Risk Factors</u>: **advanced age, Caucasian, female, sedentary lifestyle**, low BMI, corticosteroid use, smoking, chronic kidney disease, diet (low calcium and vitamin D), alcohol use

Patho-physiology	• Imbalance of bone resorption (osteoblasts) and bone remodeling (osteoclasts) leads to decreased skeletal bone mass which may result in low-impact fragility fractures
Signs & Symptoms	• **Asymptomatic** • <u>Pathologic Fracture</u>: fracture from **low-impact mechanism of vertebrae** (most common), hip, distal radius, humerus, pelvis • <u>Spinal Compression</u>: **loss of vertebral height, kyphosis** (exaggerated forward rounding of upper back), **back pain**

Diagnosis	• <u>Dual-Energy X-ray Absorptiometry (DEXA)</u>: **diagnostic test of choice**; screening and treatment monitoring, quantitative measure of bone loss, fracture risk prediction
	  • **Normal**: T score >1.0
	  • **Osteopenia**: T score between -1 and -2.5
	  • **Osteoporosis**: T score less than -2.5
	• <u>X-Ray</u>: evaluate for pathologic fractures; may show decreased radiodensity, loss of trabecular structure, and/or loss of vertebral height
	• <u>Labs</u>: evaluate for secondary cause with calcium, phosphorus, parathyroid, alkaline phosphatase, vitamin D, testosterone

Treatment	• <u>Lifestyle Modifications</u>: **vitamin D and calcium supplementation**, resistance and weight bearing exercise, proper diet, smoking and alcohol cessation, fall prevention • <u>Bisphosphonates</u>: **alendronate, risedronate; first-line medication for treatment and prevention**; inhibits osteoclast-mediated resorption to preserve bone mass <u>Selective Estrogen Receptor Modulators</u>: raloxifene; estrogen receptor agonist on bones to reduce osteoclast resorption • <u>Anabolic Recombinant form of Parathyroid Hormone</u>: teriparatide; stimulates osteoblasts to produce more bone; used in severe osteoporosis • <u>RANKL inhibitors</u>: denosumab; RANKL binding antagonism leads to inhibition of osteoclast activation; used as alternative to those that fail bisphosphonate therapy • <u>Calcitonin</u>: may provide short term analgesia for acute fracture; should not be used regularly to treat osteoporosis
Key Words & Most Common	• Loss of bone mineral density that may lead to low-impact fragility fractures • Most common in postmenopausal women; sedentary lifestyle, chronic steroid use, hyperparathyroidism • Asymptomatic; often presents as pathological fracture • DEXA scan is diagnostic test of choice • Vitamin D and calcium supplements, resistance exercise • Bisphosphonates are first-line

Disc Herniation

Etiology & Risk Factors	• Spinal condition in which the annulus fibrosis is damaged resulting in herniation of the nucleus pulposus • **Most common at L5-S1 space** due to mobile/non-mobile spinal junction; Lumbar>cervical>thoracic • <u>Etiology</u>: **trauma**, lifting heavy object, twisting with axial load, degenerative changes
Patho-physiology	• Mechanical compression of the nerve secondary to a herniated nucleus pulposus results in a local release of inflammatory chemokines

Signs & Symptoms	• <u>Radicular Back Pain:</u>
	  • Usually **unilateral +/- paresthesia** down leg following dermatome
	  • **Relieved with rest** and activity modification
	  • Worse with coughing, sneezing, bending forward, sitting
	• <u>Physical Exam:</u>
	  • **Positive straight leg raise** (*see next slide for nerve distributions*)
	  • May have gait disturbances or poor posture

Diagnosis	• <u>X-Ray</u>: may show loss of disc heigh or degenerative changes, loss of lumbar lordosis secondary to muscle spasm • <u>MRI</u>: **imaging study of choice** to visual herniated disc; may be used for preprocedural planning

Treatment	• <u>Conservative</u>: **heat, activity modifications** (bed rest often contraindicated), physical therapy
	• <u>Medications:</u>
	  • **NSAIDs: first-line for pain control**
	  • <u>Muscle Relaxers</u> (cyclobenzaprine): limited efficacy; may provide symptomatic relief
	  • <u>Corticosteroids</u>: oral or IM; may relieve pain/inflammation
	• <u>Corticosteroid Injections</u>: translaminar epidural injections and selective nerve root blocks for those refractory to conservative therapy
	• <u>Surgery</u>: laminectomy with discectomy reserved for those with ongoing severe symptoms not responding to non-operative measures

Key Words & Most Common	• Herniation of nucleus pulposus through annulus fibrosis often by traumatic mechanism • Most common at L5-S1 space • Radicular back pain +/- paresthesia • Relieved with rest; worse with coughing, bending forward, sitting • MRI is diagnostic test of choice • Heat + activity modifications • NSAIDs → steroids → steroid injections → surgery

L4-L5 disc herniation

Cervical

	C5	C6	C7	C8	T1
Pain	• Neck, shoulder, scapula pain	• Neck, shoulder, scapula, lateral arm, forearm pain	• Neck, shoulder, middle finger pain	• Neck, shoulder, medial forearm pain	• Neck, medial arm, forearm pain
Numbness	• Lateral arm numbness	• Lateral forearm, thumb, index finger numbness	• Index, middle finger, palm numbness	• Medial forearm, medial hand numbness	• Anterior arm, medial forearm numbness
Weakness	• Shoulder abduction, external rotation, elbow flexion, forearm supination	• Shoulder abduction, external rotation, elbow flexion, forearm supination and pronation	• Elbow, wrist, forearm pronation	• Finger and wrist extension, distal finger flexion/extension/abduction/adduction	• Thumb abduction, distal thumb flexion, finger abduction/adduction
Diminished Reflex	• Biceps, brachioradialis	• Biceps, brachioradialis	• Triceps	• N/A	• N/A

Lumbar

	L1	L2-L4	L5	S1	S2-S4
Pain	• Inguinal pain	• Low back pain radiating to anterior thigh, medial lower leg	• Low back pain radiating to buttock, lateral thigh, lateral calf, dorsum of foot, great toe	• Low back pain radiating to buttock, lateral/posterior thigh, posterior calf, lateral/plantar foot	• Sacral/buttock pain radiating to posterior thigh or perineum
Numbness	• Inguinal numbness	• Anterior thigh, medial lower leg numbness	• Lateral calf, dorsum of foot, 1st and 2nd toe webspace numbness	• Posterior calf, lateral/plantar foot numbness	• Medial buttock, perineal, perianal region numbness
Weakness	• Hip flexion	• Hip flexion, hip adduction, knee extension	• Hip abduction, knee flexion, foot dorsiflexion, toe extension/flexion, foot inversion/eversion	• Hip extension, knee flexion, plantar flexion of the foot	• N/A
Diminished Reflex	• N/A	• Patellar	• Semitendinosus/semimembranosus	• Achilles tendon, perineal, perianal region • May have sexual dysfunction or urinary/fecal incontinence	• Absent bulbocavernosus, anal wink

Cauda Equina Syndrome

Etiology & Risk Factors	• Constellation of symptoms occurring when nerve roots at caudal end of the cord are compressed/damaged resulting in nerve pathways to lower extremities/bladder • **Neurosurgical emergency** • <u>Etiology</u>: **disc herniation is most common**, spinal stenosis, tumors, trauma, epidural abscess or hematoma, vertebral fractures
Patho-physiology	• Cauda equina is group of nerves and nerve roots originating from distal spinal cord (level L1-L5) containing nerve axons responsible for motor and sensory innervation of legs, bladder, anus, and perineum; compression to these nerves leads to disruption of neurological function
Signs & Symptoms	• **Back pain and sciatica** • <u>Radiculopathy</u>: **lower extremity radiation of pain and weakness, decreased sensation** • <u>Saddle Anesthesia</u>: **decreased sensation to buttocks, perineum, medial thigh** • <u>Bowel/Bladder Dysfunction</u>: **spontaneous incontinence or retention** • <u>Sexual Dysfunction</u>: erectile dysfunction in men • <u>Physical Exam</u>: lower extremity motor/sensory deficits; hypotonia, saddle anesthesia, absent/decreased rectal tone or bulbocavernosus reflex
Diagnosis	• **MRI: imaging test of choice**; should be obtained urgently • <u>CT Myelogram</u>: if MRI is contraindicated (metal implants, pacemaker) • <u>Bladder Scan</u>: evaluate for urinary retention
Treatment	• **<u>Neurosurgery and/or Orthopedic Consult</u>: emergent decompression indicated; considered neurosurgical emergency** • Surgical decompression via laminectomy +/- subsequent discectomy • <u>Corticosteroids</u>: decrease inflammation and provide pain relief
Key Words & Most Common	• Neurosurgical emergency when nerve roots are compressed/damaged disruption lower extremity/bladder neurological function • Disc herniation is most common cause • Back pain + radiculopathy • Saddle Anesthesia • Bowel/bladder incontinence • MRI • Neurosurgery/Ortho consult • Surgical decompression

Cauda equina secondary to abscess in the posterior epidural space

Vertebral Compression Fracture

Etiology & Risk Factors	• Biomechanical failure of the vertebral column occurring secondary to axial/compressive load
	• <u>Etiology</u>: bimodal distribution
	  • <u>Younger</u>: secondary to fall/jump from height or motor vehicle accident
	  • <u>Elderly</u>: secondary to osteoporosis, systemic illness or malignancy

Patho-physiology	• During fall or trauma, axial or compressive load is applied to vertebral column with concomitant rotation around a center axis applies more force than the vertebral body can handle resulting in compression fracture; excessive force leads to a "burst" fracture seen with high energy traumas

Signs & Symptoms	• <u>**Back Pain**</u>: **localized at level of fracture**
	  • May have radiation of symptoms if nerve root impingement present
	  • May have paraspinal muscle spasm
	• <u>Spinal Compression</u>: **loss of vertebral height, kyphosis** (exaggerated forward rounding of upper back), **back pain**
	• <u>Physical exam</u>: loss of height, kyphosis, focal midline tenderness

Diagnosis	• <u>Spine X-Ray</u>: may be incidental finding during chronic back pain workup • Shows loss of vertebral height; may show osteoporotic changes (decreased radiodensity, loss of trabecular structure, and/or loss of vertebral height) • <u>Spine CT Scan</u>: indicated if high-energy or traumatic mechanism • <u>Spine MRI</u>: if neurological deficits present

Treatment	• <u>Neurosurgical and/or Orthopedic Consult</u>: indicated if traumatic mechanism
	• <u>Conservative</u>: if small fracture with no neurologic deficits or significant trauma
	  • Observation, **analgesia** (NSAIDs/Acetaminophen), **orthosis/bracing modalities**, physical therapy
	  • Treat underlying cause (bisphosphonates for osteoporosis
	• <u>Surgery</u>: **kyphoplasty** or vertebroplasty for severe or persistent pain

Key Words & Most Common	• Axial/compressive load leads to vertebral fracture • Young: fall from heigh; elderly: osteoporosis • Focal back pain +/- radicular symptoms • Kyphosis possible • X-ray; CT if traumatic • Neuro/ortho consult • Analgesia +/- bracing • Kyphoplasty if severe/persistent pain

T12 Compression Fracture

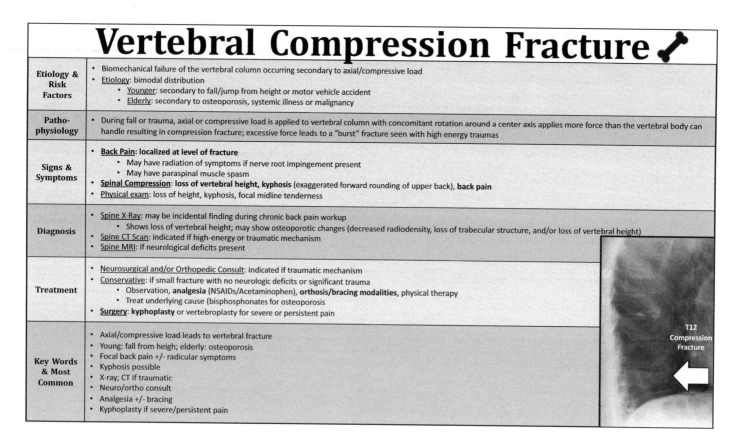

Spinal Stenosis

Etiology & Risk Factors	• Condition characterized by narrowing of vertebral spinal canal causing compression and impingement of nerve resulting in pain, weakness, and paresthesia • **Cervical and lumbar regions most commonly affected** • <u>Etiology</u>: **degenerative disk disease (arthritis) and spondylolysis most common**, iatrogenic (post-surgical changes), congenital, inflammatory, trauma (disc herniation) • <u>Risk Factors</u>: **age (>65 years old most common)**, history of trauma or surgery
Patho-physiology	• Narrowing of the vertebral spinal canal and lateral recesses by an above etiology leads to compression and impingement of the nerve

Signs & Symptoms	• **Back pain**
	• **Radiculopathy/Paresthesia**
	    • <u>Lumbar</u>: radiation to buttocks and thighs
	    • <u>Cervical</u>: radiation to shoulder, trapezius, and proximal arm
	• Weakness
	• **Pain worse with extension**; prolonged standing, walking, lifting, walking downhill
	• **Pain relieved with forward flexion**; sitting, leaning over for support (using walker/cane, leaning on grocery cart etc.), walking uphill

Diagnosis	• <u>Spine X-Ray</u>: nonspecific; shows degenerative changes, disc space narrowing • <u>Spine MRI</u>: **gold-standard and imaging test of choice** • Demonstrates intrinsic cord abnormalities, degree of stenosis, and may differentiate other etiologies (tumor, abscess) • <u>CT Myelogram</u>: If MRI is contraindicated (metal implants, pacemaker)
Treatment	• <u>Conservative</u>: Observation, **analgesia (NSAIDs/Acetaminophen)**, **orthosis/bracing modalities**, physical therapy, oral corticosteroids • **Corticosteroid Injections**: foraminal or epidural steroid injections for those refractory to conservative therapy • **Surgery**: **decompressive laminectomy** for severe or persistent pain
Key Words & Most Common	• Cervical/lumbar spinal canal narrowing causing impingement of nerves • Degenerative disk disease (arthritis) and spondylolysis most common • Age >65 • Back pain + paresthesia + weakness • Pain worse with extension, relieved with forward flexion • MRI gold-standard imaging test • Conservative measures → steroid injections → surgery

Spinal stenosis secondary to spondylosis with degenerative discopathy and posterior arthropathy

Mechanical Back Strain

Etiology & Risk Factors	• Acute or chronic strain, tear, or spasm of the paraspinal muscles • **Most common cause of back pain** • 80% of people will experience back pain during lifetime • <u>Etiology</u>: **twisting or lifting injury**, muscle spasm from poor posture or sleep position
Patho-physiology	• Muscle fibers are unable to meet the physical demand while performing an exercise or maneuver • Poor posture leads to increased stress on muscle fibers

Signs & Symptoms	• **Back pain +/- paraspinal muscle spasm**
	    • **Worse with activity**
	    • **Positional**
	    • **No radicular symptoms**
	• **Back stiffness** and inability to bend
	• <u>Physical Exam</u>:
	    • Focal tenderness of paraspinal muscle
	    • No midline bony tenderness

Diagnosis	• **Clinical diagnosis** • <u>X-Ray</u>: not routinely required unless symptoms persistent or suspicion of fracture

Treatment	• <u>Conservative</u>: **heat, continuation of normal activity +/- activity modifications** (bed rest often contraindicated), physical therapy
	• <u>Medication Management</u>:
	    • <u>NSAIDs</u>: **first-line for pain control**
	    • <u>Muscle Relaxers (cyclobenzaprine)</u>: limited efficacy; may provide symptomatic relief with spasm
	    • <u>Corticosteroids</u>: oral or IM; may relieve pain/inflammation

Key Words & Most Common	• Most common cause of back pain • Twisting/lifting etiology; poor posture • Back pain/stiffness, muscle spasm • Worse with activity, no radiculopathy • Clinical diagnosis • Heat, continuation of activity • NSAIDs

151

Spinal Epidural Abscess

Etiology & Risk Factors	• Infection of the central nervous system characterized by a collection of pus within the epidural adipose tissue of the spine • <u>Etiology</u>: *Staphylococcus aureus* most common (60%), *S. epidermis* (implantable devices, prosthesis), *E. coli* (urinary spread), *Pseudomonas* (IV drug users) • <u>Risk Factors</u>: **IV drug user, immunocompromised** (HIV, immunosuppressive medication, **diabetes**), alcohol abuse, malignancy, **history of spinal surgery**, recent fracture of spine, indwelling catheter, epidural catheter placement, chronic renal failure
Patho-physiology	• Contiguous spread or hematogenous seeding of bacteria from a remote infection enters the epidural space and colonizes the area between the dura mater and vertebral wall of the spinal canal leading to pyogenic infection • Underlying infection often present (osteomyelitis, pressure ulcer, retroperitoneal abscess) • **Posterior most common; most common site is lumbar and thoracic spine** • Often spans 3-5 vertebral spaces
Signs & Symptoms	• <u>**Triad**</u>: **fever + localized back pain + neurological deficit** • <u>Back Pain</u>: focal and severe • <u>Radicular Symptoms</u>: occur as spinal nerve roots are compressed • <u>Neurological Deficits</u>: motor/sensory impairment, bowel/bladder incontinence, saddle anesthesia, motor weakness, paralysis; symptoms occur over hours to days
Diagnosis	• <u>Labs</u>: increased ESR/CRP, elevated WBC count, **blood cultures to identify source organism** • <u>Lumbar Puncture</u>: **contraindicated due to risk of spinal cord herniation** • <u>**Spine MRI with Gadolinium Contrast**</u>: **imaging test of choice; shows ring-enhancing lesion** • <u>Spine CT Scan</u>: if MRI is contraindicated (metal implants, pacemaker)
Treatment	• **Emergent spinal surgery consult** • <u>**Parenteral Needle Aspiration**</u>: for decompression and diagnosis (culture of aspirate to guide antibiotic therapy) • <u>Antibiotics</u>: empiric regimen until bacterial etiology and susceptibility obtained; treatment for 4-8 weeks • **Vancomycin PLUS 3rd/4th generation cephalosporin (cefotaxime, ceftriaxone**; cefepime or ceftazidime if *Pseudomonas* suspected)
Key Words & Most Common	• Contiguous or hematogenous spread of bacteria leads to infection of CNS • S. aureus most common • IVDU, immunocompromised • <u>Triad</u>: fever + focal back pain + neurological deficits • MRI with contrast • Antibiotics (Vanco + 3rd/4th gen cephalosporin) +/- needle aspiration

Cauda equina secondary to abscess in the posterior epidural space

Scoliosis

Etiology & Risk Factors	• **Lateral curvature of the spine** • May have associated **kyphosis** (exaggerated, forward rounding of the upper back) or **lordosis** (excessive inward curvature of the spine) • <u>Etiology</u>: not fully understood • <u>Risk Factors</u>: **female** (adolescent girls are 10x more likely to develop and require treatment), **family history, age (10-18 years old most common)**
Patho-physiology	• No identifiable etiology; potential theories include hormones, asymmetrical growth, muscular imbalances, and genetic factors • Must have Cobb angle of at least 10 degrees in the coronal plane
Signs & Symptoms	• Often asymptomatic • **Back pain/fatigue with prolonged standing or sitting** • Asymmetry of shoulder height
Diagnosis	• <u>**Adams Forward Bend Test**</u>: unilateral thoracic/lumbar prominence with curvature • <u>**Spine X-Ray**</u>: lateral curvature of spine; Cobb angle >10° • **Cobb Angle**: AP view; angle formed when a line is drawn from the top of the most tilted superior vertebra and line drawn from the bottom of the most tilted inferior vertebra • <u>Spine MRI/CT</u>: may be included for pre-operative workup

Treatment	• <u>Orthopedic Referral</u>: treatment depends on skeletal maturity and severity/progression of curvature
	• <u>**Observation**</u>: serial monitoring with x-ray
	    • Indicated for Cobb angle between 10° and 25°
	• <u>Bracing</u>: may be used to slow progression in skeletally immature patient
	    • Indicated for Cobb angle between 25° and 40°
	    • Contraindicated if Cobb angle >40° or skeletally mature
	• <u>Surgery</u>: for severe cases; **spinal fusion with rod placement** (major surgery)
	    • Indicated for Cobb angle >40°

Key Words & Most Common	• Lateral curvature of the spine most common in adolescent females • Asymptomatic or back pain/fatigue with prolonged standing/sitting • Adams forward bend test • <u>X-ray</u>: Cobb angle >10° • Observation +/- bracing • Surgery for severe cases

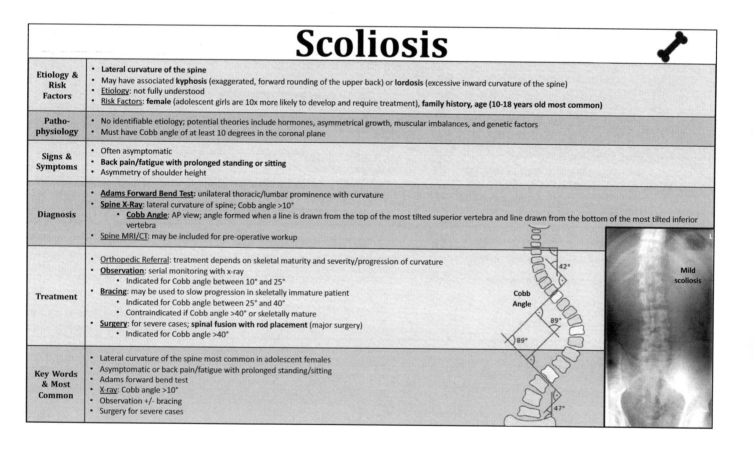

Cobb Angle — 42° — 89° — 89° — 47°

Mild scoliosis

Thoracic Outlet Syndrome

Etiology & Risk Factors	• Idiopathic compression of the neurovascular structures (brachial plexus, subclavian vein, or subclavian artery) as they pass through the thoracic outlet • Thoracic outlet is comprised of the first rib, scalene muscles, and clavicle • Etiology: neck/shoulder position (elevation, abduction, external rotation; sleeping on side with arm up), space occupying lesions (tumors, cysts), muscular overuse, trauma, trapezius muscle deficiency, clavicle fracture • Risk Factors: female, age (35-55 years old most common), poor posture
Patho-physiology	• Compression of neurovascular structures (brachial plexus, subclavian vein, subclavian artery) as they pass through the thoracic outlet • Thoracic outlet is comprised of the first rib, scalene muscles, and clavicle

Signs & Symptoms	• Nerve Compression: ulnar neuropathy, pain/paresthesia starting at neck or shoulder extending to medial aspect of arm and hand
	• Vascular Compression:
	   • Arterial Compression: hand ischemia (pain, pallor, paresthesia, cold)
	   • Venous Compression: erythema, edema, cyanosis, claudication, pain
	• Neck rotation, arm elevation/abduction or upper extremity external rotation may exacerbate symptoms
	• Adson's Sign: loss of radial pulse when head is rotated to ipsilateral side with an extended neck

Diagnosis	• Clinical Diagnosis • X-Ray: CXR or cervical spine; identifies anatomical risk factors • Doppler Ultrasound: may assist in diagnosing vascular compression • MRI: shows anatomy and identifies soft tissue and brachial plexus compression
Treatment	• Conservative: physical therapy, analgesia (NSAIDs), ergonomic desk setup, posture correction • Surgery: reserved for significant or progressive neurovascular deficits or failed conservative treatments
Key Words & Most Common	• Compression of neurovascular structures as they pass through thoracic outlet • Most common from neck/shoulder position (sleeping on side with arm abducted) • Pain/paresthesia from neck/shoulder to medial arm/hand • Erythema, edema, cyanosis from venous compression • Adson's Sign: loss of radial pulse with head rotation • Clinical diagnosis; confirmed with MRI • Conservative treatment

Spondylolysis

Etiology & Risk Factors	• Defect of the pars interarticularis with or without vertebral body slippage as a result of repetitive trauma • Most commonly occurs at L5-S1 • Etiology: stress fracture or fatigue most common; non-union, repetitive use (lumbar hyperextension with rotation) • Risk Factors: male, family history, sport participation, other pathologies (Marfan syndrome, spina bifida, osteogenesis imperfecta, osteoporosis), lumbar lordosis
Patho-physiology	• Repetitive trauma with axial load and/or lumbar hyperextension and rotation leads to excessive stress on vertebral body • Gymnastics, dance, football, weightlifting, wrestling, cheerleading, martial arts

Signs & Symptoms	• Mostly asymptomatic
	• Dull, achy, low back pain worse with activity
	   • May radiate to buttocks and posterior thigh
	• Physical Exam:
	   • Lumbar lordosis
	   • Hamstring inflexibility
	   • Focal tenderness
	   • Limited trunk range of motion
	   • Stork Test: patient stands on one leg with opposite leg elevated and performs lumbar extension; positive if pain is produced at site of defect

Diagnosis	• Spine X-Ray: initial imaging test
	   • Lateral View: radiolucent defect of pars interarticularis
	   • Oblique View: "Collar on a Scotty Dog"; bony defect between the inferior articular surface and the superior articular surface of the vertebra
	     • Normal lumbar spine resembles a "scotty dog" if spondylolysis present, the defect of the pars interarticularis resembles a dog collar
	• Spine CT/MRI: may be used for definitive diagnosis; not routinely ordered

Treatment	• Asymptomatic: conservative treatment with observation and maintaining regular activity if low-grade or asymptomatic • Symptomatic: physical therapy (focus on flexibility of hip flexors, hamstrings; back and core strength), analgesia (NSAIDs), activity modifications or restrictions • Spinal bracing if stress reaction or symptoms refractory to physical therapy
Key Words & Most Common	• Pars interarticularis defect as result of repetitive trauma from axial load +/- lumbar hyperextension • Mostly asymptomatic • Dull, achy, low back pain • X-Ray: collar on scotty dog (defect between inferior and superior articular surface of vertebra) • Conservative treatment +/- physical therapy

L5/S1
Spondylolysis

Spondylolisthesis

Etiology & Risk Factors	• Occurs due to forward slipping of one vertebral body with respect to the adjacent vertebral body leading to pain and mechanical or radicular symptom • **Most commonly occurs at L5-S1** (anterior translation of L5 vertebral body on S1 vertebral body) • Etiology: **complication of spondylolysis is most common cause**; degenerative disc disease (arthritis), repetitive use (lumbar hyperextension with rotation)
Patho-physiology	• Repetitive trauma with axial load and/or lumbar hyperextension and rotation leads to excessive stress on vertebral body resulting in bilateral fracture/defect of the pars interarticularis; this allows for forward slipping of the vertebral body leading to nerve impingement
Signs & Symptoms	• Most cases **asymptomatic** • **Low Back Pain: most common symptom** • Nerve Impingement: leads to **radiculopathy**, paresthesia, weakness, sciatica; bowel/bladder dysfunction or neurological deficits if severe
Diagnosis	• **Spine X-Ray: standard imaging for diagnosis** • Demonstrates **anterior slipping of the vertebra**; lateral views utilized for grading • Spine CT Scan: provides highest sensitivity/specificity; not routinely ordered • Spine MRI: indicated to identify soft tissue or disc abnormalities

Treatment	• Asymptomatic: **conservative treatment** with observation and maintaining regular activity if low-grade or asymptomatic
	• Symptomatic: **physical therapy (focus on flexibility of hip flexors, hamstrings; back and core strength)**, analgesia (NSAIDs), activity modifications or restrictions
	   • Spinal bracing if stress reaction or symptoms refractory to physical therapy
	• Surgery: reserved for severe cases refractory to all non-surgical treatment or instability
	   • Combination of decompression, fusion +/- instrumentation, or interbody fusion

Key Words & Most Common	• Forward slipping of vertebral body secondary to bilateral fracture/defect of pars interarticularis • Most common at L5-S1 • Asymptomatic • Low back pain +/- radiculopathy • X-Ray is standard imaging; shows anterior slipping of vertebra • Conservative treatment +/- physical therapy → surgery Forward slipping of L4-L5

Glenohumeral Dislocation

Etiology & Risk Factors	• Injury in which the humerus separates from the scapula at the glenohumeral joint
	• **Anterior is most common (97%)**; may also be posterior or inferior
	• Shoulder joint is most commonly dislocated joint in the body
	   • Patients with previous dislocation are prone to repeat dislocation
	   • Shoulder is an unstable joint as the shallow glenoid articulates with only a small portion of the humeral head
	• Etiology: **trauma, contact sports injuries**, motor vehicle accidents	

	Anterior	**Posterior**

Patho-physiology	• Mechanism: **blow to abducted, externally rotated, extended extremity**
	   • Posterior force or fall on outstretched arm
		• Mechanism: **blow to anterior shoulder and axial loading of adducted and internally rotated extremity**
		   • Violent muscle contractions (**seizure**, electrocution)

Signs & Symptoms	• Sudden onset of pain and decreased range of motion; may have audible pop
	• Physical Exam:
	   • **Arm is abducted and externally rotated**
	   • Humeral head is palpated anteriorly
	   • **Loss of deltoid contour "squared off shoulder"**
		• Sudden onset of pain and decreased range of motion; may have audible pop
		• Physical Exam:
		   • **Arm is adducted and internally rotated**
		   • May appear that patient is guarding extremity

Diagnosis	• Evaluate neurovascular function; **axillary nerve injury is most common**
	   • Axillary nerve innervates posterior deltoid, teres minor, and provides sensation to lateral shoulder
	• X-Ray: initial imaging test; axillary and scapular "Y" view
	   • **Hill-Sachs Lesion:** compression "groove" fracture of the posterolateral humeral head
	   • **Bankart Lesion:** avulsion rim fracture of anterior glenoid from labral tear
		• Evaluate neurovascular function; **axillary nerve injury is most common**
		   • Axillary nerve innervates posterior deltoid, teres minor, and provides sensation to lateral shoulder
		• X-Ray: initial imaging test; axillary and scapular "Y" view
		   • **"Light Bulb" Sign:** humeral head looks like light bulb or ice cream cone on AP view
		   • **Reverse Hill-Sachs Lesion:** impact fracture of anteromedial humeral head

Treatment	• **Reduction and Immobilization:** sling • **Assess axillary nerve** pre-and post-reduction (deltoid pinprick sensation) • **Orthopedic Follow-Up:** physical therapy vs surgical repair of labrum	
Key Words & Most Common	• Anterior shoulder dislocation significantly more common; axillary nerve most commonly injured nerve • Anterior: abducted, externally rotated; Hill-Sachs lesion, Bankart lesion on x-ray • Posterior: adducted and internally rotated; "light bulb" sign, reverse Hill-Sachs lesion on x-ray • Reduction and immobilization + orthopedic follow-up	Anterior shoulder dislocation

Acromioclavicular Joint Injury

Etiology & Risk Factors	• Injury of the clavicle articulation with the acromion process; common among athletes and young individuals
	• **Joint is stabilized by the acromioclavicular ligament** (comprised of anterior, posterior, inferior, superior components) which provides horizontal stability
	  • **Superior portion of AC ligament is most crucial for AC joint stability**
	  • Coracoclavicular ligaments provide vertical stability
	• Etiology: **common sports related injury (football, hockey most common**; skiing, lacrosse), trauma, motor vehicle accident

Patho-physiology	• Mechanism: **direct trauma to lateral aspect of shoulder when arm is adducted**; falling on outstretched hand or elbow possible

Signs & Symptoms	• **Shoulder Pain: anterosuperior shoulder most common**
	  • **Pain worse with movement** (elevation of extremity)
	  • **Difficulty sleeping on affected shoulder**
	• Physical Exam:
	  • Swelling, bruising
	  • **Deformity (step-off) at AC joint**
	  • "Piano Key" Sign: elevation of clavicle that rebounds after inferior compression of lateral clavicle

Diagnosis	• **X-Ray: AP view of bilateral clavicle for comparison**
	  • Grade I: no joint disruption
	  • Grade II: subluxation with slight widening (acromioclavicular ligament rupture; coracoclavicular ligament sprained)
	  • Grade III: complete disruption and significant widening (acromioclavicular and coracoclavicular ligaments ruptured); *type IV-VI are variations of type III*
	    • Grade IV: posterior displacement of distal clavicle
	    • Grade V: superior displacement of distal clavicle
	    • Grade VI: inferior displacement of distal clavicle

Treatment	• Conservative: indicated for type I, II and most type III
	  • Ice, analgesia, **immobilization (sling)**, with range of motion and strengthening exercise as soon as tolerated
	  • Orthopedic referral for type III
	• Surgery: indicated for most type IV-VI injuries

Key Words & Most Common	• Injury of acromioclavicular joint through lateral impact trauma to adducted arm • Commonly seen in football/hockey • Pain to anterosuperior shoulder worse with movement • May have visible deformity (step-off) • X-ray shows degree of separation • Conservative with sling immobilization → early ROM and strengthening

Grade 3 AC joint separation

Rotator Cuff Injury

Etiology & Risk Factors	• Spectrum of injury from tendinopathy to partial or complete tear of one or more of the rotator cuff tendons (supraspinatus, infraspinatus, subscapularis, teres minor) • **Supraspinatus is most commonly injured rotator cuff tendon** • Risk Factors: **occupation or activity involving repetitive overhead activity, age (>40 years old)**, poor posture, smoking, trauma, hypercholesterolemia, family history
Patho-physiology	• Macro trauma from an acute injury leads to acute tear of rotator cuff tendon • Micro-trauma from repetitive or chronic use results in degeneration of tissue and, with insufficient healing, can lead to degenerative tear of rotator cuff tendon

Signs & Symptoms	• **Anterolateral shoulder pain**
	  • **Painful arc of motion** (pain worse between 60° and 120° of shoulder abduction or flexion)
	• **Decreased range of motion** (especially overhead, external rotation or abduction)
	• Inability to sleep on affected side
	• Marked weakness, atrophy, and constant pain present if tear
	• Physical Exam: (subacromial lidocaine injection can enhance specificity of tendinopathy vs tears of the following tests)
	  • **Supraspinatus Test**: "Empty Can Test" test for pain/weakness to resisted abduction to an abduct arm to 90°, forward flexed to 30° with thumb down
	    • **Drop Arm Test**: patient is unable to hold empty can test position
	  • Infraspinatus/Teres Minor Test: test for pain/weakness to resisted external rotation with patient's arm bent to 90° with elbow at waist
	  • Subscapularis Test: patient places dorsum of hand on lower back; test for pain/weakness when trying to move push hand away from back with resistance
	  • **Impingement Tests**: positive Hawkins, Neer, and/or drop arm test
	    • **Hawkins Test**: elbow and shoulder flexed to 90°; sharp anterior shoulder pain with forced internal rotation
	    • **Neer Test**: arm fully pronated (thumb down) with sharp anterior shoulder pain with forced forward flection (arm lifted overhead)

Diagnosis	• **Clinical Diagnosis** • Shoulder X-Ray: ordered to rule out bony pathology; may show degenerative changes or proximal humeral migration with chronic, large tears • **Shoulder MRI**: gold-standard imaging test; used to determine size, extent, location, retraction and atrophy of tendon for pre-procedural planning
Treatment	• Conservative: **physical therapy** for strength and range of motion preservation, analgesia (**NSAIDs**) • Corticosteroid Injection: subacromial injection if refractory to conservative treatment • Surgery: arthroscopic rotator cuff repair indicated for full-thickness acute tear
Key Words & Most Common	• Supraspinatus most commonly injured rotator cuff tendon • Overhead activity and age are greatest risk factors • Anterolateral shoulder pain with painful arc + decreased ROM; may have weakness and inability to sleep on affected side with acute tear • Physical exam + MRI (gold-standard) for diagnosis • Physical therapy + NSAIDs +/- steroid injection → surgery

Proximal humeral migration seen with chronic tear

Humerus Fracture

Etiology & Risk Factors	• Fracture of the humerus that can be classified as proximal/humeral head, humeral shaft, or distal humerus fractures
	• May have neurovascular compromise
	  • <u>Proximal/Humeral Head</u>: **axillary nerve**
	  • <u>Humeral Shaft</u>: radial nerve
	  • <u>Distal (supracondylar) Humerus</u>: ulnar and radial nerve, brachial artery
	• <u>Etiology</u>: **trauma**, metastatic disease (breast cancer)

Patho-physiology	• <u>Mechanism</u>: fall on an outstretched hand, direct trauma, or pathologic fractures in metastatic disease • Result of high-energy trauma in younger population; result of ground-level fall in elderly population
Signs & Symptoms	• **Pain, swelling, ecchymosis to arm** • **Inability to move arm** • Adducted arm; patient often presents using non-injured arm to support elbow of injured arm • <u>Physical Exam</u>: **must rule out nerve injury** (proximal=axillary; shaft=radial; distal=ulnar/radial) • **Volkmann <u>Contracture</u>**: claw-like deformity secondary to ischemia (brachial artery injury from supracondylar humerus fracture)
Diagnosis	• <u>Humeral X-Ray</u>: initial imaging test • **Displaced anterior fat pad sign or posterior fat pad sign implicates fracture (hemarthrosis)** • <u>Humeral/Shoulder CT Scan</u>: utilized if fracture poorly visualized on x-ray or for pre-procedural planning

Treatment	• **<u>Conservative</u>**: indicated for small, non-displaced, non-comminuted fractures with no neurovascular compromise
	  • **Analgesia, immobilization (sling or splint), orthopedic referral**
	• <u>Surgical</u>: indicated for complex, displaced or comminuted fractures
	  • ORIF vs intermedullary nailing vs hemiarthroplasty (elderly)

Key Words & Most Common	• Fracture of humerus typically from traumatic mechanism (FOOSH) • Pain, swelling, bruising to arm • Inability to move arm • Arm adducted to side • X-ray → CT • Conservative: pain control, sling → ortho • Surgical: if complex

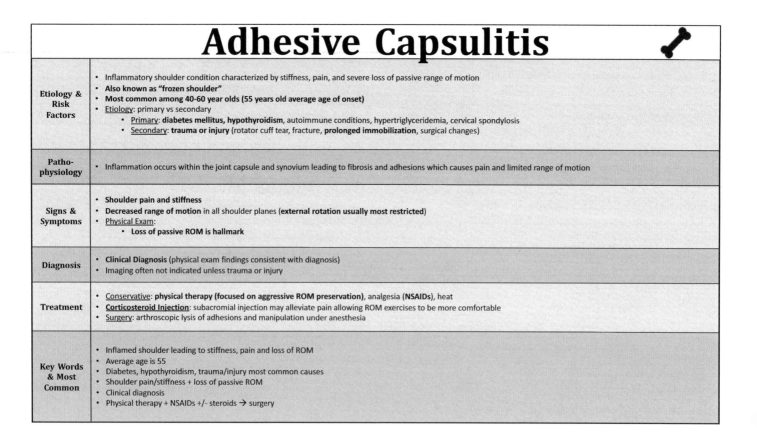

Supracondylar fracture with anterior/posterior fat pad sign

Proximal humerus fracture

Adhesive Capsulitis

Etiology & Risk Factors	• Inflammatory shoulder condition characterized by stiffness, pain, and severe loss of passive range of motion
	• **Also known as "frozen shoulder"**
	• **Most common among 40-60 year olds (55 years old average age of onset)**
	• <u>Etiology</u>: primary vs secondary
	  • <u>Primary</u>: **diabetes mellitus, hypothyroidism**, autoimmune conditions, hypertriglyceridemia, cervical spondylosis
	  • <u>Secondary</u>: **trauma or injury** (rotator cuff tear, fracture, **prolonged immobilization**, surgical changes)

Patho-physiology	• Inflammation occurs within the joint capsule and synovium leading to fibrosis and adhesions which causes pain and limited range of motion
Signs & Symptoms	• **Shoulder pain and stiffness** • **Decreased range of motion** in all shoulder planes (**external rotation usually most restricted**) • <u>Physical Exam</u>: • **Loss of passive ROM is hallmark**
Diagnosis	• **Clinical Diagnosis** (physical exam findings consistent with diagnosis) • Imaging often not indicated unless trauma or injury
Treatment	• <u>Conservative</u>: **physical therapy (focused on aggressive ROM preservation)**, analgesia (**NSAIDs**), heat • **<u>Corticosteroid Injection</u>**: subacromial injection may alleviate pain allowing ROM exercises to be more comfortable • <u>Surgery</u>: arthroscopic lysis of adhesions and manipulation under anesthesia
Key Words & Most Common	• Inflamed shoulder leading to stiffness, pain and loss of ROM • Average age is 55 • Diabetes, hypothyroidism, trauma/injury most common causes • Shoulder pain/stiffness + loss of passive ROM • Clinical diagnosis • Physical therapy + NSAIDs +/- steroids → surgery

Clavicle Fracture

Etiology & Risk Factors	• **Most common childhood fracture**; also common among adolescents or newborns during birth
	• <u>Etiology</u>: **trauma or injury (sports or motor vehicle accident)**; consider child abuse if present in children <2yo, malignancy
	• <u>Classification</u>:
	  • **Type I: middle third (midshaft); 80% of fractures (most common)**
	  • <u>Type II</u>: lateral third; 15% of fractures
	  • <u>Type III</u>: medial third; 5% of fractures

Patho-physiology	• <u>Mechanism</u>: **direct trauma or fall onto lateral shoulder is most common**; fall on an outstretched hand (FOOSH) • Clavicle has multiple ligamentous and muscular attachment sites leading to increased force applied; midshaft is thinnest portion of bone with no ligamentous attachment leading to increased incidence of fracture

Signs & Symptoms	• **Focal clavicle pain**
	• Perceived "pop" or "crack" at time of injury
	• <u>Physical Exam</u>:
	  • Adducted arm held close to body
	  • **May have visible or palpable deformity at fracture site; skin tenting** signifies high risk of developing into open fracture

Diagnosis	• Proper neurovascular exam • <u>Clavicle X-Ray</u>: **initial imaging test of choice**; 2 view (AP and 45° of cephalic tilt) • <u>Clavicle/Shoulder CT Scan</u>: if high suspicion for fracture with negative x-ray

Treatment	• <u>Conservative</u>: indicated for small, non-displaced, non-comminuted fractures with no neurovascular compromise
	  • **Analgesia, immobilization (simple sling), orthopedic referral**
	• <u>Surgical</u>: indicated for complex, displaced, shortened, open or comminuted fractures
	  • ORIF or pinning

Key Words & Most Common	• Common childhood fracture secondary to trauma or injury • Middle 1/3rd is most common fracture site • Direct trauma to lateral shoulder is most common mechanism • Focal clavicle pain +/- crack/pop • May have deformity at fracture site; skin tenting=impending open fracture • X-ray • Simple sling + pain control + ortho referral • Surgical fixation if shortened, displaced, open/tenting

Type I Clavicle Fracture

Radial Head Fracture

Etiology & Risk Factors	• Fracture of the proximal end of the radius • Radial head articulates with lateral epicondyle and rotates during pronation/supination; palpable at lateral elbow • More common among adults than children • <u>Etiology</u>: **trauma or injury**
Patho-physiology	• <u>Mechanism</u>: **fall on outstretched hand (FOOSH) in pronation** • Fracture is often intraarticular
Signs & Symptoms	• **Lateral elbow pain** • **Worse with pronation/supination** • May have **ecchymosis** • <u>Physical Exam</u>: point tenderness to radial head; restricted ROM of pronation/supination, **inability to fully extend elbow**

Diagnosis	• <u>X-Ray</u>: **initial imaging test of choice**; often difficult to identify on x-ray
	  • **Displaced anterior fat pad sign or posterior fat pad sign** implicates fracture (hemarthrosis)
	  • **Disruption of radiocapitellar line** (line through midshaft of radius that normally transects middle of capitellum; disruption of line implicates fracture)

Treatment	• <u>Conservative</u>: indicated for small, non-displaced, non-comminuted fractures with no neurovascular compromise
	  • **Analgesia, immobilization (simple sling), orthopedic referral**
	  • **Early ROM often indicated**
	• <u>Surgical</u>: indicated for complex, displaced or comminuted fractures
	  • ORIF or pinning

Key Words & Most Common	• Fracture of radial head secondary to FOOSH injury • Lateral elbow pain worse with pronation/supination • Bruising • Inability to fully extend elbow • X-ray shows abnormal fat pad signs; disruption of radiocapitellar line • Pain control + simple sling + ortho referral; early ROM often indicated

Olecranon Fracture

Etiology & Risk Factors	• Fracture of the proximal articular portion of the ulna • **More common in patients >50 years old** • <u>Etiology</u>: **trauma or injury**; falls in elderly
Patho-physiology	• <u>Mechanism</u>: **direct blow to flexed elbow** (fall onto elbow) • Displacement of olecranon fracture disrupts extensor mechanism of triceps (triceps inserts onto olecranon) resulting in loss of active elbow extension • Ulnar nerve lies medially to olecranon and adjacent to ulnar artery; fractures may disrupt neurovascular function
Signs & Symptoms	• **Pain and swelling to posterior elbow** • **Loss of extensor mechanism** • <u>Physical Exam</u>: • Ulnar neuropathy (paresthesia to 4th and 5th digit)
Diagnosis	• <u>Elbow X-Ray</u>: **initial imaging test of choice**; helps determine fracture pattern • <u>Elbow CT Scan</u>: may be ordered for complex fractures or pre-procedural planning

Treatment	• <u>Conservative</u>: indicated for small, non-displaced, non-comminuted fractures with no neurovascular compromise
	  • **Analgesia, immobilization (posterior splint in slight extension), orthopedic referral**
	  • Early ROM with avoidance of active extension
	• <u>Surgical</u>: indicated for complex, displaced or comminuted fractures
	  • Open reduction internal fixation (ORIF)

Key Words & Most Common	• Fracture of proximal ulna secondary to trauma or injury • More common in elderly • Direct blow to flexed elbow (fall) • Pain/swelling to posterior elbow • Loss of extensor mechanism • Ulnar neuropathy • X-Ray • Pain control + immobilization (posterior splint in slight extension) + ortho referral • Surgery if complex, displaced or comminuted

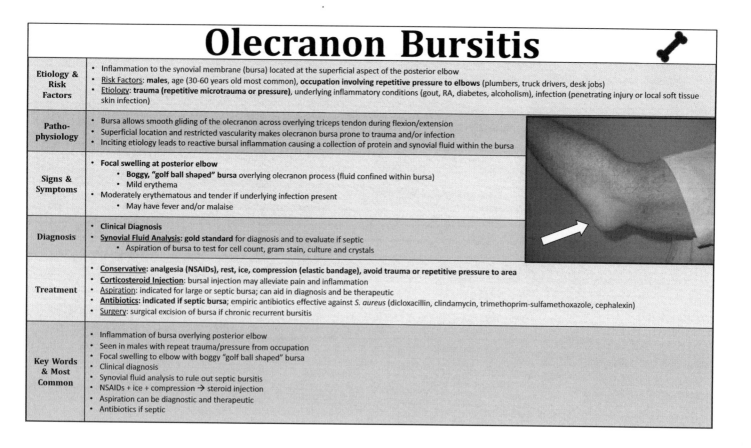

Olecranon Bursitis

Etiology & Risk Factors	• Inflammation to the synovial membrane (bursa) located at the superficial aspect of the posterior elbow • <u>Risk Factors</u>: males, age (30-60 years old most common), **occupation involving repetitive pressure to elbows** (plumbers, truck drivers, desk jobs) • <u>Etiology</u>: **trauma (repetitive microtrauma or pressure)**, underlying inflammatory conditions (gout, RA, diabetes, alcoholism), infection (penetrating injury or local soft tissue skin infection)
Patho-physiology	• Bursa allows smooth gliding of the olecranon across overlying triceps tendon during flexion/extension • Superficial location and restricted vascularity makes olecranon bursa prone to trauma and/or infection • Inciting etiology leads to reactive bursal inflammation causing a collection of protein and synovial fluid within the bursa

Signs & Symptoms	• **Focal swelling at posterior elbow**
	  • **Boggy, "golf ball shaped" bursa** overlying olecranon process (fluid confined within bursa)
	  • Mild erythema
	• Moderately erythematous and tender if underlying infection present
	  • May have fever and/or malaise

Diagnosis	• **Clinical Diagnosis** • <u>Synovial Fluid Analysis</u>: **gold standard** for diagnosis and to evaluate if septic • Aspiration of bursa to test for cell count, gram stain, culture and crystals
Treatment	• <u>Conservative</u>: analgesia (NSAIDs), rest, ice, compression (elastic bandage), avoid trauma or repetitive pressure to area • <u>Corticosteroid Injection</u>: bursal injection may alleviate pain and inflammation • <u>Aspiration</u>: indicated for large or septic bursa; can aid in diagnosis and be therapeutic • <u>Antibiotics</u>: indicated if septic bursa; empiric antibiotics effective against *S. aureus* (dicloxacillin, clindamycin, trimethoprim-sulfamethoxazole, cephalexin) • <u>Surgery</u>: surgical excision of bursa if chronic recurrent bursitis
Key Words & Most Common	• Inflammation of bursa overlying posterior elbow • Seen in males with repeat trauma/pressure from occupation • Focal swelling to elbow with boggy "golf ball shaped" bursa • Clinical diagnosis • Synovial fluid analysis to rule out septic bursitis • NSAIDs + ice + compression → steroid injection • Aspiration can be diagnostic and therapeutic • Antibiotics if septic

Galeazzi Fracture

Etiology & Risk Factors	• **Fracture of the middle to distal radius associated with dislocation/subluxation of distal radioulnar joint (DRUJ)** • <u>Etiology</u>: **fall on an outstretched hand**, direct impact trauma, sports injuries, fall from height, motor vehicle accidents
Patho-physiology	• <u>Mechanism</u>: **fall on an outstretched hand with an extended wrist and hyperpronated forearm** • Energy from trauma is transmitted along interosseous membrane resulting in damage to distal radioulnar joint leading to instability (dislocation/subluxation) and associated fracture

Signs & Symptoms	• **Focal pain and swelling to wrist/forearm**
	• **Deformity (radial side of wrist) and prominent ulna (dorsally displaced)**
	   • Assess wounds overlying fracture site (open fracture)
	• Pain or inability to pronate/supinate
	• **Assess neurovascular function (median and radial nerve distributions)**
	   • **Anterior interosseus nerve is most common complication** (cannot give "OK" sign)

Diagnosis	• <u>**Forearm X-Ray**</u>: AP, oblique, lateral • <u>Forearm CT Scan</u>: rarely performed; indicated for complex fractures or pre-procedure planning
Treatment	• <u>**General Fracture Care**</u>: analgesia (NSAIDs), Immobilization (long arm or sugar tong splint) • <u>**Urgent Orthopedic Referral**</u>: **considered unstable fracture** • <u>**Surgical**</u>: ORIF
Key Words & Most Common	• Fracture of them idle to distal radius with dislocation/subluxation of distal radioulnar joint • FOOSH with extended wrist and hyperpronated forearm • Focal pain/swelling to wrist/forearm • Deformity and prominent ulna • X-Ray • Pain control + immobilization (long arm/sugar tong splint) + urgent ortho referral • Unstable fracture requires ORIF

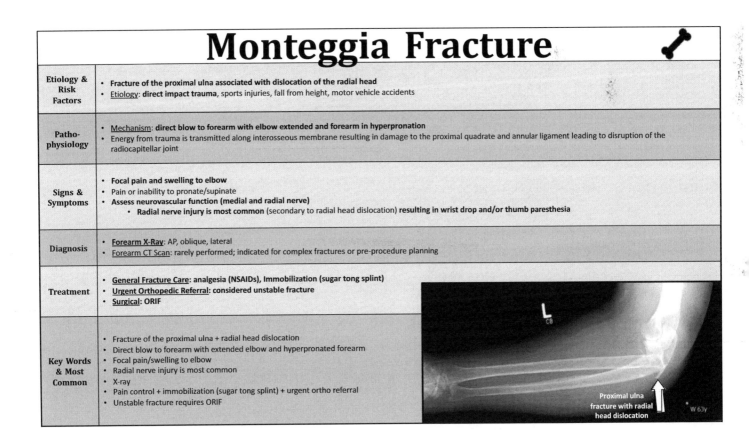

Middle radius fracture with dislocation of distal radioulnar joint

Monteggia Fracture

Etiology & Risk Factors	• **Fracture of the proximal ulna associated with dislocation of the radial head** • <u>Etiology</u>: **direct impact trauma**, sports injuries, fall from height, motor vehicle accidents
Patho-physiology	• <u>Mechanism</u>: **direct blow to forearm with elbow extended and forearm in hyperpronation** • Energy from trauma is transmitted along interosseous membrane resulting in damage to the proximal quadrate and annular ligament leading to disruption of the radiocapitellar joint
Signs & Symptoms	• **Focal pain and swelling to elbow** • Pain or inability to pronate/supinate • **Assess neurovascular function (medial and radial nerve)** • **Radial nerve injury is most common** (secondary to radial head dislocation) **resulting in wrist drop and/or thumb paresthesia**
Diagnosis	• <u>**Forearm X-Ray**</u>: AP, oblique, lateral • <u>Forearm CT Scan</u>: rarely performed; indicated for complex fractures or pre-procedure planning
Treatment	• <u>**General Fracture Care**</u>: analgesia (NSAIDs), Immobilization (sugar tong splint) • <u>**Urgent Orthopedic Referral**</u>: **considered unstable fracture** • <u>**Surgical**</u>: ORIF
Key Words & Most Common	• Fracture of the proximal ulna + radial head dislocation • Direct blow to forearm with extended elbow and hyperpronated forearm • Focal pain/swelling to elbow • Radial nerve injury is most common • X-ray • Pain control + immobilization (sugar tong splint) + urgent ortho referral • Unstable fracture requires ORIF

Proximal ulna fracture with radial head dislocation

Ulnar Shaft Fracture

Etiology & Risk Factors	• Fracture of the diaphysis of the ulna • Isolated fracture of the ulnar shaft is also known as "**nightstick fractures**" • Idea that patient is using forearm in defense posture to cover face from being struck with police baton • <u>Etiology</u>: **direct impact trauma**, sports injuries, motor vehicle accidents, fall from height
Patho-physiology	• <u>Mechanism</u>: direct blow to forearm or axial load to outstretched hand • Elderly may be prone to fracture secondary to poor bone quality as a result of osteoporosis

Signs & Symptoms	• **Focal pain and swelling** to forearm
	• Pain or inability to pronate/supinate
	• **Assess neurovascular function**
	    • <u>Anterior interosseus nerve</u>: "OK" sign
	    • <u>Posterior interosseus nerve</u>: thumbs up
	    • <u>Ulnar nerve</u>: crossing of 4th and 5th fingers

Diagnosis	• <u>Forearm X-Ray</u>: AP, oblique, lateral • <u>Forearm CT Scan</u>: rarely performed; indicated for complex fractures or pre-procedure planning

Treatment	• <u>Conservative</u>: indicated for small, non-displaced, non-comminuted fractures with no neurovascular compromise
	    • **Analgesia (NSAIDs)**
	    • **Immobilization** (short arm cast if distal 1/3 fracture; long arm cast if mid or proximal 1/3 fracture)
	    • **Orthopedic referral**
	• <u>Surgical</u>: indicated for complex, displaced or comminuted fractures
	    • Open reduction internal fixation (ORIF)

Key Words & Most Common	• Ulnar diaphysis fracture; AKA nightstick fracture • Direct impact trauma most common • Focal pain and swelling; must assess neurovascular function • X-ray • Pain control + immobilization with cast + ortho referral • Surgical ORIF if displaced

Radial Head Subluxation
Nursemaid's Elbow

Etiology & Risk Factors	• Common childhood injury resulting in **radial head subluxation under the annular ligament** • **Most common in children 1-4 years of age** • <u>Etiology</u>: **longitudinal traction**, trauma, direct impact from fall
Patho-physiology	• <u>Mechanism</u>: **longitudinal traction while forearm is pronated and extended** • **Child is swung by the arm, lifted or pulled by one arm**; parent catches child from falling by grabbing arm

Signs & Symptoms	• **Acute onset elbow pain and refusal to use affected arm**
	• Limited edema
	• <u>Physical Exam</u>:
	    • Tenderness to radial head
	    • **Arm held in extension and pronation**
	    • Refusal to supinate or flex elbow

Diagnosis	• **Clinical Diagnosis** • <u>Elbow X-Ray</u>: ordered if suspected fracture from traumatic mechanism

Treatment	• **Closed Reduction: Supination/Flexion Method**
	    • Pressure applied to radial head using thumb of one hand while supporting elbow
	    • Opposite hand grasps patient's distal forearm while in pronation
	    • Patient's forearm should be supinated and fully flexed with gentle traction
	    • Click may be heard/felt if successful
	    • After 5-10minutes, test success by having child reach for object (sucker, toy etc.)
	• If no improvement with closed reduction, consider x-ray and/or orthopedic referral
	• Avoid axial traction activities (lifting, swinging, monkey bars) to avoid reinjury

Key Words & Most Common	• Radial head subluxation under annular ligament • Most common age 1-4yo • Longitudinal traction (child swung or lifted by arm) • Elbow pain + refusal to use arm • Arm held in extension/pronation • Clinical Diagnosis • Closed reduction using supination/flexion technique

Tennis Elbow	# Lateral Epicondylitis
Etiology & Risk Factors	• Overuse injury occurring secondary to eccentric overload of the common extensor/supinator tendon at the origin of the extensor carpi radialis brevis tendon • <u>Etiology</u>: **repetitive supination, gripping and wrist extension** • <u>Risk Factors</u>: **occupation or sports requiring gripping and repetitive wrist extension**, smoking, obesity, strenuous/repetitive lifting, poor technique • Tennis, squash, badminton players; hairdressers, waiters/waitresses, plumbers, carpenters, butchers
Patho-physiology	• <u>Mechanism</u>: **repetitive gripping, wrist extension, forearm supination** • Degenerative overuse process leads to granulation tissue formation, unstructured collagen deposition, vascular hyperplasia within the tissue and repetitive micro-tearing of the tendon origin; often lacks inflammatory cells (macrophages, lymphocytes, neutrophils)

Signs & Symptoms	• **Lateral elbow pain**
	    • Worse with activity, improves with rest
	    • **May be insidious in onset** or acute-on-chronic
	    • Pain can be excruciating (unable to grip coffee mug)
	• <u>Physical Exam</u>:
	    • **Focal tenderness 1-2cm distal to lateral epicondyle**
	    • **Reproducible pain with resisted wrist extension, resisted forearm supination**, resisted extension of middle finger

Diagnosis	• **Clinical Diagnosis** • <u>Elbow X-Ray</u>: may be ordered to rule out fracture • <u>Elbow MRI/US</u>: if patient refractory to conservative treatment or pre-procedural planning
Treatment	• <u>Conservative</u>: activity modifications, rest, **forearm counterforce straps** (tennis elbow strap), **physical therapy**, analgesia (**NSAIDs**) • <u>**Corticosteroid Injection**</u>: injection to extensor/supinator tendon origin if refractory to conservative treatment • <u>Surgery</u>: scar/degenerative tissue excision from extensor tendon if severe or refractory to all other conservative treatments
Key Words & Most Common	• Overuse injury to common extensor/supinator tendon • Repetitive supination, gripping, wrist extension • Lateral elbow pain; may be insidious onset • Focal pain 1-2cm distal to lateral epicondyle • Pain with resisted wrist extension, forearm supination, middle finger extension • Clinical diagnosis • Rest + NSAIDs + tennis elbow strap + PT → steroid injection → surgery

Golfer's Elbow	# Medial Epicondylitis

Etiology & Risk Factors	• Overuse injury occurring secondary to repetitive stress or overuse of the flexor/pronator tendon at the origin of the pronator teres and common flexor tendon group
	• <u>Etiology</u>: **repetitive pronation, gripping and wrist flexion**
	• <u>Risk Factors</u>: **occupation or sports requiring gripping and repetitive wrist extension or throwing**, smoking, obesity, diabetes, repetitive lifting, poor technique
	    • Baseball pitchers, **golfers**; carpenters, utility workers, butchers, caterers, waiters/waitresses
	    • More common among 40-60 years old

Patho-physiology	• <u>Mechanism</u>: **repetitive wrist flexion, forearm pronation, or gripping** • Degenerative overuse process leads to granulation tissue formation, unstructured collagen deposition, vascular hyperplasia within the tissue and repetitive micro-tearing of the tendon origin; often lacks inflammatory cells (macrophages, lymphocytes, neutrophils)

Signs & Symptoms	• **Medial elbow pain**
	    • Worse with activity, improves with rest
	    • **May be insidious in onset** or acute-on-chronic
	    • Pain may radiate to forearm or wrist
	• May have associated **paresthesia in ulnar nerve distribution** due to proximity
	• <u>Physical Exam</u>:
	    • **Focal tenderness 0.5-1cm distal to medial epicondyle**
	    • **Reproducible pain with resisted wrist flexion, resisted forearm pronation**
	    • Ulnar neuritis with Tinel's sign (tapping of cubital tunnel)

Diagnosis	• **Clinical Diagnosis** • <u>Elbow X-Ray</u>: may be ordered to rule out fracture • <u>Elbow MRI/US</u>: if patient refractory to conservative treatment or pre-procedural planning
Treatment	• <u>Conservative</u>: activity modifications, rest, **forearm counterforce straps** (golfer elbow strap), **physical therapy**, analgesia (**NSAIDs**) • <u>**Corticosteroid Injection**</u>: injection to flexor/pronator tendon origin if refractory to conservative treatment • <u>Surgery</u>: scar/degenerative tissue excision from extensor tendon if severe or refractory to all other conservative treatments
Key Words & Most Common	• Overuse injury to common flexor/pronator tendon • Repetitive pronation, gripping, wrist flexion • Medial elbow pain; Focal pain 0.5-1cm distal to medial epicondyle • Pain with resisted wrist flexion, forearm pronation; may have ulnar neuritis • Clinical diagnosis • Rest + NSAIDs + golfer elbow strap + PT → steroid injection → surgery

Elbow Dislocation

Etiology & Risk Factors	• Disruption of the articulation of the distal humerus and proximal radius and ulna • **Posterior dislocation is most common** • <u>Etiology</u>: **trauma**, sports injury, (football, skateboarding, rollerblading) fall; **most common when falling backwards on outstretched hand**
Patho-physiology	• <u>Mechanism</u>: **fall on an outstretched hand (FOOSH) with elbow hyperextension and axial loading** • Axial loading during a fall onto an outstretched hand will cause the arm to experience a supination moment as the body rotates during the fall. This period of supination leads to valgus force to the elbow, disrupting the articulation and causing dislocation • Ulnar and radial nerve or brachial artery may be injured

Signs & Symptoms	• **Severe elbow pain** following injury
	• **Significant swelling**
	• May have paresthesia if nerve injury
	• Loss of elbow range of motion
	• <u>Physical Exam</u>:
	   • Significant swelling, **visible deformity** (olecranon prominent posteriorly), elbow held at 45° of flexion
	   • Assess for open fracture/compartment syndrome
		• Must assess neurovascular function
		   • <u>Anterior interosseus nerve</u>: "OK" sign
		   • <u>Posterior interosseus nerve</u>: thumbs up
		   • <u>Median nerve</u>: make a fist
		   • <u>Ulnar nerve</u>: crossing of 4th and 5th fingers
		   • <u>Radial nerve</u>: wrist drop, numbness of thumb	

Diagnosis	• <u>Elbow X-Ray</u>: determines direction of dislocation; pre- and post-reduction films are necessary • <u>Elbow CT Scan</u>: aids in identifying associated fractures/injuries (radial head and coronoid fracture)	
Treatment	• <u>Emergent Reduction</u>: considered orthopedic emergency • Pre- and post-reduction films and neurovascular status necessary • <u>Analgesia</u>: **NSAIDs** • <u>Immobilization</u>: **long-arm splint with elbow at 90° of flexion** • <u>Surgical</u>: ORIF if unstable	**Elbow Dislocation**
Key Words & Most Common	• FOOSH with axial loading and elbow hyperextended (falling backwards) • Posterior dislocation most common • Severe elbow pain and swelling • Visible deformity, loss of range of motion • Assess neurovascular function • X-Ray • Emergent reduction + long-arm splint with elbow at 90°	

Cubital Tunnel Syndrome

Etiology & Risk Factors	• Neuropathy of the ulnar nerve secondary to compression of the nerve as it passes through the cubital tunnel at the medial side of the elbow • <u>Etiology</u>: **trauma/pressure** (hitting elbow on hard surface), **stretching** (prolonged elbow flexion during sleep), **injuries resulting in swelling** (fracture, sprain, dislocations)
Patho-physiology	• Ulnar nerve traverses along medial aspect of the triceps before entering cubital tunnel and travels between medial epicondyle of the humerus and the olecranon • Compression most likely to occur at level of cubital tunnel due to narrow anatomy and location

Signs & Symptoms	• **Paresthesia along ulnar nerve distribution**
	   • **Numbness/tingling of forearm, hand, and ulnar side of 4th/5th digit**
	• May have pain
	• <u>Physical Exam</u>:
	   • **Reduced sensation of palmar and ulnar side of 5th digit and ulnar side of 4th digit; worse with elbow flexion**
	   • May have weakness of interosseous muscles
	   • <u>Tinel's Sign</u>: tapping of ulnar nerve at cubital tunnel produces paresthesia
	   • <u>Froment's Sign</u>: patient grasps piece of paper with thumb and side of index finger; positive test if thumb flexes at interphalangeal joint when paper is attempted to be withdrawn

Diagnosis	• **Clinical Diagnosis** • <u>Nerve Conduction Study</u>: confirms diagnosis • <u>Elbow X-Ray</u>: evaluate other bony pathologies • <u>Elbow MRI/US</u>: evaluates soft tissue pathologies that may cause compression
Treatment	• <u>Conservative</u>: activity and posture modifications, **elbow splint (especially at night)**, rest, **physical therapy**, analgesia (**NSAIDs**) • <u>Surgery</u>: decompression of the nerve
Key Words & Most Common	• Ulnar nerve neuropathy secondary to nerve compression from pressure, stretching, or injury • Paresthesia along ulnar nerve (forearm, hand, ulnar side of 4th/5th digit) • Tinel's and Froment's Sign • Clinical diagnosis; confirmed with nerve conduction study • Conservative treatment

Pronator Teres Syndrome

Etiology & Risk Factors	• **Compression of the median nerve by the pronator teres muscle in the forearm** • Etiology: **repetitive grasping/pronation movements** (hammering, scooping of food, clerical work, washing dishes, tennis/golf), forearm hypertrophy (athletes) • Risk Factors: female, age (40-50 years old most common)
Patho-physiology	• Compression of median nerve as it traverses between the two heads of the pronator teres muscle produces pain and paresthesia

Signs & Symptoms	• **Paresthesia of 1st/2nd/3rd and lateral 4th digit**
	• **Proximal forearm pain** (volar aspect)
	• **Typically does not feature nocturnal exacerbation** (compared to carpal tunnel syndrome)
	• Physical Exam:
	   • **Pain worse with resisted pronation and elbow flexion**
	   • Grip weakness

Diagnosis	• **Can be clinical diagnosis** • Nerve Conduction Study: may be used to rule out other neuropathies • Elbow X-Ray: usually no gross pathology • Elbow US/MRI: more sensitive for diagnosis
Treatment	• Conservative: **activity modifications**, physical therapy, analgesia (NSAIDs) • **Corticosteroid Injection**: injection if refractory to conservative treatment • Surgery: decompression if severe or refractory to all other conservative treatments
Key Words & Most Common	• Median nerve compression by pronator teres muscle • Repetitive grasping/pronation movements • Paresthesia of 1st/2nd/3rd and lateral 4th digit • Proximal forearm pain (worse with pronation) • NO night pain • Activity modifications + pain control → steroid injection → surgery

Ulnar Collateral Ligament Sprain

Etiology & Risk Factors	• **Sprain/tear of ulnar collateral ligament of the thumb** leading to instability of the metacarpophalangeal (MCP) joint; can be acute or chronic • Also known as gamekeeper's thumb or skier's thumb • Etiology: **trauma, athletic injury** (fall onto ski pole; hockey, basketball, volleyball)
Patho-physiology	• Mechanism: **forced abduction/valgus stress of the thumb causes sprain of the ulnar collateral ligament (UCL)**, the primary stabilizer ligament against valgus force

Signs & Symptoms	• **Pain and swelling along ulnar border of the thumb MCP joint**
	• Physical Exam:
	   • **UCL laxity with radial deviation (valgus) stress testing of thumb**
	   • **Weakness in pinch strength**
	   • MCP tenderness

Diagnosis	• **Elbow X-Ray**: perform before stress testing • May show **avulsion fracture at base of the proximal phalanx**
Treatment	• **Immobilization: thumb spica splint for 4-6 weeks** • Orthopedic Hand Surgeon Referral • Surgery may be required if ruptured
Key Words & Most Common	• Sprain of UCL of thumb • Traumatic etiology (fall onto ski pole or hockey stick) • Forced abduction/valgus stress • Pain/swelling at ulnar border of thumb MCP • Laxity with radial deviation of thumb • Weak pinch • X-ray before stress test to r/o avulsion fracture • Thumb spica immobilization → orthopedic hand follow-up

Scaphoid Fracture

Etiology & Risk Factors	• **Most commonly fractured carpal bone** • Predominantly affect younger patients (average age 29 years old) • <u>Etiology</u>: **fall on an outstretched hand (FOOSH)**; trauma, sports related injury, motor vehicle accident

Patho-physiology	• Scaphoid is largest of carpal bones and has a waist portion of bone between a proximal and distal pole
	  • Blood supply is from radial artery branches; proximal pole is supplied by retrograde blood flow
	    • If fracture occurs at the waist, there is disruption of retrograde blood flow to proximal pole of scaphoid resulting in avascular necrosis

Signs & Symptoms	• **Pain and swelling at the base of the thumb/radial surface of wrist (anatomical snuffbox)** • Restricted wrist range of motion

Diagnosis	• <u>Wrist X-Ray</u>: AP, lateral, scaphoid views (30° wrist extension and 20° ulnar deviation)
	  • 25% of scaphoid fractures are not visualized on initial x-ray
	  • **Fracture may not be seen on plain x-ray for up to 2 weeks**
	• <u>Wrist CT/MRI</u>: more sensitive/specific; **MRI is gold standard**

Treatment	• <u>General Fracture Care</u>: indicated for nondisplaced fracture or any snuffbox tenderness with negative x-ray
	  • **Fracture may not be apparent for up to 2 weeks; repeat x-rays indicated 7-14 days after injury if still experiencing symptoms**
	  • Analgesia (NSAIDs)
	  • **Immobilization (thumb spica splint)**
	• <u>Surgical</u>: ORIF or percutaneous pins indicated for complex, displaced, or comminuted fractures or nonunion/avascular necrosis

Key Words & Most Common	• Most common carpal bone fracture • FOOSH • Pain/swelling to base of thumb/radial side of wrist (anatomical snuffbox) • X-ray; fracture may not be visualized for up to 2 weeks • MRI gold standard • Pain control + immobilization with thumb spica splint (with snuffbox tenderness even if negative x-ray) • May require surgery if risk for nonunion/AVN

Fracture across waist of scaphoid bone

Osteogenesis Imperfecta

Etiology & Risk Factors	• Genetic connective tissue disorder caused by **abnormal synthesis of type I collagen** • **Autosomal dominant** • Also known as "brittle bone disease" • <u>Etiology</u>: mutations in the *COL1A1* and *COL1A2* genes is most common
Patho-physiology	• Type I collagen assembles to form the structural matrix of bone, skin, tendons, cornea, blood vessels walls and connective tissue • Genetic defect results in abnormalities of type I collagen molecules resulting in clinical manifestation of the above tissues

Signs & Symptoms	• **Hearing loss is present in 50-65% of all patients with OI**
	• **Severe premature osteoporosis resulting in multiple recurrent fractures**
	• <u>Type I</u>: most mild
	  • **Blue sclerae**, musculoskeletal pain, hypermobility, recurrent fractures
	• <u>Type II</u>: most severe and lethal
	  • Congenital fractures, shortened extremities, blue sclerae, soft skull (trauma during delivery may result in intracranial hemorrhage or stillbirth)
	• <u>Type III</u>: most severe non-lethal form
	  • Short stature, spinal curvature, multiple recurrent fractures; macrocephaly
	• <u>Type IV</u>: intermediate
	  • Easily fractured bones, moderate to short stature, sclerae typically normal

Diagnosis	• **Clinical Diagnosis** • Cultured fibroblasts (skin biopsy) or genetic sequency can confirm diagnosis
Treatment	• <u>Growth Hormone</u>: growth responsive children (types I and IV) • <u>**Bisphosphonates**</u>: reduce bone pain and fracture risk • <u>**Cochlear Implant**</u>: for hearing loss • Orthopedic surgery, physical/occupational therapy may help improve function
Key Words & Most Common	• Autosomal dominant genetic connective tissue disease resulting in abnormal type I collagen synthesis • "brittle bone disease" • Hearing loss, multiple fractures, blue sclerae are hallmarks • Clinical diagnosis • Bisphosphonates, cochlear implants, physical therapy

Complex Regional Pain Syndrome (CRPS)

Etiology & Risk Factors	• Neuropathic pain disorder characterized by ongoing pain disproportionate to degree of bone or soft tissue injury (trauma, surgery, fracture)
	  • **Sensory, motor, and autonomic dysfunction**
	• <u>Etiology</u>: **fracture (most common)**, trauma, surgery, sprains, contusions, crush injuries, procedure sites, amputation
	  • **Upper extremity most common**
	• <u>Risk factors</u>: **female, age (60-70 years old most common)**, asthma, ACEI use, menopause, osteoporosis, migraine, smoking

Patho-physiology	• Not fully understood • Central sympathetic sensitization, peripheral nociceptor sensitization, and neuropeptide release leads to ongoing pain and inflammation
Signs & Symptoms	• <u>Sensory</u>: **regional pain (burning/aching) is hallmark symptom**; **hyperalgesia** (extreme sensitivity to pain), **allodynia** (pain to stimulus that does not usually provoke pain) • <u>Cutaneous Changes</u>: **edema, dry or hyperhidrotic skin**, red/mottled skin, increased/decreased temperature • <u>Trophic Changes</u>: shiny, atrophic skin; cracking or excessive growth of nails, hair loss • <u>Motor Abnormalities</u>: **decreased range of motion, weakness**, tremors, spasms • <u>Psychologic Stress</u>: **depression, anxiety, anger** (often secondary to frustration of unclear cause or prolonged course)

Diagnosis	• **Clinical Diagnosis**
	• <u>X-Ray</u>: may show bone demineralization
	• <u>Bone Scintigraphy</u>: increased uptake/activity
	
	• <u>Budapest Criteria</u> (1 symptom in three of the four categories)
	  • <u>Sensory</u>: hyperalgesia or allodynia
	  • <u>Vasomotor</u>: temperature or skin color asymmetry to contralateral side
	  • <u>Sudomotor/Edema</u>: sweating changes, sweating asymmetry, edema
	  • <u>Motor/Trophic</u>: trophic changes to hair/skin/nails; ↓ ROM, motor dysfunction (weakness, tremor, dystonia)

Treatment	• <u>Conservative</u>: analgesia (**NSAIDs**), physical/occupational therapy, desensitization therapy, transcutaneous electrical nerve stimulation, acupuncture
	  • Vitamin C prophylaxis has been hypothesized to lower risk of CRPS after fractures
	  • Behavioral therapy for psychologic stress
	• <u>Medication Management</u>: oral corticosteroids, tricyclic antidepressants, antiseizure medications may be attempted
	  • Gabapentin often has greatest benefit
	  • Ketamine infusion may aid in acute flare

Key Words & Most Common	• Sensory, motor, and autonomic dysfunction most common after fracture • Hyperalgesia/allodynia, temperature/skin color asymmetry; sweating asymmetry or edema; changes to hair/skin/nails and motor dysfunction • Clinical diagnosis • NSIADs + physical therapy • Gabapentin vs TCAs vs Gabapentin

Smith's Fracture

Etiology & Risk Factors	• **Extraarticular distal radius fracture with volar displacement or angulation** • Most common in young males or elderly females • <u>Etiology</u>: **fall on an outstretched hand with wrist flexed**, direct impact **trauma to dorsal side of wrist**, **sports injuries**, fall from height, motor vehicle accidents
Patho-physiology	• <u>Mechanism</u>: **fall onto a dorsiflexed wrist or blow to dorsal aspect of wrist** • Flexed wrist trauma causes force to be transmitted ventrally resulting in the volar displacement/angulation of radius • Low bone mineralization during puberty in adolescents and osteopenia/osteoporosis in elderly increases fracture risk

Signs & Symptoms	• **Wrist pain and swelling**
	• Restricted range of motion
	• <u>Physical Exam</u>:
	  • Bruising and swelling often present
	  • May have palmar paresthesia (median nerve compression)
	  • **Volar deformity with prominent ulna along dorsum of wrist ("garden spade deformity"**: supinated wrist looks like a garden hoe with spade side down)

Diagnosis	• Assess neurovascular status • <u>Wrist X-Ray</u>: initial imaging test of choice; lateral view demonstrates **ventrally displaced or angulated extraarticular fracture of the distal radius** • <u>Wrist CT Scan</u>: may be used for occult fractures or preprocedural planning Ventrally displaced distal radius
Treatment	• <u>Closed Reduction</u>: traction and dorsal force to radius • <u>General Fracture Care</u>: analgesia (**NSAIDs**); Immobilization (sugar tong splint) • <u>Surgical</u>: ORIF if unstable fracture (>20° of angulation, shortening of radius, intra-articular involvement, comminution)
Key Words & Most Common	• Distal radius fracture with volar displacement/angulation • FOOSH with wrist flexed • Wrist pain/swelling + volar deformity (prominent ulna at dorsal wrist) • "Garden spade deformity" • X-Ray shows ventrally displaced/angulated fracture of distal radius • Closed reduction + pain control + immobilization (sugar tong splint) • Ortho referral for ORIF often required

Colles' Fracture

Etiology & Risk Factors	• **Distal radial metaphysis fracture that is dorsally displaced and angulated** 　• Ulnar styloid fracture seen in ~60% • **More common in adolescents or elderly** (age 20-50 least common age group) • <u>Etiology</u>: **fall on an outstretched hand**, direct impact **trauma**, **sports injuries**, fall from height, motor vehicle accidents
Patho-physiology	• <u>Mechanism</u>: **fall on an outstretched hand with wrist in dorsiflexion** • Low bone mineralization during puberty in adolescents and osteopenia/osteoporosis in elderly increases fracture risk
Signs & Symptoms	• **Wrist pain and swelling** • Restricted range of motion • <u>Physical Exam</u>: 　• Bruising and swelling often present 　• May have palmar paresthesia (median nerve compression) 　• **Dorsiflexion deformity ("dinner fork deformity":** supinated wrist looks like a fork with tine side down)
Diagnosis	• Assess neurovascular status • <u>Wrist X-Ray</u>: **initial imaging test of choice**; lateral view demonstrates **dorsally displaced or angulated fracture of the distal radius** • <u>Wrist CT Scan</u>: may be used for occult fractures or preprocedural planning
Treatment	• **Closed Reduction**: traction and volar/medial force to radius • **General Fracture Care:** analgesia **(NSAIDs); Immobilization (sugar tong splint)** • <u>Surgical</u>: **ORIF** if unstable fracture (>20° of angulation, shortening of radius, intra-articular involvement, comminution)
Key Words & Most Common	• Distal radius fracture with dorsal angulation • FOOSH injury • Wrist pain/swelling + bruising • Dorsiflexion "dinner fork" deformity • X-ray shows dorsally displaced/angulated fracture of distal radius • Closed reduction + pain control + immobilization (sugar tong splint) • Ortho referral for ORIF if unstable

Dorsally displaced distal radius

Lunate Dislocation

Etiology & Risk Factors	• Perilunate dislocations and lunate dislocations are rare high-energy wrist injuries 　• <u>Perilunate dislocation</u>: no articulation with capitate; articulation with radius preserved 　• <u>Lunate dislocation</u>: no articulation with capitate or radius • <u>Etiology</u>: **high-energy injury**; trauma, motor vehicle accident, athletic injury, industrial accidents
Patho-physiology	• <u>Mechanism</u>: **high-energy injury with wrist in forced hyperextension and ulnar deviation** • Perilunate ligaments rupture during injury allowing dislocation of the joint
Signs & Symptoms	• **Acute wrist pain and swelling** • Restricted range of motion • <u>Physical Exam</u>: 　• **May have palmar paresthesia (median nerve compression)** 　• Palpable bony prominence
Diagnosis	• <u>Wrist X-Ray</u>: PA, oblique, lateral, scaphoid views 　• <u>PA</u>: triangular appearance due to rotation (**"piece of pie"** sign) 　• <u>Lateral</u>: volar dislocation and tilt of lunate (**"spilled teacup"** sign) • <u>Wrist CT</u>: may aid in preprocedural planning
Treatment	• **Emergent closed reduction and splint immobilization** 　• Considered orthopedic emergency • <u>Surgery</u>: ORIF within 2 months
Key Words & Most Common	• Perilunate dislocation: radius articulation; no capitate articulation • Lunate dislocation: no articulation with capitate or radius • High-energy injury forcing hyperextension and ulnar deviation • Acute wrist pain/swelling +/- palm paresthesia (median nerve) • X-Ray • Emergent reduction + splint immobilization → ORIF

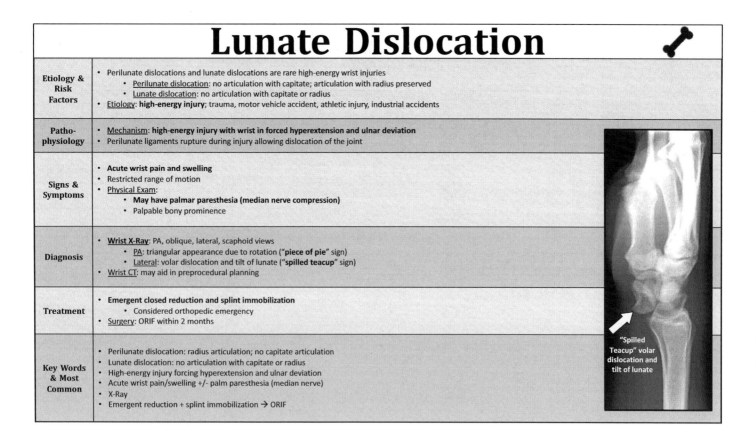

"Spilled Teacup" volar dislocation and tilt of lunate

Carpal Tunnel Syndrome

Etiology & Risk Factors	• Entrapment neuropathy caused by compression of the median nerve as it travels through the carpal tunnel in the wrist • <u>Etiology</u>: **repetitive wrist flexion/extension** (drawing, typing, video games), trauma, edema • <u>Risk Factors</u>: **females**, **age (40-60yo most common)**, **diabetes**, **pregnancy**, hypothyroidism, occupations with repetitive wrist flexion/extension, obesity, autoimmune disorders
Patho-physiology	• Increased pressure, local edema, or tendinous inflammation leads to compression of the median nerve as it travels through the carpal tunnel causing entrapment neuropathy

Signs & Symptoms	• **Burning/aching pain and paresthesia in median nerve distribution**
	   • Palmar aspect of thumb, index, middle and radial aspect of ring finger
	• **Waking at night** (patient may report shaking hand to restore sensation)
	• <u>Physical Exam</u>:
	   • **Tinel Sign**: paresthesia is reproduced by tapping the volar aspect of wrist
	   • **Phalen Sign**: paresthesia is reproduced by holding flexion of both wrists for 30-60 seconds
	   • <u>Carpal Compression Test</u>: paresthesia is reproduced by applying direct, firm pressure to carpal tunnel of the wrist in neutral position
	   • **Thenar atrophy** and weakness occurs in advanced cases

Diagnosis	• **Clinical Diagnosis** • <u>Electrophysiologic Testing</u>: gold standard; often not required for diagnosis
Treatment	• <u>Conservative</u>: **activity modifications, proper hand ergonomics** (keyboard at proper height), physical therapy, analgesia (NSAIDs) • **Immobilization: volar splint is initial management; especially beneficial at night** • **Corticosteroid Injection**: indicated if refractory to conservative treatment • <u>Surgery</u>: carpal tunnel release if severe or refractory to all other conservative treatments
Key Words & Most Common	• Median nerve entrapment as it travels through the carpal tunnel • Repetitive wrist use • Female, middle age, pregnancy, occupation • Burning/aching pain + paresthesia • Night symptoms • + Tinel; + Phalen sign • Clinical diagnosis • Wrist splint + activity/ergonomic modifications → steroid injection → surgery Thenar Atrophy

De Quervain Tenosynovitis

Etiology & Risk Factors	• First dorsal compartment stenosis of the wrist leading to tendon entrapment and inflammation • <u>Etiology</u>: **repetitive wrist and thumb motion**; thumb abduction and extension and radial wrist deviation • <u>Risk Factors</u>: golfers, clerical workers, **new mothers (lifting a child with thumbs under arms)**, diabetics, **carpenter/roofer (using hammer)**, excessive texting
Patho-physiology	• <u>Mechanism</u>: **repetitive use with thumb abduction and extension with radially deviated wrist** • Thickening of abductor pollicis longus and extensor pollicis brevis tendons secondary to overuse or trauma leads to entrapment of the tendon and inflammation

Signs & Symptoms	• **Acute wrist pain**
	   • **Radial aspect/base of thumb**; may radiate to forearm
	   • **Worse with thumb extension/gripping** or wrist motion
	• Pain with specific tasks (**picking up child, opening jar**)
	• <u>Physical Exam</u>:
	   • Tenderness/swelling over radial styloid and first dorsal compartment
	   • **Finkelstein Test**: sharp pain with ulnar deviation of wrist while thumb is flexed and held in a fist

Diagnosis	• **Clinical Diagnosis** • <u>Wrist X-Ray</u>: may be ordered to rule out other bony pathology (arthritis) Finkelstein Test
Treatment	• <u>Conservative</u>: **immobilization (thumb spica) is initial management**, analgesia (**NSAIDs**), physical therapy • **Corticosteroid Injection**: injection to tendon sheath if refractory to conservative treatment • <u>Surgery</u>: first dorsal compartment release if severe or refractory to all other conservative treatments
Key Words & Most Common	• Wrist tendon entrapment secondary to repetitive thumb abduction/extension with radially deviated wrist • Most common in new mothers (picking child up from underarms) or carpenter/roofers (using hammer repetitively) • Acute radial sided wrist pain, worse with thumb extension/gripping • Pain picking up child or opening jar • <u>Finkelstein Test</u>: sharp pain with ulnar deviation of wrist with thumb flexion held in fist • Clinical diagnosis • Thumb spica immobilization + NSAIDs → steroid injection → surgery

Mallet Finger

Etiology & Risk Factors	• **Flexion, "hammer-like" deformity of fingertip caused by avulsion injury of the extensor tendon from the distal phalanx** • Also known as "baseball finger" • <u>Etiology</u>: **trauma, athletic injury** (baseball, football, volleyball), household chores (tucking in sheet, tucking in shirt), occupation related activity, laceration
Patho-physiology	• <u>Mechanism</u>: **distal tip of finger is struck causing avulsion of the extensor tendon leading to forced flexion of an extended finger** • Disruption of extensor mechanism leads to distal flexed deformity
Signs & Symptoms	• **Pain and swelling over distal tip of finger** (may have associated subungual hematoma) • Inability to extend distal interphalangeal joint (DIPJ) • <u>Physical Exam</u>: • **Inability to actively extend the DIPJ** • **"Hammer-like" flexion deformity at DIPJ**
Diagnosis	• **Clinical diagnosis** • <u>Finger X-Ray</u>: • **May be normal** • May show **avulsion fracture at the tendon insertion site** • May show volar (palmar) subluxation of distal phalanx
Treatment	• **Immobilization**: splint of DIPJ in extension or slight hyperextension for 6-8 weeks (uninterrupted) • <u>Surgical</u>: indicated if displaced fracture, subluxation of DIPJ, open fracture • Closed reduction with percutaneous pinning vs ORIF; surgical reconstruction of tendon if severe injury
Key Words & Most Common	• "Hammer-like" flexion deformity of DIPJ secondary to extensor tendon avulsion injury Athletic injury trauma most common (ball strikes distal tip of finger) • Pain/swelling at distal tip • Inability to actively extend DIPJ • Clinical diagnosis + x-ray to determine avulsion fracture/subluxation • Splint of DIPJ in extension

"Hammer-like" flexion deformity at DIPJ

Boutonniere Deformity

Etiology & Risk Factors	• Flexion of the proximal interphalangeal joint (PIPJ) accompanied by hyperextension of the distal interphalangeal joint (DIPJ) • <u>Etiology</u>: **forced flexion of an actively extended finger** • **Trauma, sports injury** (basketball, football most common), **tendon laceration**, dislocation/fracture, osteoarthritis, rheumatoid arthritis
Patho-physiology	• <u>Mechanism</u>: force to tip of partially extended finger leads to disruption of extensor tendon at base of middle phalanx causing hyperflexion at the PIP joint and hyperextension at the DIP joint
Signs & Symptoms	• **Pain and swelling of finger** • <u>Physical Exam</u>: • **Deformity with finger flexed at PIP joint and hyperextended at DIP joint** • <u>Elson's Test</u>: bend PIP joint to 90° over edge of table, extend middle phalanx against resistance. Will have weak PIP extension and rigid hyperextension of DIP
Diagnosis	• **Clinical diagnosis** • <u>Finger X-Ray</u>: • **May be normal** • May show **avulsion fracture at middle phalanx**
Treatment	• <u>Immobilization</u>: splint of PIPJ in extension for 4-6 weeks • <u>Orthopedic Hand Surgeon Referral</u>
Key Words & Most Common	• Flexion of PIPJ with hyperextension of DIPJ • Forced flexion of extended finger (jammed finger) • Pain/swelling • Deformity (flexed PIPJ and hyperextended DIPJ) • Clinical diagnosis + x-ray to rule out fracture • Splint PIPJ in extension + orthopedic hand follow-up

Flexed PIPJ and hyperextended DIPJ

Pyogenic Flexor Tenosynovitis

Etiology & Risk Factors	• Severe bacterial infection within the digital flexor tendon synovial sheath; surgical emergency
	• <u>Etiology</u>: **penetrating trauma is most common**; contiguous spread from adjacent infected tissue
	• <u>Organism</u>: ***Staphylococcus aureus* most common bacteria**; other bacteria include *Staphylococcus epidermis*, group A *Streptococcus*, *Pseudomonas*
	   • *Eikenella corrodens* with penetrating human bites
	   • *Pasteurella multocida* with penetrating animal bites

Patho-physiology	• Penetrating trauma introduces bacteria to enclosed space of digital flexor tendon sheath which may lead to necrosis and devitalization of finger(s) • Infection causes adhesions within the synovial sheath and severely restricts range of motion

Signs & Symptoms	• **Pain and swelling to affected finger (worse at palmar aspect)**
	• May have evidence of trauma (penetrating injury; bite mark)
	• <u>Kanavel's Signs</u>:
	   1. **Pain with passive extension**
	   2. **Percussion tenderness** (diffuse tenderness to flexor tendon sheath)
	   3. **Fusiform swelling** (swelling along flexor tendon sheath)
	   4. **Flexion posture** (passive flexion of digit to reduce pain)

Diagnosis	• **Clinical diagnosis** • <u>Labs</u>: **elevated WBC count**, elevated ESR/CRP; local wound culture; blood cultures if signs of sepsis or hematogenous spread • <u>Finger X-Ray</u>: **ordered to rule out retained foreign body, osteomyelitis, or fracture** • <u>Finger Ultrasound/MRI</u>: may be sued to visualize flexor tendon sheath and fluid collection; non-specific
Treatment	• Emergent hand surgery consult • **Surgical debridement and irrigation** • <u>Antibiotics</u>: **broad-spectrum** initially then guided therapy based on culture • Vancomycin PLUS Ampicillin/Sulbactam OR cefoxitin OR piperacillin/tazobactam
Key Words & Most Common	• Bacterial infection of flexor tendon sheath from penetrating trauma • *S. aureus* most common; *Eikenella*=human bites; *Pasteurella multocida*=animal bites • Pain and swelling to affected finger (worse at palmar aspect) • Clinical diagnosis • X-ray to rule out foreign body or osteomyelitis • Surgical clean out procedure + broad-spectrum antibiotics

Flexor Tenosynovitis

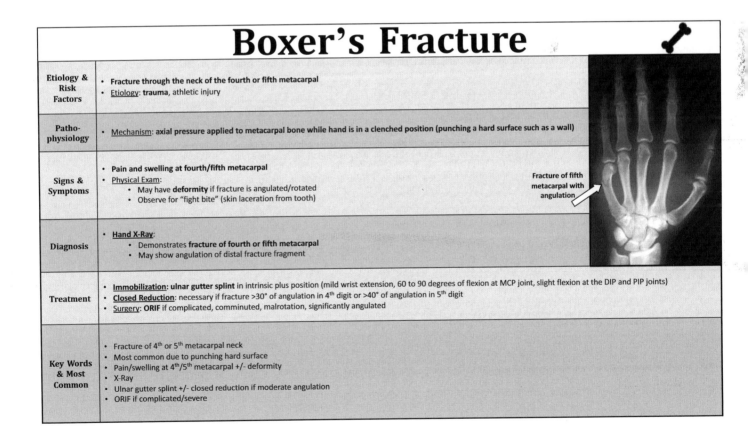

Boxer's Fracture

Etiology & Risk Factors	• **Fracture through the neck of the fourth or fifth metacarpal** • <u>Etiology</u>: **trauma**, athletic injury
Patho-physiology	• <u>Mechanism</u>: axial pressure applied to metacarpal bone while hand is in a clenched position (punching a hard surface such as a wall)

Signs & Symptoms	• **Pain and swelling at fourth/fifth metacarpal**
	• <u>Physical Exam</u>:
	   • May have **deformity** if fracture is angulated/rotated
	   • Observe for "fight bite" (skin laceration from tooth)

Diagnosis	• **Hand X-Ray**:
	   • Demonstrates **fracture of fourth or fifth metacarpal**
	   • May show angulation of distal fracture fragment

Treatment	• **Immobilization**: ulnar gutter splint in intrinsic plus position (mild wrist extension, 60 to 90 degrees of flexion at MCP joint, slight flexion at the DIP and PIP joints) • **Closed Reduction**: necessary if fracture >30° of angulation in 4th digit or >40° of angulation in 5th digit • <u>Surgery</u>: **ORIF** if complicated, comminuted, malrotation, significantly angulated
Key Words & Most Common	• Fracture of 4th or 5th metacarpal neck • Most common due to punching hard surface • Pain/swelling at 4th/5th metacarpal +/- deformity • X-Ray • Ulnar gutter splint +/- closed reduction if moderate angulation • ORIF if complicated/severe

Fracture of fifth metacarpal with angulation

Thumb Fractures

Etiology & Risk Factors	• Metacarpal fractures involving base of the thumb • <u>**Bennet fracture**</u>: **non-comminuted fracture/dislocation** of base of the metacarpal • <u>**Rolando fracture**</u>: **comminuted fracture** of base of the metacarpal • <u>Etiology</u>: **trauma**, athletic injury, fall
Patho-physiology	• <u>Mechanism</u>: **axial loading to a flexed thumb (punch with thumb tucked into fist)** • Axial load to thumb with metacarpal force to opposite direction leads to fracture line along point of weakness; shaft often subluxed/displaced due to pull of abductor pollicis longus, extensor pollicis longus, extensor pollicis brevis, and the adductor pollicis brevis on insertion point
Signs & Symptoms	• **Pain/swelling to base of thumb** • May have ecchymosis

Diagnosis	• <u>**Thumb X-Ray**</u>:
	  • <u>**Bennet fracture**</u>: **small fragment of first MCP base fracture articulates with trapezium**
	  • <u>**Rolando fracture**</u>: **comminuted fracture at the base of the first MCP** with a maintained volar carpal ligament; fracture typically "T" or "Y" shaped

Treatment	• <u>**Immobilization**</u>: **thumb spica splint** • <u>Closed Reduction</u>: fractures >20-30° of angulation • <u>Surgery</u>: ORIF vs closed reduction and percutaneous pinning • Rolando are more unstable fractures
Key Words & Most Common	• Base of thumb fracture Bennet: non-comminuted fracture • Rolando: comminuted fracture • Pain/swelling to base of thumb • X-Ray • Thumb spica splint → orthopedic hand follow-up

Rolando Fracture   Bennet Fracture

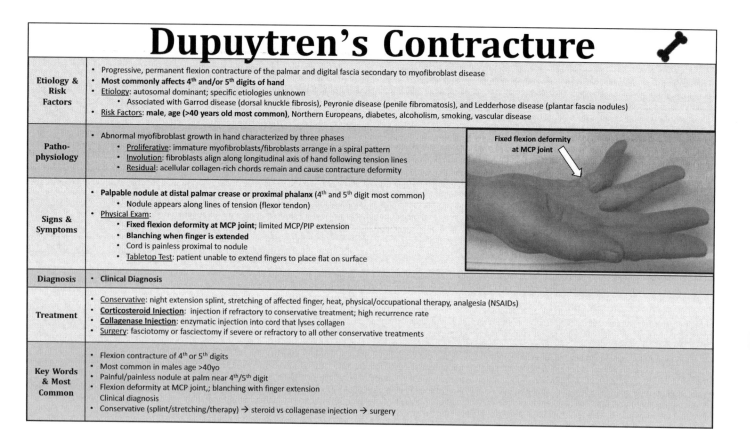

Dupuytren's Contracture

Etiology & Risk Factors	• Progressive, permanent flexion contracture of the palmar and digital fascia secondary to myofibroblast disease • **Most commonly affects 4th and/or 5th digits of hand** • <u>Etiology</u>: autosomal dominant; specific etiologies unknown • Associated with Garrod disease (dorsal knuckle fibrosis), Peyronie disease (penile fibromatosis), and Ledderhose disease (plantar fascia nodules) • <u>Risk Factors</u>: **male, age (>40 years old most common)**, Northern Europeans, diabetes, alcoholism, smoking, vascular disease

Patho-physiology	• Abnormal myofibroblast growth in hand characterized by three phases
	  • <u>Proliferative</u>: immature myofibroblasts/fibroblasts arrange in a spiral pattern
	  • <u>Involution</u>: fibroblasts align along longitudinal axis of hand following tension lines
	  • <u>Residual</u>: acellular collagen-rich chords remain and cause contracture deformity

Signs & Symptoms	• **Palpable nodule at distal palmar crease or proximal phalanx** (4th and 5th digit most common)
	  • Nodule appears along lines of tension (flexor tendon)
	• <u>Physical Exam</u>:
	  • **Fixed flexion deformity at MCP joint**; limited MCP/PIP extension
	  • **Blanching when finger is extended**
	  • Cord is painless proximal to nodule
	  • <u>Tabletop Test</u>: patient unable to extend fingers to place flat on surface

Diagnosis	• **Clinical Diagnosis**
Treatment	• <u>Conservative</u>: night extension splint, stretching of affected finger, heat, physical/occupational therapy, analgesia (NSAIDs) • <u>**Corticosteroid Injection**</u>: injection if refractory to conservative treatment; high recurrence rate • <u>**Collagenase Injection**</u>: enzymatic injection into cord that lyses collagen • <u>Surgery</u>: fasciotomy or fasciectomy if severe or refractory to all other conservative treatments
Key Words & Most Common	• Flexion contracture of 4th or 5th digits • Most common in males age >40yo • Painful/painless nodule at palm near 4th/5th digit • Flexion deformity at MCP joint,; blanching with finger extension Clinical diagnosis • Conservative (splint/stretching/therapy) → steroid vs collagenase injection → surgery

Fixed flexion deformity at MCP joint

References

1. Osteomyelitis of Tibia in Child.jpg. (2023, April 5). *Wikimedia Commons*. Retrieved 23:06, August 10, 2023 from https://commons.wikimedia.org/w/index.php?title=File:Osteomyelitis_of_Tibia_in_Child.jpg&oldid=747138218.
2. Osteoarthritis on X-ray.jpg. (2023, April 5). *Wikimedia Commons*. Retrieved 23:17, August 10, 2023 from https://commons.wikimedia.org/w/index.php?title=File:Osteoarthritis_on_X-ray.jpg&oldid=747138193.
3. Rheumatoid Arthritis.JPG. (2023, May 23). *Wikimedia Commons*. Retrieved 23:38, August 10, 2023 from https://commons.wikimedia.org/w/index.php?title=File:Rheumatoid_Arthritis.JPG&oldid=766166658.
4. Dislocated hip.jpg. (2023, May 19). *Wikimedia Commons*. Retrieved 23:50, August 10, 2023 from https://commons.wikimedia.org/w/index.php?title=File:Dislocated_hip.jpg&oldid=764912887.
5. AcetabularfracX.png. (2023, July 7). *Wikimedia Commons*. Retrieved 23:54, August 10, 2023 from https://commons.wikimedia.org/w/index.php?title=File:AcetabularfracX.png&oldid=781169579.
6. HipdisX.png. (2020, October 22). *Wikimedia Commons*. Retrieved 23:57, August 10, 2023 from https://commons.wikimedia.org/w/index.php?title=File:HipdisX.png&oldid=497177067.
7. Cdm hip fracture 343.jpg. (2020, September 14). *Wikimedia Commons*. Retrieved 15:07, August 13, 2023 from https://commons.wikimedia.org/w/index.php?title=File:Cdm_hip_fracture_343.jpg&oldid=458726624.
8. Roe-perthes.jpg. (2021, March 8). *Wikimedia Commons*. Retrieved 15:11, August 13, 2023 from https://commons.wikimedia.org/w/index.php?title=File:Roe-perthes.jpg&oldid=540629774.
9. SCFE FROG B&W.jpg. (2020, November 22). *Wikimedia Commons*. Retrieved 15:22, August 13, 2023 from https://commons.wikimedia.org/w/index.php?title=File:SCFE_FROG_B%26W.jpg&oldid=514016855.
10. Osteonecrosis femur 2img.jpg. (2020, October 5). *Wikimedia Commons*. Retrieved 15:25, August 13, 2023 from https://commons.wikimedia.org/w/index.php?title=File:Osteonecrosis_femur_2img.jpg&oldid=481195264.
11. Knee medial view.gif. (2022, July 2). *Wikimedia Commons*. Retrieved 15:43, August 13, 2023 from https://commons.wikimedia.org/w/index.php?title=File:Knee_medial_view.gif&oldid=670794191.
12. VKB-Riss MRT T1 PDW sag.jpg. (2022, March 30). *Wikimedia Commons*. Retrieved 15:52, August 13, 2023 from https://commons.wikimedia.org/w/index.php?title=File:VKB-Riss_MRT_T1_PDW_sag.jpg&oldid=645327944.
13. MRI meniscus tear.jpg. (2022, November 6). *Wikimedia Commons*. Retrieved 16:22, August 13, 2023 from https://commons.wikimedia.org/w/index.php?title=File:MRI_meniscus_tear.jpg&oldid=703070053.
14. Fracpetella.PNG. (2022, June 2). *Wikimedia Commons*. Retrieved 16:27, August 13, 2023 from https://commons.wikimedia.org/w/index.php?title=File:Fracpetella.PNG&oldid=660822155.
15. PetellardislocationChildMark.png. (2020, October 29). *Wikimedia Commons*. Retrieved 16:31, August 13, 2023 from https://commons.wikimedia.org/w/index.php?title=File:PetellardislocationChildMark.png&oldid=506137331.
16. Osgood.jpg. (2020, September 17). *Wikimedia Commons*. Retrieved 16:36, August 13, 2023 from https://commons.wikimedia.org/w/index.php?title=File:Osgood.jpg&oldid=463157508.
17. Patellarsehenruptur Quadrizepssehnenruptur Roe.jpg. (2022, March 30). *Wikimedia Commons*. Retrieved 16:39, August 13, 2023 from https://commons.wikimedia.org/w/index.php?title=File:Patellarsehenruptur_Quadrizepssehnenruptur_Roe.jpg&oldid=645369541.
18. PosteriorKneeDislocation.jpg. (2023, January 10). *Wikimedia Commons*. Retrieved 16:44, August 13, 2023 from https://commons.wikimedia.org/w/index.php?title=File:PosteriorKneeDislocation.jpg&oldid=724238288.
19. Lateral Tibial Plateau fracture XRay with Depression 2.jpg. (2022, December 6). *Wikimedia Commons*. Retrieved 16:50, August 13, 2023 from https://commons.wikimedia.org/w/index.php?title=File:Lateral_Tibial_Plateau_fracture_XRay_with_Depression_2.jpg&oldid=712971888.
20. Rupture tendon achiléen.jpg. (2023, March 4). *Wikimedia Commons*. Retrieved 17:01, August 13, 2023 from https://commons.wikimedia.org/w/index.php?title=File:Rupture_tendon_achil%C3%A9en.jpg&oldid=737692402.
21. Stress fracture of the second metatarsal bone1.jpg. (2021, December 16). *Wikimedia Commons*. Retrieved 17:25, August 13, 2023 from https://commons.wikimedia.org/w/index.php?title=File:Stress_fracture_of_the_second_metatarsal_bone1.jpg&oldid=614418898.
22. Projectional radiography of calcaneal spur.jpg. (2023, January 31). *Wikimedia Commons*. Retrieved 17:28, August 13, 2023 from https://commons.wikimedia.org/w/index.php?title=File:Projectional_radiography_of_calcaneal_spur.jpg&oldid=729135129.
23. Tarsal tunnel syndrome.png. (2023, February 8). *Wikimedia Commons*. Retrieved 17:33, August 13, 2023 from https://commons.wikimedia.org/w/index.php?title=File:Tarsal_tunnel_syndrome.png&oldid=730872711.
24. Hallux Valgus-Aspect pré op décharge.JPG. (2022, April 26). *Wikimedia Commons*. Retrieved 17:54, August 13, 2023 from https://commons.wikimedia.org/w/index.php?title=File:Hallux_Valgus-Aspect_pr%C3%A9_op_d%C3%A9charge.JPG&oldid=651940763.
25. Hammerzehe vor dem OP.JPG. (2020, October 4). *Wikimedia Commons*. Retrieved 18:00, August 13, 2023 from https://commons.wikimedia.org/w/index.php?title=File:Hammerzehe_vor_dem_OP.JPG&oldid=480589565.
26. Charcot arthropathy X-ray.jpg. (2020, October 4). *Wikimedia Commons*. Retrieved 18:09, August 13, 2023 from https://commons.wikimedia.org/w/index.php?title=File:Charcot_arthropathy_X-ray.jpg&oldid=480051361.
27. Neuroma de Morton.jpg. (2023, August 6). *Wikimedia Commons*. Retrieved 18:24, August 13, 2023 from https://commons.wikimedia.org/w/index.php?title=File:Neuroma_de_Morton.jpg&oldid=790590316.
28. Proximal fractures of 5th metatarsal.jpg. (2020, October 28). *Wikimedia Commons*. Retrieved 19:00, August 13, 2023 from https://commons.wikimedia.org/w/index.php?title=File:Proximal_fractures_of_5th_metatarsal.jpg&oldid=505243081.

References

29. LisFrancArrow.png. (2023, March 21). *Wikimedia Commons*. Retrieved 19:10, August 13, 2023 from https://commons.wikimedia.org/w/index.php?title=File:LisFrancArrow.png&oldid=742438808.
30. 612 Types of Fractures.jpg. (2023, June 1). *Wikimedia Commons*. Retrieved 19:18, August 13, 2023 from https://commons.wikimedia.org/w/index.php?title=File:612_Types_of_Fractures.jpg&oldid=769569737.
31. SalterHarris.svg. (2020, October 18). *Wikimedia Commons*. Retrieved 19:28, August 13, 2023 from https://commons.wikimedia.org/w/index.php?title=File:SalterHarris.svg&oldid=493482850.
32. Osteosarcoma of the tibia.png. (2020, October 19). *Wikimedia Commons*. Retrieved 19:32, August 13, 2023 from https://commons.wikimedia.org/w/index.php?title=File:Osteosarcoma_of_the_tibia.png&oldid=494518018.
33. Condrosarcoma-RX-TC.jpg. (2020, September 15). *Wikimedia Commons*. Retrieved 19:40, August 13, 2023 from https://commons.wikimedia.org/w/index.php?title=File:Condrosarcoma-RX-TC.jpg&oldid=459890480.
34. Ewing sarcoma tibia child.jpg. (2021, May 30). *Wikimedia Commons*. Retrieved 19:46, August 13, 2023 from https://commons.wikimedia.org/w/index.php?title=File:Ewing_sarcoma_tibia_child.jpg&oldid=566040803.
35. Osteochondroma X-ray.jpg. (2021, December 22). *Wikimedia Commons*. Retrieved 19:52, August 13, 2023 from https://commons.wikimedia.org/w/index.php?title=File:Osteochondroma_X-ray.jpg&oldid=615656776.
36. Osteoidosteom Roentgen-MRT.png. (2022, March 30). *Wikimedia Commons*. Retrieved 20:03, August 13, 2023 from https://commons.wikimedia.org/w/index.php?title=File:Osteoidosteom_Roentgen-MRT.png&oldid=645371390.
37. Tender points fibromyalgia.svg. (2020, November 24). *Wikimedia Commons*. Retrieved 20:11, August 13, 2023 from https://commons.wikimedia.org/w/index.php?title=File:Tender_points_fibromyalgia.svg&oldid=514649381.
38. Polymyalgia rheumatica man.svg. (2021, March 31). *Wikimedia Commons*. Retrieved 20:17, August 13, 2023 from https://commons.wikimedia.org/w/index.php?title=File:Polymyalgia_rheumatica_man.svg&oldid=548551588.
39. Dermatomyositis.jpg. (2020, September 11). *Wikimedia Commons*. Retrieved 20:39, August 13, 2023 from https://commons.wikimedia.org/w/index.php?title=File:Dermatomyositis.jpg&oldid=455068180.
40. Lupus pernio 01.jpg. (2020, October 16). *Wikimedia Commons*. Retrieved 20:43, August 13, 2023 from https://commons.wikimedia.org/w/index.php?title=File:Lupus_pernio_01.jpg&oldid=491050329.
41. Sjogrens Syndrome.jpg. (2020, October 30). *Wikimedia Commons*. Retrieved 20:49, August 13, 2023 from https://commons.wikimedia.org/w/index.php?title=File:Sjogrens_Syndrome.jpg&oldid=506999226.
42. Henoch-schonlein-purpura.jpg. (2020, September 22). *Wikimedia Commons*. Retrieved 21:28, August 13, 2023 from https://commons.wikimedia.org/w/index.php?title=File:Henoch-schonlein-purpura.jpg&oldid=467904328.
43. Psoriasisarthritis distales Interphalangealgelenk 79M - CR seitlich - 001.jpg. (2022, March 30). *Wikimedia Commons*. Retrieved 21:40, August 13, 2023 from https://commons.wikimedia.org/w/index.php?title=File:Psoriasisarthritis_distales_Interphalangealgelenk_79M_-_CR_seitlich_-_001.jpg&oldid=645349122.
44. Ankylosing spondylitis lumbar spine.jpg. (2020, September 20). *Wikimedia Commons*. Retrieved 21:51, August 13, 2023 from https://commons.wikimedia.org/w/index.php?title=File:Ankylosing_spondylitis_lumbar_spine.jpg&oldid=466407348.
45. Feet-Reiters syndrome.jpg. (2020, September 28). *Wikimedia Commons*. Retrieved 21:54, August 13, 2023 from https://commons.wikimedia.org/w/index.php?title=File:Feet-Reiters_syndrome.jpg&oldid=474281691.
46. Fluorescent uric acid.JPG. (2020, August 30). *Wikimedia Commons*. Retrieved 14:43, August 14, 2023 from https://commons.wikimedia.org/w/index.php?title=File:Fluorescent_uric_acid.JPG&oldid=445683152.
47. Pseudogout crystals (calcium pyrophosphate dihydrate crystal).png. (2022, August 6). *Wikimedia Commons*. Retrieved 14:43, August 14, 2023 from https://commons.wikimedia.org/w/index.php?title=File:Pseudogout_crystals_(calcium_pyrophosphate_dihydrate_crystal).png&oldid=680597289.
48. L4-l5-disc-herniation.png. (2022, May 30). *Wikimedia Commons*. Retrieved 14:57, August 14, 2023 from https://commons.wikimedia.org/w/index.php?title=File:L4-l5-disc-herniation.png&oldid=660100222.
49. MRI of the lumbar spine with abscess in the posterior epidural space, causing cauda equina syndrome.jpg. (2022, November 6). *Wikimedia Commons*. Retrieved 15:03, August 14, 2023 from https://commons.wikimedia.org/w/index.php?title=File:MRI_of_the_lumbar_spine_with_abscess_in_the_posterior_epidural_space,_causing_cauda_equina_syndrome.jpg&oldid=703046845.
50. T12compressionfracMark.png. (2020, October 4). *Wikimedia Commons*. Retrieved 15:14, August 14, 2023 from https://commons.wikimedia.org/w/index.php?title=File:T12compressionfracMark.png&oldid=480218494.
51. Lumbar spinal stenosis 1 8.png. (2021, June 14). *Wikimedia Commons*. Retrieved 15:24, August 14, 2023 from https://commons.wikimedia.org/w/index.php?title=File:Lumbar_spinal_stenosis_1_8.png&oldid=569116960.
52. Scoliosis cobb.svg. (2021, December 11). *Wikimedia Commons*. Retrieved 15:37, August 14, 2023 from https://commons.wikimedia.org/w/index.php?title=File:Scoliosis_cobb.svg&oldid=613227621.
53. Scoliosis.jpg. (2020, November 1). *Wikimedia Commons*. Retrieved 15:37, August 14, 2023 from https://commons.wikimedia.org/w/index.php?title=File:Scoliosis.jpg&oldid=508821094.
54. Spondylolyse L5S1 LWS seitlich 002.jpg. (2022, March 30). *Wikimedia Commons*. Retrieved 15:47, August 14, 2023 from https://commons.wikimedia.org/w/index.php?title=File:Spondylolyse_L5S1_LWS_seitlich_002.jpg&oldid=645338180.
55. Spondylolisthesis.jpg. (2020, October 4). *Wikimedia Commons*. Retrieved 15:52, August 14, 2023 from https://commons.wikimedia.org/w/index.php?title=File:Spondylolisthesis.jpg&oldid=480713732.

References

56. Dislocated shoulder X-ray 10.png. (2022, March 31). *Wikimedia Commons*. Retrieved 15:56, August 14, 2023 from https://commons.wikimedia.org/w/index.php?title=File:Dislocated_shoulder_X-ray_10.png&oldid=645454402.

57. Grade3ACsepMark.png. (2020, October 28). *Wikimedia Commons*. Retrieved 16:26, August 14, 2023 from https://commons.wikimedia.org/w/index.php?title=File:Grade3ACsepMark.png&oldid=505405677.

58. Rot cuff tear x-ray.jpg. (2021, May 19). *Wikimedia Commons*. Retrieved 16:28, August 14, 2023 from https://commons.wikimedia.org/w/index.php?title=File:Rot_cuff_tear_x-ray.jpg&oldid=561739947.

59. SupracondylarfracMark.png. (2020, October 2). *Wikimedia Commons*. Retrieved 17:51, August 14, 2023 from https://commons.wikimedia.org/w/index.php?title=File:SupracondylarfracMark.png&oldid=478163791.

60. ProxHumeralFracture.png. (2022, April 22). *Wikimedia Commons*. Retrieved 17:47, August 14, 2023 from https://commons.wikimedia.org/w/index.php?title=File:ProxHumeralFracture.png&oldid=650835176.

61. Clavicle Fracture Left.jpg. (2022, April 23). *Wikimedia Commons*. Retrieved 17:58, August 14, 2023 from https://commons.wikimedia.org/w/index.php?title=File:Clavicle_Fracture_Left.jpg&oldid=651099043.

62. Olecranon Fracture.jpg. (2020, October 28). *Wikimedia Commons*. Retrieved 18:05, August 14, 2023 from https://commons.wikimedia.org/w/index.php?title=File:Olecranon_Fracture.jpg&oldid=504901461.

63. Bursitis Elbow WC.JPG. (2022, December 18). *Wikimedia Commons*. Retrieved 18:08, August 14, 2023 from https://commons.wikimedia.org/w/index.php?title=File:Bursitis_Elbow_WC.JPG&oldid=716983051.

64. Monteggia Fracture.jpg. (2020, October 16). *Wikimedia Commons*. Retrieved 18:26, August 14, 2023 from https://commons.wikimedia.org/w/index.php?title=File:Monteggia_Fracture.jpg&oldid=491929959.

65. Monteggia LAT.jpg. (2020, June 15). *Wikimedia Commons*. Retrieved 18:29, August 14, 2023 from https://commons.wikimedia.org/w/index.php?title=File:Monteggia_LAT.jpg&oldid=426479595.

66. Galeazzi Fracture of Distal Radius.jpg. (2022, November 28). *Wikimedia Commons*. Retrieved 18:33, August 14, 2023 from https://commons.wikimedia.org/w/index.php?title=File:Galeazzi_Fracture_of_Distal_Radius.jpg&oldid=710674676.

67. Elbow1.jpg. (2020, October 13). *Wikimedia Commons*. Retrieved 18:51, August 14, 2023 from https://commons.wikimedia.org/w/index.php?title=File:Elbow1.jpg&oldid=488946348.

68. X-ray of scaphoid fracture.png. (2020, October 4). *Wikimedia Commons*. Retrieved 18:58, August 14, 2023 from https://commons.wikimedia.org/w/index.php?title=File:X-ray_of_scaphoid_fracture.png&oldid=480912606.

69. Collesfracture.jpg. (2021, February 21). *Wikimedia Commons*. Retrieved 19:03, August 14, 2023 from https://commons.wikimedia.org/w/index.php?title=File:Collesfracture.jpg&oldid=534768306.

70. Smith2019Frac.jpg. (2023, May 2). *Wikimedia Commons*. Retrieved 19:06, August 14, 2023 from https://commons.wikimedia.org/w/index.php?title=File:Smith2019Frac.jpg&oldid=757902621.

71. LunatedislocationL.jpg. (2020, October 16). *Wikimedia Commons*. Retrieved 19:09, August 14, 2023 from https://commons.wikimedia.org/w/index.php?title=File:LunatedislocationL.jpg&oldid=491732471.

72. Untreated Carpal Tunnel Syndrome.JPG. (2020, September 25). *Wikimedia Commons*. Retrieved 19:24, August 14, 2023 from https://commons.wikimedia.org/w/index.php?title=File:Untreated_Carpal_Tunnel_Syndrome.JPG&oldid=470760641.

73. Finkelstein Test Arrow.jpg. (2020, September 22). *Wikimedia Commons*. Retrieved 19:27, August 14, 2023 from https://commons.wikimedia.org/w/index.php?title=File:Finkelstein_Test_Arrow.jpg&oldid=467520994.

74. Mallet Finger Injury.jpg. (2022, August 28). *Wikimedia Commons*. Retrieved 19:29, August 14, 2023 from https://commons.wikimedia.org/w/index.php?title=File:Mallet_Finger_Injury.jpg&oldid=685472493.

75. Boutonnière deformity.jpg. (2020, October 11). *Wikimedia Commons*. Retrieved 19:32, August 14, 2023 from https://commons.wikimedia.org/w/index.php?title=File:Boutonni%C3%A8re_deformity.jpg&oldid=486555849.

76. Flexor Tenosynovitis.jpg. (2022, June 22). *Wikimedia Commons*. Retrieved 19:34, August 14, 2023 from https://commons.wikimedia.org/w/index.php?title=File:Flexor_Tenosynovitis.jpg&oldid=667431167.

77. Location of UCL injury.jpg. (2022, November 28). *Wikimedia Commons*. Retrieved 19:37, August 14, 2023 from https://commons.wikimedia.org/w/index.php?title=File:Location_of_UCL_injury.jpg&oldid=710594887.

78. Boxers fracture.JPG. (2020, August 26). *Wikimedia Commons*. Retrieved 19:42, August 14, 2023 from https://commons.wikimedia.org/w/index.php?title=File:Boxers_fracture.JPG&oldid=443534378.

79. Rolando fracture.jpg. (2022, March 29). *Wikimedia Commons*. Retrieved 19:52, August 14, 2023 from https://commons.wikimedia.org/w/index.php?title=File:Rolando_fracture.jpg&oldid=645124240.

80. Bennett-Faktur seitlich cropped.jpg. (2023, January 2). *Wikimedia Commons*. Retrieved 19:54, August 14, 2023 from https://commons.wikimedia.org/w/index.php?title=File:Bennett-Faktur_seitlich_cropped.jpg&oldid=722021033.

81. Dupuytren's2010.JPG. (2020, October 1). *Wikimedia Commons*. Retrieved 19:56, August 14, 2023 from https://commons.wikimedia.org/w/index.php?title=File:Dupuytren%27s2010.JPG&oldid=476895980.

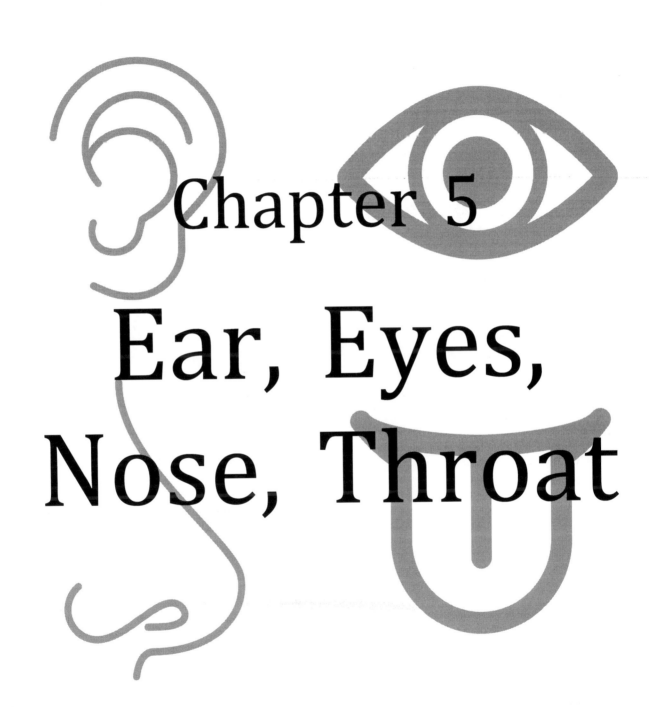

Chapter 5
Ear, Eyes, Nose, Throat

Entropion and Ectropion ◉

	Entropion	Ectropion
Etiology & Risk Factors	• **Inversion of the eyelid (eyelid and lashes turned *inward*)** • Lower eyelid more common • Etiology: involutional change (**aging**) is most common, post-surgical • Risk Factors: **age**, recent intraocular surgery, female, infection, inflammation, **blepharospasm**	• **Eversion of the eyelid (eyelid and lashes turned *outward*)** • Lower eyelid more common • Etiology: involutional change (**aging**) most common, post-surgical • Risk Factors: **age**, CNVII (facial) palsy, recent blepharoplasty, trauma, post-infection, sun exposure
Patho-physiology	• Weakening of lower lid retractors, orbicularis, tarsus, and canthal tendons (eyelid stabilizers) secondary to age-related tissue relaxation • Ocular irritation can lead to sustained orbicularis oculi muscle spasm leading to inward rotation of eyelid margin	• Horizontal eyelid laxity and disinsertion of eyelid retractors secondary to age-related tissue relaxation
Signs & Symptoms	• **Eye pain and erythema** • Irritation/sensitivity of eye • **Foreign body sensation (corneal abrasion secondary to inversion of eyelashes)** • **Excessive tearing**	• **Sagging of eyelid outward** • Irritation/sensitivity of eye • **Ocular dryness** • **Excessive tearing** (nasolacrimal system may no longer contact eye)
Diagnosis	• **Clinical Diagnosis**	• **Clinical Diagnosis**
Treatment	• Lubrication: **artificial tears**; gels or ointments provide moisture shields • Contact Lenses: may provide protection of ocular surface from eyelashes • Botulinum Toxin Injection: Botox injection if spastic etiology • Surgery: definitive management	• Lubrication: artificial tears; gels or ointments provide moisture shields • Surgery: definitive management
Key Words & Most Common	• Inversion of eyelid • Age related condition • Eye pain/erythema • Foreign body sensation (corneal abrasion from eyelashes) • Clinical diagnosis • Lubrication +/- contact lenses for protection → surgery	• Eversion of eyelid • Age related condition • Eyelid sagging outward • Ocular dryness • Clinical Diagnosis • Lubrication → surgery

Subconjunctival Hemorrhage ◉

Etiology & Risk Factors	• Bleeding of the ocular conjunctival blood vessels into the subconjunctival space
	• Etiology: traumatic or spontaneous
	  • Trauma: **rubbing eyes**, foreign body, direct impact
	  • Spontaneous: **related to elevated venous pressures; hypertension, Valsalva (coughing, straining, sneezing)**, vomiting, strenuous/heavy lifting
	• Risk Factors: **hypertension is greatest risk factor**, diabetes, hyperlipidemia, **anticoagulation therapy (warfarin, heparin, etc.)**, NSAID/aspirin/clopidogrel use

Patho-physiology	• Elastic and connective tissue of blood vessels become weak due to age or comorbidities • Periods of elevated venous pressure or trauma cause bleeding from the conjunctival or episcleral blood vessels to leak into the subconjunctival space

Signs & Symptoms	• **Painless red eye**
	  • *May be alarming to patient*
	• **Focal, flat, red region of ocular surface**
	• **No change in visual acuity**
	• Possible foreign body sensation
	• Physical Exam:
	  • **Bleeding between sclera and conjunctiva (bleeding on white sclera with clear borders)**

Diagnosis	• **Clinical Diagnosis** • Consider fluorescein stain to rule out foreign body or corneal abrasion if history suggests
Treatment	• Reassurance: adequate therapy; often resolve spontaneously within 7-14 days • **Hypertension and anticoagulation medication management as indicated** • *Topical corticosteroids, antibiotics, vasoconstrictors, and warm/cool compresses do not speed reabsorption*
Key Words & Most Common	• Bleeding into subconjunctival space • Elevated venous pressure (HTN, sneezing, vomiting, lifting, straining) • Hypertension greatest risk factor; anticoagulation therapy • Painless red eye • No change in visual acuity • Bleeding on white sclera with clear borders • Clinical diagnosis • Reassurance

Bleeding on sclera with clear borders

Cranial Nerve III Palsy

Etiology & Risk Factors	<ul><li>Oculomotor (CNIII) nerve palsy</li><li><u>Etiology</u>: may involve or spare the pupil vascular ischemia, trauma, intracranial neoplasm, congenital, idiopathic<ul><li><u>Pupil Involvement</u>: **aneurysm (posterior communicating artery)**, trauma, **intracranial neoplasm**, uncal herniation</li><li><u>Pupil Sparing</u>: **CNIII ischemia** (secondary to hypertension or diabetes)</li></ul></li><li><u>Risk Factors</u>: **hypertension, diabetes**</li></ul>
Patho-physiology	<ul><li>Oculomotor nerve lies lateral to the posterior communicating artery; innervates eyelid muscles and external ocular muscles (except lateral rectus and superior oblique)</li><li>Lesions (aneurysm, neoplasm) cause compression of oculomotor nerve</li></ul>
Signs & Symptoms	<ul><li>**Affected eye deviates *laterally* and *down* ("down and out")**</li><li>**Ptosis**</li><li>**Diplopia**</li><li>**Headache (if due to aneurysm)**</li><li><u>Physical Exam</u>:<ul><li>**If pupil is dilated or nonreactive, indicates space occupying lesion (aneurysm, mass, herniation)**</li><li>**If pupil is spared, indicates ischemic etiology**</li></ul></li></ul>
Diagnosis	<ul><li><u>**CT Angiography of Brain**</u>: **urgently performed if exam suggests aneurysm (headache + dilated pupil)**</li><li><u>MRI</u>: more sensitive to identify cranial nerve</li></ul>
Treatment	<ul><li><u>**Aneurysm or Space-Occupying Lesion**</u>: **urgent neurosurgery consult**</li><li><u>Ischemic</u>: medical management +/- aspiring; ophthalmology follow-up</li></ul>
Key Words & Most Common	<ul><li>Oculomotor nerve palsy</li><li>Pupil involvement: aneurysm, neoplasm</li><li>Pupil sparing: ischemia</li><li>Eye deviates *down* and out</li><li>Dilated/nonreactive pupil = space occupying lesion</li><li>Spared pupil = ischemia</li><li>CTA</li><li>Urgent neurosurgeon consult (aneurysm, lesion)</li><li>Medical management if ischemic</li></ul>

Cranial Nerve IV Palsy

Etiology & Risk Factors	<ul><li>Trochlear (CNIV) nerve palsy</li><li>**Most common cause of vertical diplopia**</li><li><u>Etiology</u>: **head trauma most common, congenital**, idiopathic, increased intraocular pressure, herpes zoster ophthalmicus, meningitis, **diabetic neuropathy**, infarction</li><li><u>Risk Factors</u>: hypertension, **diabetes**</li></ul>
Patho-physiology	<ul><li>Trochlea innervates superior oblique muscle</li><li>Frontolateral head trauma leads to cranial nerve injury</li></ul>
Signs & Symptoms	<ul><li>**Vertical diplopia**</li><li>**Hypertropia (eye is deviated upwards)**<ul><li>**Inability to move eye down and in**</li></ul></li><li>Difficulty going downstairs</li><li><u>Physical Exam</u>:<ul><li>**Compensatory head tilt *away* from affected side**</li></ul></li></ul>
Diagnosis	<ul><li>**Clinical Diagnosis**</li><li><u>Labs</u>: point of care glucose, CBC depending on suspected etiology</li><li><u>CT Head</u>: if traumatic and/or subarachnoid hemorrhage or stroke suspected</li><li><u>MRI Head</u>: most sensitive imaging test</li></ul>
Treatment	<ul><li><u>Address Underlying Etiology</u>:</li><li><u>**Prism Glasses**</u>: **restores concordant vision**</li><li><u>Surgery</u>: **surgical correction required in many cases**; inferior oblique weakening with vertical and horizontal rectus surgery is most common procedure</li></ul>
Key Words & Most Common	<ul><li>Trochlear (CNIV) nerve palsy</li><li>Head trauma is most common cause; congenital</li><li>Vertical diplopia</li><li>Hypertropia (eye deviated upwards)</li><li>Inability to look down and in</li><li>Compensatory head tilt away from affected side</li><li>Clinical diagnosis</li><li>Prism glasses → surgical correction</li></ul>

Cranial Nerve VI Palsy

Etiology & Risk Factors	• Abducens (CNVI) nerve palsy • **Most common ocular nerve palsy** • <u>Etiology</u>: **increased intracranial pressure most common, vasculopathy (diabetes), congenital**, aneurysm, **idiopathic, ischemia**, iatrogenic (post-lumbar puncture, spinal anesthesia), inflammatory conditions (lupus, sarcoidosis, giant cell arteritis), lesion of cavernous sinus/orbit/base of skull, infection (Lyme disease, syphilis, meningitis) • <u>Risk Factors</u>: **diabetes is greatest risk factor (especially uncontrolled)**, hypertension
Patho-physiology	• Abducens nerve innervates the ipsilateral lateral rectus muscle which controls eye abduction • Esotropia (inward eye movement) of the affected eye is secondary to the unopposed action of the medial rectus muscle

Signs & Symptoms	• **Horizontal diplopia (double vision when attempting lateral gaze)**
	• **Esotropia (eye deviated inwards)**
	    • **Inability to abduct the eye**
	• <u>Physical Exam</u>:
	    • **Compensatory head turn *toward* the affected eye**

Diagnosis	• **Workup dependent on suspected etiology** • <u>Neuroimaging</u>: CT or MRI; MRI preferred • <u>Lumbar Puncture</u>: if meningitis or benign intracranial hypertension suspected • <u>Labs</u>: consider point of care glucose, CBC, ESR/CRP, fluorescent treponemal antibody-absorption test (syphilis), Lyme titer, thyroid function tests, antinuclear antibody test
Treatment	• **Treat underlying etiology** • <u>Child</u>: **alternating patches (prevents amblyopia), prism therapy**, strabismus surgery • <u>Adult</u>: **observation; often self-limited**; strabismus surgery
Key Words & Most Common	• Abducens (CNVI) nerve palsy • Increased ICP most common, vasculopathy (diabetes), idiopathic, ischemia, congenital • Diabetes is greatest risk factor • Horizontal diplopia • Isotropic (eye deviated inward) • Compensatory head turn toward affected eye • Workup and treatment dependent on underlying etiology • Alternating patches or prism therapy if child

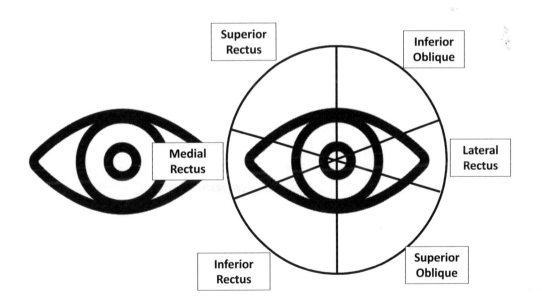

Dacryocystitis

Etiology & Risk Factors	• Inflammatory state of the nasolacrimal sac leading to obstruction and stagnation of tears within sac • <u>Etiology</u>: **infection (*Staphylococcus* and *Streptococcus* species most common**; *Pseudomonas, Haemophilus influenzae*), chronic debris in eye, trauma, surgery, medications, neoplasm
Patho-physiology	• Obstruction of nasolacrimal system results in stagnation of tears provides environment for infection to propagate and debris to collect leading to further inflammation

Signs & Symptoms	• **Signs of infection at medial canthus overlying the lacrimal space** (lower nasal-side corner of eyelid)
	  • **Tenderness, erythema, warmth, edema**
	    • May have purulent discharge or signs of abscess formation
	• May have increased tear production

Diagnosis	• **Clinical diagnosis** • Culture of purulent drainage

Treatment	• <u>Conservative</u>: **warm compresses, nasolacrimal massage**, decongestants
	• <u>Antibiotics</u>: broad-spectrum covering *Staph/Strep*
	  • <u>Mild</u>: **clindamycin**
	    • <u>Severe</u>: IV cephalosporin (cefuroxime or ceftriaxone or cefazolin); IV clindamycin; add Vancomycin if MRSA suspected

Key Words & Most Common	• Obstruction of nasolacrimal sac leading to stagnation and infection • *Staph* and *Strep* spp. most common • Pain, swelling, redness, warmth to lower nasal-side corner of eye • +/- purulent drainage • Clinical diagnosis • Warm compresses + massage • <u>Antibiotics</u>: oral clindamycin if mild → IV cephalosporin or clindamycin • Vancomycin if MRSA

Blepharitis

Etiology & Risk Factors	• **Inflammation of the eyelid margins**
	• Can be acute or chronic; chronic more common
	• <u>Etiology</u>:
	  • <u>Acute</u>: **bacterial infection (*Staphylococcus aureus* or *Staphylococcus epidermis*) is most common**, viral infection (*Herpes simplex* or *Varicella zoster*)
	    • <u>Chronic</u>: **meibomian gland dysfunction (most common type)**, seborrheic blepharitis, atopy/seasonal
	• <u>Risk Factors</u>: female, age (>40yo), atopic dermatitis, seborrheic dermatitis, Down syndrome

Patho-physiology	• Chronic, low-grade infection of the ocular surface or inflammatory skin conditions lead to inflammation of eyelid margins • Meibomian gland over-secretion of oily substance leads to clogged/engorged duct
Signs & Symptoms	• **Burning, itching, crusting of eyelids** • **Inflammation of eyelid margins** • Matted eyelashes
Diagnosis	• **Clinical Diagnosis** • <u>Slit Lamp</u>: may be used to determine anterior (infectious) vs posterior (Meibomian gland dysfunction)

Treatment	• <u>Eyelid Hygiene</u>: **mainstay of treatment**
	  • **Eyelid massage** (expresses oil from meibomian gland)
	  • **Warm compress** (softens debris and oils, dilates meibomian gland)
	  • **Eyelid washing** (diluted baby shampoo to remove debris and oil)
	• <u>Lubrication</u>: artificial tears
	• <u>Acute Blepharitis</u>: topical bacitracin or erythromycin
	  • <u>Severe or refractory</u>: oral tetracycline or macrolide (azithromycin)

Key Words & Most Common	• Inflammation of eyelid margin • Bacterial infection (acute) vs Meibomian gland dysfunction (chronic) • Burning, itching, crusting, inflammation of eyelids • Clinical diagnosis • Eyelid hygiene (massage → warm compress → washing) • Topical bacitracin or erythromycin for acute infections → oral antibiotics if severe

Inflammation of eyelid margins

Hordeolum (Stye)

Etiology & Risk Factors	• **Acute bacterial infection of the eyelid margin**
	   • <u>Internal</u>: blockage/infection of meibomian gland; deep from palpebral margin under eyelid
	   • <u>External</u>: blockage/infection of Zeis (sebaceous) or Moll (sweat) glands; near eyelid margin
	• <u>Etiology</u>: **bacterial infection of eyelash follicle (*Staphylococcus aureus* most common cause)**
	• <u>Risk Factors</u>: **blepharitis, seborrheic dermatitis**, rosacea, diabetes, hyperlipidemia, use of makeup

Patho-physiology	• Thickening or stasis of Zeis, Moll, or Meibomian gland secretion leads to blockage of gland, impairing ocular defense mechanisms • Stasis leads to infection with bacteria (*Staphylococcus aureus*) causing localized inflammation and leukocyte infiltration leading to purulent abscess
Signs & Symptoms	• **Pain, edema and erythema of eyelid** • May have **pustule at eyelid margin**
Diagnosis	• **Clinical Diagnosis**
Treatment	• <u>**Warm Compresses**</u>: **mainstay of treatment**; softens debris and oils, dilates glands • <u>**Eyelid Massage**</u>: expresses purulent drainage from infected glands • <u>Incision and Drainage</u>: may be necessary for large abscesses without spontaneous drainage • <u>**Topical Antibiotics**</u>: erythromycin or bacitracin ointment
Key Words & Most Common	• Acute bacterial infection of eyelid margin • Bacterial (S. aureus) most common • Pain, edema, erythema of eyelid +/- pustule at eyelid margin • Clinical diagnosis • Warm compress + massage → topical erythromycin → I&D if severe/refractory

Pustule on eyelid margin

Chalazion

Etiology & Risk Factors	• **Chronic, sterile, lipogranuloma of the internal Meibomian sebaceous gland** • More commonly affects upper eyelid • <u>Etiology</u>: **inflammation or obstruction of eyelid sebaceous glands**
Patho-physiology	• Abnormally thick secretions lead to obstruction of the Zeis or Meibomian glands causing a granulomatous inflammatory response as lipid breakdown products infiltrate surrounding tissue
Signs & Symptoms	• **Eyelid swelling and erythema of the conjunctival surface of eyelid** • **Progresses to painless nodular lesion** • Often **slow growing** over weeks to months
Diagnosis	• **Clinical Diagnosis**

Treatment	• <u>**Eyelid Hygiene**</u>: **mainstay of treatment**
	   • **Eyelid massage** (expresses oil from meibomian gland)
	   • **Warm compress** (softens debris and oils, dilates meibomian gland)
	   • **Eyelid washing** (diluted baby shampoo to remove debris and oil)
	• <u>Ophthalmology Referral</u>: for refractory cases; may require intralesional steroid injection or surgical curettage
	• Antibiotics often not indicated (granulomatous condition)

Key Words & Most Common	• Lipogranuloma of internal Meibomian sebaceous gland • Eyelid swelling/erythema of internal eyelid → painless nodule • Slow growing • Clinical Diagnosis • Eyelid massage + warm compress + eyelid washing → ophthalmology referral • Antibiotics often not indicated

Eyelid swelling and erythema with nodular lesion

Pinguecula and Pterygium

	Pinguecula	Pterygium
Etiology & Risk Factors	• Benign scleral growth characterized by slow-growing, thickening of the bulbar conjunctiva • Risk Factors: **sunlight**, trauma, **wind/dust/sand exposure**, **males**, advanced age, contact lens wearer	• Fibrovascular overgrowth of conjunctival tissue • Risk Factors: **sunlight**, trauma, **wind/dust/sand exposure**, **males**, advanced age, smoking
Patho-physiology	• Exposure to UV light, wind, dust, or sand causes chronic inflammation and leads to collagen degeneration and fibroblastic proliferation • Scleral growth consists of fat, protein, and calcium	• Exposure to UV light, wind, dust, or sand causes chronic inflammation and leads to collagen degeneration and fibroblastic proliferation • Benign scleral growth starts at medial canthus and grows laterally

Signs & Symptoms	• Commonly asymptomatic
	• **Whitish/yellow, slightly elevated nodule on the sclera**
	  • More common on nasal side of bulbar conjunctiva
	• **Foreign body sensation** (irritation, tearing, dryness)
	• **Does *not* grow into the cornea**
	• **Does *not* affect visual acuity**
		• **Triangular, whitish/yellow, slightly elevated mass on the sclera**
		  • Begins medially (nasal side) and extends laterally
		• **Foreign body sensation** (irritation, tearing, dryness)
		• **Can grow and affect cornea**
		• **Can affect visual acuity** (astigmatism or altered refractive power)

Diagnosis	• **Clinical Diagnosis**	• Clinical Diagnosis

Treatment	• Prevention: **sun protection** (sunglasses, wide brimmed hat), **eye protection**,
	• Supportive: artificial tears, cold compresses
	  • Topical NSAIDs (ketorolac drops) if inflammation/irritation persists
	• Surgery: surgical resection for cosmesis or if chronically inflamed
		• Prevention: **sun protection** (sunglasses, wide brimmed hat), **eye protection**,
		• Supportive: artificial tears, cold compresses
		  • Topical NSAIDs (ketorolac drops) if inflammation/irritation persists
		• Surgery: surgical resection for cosmesis or if vision is impaired

Key Words & Most Common	• Slow-growing, benign scleral growth • Sunlight, wind, dust, sand exposure • White/yellow, mass on nasal side of sclera • Does NOT grow into cornea • Does NOT affect visual acuity • Clinical diagnosis • Conservative treatment Nodule on sclera	• Benign fibrovascular overgrowth of conjunctival tissue • Sunlight, wind, dust, sand, smoking exposure • Triangular, whitish/yellow, mass on nasal side of sclera • CAN grow and affect cornea • CAN affect visual acuity • Clinical diagnosis • Conservative treatment → surgery if vision is impaired Triangular mass on sclera

Globe Rupture

Etiology & Risk Factors	• Blunt or penetrative trauma results in full thickness disruption of the other ocular membrane (sclera or cornea)
	• **Vision-threatening ophthalmologic emergency**
	• Etiology: **trauma (blunt or penetrative)**, occupational injury, motor vehicle accident, athletic injury, shotgun or bb pellets
	  • **Scissors** are most common cause in children
	  • **Foreign body** (metal-on-metal shards from grinder/drilling, wood shavings, lawn mower) most common cause in adults

Patho-physiology	• Trauma to eye causes and acute rise in intraocular pressure resulting in rupture of ocular membranes at the weakest point

Signs & Symptoms	• **Acute eye pain and decreased visual acuity**
	• Physical Exam:
	  • **Teardrop shaped pupil**
	  • Prolapse of ocular tissue from sclera/corneal opening
	  • **Severe, diffuse subconjunctival hemorrhage involving entire sclera**
	  • **Hyphema** (blood in anterior chamber)

Diagnosis	• **Clinical diagnosis** • Slit Lamp Exam: may aid in diagnosis; contraindicated if obvious globe rupture • Seidel's Test: leakage of aqueous humor from anterior chamber when performing fluorescein stain; contraindicated if obvious globe rupture • Maxillofacial CT: preferred imaging to detect foreign body Hyphema of anterior chamber
Treatment	• **Emergent Ophthalmology Consult: vision-threatening ocular emergency** • **Eye Protection: metal shield** (Fox shield) or cup to prevent further injury/pressure to eye • Minimize rise in intraocular pressure (**elevate head of bed**, strict bed rest, antiemetics) • Tetanus Prophylaxis: if indicated • Surgery: foreign body removal + corneal/scleral wound repair
Key Words & Most Common	• Ophthalmologic emergency • Trauma (blunt or penetrative) • Scissors most common in kids; foreign body most common in adults • Acute eye pain + ↓visual acuity • Teardrop shaped pupil; hemorrhage; hyphema • Clinical diagnosis • Emergent ophthalmology consult + eye protection → surgery

Orbital Fracture

Etiology & Risk Factors	• Fracture of the orbital floor or medial orbital wall (**blowout fracture**) that may lead to trapping of ocular structures • **Etiology: blunt force trauma**; falls, high-velocity **ball-related sports** (baseball), motor vehicle accidents, **assault/violence**		
Patho-physiology	• Acute trauma leads to sharp increase in intraorbital pressure • Impact energy is transferred to bony structures within orbit • Posterior medial aspect of orbit is most commonly affected • Adipose tissue, inferior rectus or inferior oblique muscles can entrap within maxillary or ethmoid sinus	**Anatomy**	Frontal, ethmoidal, sphenoid, zygomatic, and lacrimal bones form the bony structures of the orbit • Medial Wall: maxillary, lacrimal and ethmoid bones (lamina papyracea) • Posterior Wall: sphenoid bone • Lateral Wall: zygomatic bone • Superior/Inferior Wall: frontal and maxillary bones

Signs & Symptoms	**Eyes**	**Face**
	• **Decreased visual acuity** • **Painful or restricted extraocular movements** • **Diplopia with upward gaze** (inferior rectus muscle entrapment) • Enophthalmos (posterior displacement of eyeball; indicates globe herniation) • Exophthalmos (anterior protrusion of eyeball; indicates swelling behind globe)	• **Orbital rim bony step-off** • **Infraorbital** (anteromedial cheek) **anesthesia due to infraorbital nerve damage** • Hyperalgesia to cheek and upper lid • Epistaxis • Subcutaneous emphysema (fracture involving maxillary sinus) • Eyelid swelling after blowing nose

Diagnosis	• **Orbital CT: imaging study of choice to localize fracture** • **Teardrop Sign**: inferior herniation of orbital fat or inferior rectus muscle into the maxillary sinus

Treatment	• Supportive: **nasal decongestants** (decreases pain), **avoiding blowing nose or Valsalva** (can worsen orbital emphysema) • Medications: • Oxymetazoline (vasoconstrictor) for epistaxis • Corticosteroids to alleviate edema • **Antibiotics**: considered open fracture; amoxicillin-clavulanate, clindamycin, cephalexin vs IV ampicillin-sulbactam • Surgery: indicated for severe cases with enophthalmos or persistent diplopia

Inferior orbital (blow out) fracture

Key Words & Most Common	• Fracture of orbital secondary to blunt force trauma • Decreased visual acuity + painful/restricted EOM + diplopia • Infraorbital numbness or hyperalgesia (infraorbital nerve) • Orbital CT • Decongestants + avoid blowing nose/Valsalva +/- antibiotics → surgery if severe

Retinoblastoma

Etiology & Risk Factors	• Most common primary intraocular malignancy in childhood • **Most often diagnosed before age of 2** (90% of cases present before age 3) • Etiology; • Heritable: family history (autosomal dominant); may develop bilateral retinoblastoma • Non-heritable: no positive family history; 90% of unilateral retinoblastoma are non-heritable

Patho-physiology	• Heritable: germline mutations of the RB1 gene (tumor suppressor gene on chromosome 13) • Non-heritable: somatic mutation of the RB1 gene

Signs & Symptoms	• **Leukocoria (white reflex of pupil) is most common presenting feature** • **Strabismus** is second most common presenting feature • Ocular inflammation or impaired vision (rare)

Diagnosis	• **Indirect Ophthalmoscopy**: under general anesthesia with pupils widely dilated; may show single or multiple grayish/white elevations of retina • CT: detects calcifications • MRI: evaluates optic nerve and extraocular extension • Genetic Testing: for patient, parents and/or siblings

Treatment	• **Chemotherapy: mainstay treatment**; carboplatin, etoposide, vincristine • Enucleation: removal of eye if unilateral; severe, recurrent, refractory to chemotherapy • Secondary Malignancy Screening: may be associated with osteosarcoma • 95% survival rate if treated promptly; fatal if untreated

Leukocoria (white reflex of pupil)

Key Words & Most Common	• Most common intraocular malignancy in childhood • Often diagnosed before age 2-3yo • Leukocoria (white reflex of pupil) + strabismus • Indirect ophthalmoscopy → CT/MRI • Chemotherapy • Enucleation if unilateral • Associated with osteosarcoma

Macular Degeneration

Etiology & Risk Factors	• **Age-related macular degeneration (ARMD) is the leading cause of irreversible central vision loss in older patients** (especially >60 years of age) • <u>Risk Factors</u>: **age**, genetic variants, family history, smoking, **cardiovascular disease, hypertension**, obesity, sun exposure, poor diet
Patho-physiology	• <u>**Dry (nonexudative or atrophic)**</u>: most common type; accumulation of rod/cone waste products changes retinal pigment epithelium results in progressive vision loss • <u>**Wet (exudative or neovascular)**</u>: abnormal blood vessels develop leading to macular edema or hemorrhage causing retinal pigment epithelial detachment

	Dry (atrophic)	Wet (neovascular)

Signs & Symptoms	• *Progressive* **(years)** loss of central vision
	• Non-painful
	• **Bilateral**
	• Central vision spots (scotoma) occur later in course
	• <u>**Fundoscopic Exam**</u>:
	   • <u>**Drusen Bodies**</u>: small, round, yellowish/white spots under the retina; extracellular (lipid and protein) deposits
	   • Retinal pigment epithelium changes
	   • Chorioretinal atrophy
		• *Rapid* **(days to weeks)** loss of central vision
		• Central vision spots (scotoma) and curving of straight lines (metamorphopsia) often first initial symptom
		• Usually **unilateral**
		• Peripheral and color vision generally unaffected
		• <u>**Fundoscopic Exam**</u>:
		   • **Subretinal hemorrhage** (secondary to abnormal blood vessel formation)
		   • **Retinal edema**
		   • Retinal pigment epithelium detachment
		   • Gray/green macular discoloration
		Drusen Bodies

Diagnosis	• **Fundoscopic Exam** • <u>Amsler Grid</u>: horizontal/vertical lines (looks like graph paper) to detect if straight lines look curved or distorted • <u>Fluorescein Angiography</u>: used for wet macular degeneration to identify neovascular areas	

Treatment	• <u>**Proper Nutrition + Dietary Supplementation**</u>:
	   • **Zinc**, copper, **vitamin C, vitamin E**, lutein, omega-3 fatty acids, zeaxanthin
	   • Does not reverse changes but may slow progression
		• **Intravitreal injection of antivascular endothelial growth factor (anti-VEGF) drugs**
		   • Bevacizumab, ranibizumab, aflibercept
		   • Decreases new vessel formation
		• Laser Photocoagulation

Key Words & Most Common	• Age related • Progressive, bilateral loss of central vision • Fundoscopic exam shows Drusen bodies (yellow/white spots on retina) • Supplementation with zinc, vitamin C/E to slow progression	• Age related • Rapid, unilateral loss of central vision • Central vision spots (scotoma) and straight-line distortion (metamorphopsia • Fundoscopic exam show subretinal hemorrhages and retinal edema • Intravitreal injection of anti-VEGF medications → laser photocoagulation

Diabetic Retinopathy

Etiology & Risk Factors	• Microvascular condition occurring secondary to long-term effects of diabetes mellitus • **Most common cause of new, severe vision loss in working-age adults** • <u>Etiology</u>: **diabetes mellitus** • <u>Risk Factors</u>: **advanced age, poor-glycemic control, hypertension**, obesity, vitamin D deficiency, dyslipidemia
Patho-physiology	• Chronic hyperglycemia and oxidative stress leads cellular and tissue damage • <u>Nonproliferative</u>: increased capillary permeability, microaneurysms, hemorrhage, ischemia and edema leads to retinal thickening secondary to fluid leakage • <u>Proliferative</u>: abnormal neovascularization (new vessel formation) of retina and vitreous cavity leads to vitreous hemorrhage and/or traction retinal detachment
Signs & Symptoms	• **Blurred vision, floaters** (black spots), or **flashing lights** (photopsia) • **Partial or total vision loss (painless)**

	Nonproliferative Fundoscopy	Proliferative Fundoscopy

Diagnosis	• **Capillary microaneurysms**
	• <u>**Blot and Dot Retinal Hemorrhages**</u>: deep retinal layer hemorrhage
	• <u>**Flame-Shaped Hemorrhages**</u>: nerve fiber layer hemorrhage
	• <u>**Cotton Wool Spots**</u>: microinfarction of retinal nerve layer
	   • **Fuzzy-edged, gray/white spots** that obscure underlying layer
	• <u>**Hard Exudates**</u>: suggestive of chronic edema; lipid and lipoprotein deposits
	   • **Discrete, yellow spots with sharp margins**
		• <u>**Neovascularization**</u>: new, abnormal blood vessel formation
		   • Visible on optic nerve or retinal surface
		• Vitreous Hemorrhage or tractional retinal detachment
		• Macular edema

Treatment	• **Strict control of blood glucose**
	• Focal laser photocoagulation
		• **Strict control of blood glucose and blood pressure**
		• **Intravitreal injection of antivascular endothelial growth factor (anti-VEGF) drugs**
		   • Bevacizumab, ranibizumab, aflibercept
		   • Decreases new vessel formation
		• Focal laser photocoagulation
		Hard Exudates

Key Words & Most Common	• Vision loss secondary to poorly controlled diabetes • Blurred vision, floaters, flashing lights; partial/full vision loss (painless) • Nonproliferative: cotton wool spots, hard exudates, flame-shaped hemorrhage, blot and dot hemorrhage, capillary microaneurysms • Proliferative: neovascularization • Strict blood glucose control → laser photocoagulation; Injected anti-VEGF for proliferative	*Small hemorrhages* A

Hypertensive Retinopathy

Etiology & Risk Factors	• Retinal vascular damage secondary to elevated blood pressure • Considered end-organ damage • Etiology: acute or chronic elevated blood pressure (often untreated) • Risk Factors: **chronic kidney disease (most significant risk factor)**, smoking, diabetes
Patho-physiology	• Acute blood pressure elevation causes retinal blood vessel vasoconstriction eventually leading to endothelial damage and necrosis
Signs & Symptoms	• **Often asymptomatic** until later in disease course • **Blurred vision** • **Visual field defects**

Diagnosis	Mild	Moderate	Severe
Fundoscopic Exam	• **Arterial narrowing**: abnormal light reflex on dilated, tortuous arteriole • **Arteriovenous (AV) Nicking**: venous compression at arterial-venous junction • **Arteriosclerosis**: moderate vascular wall changes (copper wiring) or severe vascular wall hyperplasia and thickening (silver wiring)	• **Flame-Shaped Hemorrhages**: nerve fiber layer hemorrhage • **Cotton Wool Spots**: microinfarction of retinal nerve layer (**Fuzzy-edged, gray/white spots** that obscure underlying layer) • **Hard Exudates**: suggestive of chronic edema; lipid and lipoprotein deposits (**Discrete, yellow spots with sharp margins**)	• **Papilledema**: optic disc becomes congested and edematous (ophthalmologic emergency)

Treatment	• **Adequate blood pressure control** • Intravitreal injection of antivascular endothelial growth factor (anti-VEGF) drugs (Decreases new vessel formation) • Bevacizumab, ranibizumab, aflibercept • Focal laser photocoagulation • **Papilledema is ophthalmologic emergency and requires controlled blood pressure reduction**
Key Words & Most Common	• Retinal vascular damage secondary to elevated BP • CKD is most significant risk factor • Asymptomatic → blurred vision, visual field defects • Fundoscopy • Strict BP control

Retinal Detachment

Etiology & Risk Factors	• Separation of the neurosensory retina from the underlying retinal pigment epithelium
	• Etiology: **advanced age**
	    • Rhegmatogenous: **myopia, previous cataract surgery**, ocular trauma, lattice retinal degeneration
	    • Exudative: **neoplasm**, inflammatory conditions, hypertension, preeclampsia
	    • Tractional: **proliferative diabetic retinopathy**, sickle cell disease, trauma

Patho-physiology	• Rhegmatogenous: full-thickness retinal tear allows vitreous to enter space below the neurosensory retina leading to detachment from the retinal pigment epithelium • Exudative: subretinal fluid accumulates below the retina without retinal tear • Tractional: acquired fibrocellular bands in the vitreous contract to separate the retina from the base

Signs & Symptoms	• **Photopsia** (flashing lights)
	• **Floaters** (black spots in visual fields)
	• **Progressive unilateral vision loss** (painless)
	    • **Starts at periphery and moves centrally**
	    • May be described as a "shadow" or **"curtain coming down"** in periphery

Diagnosis	• **Fundoscopy with Pupillary Dilation:**
	    • **May show retinal tear** (detached, suspended retina "flapping" in vitreous humor)
	    • Elevated retina will appear hazy/out of focus
	    • Shafer's Sign: liquified vitreous breaks down intercellular bonds of retinal pigment epithelium releasing brown-colored pigment (pathognomonic)
	• B-Scan Ocular Ultrasound: ordered if view is obstructed or to confirm diagnosis

Treatment	• **Ophthalmologic Emergency**
	• **Position patient so area of retinal detachment lies flat**
	    • Superior Detachment: lie patient supine
	    • Inferior Detachment: elevate head
	• **Ocular Surgery**: surgical reattachment of retina often required

Key Words & Most Common	• Separation of retina from underlying retinal epithelium • Myopia, previous cataract surgery, advanced age, trauma • Flashing lights + floaters + progressive painless unilateral vision loss • Peripheral → central vision loss • Fundoscopy • Emergent ophthalmologic consult → position patient so retinal detachment lies flat while awaiting consult → ocular surgery

Retinal detachment seen on ocular ultrasound

Ophthalmia Neonatorum

Etiology & Risk Factors	• Neonatal conjunctivitis often contracted during vaginal delivery
	• Etiology: bacterial, viral, or chemical
	   • Bacterial: ***Chlamydia trachomatis* (most common)**, *Neisseria gonnorhoaea, Streptococcal pneumoniae, Haemophilus influenzae*
	   • Viral: herpes simplex virus type 1 and 2, adenovirus
	   • Chemical: secondary to topical therapy for ocular prophylaxis (**silver nitrate most common**)

Patho-physiology	• Exposure to infection during passage through birth canal during vaginal delivery

Signs & Symptoms	• Chemical: occurs in **first day of life** and resolves within 48 hours
	   • Secondary to **silver nitrate** prophylaxis
	• Gonococcal: presents day 2-5 of life
	   • **Profuse bilateral purulent conjunctivitis with significant erythema and swelling of eyelids**
	• Chlamydia: presents day 5-7 of life, peaks 1 week to 1 month after birth
	   • **Mild bilateral purulent conjunctivitis with mild erythema and swelling of eyelids**
	• Herpetic: presents day 6-14 of life
	   • Bilateral inflammation and edema of eyelids without purulent discharge; assess infant and mother for mucocutaneous lesions

Diagnosis	• Gram stain/culture or nucleic acid amplification test (NAAT) of conjunctival material
Treatment	• Chemical: observation; artificial tears may be helpful • **Gonococcal: IV/IM cefotaxime or ceftriaxone**; irrigate eyes with sterile saline • **Chlamydia: erythromycin ophthalmic ointment + oral azithromycin or erythromycin** • Herpetic: IV acyclovir + topical antiviral ointment + neonatal sepsis evaluation • **Prophylaxis: erythromycin ophthalmic ointment given immediately after birth** (not effective to prevent chlamydial conjunctivitis)
Key Words & Most Common	• Neonatal conjunctivitis contracted during vaginal delivery • Chemical: day 1; secondary to silver nitrate prophylaxis → observation • Chlamydia: day 5-7; mild purulent conjunctivitis → erythromycin ointment + oral azithromycin/erythromycin • Gonococcal: day 2-5; severe purulent conjunctivitis → IV/IM cefotaxime or ceftriaxone • Herpetic: day 6-14; inflammation/edema without purulent discharge → IV acyclovir + topical antiviral • Prophylaxis: erythromycin ointment

Ocular Foreign Body and Corneal Abrasion

Etiology & Risk Factors	• Common ocular trauma that is typically superficial and benign • Etiology: **high-risk activity without eye protection** • **Grinding, hammering**, drilling, welding, metal-on-metal mechanism, **landscaping/lawncare, wind-blown debris while driving or walking**
Patho-physiology	• Foreign body contacts with and disrupts the cornea, the outer surface of the eye. Foreign body may become lodged within any of the 5 layers of the eye
Signs & Symptoms	• **Sudden onset foreign body sensation** • **Copious tearing** • **Red/painful eye** (pain relieved with topical analgesic drops) • **Blepharospasm** (difficulty keeping eye open) • Photophobia and blurred vision may be present • Physical Exam: eyelid edema, focal conjunctival injection

Diagnosis	• Thorough ocular exam following topical analgesic drops (**proparacaine**)
	   • Evert eyelid to check for subtarsal foreign bodies
	   • **Visual Acuity**
	• **Fluorescein Stain**: with cobalt light illumination; renders corneal abrasion and nonmetallic foreign bodies more apparent
	• Slit-Lamp Exam: should be performed with and without fluorescein stain
	• Intraocular Pressure: contraindicated for globe perforation/rupture

Treatment	• Analgesia: pain control with topical NSAIDs (ophthalmic ketorolac)
	• **Foreign Body Removal**: sterile irrigation, lift with moistened sterile cotton swab or lift with sterile needle under loupe or slit-lamp magnification (if experienced)
	   • Rust Ring: metallic foreign bodies can create rust rings that are toxic to corneal tissue; removal with low-speed rotary burr by ophthalmologist
	• Topical Antibiotics: indicated for corneal abrasion and foreign bodies
	   • **Contact Lens Wearers: topical moxifloxacin drops for Pseudomonal coverage**
	   • Non-contact Lens Wearers: erythromycin ointment, polymyxin-trimethoprim drops
	• 24 Hour Ophthalmology Follow-Up

Key Words & Most Common	• Ocular trauma following high-risk activity without eye protection (metal-on-metal grinding/hammering most common) • Sudden onset red/painful eye + tearing + inability to keep eye open • Topical analgesia → visual acuity → fluorescein stain → slit-lamp exam • Foreign body removal with irrigation or manually + topical antibiotics (moxifloxacin if contact lens wearer) • Rust ring may develop if metallic foreign body

Bacterial Conjunctivitis

Etiology & Risk Factors	• Common bacterial infection of the eye; also known as **"pink eye"** • Etiology: ***Staphylococcus aureus* most common in adults**; ***Haemophilus influenzae* most common in children**; *Streptococcus pneumoniae, Moraxella catarrhalis* • *Neisseria gonorrhoeae* and *Chlamydia trachomatis* possible in neonates or sexually active adolescents/adults
Patho-physiology	• Direct transmission of pathogens to conjunctiva compromises the epithelial layer and results in infectious conjunctivitis • Transmission through hand to eye, eye contact with fomite, and/or person-to-person through respiratory droplets; autoinoculation possible
Signs & Symptoms	• **Unilateral purulent discharge** • **Eyelid crusting (eye "stuck shut" first thing in morning)** • **Chemosis (edema of conjunctiva)** • **Erythema/injection of conjunctiva** • No significant vision changes; pruritis is rare
Diagnosis	• **Clinical diagnosis** • <u>Fluorescein Stain</u>: may be used to detect keratitis or corneal abrasion • <u>Culture and Gram Stain</u>: of purulent discharge if recurrent

Treatment	• <u>Proper Hygiene</u>: **washing hands**, changing pillowcases and towels, disinfecting high-traffic contact surfaces
	• <u>Topical Antibiotics</u>: indicated for corneal abrasion and foreign bodies
	  • <u>Contact Lens Wearers</u>: **topical moxifloxacin drops for Pseudomonal coverage**
	    • <u>Non-contact Lens Wearers</u>: erythromycin ointment, **polymyxin B/trimethoprim drops**, ofloxacin drops
	• <u>Gonococcal/Chlamydia Conjunctivitis</u>: IM ceftriaxone PLUS oral azithromycin OR doxycycline

Key Words & Most Common	• S. aureus most common cause in adults; H. influenzae most common cause in kids • Unilateral purulent discharge and eyelid crusting • Erythema and edema of conjunctiva • Clinical diagnosis • Hand hygiene • Antibiotics: topical moxifloxacin for pseudomonal coverage (contacts) or polymyxin B/trimethoprim drops or erythromycin ointment (no contacts) • G/C: IM ceftriaxone + azithromycin OR doxycycline

Purulent ocular discharge

Viral Conjunctivitis

Etiology & Risk Factors	• Common viral infection of the conjunctiva • **Often preceded by upper respiratory infection** • Children are most susceptible to viral conjunctivitis • <u>Etiology</u>: **adenovirus is most common cause (90%)**; enterovirus and herpes simplex virus
Patho-physiology	• Transmission occurs through direct contact with virus, airborne transmission or contact with reservoir (swimming pool) • Highly contagious for 10-14 days
Signs & Symptoms	• **Sudden onset foreign body sensation, pruritis, burning, grittiness** • **Watery discharge** • **Unilateral conjunctival injection progressing to *bilateral involvement* within 24-48 hours** • Chemosis (edema of conjunctiva) • May have other constitutional viral symptoms • <u>Physical Exam</u>: • **Preauricular lymphadenopathy**, copious watery discharge
Diagnosis	• **Clinical diagnosis** • <u>Nucleic Acid Amplification Test (NAAT)</u>: may diagnose adenovirus (to rule out other diagnosis such as orbital cellulitis) • <u>Slit-Lamp Exam</u>: inferior palpebral conjunctival follicles; **punctate fluorescein staining of cornea**

Treatment	• <u>Supportive</u>: **cool compresses, artificial tears**
	• <u>Proper Hygiene</u>: **washing hands**, changing pillowcases and towels, disinfecting high-traffic contact surfaces, **avoid swimming pools**
	• <u>Topical Antihistamines</u>: for symptomatic relief
	  • <u>Pheniramine-Naphazoline</u>: antihistamine and ocular decongestant
	  • <u>Olopatadine or Ketotifen</u>: antihistamine and mast cell stabilizer

Key Words & Most Common	• Viral infection of the conjunctiva most commonly caused by adenovirus • Sudden onset foreign body sensation, pruritis, burning • Watery discharge • Unilateral conjunctival injection → bilateral involvement • Preauricular lymphadenopathy • Clinical diagnosis • Supportive + proper hygiene → topical antihistamines for symptomatic relief

Conjunctival injection

Allergic Conjunctivitis

Etiology & Risk Factors	• Acute or chronic conjunctival inflammation in response to airborne allergens
	• Etiology:
	    • <u>Seasonal</u>: **mold spores, pollen, grasses/weeds**; peak during spring and late summer/early fall
	    • <u>Perennial</u>: **dust mites, animal dander**; tend to cause symptoms year-round
	    • <u>Vernal Keratoconjunctivitis</u>: more severe conjunctivitis **associated with atopy** (seasonal allergies, eczema and asthma); worst during spring

Patho-physiology	• Allergic conjunctivitis (acute, seasonal, and perennial) is an immunoglobulin E (IgE) mediated hypersensitivity reaction (type I) and subsequent mast cell degranulation is secondary to ocular surface contact with an airborne allergen
Signs & Symptoms	• **Bilateral mild to severe ocular pruritis** • **Watery discharge** • **Conjunctival erythema** (red eyes) • **Rhinitis is common** (nasal congestion, sneezing, rhinorrhea) • Physical Exam: • **Cobblestone papillae of the inner upper eyelid**, erythema, injected conjunctiva, watery discharge; no visual acuity changes
Diagnosis	• **Clinical diagnosis** • Fluorescein stain to rule out foreign body if indicated

Treatment	• <u>Supportive</u>: cool compresses, eye irrigation (to remove allergens), artificial tears
	• <u>Topical Antihistamines</u>: for symptomatic relief
	    • **Pheniramine-Naphazoline**: antihistamine and ocular decongestant
	    • **Olopatadine or Ketotifen: antihistamine and mast cell stabilizer**
	• <u>Topical NSAIDs</u>: ketorolac for symptomatic relief
	• <u>Oral Antihistamines</u>: helpful if patients have other symptoms (rhinitis)

Key Words & Most Common	• Acute/chronic conjunctivitis due to airborne allergens (mold, pollen, grass, dust mites, animal dander) • Bilateral ocular pruritis, watery discharge, erythema • Rhinitis common (congestion, sneezing) • Cobblestone papillae of inner/upper eyelid • Clinical diagnosis • Supportive → topical antihistamines → oral antihistamines

Watery discharge and conjunctival erythema

Ocular Burns

Etiology & Risk Factors	• Acute burn to the eye that constitutes an **ophthalmologic emergency**
	• Etiology:
	    • <u>Thermal</u>: exposure to flame, **explosion or fireworks, hot water, hot cooking oil**, curling iron
	    • <u>Chemical</u>: drain cleaner, **detergent**, batteries, bleach, **cleaning products**, occupational exposure (fertilizer, lye, lime, cement), swimming pool chemicals

Patho-physiology	• <u>Thermal burns</u>: often less severe due to blink reflex and minimal contact time; skin of eyelid usually receives most of the heat energy • <u>Alkali burns</u>: more severe than acidic burns; alkali substances are lipophilic and disrupt proteins so deeper penetration and cause **liquefactive necrosis** of the tissue • <u>Acidic burns</u>: coagulate proteins in superficial structures and can cause **coagulative necrosis**
Signs & Symptoms	• **Severe ocular pain** • **Conjunctival injection or blanching** • Reduced visual acuity • **Significant blepharospasms** (inability to open eyelids) • Photosensitivity/**photophobia** • Physical Exam: perilimbal ischemia possible (white ring around iris)
Diagnosis	• **Clinical Diagnosis**

Treatment	• <u>Immediate Irrigation</u>: **most important initial treatment**; type of irrigation is less important than timing
	    • **Normal saline or lactated ringers** (lactated ringers preferred as closer to normal pH and less irritating); tap water acceptable in non-medical setting
	    • **Goal is to restore neutral pH** (7.0-7.2)
	• <u>Foreign Body Removal</u>: as indicated; evert eye lids
	• <u>Topical Anesthetic</u>: prilocaine or tetracaine for pain relief to allow proper irrigation and exam
	• <u>**Topical Antibiotics**</u>: **erythromycin ointment for mild burns, moxifloxacin drops for more severe burns**
	• <u>**Ophthalmology Consult**</u>: for all burns unless extremely mild

Key Words & Most Common	• Acute burn to eye; ophthalmologic emergency • Fireworks, hot water, cooking oil, detergents, cleaning products • Severe ocular pain + reduced visual acuity • Unable to hold eyes open • Change in vision + light sensitivity • Clinical diagnosis • Immediate irrigation → topical anesthetic → thorough irrigation → topical antibiotics → ophthalmology

Strabismus

Etiology & Risk Factors	• **Misalignment of one or both eyes**; may be referred as "squinty eyes", "crossed eyes" or "walled eyes" • Etiology: **refractive error, neuromuscular imbalance**, binocular fusion abnormalities • Risk Factors: **family history, genetic disorders (trisomy 21)**, prenatal drug exposure (alcohol), prematurity or low birth weight, cerebral palsy, head trauma
Patho-physiology	• Primary motor dysfunction leads to poor sensory status which may progress to strabismus if left untreated • Amblyopia (reduction in visual acuity of one eye) may occur secondary to cortical suppression of unilateral vision to avoid confusion and diplopia • Eso- (nasal deviation), Exo- (temporal deviation), Hyper- (upward deviation), Hypo- (downward deviation)
Signs & Symptoms	• **Asymptomatic** • **Asthenopia** (eye strain) • **Diplopia** (double vision) • Scotomas (loss of visual field; "blind spot") • **Amblyopia** (reduction in visual acuity of one eye) • Physical Exam: • **Corneal Light Reflex Test**: initial screening test; asymmetry of corneal light reflex in one eye • **Cover Test**: child fixates on an object then one eye is covered; if properly aligned there will be no eye movement; strabismus present if one eye shifts to stay focused when opposite is covered • **Cover-Uncover Test**: child fixates on an object; one eye is covered then the other (back and forth) • Eye with strabismus will shift after being uncovered
Diagnosis	• **Clinical Diagnosis** • Neuroimaging necessary if cranial nerve palsy suspected
Treatment	• **Eye Patch Therapy: first-line**; patch applied to normal eye to stimulate and strengthen the affected eye • Optimize and restore vision (atropine drops may also be used) • **Contact Lenses or Eyeglasses**: to correct refractive error • Surgery: if unresponsive or severe misalignment; involves loosening or tightening horizontal rectus muscles • Referral necessary if persists beyond 4-6 months of age to reduce risk of amblyopia
Key Words & Most Common	• Misalignment of one or both eyes as a result of refractive error or neuromuscular imbalance • Eye strain, double vision, unilateral reduced visual acuity • Corneal light reflex test (initial screening test); cover test; cover-uncover test • Eye patch therapy first-line • Contact lenses/eyeglasses if refractive error • Surgery if severe

Esotropia (eyes crossed)

Exotropia (eyes diverged)

Hypertropia (eyes diverged upward)

Bacterial Keratitis

Etiology & Risk Factors	• Bacterial infection of the corneal tissue that can rapidly progress and become a sight-threatening emergency • Also known as **corneal ulcer** • Etiology: • **Improper contact lens use** (overnight wear, inadequate cleaning, rinsing with tap water, swimming in lenses) • Dry eyes (conditions causing inability to close eyes fully such as Bell's palsy or ectropion) • Trauma or foreign body • Immunosuppression
Patho-physiology	• Corneal epithelial defect leads to infiltration of bacteria leading to infection, inflammation, and necrosis of the corneal stroma • Pathogens include *Staphylococcus aureus*, *Streptococcal* spp. and ***Pseudomonas aeruginosa* (contact lens wearers)**
Signs & Symptoms	• **Eye pain and erythema** • **Foreign body sensation + blepharospasm** (difficulty keeping eye open) • Impaired visual acuity • **Excessive tearing, discharge** • **Photophobia** • Physical Exam: • **Ciliary injection (limbal flush)** • **Hazy/dull cornea (corneal opacification)** • Hypopyon (WBCs in anterior chamber) in severe cases
Diagnosis	• **Slit-Lamp Exam: corneal infiltrate with epithelial defect and increased fluorescein uptake** • Corneal Culture: scraping of tissue with #15 blade or jeweler's forceps (performed by ophthalmologist)
Treatment	• **Topical Fluoroquinolone Antibiotics: moxifloxacin**, gatifloxacin (covers for *Pseudomonas*) • **Patching: contraindicated** (creates warm, stagnant environment for bacterial growth)
Key Words & Most Common	• Bacterial infection of corneal tissue (corneal ulcer) • Most common with improper contact lens use • Eye pain/erythema + foreign body sensation and difficulty keeping eye open • Impaired vision + photophobia • Excessive tearing • Slit-lamp exam shows corneal infiltrate with epithelial defect + ↑fluorescein uptake • Topical fluoroquinolone antibiotics (moxifloxacin) • Patching contraindicated

Ciliary injection

Orbital (Septal) Cellulitis 👁

Etiology & Risk Factors	• Infection of fat and ocular muscles within the orbit posterior to the orbital septum (post-septal cellulitis) • <u>Etiology</u>: **secondary to acute bacterial sinusitis (ethmoid) most common**; trauma (insect or animal bite), dental/middle ear infection, ophthalmic surgery • <u>Polymicrobial</u>: *Streptococcus pneumoniae* **(sinus infection) is most common**, *Staphylococcus aureus* and *Staphylococcus pyogenes* (trauma), *H. influenzae*
Patho-physiology	• Rare complication of acute bacterial sinusitis in which fulminant infection of the sinus may traverse beyond the thin ethmoid bone leading to extensive and severe infection posterior to the orbital septum
Signs & Symptoms	• **Erythema and edema of eyelid and surrounding soft tissue** • **Decreased ocular motility** • **Ocular pain (especially with extraocular movements)** • **Decreased visual acuity** • **Proptosis (bulging of eyes) secondary to swelling** • Signs of primary infection (nasal congestion, mucopurulent nasal discharge, sinus pressure, etc.)
Diagnosis	• **Clinical Diagnosis** • <u>Orbital CT with IV Contrast</u>: confirms diagnosis; shows proptosis, post-septal fat and ocular muscle inflammation, subperiosteal or orbital abscess • <u>Blood Cultures</u>: prior to starting antibiotics

Treatment	• <u>**Inpatient Admission**</u>: ophthalmology consult with close follow-up
	• <u>**Antibiotics**</u>: Vancomycin PLUS one of the following
	    • **Ceftriaxone, cefotaxime**, ampicillin-sulbactam, piperacillin-tazobactam
	    • Consider metronidazole if secondary to dental infection

Key Words & Most Common	• Infection of tissue posterior to orbital septum • Secondary to bacterial sinusitis (ethmoid) • S. pneumoniae is most common bacteria; often polymicrobial • Erythema/edema of eye + bulging • ↓eye motility • Pain with eye movement • Clinical diagnosis + orbital CT to confirm Admit → ophthalmology consult → antibiotics (vancomycin + ceftriaxone, cefotaxime, ampicillin-sulbactam)

Erythema and edema of eyelid and surrounding soft tissue

Periorbital (Preseptal) Cellulitis 👁

Etiology & Risk Factors	• Infection of the skin and soft tissue of the eyelid and periocular area anterior to the orbital septum • **More common in children (<10yo most common)** • <u>Etiology</u>: **contiguous infection of soft tissue of eyelids/face**; trauma, insect/animal bites, **bacterial sinusitis, chalazion, impetigo** • Pathogens include *Staphylococcus aureus* (MRSA possible), *Streptococcal* spp. and anaerobes
Patho-physiology	• Bacterial inoculation secondary to break in skin barrier from trauma, bites or contiguous/hematogenous spread from sinusitis, chalazion, impetigo leads to infection of the surrounding soft tissue

Signs & Symptoms	• **Erythema and edema of eyelid and surrounding soft tissue**
	• **May have low-grade fever**
	• <u>**ABSENCE OF**</u>: (differentiates between septal and preseptal cellulitis)
	    • **Proptosis (bulging of eye)**
	    • **Ophthalmoplegia (decreased ocular motility)**
	    • **Pain with extraocular movements**
	    • **Vision loss/changes**

Diagnosis	• **Clinical Diagnosis** • <u>Orbital CT with IV Contrast</u>: distinguishes preseptal vs postseptal cellulitis if diagnosis is clinically unclear

Treatment	• Can often be managed outpatient especially if mild
	• <u>**Antibiotics**</u>: should include MRSA coverage
	    • **Clindamycin (monotherapy; antibiotic of choice)**
	    • Trimethoprim-sulfamethoxazole PLUS amoxicillin-clavulanic acid OR cefpodoxime OR cefdinir

Key Words & Most Common	• Infection of area surrounding eye/eyelid anterior to orbital septum • More common in children • Sinusitis, chalazion, impetigo, insect/animal bites • Redness/swelling of eyelid and surrounding tissue • NO bulging of eye, NO decreased ocular motility, NO pain with EOM • Clinical diagnosis → CT if unsure • Antibiotics with MRSA coverage (Clindamycin preferred; trimethoprim-sulfamethoxazole + amoxicillin-clavulanic acid)

Periorbital cellulitis

Herpes Simplex Keratitis

Etiology & Risk Factors	• Infection and inflammation of the cornea secondary by herpes simplex virus • Leading cause of infection-related blindness worldwide • <u>Etiology</u>: primary infection or reactivation of herpes simplex virus in trigeminal ganglion
Patho-physiology	• <u>Primary HSV-1</u>: infection of face, lips, eyes; direct infection to eye • <u>Primary HSV-2</u>: infection of genitalia; transmitted to eye through contact with infected secretions • <u>Reactivation</u>: latent infection may be reactivated secondary to stress (physical/emotional stress, trauma, fever, hormonal change, immunosuppression, UV light)
Signs & Symptoms	• **Blurred vision** • **Eye pain and erythema** • **Excessive tearing** • **Photophobia** • Vesicles may be present in primary disease
Diagnosis	• <u>Slit-Lamp Exam/Fluorescein Stain</u>: characteristic dendritic corneal ulceration (branching or serpentine) is hallmark
Treatment	• <u>**Topical Antivirals:**</u> • **Acyclovir 3% ophthalmic ointment** • **Ganciclovir ointment** • Trifluridine • <u>**Oral Antivirals**</u> • **Acyclovir or valacyclovir** • Topical corticosteroids contraindicated • Ophthalmology follow-up
Key Words & Most Common	• Primary or reactivated infection of HSV in trigeminal ganglion • Blurred vision + photophobia • Eye pain/erythema, tearing • Slit-lamp/fluorescein: dendritic (branching) corneal ulcer • Topical antivirals (acyclovir or ganciclovir ointment) • Oral antivirals (acyclovir or valacyclovir)

Dendritic ulcer on fluorescein stain

Uveitis

Etiology & Risk Factors	• Inflammation of the uveal tract containing iris, ciliary body, and choroid • Etiology: • **Inflammatory: HLA-B27-associated conditions** (ankylosing spondylitis, psoriatic/reactive arthritis, IBD), sarcoidosis, multiple sclerosis • <u>Environmental</u>: trauma, UV keratitis, corneal foreign body • <u>Infections</u>: uncommon; bacterial (syphilis, TB), viral (HSV, HIV, VZV), parasitic (toxoplasmosis, Lyme)
Patho-physiology	• <u>Anterior Uveitis</u>: localized inflammation to anterior eye segment; includes iritis (anterior chamber inflammation), iridocyclitis (anterior chamber and anterior vitreous inflammation) • <u>Posterior Uveitis</u>: inflammation of retina, choroid, or optic disk

Signs & Symptoms	• Anterior: • **Sudden eye pain/erythema (deep ache); worse with extraocular movements** • **Ciliary flush** (marked injection at limbus compared to perilimbal sparing in conjunctivitis) • **Constricted, poorly reactive pupil** • Photophobia • Vision changes	• Posterior: • **Floaters** (black spots in visual fields) • **Painless vision change (blurry)** • Blind spots • Photopsia (flashing lights)

Diagnosis	• <u>Slit-Lamp Exam</u>: inflammatory cell and flare • <u>Cell</u>: white blood cells in anterior chamber (white hypopyon) • <u>Flare</u>: increased protein within the vitreous humor	

Treatment	• Anterior: • <u>**Topical Corticosteroids**</u>: prednisolone to relieve inflammation • <u>Mydriatics (sympathomimetics)</u>: cyclopentolate or homatropine; dilates iris to prevent adhesions • <u>Cycloplegics</u>: scopolamine to relieve pain	• Posterior: • Ophthalmology consult • Systemic corticosteroids may be indicated

Key Words & Most Common	• Inflammation of iris, ciliary body, and choroid most commonly secondary to inflammatory condition • <u>Anterior</u>: sudden eye pain/redness, photophobia, ciliary injection + constricted pupil • <u>Posterior</u>: floaters, painless vision change • <u>Slit-Lamp Exam</u>: inflammatory cell (WBCs in anterior chamber) and flare (protein within vitreous humor) • <u>Anterior</u>: topical steroids (prednisolone) • <u>Posterior</u>: ophthalmology consult +/- systemic steroids		

Cataract

Etiology & Risk Factors	• Congenital or degenerative opacification of the lens in one/both eyes leading to decreased visual acuity • Leading cause of blindness worldwide • <u>Etiology</u>: **age-related changes most common** • <u>Risk Factors</u>: **age (most common >60 years old)**, trauma, smoking, alcoholism, radiation exposure, corticosteroid use, diabetes mellitus, UV light, malnutrition
Patho-physiology	• Age-related degenerative processes denature and coagulate lens proteins leading to loss of lens transparency and opacification

Signs & Symptoms	• **Painless vision loss over months to years (slow progressive)**
	• **Cloudy/blurry vision**
	• **Difficulty with night-time vision**
	• **Colors appear faded** (difficulty telling difference between navy and black)
	• **Visual glare** (appearance of halo or starbursts around lights)
	• <u>Physical Exam</u>:
	    • **Lens opacification**
	    • **Absent or darkened red reflex**

Diagnosis	• **Clinical Diagnosis with ophthalmoscopy** • <u>Slit-Lamp Exam</u>: confirms diagnosis and details location, character, and extent of lens opacification
Treatment	• <u>Observation</u>: if mild; monitor with routine evaluation • <u>Supportive</u>: corrective lens prescription changes, use of brighter lights, anti-glare sunglasses, magnifying glass for small-print reading • <u>Surgery</u>: **definitive treatment**; indicated if visual changes affect activities of daily living • Opacified lens removed and replaced with clear artificial lens
Key Words & Most Common	• Age-related changes • Painless vision loss • Progressive over months-years • Poor night and color vision • Vision glare (halos around lights) • Physical Exam: lens opacification; absent/darkened red reflex • Clinical diagnosis • Observation + supportive treatment → surgery

Lens opacification

Papilledema

Etiology & Risk Factors	• Swelling of the optic disc secondary to elevated intracranial pressure (ICP) • Most common bilaterally • <u>Etiology</u>: **space-occupying lesion (brain tumor or abscess), malignant hypertension**, cerebral trauma or hemorrhage, meningitis, idiopathic intracranial hypertension
Patho-physiology	• Elevated intracranial pressure disrupts the normal pressure gradient across the intraocular and orbital optic nerve leading to disc edema and optic neuropathy • May be related to mechanical compression or ischemia to nerve axons
Signs & Symptoms	• **Headache (worse in morning or while supine)** • **Nausea and vomiting** • **Preservation of visual acuity** • May have brief (seconds) of blurry/gray vision, double vision, or flickering

Diagnosis	• <u>Fundoscopy</u>:
	    • **Engorged and tortuous retinal veins**
	    • **Hyperemic (excess blood) and swollen optic disc**
	    • **Disc margin blurring**
	    • Loss of venous pulsations
	• <u>MRI/CT</u>: rule out space-occupying lesion
	• <u>Lumbar Puncture</u>: measurement and analysis of cerebrospinal fluid (CSF) if mass-effect ruled out; opening pressure >25 is abnormal

Treatment	• **Treat underlying cause** • <u>Acetazolamide</u>: decreases CSF and aqueous humor production; indicated if no structural or localizing causes present
Key Words & Most Common	• Optic disc edema due to elevated ICP • Space-occupying lesion (brain tumor/abscess), malignant hypertension • Headache (morning or while lying down) • Nausea/vomiting • Visual acuity intact • Fundoscopy: engorged retinal veins with swollen optic disc and blurred margins • MRI/CT rule out mass effect → lumbar puncture • Treat underlying cause • Acetazolamide decreases CSF and aqueous humor production

Hyperemic and swollen optic disc with blurring of disc margin

Acute Closed-Angle Glaucoma 👁

Etiology & Risk Factors	• Ocular emergency characterized by a rapid increase in intraocular pressure secondary to an aqueous humor outflow obstruction • <u>Etiology</u>: anatomic variants (shallow anterior chamber angle), **mydriasis** (pupillary dilation), **dim/dark lights, sympathomimetics, anticholinergics** • <u>Risk Factors</u>: **advanced age (>60 years most common)**, hyperopes (far-sighted vision), female, family history, Asians
Patho-physiology	• Lens continues to grow as people age causing iris to be pushed forward, narrowing distance between iris and the lens which prevents aqueous passage • Obstruction of aqueous outflow tract leads to rapid increase in intraocular pressure causing damage to optic nerve and results in vision loss

Signs & Symptoms	• **Sudden onset of severe, unilateral eye pain**
	• Headache
	• Blurred vision and **loss of peripheral vision**
	• **Vision glare (rainbow-colored halo around bright lights)**
	• Nausea/vomiting
	
	• <u>Physical Exam</u>:
	  • **Hazy/cloudy cornea with conjunctival injection**
	  • **Fixed, mid-dilated pupil (reacts poorly to light)**
	  • Hard globe on palpation

Diagnosis	• **Clinical findings + tonometry** • <u>Tonometry</u>: **increased intraocular pressure (>20 mmHg)** • <u>Slit-Lamp Exam</u>: optic disc blurring and shallow anterior chamber

Treatment	• <u>Emergent Ophthalmology Consult</u>
	• <u>Supportive</u>: **elevate head of bead (reduces IOP)**, place patient in well-lit room (prevents pupillary dilation)
	• <u>Topical Beta-Blocker + Alpha-Agonist</u>
	  • <u>Timolol</u>: blocks beta receptors on ciliary epithelium and reduces aqueous humor production
	  • <u>Apraclonidine</u>: alpha-2 agonist to increase trabecular outflow
	  • <u>Pilocarpine</u>: facilitates outflow of aqueous humor by contracting iris sphincter muscle; not effective if IOP>40-50 mmHg
	• <u>Acetazolamide</u>: carbonic anhydrase inhibitor to **decrease aqueous humor production**
	• <u>Mannitol</u>: reduces volume of aqueous humor
	• <u>Iridotomy</u>: **definitive treatment**; laser (preferred) vs surgical

Key Words & Most Common	• Rapid increase in IOP secondary to aqueous humor outflow obstruction • Advanced age biggest risk factor, dilated pupils, sympathomimetics/anticholinergics • Sudden onset severe unilateral eye pain • Loss of peripheral vision + Halo around bright lights • Tonometry: increase IOP (>20 mmHg) • Ocular emergency → consult ophthalmology • Topical beta-blocker (timolol) + alpha-agonist (apraclonidine) + acetazolamide → iridotomy

Fixed, mid-dilated pupil that reacts poorly to light

Chronic Open-Angle Glaucoma 👁

Etiology & Risk Factors	• Chronic, progressive, irreversible optic neuropathy characterized by an open anterior chamber angle and elevated/average intraocular pressure (IOP) • <u>Etiology</u>: anatomic and **genetic variants** • <u>Risk Factors</u>: **advanced age (>40 years old most common), family history, African-Americans**, diabetes mellitus, systemic hypertension, myopia, migraines, OCP use
Patho-physiology	• Abnormality of the trabecular meshwork within the extracellular matrix leads to inadequate aqueous humor drainage which gradually increases intraocular pressure • Vascular disorder or vasospasm may compromise blood flow to optic nerve while maintaining a normal intraocular pressure

Signs & Symptoms	• **Asymptomatic in early stages**
	• **Slow, progressive, painless, peripheral vision loss (tunnel vision)**
	  • Patient may complain of missing stairs (inferior peripheral vision loss), noticing portions of words missing while reading, difficulty with driving, or bumping into objects while walking
	• <u>Physical Exam</u>:
	  • <u>Fundoscopy</u>: **cupping of optic discs (increased cup:disc ratio), thinning of neurosensory rim**, pitting or notching of the disc rim
	  • <u>Visual Field Defects</u>: asymmetry of visual field between eyes, paracentral scotoma

Diagnosis	• **Clinical diagnosis with visual field testing and fundoscopy** • <u>Tonometry</u>: may be normal or elevated; difference of >3 mmHg between eyes suggests glaucoma • <u>Optic Disc Photography</u>: helpful to monitor progression

Treatment	• <u>Reduce Intraocular Pressure</u>: combination drug therapy
	  • <u>Topical Prostaglandin Analogs</u>: **first-line medication (Latanoprost)**; increases outflow of aqueous humor to decrease intraocular pressure
	  • <u>Topical Beta-Blockers</u>: **(Timolol)** blocks beta receptors on ciliary epithelium and reduces aqueous humor production
	  • <u>Alpha-2 Agonist</u>: (Apraclonidine) increases trabecular outflow and decreases aqueous humor production
	  • <u>Carbonic Anhydrase Inhibitors</u>: **(Acetazolamide) decreases aqueous humor production**
	• <u>Laser Trabeculoplasty</u>: **indicated if refractory to medical therapy**; increases aqueous outflow via trabecular meshwork
	• <u>Surgery</u>: trabeculectomy or bypass procedure reserved as last-resort

Key Words & Most Common	• Chronic progressive optic neuropathy with open anterior chamber angle +/- elevated IOP • Most common in African Americans >40yo • Asymptomatic → slow painless peripheral vision loss (tunnel vision) • Fundoscopy: cupping of optic discs with increased cup:disc ration + visual field defects • Visual field testing + fundoscopy; tonometry may show normal or elevated IOP • Latanoprost (prostaglandin analog) + timolol (topical beta-blocker) • Laser trabeculoplasty vs surgery

Optic Neuritis

Etiology & Risk Factors	• Acute inflammatory demyelination of the optic nerve • <u>Etiology</u>: **multiple sclerosis is most common**, autoimmune conditions, post-childhood vaccination, viral infection, sinusitis, meningitis, **medications (ethambutol)** • <u>Risk Factors</u>: **age (20-40 years old most common)**, female, Caucasian
Patho-physiology	• Central nervous system inflammation leads to demyelination of the optic nerve and the resultant loss of vision

Signs & Symptoms	• **Acute, unilateral vision loss** (occurs over hours to days)
	   • Painful (with extraocular movement)
	• **Retro-orbital headache**
	• **Loss of color vision** (desaturation of color out of proportion to loss of visual acuity)
	• Visual field defects (central scotoma)
	• <u>Physical Exam</u>:
	   • **Marcus-Gunn Pupil**: unilateral unequal pupillary response to light (pupils appear to dilate when swinging flashlight from unaffected eye to affected eye)

Diagnosis	• <u>Fundoscopy</u>: optic disc swelling/blurring (papillitis) • <u>MRI with Gadolinium Contrast</u>: confirms diagnosis if multiple sclerosis suspected etiology; may show enlarged optic nerve or demyelinating lesions
Treatment	• <u>Corticosteroids</u>: **first-line management;** IV methylprednisolone followed by oral corticosteroids (high-dose) • Treat underlying cause
Key Words & Most Common	• Inflammatory demyelination of optic nerve • Multiple sclerosis • Female age 20-40 • Acute vision loss + retro-orbital headache • Color vision loss (out of proportion to visual acuity loss) • MRI confirms diagnosis if MS • Corticosteroids (methylprednisolone → oral prednisone)

Optic disc swelling/blurring

Amaurosis Fugax

Etiology & Risk Factors	• Transient monocular vision loss lasting seconds to minutes with complete recovery • <u>Etiology</u>: **thromboembolism or hypoperfusion most common** (carotid artery disease), vasospasm (migraine or cocaine), giant cell arteritis, central retinal artery occlusion, systemic lupus erythematosus • <u>Risk Factors</u>: **carotid artery disease, age (>50 years old)**, hypertension, **hyperlipidemia**, history of transient ischemic attack (TIA), **smoking**, cocaine use
Patho-physiology	• Thromboembolism (carotid artery atherosclerotic plaque rupture) or hypoperfusion (carotid artery stenosis) or vasospasm (migraine/cocaine use) causes retinal ischemia and subsequent vision loss

Signs & Symptoms	• **Sudden, monocular vision loss**
	   • **Described as descending vision loss; "curtain or shade coming down over field of vision"**
	   • Resolves within 1 hour (usually seconds to minutes)
	   • May be partial or complete

Diagnosis	• **Workup determined by suspected etiology** • <u>Labs</u>: CBC, CMP, lipid profile, PT/PTT, ESR/CRP often ordered • <u>**Carotid Doppler Ultrasound**</u>: **non-invasive test to determine patency of carotid arteries** • <u>ECG/Echocardiogram</u>: determine embolic source • <u>MRI</u>: helps determines carotid artery patency; order if suspicious for cerebral vascular accident (CVA), multiple sclerosis, or mass effect
Treatment	• **Treat underlying vascular risk factors** • Hypertension, diabetes, hyperlipidemia management; smoking cessation • <u>Antiplatelet/Anticoagulation</u>: warfarin, aspirin, clopidogrel if cardiac source of embolism • **Carotid Stenting vs Endarterectomy if high risk or recurrent symptoms**
Key Words & Most Common	• Monocular vision loss secondary to thromboembolism or hypoperfusion • Carotid artery disease greatest risk factor (high cholesterol and smoking) • Sudden, unilateral vision loss • "Curtain coming down over visual field" • Carotid doppler ultrasound • Treat underlying cause → carotid stenting or endarterectomy

Central Retinal Artery Occlusion 👁

Etiology & Risk Factors	• Sudden occlusion of central retinal artery by thrombus or embolus resulting in retinal hypoperfusion, ischemia, and vision loss (ophthalmologic emergency) • <u>Etiology</u>: **embolism from carotid artery atherosclerotic plaque rupture most common; cardiogenic emboli**, vasculitis (SLE, giant cell arteritis), vasospasm • <u>Risk Factors</u>: **carotid artery disease, age (50-80 years old)**, hypertension, **hyperlipidemia**, **smoking**, hypercoagulable states, male, sickle cell disease
Patho-physiology	• First branch of the internal carotid artery is ophthalmic artery • Embolism results in occlusion of central retinal artery leading to retinal ischemia, vision loss and eventually necrosis

Signs & Symptoms	• **Acute, painless, monocular vision loss**
	    • **Often preceded by episodes of amaurosis fugax**
	• <u>Physical Exam</u>:
	    • **May have carotid bruit**
	    • **Relative afferent pupillary defect**; pupil responds poorly to light but constricts when contralateral eye is illuminated

Diagnosis	• **Clinical diagnosis + fundoscopy**
	• <u>Fundoscopy</u>: confirmatory; **shows evidence of retinal ischemia**
	    • **Pale retina with cherry-red macula**
	    • **Boxcar segmentation** of retinal blood vessels (segmentation of vascular flow)
	• <u>Electrocardiogram/Echocardiogram</u>: determine embolic source

Treatment	• **No evidence supporting optimal treatment** • <u>Ocular Massage</u>: dilates ocular blood vessels and creates pressure gradient in effort to dislodge clot • <u>Hyperventilation Into Paper Bag</u>: increases pCO_2 leading to retinal artery vasodilation and increased blood flow • <u>Reduction of Intraocular Pressure</u>: decompression of anterior chamber with topical timolol or oral acetazolamide • <u>Antiplatelet/Anticoagulation</u>: warfarin, aspirin, clopidogrel if cardiac source of embolism • <u>High-Dose Corticosteroids</u>: if giant cell arteritis suspected etiology
Key Words & Most Common	• Central retinal artery occlusion secondary to embolism • Carotid artery atherosclerotic plaque rupture most common etiology • Acute, painless, monocular vision loss • May have carotid bruit • <u>Fundoscopy</u>: pale retina with cherry-red macula + boxcar segmentation • No definitive optimal treatment

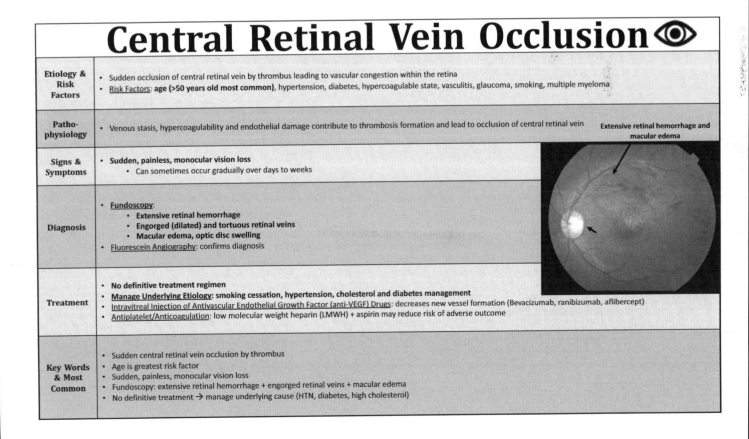

Boxcar segmentation — Pale retina with cherry-red macula

Central Retinal Vein Occlusion 👁

Etiology & Risk Factors	• Sudden occlusion of central retinal vein by thrombus leading to vascular congestion within the retina • <u>Risk Factors</u>: **age (>50 years old most common)**, hypertension, diabetes, hypercoagulable state, vasculitis, glaucoma, smoking, multiple myeloma
Patho-physiology	• Venous stasis, hypercoagulability and endothelial damage contribute to thrombosis formation and lead to occlusion of central retinal vein
Signs & Symptoms	• **Sudden, painless, monocular vision loss** • Can sometimes occur gradually over days to weeks

Diagnosis	• <u>Fundoscopy</u>:
	    • **Extensive retinal hemorrhage**
	    • **Engorged (dilated) and tortuous retinal veins**
	    • **Macular edema, optic disc swelling**
	• <u>Fluorescein Angiography</u>: confirms diagnosis

Treatment	• **No definitive treatment regimen** • **Manage Underlying Etiology: smoking cessation, hypertension, cholesterol and diabetes management** • <u>Intravitreal Injection of Antivascular Endothelial Growth Factor (anti-VEGF) Drugs</u>: decreases new vessel formation (Bevacizumab, ranibizumab, aflibercept) • <u>Antiplatelet/Anticoagulation</u>: low molecular weight heparin (LMWH) + aspirin may reduce risk of adverse outcome
Key Words & Most Common	• Sudden central retinal vein occlusion by thrombus • Age is greatest risk factor • Sudden, painless, monocular vision loss • Fundoscopy: extensive retinal hemorrhage + engorged retinal veins + macular edema • No definitive treatment → manage underlying cause (HTN, diabetes, high cholesterol)

Extensive retinal hemorrhage and macular edema

Scleritis

Etiology & Risk Factors	• Severe ocular inflammatory condition involving the deep episclera and sclera that can be vision threatening • <u>Etiology</u>: **underlying autoimmune condition (inflammatory bowel disease, rheumatoid arthritis, granulomatosis with polyangiitis)**, infection (viral, bacterial, fungal) • <u>Risk Factors</u>: **history of autoimmune condition, female, age (45-60 years old most common)**
Patho-physiology	• Scleral anatomical structure is made up of collagen, elastin and proteoglycans which are similar makeup to joint tissue leading to susceptibility by inflammatory conditions (rheumatoid arthritis) • Inflammation of sclera can lead to adhesion to dura mater and arachnoid sheath of optic nerve leading to visual complications

Signs & Symptoms	• **Scleral edema and marked erythema (hyperemic patches)**
	• **Intense ocular pain**
	   • **Described as a deep ache**
	   • May affect sleep and appetite
	• Photophobia
	• <u>Physical Exam</u>:
	   • Pain with extraocular movement (extraocular muscles insert into sclera)
	   • Globe tenderness to palpation

Diagnosis	• **Clinical Diagnosis + Slit-Lamp Exam** • <u>Ocular CT/Ultrasound</u>: confirms diagnosis; shows thickening of sclera • Evaluate for underlying etiology

Treatment	• <u>Systemic Corticosteroids</u>:
	   • **Oral prednisone taper is initial therapy**
	   • IV/IM methylprednisolone if inflammation returns

Key Words & Most Common	• Ocular inflammation involving episclera and sclera • Most common secondary to autoimmune conditions • Scleral edema/erythema • Intense ocular pain (deep ache) affecting sleep • Photophobia • Clinical diagnosis + slit-lamp exam → CT/US to confirm • Systemic steroids: oral prednisone → IV/IM methylprednisolone

Scleral edema and marked hyperemic patch

Otitis Externa

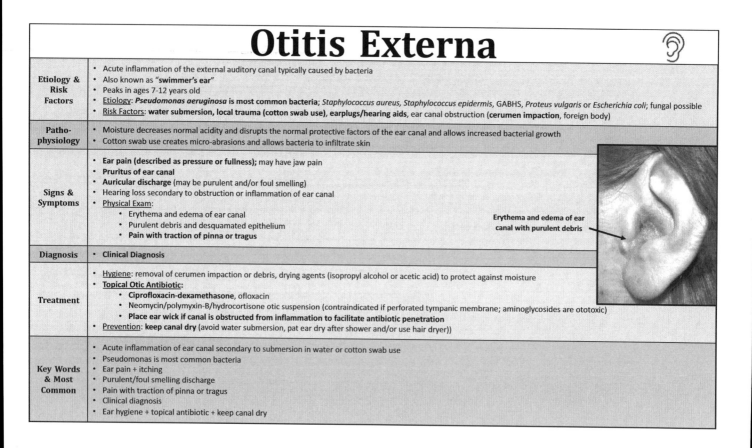

Etiology & Risk Factors	• Acute inflammation of the external auditory canal typically caused by bacteria • Also known as **"swimmer's ear"** • Peaks in ages 7-12 years old • <u>Etiology</u>: ***Pseudomonas aeruginosa* is most common bacteria**; *Staphylococcus aureus, Staphylococcus epidermis*, GABHS, *Proteus vulgaris* or *Escherichia coli*; fungal possible • <u>Risk Factors</u>: **water submersion, local trauma (cotton swab use), earplugs/hearing aids**, ear canal obstruction (**cerumen impaction**, foreign body)
Patho-physiology	• Moisture decreases normal acidity and disrupts the normal protective factors of the ear canal and allows increased bacterial growth • Cotton swab use creates micro-abrasions and allows bacteria to infiltrate skin

Signs & Symptoms	• **Ear pain (described as pressure or fullness);** may have jaw pain
	• **Pruritus of ear canal**
	• **Auricular discharge** (may be purulent and/or foul smelling)
	• Hearing loss secondary to obstruction or inflammation of ear canal
	• <u>Physical Exam</u>:
	   • Erythema and edema of ear canal
	   • Purulent debris and desquamated epithelium
	   • **Pain with traction of pinna or tragus**

Diagnosis	• **Clinical Diagnosis**

Treatment	• <u>Hygiene</u>: removal of cerumen impaction or debris, drying agents (isopropyl alcohol or acetic acid) to protect against moisture
	• <u>Topical Otic Antibiotic</u>:
	   • **Ciprofloxacin-dexamethasone**, ofloxacin
	   • Neomycin/polymyxin-B/hydrocortisone otic suspension (contraindicated if perforated tympanic membrane; aminoglycosides are ototoxic)
	   • **Place ear wick if canal is obstructed from inflammation to facilitate antibiotic penetration**
	• <u>Prevention</u>: **keep canal dry** (avoid water submersion, pat ear dry after shower and/or use hair dryer))

Key Words & Most Common	• Acute inflammation of ear canal secondary to submersion in water or cotton swab use • Pseudomonas is most common bacteria • Ear pain + itching • Purulent/foul smelling discharge • Pain with traction of pinna or tragus • Clinical diagnosis • Ear hygiene + topical antibiotic + keep canal dry

Erythema and edema of ear canal with purulent debris

Malignant Otitis Externa

Etiology & Risk Factors	• Invasive infection of the base of the skull and surrounding soft tissue secondary to external auditory canal infection • <u>Etiology</u>: ***Pseudomonas aeruginosa* is most common (>95%)**, methicillin-resistant *Staphylococcus aureus* (MRSA) • <u>Risk Factors</u>: **advanced age, diabetes, immunocompromised**, corticosteroid use, chemotherapy
Patho-physiology	• Infection begins as simple otitis externa and can spread to infect surrounding soft tissue and base of skull leading to life-threatening osteomyelitis
Signs & Symptoms	• **Otitis externa that has not resolved in 2-3 weeks despite antibiotic use** • **Severe ear pain** (out of proportion to typical otitis externa pain) • **Auricular discharge** • **Cranial nerve palsies (CN VII most common)** as osteomyelitis spreads • <u>Physical Exam</u>: • Severe auricular pain with traction of pinna or tragus
Diagnosis	• <u>CT or MRI</u>: **confirms diagnosis, MRI is more sensitive**

Treatment	• **Inpatient admission**
	• <u>**Antibiotics**</u>:
	   • **IV ciprofloxacin is first-line**
	   • Topical ciprofloxacin-dexamethasone

Key Words & Most Common	• Invasive osteomyelitis of skull secondary to otitis externa • Pseudomonas most common bacteria • Elderly diabetic is most common • Refractory otitis externa despite antibiotic use • Severe ear pain + discharge → CN palsy • CT/MRI • Admit → IV ciprofloxacin + topical ciprofloxacin

Mastoiditis

Etiology & Risk Factors	• Infection of the mastoid air cells of the temporal bone as a result of acute otitis media • <u>Etiology</u>: **complication of acute otitis media** • ***Streptococcus pneumoniae* most common**, *Streptococcus pyogenes, Staphylococcus aureus, Haemophilus influenzae, Pseudomonas aeruginosa* • <u>Risk Factors</u>: **age (less than 2 years old)**, immunocompromised, recurrent otitis media
Patho-physiology	• Infection and inflammation of the middle ear cavity from acute otitis media extends to the mastoid air cells

Signs & Symptoms	• **Deep, throbbing ear pain**
	   • Worse at night
	   • Begins days to weeks after otitis media infection
	• **Fever**, fatigue, lethargy
	• <u>Physical Exam</u>:
	   • **Bulging, erythematous tympanic membrane**
	   • **Postauricular (mastoid) tenderness, edema, erythema**
	   • Lateral and inferior displacement of pinna; **protrusion of auricle**

Diagnosis	• **Clinical Diagnosis** • <u>**CT Mastoid with IV Contrast**</u>: **first-line diagnostic test**; determines extent of bone involvement and abscess formation

Treatment	• Inpatient admission
	• <u>**IV Antibiotics**</u>:
	   • **IV Ceftriaxone initial drug of choice** (good CNS penetration) **if uncomplicated**
	   • Vancomycin AND ceftriaxone OR piperacillin-tazobactam if MRSA suspected or complicated
	• <u>Mastoidectomy</u>: if severe/refractory or subperiosteal abscess present

Key Words & Most Common	• Infection of mastoid air cells of temporal bone secondary to acute otitis media • *Streptococcus pneumoniae* most common pathogen • Age>2yo with recurrent otitis media • Deep/throbbing pain + fever • Otitis media findings + postauricular (mastoid) tenderness, swelling, redness • CT with IV contrast • IV antibiotics (ceftriaxone vs vanco + ceftriaxone) → mastoidectomy

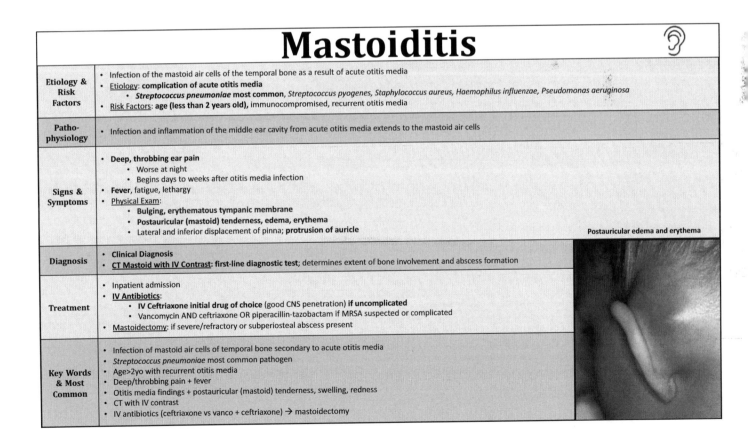

Postauricular edema and erythema

Chronic Suppurative Otitis Media 👂

Etiology & Risk Factors	• **On-going chronic infection of the middle ear with perforated tympanic membrane**
	• Chronic/persistent symptoms for 2-6+ weeks
	• Etiology: **complication of acute otitis media**, trauma, cholesteatoma, eustachian tube obstruction, iatrogenic (tympanostomy tubes)
	   • Polymicrobial: *Staphylococcus aureus, Pseudomonas aeruginosa, Proteus* spp., *Klebsiella* spp.
	• Risk Factors: **age (2-3 years old most common)**, poor hygiene, pollution exposure **(secondhand smoke)**
	   • **May be worse after upper respiratory infection or water exposure (bathing, swimming)**

Patho-physiology	• Bacterial pathogens invade middle ear through the external canal leading to inflammatory reaction and spontaneous perforation of the tympanic membrane • May be iatrogenic from tympanostomy tube placement

Signs & Symptoms	• **Otorrhea (ear drainage)**
	• **Conductive hearing loss**
	• Often *painless*
	• Physical Exam:
	   • **Perforated tympanic membrane**
	   • Macerated auditory canal with granulation tissue

Diagnosis	• **Clinical Diagnosis**
Treatment	• Removal of auditory canal debris and granulation tissue • **Topical Otic Antibiotics: first-line medication; ciprofloxacin-dexamethasone or ofloxacin** • Neomycin/polymyxin-B/hydrocortisone otic suspension is contraindicated (aminoglycosides are ototoxic) • **Oral Antibiotics: reserved for severe cases; amoxicillin or 3rd generation cephalosporin** • Surgery: tympanoplasty if refractory or cholesteatoma present
Key Words & Most Common	• Chronic middle ear infection + TM perforation • Age 2-3 most common • Worse after URI or bathing/swimming • Ear drainage + hearing loss • Painless • Perforated TM • Clinical diagnosis • Debris removal → topical antibiotics (ciprofloxacin-dexamethasone drops) → oral antibiotics → tympanoplasty

Acute Otitis Media 👂

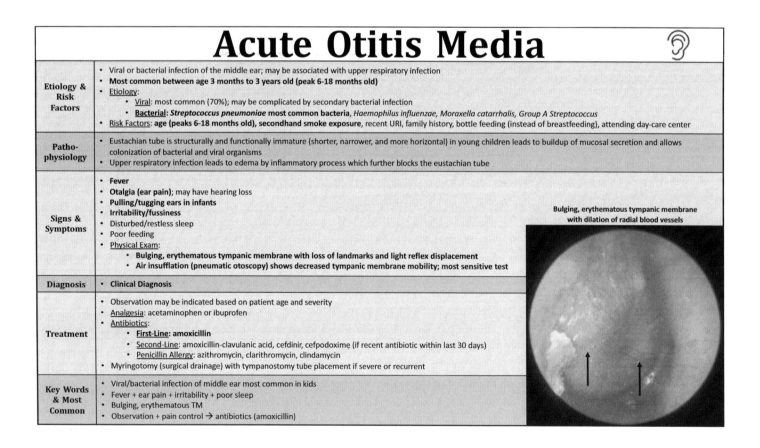

Etiology & Risk Factors	• Viral or bacterial infection of the middle ear; may be associated with upper respiratory infection
	• **Most common between age 3 months to 3 years old (peak 6-18 months old)**
	• Etiology:
	   • Viral: most common (70%); may be complicated by secondary bacterial infection
	   • **Bacterial:** *Streptococcus pneumoniae* **most common bacteria**, *Haemophilus influenzae, Moraxella catarrhalis, Group A Streptococcus*
	• Risk Factors: **age (peaks 6-18 months old), secondhand smoke exposure**, recent URI, family history, bottle feeding (instead of breastfeeding), attending day-care center

Patho-physiology	• Eustachian tube is structurally and functionally immature (shorter, narrower, and more horizontal) in young children leads to buildup of mucosal secretion and allows colonization of bacterial and viral organisms • Upper respiratory infection leads to edema by inflammatory process which further blocks the eustachian tube

Signs & Symptoms	• **Fever**
	• **Otalgia (ear pain)**; may have hearing loss
	• **Pulling/tugging ears in infants**
	• **Irritability/fussiness**
	• **Disturbed/restless sleep**
	• Poor feeding
	• Physical Exam:
	   • **Bulging, erythematous tympanic membrane with loss of landmarks and light reflex displacement**
	   • **Air insufflation (pneumatic otoscopy) shows decreased tympanic membrane mobility; most sensitive test**
	
	Bulging, erythematous tympanic membrane with dilation of radial blood vessels

Diagnosis	• **Clinical Diagnosis**

Treatment	• Observation may be indicated based on patient age and severity
	• Analgesia: acetaminophen or ibuprofen
	• Antibiotics:
	   • **First-Line: amoxicillin**
	   • Second-Line: amoxicillin-clavulanic acid, cefdinir, cefpodoxime (if recent antibiotic within last 30 days)
	   • Penicillin Allergy: azithromycin, clarithromycin, clindamycin
	• Myringotomy (surgical drainage) with tympanostomy tube placement if severe or recurrent

Key Words & Most Common	• Viral/bacterial infection of middle ear most common in kids • Fever + ear pain + irritability + poor sleep • Bulging, erythematous TM • Observation + pain control → antibiotics (amoxicillin)

Serous Otitis Media

Etiology & Risk Factors	• Evidence of middle ear fluid without signs or symptoms of acute infection (fever, pain, erythema/bulging of TM) • Etiology: **sequela to acute otitis media; eustachian tube dysfunction**, allergies, environmental barometric pressure changes
Patho-physiology	• Eustachian tube obstruction secondary to inflammation of the nasopharynx creates a relative negative pressure within the middle ear leading to fluid accumulation • Fluid accumulation inhibits normal vibration of tympanic membrane and sound transmission

Signs & Symptoms	• May be asymptomatic
	• **Hearing loss**
	• **Ear pressure/fullness**
	• **Ear popping** with swallowing
	• Ear pain is rare
	• Physical Exam: Otoscopic Exam
	  • Opacification of tympanic membrane, loss of light reflex, hypomobility with insufflation
	  • **Retracted or flat tympanic membrane with effusion**
	  • **Air fluid level or air bubbles visible through tympanic membrane**

Diagnosis	• **Clinical Diagnosis** with otoscopic exam
Treatment	• **Observation: most resolve spontaneously** • Supportive: antihistamines or nasal corticosteroids if allergy related, Valsalva maneuver to temporarily ventilate middle ear • Tympanostomy Tube: if persistent, affecting child's hearing, or causing developmental delays
Key Words & Most Common	• Middle ear fluid without signs of infection • Asymptomatic • Hearing loss • Ear pressure/fullness (no pain) • Otoscopic exam: retracted/flat TM with effusion; air fluid level/air bubbles • Clinical diagnosis • Observation + supportive treatment → tympanostomy tube • Eustachian Tube Dysfunction = inability to open eustachian tube; serous otitis media = accumulation of fluid in middle ear space

Flat tympanic membrane and visible landmarks

Eustachian Tube Dysfunction

Etiology & Risk Factors	• Failure of middle ear to maintain proper pressure equalization • Etiology: **sequela of viral URI or allergic rhinitis**, sinusitis, tumor, **allergies, atmospheric barometric pressure changes**, airplane travel, GERD, hypertrophic adenoids
Patho-physiology	• Inability of the eustachian tube to open creates a relative negative pressure within the middle ear leading to fluid accumulation • Fluid accumulation inhibits normal vibration of tympanic membrane and sound transmission

Signs & Symptoms	• **Ear-ache (may radiate to jaw)**
	• **Ear fullness/pressure**
	• **Ear popping**
	• **Disequilibrium**
	• **Muffled hearing** (conductive hearing loss)
	• Tinnitus
	• Physical Exam: may be normal
	  • **Air fluid level or air bubbles visible through tympanic membrane**
	  • **Opacification of tympanic membrane**, loss of light reflex, hypomobility with insufflation

Diagnosis	• **Clinical Diagnosis**

Treatment	• **Treat underlying cause** (GERD management, avoid allergens, weight reduction)
	• **Autoinsufflation: swallowing, yawning, Valsalva maneuver** (temporarily ventilates middle ear by opening Eustachian tube), chewing
	• Medications:
	  • **Antihistamines and nasal corticosteroids** if related to allergic rhinitis
	  • **Decongestants** (pseudoephedrine, phenylephrine) or topical vasoconstrictors (oxymetazoline) if nasal congestion present
	• Surgery: surgical dilation of Eustachian tube if refractory and persistent

Key Words & Most Common	• Inadequate middle ear pressure equalization • Viral URI, allergies, change in pressure • Ear fullness/pressure, popping • Disequilibrium • Normal or signs of fluid in middle ear • Clinical diagnosis • Autoinsufflation → antihistamines + nasal corticosteroids → decongestants • Eustachian Tube Dysfunction = inability to open eustachian tube; serous otitis media = accumulation of fluid in middle ear space

Otic Barotrauma

Etiology & Risk Factors	• Physical damage to the tympanic membrane secondary to rapid change in pressure
	• Etiology: **rapid altitude change most common**
	    • Ascent: **scuba diving**, mountain climbing
	    • Descent: **airplane travel, skiing**
	• Risk Factors: asthma, **sinusitis, concurrent URI**, vertigo, Eustachian tube dysfunction, inexperience with activity

Patho-physiology	• Changes in environmental barometric pressure causes middle ear pressure to fall below ambient pressure (retraction of tympanic membrane) or rise above ambient pressure (bulging of tympanic membrane) • Compressive/expansive forces lead to shear stress on the tympanic membrane and possible tympanic membrane rupture

Signs & Symptoms	• **Ear pain, fullness, pressure**
	• **Hearing loss**
	• **Vertigo**
	• Physical Exam:
	    • **Bloody auricular discharge if tympanic membrane rupture**
	    • **Middle ear effusion** or hemorrhage if TM visualized

Diagnosis	• **Clinical Diagnosis**
Treatment	• **Avoidance of triggering activity**; avoid airplane travel with URI • **Mechanical autoinsufflation: swallowing, yawning** (temporarily ventilates middle ear by mechanically opening Eustachian tube), chewing • *Avoid* Valsalva or blowing nose (pressure difference can cause TM rupture) • **Decongestants** (pseudoephedrine, phenylephrine) or topical vasoconstrictors (oxymetazoline) if nasal congestion present • Consider antibiotics and ENT referral if TM rupture
Key Words & Most Common	• Tympanic membrane damage secondary to rapid change in pressure • Scuba diving, airplane travel • Ear pain, fullness, pressure • Hearing loss • Vertigo • Signs of TM rupture • Clinical Diagnosis • Avoid triggering activity • Manual autoinsufflation (avoid Valsalva and blowing nose) + decongestants

Cerumen Impaction

Etiology & Risk Factors	• Build up of cerumen (ear wax) within the external auditory canal leads to obstruction • Etiology: excessive cerumen production • Risk Factors: **use of hearing aids or ear plugs**, anatomical abnormalities of ear canal, hair within ear canal
Patho-physiology	• Cerumen production is normal body process; self-cleaning mechanism of the ear may fail or become obstructed leading to build-up of wax within the external auditory canal

Signs & Symptoms	• **Conductive hearing loss**
	• **Ear fullness**
	• Ear canal pruritus
	• Physical Exam: otoscopic exam
	    • Direct visualization of cerumen impaction
	    • **Conductive hearing loss: lateralization to affected ear with Weber testing**

Diagnosis	• **Clinical Diagnosis**

Treatment	• Cerumenolytic Agents: soften cerumen to facilitate removal
	    • **Hydrogen peroxide**, sterile saline, carbamide peroxide
	• **Irrigation: after wax is softened**
	    • **Syringe with warm water** and soft catheter tubing
	    • Gentle jet lavage until wax is flushed out
	    • **Contraindicated if TM rupture**
	• Manual Removal:
	    • Removal with cerumen spoon/curette under direct visualization

Key Words & Most Common	• Ear wax obstruction within the external auditory canal • Use of hearing aids/ear plugs • Conductive hearing loss • Ear fullness • Clinical diagnosis • Hydrogen peroxide solution to soften wax → syringe irrigation • Manual removal with curette

Tympanic Membrane Perforation 🕉

Etiology & Risk Factors	• Rupture of the tympanic membrane (TM) leads to connection between external auditory canal and middle ear • Etiology: **blunt trauma** (direct impact blow to ear), **penetrating trauma (cotton swab)**, **complication of acute otitis media**, iatrogenic (foreign body or cerumen removal), barotrauma (**gun shot**, blast injury, scuba diving) • Risk Factors: prior or current acute otitis media, severe otitis externa, prior ear surgery
Patho-physiology	• Barotrauma creates large, rapid and unequal changes of the pressure gradient between external and middle ear causing stress to the tympanic membrane • Direct penetration of tympanic membrane most commonly causes perforation at the **pars tensa** (largest and thinnest area of tympanic membrane)

Signs & Symptoms	• **Sudden onset ear pain and hearing loss**
	• **Vertigo**
	• **Tinnitus**
	• **Bloody otorrhea**
	• *If associated with acute otitis media, patients may experience **rising pain with sudden pain relief and bloody auricular discharge** as perforation relieves pressure*
	• Physical Exam: otoscopic exam
	   • **Perforated tympanic membrane seen under direct visualization**
	     • May have conductive hearing loss (lateralization to affected ear with Weber test; bone>air conduction with Rinne test)

Diagnosis	• **Clinical Diagnosis**
Treatment	• Supportive: most TM perforations heal spontaneously; **keep ear dry (avoid water)**, avoid forceful Valsalva • **Topical Otic Antibiotics: ofloxacin otic drops (if contaminated)** • *Avoid* ciprofloxacin (can damage inner ear) and Neomycin/polymyxin-B/hydrocortisone (aminoglycosides are ototoxic) • Oral Antibiotics: indicated if rupture secondary to acute otitis media • Otolaryngology Referral: if vertigo or hearing loss present
Key Words & Most Common	• Blunt/penetrating trauma, acute otitis media, barotrauma • Sudden onset ear pain + hearing loss + bloody auricular discharge • Rising pain + sudden pain relief + bloody discharge if secondary to acute otitis media • Clinical diagnosis with direct visualization

Cholesteatoma 🕉

Etiology & Risk Factors	• Abnormal collection of keratinized squamous epithelium within the middle ear • Etiology: **Eustachian tube dysfunction (retracts TM)**, chronic otitis media or other middle ear conditions,
Patho-physiology	• Chronic retraction of tympanic membrane results in a retraction pocket in which keratinized squamous cells accumulate leading to an expanding mass which may expand into the middle ear and damage the bony ossicles

Signs & Symptoms	• **Painless otorrhea (malodorous, brownish/yellow ear discharge)**
	• **Conductive hearing loss**
	• Peripheral vertigo
	• Tinnitus
	• Cranial nerve palsy (CNVII most commonly affected)
	• Physical Exam:
	   • **Collection of white granulation tissue debris** (posterosuperior quadrant most common)
	   • Malodourous otorrhea
	   • Retraction of tympanic membrane; perforated tympanic membrane
	   • **Conductive hearing loss** (lateralization to affected ear with Weber test; bone>air conduction with Rinne test)

Diagnosis	• **Clinical Diagnosis** • CT: evaluates for ossicle encasement

Treatment	• Surgery: **surgical excision of cholesteatoma and granular debris**
	   • Does not restore hearing
	   • High recurrence rate

Key Words & Most Common	• Keratinized squamous epithelium collection in inner ear • Secondary to chronic middle ear conditions (eustachian tube dysfunction most common) • Painless otorrhea (malodourous, brown/yellow discharge) • Conductive hearing loss • Granulation tissue debris at tympanic membrane • Clinical diagnosis • Surgical excision

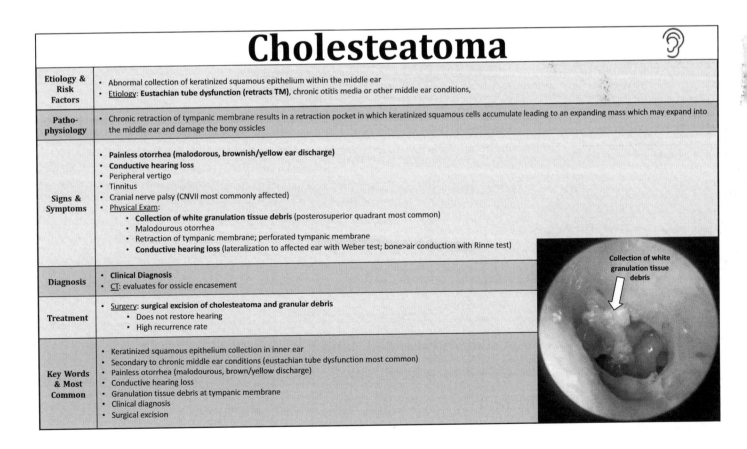

Collection of white granulation tissue debris

Otosclerosis

Etiology & Risk Factors	• Abnormal middle ear bone remodeling and accumulation of new bone within the oval window leading to fixation of the stapes • Etiology: **genetic predisposition (autosomal dominant)**, anatomic abnormality • <u>Risk Factors</u>: **family history**, female, age (20-30 years old most common), Paget disease
Patho-physiology	• Bone remodeling (bone resorption and subsequent bone deposition) causes focal lesions that replace normal bone with sclerotic bone resulting in entrapment and restriction of the stapes and conductive hearing loss

Signs & Symptoms	• **Slow, progressive, conductive hearing loss**
	  • **Low-frequency sounds most affected** (unable to hear whispering)
	• Tinnitus
	• Vertigo (uncommon)
	• <u>Physical Exam</u>: often normal
	  • **Conductive hearing loss** (lateralization to affected ear with Weber test; bone>air conduction with Rinne test)

Diagnosis	• <u>Pure Tone Audiometry</u>: reveals low-frequency hearing loss of air conduction; bone conduction normal • <u>High-Contrast CT</u>: **standard diagnostic study; shows thickening of footplate of stapes bone**
Treatment	• <u>Hearing Aids</u>: may improve hearing • <u>Surgery</u>: **stapedectomy with prosthesis in severe cases**; may still require hearing aids
Key Words & Most Common	• Middle ear bone remodeling leading to fixation of stapes bone • Family history • Conductive hearing loss (low-frequency) • High-contrast CT • Hearing aids → surgery

Benign Paroxysmal Positional Vertigo

Etiology & Risk Factors	• Peripheral vertigo most commonly due to **canalolithiasis (migration of otolith particles within semicircular canal)** • **Most common cause of peripheral vertigo** • <u>Etiology</u>: **otoconial crystals displacement, head trauma**, migraine, otitis media, recent viral infection, head trauma, prolonged anesthesia or bed rest • <u>Risk Factors</u>: age (50-70 years old most common), female, history of ear surgery
Patho-physiology	• Otoconial crystals (calcium carbonate) are displaced which stimulates hair cells within the semicircular canal which creates the illusion of motion through disequilibrium

Signs & Symptoms	• **Sudden onset vertigo**
	  • **Triggered by specific head movements** (rolling over in bed, bending over to pick something up, turning to check blind spot in car, looking up, etc.)
	  • **Lasts 60 seconds or less**
	  • Worse in morning and may improve throughout day
	• Nausea/vomiting
	• **Not associated with hearing loss or tinnitus**

Diagnosis	• <u>Dix-Hallpike Maneuver</u>: • Patient sits upright with head rotated 45° to one side → patient quickly lies down with pillow under shoulders (head remains rotated) → observe eyes for 45 seconds for nystagmus → **positive if rotational (torsional) nystagmus present** toward affected ear (ear closest to ground when lying)

Treatment	• <u>Epley Maneuver</u>: **canalith repositioning procedure; first-line treatment**
	  • Begins after last step of Dix-Hallpike → patient holds position for 2 minutes → head rotated 90° (unaffected ear faces ground) → patient rolls onto unaffected side shoulder and looks downward at 45° angle and holds for 1 minute → patient is sat up with head held in 45° of rotation → patient may slowly bring gaze to midline
	• <u>Medication Management</u>: episodes are brief and medications are rarely indicated
	  • <u>Antihistamines</u>: **meclizine first-line medication**, diphenhydramine
	  • <u>Anticholinergics</u>: scopolamine
	  • <u>Benzodiazepines</u>: lorazepam or diazepam if severe or refractory
	  • <u>Antiemetics</u>: ondansetron, metoclopramide or promethazine as needed

Key Words & Most Common	• Otolith particles within semicircular canal • Sudden onset vertigo triggered by head movement lasting <60 seconds • NOT associated with hearing loss/tinnitus • Dix-Hallpike maneuver to diagnose • Epley maneuver repositions canalith • Medications rarely indicated; meclizine first-line as necessary Epley Maneuver

Vestibular Neuritis and Labyrinthitis 👂

Etiology & Risk Factors	• <u>Vestibular Neuritis</u>: inflammation of the vestibular division of CNVIII • <u>Labyrinthitis</u>: inflammation of the vestibular and cochlear portion of CNVIII • <u>Etiology</u>: idiopathic; **may be viral or post-viral inflammation**
Patho-physiology	• Viral or post-viral inflammation of vestibulocochlear cranial nerve

Signs & Symptoms	• **Vestibular Neuritis:**
	   • **Acute, constant, severe vertigo lasting several days**
	   • **Nausea and vomiting**
	   • **Horizontal/rotary nystagmus toward affected side**
	   • **NO hearing loss or tinnitus**
	• **Labyrinthitis:**
	   • **Above symptoms WITH hearing loss and/or tinnitus**

Diagnosis	• **Clinical Diagnosis** • <u>CT/MRI</u>: ordered to rule out other causes of symptoms if diagnosis unclear; MRI may show inflammatory enhancement of vestibular nerve

Treatment	• <u>Medications</u>: **symptoms-based treatment**
	   • <u>Antihistamines</u>: **meclizine**, diphenhydramine
	   • <u>Anticholinergics</u>: scopolamine
	   • <u>Benzodiazepines</u>: lorazepam or diazepam if severe or refractory
	   • <u>Antiemetics</u>: ondansetron, metoclopramide or promethazine as needed
	   • <u>**Corticosteroids**</u>: **IM methylprednisolone and/or oral prednisone taper for nerve inflammation**

Key Words & Most Common	• Viral or post-viral inflammation of vestibulocochlear nerve (CNVIII) • Vestibular Neuritis: acute, constant vertigo lasting for days *WITHOUT* hearing loss • Labyrinthitis: acute, constant vertigo lasting days *WITH* hearing loss • Clinical diagnosis • Symptom-based treatment with meclizine, steroids, benzodiazepines

Ménière's Disease 👂

Etiology & Risk Factors	• **Idiopathic collection of endolymphatic fluid within the cochlea and vestibular organs** (idiopathic endolymphatic hydrops) • **<u>Etiology</u>: not fully understood** • <u>Risk Factors</u>: preexisting autoimmune condition, migraines, allergies, trauma to ear, age (20-50 years most common)
Patho-physiology	• Unknown; may be related to imbalance between secretion and resorption of endolymphatic fluid within the cochlea
Signs & Symptoms	• **Sudden episodic peripheral vertigo** • **Lasts minutes to hours** (usually 2-8 hours) • **Pressure/fullness in affected ear** • **Tinnitus in affected ear** • **Diminished hearing (typically low-frequency)** • Nausea/vomiting
Diagnosis	• **Clinical Diagnosis** • <u>**Audiogram**</u>: **shows low-frequency sensorineural hearing loss in affected ear** • <u>MRI</u>: rules out lesions • Confirmed via glycerol testing or vestibular-evoked potentials by ENT

Treatment	• <u>Supportive</u>: dietary modifications (**low-salt diet; avoid caffeine**, nicotine, chocolate, alcohol)
	• <u>Medications</u>: **symptoms-based treatment**
	   • <u>Antihistamines</u>: **meclizine**, diphenhydramine
	   • <u>Anticholinergics</u>: scopolamine
	   • <u>Benzodiazepines</u>: lorazepam or diazepam if severe or refractory
	   • <u>**Antiemetics**</u>: **prochlorperazine or promethazine as needed**; ondansetron second-line
	   • <u>**Corticosteroids**</u>: IM methylprednisolone and/or oral prednisone taper
	   • <u>**Diuretics**</u>: **hydrochlorothiazide or acetazolamide; avoid loop diuretics) reduces endolymphatic pressure**
	• <u>Surgery</u>: endolymphatic sac decompression; surgical labyrinthectomy or intraaural gentamicin (chemical labyrinthectomy) if severe

Key Words & Most Common	• Collection of endolymphatic fluid within cochlea of unknown etiology Sudden, episodic vertigo lasting minutes to hours • Pressure/fullness • Tinnitus • Diminished low-frequency hearing • Low-salt diet; avoid caffeine + antihistamines, antiemetics, steroids, diuretics (hydrochlorothiazide)

Acoustic Neuroma

Etiology & Risk Factors	• **Benign tumor developing from the sheath of Schwann cells on the vestibular division of CNVIII**; also known as vestibular schwannoma • <u>Etiology</u>: may be related to neurofibromatosis type 2; radiation exposure (chronic mobile phone use may be implicated)
Patho-physiology	• Schwann cell tumor arises from vestibular division of CNVIII which further expands and projects into the cerebellopontine angle and compress CN VII and VIII
Signs & Symptoms	• **Unilateral sensorineural hearing loss** • May be slow progressive or abrupt • **Vertigo** • **Unilateral tinnitus** • **Facial numbness or paresis** (facial and trigeminal nerve compression)
Diagnosis	• **Audiogram: initial test; reveals asymmetric sensorineural hearing loss** • <u>MRI</u>: **imaging test of choice**; contrast enhancement at vestibular division of CNVIII
Treatment	• <u>Observation</u>: small or nongrowing schwannoma • Stereotactic radiation therapy vs microsurgery (depends on residual hearing, tumor size, patient age and health)
Key Words & Most Common	• Benign tumor on Schwann cells of CNVIII • Unilateral sensorineural hearing loss • Vertigo, tinnitus • Facial numbness • Audiogram • MRI • Observation → surgery vs radiation therapy

Vestibular Schwannoma

Tinnitus

Etiology & Risk Factors	• Perception of high-pitched ringing or buzzing without external stimulation
	• <u>Etiology</u>: may be subjective or objective
	  • <u>Subjective</u>: **noise trauma is most common cause, sensorineural hearing loss, ototoxic medications (aspirin**, NSAIDs, loop diuretics, aminoglycoside antibiotics), **caffeine toxicity, otitis media**, Ménière's disease, labyrinthitis, head trauma, barotrauma, migraines
	  • <u>Objective</u>: enlarged Eustachian tube, vascular (arterial bruit, carotid stenosis), arteriovenous malformation

Patho-physiology	• <u>Subjective Tinnitus</u>: normal input from the auditory pathway is disrupted or altered leading to abnormal neuronal activity in the auditory cortex • <u>Objective Tinnitus</u>: noise generated by anatomical cause occurring near the middle ear; may be heard by examiner

Signs & Symptoms	• **Described as high-pitched ringing, buzzing, whistling, hissing**
	• **Most noticeable in quiet environments** with absence of distracting stimuli
	  • Lying in bed to go to sleep, sitting in quiet waiting room, etc.
	• May be continuous or intermittent
	• May be exacerbated by stress
	• <u>Physical Exam</u>:
	  • Evaluate inspect tympanic membrane for signs of infection, inspect ear canal for discharge, cerumen impaction or foreign body, auscultate carotid artery for bruit

Diagnosis	• **Clinical Diagnosis** • <u>Audiogram</u>: determines hearing loss • Exact source may require extensive otolaryngologist workup
Treatment	• **Treat underlying etiology** • <u>Supportive</u>: reassurance, stress management techniques, caffeine cessation, masking symptoms (white noise, low-volume music) • <u>Correct Hearing Loss</u>: hearing aid; provides relief in ~50% of patients
Key Words & Most Common	• Noise trauma most common cause leading to sensorineural hearing loss • Ototoxic medications (aspirin and aminoglycosides most common) • High-pitched ringing, buzzing • Continuous or intermittent • Clinical diagnosis (exact etiology requires extensive workup) • Treat underlying etiology • Supportive measures → hearing aids if indicated

Herpes Zoster Oticus

Etiology & Risk Factors	• Complication of reactivation of varicella-zoster virus resulting in inflammation of geniculate ganglion of facial cranial nerve (CNVII) • **Also known as Ramsay-Hunt Syndrome** • <u>Etiology</u>: **reactivation of varicella-zoster virus** • <u>Risk Factors</u>: **immunocompromised** (chemotherapy/radiation therapy, HIV infection, diabetes), **physiologic stress**, infection, malnutrition
Patho-physiology	• Varicella zoster virus remains latent in dorsal root ganglion or in the geniculate ganglion; upon reactivation, symptoms involve the facial and vestibulocochlear cranial nerves

Signs & Symptoms	• <u>**Classic Triad**</u>:
	   • **Ipsilateral facial paralysis**
	   • **Otalgia (ear pain)**
	   • **Painful vesicles on auricle**
	• Ear pain radiating from deep within ear to pinna
	• Upper respiratory symptoms may precede triad by 1-3 days
	• May have vertigo or hearing loss
	• <u>Physical Exam</u>:
	   • **Vesicles of pinna and external auditory canal** following sensory branch distribution of facial nerve

Diagnosis	• **Clinical Diagnosis**
Treatment	• <u>**Antivirals**</u>: **acyclovir or valacyclovir** • <u>**High-Dose Corticosteroids**</u>: **prednisone** • <u>Oral Analgesia</u>: NSAIDs, acetaminophen
Key Words & Most Common	• Complication of varicella-zoster virus reactivation; aka Ramsay-Hunt Syndrome • Reactivation secondary to physiologic stress or immunocompromised • Classic Triad: ipsilateral facial paralysis, ear pain, painful vesicles on auricle • Clinical diagnosis • Antivirals (acyclovir/valacyclovir) + high-dose corticosteroids

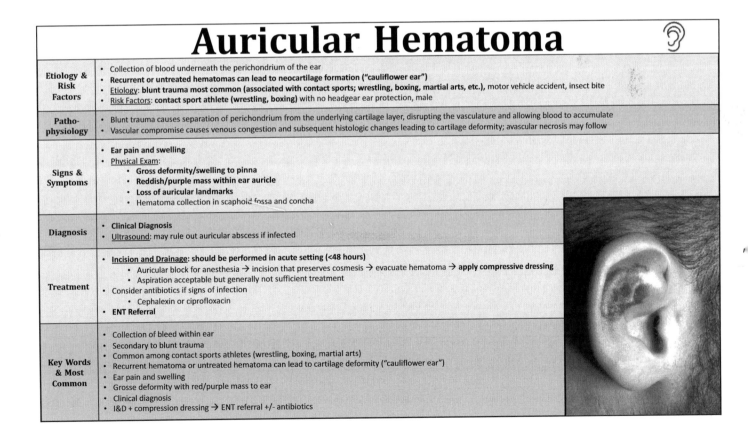

Vesicles of pinna and external auditory canal   Ipsilateral facial paralysis

Auricular Hematoma

Etiology & Risk Factors	• Collection of blood underneath the perichondrium of the ear • **Recurrent or untreated hematomas can lead to neocartilage formation ("cauliflower ear")** • <u>Etiology</u>: **blunt trauma most common (associated with contact sports; wrestling, boxing, martial arts, etc.)**, motor vehicle accident, insect bite • <u>Risk Factors</u>: **contact sport athlete (wrestling, boxing)** with no headgear ear protection, male
Patho-physiology	• Blunt trauma causes separation of perichondrium from the underlying cartilage layer, disrupting the vasculature and allowing blood to accumulate • Vascular compromise causes venous congestion and subsequent histologic changes leading to cartilage deformity; avascular necrosis may follow

Signs & Symptoms	• **Ear pain and swelling**
	• <u>Physical Exam</u>:
	   • **Gross deformity/swelling to pinna**
	   • **Reddish/purple mass within ear auricle**
	   • **Loss of auricular landmarks**
	   • Hematoma collection in scaphoid fossa and concha

Diagnosis	• **Clinical Diagnosis** • <u>Ultrasound</u>: may rule out auricular abscess if infected

Treatment	• <u>**Incision and Drainage**</u>: **should be performed in acute setting (<48 hours)**
	   • Auricular block for anesthesia → incision that preserves cosmesis → evacuate hematoma → **apply compressive dressing**
	   • Aspiration acceptable but generally not sufficient treatment
	• Consider antibiotics if signs of infection
	   • Cephalexin or ciprofloxacin
	• **ENT Referral**

Key Words & Most Common	• Collection of bleed within ear • Secondary to blunt trauma • Common among contact sports athletes (wrestling, boxing, martial arts) • Recurrent hematoma or untreated hematoma can lead to cartilage deformity ("cauliflower ear") • Ear pain and swelling • Grosse deformity with red/purple mass to ear • Clinical diagnosis • I&D + compression dressing → ENT referral +/- antibiotics

Perichondritis

Etiology & Risk Factors	• Infection of ear connective tissue that covers the auricle • May lead to avascular necrosis and deformed auricle ("cauliflower ear") • <u>Etiology</u>: **trauma (blunt trauma, burns or laceration), insect bites, ear piercings through cartilage,** herpes zoster infection • *Pseudomonas aeruginosa* **most common causative organism (95%)**; may have coinfection with *E. coli* or *S. aureus* • <u>Risk Factors</u>: **at-home ear piercing** (unsterile equipment), **immunocompromised** (HIV, diabetes, Non-Hodgkin's lymphoma), systemic inflammatory conditions
Patho-physiology	• Perichondrium is a layer of dense connective tissue that surrounds the cartilage with minimal blood supply allowing increased susceptibility to infection • If infection is left untreated, can lead to cartilage deformity to auricle ("cauliflower ear") or abscess formation

Signs & Symptoms	• **Ear pain and swelling**
	   • Ranges from dull to severe pain
	• <u>Physical Exam</u>:
	   • **Erythema, warmth, edema to auricle**
	   • May have **purulent discharge** (especially if insect bite or ear-piercing infection)
	   • **No lobule involvement** (differentiates from otitis externa)

Diagnosis	• **Clinical Diagnosis** • <u>Wound Culture</u>: of purulent discharge to guide antibiotic treatment
Treatment	• **Oral Antibiotics:** mainstay of treatment • **Ciprofloxacin is first-line antibiotic**; good *Pseudomonas* and *Staphylococcus* coverage and cartilage penetration • <u>Pain Control</u>: NSAIDs, acetaminophen • <u>Urgent ENT Referral</u>: monitoring +/- incision and drainage procedure to preserve cosmesis
Key Words & Most Common	• Infection of ear auricle • Trauma (burns, lacerations), insect bites, ear piercings are most common cause • *Pseudomonas aeruginosa* most common bacteria • Ear pain + swelling • Erythema, warmth, edema to auricle +/- purulent discharge • Clinical diagnosis • Antibiotics (ciprofloxacin) first-line → ENT referral

Acute Sinusitis

Etiology & Risk Factors	• Acute inflammation of the nasal cavity and paranasal sinuses due to viral, bacterial or fungal infections or allergic reactions
	• Acute (<4 weeks); subacute (4-12 weeks); chronic (>12 weeks)
	• <u>Etiology</u>:
	   • <u>Viral</u>: most common cause (98-99%); rhinovirus, adenovirus, influenza virus, parainfluenza virus
	   • <u>Bacterial</u>: *Streptococcus pneumoniae* **(most common bacteria)**, *Haemophilus influenzae* and *Moraxella catarrhalis*
	• <u>Risk Factors</u>: **viral URI**, obstruction of normal sinus drainage (**allergic rhinitis, nasal polyps**), **immunocompromised states**, prolonged ICU stay, smoking, cystic fibrosis

Patho-physiology	• Viral nasal mucosal inflammation obstructs paranasal sinus ostium creating a relative negative pressure and transudate accumulation within the sinus • Excess transudate serves as medium for bacteria to colonize leading to secondary bacterial infections

Signs & Symptoms	• **Facial pain or pressure**
	   • **Worse when bending over or leaning forward**
	• **Nasal congestion** +/- **purulent nasal discharge**
	• **Headache**
	• Malaise
	• Halitosis (bad breath) and hyposmia (decreased sense of smell)
	• *May have associated URI symptoms (cough, sore throat)*
		• **Clinical Features of Bacterial Sinusitis**
		   • Symptoms persisting >10 days
		   • Bimodal course (patient feels improvement then regresses and worsens)
		   • Fever (>102.2°F)
		   • Purulent rhinorrhea >3 days
		   • Maxillary/teeth pain for 3+ consecutive days
		   • History of diabetes

Diagnosis	• **Clinical Diagnosis** • <u>CT Scan</u>: imaging only indicated for toxic patients; ordered to rule out bone, soft tissue, or dental abnormalities or chronic sinusitis

Treatment	• <u>Supportive</u>: if symptoms <10 days
	   • **Decongestants** (pseudoephedrine), intranasal vasoconstrictors (oxymetazoline; use <3 days), analgesics, antihistamines, mucolytics, intranasal glucocorticoids
	   • Saline nasal irrigation
	• <u>Antibiotics</u>: **indicated if symptoms >10-14 days** or worsening
	   • <u>First-line</u>: **amoxicillin-clavulanic acid**
	   • <u>Second-line</u>: **doxycycline**, respiratory fluoroquinolone (moxifloxacin, levofloxacin); cefdinir may be used if penicillin allergic (not anaphylactic)

Key Words & Most Common	• Acute inflammation of sinuses; viral most common → may progress to secondary bacterial infection • Facial pain/pressure + nasal congestion + headache • Bacterial sinusitis: symptoms >10 days or worsening • Clinical diagnosis • Supportive: decongestants, analgesics, antihistamines, sinus rinses • Antibiotics: amoxicillin-clavulanic acid first-line

Chronic Sinusitis

Etiology & Risk Factors	• Chronic inflammation of the nasal cavity and paranasal sinuses for 12 or more consecutive weeks
	• Etiology: infectious (bacterial/fungal), allergy, exposure, anatomy
	   • <u>Bacterial</u>: ***Staphylococcus aureus*** (most common bacteria), ***Streptococcus pneumoniae***, *Haemophilus influenzae*, *Moraxella catarrhalis*, *Pseudomonas aeruginosa*
	   • <u>Fungal</u>: ***Aspergillus*** (most common fungal), *Mucormycosis*; typically affect elderly or immunocompromised
	   • <u>Allergy/Exposure</u>: dust, **mold**, cigarette smoke, airborne irritants, fragrance, occupational exposures
	   • <u>Anatomy</u>: nasal polyps, deviated septum

Patho-physiology	• Chronic inflammation causes obstruction of the nasal passages prevents normal sinus drainage, allowing bacteria to colonize
Signs & Symptoms	• **Symptoms ≥12 weeks** • **Facial pain or pressure; dental pain** • **Worse when bending over or leaning forward** • **Nasal congestion** • **Purulent nasal discharge** • **Headache**, malaise, fatigue, cough • Halitosis (bad breath) and **hyposmia** (decreased sense of smell)
Diagnosis	• Clinical Diagnosis • <u>**Nasal Endoscopy + Culture**</u>: preferred test to identify inflammation through direct visualization; culture identifies organism and can guide treatment • <u>CT Scan</u>: confirms inflammation presence; most sensitive but most expensive

Treatment	• <u>Supportive</u>: symptomatic relief
	   • **Saline nasal irrigation (high-volume), decongestants, intranasal glucocorticoids**, antihistamines (if allergy related)
	• <u>Antibiotics</u>: if bacterial; may be given up to 3 weeks
	   • **Amoxicillin-clavulanic acid**, doxycycline
	• **Oral corticosteroids**; antifungals as indicated
	• <u>Surgery</u>: functional endoscopic sinus surgery if failed conservative therapy

Key Words & Most Common	• Chronic inflammation of sinuses for ≥12 weeks • Facial pain/pressure + congestion + purulent discharge + hyposmia • Clinical diagnosis → nasal endoscopy + culture preferred • Saline irrigation + intranasal steroids + decongestants +/- antibiotics +/- oral steroids • Surgery if refractory

Inflammation and filling of right sinus with sclerotic bone

Mucormycosis

Etiology & Risk Factors	• Opportunistic invasive fungal infection affecting the sinuses and respiratory tract of immunocompromised patients • <u>Etiology</u>: fungi (*Mucorales*) found in soil, bread mold, decomposing fruit matter • <u>Risk Factors</u>: **immunocompromised (leukemia, organ/bone-marrow transplant, HIV, chemotherapy) or uncontrolled diabetes mellitus**
Patho-physiology	• Spores are inhaled and adhere to the nasal mucosa and paranasal sinuses of an immunocompromised patient • Subsequent invasion of nasal septum, bone, and palate occurs leading to rapidly progressive necrosis that may infiltrate the brain (**rhino-orbital-cerebral form**)

Signs & Symptoms	• **Severe sinusitis symptoms** (facial pain/pressure, headache, purulent nasal discharge etc.)
	• **Fever**
	• **Orbital cellulitis**
	• **Rapid progression spreading to orbits**, naso- and oropharynx, brain and vasculature
	   • May cause change in vision, headache, cranial nerve defects
	• <u>Physical Exam</u>:
	   • **Black discoloration of palate, nasal mucosa or face indicates necrosis**

Diagnosis	• <u>**Tissue Biopsy and Histopathology**</u>: large non-septate hyphae with irregular diameters and right-angle (90°) branching patterns; necrotic tissue may not contain organisms • <u>CT</u>: determine extent of bone destruction
Treatment	• <u>**Antifungals**</u>: IV Amphotericin B is first-line medication • <u>**Surgical Debridement**</u>: aggressive surgical debridement of necrotic tissue is critical
Key Words & Most Common	• Fungal infection of sinuses/respiratory tract of immunocompromised • Immunocompromised (leukemia or bone-marrow transplant most common) or poorly-controlled diabetics • Severe sinusitis + fever + cellulitis → progressive to involve orbits • Black discoloration of palate or face • Tissue biopsy + histopathology: large non-septate hyphae with irregular diameters and right-angle branching patterns • IV amphotericin B + surgical debridement

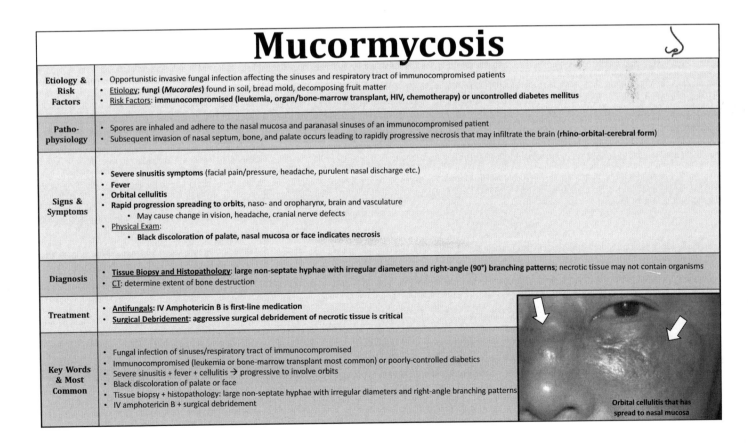

Orbital cellulitis that has spread to nasal mucosa

Allergic Rhinitis

Etiology & Risk Factors	• Seasonal or perennial inflammation of nasal mucosa secondary to airborne allergens (also known as hay fever) • Etiology: **plant allergens most common (tree, grass, or weed pollen)**; dust, cockroaches, animal dander, cigarette smoke, cold air exposure • Risk Factor: **atopy (asthma, atopic dermatitis, allergic rhinitis)**, family history, male, secondhand smoke exposure as child
Patho-physiology	• Exposure to allergen creates IgE-mediated mast cell histamine release resulting in inflammation and mucous gland stimulation • Other immune modulators (leukotrienes, prostaglandins) act on blood vessels to induce nasal congestion

Signs & Symptoms	• **Thin and clear (watery) rhinorrhea**
	• **Nasal congestion**
	• **Itching of nose, eyes, mouth**
	• **Sneezing**
	• Ear fullness ("clogged" feeling)
	• *Absence of fever*
	• Physical Exam:
	   • **Infraorbital edema and darkening ("allergic shiner")**
	   • **Transverse nasal bridge crease** (from chronic wiping or rubbing of nose)
	   • **Cobblestoning of posterior oropharynx** (post-nasal drip)
	   • Pale or **boggy nasal turbinates**

Diagnosis	• **Clinical Diagnosis** • Serum testing for allergen-specific IgE or allergy skin testing to determine etiology if unclear

Treatment	• Supportive:
	   • **Reduce Exposure to Allergen:** sleep with window closed, air purifier, change furnace filters, change clothes and shower after being outdoors
	   • **Saline Nasal Irrigation:** washes out allergens
	• Medication Management:
	   • **Topical Intranasal Corticosteroids: fluticasone propionate is first-line**; decreases inflammation of nasal turbinates and sinuses to relieve obstruction
	   • Oral antihistamines (diphenhydramine, loratadine, etc.), leukotriene receptor antagonists (montelukast), or decongestants (pseudoephedrine) for symptomatic relief

Key Words & Most Common	• Exposure to airborne allergen produces nasal mucosa inflammation • Plant allergens (weed pollen), dust, animal dander, and cigarette smoke most common • Atopic triad (asthma, atopic dermatitis, allergic rhinitis) • Thin/clear rhinorrhea + nasal congestion + itching of nose + sneezing; infraorbital edema/darkening • Clinical Diagnosis • Reduce allergen exposure + saline nasal irrigation → topical intranasal corticosteroids

Nasal Polyps

Etiology & Risk Factors	• Benign inflammatory and hyperplastic growths of the sinonasal mucosa • Etiology: secondary to inflammatory process and **impaired clearance of irritants**; result of foreign body • Risk Factors: **allergic rhinitis, acute/chronic sinusitis, cystic fibrosis**, aspirin allergy
Patho-physiology	• Sinonasal mucosal atrophy, decreased mucous secretions and chronic exposure to irritants leads to inflammation and cell/tissue hypertrophy

Signs & Symptoms	• **Nasal congestion and obstruction**
	• **Thick nasal discharge**
	• **Post-nasal drainage**
	• Hyposmia (decreased sense of smell)
	• Sneezing, ocular itching, asthma
	• Physical Exam: may use nasal speculum
	   • **Pale (gray) boggy tear-drop shaped mass of the nasal mucosa**
	   • **Cobblestoning of posterior oropharynx** (post-nasal drip)

Nasal polyp of right nostril |
Diagnosis	• **Clinical Diagnosis**

Treatment	• Supportive: managing underlying etiology; reduce exposure to allergens, nasal saline irrigation, antihistamines, leukotriene receptor antagonists
	• Medication Management:
	   • **Topical Intranasal Corticosteroids: first-line**; decreases inflammation of nasal turbinates and sinuses to relieve obstruction
	   • Oral Corticosteroids: reserved for refractory cases
	• Surgery: nasal endoscopic polypectomy if large, severe or refractory

Key Words & Most Common	• Risk Factors: allergic rhinitis, acute/chronic sinusitis • Nasal congestion/obstruction + post-nasal drainage + thick nasal discharge • Pale boggy tear-drop shaped mass of nasal mucosa • Clinical Diagnosis • Allergen reduction • Topical intranasal corticosteroids is first-line → surgery

Epistaxis

	Anterior	Posterior
Etiology & Risk Factors	• Rupture of blood vessels within the anterior nasal mucosa • Etiology: **nasal trauma (nose picking in children is most common), blowing nose, low humidity or hot/dry environment** • Risk Factors: deviated septum, nasal neoplasm, polyps, cocaine use, foreign body	• Rupture of blood vessels within the posterior nasal mucosa • Etiology: **hypertension**, nasal trauma, blowing nose, dry environment • Risk Factors: **hypertension, atherosclerosis, anticoagulant use**, age, **coagulopathy**
Patho-physiology	• **Kiesselbach venous plexus is most common site**	• **Nasopalatine branch of the sphenopalatine artery** (Woodruff's plexus) is most common site

Signs & Symptoms	• **Nasal bleeding more likely from *one* nare**
	  • *Can* often be visualized
		• **Posterior: nasal bleeding more likely from *both* nares**
		  • *Cannot* visualize without endoscope
		  • Significant hemorrhage may be visible in posterior nasopharynx
		  • Posterior epistaxis is an emergency

Diagnosis	• **Clinical Diagnosis** (equipment should include light, nasal speculum, suction, packing gauze, vasoconstrictors, airway equipment) • **Anterior rhinoscopy can aid diagnosis** • Labs: coagulation studies if on anticoagulants	• **Clinical Diagnosis** (equipment should include light, nasal speculum, suction, packing gauze, vasoconstrictors, airway equipment) • **Posterior can be diagnosed when measures to control anterior bleed fail** • **Endoscopy (posterior) can aid diagnosis** • Labs: coagulation studies if on anticoagulants
Treatment	• **Direct Nasal Pressure: first-line therapy**; pressure applied for 5-15 minutes while in a seated and leaning forward position • **Topical Vasoconstrictors: oxymetazoline**; may spray directly or soak gauze • **Cauterization**: electrocautery or silver nitrate if bleeding site can be visualized • **Anterior Nasal Packing**: indicated if direct nasal pressure, topical vasoconstrictor and cauterization fail • Prevention: nasal mucosa hydration (saline nasal spray, humidifier, petroleum gauze)	• **Posterior Nasal Packing**: indicated if direct nasal pressure, topical vasoconstrictor and cauterization fail • Admission to inpatient for monitoring • Management of underlying etiology
Key Words & Most Common	• Nasal trauma (nose picking) is most common etiology; blowing nose, dry environment • Kiesselbach venous plexus • Nosebleed from one nare • Clinical diagnosis + rhinoscopy • Direct nasal pressure → vasoconstrictors → cauterization → nasal packing	• Hypertension and anticoagulant use • Palatine artery • Nosebleed from both nares • Clinical diagnosis + endoscopy • Posterior nasal packing → admit

Nasal Foreign Body

Etiology & Risk Factors	• Foreign body within nasal cavity • Etiology: **food (beans, nuts, gum)**, marbles, pebbles, **beads**, tissue, batteries, magnets, toys, cotton • Risk Factors: **most common among children** or adults with psychiatric illness or developmental disabilities
Patho-physiology	• Most common location is at the floor of the inferior turbinate or anterior to the middle turbinate. • Foreign body leads to nasal mucosal erosion, irritation, and epistaxis; can lead to infectious sinusitis

Signs & Symptoms	• **Unilateral epistaxis with mucopurulent nasal discharge**
	• **Foul-smelling nasal discharge**
	• **Nasal obstruction (mouth breathing)**
	• Physical Exam:
	  • **Direct visualization of foreign body on exam**
	  • May require nasal speculum

Diagnosis	• **Clinical Diagnosis** • Rigid or Flexible Fiberoptic Endoscopy: helpful to obtain direct visualization • X-Ray: only if foreign body is button battery, radiopaque and/or unable to be visualized
Treatment	• **Topical Vasoconstrictors: oxymetazoline**; apply prior to removal attempts to reduce inflammation • **Positive Pressure Technique**: have patient attempt to blow nose with contralateral nare occluded • "Mother's kiss": parent occludes contralateral nare, forms tight seal over mouth (mouth to mouth), and blows air quickly and sharply • **Manual Removal: alligator forceps or curette if able to be visualized; urgent removal of button batteries (can cause septal perforation in <4 hours)** • ENT Referral: if unable to be visualized or removed • Antibiotics: if signs of sinusitis and foreign body present for extended period of time
Key Words & Most Common	• Food, beads, marbles, toys most common • Unilateral nosebleed with purulent nasal discharge (foul-smelling) • Nasal obstruction (mouth breathing) • Clinical diagnosis • Topical vasoconstrictors → positive pressure technique • Manual removal if visualized • ENT referral if unable to be visualized

Acute Pharyngitis ᕫ

Etiology & Risk Factors	• Acute inflammation of the mucous membranes of the oropharynx
	• **Etiology: infectious (bacterial or viral)**; allergies (post-nasal drip), trauma, GERD, burns
	  • <u>Viral</u>: **most common cause**; rhinovirus, influenza, coronavirus, adenovirus, parainfluenza, Epstein-Barr virus (EBV), HIV, herpes simplex virus
	  • <u>Bacterial</u>: **Group A *Streptococcus* (*S. pyogenes*) most common bacterial cause**; Group B & C streptococci, *C. pneumoniae*, *M. pneumoniae*, *H. influenzae*, *Candida*
	• <u>Risk Factors</u>: **age (5-15 years old most common**; uncommon before age 3)

Patho-physiology	• Infectious pathogens cause direct invasion of the pharyngeal mucosa resulting in inflammation, excess mucous secretions and pharyngeal edema

Signs & Symptoms	• **Sore throat worse with swallowing (dysphagia)**
	• **Fever**
	• **Rhinorrhea and cough (indicate viral etiology)**
	• Referred ear pain
	• Malaise, headache, body aches
	• **GI upset**
	• <u>Physical Exam</u>:
	  • Cobblestoning of posterior pharynx
	  • **Tonsillar edema and erythema**
	  • **Tonsillar exudate** (marked bilateral exudate in EBV)

Diagnosis	• **Clinical Diagnosis** • <u>Rapid Antigen Test</u>: high specificity, low sensitivity; used to detect bacterial etiology • <u>Throat Culture</u>: gold standard to diagnose bacterial etiology

Treatment	• <u>**Supportive: mainstay of treatment**</u>; rest, hydration, warm saltwater gargles, throat lozenges, warm liquids
	• <u>Medication</u>: *antibiotics reserved for bacterial etiology*
	  • Topical analgesia (viscous lidocaine), throat sprays
	  • Oral analgesia (NSAIDs)
	  • Dexamethasone: single dose; shortens symptom duration without affecting rates of relapse or adverse effects

Key Words & Most Common	• Viral more common; bacteria (Group A Strep) • Sore throat with swallowing +/- fever • Rhinorrhea/cough indicate viral etiology • Clinical diagnosis → rapid antigen and throat culture to determine bacterial etiology • Supportive → topical/oral analgesia

Cobblestoning of posterior pharynx

Streptococcal Pharyngitis ᕫ

Etiology & Risk Factors	• Acute inflammation of the mucous membranes of the oropharynx • <u>Etiology</u>: **Group A *Streptococcus* (*S. pyogenes*)** • <u>Risk Factors</u>: **age (5-15 years old most common**; uncommon before age 3), previous streptococcal pharyngitis infection
Patho-physiology	• Group A *Streptococcus* bacteria cause direct invasion of the pharyngeal mucosa resulting in inflammation, excess mucous secretions and pharyngeal edema • Uncommon before age 3 because immature immune system rarely develops anti-streptolysin O (ASO) antibodies

Signs & Symptoms	• **Sore throat worse with swallowing (dysphagia)**
	• **Fever**
	• **Lack of viral symptoms (cough, hoarse voice, rhinorrhea, conjunctivitis, diarrhea)**
	• <u>Physical Exam</u>:
	  • **Pharyngeal edema**
	  • Tonsillar edema, erythema and **exudate**
	  • **Palatal petechiae**
	  • **Anterior cervical lymphadenopathy**

Centor Criteria (one point for each)	Probability of Streptococcal Pharyngitis
Fever (>100.4°F)	≤1 Point: Unlikely
Tonsillar exudate or edema	2 Points: Should be tested
Swollen/tender cervical lymph nodes	3 or 4 points: should be tested and may be treated empirically
Absence of cough	

Diagnosis	• <u>**Centor Criteria**</u>: **determines pretest probability** and may help clinically diagnose • <u>**Rapid Antigen Test**</u>: **best initial test**; high specificity, low sensitivity • <u>**Throat Culture**</u>: **gold-standard**; confirmatory test; should be obtained if antigen test negative

Treatment	• <u>**Supportive: mainstay of treatment**</u>; rest, hydration, warm saltwater gargles, throat lozenges, warm liquids
	• <u>Medication</u>:
	  • Topical analgesia or oral analgesia (NSAIDs)
	  • Dexamethasone: single dose; shortens symptom duration without affecting rates of relapse or adverse effects
	• <u>Antibiotics</u>:
	  • <u>**Penicillin: first-line treatment**</u> (penicillin V is considered drug of choice, amoxicillin is more palatable for children in liquid form)
	  • <u>Penicillin allergy</u>: macrolides (azithromycin, clindamycin) or cephalosporins (cefuroxime or cefdinir; do not use if anaphylactic to PCN)
	• <u>Recurrence prevention</u>: hydrogen peroxide/water (1:1 ratio) gargles help with debridement, proper oral hygiene (change toothbrushes)

Key Words & Most Common	• Group A *Streptococcus* (*S. pyogenes*) • Sore throat with swallowing + fever + lack of viral symptoms • Pharyngeal edema + petechiae of palate + cervical lymphadenopathy • Rapid antigen test → throat culture • Supportive + pain control • Antibiotics: penicillin first-line (PCN V or amoxicillin) → macrolides or cephalosporins if PCN allergic

Tonsillar edema with exudate

Laryngitis

Etiology & Risk Factors	• Acute inflammation of the larynx
	• Etiology: may be infectious or overuse
	   • **Viral: viral upper respiratory tract is most common cause** (rhinovirus, influenza, coronavirus, adenovirus, parainfluenza)
	   • Bacterial: *Moraxella catarrhalis, Haemophilus influenzae, Streptococcus pneumoniae*
	   • Overuse: **excessive vocal strain (singing, loud speaking), excessive coughing**
	   • Exposures: cigarette smoke, aerosolized irritants, fragrances, allergies, GERD

Patho-physiology	• Local inflammation to the vocal folds and surrounding tissue secondary to infectious or non-infectious etiology increases the phonation pressure threshold resulting in hoarse voice and difficulty to talk
Signs & Symptoms	• **Hoarse voice is hallmark symptom** • "Tickling, rawness, urge to clear throat" may be described • **Marked decrease in voice volume** • **Aphonia** (inability to speak) if severe • Rhinorrhea, dry cough, sore throat may be present if viral etiology
Diagnosis	• **Clinical Diagnosis**

Treatment	• Supportive: **mainstay of treatment**; rest, hydration, **vocal rest, humidification, steam inhalation**, warm saltwater gargles, throat lozenges, warm liquids, avoidance of irritants
	   • Dietary modification if related to GERD
	• Medication: *antibiotics reserved for bacterial etiology*
	   • Oral analgesia (NSAIDs)

Key Words & Most Common	• Viral most common cause • Excessive vocal strain (singing, loud speaking) or excessive coughing • Hoarse voice • Marked decrease in voice volume • Aphonia possible • Clinical diagnosis • Supportive (vocal rest, humidification, steam inhalation)

Peritonsillar Abscess

Etiology & Risk Factors	• Localized collection of pus in the peritonsillar space • Etiology: **complication of bacterial pharyngitis/tonsillitis** • **Polymicrobial: Group A *Streptococcus* (*S. pyogenes*) is most common bacterial cause**; staphylococcal, pneumococcal, and hemophilic organisms • Risk Factors: **age (15-30 years old most common)**; recent bacterial pharyngitis/tonsillitis, **smoking, chronic periodontal disease**	
Patho-physiology	• The peritonsillar space between the superior constrictor muscle and tonsillar capsule is comprised of loose connective tissue making it highly susceptible to abscess formation	

Signs & Symptoms	• **Severe, unilateral sore throat**
	• **Dysphagia**
	• **High fever**
	• **Muffled "hot potato" voice** (speaking as if hot food was in mouth)
	• **Inability to handle secretions (drooling)**
	• Severe halitosis (bad breath)
		• Physical Exam:
		   • **Swollen/fluctuant tonsil causing uvular deviation to the contralateral side**
		   • **Trismus** (muscle spasms of temporomandibular joint; aka "lockjaw")
		   • **Bulge of posterior soft palate**
		   • Cervical lymphadenopathy

Diagnosis	• **Clinical diagnosis** • Ultrasound: confirms diagnosis; may aid in needle aspiration procedure • CT Scan *with* Contrast: imaging test of choice if diagnosis unclear	 Right peritonsillar abscess with uvular deviation to contralateral side

Treatment	• Drainage: indicated for large abscesses; **needle aspiration vs incision and drainage**
	   • **Needle aspiration is preferred**; aspirated pus can be sent for culture
	• Antibiotics: oral vs parenteral
	   • Oral: **clindamycin or amoxicillin-clavulanic acid**
	   • Parenteral: ampicillin-sulbactam, clindamycin, piperacillin-tazobactam
	• Corticosteroids: methylprednisolone or dexamethasone decreases duration and severity of pain
	• Surgery: tonsillectomy may be necessary if refractory to treatment or severe	

Key Words & Most Common	• Polymicrobial (Group A *Strep* most common) • Severe, unilateral sore throat + fever + dysphagia + muffled voice + drooling • Swollen/fluctuant tonsil with uvular deviation + trismus • Clinical diagnosis • Needle aspiration +/- antibiotics	

Retropharyngeal Abscess

Etiology & Risk Factors	• Deep neck space infection and abscess of space between posterior pharyngeal wall and prevertebral fascia
	• Etiology: bacterial or trauma
	  • Often polymicrobial; **Group A *Streptococcus* (*S. pyogenes*) is most common bacterial cause**; staphylococcal, pneumococcal, and hemophilic organisms
	  • **Penetrating trauma** (swallowing chicken or fish bone; child falling with stick in mouth, dental instrumentation)
	• Risk Factors: **age (2-4 years old most common)**, poor oral hygiene, diabetes, immunocompromised

Patho-physiology	• Upper respiratory infection causes suppurative adenitis of retropharyngeal lymph nodes which can lead bacterial seeding and abscess formation

Signs & Symptoms	• **Sore throat, fever, dysphagia, drooling**
	• Muffled "hot potato" voice
	• **Torticollis** (twisting of head/neck to one side secondary to pain or muscle spasm)
	• **Neck stiffness**
	• Physical Exam:
	  • **Midline or unilateral posterior pharyngeal wall edema**
	  • **Pain with neck extension** (patient holds neck in flexion for comfort)

Diagnosis	• <u>Lateral Neck Soft-Tissue X-Ray</u>: initial test if low suspicion; shows focal widening of prevertebral soft tissue • **<u>Neck CT Scan *with* Contrast</u>: gold-standard imaging test**
Treatment	• **<u>Secure Airway</u>**: endotracheal intubation often required as rupture of abscess can result in asphyxiation • **<u>Antibiotics</u>**: broad spectrum; **IV ampicillin-sulbactam OR clindamycin OR cephalosporin** (ceftriaxone) • **<u>Emergent ENT Consult</u>: most patients require incision and drainage in operating room**
Key Words & Most Common	• Group A Strep most common bacterial cause • Penetrating trauma (swallowing chicken/fish bone, child falling with stick in mouth) • Age 2-4 most common • Sore throat + fever + drooling • Torticollis and neck stiffness • Midline/unilateral posterior pharyngeal wall edema + pain with neck extension • Neck CT w/ contrast • Secure airway → broad spectrum antibiotics → emergent ENT consult for I&D

Large retropharyngeal abscess

Oral Lichen Planus

Etiology & Risk Factors	• Idiopathic, chronic, T-cell mediated autoimmune reaction affecting skin and mucous membranes • Oral involvement in 50% of all lichen planus cases • Etiology: **idiopathic most common**, trauma, dental plaque, stress, drug induced (beta-blockers, NSAIDs, ACEI, penicillamines, thiazides • Risk Factors: **increased incidence with hepatitis C infection, age (30-60 years old most common)**
Patho-physiology	• Activation of CD4+ helper T cells releases pro-inflammatory cytokines resulting in cytotoxic reaction of epidermal basement membrane and keratocyte apoptosis

Signs & Symptoms	• **Painful oral mucosa (often described as "rough" or "tight")**
	  • May involve buccal mucosa, tongue, gingiva, and labial mucosa
	• **Sensitivity to spicy or acidic foods**
	• Physical Exam:
	  • **<u>Wickham's Striae</u>: hallmark sign**; reticular, bluish-white, linear lesions on oral/buccal mucosal surface
	  • **<u>Koebner's Reaction</u>**: lesions appear in areas of trauma (lip/tongue biting, trauma from dental restorations)

Diagnosis	• **Clinical Diagnosis** • <u>Biopsy</u>: confirms diagnosis
Treatment	• **No definitive cure; symptom-guided treatment** • **<u>Topical Corticosteroids</u>: first-line medication; triamcinolone acetonide gel or clobetasol propionate** (higher potency), dexamethasone elixir (swish and spit) • <u>Topical Analgesics</u>: viscous lidocaine provides pain relief • <u>Oral Corticosteroids</u>: prednisone; reserved for severe or recalcitrant cases • Oral dapsone, hydroxychloroquine or cyclosporin may be considered if fails corticosteroid treatment
Key Words & Most Common	• T-cell mediated autoimmune reaction of oral mucosa • Increased incidence with hepatitis C infection • Painful oral mucosa • Sensitivity to spicy/acidic floods • <u>Wickham's Striae</u>: reticular, white network of oral mucosa • Clinical diagnosis → biopsy • Topical corticosteroids (triamcinolone acetonides, clobetasol propionate, dexamethasone) first-line

Wickham's Striae

Ludwig's Angina

Etiology & Risk Factors	• Acute bilateral soft tissue cellulitis of the submental, submandibular and sublingual space (floor of mouth) • Can be rapidly progressive with potential to obstruct airway; can be life-threatening • Etiology: **odontogenic infection (periapical abscesses) of the 2nd/3rd molars is most common**; trauma/laceration to floor of mouth, oral piercing, sialadenitis or sialolithiasis • Polymicrobial infection (oral flora); *Staphylococcus, Streptococcus, Peptostreptococcus, Fusobacterium, Bacteroides,* and *Actinomyces* • Risk Factors: **poor dental hygiene, recent dental extraction**, diabetes, malnutrition, immunocompromised
Patho-physiology	• Dental infection of the 2nd/3rd molars begins in subgingival pocket and extends to the submental, submandibular, and sublingual space **Right submandibular soft tissue cellulitis**

Signs & Symptoms	• Early Signs:
	  • **Dental pain**
	  • **Dysphagia, odynophagia**
	  • **Trismus**
	• Physical Exam:
	  • **Tender, symmetrical edema of upper neck, chin and floor of mouth → tongue protrusion**
	  • **"Woody" or brawny texture to floor of mouth with visible erythema and edema**
	  • *No lymphadenopathy or abscess formation*

Diagnosis	• **Clinical Diagnosis** • CT Scan with Contrast: **imaging test of choice**; confirms diagnosis and determines area of infection (should not delay airway management to obtain imaging)

Treatment	• Airway Management: **maintaining airway is first priority** and tongue swelling can compromise airway; intubation can be difficult with trismus and tongue edema
	  • Flexible fiberoptic nasal intubation is preferred method with setup for emergent cricothyrotomy ready
	  • Admit to ICU
	• IV Antibiotics: **broad spectrum**
	  • Immunocompetent: **ampicillin-sulbactam** OR clindamycin OR penicillin G + metronidazole
	  • Immunocompromised: **cefepime + metronidazole** OR meropenem OR piperacillin-tazobactam; add vancomycin if concern for MRSA
	• Surgery: surgical I&D if suppurative infection; **dental extraction** if source of infection is odontogenic

Key Words & Most Common	• Bilateral soft tissue cellulitis of floor of mouth • Odontogenic infection of 2nd/3rd molars most common • Dental pain + dysphagia + trismus → neck pain/swelling + drooling + muffled voice • Symmetrical edema of neck, chin and floor of mouth; "Woody" or brawny texture of floor of mouth • Clinical Diagnosis + CT scan confirmation • Airway management + IV antibiotics (ampicillin-sulbactam)

Oropharyngeal Candidiasis (Thrush)

Etiology & Risk Factors	• Infection of the oral cavity by *Candida albicans*; also known as thrush
	• Etiology: **pathologic overgrown of *Candida albicans* secondary to immunosuppressed state**
	• Risk Factors: **secondary to immunosuppression (local or systemic)**, extremes of age (**newborn** or advanced age), malnourished, vitamin deficiencies, metabolic disease
	  • Local immunosuppression: **inhaled corticosteroids**
	  • Systemic immunosuppression: **HIV/AIDS**, diabetes, **chronic systemic corticosteroids, chronic antibiotic use**

Patho-physiology	• *Candida albicans* is part of the normal oral flora; immunosuppression disrupts normal host immunity leading to pathogenic overgrowth and formation of a pseudomembrane • Neonates may contract through colonized breasts when breastfeeding

Signs & Symptoms	• Mild mouth/throat discomfort with swallowing
	• **Loss of taste**
	• **Cotton-like sensation in mouth**
	• Physical Exam:
	  • **White, curd-like (pseudomembranous) plaques of the oral mucosa, tongue,** palate or oropharynx
	    • **Easily removed when scraped with gauze or tongue depressor leaving erythematous and friable mucosal base**
	  • **Angular cheilitis** (painful, cracked sores at corners of mouth)

Diagnosis	• **Clinical Diagnosis** • Potassium Hydroxide Wet Mount: smear of scrapings of lesion; **show budding yeast and pseudohyphae**

Treatment	• Topical Antifungals: **first-line medications**; used in mild cases
	  • **Nystatin oral suspension (100,000units/mL) swish and swallow**; 14+ day treatment
	  • **Clotrimazole troches** 5x per day for 14 days
	• Systemic Antifungals: reserved for refractory or severe cases
	  • **Oral fluconazole**

Key Words & Most Common	• Candida albicans overgrowth within oral cavity • Immunosuppression (HIV/AIDs, chronic steroid or antibiotic use, steroid inhaler) • Loss of taste + cotton-like sensation in mouth • White, curdy plaques of oral mucosa/tongue • Easily removed leaving erythematous base • Clinical diagnosis + KOH wet mount to confirm (shows budding yeast and pseudohyphae) • Topical antifungals (nystatin or clotrimazole) → oral antifungals (fluconazole)

Oral Leukoplakia

Etiology & Risk Factors	• **Hyperkeratosis of the oral cavity that is potentially malignant** • Up to 6% can be dysplastic or squamous cell carcinoma • <u>Etiology</u>: idiopathic, **chronic irritation/inflammation** • <u>Risk Factors</u>: **tobacco use (smoking or smokeless) is greatest risk factor**, alcohol, dentures, HPV infection
Patho-physiology	• Chronic exposure to carcinogens and irritation leads to cellular hyperplasia and resultant cellular degeneration; this eventually causes irrevocable cell damage and malignancy • Lesions appear white due to thickened layers of keratin as result of chronic irritation

Signs & Symptoms	• Mostly asymptomatic
	• **White, hyperkeratotic, patchy lesions of oral mucosa**
	  • **Lesions are painless and cannot be scraped off** (differentiates from oropharyngeal candidiasis (thrush) which is *painful* and *can* be scraped off)
	  • Common on lateral or ventral sides of tongue

Diagnosis	• <u>Lesion Biopsy</u>: **gold-standard for diagnosis**; shows hyperkeratinization of epithelium and cellular dysplasia • Used to rule out squamous cell carcinoma
Treatment	• <u>Avoidance of Irritant</u>: **tobacco cessation**, alcohol cessation • <u>Surgery</u>: **surgical excision or laser ablation** • Indicated for severe dysplasia or risk of malignancy or if lesion located on lateral/ventral side of tongue, soft palate, floor of mouth, or oropharynx
Key Words & Most Common	• Hyperkeratosis of oral cavity secondary to chronic irritation exposure • Tobacco use (smoking or smokeless) is greatest risk factor • White, hyperkeratotic, patchy lesions of oral mucosa • Painless and cannot be scraped off • Biopsy is gold-standard • Smoking cessation → surgical excision or laser ablation

White hyperkeratotic patchy lesion

Hairy Oral Leukoplakia

Etiology & Risk Factors	• Total or focal oral mucocutaneous changes secondary to Epstein-Barr Virus (human herpesvirus-4) infection • <u>Etiology</u>: **manifestation of Epstein-Barr Virus (human herpesvirus-4)** • <u>Risk Factors</u>: **immunocompromised (HIV/AIDs most common)**, smoking, organ or bone marrow transplant, hematologic malignancy
Patho-physiology	• Impaired immune status of host leads to EBV establishment within basal cells of the oral epithelium; mechanical trauma to side of tongue results in mucocutaneous changes • Hyperkeratosis and epithelial hyperplasia causes the white plaque appearance

Signs & Symptoms	• **Often asymptomatic**; patients often present due to cosmetic concern
	• <u>Physical Exam</u>:
	  • **Non-tender, white plaque on lateral side(s) of tongue**
	    • **Plaques *cannot* be scraped off** (differentiates from oropharyngeal candidiasis)
	    • Lesions range from smooth and flat to having a **"hairy" or "feathered" appearance**

Diagnosis	• **Clinical Diagnosis** • <u>Labs</u>: EBV testing (polymerase chain reaction, electron microscopy, in-situ hybridization), consider HIV testing if risk factors present
Treatment	• <u>Reassurance</u>: **benign condition that resolves spontaneously** • <u>Oral Antivirals</u>: **high-dose acyclovir or valacyclovir**; relief is temporary, and condition often recurs after cessation of treatment • <u>Topicals</u>: retinoic acid or tretinoin; inhibit viral replication
Key Words & Most Common	• Oral mucocutaneous change secondary to Epstein-Barr Virus • Most common in immunocompromised (HIV/AIDS) • Asymptomatic • Non-tender, "hairy" white plaques on lateral sides of tongue • Lesions *cannot* be scraped off • Clinical Diagnosis • Reassurance

White plaque on lateral side of tongue

Oral Mucosa Cancer

Etiology & Risk Factors	• Cancer occurring on the mucosal lining of the lips, cheeks, gingiva (gums), anterior two-thirds of the tongue, floor of the mouth, or palate • <u>Etiology</u>: **chronic irritation of oral mucosa** (overuse of mouthwash, dental caries, tobacco), **oral human papillomavirus (HPV)** (viral oral-to-genital contact) • <u>Risk Factors</u>: **tobacco use (smoking or chewing tobacco), alcohol use**
Patho-physiology	• Chronic irritation of oral mucosa leads to cellular dysplasia and eventually causes irrevocable cell damage and malignancy
Signs & Symptoms	• **Irregular white/red patches on oral mucosa** • **Raised nodule with ulcerated surface on oral mucosa** • <u>Systemic signs</u>: may be present with advanced disease; **dysphagia, odynophagia, hoarse voice, unintentional weight loss**, lymphadenopathy, ear pain
Diagnosis	• <u>**Tissue Biopsy**</u>: **initial diagnostic test** • <u>Endoscopy</u>: used to identify lesions involving pharynx and larynx
Treatment	• <u>**Surgical Excision**</u>: **mainstay of treatment**; wide local excision +/- lymph node excision • <u>Chemoradiotherapy</u>: chemotherapy or radiation therapy (or combination) may be used with surgical excision to prevent further malignancy
Key Words & Most Common	• Cancer of the oral mucosa • Chronic irritation (mouthwash, poor dentition, tobacco use), oral HPV most common causes • Tobacco and alcohol use greatest risk factors • Irregular white/red patches or raised nodule on oral mucosa • Systemic signs of dysphagia, hoarse voice, weight loss with advanced disease • Tissue Biopsy • Surgical excision +/- chemoradiotherapy

Irregular white/red patches on oral mucosa

Aphthous Ulcers

Etiology & Risk Factors	• Recurrent ulcers occurring on the oral mucosa; **also known as canker sores or ulcerative stomatitis** • <u>Etiology</u>: **unknown etiology**; may be associated with human herpes virus 6 • <u>Risk Factors</u>: **stress**, hormonal changes, **certain foods** (citrus fruits, coffee, sour candy, salty/spicy foods), **oral trauma (toothbrushing, braces, biting tongue/cheek)**, **nutritional deficiency (iron, vitamin D, zinc, folate or vitamin b6)**, sensitivities (sodium lauryl sulfate in toothpaste), alterations of oral microbiome (mouthwash, antibiotics) • *May be seen as manifestation of systemic conditions such as inflammatory bowel disease (Crohn disease), systemic lupus erythematous*
Patho-physiology	• T-cell mediated immune dysfunction leads to neutrophil and mast cell mediated mucosal epithelium damage

Signs & Symptoms	• **Small, painful, shallow round or oval-shaped ulcers**
	   • **White/yellow/gray pseudomembrane exudate with erythematous halo and slightly raised erythematous margins**
	   • Occurs on non-keratinized mucosa **(labial or buccal mucosa most common)**

Diagnosis	• **Clinical Diagnosis**

Treatment	• <u>Supportive</u>: avoidance of triggers; change toothpaste, avoid certain foods, stress management
	• <u>**Topical Corticosteroids**</u>: **first-line medication**
	   • **Dexamethasone elixir (swish and spit)**
	   • Betamethasone syrup
	   • Fluocinonide gel applied directly to lesion
	• <u>Topical Antiseptics</u>: chlorhexidine gluconate mouthwash
	• <u>Oral Corticosteroids</u>: prednisone; if refractory to topical corticosteroids
	• <u>**Dietary Supplementation**</u>: **vitamin B complex, iron, folate supplementation if deficient**

Key Words & Most Common	• Canker sores or ulcerative stomatitis are ulcers of the oral mucosa • Stress, certain foods (pineapple, salty/sour, coffee), oral trauma (toothbrush, braces), or nutritional deficiencies • Small, painful ulcers of labial or buccal mucosa • White/yellow/gray ulcer with erythematous halo and margins • Clinical diagnosis • Topical steroids are first-line (dexamethasone elixir)

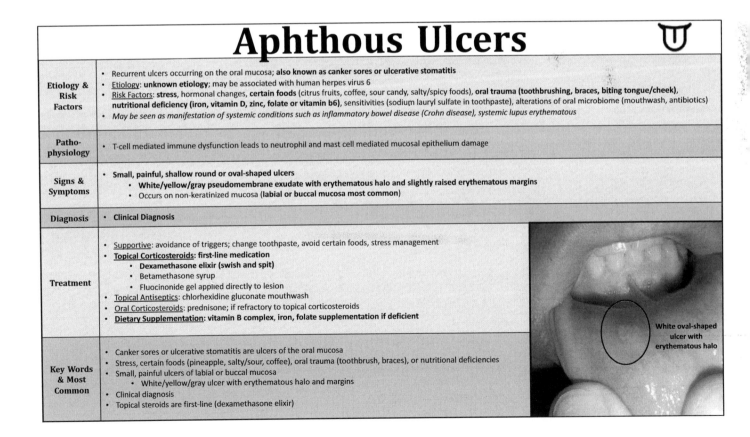

White oval-shaped ulcer with erythematous halo

Sialolithiasis

Etiology & Risk Factors	• Formation of stone within the major salivary glands or ducts (submandibular, parotid, sublingual) • <u>Etiology</u>: **stone within the submandibular gland duct (Wharton's duct) is most common**; also occurs within parotid gland duct (Stensen's duct) • <u>Risk Factors</u>: **salivary stasis (dehydration, anticholinergic medications**, reduced oral intake, diuretics), tobacco smoke, **Sjögren's syndrome**, malnutrition or anorexia
Patho-physiology	• Microcalculi consisting of calcium carbonate or calcium phosphate forms and is secreted within a stagnant salivary gland; microcalculi acts as nidus for larger stone formation • Bacteria or food debris of the oral cavity may collect within salivary gland ducts
Signs & Symptoms	• **Unilateral pain and swelling of salivary gland** • *May resemble parotitis* • **Pain/swelling worse while eating or anticipation of eating** (salivary gland stimulation) • <u>Physical Exam</u>: • Tenderness to palpation of submandibular or parotid gland • Firmness of salivary gland if stone present
Diagnosis	• **Clinical Diagnosis** • <u>X-Ray</u>: minimally invasive and less radiating imaging modality; 80% of stones are radiopaque • <u>CT or Ultrasound</u>: confirms diagnosis; allows visualization of duct and stone
Treatment	• <u>Supportive</u>: hydration, analgesia (NSAIDs), ductal/glandular massage, manual expression, moist heat, good oral hygiene, discontinue anticholinergic medications if possible • <u>Sialagogues</u>: **first-line therapy; used to stimulate salivary flow** • **Suck on lemon wedge or sour candy every 2-3 hours** (tart candies, gum, candy also acceptable) • <u>Minimally Invasive Procedures</u>: external shockwave lithotripsy or sialoendoscopy; reserved for recurrent cases failing conservative treatment • <u>Surgery</u>: surgical excision of salivary gland (sialoadenectomy) for recurrent or severe cases; last resort
Key Words & Most Common	• Formation of stone within submandibular gland most common (80%) • Unilateral pain/swelling of salivary gland (may resemble parotitis) • Symptoms worse while eating • Clinical diagnosis • Sialagogues are first-line to stimulate salivary flow + moist heat + massage

Sialadenitis

Etiology & Risk Factors	• Bacterial infection of the submandibular or parotid salivary glands • **Parotid gland is most commonly affected** • <u>Etiology</u>: **bacterial infection secondary to salivary gland obstruction from a stone (sialolithiasis) most common**; hyposecretion of salivary gland • ***Staphylococcus aureus* most common**, *S. pneumoniae, S. viridans, H. influenzae, Enterobacteriaceae* spp. and anaerobes • <u>Risk Factors</u>: **salivary stasis (dehydration, anticholinergic medications**, reduced oral intake, diuretics), tobacco smoke, **Sjögren's syndrome**, malnutrition or anorexia, radiation therapy of oral cavity or radioactive iodine therapy for thyroid cancer
Patho-physiology	• Hyposecretion of saliva or obstruction of salivary gland leads to bacterial contamination and infection of the salivary gland/ducts and parenchymal tissue
Signs & Symptoms	• **Unilateral pain and swelling of salivary gland** • *May resemble parotitis* • **Fever and chills** (indicate infection)**, dysphagia, trismus** • **Purulent drainage of salivary gland** • <u>Physical Exam</u>: • **Firm and diffusely tender salivary gland** • Erythema and edema of overriding soft tissue • Focal enlargement of salivary gland (may indicate abscess)
Diagnosis	• **Clinical Diagnosis** • <u>Gram Stain and Culture</u>: if purulence can be expressed to determine antibiotic therapy • <u>CT Scan</u>: **definitive diagnosis**; used to determine extent of tissue involvement or presence of abscess
Treatment	• <u>Supportive</u>: hydration, analgesia (NSAIDs), ductal/glandular massage, manual expression, moist heat, good oral hygiene, discontinue anticholinergic medications if possible • <u>Sialagogues</u>: **used to stimulate salivary flow** • **Suck on lemon wedge or sour candy every 2-3 hours** (tart candies, gum, candy also acceptable) • <u>Antibiotics</u>: broad spectrum anti-staphylococcal antibiotics; guided by culture and sensitivity • **Amoxicillin-clavulanate or dicloxacillin or clindamycin**
Key Words & Most Common	• Bacterial infection of salivary gland (parotid most common) secondary to obstruction or hyposecretion • Dehydration, anticholinergic medications, Sjögren's syndrome • Unilateral pain/swelling of salivary gland + fever/chills + dysphagia • Purulent drainage of salivary gland • Clinical diagnosis; CT scan definitive • Supportive + sialagogues + antibiotics (amoxicillin-clavulanate, dicloxacillin, clindamycin)

Viral Parotitis

Etiology & Risk Factors	• Acute inflammation of the parotid gland • <u>Etiology</u>: **paramyxovirus (mumps) is most common; influenza**, parainfluenza, coxsackie • <u>Risk Factors</u>: **age (<15 years old most common)**, immunosuppression, **unimmunized or partially immunized (MMR)**, congregate settings (college campus/dorms)
Patho-physiology	• Virus enters upper respiratory tract through nose or mouth; following exposure, virus spreads to parotid gland causing local inflammation
Signs & Symptoms	• **Prodrome of fever, headache, arthralgias/myalgias, malaise** • **Unilateral or bilateral parotid gland pain and swelling** • May have pain with chewing • **Unilateral orchitis** (20-30% of male patients)
Diagnosis	• **Clinical Diagnosis** • <u>Mumps immunoglobulin (IgM and IgG) or Polymerase Chain Reaction (PCR)</u>: **confirms diagnosis**; may require reporting to local health department • <u>Testicular Ultrasound</u>: if concern for orchitis
Treatment	• <u>Supportive</u>: **mainstay of treatment**; rest, hydration, analgesia (NSAIDs), soft diet • <u>Testicular Support</u>: scrotal sling or supportive, non-restrictive underwear to minimize tension, ice packs
Key Words & Most Common	• Acute inflammation of parotid gland • Paramyxovirus (mumps) most common; influenza • Unimmunized/partially immunized against MMR • Prodrome of fever, headache, body/muscle aches • Unilateral/bilateral parotid gland pain and swelling • Orchitis • Clinical diagnosis + Mumps immunoglobulin or PCR to confirm diagnosis • Testicular ultrasound as indicated • Supportive care

Unilateral parotid gland swelling

Dental Infection

Etiology & Risk Factors	• Infection originating in tooth or surrounding structures • May become periapical or periodontal abscess • <u>Etiology</u>: **bacterial infection (*Streptococcus mutans* most common bacteria**, *Lactobacilli*); dental caries (tooth decay), pulpitis (inflammation of pulp), dental trauma • <u>Risk Factors</u>: **poor dental hygiene**, trauma, dental procedure
Patho-physiology	• Dental plaque biofilm is broken down which disrupts oral microbial homeostasis leading to overgrowth of acid-producing and acid-tolerating bacteria • Enamel demineralization occurs resulting in bacterial invasion of tooth and surrounding structures

Signs & Symptoms	• **Acute pain and swelling of tooth and surrounding gingiva**
	• **Increased sensitivity with pressure** (clenching, chewing) **or stimuli** (hot/cold drinks or food)
	• May have spontaneous drainage if abscess
	• <u>Physical Exam</u>:
	  • **Brown/yellow teeth with black cavities** (dental caries)
	  • **Erythematous, swollen gingiva with bleeding while probing** (gingivitis)
	  • **Palpable swelling at gumline** (periapical abscess)

Diagnosis	• **Clinical Diagnosis** • <u>CT Scan</u>: if large or deep abscess • <u>MRI</u>: if concern for underlying osteomyelitis

Treatment	• <u>Analgesia</u>: **NSAIDs**, acetaminophen or **topical anesthetics** (viscous lidocaine, benzocaine gel)
	• <u>Oral Antiseptics</u>: chlorhexidine gluconate mouth rinse or hypertonic saline soak
	• <u>Antibiotics</u>: broad-spectrum
	  • **Amoxicillin-clavulanate first-line**
	  • **Clindamycin second-line**; preferred if penicillin allergic
	• <u>Urgent Dental Follow-Up</u>: **within 48 hours; dental extraction may be necessary if infection severe or compromised tooth**
	• <u>Incision and Drainage</u>: may be performed if abscess present depending on experience level of provider

Key Words & Most Common	• Infection of tooth and surrounding structures • Bacterial infection (S. mutans most common) • Poor dental hygiene, trauma, dental procedure • Acute pain/swelling of tooth and gingiva • Dental caries, gingivitis, abscess on exam • Clinical Diagnosis • Pain control → antibiotics (amoxicillin-clavulanate vs clindamycin) → dentist referral

Periapical Abscess

References

1. SubconjunctivalHaemorrhage.jpeg. (2023, June 26). *Wikimedia Commons*. Retrieved 21:02, August 14, 2023 from https://commons.wikimedia.org/w/index.php?title=File:SubconjunctivalHaemorrhage.jpeg&oldid=777462636.
2. Blepharitis.JPG. (2023, May 14). *Wikimedia Commons*. Retrieved 21:28, August 14, 2023 from https://commons.wikimedia.org/w/index.php?title=File:Blepharitis.JPG&oldid=763132458.
3. Stye02.jpg. (2023, January 27). *Wikimedia Commons*. Retrieved 21:31, August 14, 2023 from https://commons.wikimedia.org/w/index.php?title=File:Stye02.jpg&oldid=728330400.
4. Chalazion.JPG. (2023, May 24). *Wikimedia Commons*. Retrieved 21:33, August 14, 2023 from https://commons.wikimedia.org/w/index.php?title=File:Chalazion.JPG&oldid=766513644.
5. Large Pterygium.jpg. (2021, October 20). *Wikimedia Commons*. Retrieved 21:36, August 14, 2023 from https://commons.wikimedia.org/w/index.php?title=File:Large_Pterygium.jpg&oldid=600464389.
6. PRE-OPERATIVE PINGUECULA.JPG. (2020, October 10). *Wikimedia Commons*. Retrieved 21:37, August 14, 2023 from https://commons.wikimedia.org/w/index.php?title=File:PRE-OPERATIVE_PINGUECULA.JPG&oldid=486165782.
7. Pblowoutfracture.png. (2022, June 1). *Wikimedia Commons*. Retrieved 21:43, August 14, 2023 from https://commons.wikimedia.org/w/index.php?title=File:Pblowoutfracture.png&oldid=660596507.
8. Rb whiteeye.PNG. (2022, May 15). *Wikimedia Commons*. Retrieved 21:46, August 14, 2023 from https://commons.wikimedia.org/w/index.php?title=File:Rb_whiteeye.PNG&oldid=656109608.
9. Intermediate age related macular degeneration.jpg. (2020, September 21). *Wikimedia Commons*. Retrieved 21:49, August 14, 2023 from https://commons.wikimedia.org/w/index.php?title=File:Intermediate_age_related_macular_degeneration.jpg&oldid=467096758.
10. Fundus - diabetic retinopathy.png. (2022, October 30). *Wikimedia Commons*. Retrieved 21:54, August 14, 2023 from https://commons.wikimedia.org/w/index.php?title=File:Fundus_-_diabetic_retinopathy.png&oldid=700485119.
11. Retinal Detachment.jpg. (2022, July 24). *Wikimedia Commons*. Retrieved 21:59, August 14, 2023 from https://commons.wikimedia.org/w/index.php?title=File:Retinal_Detachment.jpg&oldid=677345672.
12. Gonococcal ophthalmia neonatorum.jpg. (2020, November 5). *Wikimedia Commons*. Retrieved 22:01, August 14, 2023 from https://commons.wikimedia.org/w/index.php?title=File:Gonococcal_ophthalmia_neonatorum.jpg&oldid=510334756.
13. Swollen eye with conjunctivitis.jpg. (2023, January 2). *Wikimedia Commons*. Retrieved 22:04, August 14, 2023 from https://commons.wikimedia.org/w/index.php?title=File:Swollen_eye_with_conjunctivitis.jpg&oldid=722068045.
14. Conjunctivitis disease.jpg. (2021, November 27). *Wikimedia Commons*. Retrieved 22:06, August 14, 2023 from https://commons.wikimedia.org/w/index.php?title=File:Conjunctivitis_disease.jpg&oldid=610290022.
15. Allergicconjunctivitis.jpg. (2023, August 2). *Wikimedia Commons*. Retrieved 22:07, August 14, 2023 from https://commons.wikimedia.org/w/index.php?title=File:Allergicconjunctivitis.jpg&oldid=789310902.
16. Depiction of a person suffering from Strabismus or crossed-eyes.png. (2021, May 28). *Wikimedia Commons*. Retrieved 22:20, August 14, 2023 from https://commons.wikimedia.org/w/index.php?title=File:Depiction_of_a_person_suffering_from_Strabismus_or_crossed-eyes.png&oldid=565653007.
17. Celulitis Periorbitaria (Preseptal).JPG. (2020, September 26). *Wikimedia Commons*. Retrieved 22:22, August 14, 2023 from https://commons.wikimedia.org/w/index.php?title=File:Celulitis_Periorbitaria_(Preseptal).JPG&oldid=472060923.
18. Clare-314.jpg. (2023, January 22). *Wikimedia Commons*. Retrieved 23:06, August 14, 2023 from https://commons.wikimedia.org/w/index.php?title=File:Clare-314.jpg&oldid=726956193.
19. Dendritic corneal ulcer.jpg. (2020, October 30). *Wikimedia Commons*. Retrieved 23:08, August 14, 2023 from https://commons.wikimedia.org/w/index.php?title=File:Dendritic_corneal_ulcer.jpg&oldid=506938922.
20. Cataract in human eye.png. (2022, October 17). *Wikimedia Commons*. Retrieved 23:11, August 14, 2023 from https://commons.wikimedia.org/w/index.php?title=File:Cataract_in_human_eye.png&oldid=696873444.
21. Papilledema.jpg. (2020, October 14). *Wikimedia Commons*. Retrieved 23:14, August 14, 2023 from https://commons.wikimedia.org/w/index.php?title=File:Papilledema.jpg&oldid=489777474.
22. Optic-neuritis-in-the-right-eye.jpg. (2023, June 6). *Wikimedia Commons*. Retrieved 23:16, August 14, 2023 from https://commons.wikimedia.org/w/index.php?title=File:Optic-neuritis-in-the-right-eye.jpg&oldid=771652234.
23. Acute angle closure glaucoma.JPG. (2023, July 9). *Wikimedia Commons*. Retrieved 23:19, August 14, 2023 from https://commons.wikimedia.org/w/index.php?title=File:Acute_angle_closure_glaucoma.JPG&oldid=781841616.
24. Cherry red spot in patient with central retinal artery occlusion (CRAO).jpg. (2022, July 5). *Wikimedia Commons*. Retrieved 23:27, August 14, 2023 from https://commons.wikimedia.org/w/index.php?title=File:Cherry_red_spot_in_patient_with_central_retinal_artery_occlusion_(CRAO).jpg&oldid=671361114.
25. Branch retinal vein occlusion.jpg. (2020, October 8). *Wikimedia Commons*. Retrieved 23:31, August 14, 2023 from https://commons.wikimedia.org/w/index.php?title=File:Branch_retinal_vein_occlusion.jpg&oldid=484092628.
26. Scleritis.png. (2022, September 26). *Wikimedia Commons*. Retrieved 23:33, August 14, 2023 from https://commons.wikimedia.org/w/index.php?title=File:Scleritis.png&oldid=692128177.
27. Otitis externa.jpg. (2021, January 21). *Wikimedia Commons*. Retrieved 23:37, August 14, 2023 from https://commons.wikimedia.org/w/index.php?title=File:Otitis_externa.jpg&oldid=527351195.
28. Mastoiditis1.jpg. (2020, September 9). *Wikimedia Commons*. Retrieved 23:40, August 14, 2023 from https://commons.wikimedia.org/w/index.php?title=File:Mastoiditis1.jpg&oldid=452681973.
29. Acute Otitis Media Stage of Resolution.jpg. (2023, July 9). *Wikimedia Commons*. Retrieved 23:45, August 14, 2023 from https://commons.wikimedia.org/w/index.php?title=File:Acute_Otitis_Media_Stage_of_Resolution.jpg&oldid=781841451.

References

30. Adult Serous Otitis Media.jpg. (2023, July 11). *Wikimedia Commons*. Retrieved 23:48, August 14, 2023 from https://commons.wikimedia.org/w/index.php?title=File:Adult_Serous_Otitis_Media.jpg&oldid=782452905.
31. Traumatic Perforation of the Tympanic Membrane.jpg. (2020, September 27). *Wikimedia Commons*. Retrieved 23:57, August 14, 2023 from https://commons.wikimedia.org/w/index.php?title=File:Traumatic_Perforation_of_the_Tympanic_Membrane.jpg&oldid=472922076.
32. Cholesteatoma and large perforation left ear.jpg. (2023, July 16). *Wikimedia Commons*. Retrieved 23:58, August 14, 2023 from https://commons.wikimedia.org/w/index.php?title=File:Cholesteatoma_and_large_perforation_left_ear.jpg&oldid=783915831.
33. Epley maneuver.jpg. (2022, May 17). *Wikimedia Commons*. Retrieved 12:40, August 15, 2023 from https://commons.wikimedia.org/w/index.php?title=File:Epley_maneuver.jpg&oldid=656906267.
34. Vestibular-schwannoma-003.jpg. (2022, April 3). *Wikimedia Commons*. Retrieved 12:45, August 15, 2023 from https://commons.wikimedia.org/w/index.php?title=File:Vestibular-schwannoma-003.jpg&oldid=646376958.
35. Ramsey Hunt Syndrome.png. (2020, September 29). *Wikimedia Commons*. Retrieved 12:49, August 15, 2023 from https://commons.wikimedia.org/w/index.php?title=File:Ramsey_Hunt_Syndrome.png&oldid=475480015.
36. Hematoma ear.jpg. (2021, January 21). *Wikimedia Commons*. Retrieved 12:50, August 15, 2023 from https://commons.wikimedia.org/w/index.php?title=File:Hematoma_ear.jpg&oldid=527349982.
37. Perichondritis1.JPG. (2020, October 8). *Wikimedia Commons*. Retrieved 12:53, August 15, 2023 from https://commons.wikimedia.org/w/index.php?title=File:Perichondritis1.JPG&oldid=484032742.
38. CT of chronic sinusitis.jpg. (2022, November 25). *Wikimedia Commons*. Retrieved 12:58, August 15, 2023 from https://commons.wikimedia.org/w/index.php?title=File:CT_of_chronic_sinusitis.jpg&oldid=709324295.
39. Mucormycosis.jpg. (2021, May 22). *Wikimedia Commons*. Retrieved 13:01, August 15, 2023 from https://commons.wikimedia.org/w/index.php?title=File:Mucormycosis.jpg&oldid=562837846.
40. Polype nasal.jpg. (2023, January 31). *Wikimedia Commons*. Retrieved 13:04, August 15, 2023 from https://commons.wikimedia.org/w/index.php?title=File:Polype_nasal.jpg&oldid=729153726.
41. Orbital cellulitis.jpg. (2020, October 14). *Wikimedia Commons*. Retrieved 13:10, August 15, 2023 from https://commons.wikimedia.org/w/index.php?title=File:Orbital_cellulitis.jpg&oldid=489295380.
42. Pharyngitis.jpg. (2023, April 10). *Wikimedia Commons*. Retrieved 13:22, August 15, 2023 from https://commons.wikimedia.org/w/index.php?title=File:Pharyngitis.jpg&oldid=749160557.
43. Pos strep.JPG. (2023, January 13). *Wikimedia Commons*. Retrieved 13:24, August 15, 2023 from https://commons.wikimedia.org/w/index.php?title=File:Pos_strep.JPG&oldid=724944346.
44. PeritonsilarAbsess.jpg. (2020, October 29). *Wikimedia Commons*. Retrieved 13:27, August 15, 2023 from https://commons.wikimedia.org/w/index.php?title=File:PeritonsilarAbsess.jpg&oldid=506423741.
45. LargeRetroAbsMarkTra.png. (2020, September 27). *Wikimedia Commons*. Retrieved 13:30, August 15, 2023 from https://commons.wikimedia.org/w/index.php?title=File:LargeRetroAbsMarkTra.png&oldid=473717233.
46. Lichen planus.jpg. (2023, June 29). *Wikimedia Commons*. Retrieved 13:32, August 15, 2023 from https://commons.wikimedia.org/w/index.php?title=File:Lichen_planus.jpg&oldid=778338208.
47. Ludwig angina.jpg. (2020, October 18). *Wikimedia Commons*. Retrieved 13:35, August 15, 2023 from https://commons.wikimedia.org/w/index.php?title=File:Ludwig_angina.jpg&oldid=493688154.
48. Human tongue infected with oral candidiasis.jpg. (2022, October 31). *Wikimedia Commons*. Retrieved 13:37, August 15, 2023 from https://commons.wikimedia.org/w/index.php?title=File:Human_tongue_infected_with_oral_candidiasis.jpg&oldid=701228515.
49. Leukoplakia02-04-06.jpg. (2021, November 6). *Wikimedia Commons*. Retrieved 13:39, August 15, 2023 from https://commons.wikimedia.org/w/index.php?title=File:Leukoplakia02-04-06.jpg&oldid=605877410.
50. Leukoplakiaaitor.jpg. (2023, July 21). *Wikimedia Commons*. Retrieved 13:43, August 15, 2023 from https://commons.wikimedia.org/w/index.php?title=File:Leukoplakiaaitor.jpg&oldid=785499914.
51. ZungenCa2a.jpg. (2020, December 31). *Wikimedia Commons*. Retrieved 13:45, August 15, 2023 from https://commons.wikimedia.org/w/index.php?title=File:ZungenCa2a.jpg&oldid=522641378.
52. Aphthe Unterlippe.jpg. (2021, September 9). *Wikimedia Commons*. Retrieved 13:49, August 15, 2023 from https://commons.wikimedia.org/w/index.php?title=File:Aphthe_Unterlippe.jpg&oldid=589954133.
53. Salivary stone in submandibular salivary duct.jpg. (2020, October 25). *Wikimedia Commons*. Retrieved 13:55, August 15, 2023 from https://commons.wikimedia.org/w/index.php?title=File:Salivary_stone_in_submandibular_salivary_duct.jpg&oldid=501136997.
54. Parotiditis (Parotitis; Mumps).JPG. (2020, October 10). *Wikimedia Commons*. Retrieved 14:03, August 15, 2023 from https://commons.wikimedia.org/w/index.php?title=File:Parotiditis_(Parotitis;_Mumps).JPG&oldid=485515925.
55. Abces parulique.jpg. (2023, July 2). *Wikimedia Commons*. Retrieved 14:06, August 15, 2023 from https://commons.wikimedia.org/w/index.php?title=File:Abces_parulique.jpg&oldid=779764280.
56. Hyphema - occupying half of anterior chamber of eye.jpg. (2022, October 25). *Wikimedia Commons*. Retrieved 14:09, August 15, 2023 from https://commons.wikimedia.org/w/index.php?title=File:Hyphema_-_occupying_half_of_anterior_chamber_of_eye.jpg&oldid=698970649.

Chapter 6

Reproductive

Acute Mastitis

Etiology & Risk Factors	• Inflammation of breast tissue • **Most common in lactating women (first 6 weeks postpartum most common)** • <u>Etiology</u>: **nipple trauma** (allows bacterial inoculation), clogged ducts lead to engorgement • *Staphylococcus aureus* **most common bacteria**; *Streptococcus pyogenes, Escherichia coli, Bacteroides* spp. • <u>Risk Factors</u>: history of mastitis, **nipple cracks/fissures**, inadequate milk drainage (**clogged ducts**), lack of sleep, maternal stress, **tight-fitting bras**
Patho-physiology	• Infrequent feedings, milk oversupply or clogged duct leads to build up of breast milk causes engorgement of breast tissue, inflammation and stagnation of milk • Bacteria from infant's mouth or mother's skin colonizes breast tissue through nipple cracks or fissures
Signs & Symptoms	• **Unilateral, localized breast pain and swelling** • **Focal area of erythema and firmness (induration)** • **Fever**/chills, myalgia, malaise • **Cracked or fissured nipples** • Purulent nipple discharge or fluctuance (indicates breast abscess)
Diagnosis	• **Clinical Diagnosis** • <u>Breast Ultrasound</u>: ordered to rule out breast abscess • <u>Culture of Breast Milk</u>: can guide antibiotic treatment; indicated for cases refractory to initial treatment

Treatment	• <u>Supportive</u>: warm compresses (encourage milk let-down), cool compresses (after emptying breast), breast massage, supportive bras, analgesia (NSAIDs, acetaminophen)
	• <u>Milk Expression</u>: **continue to breastfeed, pump, or manually express**; no need to dispose of breastmilk
	• <u>Oral Antibiotics</u>: **anti-staphylococcal coverage**
	   • **Dicloxacillin is first-line**
	   • **Cephalexin** *OR* **clindamycin** *OR* **amoxicillin-clavulanate**
	   • <u>MRSA Concern</u>: cephalexin + trimethoprim-sulfamethoxazole *OR* clindamycin

Key Words & Most Common	• Inflammation of breast tissue in lactating women (first 6 weeks postpartum most common) • Nipple trauma + clogged ducts; *S. aureus* most common bacteria • Unilateral, localized breast pain/swelling + focal erythema + cracked/fissured nipples • Clinical diagnosis • Supportive + milk expression • Oral antibiotics (dicloxacillin first line)

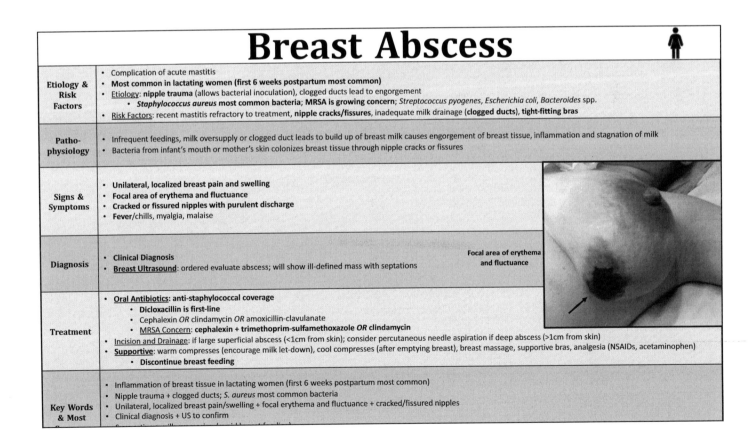

Focal erythema of underside of breast

Breast Abscess

Etiology & Risk Factors	• Complication of acute mastitis • **Most common in lactating women (first 6 weeks postpartum most common)** • <u>Etiology</u>: **nipple trauma** (allows bacterial inoculation), clogged ducts lead to engorgement • *Staphylococcus aureus* **most common bacteria; MRSA is growing concern**; *Streptococcus pyogenes, Escherichia coli, Bacteroides* spp. • <u>Risk Factors</u>: recent mastitis refractory to treatment, **nipple cracks/fissures**, inadequate milk drainage (**clogged ducts**), tight-fitting bras
Patho-physiology	• Infrequent feedings, milk oversupply or clogged duct leads to build up of breast milk causes engorgement of breast tissue, inflammation and stagnation of milk • Bacteria from infant's mouth or mother's skin colonizes breast tissue through nipple cracks or fissures
Signs & Symptoms	• **Unilateral, localized breast pain and swelling** • **Focal area of erythema and fluctuance** • **Cracked or fissured nipples with purulent discharge** • **Fever**/chills, myalgia, malaise
Diagnosis	• **Clinical Diagnosis** • <u>Breast Ultrasound</u>: ordered evaluate abscess; will show ill-defined mass with septations

Treatment	• <u>Oral Antibiotics</u>: **anti-staphylococcal coverage**
	   • **Dicloxacillin is first-line**
	   • Cephalexin *OR* clindamycin *OR* amoxicillin-clavulanate
	   • <u>MRSA Concern</u>: **cephalexin + trimethoprim-sulfamethoxazole** *OR* **clindamycin**
	• <u>Incision and Drainage</u>: if large superficial abscess (<1cm from skin); consider percutaneous needle aspiration if deep abscess (>1cm from skin)
	• <u>Supportive</u>: warm compresses (encourage milk let-down), cool compresses (after emptying breast), breast massage, supportive bras, analgesia (NSAIDs, acetaminophen)
	   • **Discontinue breast feeding**

Key Words & Most	• Inflammation of breast tissue in lactating women (first 6 weeks postpartum most common) • Nipple trauma + clogged ducts; *S. aureus* most common bacteria • Unilateral, localized breast pain/swelling + focal erythema and fluctuance + cracked/fissured nipples • Clinical diagnosis + US to confirm

Focal area of erythema and fluctuance

Fibrocystic Breast Changes

Etiology & Risk Factors	• Non-malignant, fluid-filled breast cysts secondary to hormonal fluctuations • Most common benign breast disease among reproductive age women; symptoms may subside after menopause • Etiology: hormonal fluctuations (estrogen or anti-estrogen treatment, monthly menstrual cycle) • Risk Factors: early menarche, advanced maternal age, nulliparous, anovulation, iodine deficiency
Patho-physiology	• Chronic hormonal fluctuation amplify or regulate breast tissue cell growth which eventually produce small cysts or areas of dense/fibrotic tissue within the breast

Signs & Symptoms	• Multiple painful or painless breast masses
	  • May increase or decrease in size with monthly menstrual cycle
	• Physical Exam:
	  • Nodular, mobile, smooth, round, rubber-like masses within breast tissue
	  • Often multiple and bilateral
	  • Most common in superolateral ("upper-outer") quadrant of breast
	  • Not usually associated with axillary lymphadenopathy

Diagnosis	• Ultrasound: initial imaging test of choice • Fine-Needle Aspiration: not commonly performed; straw-colored or light green fluid (no blood) • Mammogram: indicated if recurrent/persistent cysts or suspicious lesion
Treatment	• Supportive: observation (regular self-breast exams), analgesia (NSAIDs, acetaminophen), warm or cool compresses, supportive bra, evening primrose oil may be effective • Dietary Modification: reduce caffeine/chocolate intake, avoid soy-based food products, iodine supplementation • Oral Contraceptives: may improve or worsen symptoms • Fine-Needle Aspiration: may be diagnostic and therapeutic
Key Words & Most Common	• Non-malignant breast cyst secondary to hormone fluctuation • Multiple, painful or painless breast masses • Mobile, smooth, round, rubber-like masses • Bilateral, multiple • Most common in superolateral ("upper-outer") quadrant • Ultrasound → FNA or mammogram • Observation

Nodular, round, rubber-like masses within breast tissue

Breast Fibroadenoma

Etiology & Risk Factors	• Marble-like, benign, solid mass comprising of epithelial and stromal tissue located just under the skin of the breast • Second most common benign breast mass in reproductive age women; most common benign mass in women <30 years old • Etiology: hormonal fluctuation (increased size during pregnancy, decreased size during menopause) • Risk Factors: long-term oral contraceptive use (20+ years), age (14-35 years old most common)
Patho-physiology	• Stromal and epithelial tissues of breast have estrogen and progesterone receptors; hormonal sensitivity increases proliferation of breast connective tissues

Signs & Symptoms	• Painless breast mass
	  • May become tender prior to menstruation
	• Does not change in size during menstrual cycle
	• Physical Exam:
	  • Firm, solitary, non-tender, well-circumscribed, mobile, rubber-like breast mass
	  • Usually 2-3cm in size
	  • Not usually associated with axillary lymphadenopathy

Diagnosis	• Ultrasound: initial imaging test of choice for women <35 years old; shows solid, well-circumscribed, round mass with uniform hypoechogenicity • Mammogram: indicated in women >35 years old; well-circumscribed, discrete oval mass that is hypodense or isodense • Core-Needle Biopsy: definitive diagnosis

Treatment	• Observation: most small masses will shrink and disappear with time; repeat ultrasound in 3-6 months to monitor size; self breast exams
	• Surgery: indicated if large size (>2-3cm), rapid growth, patient request
	  • Lumpectomy: surgical excision of fibroadenoma; can distort shape of breast if large mass removed
	  • Cryoablation: freezes and destroys cellular structure (<4cm)

Key Words & Most Common	• Epithelial and stromal tissue within the breast • Hormone fluctuation most common cause (grows with pregnancy) • Most common in mid to late adolescents (age 14-35 most common); long-term OCP use • Painless breast mass • Firm, well-circumscribed, highly mobile, rubber-like breast mass • US if <35 yo; mammogram if >35 • Observation with repeat US • Surgery if large, rapid growth, or patient request

Solid, well-circumscribed, round mass with uniform hypoechogenicity

Gynecomastia

Etiology & Risk Factors	• Enlargement of glandular breast and adipose tissue in males
	• Etiology: **idiopathic most common; hormone imbalance (increased estrogen and decreased testosterone)**, **medications** (digoxin, **thiazides**, cimetidine, **spironolactone**, ketoconazole, and **finasteride**), **physiologic (age-related)**
	  • Neonates: due to increased level of circulating maternal estrogens
	  • Adolescents: imbalance of estradiol and testosterone during puberty
	  • Elderly: testosterone decline with a shift in the ratio of testosterone to estrogen
	• Risk Factors: **medications**, breast or lung cancer, **obesity**, **hypogonadism**, adrenal disease, thyroid disease, cirrhosis, renal failure, malnutrition, **marijuana or alcohol abuse**

Patho-physiology	• Estrogen is responsible for glandular breast tissue growth and suppresses luteinizing hormone which blocks testicular secretion of testosterone • This hormonal imbalance leads to enlargement of breast tissue in males

Signs & Symptoms	• **Symmetrical, centrally-located, palpable rim of tissue located just under the nipple**
	  • Approximately **0.5-1cm** in diameter
	  • May be tender to palpation
	• **Circumferential fat in the subareolar area**

Diagnosis	• **Clinical Diagnosis**
	• Labs: **serum testosterone, luteinizing hormone, estradiol, DHEA**, follicle-stimulating hormone, renal/liver function tests
	• Imaging:
	  • Testicular Ultrasound: if testicular mass present
	  • Mammogram or Breast Ultrasound: if breast mass present

Treatment	• **Supportive: observation** if early in disease course (<6 months) or physiologic etiology (age-related); **discontinue offending medications** • Tamoxifen: antagonizes estrogen within the breast; for men treated with high-dose antiandrogen (bicalutamide) for prostate cancer • Surgery: reserved for large breasts, cosmetically unappealing, fibrosis, or severe cases refractory to conservative measure (>12 months) • Surgical removal of excess breast tissue (suction lipectomy with or without cosmetic surgery)
Key Words & Most Common	• Enlargement of glandular breast/adipose tissue in males • Hormone imbalance, medications (thiazides, spironolactone, finasteride), physiologic (age-related) • Symmetrical, rim of tissue 0.5-1cm in diameter located under nipple • Fat of subareolar area • Clinical diagnosis • Labs to confirm hormone imbalance • Supportive → surgery to remove breast tissue

Circumferential fat in subareolar area

Breast Cancer

Etiology & Risk Factors	• Epithelial tumors involving the ducts and lobules of the breast • **Most commonly diagnosed cancer in women** (1 in 10 new cancer diagnosis per year) and second most common cause of cancer related death in women (lung most common) • Risk Factors: **age is strongest risk factor (60 years old median age)**, family history, genetic (*BRCA1* and *BRCA2* genetic mutation increases risk by about 70%), gynecologic history (**nulliparity, early menarche**, late first full-term pregnancy), **increased estrogen exposure (postmenopausal hormone replacement therapy, use of oral contraceptives**, obesity, alcohol use), late menopause
Patho-physiology	• DNA damage and genetic mutations that are influenced by hormone exposure cause uncontrollable cell growth • Classified based on proteins on/in cancer cells (estrogen receptor (ER), progesterone receptor (PR), or human epidermal growth factor 2 (HER2)) • Cancer cells may invade locally and spread through regional lymph nodes and/or bloodstream to become metastatic • Most common metastatic sites are bone (pathological fracture of vertebrae, ribs, pelvis, femur), lungs (dyspnea, cough), liver (abdominal pain, nausea, jaundice), or brain

Signs & Symptoms	• **Painless, hard, immobile breast mass; often found incidentally or during routine physical exam**
	• Nipple inversion, nipple discharge; may present with signs of metastatic disease (pathologic fracture, abdominal pain, jaundice, dyspnea)
	• Physical Exam:
	  • **Palpable breast mass most common in superolateral (upper-outer) quadrant (65%)**; deep to areola
	  • Skin Changes: **erythema of breast, skin thickening**, skin ulceration or retraction, breast size and contour changes, inversion of the nipple
	  • **Axillary lymphadenopathy** in locally advanced disease

Diagnosis	• **Mammography: initial imaging modality in women >40 years old**; shows soft tissue mass/density and grouped microcalcifications • **Ultrasound: initial imaging modality in women <40 years old due to breast tissue density**; may be used to guide fine needle aspiration with biopsy • MRI: indicated for occult lesions, or suspicion of multifocal/bilateral malignancy or to monitor response to neoadjuvant chemotherapy; shows irregular, spiculated mass • **Tissue Biopsy: definitive histologic diagnosis**; fine-needle aspiration cytology, core biopsy and incisional or excisional biopsy

Treatment	• **Surgical Oncology: mastectomy or breast-conserving surgery + lymph node evaluation**
	  • **Mastectomy**: removal of the entire breast
	  • **Breast-Conserving Surgery**: lumpectomy; removal of tumor and required margins
	• **Radiation Oncology**: local disease control after breast-conserving surgery external beam radiation, brachytherapy, or a combination
	  • Indicated for large tumors (>5cm), invasion of chest wall or skin, or lymph node involvement
	• **Medical Oncology**: chemotherapy, hormone therapy, and targeted therapy
	  • First-Generation Chemotherapy: cyclophosphamide, methotrexate, and 5-fluorouracil (CMF)
	  • Anthracycline: doxorubicin or epirubicin
	  • Selective Estrogen Receptor Modulator Therapy: **tamoxifen is mainstay of treatment for *pre*menopausal women with hormone receptor positive (HR+) breast cancer**
	  • Aromatase Inhibitors: anastrozole; indicated for *post*menopausal women with HR+ breast cancer.
	  • Anti-HER2 Therapy: **trastuzumab**; humanized monoclonal antibody that improves survival with lymph node involvement

Carcinoma In Situ

Etiology & Risk Factors	• **Non-invasive breast cancer involving proliferation of abnormal epithelial cells within the breast ducts and lobules and *without* invasion of surrounding stromal tissue** • 2 Types: Ductal or Lobular • Comprises 20-25% of new breast cancer diagnoses • <u>Etiology</u>: **unknown**; genetic predisposition (*BRCA1* and *BRCA2* mutations) • <u>Risk Factors</u>: **age is strongest risk factor (50-64 years old most common), family history of breast cancer, genetic predisposition, gynecologic history (nulliparity, early menarche**, late first full-term pregnancy), **increased estrogen exposure (postmenopausal hormone replacement therapy, use of oral contraceptives**, obesity, alcohol use)
Patho-physiology	• DNA damage and genetic mutations that are influenced by estrogen exposure • Proliferation of abnormal epithelial cells remain in normal location (in situ) within ducts and lobules of breast that does not invade basement membrane • Considered pre-malignant
Signs & Symptoms	• **Mostly asymptomatic** • Discovered during routine mammogram or breast exam • **Painless, hard, immobile breast mass**
Diagnosis	• <u>**Mammography**</u>: **most commonly found incidentally during screening mammogram (90% of cases); Initial imaging modality in women >40 years old** • Demonstrate clustered macrocalcification or microcalcifications appearing in linear branching patterns or segmental types of pleomorphic calcifications • <u>**Image-Guided Core Needle Biopsy**</u>: provides histologic diagnosis and evaluate for hormone receptor status • <u>Breast Ultrasound</u>: initial imaging modality in women <40 years old due to breast tissue density; may be used to guide fine needle aspiration with biopsy
Treatment	• <u>**Breast-Conserving Surgery with Partial Mastectomy and Radiation**</u>: **recommended treatment approach as less invasive surgery** • Carcinoma in situ is noninvasive and rarely involves axillary lymph nodes • <u>**Mastectomy**</u>: **total mastectomy is curative in 98% of cases** • <u>Endocrine Therapy</u>: tamoxifen prevents recurrence if DCIS specimen positive for estrogen and/or progesterone receptors (contraindicated if bilateral mastectomy) • <u>Chemotherapy</u>: not indicated in patients with ductal carcinoma in situ after surgical treatment
Key Words & Most Common	• Non-invasive breast cancer within ducts and lobules without invading basement membrane • Unknown etiology; (*BRCA1* and *BRCA2* mutations) implicated • Age + family history + genetic predisposition; early menarche, estrogen exposure • Mostly asymptomatic (90% found on screening mammogram) • Mammogram → core needle biopsy • Breast conserving surgery with partial mastectomy and radiation

Invasive Carcinoma

Etiology & Risk Factors	• **Invasive breast cancer involving proliferation of abnormal epithelial cells within the breast ducts and lobules *with* invasion of surrounding stromal tissue**
	    • Primarily adenocarcinoma
	    • 80% is infiltrating ductal; most of the remaining are infiltrating lobular
	• <u>Etiology</u>: genetic predisposition (*BRCA1* and *BRCA2* mutations)
	• <u>Risk Factors</u>: **age is strongest risk factor (50-64 years old most common), family history of breast cancer, genetic predisposition, gynecologic history (nulliparity, early menarche**, late first full-term pregnancy), **increased estrogen exposure (postmenopausal hormone replacement therapy, use of oral contraceptives**, obesity, alcohol use)

Patho-physiology	• DNA damage and genetic mutations that are influenced by estrogen exposure • Proliferation of abnormal epithelial cells that invades surrounding tissue; cancer cells may invade locally and spread through regional lymph nodes and/or bloodstream to become metastatic
Signs & Symptoms	• **Mostly asymptomatic; often goes undiagnosed by exam or screening mammogram until advanced stages** • **Painless, hard, immobile breast mass; palpable if mass >2cm** • **May have breast swelling, thickening of skin, nipple inversion, nipple discharge** • **Metastatic spread may involve regional lymph nodes (axillary)**
Diagnosis	• <u>**Mammography**</u>: **initial imaging modality in women >40 years old**; mammograms often lack sensitivity until advanced stages • <u>**Breast Ultrasound**</u>: **initial imaging modality in women <40 years old due to breast tissue density**; may be used to guide fine needle aspiration with biopsy • <u>Breast MRI</u>: preferred imaging to detect and describe soft-tissue lesions and monitor treatment • <u>**Tissue Biopsy**</u>: **definitive histologic diagnosis**; fine-needle aspiration cytology, core biopsy or excisional biopsy

Treatment	• <u>Treatment varies by size and extent</u>
	• <u>**Surgery**</u>: **first-line treatment**
	    • **Radical mastectomy (>4cm) or lumpectomy (<4cm) is treatment of choice**
	    • **Prophylactic contralateral mastectomy may be performed in high-risk patient**
	    • **Lymph node evaluation to evaluate metastases**
	• <u>Adjuvant Therapy</u>: involves combination of radiation, chemotherapy, hormonal therapy (tamoxifen) and/or targeted therapy (trastuzumab)

Key Words & Most Common	• Invasive breast cancer of ducts and lobules with invasion of surrounding tissue Primarily adenocarcinoma • Mostly asymptomatic; often goes undiagnosed until late stage • Painless, hard, immobile mass; may have swelling, skin thickening, nipple inversion/discharge • Mammogram (>40), ultrasound (<40) → tissue biopsy • Surgery (mastectomy vs lumpectomy) + lymph node evaluation + adjuvant therapy

Inflammatory Breast Cancer

Etiology & Risk Factors	• Rare subtype (1-3% of all breast cancers) of breast cancer • **Characterized by diffuse induration of the skin with an erythematous appearance and no underlying mass** • <u>Etiology</u>: **primary** (develops in previously normal breast) or **secondary** (develops in breast with invasive cancer or after surgery for non-inflammatory breast cancer) • <u>Risk Factors</u>: **high body mass index (BMI)**, chronic inflammation, younger age at first birth, smoking; *genetic mutations and family history have no association*
Patho-physiology	• Breast erythema and swelling occurs secondary to blockage of lymph vessels by cancer cells
Signs & Symptoms	• **Pain, erythema, edema and warmth of breast** • *Commonly misdiagnosed as mastitis* • **Skin of breast may become itchy, thickened and tender** • **Nipple retraction/inversion** • *Not* **typically associated with underlying mass** • May have lymph node involvement • <u>Peau D'orange</u>: skin has erythematous and dimpled appearance resembling orange peel due to lymphatic obstruction

Diagnosis	• <u>Mammography</u>: initial imaging modality in women >40 years old
	  • May show mass, calcification, or parenchymal distortion with skin thickening
	• <u>Breast Ultrasound</u>: initial imaging modality in women <40 years old due to breast tissue density; may be used to guide fine needle aspiration with biopsy
	  • May show thickened skin, interstitial fluid, and disruption of normal tissue planes
	• Breast MRI: most accurate imaging technique to detect primary breast parenchymal lesion
	• <u>Tissue Biopsy</u>: definitive histologic diagnosis

Treatment	• **Systemic therapy prior to surgery followed by radiation is standard** • <u>Neoadjuvant Therapy</u>: anthracycline (doxorubicin) and taxane-based (paclitaxel and docetaxel) chemotherapy are commonly used • **Trastuzumab** if HER2 overexpression • <u>Surgery</u>: **radical mastectomy**; lumpectomy or breast-conserving surgery not recommended • <u>Radiation Therapy</u>: local disease control • *Often carry poor prognosis and a high risk of early recurrence*
Key Words & Most Common	• Pain, erythema, edema, warmth of breast (commonly misdiagnosed as mastitis) *without* underlying mass • Itchy, thickened skin; nipple retraction; peau d'orange • Mammogram vs ultrasound → tissue biopsy • Systemic therapy → surgery → radiation therapy • Poor prognosis with high risk of recurrence

Paget Disease of the Nipple

Etiology & Risk Factors	• Form of ductal carcinoma in situ or invasive ductal carcinoma that extends into the skin overlying the nipple and areola • Etiology: **underlying ductal carcinoma in situ or invasive ductal carcinoma** • <u>Risk Factors</u>: **age (>50)**, family history, genetic predisposition (*BRCA1* and *BRCA2)*, gynecologic history (**nulliparity, early menarche**, late first full-term pregnancy), **increased estrogen exposure (postmenopausal hormone replacement therapy, use of oral contraceptives**, obesity, alcohol use), late menopause
Patho-physiology	• Neoplastic epithelial cells of the lactiferous ducts migrate through the breast ductal system to the epidermis of the nipple and then to areola • **Presence of Paget cells on histology** (large cells with clear cytoplasm and prominent, hyperchromic nuclei found within the epidermis of the nipple)

Signs & Symptoms	• **Erythematous, crusted, scaly, thickened, plaque-like lesion on the nipple and surrounding areola**
	  • **Sharp demarcation**
	• **Areas of bleeding or oozing**
	• **Bloody nipple discharge; nipple inversion**
	• May or may not have underlying palpable mass
	• May appear eczematous
	  • *Paget disease is typically unilateral with sharp demarcation; eczema may be bilateral and not sharply demarcated*

Diagnosis	• <u>Mammography</u>: initial imaging modality • <u>Tissue Biopsy</u>: definitive histologic diagnosis
Treatment	• **Treatment of underlying ductal carcinoma in situ or invasive ductal carcinoma** • <u>Surgery</u>: **radical mastectomy often required**; breast-conserving surgery or lumpectomy indicated if cancer has not spread beyond nipple • Chemotherapy and/or radiation often required
Key Words & Most Common	• Form of ductal carcinoma in situ or invasive ductal carcinoma extending to skin of nipple and areola • Erythematous, crusted, scaly, thick, plaque-like lesion on nipple/areola • Area of bleeding/oozing (bloody nipple discharge) • Mammogram + tissue biopsy • Treat underlying cancer • Radical mastectomy often required

Breast Cancer Screening

Organization	American Academy of Family Physicians (AAFP)	American Congress of Obstetricians and Gynecologists (ACOG)	American Cancer Society (ACS)	United States Preventative Services Task Force (USPSTF)
Mammography	• Mammogram every 2 years for women 50-74 years old • Screening prior to age 50 determined by patient	• Mammogram every 1-2 years for women 40-49 years old • Mammogram annually for women 50+ years old	• Mammogram annually for women ≥40 years old	• Mammogram every 2 years for women 50-74 years old • Screening prior to age 50 determined by patient
Clinical Breast Exam	• Insufficient evidence	• Annually for all women ≥19 years old	• Every 3 years for women 20-39 years old • Annually for women ≥40 years old	• Insufficient evidence
MRI Considerations	• Insufficient evidence for MRI over film mammography		• Mammogram and MRI annually for women with >20% lifetime risk	• Insufficient evidence for MRI over film mammography
Breast Self-Exam	• Should not be taught	• Optional	• Optional for women ≥20 years old	• Should not be taught

General Recommendations for Breast Cancer Screening
• <u>Mammogram</u>: best screening modality for women >40 years old
• <u>Ultrasound</u>: best screening modality for women <40 years old (due to density of breast tissue)
• <u>Average Risk</u>: variable guidelines based on organization
  • **Mammogram every 1-2 years starting at age 40-50 years old until 74 years old**
  • Clinical breast exams have insufficient evidence to support a reduction in long-term mortality
• <u>Moderate Risk</u>: patients with a first-degree relative with breast cancer
  • Screening starting at 50 years old or **10 years prior to the age when the first-degree relative was first diagnosed with breast cancer**
• <u>High Risk</u>: patients with BRCA genetic mutation
  • Screening with MRI or Ultrasound starting at age 25-30 years old or 10 years prior to the age when the first-degree relative was first diagnosed with breast cancer
• Women with breast implants should still participate in same screening schedule

Breast Cancer Prevention
• **Chemoprophylaxis with tamoxifen** or raloxifene may be indicated in women with:
  • Age 35+ with previous lobular carcinoma in situ or atypical lobular/ductal hyperplasia
  • **Postmenopausal women that are high-risk**
  • **Presence of high-risk genetic mutations (*BRCA1* or *BRCA2*)**
  • Age 35-59 with 5-year risk of developing breast cancer >1.66% based on Gail model
    • Gail model considers current age, age at menarche, age at first live childbirth, number of 1st-degree relatives with breast cancer and results of prior breast biopsies
• **Tamoxifen is preferred**; patients should be made aware of risks such as:
  • **Endometrial cancer**
  • Thromboembolic complications (DVT/PE)
  • Cataracts
  • Possible stroke

Sperm Disorders
Infertility

Etiology & Risk Factors	• Failure to conceive after 1 year of regular unprotected sexual intercourse; **sperm disorders (abnormal spermatogenesis) in males is most common cause** • Unprotected sexual intercourse results in conception in 50% of couples within 3 months, 75% within 6 months and 90% within 1 year • Inability to conceive can lead to anxiety, sadness, depression, frustration, anger, guilt, resentment, and feeling of inadequacy • <u>Etiology</u>: **heat**, endocrine or genetic disorders, drugs (anabolic steroids), **toxins (drugs, smoking, alcohol)**, impaired sperm emission (retrograde ejaculation into bladder), **erectile dysfunction**, anatomical abnormalities (varicocele, **hypogonadism**, testicular atrophy), infection (gonorrhea or chlamydia)
Patho-physiology	• Sertoli cells regulate maturation while Leydig cells produce testosterone necessary for spermatogenesis; fructose produced in the seminal vesicles and secreted through the ejaculatory ducts
Signs & Symptoms	• **Inadequate quantity of sperm** (oligozoospermia=too few; azoospermia=none) • **Inadequate quality of sperm** (abnormal structure or motility)
Diagnosis	• <u>Semen Analysis</u>: manual masturbation into sterile cup in a laboratory setting and then examined 20-30 minutes later • Measures volume, viscosity, appearance, pH, **sperm count, sperm motility, percentage with normal morphology**, fructose, vitality, and white blood cell (WBC) count • <u>Genetic Testing</u>: standard karyotyping, polymerase chain reaction of chromosomal sites, evaluation of *CFTR* mutation • <u>Endocrine Evaluation</u>: serum total and free testosterone, follicular stimulating hormone (FSH), luteinizing hormone (LH), prolactin • <u>Infection Workup</u>: gonorrhea or chlamydia nucleic acid amplification test (NAAT) • <u>Testicular Ultrasound</u>: evaluate testicle for anatomical abnormalities such as decreased perfusion and atrophy that may impair spermatogenesis
Treatment	• <u>Lifestyle Modifications</u>: **proper nutrition**, avoidance of toxins, **exercise**, proper fitting underwear (too tight can restrict blood flow and temperature regulation) • <u>Treat Underlying Infection</u>: 500mg ceftriaxone injection and/or doxycycline (BID for 1 week) • <u>Clomiphene Citrate</u>: antiestrogen medication that stimulates sperm production • <u>Intrauterine Insemination</u>: semen samples are delivered to uterus to coincide with female ovulation • <u>Assisted Reproductive Techniques</u>: in vitro fertilization or intracytoplasmic sperm injection • <u>Surgery</u>: correction of anatomical abnormalities (varicocele)
Key Words & Most Common	• Failure to conceive after 1 year of regular unprotected sexual intercourse • Heat, toxin exposure, erectile dysfunction, endocrine/genetic disorders, infection • Inadequate quantity or quality of sperm • Semen analysis • Endocrine or genetic testing • Testicular ultrasound • Lifestyle modifications + address underlying etiology • Clomiphene citrate

1.Menstrual Phase (Days 1-5): The cycle begins with the menstrual phase, marked by the shedding of the uterine lining that wasn't needed in the previous cycle. Hormone levels, particularly estrogen and progesterone, are relatively low during this phase. This shedding results in menstrual bleeding.

2.Follicular Phase (Days 6-14): As menstruation tapers off, the body starts preparing for ovulation. The follicular phase is initiated by the hypothalamus releasing Gonadotropin-Releasing Hormone (GnRH), which stimulates the anterior pituitary gland to release Follicle-Stimulating Hormone (FSH) and Luteinizing Hormone (LH). These hormones trigger the development of follicles (fluid-filled sacs containing eggs) in the ovaries. Estrogen levels gradually rise as the follicles grow, leading to the thickening of the uterine lining.

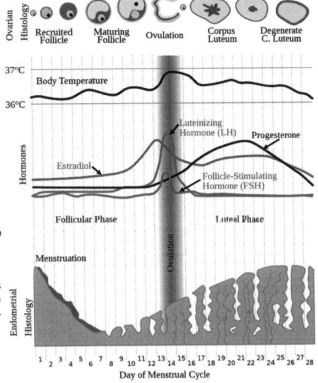

3. Ovulation (Day 14): A surge in LH triggers ovulation, where the most mature follicle ruptures, releasing a mature egg from the ovary into the fallopian tube. This typically occurs around day 14 of a 28-day cycle, but it can vary. Ovulation is the most fertile phase of the cycle, and conception can occur if sperm is present.

4. Luteal Phase (Days 15-28): After ovulation, the ruptured follicle transforms into the corpus luteum, a temporary endocrine structure that produces progesterone. Progesterone prepares the uterine lining for a possible pregnancy by making it more hospitable to a fertilized egg. If fertilization doesn't occur, the corpus luteum breaks down, leading to a drop in progesterone and estrogen levels.

5. Menstruation (Start of New Cycle): As progesterone and estrogen levels decrease, the uterine lining is no longer sustained, and it begins to break down. This marks the beginning of a new cycle, and the menstrual phase starts again, completing the cycle.

Ovulatory Dysfunction

Infertility	
Etiology & Risk Factors	• Failure to conceive after 1 year of regular unprotected sexual intercourse • Unprotected sexual intercourse results in conception in 50% of couples within 3 months, 75% within 6 months and 90% within 1 year • Inability to conceive can lead to anxiety, sadness, depression, frustration, anger, guilt, resentment, and feeling of inadequacy • **Abnormal, irregular (≤9 menses per year), or absent ovulation** • Etiology: polycystic ovary syndrome (PCOS) is most common cause; hyperprolactinemia, hypothalamic-pituitary dysfunction, **diabetes**, depression, **obesity**, **excessive exercise, excessive weight loss**, medications containing estrogen or progestins
Patho-physiology	• Hormonal imbalances do not produce enough follicles that develop into an ovule; possibly due to under-secretion of hormones from pituitary gland or hypothalamus
Signs & Symptoms	• **Menses may be absent or irregular** • Menses often not preceded by symptoms (breast tenderness, lower abdominal bloating, fatigue, headache, irritability)
Diagnosis	• **Menstrual History: menstrual period tracking**; patient may measure daily morning basal body temperature to track ovulation • **Home Testing Kits**: detect urinary luteinizing hormone (LH) which is excreted 24-36 hours prior to ovulation • Pelvic Ultrasound: monitors increase in ovarian follicle diameter and collapse of the follicle; testing should be obtained in late follicular phase • Hormone Testing: serum progesterone or urine pregnanediol glucuronide; elevated levels ~1 week before next menstrual period indicate ovulation has occurred
Treatment	• **Treatment of underlying etiology** • **Lifestyle Modifications: proper nutrition**, avoidance of toxins, **appropriate level of exercise** • **Clomiphene Citrate: selective-estrogen receptor-modulator (SERM) which induces ovulation** • Letrozole: aromatase inhibitor shown to induce ovulation particularly in obese women with PCOS • Metformin: adjunct medication used to induce ovulation in women with PCOS and insulin resistance • Exogenous Gonadotropins: human gonadotropin preparations with FSH and LH as indicated
Key Words & Most Common	• Abnormal, irregular or absent ovulation • PCOS is most common cause; diabetes, obesity, excessive exercise, excessive weight loss • Absent/irregular menses • Menstrual history • Home testing kits • Treat underlying etiology • Clomiphene citrate

Infertility Tubal Dysfunction/Pelvic Abnormalities

Etiology & Risk Factors	• Failure to conceive after 1 year of regular unprotected sexual intercourse
	• Unprotected sexual intercourse results in conception in 50% of couples within 3 months, 75% within 6 months and 90% within 1 year
	• Inability to conceive can lead to anxiety, sadness, depression, frustration, anger, guilt, resentment, and feeling of inadequacy
	• <u>Etiology</u>: tubal dysfunction or pelvic abnormalities
	   • <u>Tubal Dysfunction</u>: **pelvic inflammatory disease, ectopic pregnancy**, ruptured appendix, pelvic adhesions (prior lower abdominal surgery), inflammatory disorders
	   • <u>Pelvic Structural Abnormalities</u>: **intrauterine adhesions, fibroids**, intrauterine polyps, endometriosis

Patho-physiology	• Adhesions or anatomical abnormality leads to dysfunction of fallopian tubes by distorting, obstructing, or separating from ovary which prevents ovulation
Signs & Symptoms	• **Signs and symptoms vary based on underlying etiology**
Diagnosis	• <u>Gonorrhea/Chlamydia Nucleic Acid Amplification Test (NAAT)</u>: if pelvic inflammatory disease suspected • <u>Hysterosalpingography</u>: **evaluates tubal patency/abnormalities**; fluoroscopic imaging of uterus and fallopian tubes; performed by injecting radiopaque substance into uterus • <u>Sonohysterography</u>: further evaluates intrauterine and tubal abnormalities; performed by injecting isotonic fluid through the cervix into the uterus during ultrasound • <u>Hysteroscopy</u>: further investigation; more invasive

Treatment	• <u>Antibiotics</u>: **500mg ceftriaxone injection and/or doxycycline (BID for 1 week) if positive for gonorrhea/chlamydia or pelvic inflammatory disease or cervicitis present**
	• <u>Surgery</u>:
	   • <u>Laparoscopy</u>: **lysis of pelvic adhesions, laser ablation of endometriosis**
	   • <u>Hysteroscopy</u>: **lysis of intrauterine adhesions, removal of submucosal fibroids and intrauterine polyps**
	   • *Hysteroscopy treatment of abnormalities is often successful (60-70% pregnancy rate)*

Key Words & Most Common	• Pelvic inflammatory disease, prior ectopic pregnancy, intrauterine adhesions, fibroids • Signs and symptoms based on underlying etiology • G/C NAAT test if PID suspected • Hysterosalpingography to evaluate tubal patency • Antibiotics if PID suspected or confirmed (ceftriaxone + doxycycline) • Surgery: laparoscopy vs hysteroscopy

Infertility Abnormal Cervical Mucous

Etiology & Risk Factors	• Failure to conceive after 1 year of regular unprotected sexual intercourse • Unprotected sexual intercourse results in conception in 50% of couples within 3 months, 75% within 6 months and 90% within 1 year • Inability to conceive can lead to anxiety, sadness, depression, frustration, anger, guilt, resentment, and feeling of inadequacy • **Impaired fertility by inhibiting sperm penetration or increasing sperm destruction** • <u>Etiology</u>: **infection (gonorrhea or chlamydia, bacterial vaginosis, vulvovaginal candidiasis, trichomonas), personal lubricants**, foreign body exposure, hormonal dysfunction
Patho-physiology	• Normally, increased estradiol levels during the follicular phase leads to thin and stretchy cervical mucous • Abnormal cervical mucous may cause the mucous to be impenetrable to sperm during ovulation or promote sperm destruction (secondary to infection)
Signs & Symptoms	• **Signs and symptoms vary based on underlying etiology** • **Abnormal vaginal discharge**
Diagnosis	• <u>Gonorrhea/Chlamydia Nucleic Acid Amplification Test (NAAT)</u>: if infection suspected • <u>Cervical DNA Test</u>: test for bacterial vaginosis, trichomonas, and candidiasis

Treatment	• Avoid offending personal lubricants
	• **Treat Underlying Etiology**
	• <u>**Antibiotics**</u>:
	   • <u>Gonorrhea/Chlamydia</u>: **500mg ceftriaxone injection and/or doxycycline (BID for 1 week)**
	   • <u>Trichomonas and Bacterial Vaginosis</u>: **oral or intravaginal metronidazole**
	• <u>**Antifungals**</u>:
	   • <u>Vulvovaginal Candidiasis</u>: **oral fluconazole, intravaginal clotrimazole, miconazole, nystatin**
	• Intrauterine insemination or in vitro fertilization

Key Words & Most Common	• Impaired fertility secondary to inhibition of sperm penetration or increased sperm destruction due to cervical mucous • Infection is most common cause; personal lubricants • Abnormal vaginal discharge; s/s vary based on etiology • G/C NAAT • Cervical DNA test • Treat underlying infection

Cervical Cancer

Etiology & Risk Factors	• Most commonly due to squamous cell carcinoma (90%), adenocarcinoma (10%) • 3rd most common gynecologic cancer (#1 endometrial, #2 ovarian) • Etiology: **human papilloma virus (HPV) is associated with vast majority of cervical cancer cases (99.7%)**; diethylstilbestrol (DES) exposure (synthetic estrogen used in OCPs) • **HPV 16 and 18 are most common types implicated in invasive cervical cancer** (70%) • Risk Factors: **early sexual activity, increased number of sexual partners, unprotected sex**, smoking, DES exposure, cervical intraepithelial neoplasia, STDs, OCP use
Patho-physiology	• HPV is passed through skin-to-skin contact; may be spread through sexual intercourse, hand to genital contact, or oral sex • HPV have oncoproteins that inactivate certain tumor suppressor proteins leading to dysregulation of cell cycle and neoplastic formation of tissue (Cervical intraepithelial neoplasia) and eventually cervical cancer

Signs & Symptoms	• **Asymptomatic in early stages** (takes 2-10 years to penetrate basement membrane)
	• **Abnormal vaginal bleeding or discharge**
	   • **Postcoital bleeding is most common presenting symptom**
	   • Bleeding may occur irregularly between menses
	   • Foul-smelling discharge associated with larger cancers
	• Obstructive uropathy, back pain, leg swelling in advanced disease (due to lymphatic or venous obstruction)
	• Physical Exam:
	   • Pelvic exam may reveal exophytic necrotic cervical tumor; most cervical cancers are unable to be visualized without magnification

Diagnosis	• Papanicolaou (Pap) Test: cervical cytology evaluating for atypical or cancerous cells of the cervix; screening begins at age 21 every 3 years until age 30 then every 5 years • HPV Testing: begins at age 30 • Colposcopy with Biopsy: definitive diagnostic test; indicated if atypical/cancerous cells on pap smear or positive HPV test
Treatment	• Conservative: precancerous lesions in women <25 years old are often low-risk cervical dysplasia and resolve spontaneously • Carcinoma In Situ (Stage 0): **excision** (loop electrical excision procedure (LEEP), cold knife or conization procedure) or **ablation** (cryotherapy or laser) • Stage IA1 (_no lymphovascular space invasion_): conization indicated for women seeking to preserve fertility; simple hysterectomy preferred if no interest to preserve fertility • Stage IA1 (_with lymphovascular space invasion_) and Stage IA2: modified radical hysterectomy and pelvic lymphadenectomy +/- sentinel lymph node mapping • Stage IB1, IB2, IIA1: open radical hysterectomy with bilateral pelvic lymphadenectomy +/- sentinel lymph node mapping • Stages IB3, IIA2, IIB, III, and IVA: external pelvic radiation therapy with brachytherapy and concurrent platinum-based chemotherapy (cisplatin-based) • Stage IVB and Recurrent Cancer: systemic chemotherapy is primary treatment (cisplatin + paclitaxel)
Key Words & Most Common	• Most common cause is HPV (type 16 and 18) • Asymptomatic early → abnormal bleeding (postcoital bleeding most common) • Pap test +/- HPV test → colposcopy with biopsy • Excision or ablation • Treatment varies on staging; includes surgery, radiation therapy, and chemotherapy

Cervical Cancer Screening

Papanicolaou Smear Results					
Age Group	**Normal**	**Atypical Squamous Cells of Undetermined Significance (ASC-US)**	**Low-Grade Squamous Intraepithelial Lesion (LSIL)**	**Atypical Squamous Cells – Cannot Exclude HSIL (ASC-H)**	**High-Grade Squamous Cell Intraepithelial Lesion (HSIL)**
21-24 Years Old	• Pap smear every 3 years	• Pap smear in 1 year (preferred) _OR_ • Reflex HPV test (acceptable)	• Repeat Pap smear in 1 year	• **Colposcopy**	• Colposcopy
25-29 Years Old	• Pap smear every 3 years	• Reflex HPV testing (preferred) _OR_ • Pap smear in 1 year (acceptable)	• Colposcopy	• **Colposcopy**	• Excisional treatment _OR_ • Colposcopy
≥30 Years Old and HPV -	• HPV and Pap smear every 5 years (preferred) _OR_ • Pap smear every 3 years (acceptable)	• Repeat HPV and Pap smear in 3 years	• Repeat Pap smear in 1 year _OR_ • Colposcopy	• **Colposcopy**	• Excisional treatment _OR_ • Colposcopy
≥30 Years Old and HPV +	• HPV and Pap smear annually _OR_ • HPV genotype test	• Colposcopy	• Colposcopy	• **Colposcopy**	• Excisional treatment _OR_ • Colposcopy

General Cervical Cancer Screening		
Result	**American Cancer Society (ACS)**	**United States Preventative Task Force (USPTF)**
21-24 Years Old	• No Screening	• Cervical cytology every 3 years
25-29 Years Old	• HPV test every 5 years (preferred) _OR_ • HPV and Pap smear co-testing every 5 years (acceptable) _OR_ • Pap smear every 3 years (acceptable)	• Cervical cytology every 3 years
30-65 Years Old	• HPV test every 5 years (preferred) _OR_ • HPV and Pap smear co-testing every 5 years (acceptable) _OR_ • Pap smear every 3 years (acceptable)	• Cervical cytology every 3 years _OR_ • HPV testing every 5 years _OR_ • HPV/cervical cytology co-testing every 5 years
≥65 Years Old	• Discontinue screening if adequate negative prior screening	• Discontinue screening if adequate negative prior screening and not high-risk

Toxic Shock Syndrome

Etiology & Risk Factors	• Acute onset illness caused by exotoxins produced by *Staphylococcus aureus* or *Streptococcus pyogenes* • <u>Etiology</u>: **toxigenic strain of *Staphylococcus aureus* or Group A Strep (*Streptococcus pyogenes*) is most common cause** • <u>Risk Factors</u>: **use of high absorbency tampons is most common**; soft tissue infections and abscess, burns, post-surgical infection, **retained foreign body (nasal packing, tampon)**, dialysis catheters, intrauterine device (IUD)
Patho-physiology	• Exotoxin-producing *S. aureus* produce superantigens which activates T-cells and causes hyperactivation of cytokines and inflammatory mediators (IL-2, IL-1, TNF) • This over-activation of inflammatory cells causes **capillary leakage**, circulatory collapse, and multi-organ failure

Signs & Symptoms	• **Trio of fever, rash and hypotension**
	• <u>**Fever**</u>: **rapid onset fever (>102.2°F)**
	• <u>**Rash**</u>: **diffuse, blanching, erythroderma (diffusely erythematous macular rash)**; may resemble a sunburn
	   • **Desquamation of skin (full-thickness peeling) occurs 3-7 days later; involves palms and soles**
	   • May have mucosal involvement with hyperemia of vaginal, oropharyngeal, or conjunctival mucosa
	• <u>**Hypotension**</u>: systolic BP less than 90 mmHg
	• <u>**Multisystem Organ Failure**</u>: renal impairment (elevated BUN/creatinine), coagulopathy, liver impairment (elevated AST/ALT/bilirubin), acute respiratory distress (hypoxemia, diffuse pulmonary infiltrates), soft tissue necrosis, muscular (elevated creatine phosphokinase), CNS (altered mental status, focal neurologic deficits)
	• May have prodrome of fever and chills, nausea and vomiting, myalgias, headache, pharyngitis that progresses

Diagnosis	• **Clinical Diagnosis** • <u>Labs</u>: CBC (may show leukocytosis or leukopenia), CMP, creatine kinase (CK), coagulation studies • <u>**Culture**</u>: **blood cultures and culture of suspected source (nasal sinus, vagina) should be obtained**

Treatment	• <u>**Local Treatment**</u>: **decontamination of infection source**; irrigation of surgical incision, debridement of devitalized tissue, irrigation of colonized sites (nasal sinus, vagina), removal of retained foreign body (tampon, nasal packing)
	• <u>**Supportive**</u>: **fluid and electrolyte replacement** (due to systemic capillary leakage); circulatory, ventilation, and hemodialysis support
	• <u>**Antibiotics**</u>: **clindamycin is preferred antibiotic as it suppresses toxin synthesis**; pending culture results
	   • <u>Group A *Streptococcus*</u>: clindamycin + beta lactam
	   • <u>Methicillin-Susceptible *S. aureus* (MSSA)</u>: clindamycin + oxacillin or nafcillin
	   • <u>Methicillin-Resistant *S. aureus* (MRSA)</u>: vancomycin + clindamycin or linezolid

Key Words & Most Common	• Toxigenic S. aureus or GAS is most common cause; associated with high-absorbency tampon use, wound/burn infection, or retained foreign body (nasal packing, tampon, IUD) • Fever, rash (diffuse, blanching erythroderma with peeling), hypotension • Clinical diagnosis + labs to identify organ involvement + culture • Decontamination + fluid/electrolyte replacement + antibiotics (clindamycin preferred)

Non-Hormonal Contraceptive Methods

Name	Description or Mechanism of Action	Advantages	Disadvantages/ Side Effects	Contraindications	Reliability with Typical Use	Reliability with Perfect Use
Male Condom	• Sheath of latex, polyurethane or animal skin worn on penis to trap sperm	• Widely available • Low cost • Protects against STIs	• Careful handling and timing required • Reduced sensation	• Latex allergy	87%	98%
Female Condom	• Nitrile sheath that covers and lines the vagina and labia	• May be inserted hours prior to intercourse • Protects against STIs	• Cannot be used with male condom • Reduced sensation	• Allergy to synthetics	79%	95%
Diaphragm	• Latex or silicone cup worn over cervix to prevent sperm from entering uterus	• Comfortable • Can be worn for 24 hours	• Does not protect against STIs • Risk of UTI	• Latex or synthetics allergy • History of TSS	83%	84%
Sponge	• Soft, polyurethane foam impregnated with spermicide inserted at cervix to block sperm from entering uterus	• Widely available • Can be worn for 24 hours	• Must stay in place for 6 hours after intercourse • Does not protect against STIs	• Polyurethan or spermicide allergy • History of TSS	86%	91%
Spermicide Gel	• Cream, gel, foam, suppository inserted deep into vagina prior to intercourse • Blocks sperm motility	• Widely available • Low cost • Enhances vaginal lubrication	• May cause genital irritation • Risk of UTI/BV/yeast infection • Does not protect against STIs	• Spermicide allergy • Frequent UTIs	79%	84%
Fertility Awareness Methods	• Recording and tracking of menstrual cycle signs of ovulation (temperature, cervical mucus) • Abstinence or other contraceptive method during fertile window	• No hormonal side effects • Calendars, charts, thermometers widely available	• Requires detailed record keeping • Restricts sex to unfertile days • Less effective with irregular menses • Does not protect against STIs	• Those not committed to careful record keeping • Inability to abstain during fertile window	76%	99%
Withdrawal Method	• Withdrawing penis from vagina prior to ejaculation	• No decrease in sensation • No cost • No side effects	• Requires perfect timing • Reliance on male partner • Does not protect against STIs	• Premature ejaculation	80%	96%

Combination Hormonal Contraceptive Methods

Name	Description or Mechanism of Action	Advantages	Disadvantages/ Side Effects	Contraindications	Reliability with Typical Use	Reliability with Perfect Use
Oral Combination Pill	• Estrogen-Progestin combination • Hormones prevent ovulation and implantation (inhibits midcycle luteinizing hormone surge) • Thickens cervical mucus to prevent sperm from entering uterus • Thins endometrium of uterus	• Regular, lighter and shorter menses • Improves dysmenorrhea and irregular menses • Protective against osteoporosis, ovarian, endometrial cancers • Lowers risk of ovarian cysts, non-cancerous breast growths and ectopic pregnancy	• Increased hypercoagulability and risk of DVT, PE, stroke gallbladder stasis • Increased fluid retention, breast tenderness, nausea, headaches • Changes in weight, mood lability • Does not protect against STIs	• History of ischemic heart disease, DVT, PE, stroke • History of breast or uterine cancer • Migraine with aura • Smokers >35 years old • Severe hypertension • Breastfeeding	93%	99%
Female Condom	• Thin, plastic patch that adheres to skin and releases combination of estrogen and progestin • Patch replaced weekly for 3 weeks in a 4-week cycle • Similar mechanism of action to OCPs	• Similar advantages to OCPs • Does not require remembering to take a daily pill	• Similar disadvantages to OCPs • Local skin irritation to application site • Less effective for women >198lbs	• Similar contraindications to OCPs • Allergy to adhesive used on patch	93%	99%
Vaginal Ring	• Small, flexible ring that releases combination of estrogen and progestin • Placed into vagina once per month and stays in place for 3 weeks • Similar mechanism of action to OCPs	• Similar advantages to OCPs • Does not require remembering to take a daily pill	• Similar disadvantages to OCPs • Possible increased vaginal irritation and discharge	• Similar contraindications to OCPs • Allergy to vaginal ring	93%	99%

Progesterone-Only Contraceptive Methods

Name	Description or Mechanism of Action	Advantages	Disadvantages/ Side Effects	Contraindications	Reliability with Typical Use	Reliability with Perfect Use
Norethindrone "Mini Pill"	• Progesterone-only • Hormones prevent ovulation and implantation (inhibits midcycle luteinizing hormone surge) • Thickens cervical mucus to prevent sperm from entering uterus • Thins endometrium of uterus	• No estrogen-related side effects (minimal BP, coagulation, glucose interference) • Can be used while breastfeeding • Reduces risk of endometrial cancer • Safer for women who smoke and >35 years old, experience migraine with aura, or history of blood clots	• May cause irregular bleeding • May cause weight gain, mood lability, acne, depression, dizziness • Does not protect against STIs • Pill must be taken at same time everyday	• Women who cannot take the pill at same time everyday • Women with history of breast cancer or unexplained vaginal bleeding	93%	99%
Injectable Depot Medroxy-progesterone Acetate	• Suppresses pituitary follicle stimulation hormone and luteinizing hormone • Prevent ovulation and implantation, thins endometrium of uterus • Thickens cervical mucus to prevent sperm from entering uterus • Injection given once every 3 months	• Similar advantages to mini pill • Does not require pill to be taken at same time everyday	• Similar disadvantages to mini pill • May lead to increased calcium loss and risk of osteoporosis • Decreased bone mineral density • Possible delay in return to fertility • Not usually used for >2 years	• Similar contraindications to mini pill	96%	99%
Hormonal Implant	• Device is implanted into the arm and releases progestin for up to 3 years • Small implant (size of a matchstick)	• Similar advantages to mini pill • Lasts up to 3 years	• Similar disadvantages to mini pill • Incisional procedure (risk of infection, foreign body)	• Similar contraindications to mini pill	99%	99%

Intrauterine Device (IUD) Contraceptive Methods

Name	Description or Mechanism of Action	Advantages	Disadvantages/ Side Effects	Contraindications	Reliability with Typical Use	Reliability with Perfect Use
Levonorgestrel Intrauterine Device (IUD)	• Plastic T-shaped device inserted into uterus • Progesterone-only • Hormones prevent ovulation and implantation (inhibits midcycle luteinizing hormone surge) • Thickens cervical mucus to prevent sperm from entering uterus • Thins endometrium of uterus	• No estrogen-related side effects (minimal BP, coagulation, glucose interference) • Lower rate of hormonal release than other hormonal contraceptives • Lighter, shorter, or absent menses • **Lasts up to 3-5 years**	• May cause irregular bleeding • May cause weight gain, mood lability, acne, depression, dizziness • Does not protect against STIs • Risk of uterine perforation • **Increased risk of ectopic pregnancy and pelvic inflammatory disease**	• Women with abnormally shaped uterus • Women who have or are at-risk for pelvic inflammatory disease, STDs/STIs	99%	99%
Copper Intrauterine Device (IUD)	• Copper wrapped T-shaped device inserted into uterus • Induces foreign-body inflammation creating a hostile environment for sperm and ova; copper is toxic to sperm	• No exogenous hormones • Similar advantages to hormonal IUD • Can use while breastfeeding • **Lasts up to 10 years** • **Can be used for emergency contraception if placed within 5 days of unprotected sex**	• Similar disadvantages to hormonal IUD • Greater risk of cramping • Risk of infertility • **Increased risk of ectopic pregnancy and pelvic inflammatory disease**	• Similar contraindications to hormonal IUD	99%	99%

Emergency Contraceptive Methods

Name	Description or Mechanism of Action	Advantages	Disadvantages/ Side Effects	Contraindications	Reliability with Typical Use	Reliability with Perfect Use
Levonorgestrel or High-Dose Estrogen-Progestin Contraceptive "Morning After Pill"	• **Inhibits or delays ovulation** • Levonorgestrel is preferred method over estrogen-progestin regimen	• **Highly effective** • Gives second-chance to prevent pregnancy after failed contraception or sexual assault • Easily accessible (over the counter)	• **May cause nausea, vomiting, cramps** • Does not protect against STIs • May not be effective for overweight women	• Similar contraindications as OCPs and mini pill • Women who are already pregnant	75%	98%
Ulipristal	• **Progestin receptor modulator that delays ovulation** • Decreases uterine thickness • Must be taken within 5 days after intercourse	• **Highly effective; most effective oral emergency contraceptive** • Gives second-chance to prevent pregnancy after failed contraception or sexual assault	• Headache, nausea, vomiting, abdominal cramping • **Dysmenorrhea** • Does not protect against STIs • Prescription only	• Similar contraindications as OCPs and mini pill • Women who are already pregnant	76%	98%
Copper Intrauterine Device (IUD)	• Copper wrapped T-shaped device inserted into uterus • Induces foreign-body inflammation creating a hostile environment for sperm and ova; copper is toxic to sperm	• No exogenous hormones • Similar advantages to hormonal IUD • Can use while breastfeeding • **Lasts up to 10 years** • **Can be used for emergency contraception if placed within 5 days of unprotected sex**	• Similar disadvantages to hormonal IUD • Risk of infertility • **Increased risk of ectopic pregnancy and pelvic inflammatory disease**	• Similar contraindications to hormonal IUD	99%	99%

Pregnancy

Introduction	• In the United States, 40% of pregnancies are unintended (*unintended does not imply unwanted*) • Early prenatal care is essential to prevent poor perinatal outcomes and complications
Presenting Symptom(s)	• **Patient may present initially with fatigue, nausea/vomiting, urinary frequency, nipple/breast tenderness, increased skin pigmentation, irregular menses or amenorrhea** • **Red flags if patient presents with abdominal/pelvic pain or bleeding**

Diagnosis	• <u>Diagnosis of Pregnancy</u>: confirmed with **beta human chorionic gonadotropin (β-hCG)**
	   • <u>Urine β-hCG</u>: detects pregnancy 14 days after conception
	   • <u>Serum β-hCG</u>: blood tests to quantitatively detect pregnancy as early as 5 days after conception occurs
	     • **In first 4 weeks of pregnancy, β-hCG typically doubles every 48-72 hours (2-3 days)**
	     • After 6 weeks of pregnancy, β-hCG typically doubles every 96 hours (4 days)
	     • After 10 weeks of pregnancy, β-hCG typically peaks and remains constant for remainder of pregnancy

Initial Prenatal Visit	• <u>Thorough History</u>; necessary for risk stratification
	   • <u>Medical History</u>: diabetes, hypertension, obesity, thyroid disease, heart disease, asthma or blood disorder
	   • <u>Surgical History</u>: prior uterine or abdominal incisions including cesarean delivery
	   • <u>Family History</u>: diabetes, genetic disorders, hypertension, or complicated pregnancies
	   • <u>Obstetric History</u>: last menstrual period, preterm births, pregnancy complications, pregnancy losses
	     • <u>Gravida, Para, Abortus (GPA)</u>
	       • <u>Gravida</u>: number of pregnancies (regardless if carried to term)
	       • <u>Para</u>: number of live births or stillbirths (deaths in utero >20 weeks); **multiple gestations count as 1**
	       • <u>Abortus</u>: number of pregnancies ending in death (miscarriage, abortion)
	       • G3P2A1: 3 pregnancies, 2 births, 1 miscarriage (or abortion)
	     • <u>Full-term Births, Pre-term Births, Abortions, Living Children (TPAL)</u>; *often combined with GPA system*
	       • G5P1132: a woman who is not currently pregnant, with history of 1 full-term birth, 1 pre-term birth, 3 abortions or miscarriages, 2 living children
	       • G2P1002: a woman who is currently pregnant, with history of twins in her first pregnancy
	   • <u>Gynecologic History</u>: age of menarche, abnormal bleeding between periods, history of gynecologic infection
	   • <u>Mental Health History</u>: history of anxiety or depression, post-partum depression with prior pregnancies, medications taken
	   • <u>Social History</u>: current or past drug, tobacco, or alcohol use, safety in partnership, education level, income
	   • <u>Nutrition</u>: dietary habits, hydration intake, processed food intake
	   • <u>Exercise</u>: exercise habits prior to becoming pregnant
	   • <u>Medications</u>: daily prescription or over the counter medication use; dietary supplements and vitamins
	   • <u>Exposures</u>: home or occupational exposures to chemicals and cleaners, pollution, smoke

Education	• Education regarding family planning and counseling should be noncoercive and mother or couple provided with full disclosure of risks and benefits

Pregnancy

Physical Exam	• Full general physical exam including blood pressure, height, and weight
	• **BP and weight should be monitored at *every* prenatal visit**
	• <u>Initial Obstetric Exam</u>: **includes speculum and bimanual exam** (checks for lesions or discharge, color of cervix, obtain cervical samples for laboratory testing)
	• <u>Follow-up Obstetric Exam</u>: focus on **uterine size, fundal height, fetal heart rate and activity**; *speculum and bimanual not indicated unless discharge, bleeding, or pain*
	   • <u>Fundal Height</u>: measured in cm from symphysis pubis to top of fundus
	     • <u>12 Weeks</u>: **just above symphysis pubis**
	     • <u>16 Weeks</u>: midway between symphysis pubis and umbilicus
	     • <u>20 Weeks</u>: **at level of umbilicus**
	     • <u>20-36 Weeks</u>: **fundal height (cm) typically matches number of weeks between 20 and 36 weeks**
	     • <u>36 Weeks</u>: at xiphoid process
	     • <u>37-40 Weeks</u>: fundus drops to 36-32cm as presenting part drops into pelvis
	   • If fundal height varies by >2cm may indicate incorrect due date, slow or rapid fetal growth, abnormal amniotic fluid levels, poor maternal nutrition, molar pregnancy, multiple gestation
	• <u>Uterine Changes</u>:
	   • <u>Ladin's Sign</u>: softening of anterior uterus; occurs at 6 weeks' gestation
	   • <u>Hegar's Sign</u>: softening of uterine isthmus (portion of cervix between uterus and vaginal portion of cervix); occurs at 4-6 weeks' gestation
	   • <u>Piskacek's Sign</u>: palpable lateral bulge or soft prominence of uterine corner due to lateral implantation; occurs at 7-8 weeks' gestation
	• <u>Cervical Changes</u>:
	   • <u>Goodell's Sign</u>: softening of the vaginal portion of the cervix due to increased vascularization; occurs around 6 weeks' gestation
	   • <u>Chadwick's Sign</u>: **bluish discoloration of cervix, vagina, and vulva due to increased blood flow**; occurs around 6-8 weeks' gestation
	• <u>Other Body Changes</u>:
	   • <u>Linea Nigra</u>: pigmentation of the linea alba (darkening of the skin at the midline of the abdomen) due to hormonal changes; occurs around 20 weeks' gestation
	   • <u>Breast Changes</u>: **increased breast size; darkening of nipples and areola** due to increase in hormones
	   • <u>Stretch Marks</u>: **separation of underlying connective tissue**; dark red lines that fade to silvery-gray lines after delivery

Calculation of Due Date	• <u>Estimated Date of Delivery - Naegele's Rule</u>
	   • **1st day of last menstrual period minus 3 months, then add 1 year and 7 days**
	   • <u>Example</u>: Last menstrual period began September 9, 2022. Count back 3 months to June 9, 2022. Add 1 year and 7 days. Due date is June 16, 2023.
	   • Note this is based on a normal 28-day menstrual cycle

First Trimester Pregnancy

First Trimester	• First trimester includes week 1-12 of pregnancy • Prenatal visits usually every 4 weeks for low-risk pregnancy

Testing	• **Blood pressure and weight should be monitored at *every* prenatal visit**
	• <u>Prenatal Testing</u>: includes blood, urine and cervical specimens
	   • <u>Blood Tests</u>: **β-hCG,** complete blood count (CBC), blood typing and Rh (D) antibody level, hepatitis B serology, human immunodeficiency virus (HIV), rubella and varicella titers, syphilis serologic test, thyroid stimulating hormone (if history of thyroid disease)
	   • <u>Urine Tests</u>: urinalysis, urine protein and glucose, urine culture (if leukocytes present or concern for UTI)
	   • <u>Cervical Tests</u>: gonorrhea and chlamydia cultures, cervical Papanicolaou (Pap) test (if indicated)
	   • <u>Other Tests</u>: if at risk; tuberculosis screening, sickle cell disease, G6PD
	   • <u>Genetic Screening</u>: biochemical screening test
	      • <u>Serum Pregnancy-Associated Plasma Protein-A (PAPP-A)</u>: low with fetal Down syndrome
	      • <u>Cell-Free DNA Testing</u>: testing for aneuploidy; fetal Down syndrome, trisomy 18 and trisomy 13
	• **<u>Ultrasound</u>: transvaginal preferred**
	   • **Confirms intrauterine pregnancy**
	   • **Confirms gestational age (correlate with last menstrual period)**
	   • **Fetal heart tones may be heard at 5-6 weeks' gestation (transvaginal)** or 10-12 weeks (transabdominal)
	   • Nuchal translucency performed at 10-13 weeks to screen for trisomy 13, 18 and 21 (increased thickness abnormal); if abnormal, chorionic villous sampling offered
	• <u>Chorionic Villus Sampling</u>: chorionic villi are aspirated into a syringe and cultured
	   • **Indicated for women with increased risk of chromosomal abnormalities** (advanced maternal age, abnormal maternal screening tests, prior pregnancy lost or prior pregnancy with chromosomal abnormalities)
	   • Performed around 10-13 weeks' gestation
	   • Allows option of early termination of pregnancy if abnormal, however, is invasive and carries risk of fluid leak and spontaneous abortion

Education	• **<u>Nutrition</u>: consume a real-food, balanced diet with adequate protein**
	   • Patients may need nutritional counseling if vegetarian/vegan, dietary restrictions, allergies or religious/ethical beliefs
	• <u>Exercise</u>: regular aerobic exercise with mild resistance exercise recommended; maintain pre-pregnancy exercise routine
	   • Avoid high-risk recreation activities such as: horseback riding, contact sports (hockey, basketball, soccer, etc.), skiing
	• <u>Prenatal Vitamins</u>: ensures adequate nutrition if diet is not sufficient; **proper folate intake is essential for neural tube development**
	• <u>Recreational Drugs</u>: **recreational drugs including alcohol should be strictly avoided**; linked to various complications and developmental abnormalities
	• <u>Exposure</u>: minimizing exposure to toxins by avoiding secondhand smoke, pesticides/herbicides (consuming organic produce), toxic cleaning chemicals, radiation
	• <u>Dental Care</u>: increased hormones may cause gums to be more edematous and more likely to bleed; proper oral hygiene encouraged
	• <u>Pregnancy Classes and Birth Plan</u>: further educates patient on processes of labor and birth and interventions necessary to safely deliver the infant

Second Trimester Pregnancy

Second Trimester	• Second trimester includes weeks 13-26 of pregnancy • Prenatal visits usually every 4 weeks for low-risk pregnancy

| **Testing** | • **Blood pressure and weight should be monitored at *every* prenatal visit**
• Targeted history, physical exam and limited testing
   • Evaluation of maternal well being
   • Fetal growth and fetal heart tones
   • Targeted questions about changes and symptoms
• **<u>Quad Screening</u>: performed at 16-20 weeks' gestation to screen for aneuploidy;** includes alpha-fetoprotein (AFP), beta human gonadotropin (β-hCG), unconjugated estriol, inhibin-a
   • **<u>Alpha-Fetoprotein (AFP)</u>**: protein produced by fetus; screens for neural tube defects
   • **<u>Beta human gonadotropin (β-hCG)</u>**: hormone produced within placenta
   • **<u>Unconjugated Estriol</u>**: estrogen produced by fetus and placenta
   • **<u>Inhibin-A</u>**: protein produced by placenta and ovaries
• <u>Amniocentesis</u>: performed at 15-18 weeks' gestation
   • Measures alpha-fetoprotein and acetylcholinesterase levels in amniotic fluid
      • **Elevated AFP or presence of acetylcholinesterase may suggest neural tube defect or congenital malformation**
   • Offered to women with prior child with chromosomal abnormality, advanced maternal age (>35 years old), abnormal 1st/2nd trimester screening tests, abnormal ultrasound, or prior pregnancy loss
• <u>Ultrasound</u>: performed around 20 weeks' gestation; transabdominal ultrasound for fetal anatomy (detects congenital malformations) and confirms gestational age |

Quad Screening Results				
Aneuploidy	AFP	β-hCG	Estriol	Inhibin-A
Down Syndrome (Trisomy 21)	Low	Low	High	High
Turner Syndrome	Decreased	Decreased	Very High	Very High
Edwards' Syndrome (Trisomy 18)	Unchanged	Low	Very Low	Unchanged
Patau Syndrome (Trisomy 13)	Increased	Normal	Normal	Normal

| **Education** | • **Discussion about fetal activity**
   • **"Quickening" is small, rapid movements of fetus occurring around 18-22 weeks' gestation**
   • May be described as "butterflies" or "flutters"
   • Typically increase in strength and frequency at night or during periods of rest
   • May encouraged keeping "kick counts"; mother counts fetal movement starting in morning; may stop counting after reaching 10 movements; if noon and no fetal movement, must report to provider for further testing
   • Sudden decrease in fetal activity warrants further investigation
• General education about physiological changes in pregnancy as well as symptoms; nausea/vomiting, GERD, skin changes, bleeding gums or nosebleeds, lower extremity edema, fetal growth, Braxton Hicks contractions, round ligament pain, varicose veins, hemorrhoids, etc. |

Third Trimester Pregnancy

Second Trimester	• Second trimester includes weeks 27-delivery of infant • Prenatal visits usually every 4 weeks for low-risk pregnancy

Testing	• **Blood pressure and weight should be monitored at *every* prenatal visit**
	• Targeted history, physical exam and more specific screening
	• <u>**Gestational Diabetes Screen**</u>: **screening around 24-28 weeks' gestation**
	   • <u>**One-Hour Glucose Challenge Test**</u>: **50g** oral glucose solution; patient takes 50g glucose and has lab value drawn one-hour later
	   • <u>**Three-Hour Glucose Tolerance Test**</u>: **100g** oral glucose solution; **indicated if one-hour test is abnormal(≥130 mg/dL)**
	     • **Considered abnormal if:**
	       • **Fasting glucose >95 mg/dL**
	       • **Glucose at one hour >180 mg/dL**
	       • **Glucose at two hours >155 mg/dL**
	       • **Glucose at three hours >140 mg/dL**
	     • **Presence of 2+ abnormal results establishes gestational diabetes diagnosis**
	   • Women with confirmed gestational diabetes diagnosis should be referred to dietician and appropriate support services
	• <u>**Repeat Rh (D) Antibody**</u>: indicated for Rh-negative women; if unsensitized (Rh negative), should receive Anti-D Rh immunoglobulin at 28 weeks' gestation
	• <u>**Group B *Streptococcus* (GBS) Screening**</u>: performed at 36^{0-7}-37^{0-7} weeks' gestation
	   • GBS frequently colonizes female reproductive tract and may lead to vertical transmission to newborn during labor and delivery
	   • GBS is leading cause of neonatal infection and sepsis in newborns
	   • Rectovaginal screening culture obtained
	   • **If positive, intrapartum antibiotics are given during labor**
	     • **IV Penicillin G is first-line**; Second-line agents include ampicillin, cephalosporins (Cefazolin), clindamycin or IV vancomycin
	• <u>**Nonstress Test**</u>: indicated at 41 weeks' gestation to check amniotic fluid index
	   • Induction likely occurs if natural labor does not occur by 41 weeks' gestation
	• <u>**Other Testing**</u>: syphilis and sexually transmitted disease screening repeated in high-risk women; hemoglobin and hematocrit at 35 weeks

Education	• General education about physiological changes in pregnancy as well as symptoms; nausea/vomiting, loss of appetite, GERD, weight gain, contractions, headache, back pain, vaginal discharge, urinary symptoms, skin changes, bleeding gums or nosebleeds, lower extremity edema, round ligament pain, varicose veins, hemorrhoids, etc. • Education on signs of labor and when to present to hospital; breastfeeding education • Discussion of birth plan and/or induction plans as indicated

Hyperemesis Gravidarum

Etiology & Risk Factors	• <u>**Morning Sickness**</u>: **nausea and/or vomiting until 16 weeks' gestation (most common during first trimester)**
	   • Up to 90% of women will experience nausea during pregnancy
	• <u>**Hyperemesis Gravidarum**</u>: **intractable nausea and/or vomiting associated with weight loss and electrolyte imbalance**
	   • Develops during 1st or 2nd trimester and persists beyond 16 weeks' gestation
	• <u>Etiology</u>: unknown
	• <u>Risk Factors</u>: **primigravida (pregnant for first time)**, **multiple gestations** or molar pregnancy (larger placental mass), history of hyperemesis in previous pregnancy, use of estrogen containing medications, history of migraines, exposure to motion while pregnant

Patho-physiology	• <u>Hormonal Changes</u>: beta-hCG levels peak during first-trimester; estradiol levels increase early in pregnancy and decrease later • <u>Gastrointestinal System Changes</u>: pregnancy causes relaxation of lower esophageal sphincter which leads to increased risk of GERD and nausea
Signs & Symptoms	• **Nausea and vomiting** • **Weight loss** • <u>Physical Exam</u>: • May have dry mucous membranes, reduced skin turgor, delayed capillary refill with **volume depletion**

Diagnosis	• **Clinical Diagnosis**
	• <u>Labs</u>:
	   • <u>Blood</u>: CBC, serum electrolytes, kidney function, thyroid panel, lipase, liver function tests, magnesium, phosphorus
	     • Electrolyte imbalance secondary to vomiting; **hypokalemia, hyperchloremic metabolic alkalosis**
	   • <u>Urine</u>: **ketonuria**, elevated specific gravity

Treatment	• <u>**Lifestyle Modifications**</u>: **initial management**; **ginger supplementation**, switch prenatal vitamins to folic acid supplement only, acupressure wristbands, dietary change (high protein foods, small/frequent meals, avoid spicy/acidic/fatty foods), increased oral hydration
	• <u>**Medications**</u>:
	   • <u>**First-Line**</u>: **Pyridoxine (vitamin B6) with or without doxylamine**
	   • <u>Second-Line</u>: antihistamines (doxylamine, diphenhydramine, dimenhydrinate, meclizine)
	   • <u>Third-Line</u>: dopamine antagonists (prochlorperazine, promethazine, metoclopramide)
	   • Fourth-Line: serotonin antagonist (ondansetron)
	• <u>**Fluid and Electrolyte Replacement**</u>: IV hydration with electrolyte replacement indicated if severe volume loss

Key Words & Most Common	• Intractable nausea/vomiting associated with weight loss + electrolyte imbalance • Clinical diagnosis; vomiting + hypokalemia, ketonuria, volume depletion • Lifestyle modifications • Pyridoxine (B6) +/- doxylamine is first-line

Cervical Insufficiency

Etiology & Risk Factors	• Premature cervical dilation resulting in pregnancy loss in the absence of clinical contractions and/or labor
	   • **Usually occurs in middle to late 2nd trimester or early 3rd trimester**
	• <u>Etiology</u>: congenital or acquired
	   • <u>Congenital</u>: congenital disorders of collagen synthesis (Ehlers-Danlos Syndrome)
	   • <u>Acquired</u>: **multiple gestations**, prior cone biopsy, LEEP (loop electrosurgical excision procedure), **prior deep cervical lacerations (during vaginal or cesarean delivery)**, infection or inflammation

Patho-physiology	• The cervix undergoes extensive remodeling during gestation and parturition; if normal timing is disrupted in biological cascade, the cervix may prematurely ripen resulting in cervical insufficiency, preterm birth or miscarriage

Signs & Symptoms	• **Usually asymptomatic**
	• May have mild symptoms beginning in mid-to-late 2nd trimester
	   • **Pelvic pressure, abdominal cramping, lower backache**
	   • **Vaginal discharge** that increases in volume (clear to pink); spotting
	   • **Braxton-Hix-like contractions**
	• <u>Physical Exam</u>: digital or speculum exam
	   • **Dilation of cervix (>2cm)**
	   • **Effacement of cervix (>80%)**

Diagnosis	• **Clinical Diagnosis** • <u>**Transvaginal Ultrasound**</u>: **most accurate imaging modality** • **Shows short cervical length (≤25mm), protrusion of membranes into dilated internal cervical os** (but with a closed external cervical os)
Treatment	• <u>Conservative</u>: **activity modifications** (no heavy lifting, limited standing/walking/stairs), **modified bedrest, pelvic rest** (no sexual activity) • <u>Vaginal Pessary</u>: small, silicone ring used to provide support to cervix; supports cervical closure by deviating the uterocervical angle • <u>**Cervical Cerclage**</u>: **reinforcement of the cervical ring with nonabsorbable suture material to prevent preterm labor and delivery** • <u>17-Alpha-Hydroxyprogesterone</u>: weekly injection; prevents premature cervical ripening • <u>Corticosteroids</u>: indicated if preterm labor suspected after 22-23 weeks to accelerate fetal lung maturity
Key Words & Most Common	• Premature cervical dilation resulting in loss of pregnancy (mid to late 2nd trimester or early 3rd trimester) • Usually asymptomatic • Pelvic pressure, abdominal cramping, backache, mild contractions, vaginal discharge (may be bloody) • Dilation and effacement of cervix on exam • Clinical diagnosis → transvaginal ultrasound to confirm • Activity modifications, bedrest, pelvic rest → cervical cerclage

Multiple Gestations

Etiology & Risk Factors	• Twin births account for ~3% of all live births in United States and 97% of all multifetal pregnancies • **Considered high-risk pregnancy** • <u>Risk Factors</u>: **ovarian stimulation (clomiphene citrate** or gonadotropins), assisted reproduction (in vitro fertilization), prior multifetal pregnancy, advanced maternal age (>35 years old)

Patho-physiology	• <u>Two types</u>: monozygotic and dizygotic
	   • <u>**Monozygotic (identical)**</u>: occurs when a single ovum is fertilized by a single sperm to form one zygote which divides into two separate embryos
	   • <u>**Dizygotic (fraternal)**</u>: occurs when two ova are fertilized by two different sperm and implants to the uterine wall at the same time

Signs & Symptoms	• **Rapid maternal weight gain** • **Rapid growth of uterus** • **Preterm labor is relatively common**; overdistended uterus may initiate preterm labor • <u>Complications</u>: preeclampsia, gestational diabetes, postpartum hemorrhage, preterm delivery, intrauterine growth restriction, placental abnormalities, breech presentation, umbilical cord prolapse, stillbirth, cesarean delivery, postpartum depression
Diagnosis	• <u>**Ultrasound**</u>: **visualize the fetuses, location, and embryonic heart rate; confirms viable pregnancy** • <u>**Beta Human Chorionic Gonadotropin (hCG)**</u>: urine and/or blood to diagnose pregnancy; often higher than normal • <u>Maternal Serum Alpha-Fetoprotein</u>: higher than normal
Treatment	• <u>**Maternal Support**</u>: **adequate nutrition and hydration**, supplementation with hematinics (substances essential for blood component formation; vitamin B_{12}, folate, iron) • Core and back strengthening exercises (sacroiliac joint dysfunction common later in gestation) • **Cesarean delivery often indicated** (unless presenting twin is in vertex position)
Key Words & Most Common	• Considered high-risk pregnancy • Ovarian stimulation with clomiphene citrate most common • Monozygotic (identical): 1 egg fertilized by 1 sperm → splits to 2 separate embryos • Dizygotic (fraternal): 2 eggs fertilized by 2 sperm → 2 embryos implant to uterine wall • Rapid maternal weight gain and uterine growth • Ultrasound to confirm • Maternal support • C-section often indicated

Placenta Previa

Etiology & Risk Factors	• Implantation of placenta over or close to the internal cervical os • <u>3 Types</u>: complete, partial, marginal (placenta edge within 2cm from internal cervical os) • <u>Etiology</u>: unknown; **cervical scarring** and endometrial damage may contribute • <u>Risk Factors</u>: **history of placenta previa, history of Cesarean section, multiple gestations**, advanced maternal age (>35 years old), smoking, cocaine use, **prior uterine surgery**
Patho-physiology	• Implantation of zygote (fertilized egg) to area of uterus rich in oxygen and collagen to develop into fetal membranes and placenta; uterine scars create ideal environment • Nearly 90% of placenta previa cases where placental edge is between 2-3.5cm from cervical os will resolve as placenta migrates towards increased blood supply of fundus

Signs & Symptoms	• **Painless vaginal bleeding in 2nd or 3rd trimester is most common presentation**
	  • Most common at 28 weeks' gestation
	  • **Bleeding may be provoked by sexual intercourse, vaginal examination (speculum or bimanual exam), labor, or spontaneously**
	  • **Bleeding may be minimal to profuse and is bright-red**
	• **Absence of abdominal/pelvic pain and uterine tenderness**
	• <u>Physical Exam</u>:
	  • **Soft, nontender uterus**
	  • *Digital and speculum exam should be avoided if placenta previa suspected (may lead to massive hemorrhage)*
	  • May visualize placenta on speculum exam if cervix is dilated

Diagnosis	• <u>**Transabdominal Ultrasound**</u>: **initial screening test** • Identifies location of placenta and cervical dilation or effacement before digital or speculum exam is performed • <u>**Transvaginal Ultrasound**</u>: **confirms diagnosis; more sensitive and is considered safe** • <u>Labs</u>: type and screen, CBC (hemoglobin, hematocrit), Rh status, coagulation studies if active bleed • <u>Fetal Heart Rate Monitoring</u>: identify fetal distress (bradycardia)
Treatment	• <u>**Mild First Bleed <36 Weeks**</u>: **hospitalization** for monitoring, **activity modifications** (modified bed rest; avoid long periods of standing, walking, stairs, lifting >20lbs), **pelvic rest** (no sexual intercourse or masturbation); *may be discharged with restrictions if bleeding ceases* • <u>**Mild Second Bleed <36 Weeks**</u>: repeat hospitalization for monitoring; may be kept for observation until delivery • <u>**Mild Bleeding Between 34-36 Weeks**</u>: corticosteroids (accelerates fetal lung maturity) and magnesium sulfate (fetal neuroprotection) given prior to delivery • <u>**Cesarean Delivery**</u>: **indicated for any bleed >36 weeks' gestation, heavy or uncontrolled bleeding, fetal distress (bradycardia), maternal hemodynamic instability** • <u>Vaginal Delivery</u>: may be attempted if "low-lying placenta" (placental edge at least 1.5-2cm from cervical os), no fetal distress and provider is comfortable with method
Key Words & Most Common	• Placenta completely, partially, or marginally covers internal cervical os; most common from prior scarring (cesarean section, surgery, multiple gestations) • Painless vaginal bleeding (2nd/3rd trimester) without abdominal/pelvic pain • Avoid digital and speculum exam • Transabdominal or transvaginal ultrasound • Hospitalization, activity modifications, pelvic rest + Cesarean delivery

Internal os
Placenta is covering cervix preventing a proper birth.

Placental Abruption

Etiology & Risk Factors	• **Premature separation of the placenta from the uterine lining before the second stage of labor** (complete cervical dilation) **after 20 weeks' gestation** • Also called abruptio placentae; true obstetric emergency • <u>Etiology</u>: unknown • <u>Risk Factors</u>: **maternal hypertension is most common cause (chronic, preeclampsia, eclampsia), smoking, cocaine use**, polyhydramnios, **advanced maternal age**, placental ischemia, **trauma** (motor vehicle accident, fall, violence), multiple gestation, prior placental abruption, thrombophilia, history of Cesarean delivery
Patho-physiology	• Rupture of maternal blood vessels as placenta separates away from uterine wall; separation results in bleeding into the decidua basalis behind the placenta (retroplacental) • Blood accumulates and pushes uterine wall and placenta further apart which restricts fetal blood flow leading to fetal distress or death • Blood may also remain behind the placenta (concealed hemorrhage) or drain externally through cervix (external hemorrhage)

Signs & Symptoms	• *Severity of symptoms depends on degree of separation and amount of blood loss*
	• **Sudden onset, painful vaginal bleeding**
	  • **Often dark red**
	  • **Bleeding may be significant**
	• **Severe abdominal pain (uterine contractions)**
	• <u>Physical Exam</u>:
	  • **Tender and rigid (hypertonic) uterus**
	  • If patient has pain/tenderness out of proportion to exam or hypotension and tachycardia, consider concealed hemorrhage
	  • *Do not perform pelvic exam until ultrasound can confirm placental location (exclude placental previa)*

Diagnosis	• **Clinical Diagnosis** • <u>Fetal Heart Rate Monitoring</u>: **identify fetal distress (bradycardia)** • <u>Labs</u>: type and screen, CBC, CMP, Rh status, coagulation studies, **serum fibrinogen (most sensitive indicator)** • <u>Pelvic Ultrasound</u>: may distinguish abruption from previa; lacks sensitivity (normal ultrasound does not rule out placental abruption)
Treatment	• <u>Conservative</u>: hospitalization for observation if pregnancy not near term and mother and fetus are stable; bed rest, pelvic rest • <u>Hemodynamic Support</u>: **fluid and electrolyte replacement**; circulatory, ventilation, and hemodialysis support; **preparation for post-partum hemorrhage** • <u>Medications</u>: corticosteroids (accelerates fetal lung maturity) and magnesium sulfate (fetal neuroprotection) may be given prior to delivery if preterm • <u>**Cesarean Delivery**</u>: **prompt delivery indicated with maternal hemodynamic instability, fetal distress, term pregnancy (≥37 weeks)** • Preterm delivery may be indicated if severe risk for maternal or fetal morbidity/mortality • <u>Vaginal Delivery</u>: may be attempted if mother is stable, no signs of fetal distress and no contraindication (placenta previa)
Key Words & Most Common	• Premature separation of placenta from uterus most commonly caused by maternal hypertension or trauma • Sudden onset, painful vaginal bleeding + abdominal pain • Clinical diagnosis; abnormal coagulation studies and fetal distress supports diagnosis • Hospitalization + hemodynamic support + Cesarean delivery often indicated

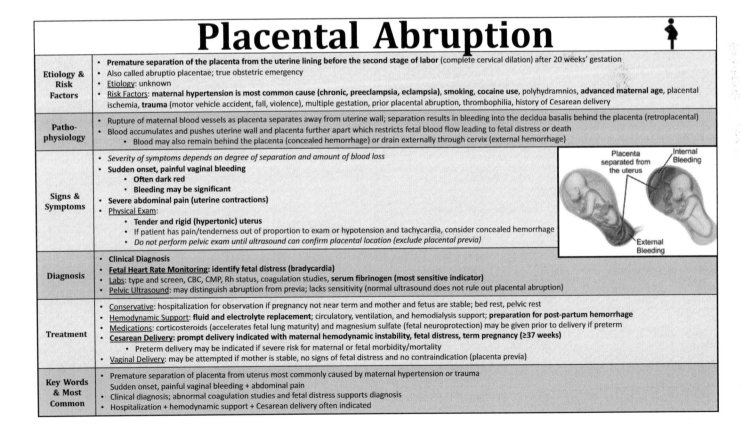

Placenta separated from the uterus
Internal Bleeding
External Bleeding

Hypertension in Pregnancy

Etiology & Risk Factors	• Blood pressure classifications include: normal (<120/80mmHg), elevated (120-129/<80mmHg), stage 1 (130-139/80-89mmHg), or stage 2 (≥140/90mmHg)
	• Hypertension during pregnancy can be classified as:
	  • **Chronic (preexisting): hypertension occurring before pregnancy or before 20 weeks' gestation**
	  • **Gestational: new onset hypertension occurring after 20 weeks' gestation (typically after 37 weeks) and resolves by 6 weeks postpartum**
	• <u>Etiology</u>: vascular insufficiency, uteroplacental blood flow restriction, multiple gestation
	• <u>Risk Factors</u>: history of preeclampsia, **pre-existing hypertension**, **diabetes**, renal disease, nulliparity, **advanced maternal age**, family history of hypertension

Patho-physiology	• Antiangiogenic factors released by placental tissue results in systemic endothelial dysfunction eventually causing systemic hypertension • Underlying etiology is multifactorial
Signs & Symptoms	• **Usually asymptomatic** • Severe features include headache, visual symptoms (blurred vision, scotoma), pulmonary edema (dyspnea, cough), renal impairment (peripheral edema), hepatic impairment (RUQ pain)

Diagnosis	• **Serial blood pressure readings at prenatal visits**
	  • <u>Chronic Hypertension</u>: BP ≥140/90 confirmed on multiple readings at least 4 hours apart occurring before pregnancy or before 20 weeks' gestation
	  • <u>Gestational Hypertension</u>: BP ≥140/90 confirmed on multiple readings at least 4 hours apart occurring after 20 weeks' gestation while pre-pregnancy BP was normal
	• <u>Ultrasound</u>: monthly monitoring of fetal growth to identify if intrauterine growth restriction present
	• <u>Preeclampsia workup</u>: urine protein, CBC (platelet level), CMP (LFTs, BUN/creatinine)

Treatment	• <u>Lifestyle Modifications</u>: proper diet and nutrition, appropriate level of activity, daily blood pressure monitoring • <u>Mild Hypertension</u>: reduction in physical activity may decrease BP and improve fetal growth; if BP does not decrease medical therapy may be necessary • <u>Medications</u>: **labetalol** (beta-blocker), **nifedipine** (calcium channel blocker) or methyldopa are first-line agents • **ACE inhibitors, angiotensin receptor blockers (ARBs) and aldosterone antagonists (spironolactone) are contraindicated in pregnancy**
Key Words & Most Common	• Chronic (preexisting): hypertension occurring before pregnancy or before 20 weeks' gestation • Gestational: new onset hypertension occurring after 20 weeks' gestation (typically after 37 weeks) and resolves by 6 weeks postpartum • Usually asymptomatic • Serial BP readings • Lifestyle modifications • Labetalol, nifedipine, or methyldopa are first-line medications • ACEI, ARBs are contraindicated

Preeclampsia

Etiology & Risk Factors	• **New onset or worsening of existing hypertension (≥140/90) with proteinuria occurring after 20 weeks' gestation +/- signs of end-organ damage** • <u>Etiology</u>: unknown; abnormal placentation may contribute • <u>Risk Factors</u>: **preexisting hypertension**, **advanced maternal age**, nulliparity, **multiple gestation**, **maternal comorbidities (diabetes, obesity, chronic hypertension**, chronic kidney disease, sleep apnea, autoimmune disorders)
Patho-physiology	• Abnormal placentation leads to vascular sclerosis and abnormal placental arteriole remodeling progresses to placental ischemia and the release of antiangiogenic and pro-inflammatory cytokines; inadequate vascular accommodation leads to hypertension and end-organ damage

Signs & Symptoms	• May be asymptomatic if mild
	• **Headache is most common presenting symptom**
	  • May be new-onset or persistent +/- **visual disturbances (photophobia, blurred vision)**
	• **Edema; may be dependent or independent; sudden weight gain (>5lbs per week)**
	  • <u>Independent</u>: **facial or hand swelling**; patient may say a "ring no longer fits"
	  • <u>Dependent</u>: lower extremity swelling; gravity-related
	• **Abdominal pain; right upper quadrant or epigastric pain with associated nausea/vomiting**
	• **Dyspnea**

Diagnosis	• **New onset or worsening of existing hypertension with proteinuria occurring after 20 weeks' gestation and/or signs of end-organ damage**
	• <u>Blood Pressure Criteria</u>: new onset or worsening of existing hypertension
	  • Systolic BP ≥140mmHg and/or diastolic BP ≥90mmHg (on 2 or more measurements taken at least 4 hours apart)
	  • Systolic BP ≥160mmHg and/or diastolic BP ≥110mmHg (at least 1 measurement)
	• <u>Proteinuria</u>: >300mg/24 hours or urine protein/creatinine ratio of ≥0.3 or dipstick 1+ to 2+
	• <u>Evidence of End-Organ Damage</u>: thrombocytopenia (platelets < 100,000/mcL), renal insufficiency (creatinine>1.1mg/dL), hepatic insufficiency (AST/ALT >2x normal limit), pulmonary edema, headache or change in vision
	• <u>Ultrasound</u>: monitoring of fetal well being (growth, intrauterine growth restriction, heart rate, movement)

Treatment	• <u>Blood Pressure Control</u>: **labetalol** (beta-blocker), **nifedipine** (calcium channel blocker) or methyldopa are first-line agents
	• <u>Delivery</u>: prompt delivery of newborn is definitive management
	  • **Indicated for pregnancy of ≥37 weeks, preeclampsia of ≥34 weeks with severe features, deteriorating cardiac/renal/pulmonary function, fetal distress, eclampsia**
	  • <u>≤34 Weeks</u>: stabilization of mother and fetus + corticosteroids for fetal lung maturation + delivery at 34 weeks' gestation or after 48 hours of steroids
	    • *Steroid administration should not delay delivery if severe features present*
	  • <u>34-37 Weeks</u>: prompt delivery in preeclampsia with severe features
	  • <u>≥37 Weeks</u>: prompt delivery + magnesium sulfate (seizure prevention) + blood pressure control

Eclampsia

Etiology & Risk Factors	• **New onset of generalized tonic-clonic seizures in a female with preeclampsia** • <u>Preeclampsia</u>: **New onset or worsening of existing hypertension (≥140/90) with proteinuria occurring after 20 weeks' gestation +/- signs of end-organ damage** • **Seizures may occur between 20 weeks' gestation to 4 weeks' postpartum** • <u>Etiology</u>: unclear • <u>Risk Factors</u>: **preexisting hypertension, advanced maternal age**, nulliparity, **multiple gestation**, maternal comorbidities (**diabetes, obesity, chronic hypertension**, chronic kidney disease, sleep apnea, autoimmune disorders)
Patho-physiology	• Preeclampsia caused by an abnormal blood supply causing uterine arterial resistance/vasoconstriction leading to placental ischemia, oxidative stress and release of antiangiogenic and pro-inflammatory cytokines that disrupt proper maternal endothelial function • Dysfunction of endothelium may occur at cerebral endothelium leading to neurological disorder

Signs & Symptoms	• **Preeclampsia + generalized tonic-clonic seizures**
	   • Usually last 60-90 seconds in duration
	   • Post-ictal state often present

Diagnosis	• **New onset or worsening of existing hypertension, proteinuria occurring after 20 weeks' gestation, signs of end-organ damage and seizures** • <u>Ultrasound</u>: monitoring of fetal well being (growth, intrauterine growth restriction, heart rate, movement)

Treatment	• <u>Secure Airway</u>: airway control to prevent aspiration of oral secretions; roll on left side + suction or intubation
	• <u>Magnesium Sulfate</u>: **first-line treatment to control convulsions and prevents seizure recurrence**
	   • May be given prophylactically to patient with severe preeclampsia
	   • Lorazepam may be used if seizures refractory to magnesium sulfate
	• <u>Blood Pressure Stabilization</u>: **IV labetalol or hydralazine first-line**
	• <u>Delivery</u>: **delivery of fetus is definitive**; delivery should be as soon as mother is stabilized

Key Words & Most Common	• New onset of generalized tonic-clonic seizures in female with preeclampsia
	• <u>Preeclampsia</u>: New onset or worsening of existing hypertension (≥140/90) with proteinuria occurring after 20 weeks' gestation +/- signs of end-organ damage
	• Preeclampsia + generalized tonic-clonic seizures
	   • Preeclampsia symptoms may include headache, edema, vision changes, abdominal pain, dyspnea
	   • Preeclampsia diagnosed with BP>140/90 + proteinuria (>300mg/24 hours or urine protein/creatinine ratio of ≥0.3 or dipstick 1+ to 2+) + end-organ damage
	• Secure airway
	• Magnesium sulfate is first-line → BP stabilization (labetalol or hydralazine) → delivery

Gestational Diabetes

Etiology & Risk Factors	• Glucose intolerance with onset or first recognition during pregnancy; usually subsides postpartum • <u>Etiology</u>: **insulin resistance secondary to placental hormone release, pancreatic beta-cell dysfunction** • <u>Risk Factors</u>: **obesity, sedentary lifestyle**, prior or family history of gestational diabetes, newborn with macrosomia, PCOS, Hgb A1c >5.7, multiple gestations
Patho-physiology	• Placental release of diabetogenic hormones; human placental lactogen provokes and alters insulin receptors which subsequently reduces glucose uptake within the tissue • Maternal hyperglycemia can translate to fetal hyperglycemia and fetal pancreas stimulation; insulin has anabolic properties which promotes fetal tissue growth (macrosomia)

Signs & Symptoms	• Disproportionate weight gain, obesity, elevated BMI
	• <u>Fetal Complications</u>:
	   • **Fetal hyperinsulinemia leads to fetal macrosomia**; macrosomia predisposes to birth injuries (**shoulder dystocia**), preterm labor, delayed fetal lung maturity, **neonatal hypoglycemia**, fetal hyperbilirubinemia, neonatal hypocalcemia and hypomagnesemia
	• <u>Maternal Complications</u>:
	   • >50% chance to develop type 2 diabetes after pregnancy and recurrence of gestational diabetes with subsequent pregnancies
	   • **Preeclampsia**, placental abruption

Diagnosis	• <u>Gestational Diabetes Screen</u>: **screening around 24-28 weeks' gestation**
	   • <u>One-Hour Glucose Challenge Test</u>: 50g oral glucose solution; patient takes 50g glucose and has lab value drawn one-hour later
	   • <u>Three-Hour Glucose Tolerance Test</u>: 100g oral glucose solution; **indicated if one-hour test is abnormal (≥130 mg/dL); diagnostic gold standard**
	      • *Presence of 2+ abnormal results establishes gestational diabetes diagnosis*
	         • **Fasting glucose >95 mg/dL**
	         • **Glucose at one hour >180 mg/dL**
	         • **Glucose at two hours >155 mg/dL**
	         • **Glucose at three hours >140 mg/dL**

Treatment	• <u>Lifestyle Modifications</u>: **diet modification** (low-carbohydrate), **exercise** (walking), **glucose monitoring** (daily fasting and postprandial glucose measure) • Women with confirmed gestational diabetes diagnosis should be referred to dietician and appropriate support services • <u>Medical Management</u>: indicated when adequate glucose levels (fasting glucose >95mg/dL and postprandial glucose >130-140mg/dL) are unachievable with diet and exercise • <u>Insulin</u>: **first-line medical therapy** (does not cross placenta); goal is fasting glucose <95mg/dL • <u>Oral Hypoglycemic Agents</u>: **metformin or glyburide** are relatively safe if patient is noncompliant or refuses insulin therapy • <u>Labor Induction</u>: occurs at 38-39 weeks in uncontrolled diabetes or evidence of macrosomia; if macrosomia present Cesarean delivery often indicated • *After delivery of placenta, most cases of gestational diabetes resolve* • Antenatal blood glucose monitoring for mother and newborn; newborn can get hypoglycemia during postpartum period

Labor and Delivery

Termin-ology	• **Braxton-Hicks Contractions:** spontaneous contractions of the uterus occurring in 2nd and 3rd trimester *without cervical dilation*; also known as prodromal or false labor pains • **Ruptured Membranes:** rupture of amniotic sac leading to leakage of amniotic fluid; also known as "water breaking" • **Lightening:** fetal head descends into pelvis in preparation of delivery; also known as "dropping" • **Bloody Show:** passage of small amount of blood or blood-tinged cervical mucus; occurs with detachment of cervical mucus plug and cervical effacement before delivery • **True Labor:** regular and painful contractions of uterine fundus leading to cervical dilation and effacement; pain may radiate to lower back, pelvis or abdomen
Cardinal Movements of Labor	**7 Cardinal Movements of Labor** 1. **Engagement:** when greatest transverse diameter (biparietal diameter) of the head in vertex presentation enters the pelvic inlet 2. **Descent:** downward movement of the fetal head deep into pelvic cavity 3. **Flexion:** fetal vertex meets resistance from cervix, pelvic floor, and walls of pelvis; flexion of fetal chin against chest to reduce diameter of presenting part 4. **Internal Rotation:** at pelvic inlet, the pelvis is widest right to left; at pelvic outlet, pelvis is widest front to back; fetal vertex rotates from sideways position to position in which the sagittal suture is parallel to the anteroposterior diameter of the pelvis 5. **Extension:** resistance from the pelvic floor causes fetal head to extend so the nuchal can pass under the pubic symphysis 6. **External Rotation:** after fetal head is delivered, the fetus externally rotates so the shoulders can be delivered 7. **Expulsion:** the rest of the body is delivered more smoothly after head and shoulders are delivered

Stages of Labor

Stage I	• **Begins with onset of true labor (regular uterine contractions) and ends with full cervical dilation to 10cm** • Labor begins when uterine contractions become strong and regularly spaced at approximately 3 to 5 minutes apart; progressive cervical effacement and dilation • **Latent Phase:** 0-6cm cervical dilation; cervical effacement (thinning) occurs with gradual cervical dilation • **Active Phase:** 6-10cm cervical dilation; more rapid cervical dilation (1.2-1.5cm per hour)
Stage II	• **Begins with cervical dilation to 10cm and ends with delivery of the neonate** • **Passive Phase:** time from complete (10cm) cervical dilation to active maternal expulsive efforts (pushing) • **Active Phase:** time from active maternal expulsive efforts (pushing) to delivery of the neonate
Stage III	• **Begins with delivery of the neonate and ends with delivery of the placenta** • Expulsion of placenta typically takes between 5-30 minutes • **Three Cardinal Signs: gush of blood at the vagina, lengthening of the umbilical cord and a globular shaped uterine fundus on palpation** • Management of the third stage includes traction applied to umbilical cord with simultaneous fundal pressure to aid in faster delivery of placenta
Stage IV	• **Begins with delivery of the placenta and ends 1-2 hours after delivery** • Recovery period where mother engages in skin-to-skin contact with neonate, initiation of breastfeeding (decreases risk of hemorrhage by facilitating uterine contractions) • Mother assessed for complications (address any hemorrhage; provider may have to repair an incision (episiotomy) or tears (lacerations) made during the delivery)

Postpartum

Postpartum Period	• Postpartum period begins following expulsion of the placenta and ends with complete physiologic recovery of organ systems
Fetal Care	• APGAR Score: Apgar scoring performed on all infants at 1 and 5 minutes after birth • Score is 1-10; ≥7 is reassuring; 4-6 is moderately abnormal; ≤3 is critically low • Vitamin K administration to prevent bleeding risk

Postpartum Changes	• Breasts: breastmilk production initiates in large amounts 2-4 days after delivery
	   • Colostrum: special yellowish milk only secreted in first 2-3 days after delivery
	     • Rich in vitamins (particularly A, E), white blood cells, and antibodies (especially IgA)
	   • Transition Milk: mature breast milk (may be bluish-white) that gradually replaces colostrum
	     • Starts 2-5 days after delivery until up to 2 weeks after delivery
	   • Mature Milk: mature breast milk to replaces transition milk (increased fat content)
	     • Starts 15 days after delivery
	• Lochia Serosa: pink/brown vaginal bleeding during postpartum period and lasts 3-4 weeks; due to decidual tissue (maternal uterine tissue)
	   • Initially red (comprised of blood and decidual tissue, endometrial tissue) lasting 1-4 days
	   • Changes to yellowish/pale brown (comprised of blood, mucus, and leukocytes) lasting 5-9 days
	   • Becomes white (comprised of mostly mucus) lasting 10-14 days; can persist up to 5 weeks postpartum
	• Menstruation/Ovulation: Patient education and contraceptive methods should be discussed
	   • Mother may be anovulatory while lactating
	   • Ovarian function may return within 3 weeks postpartum (typically 6-8 weeks) if not breastfeeding
	• Uterus: uterine fundus at umbilicus after delivery and continues to shrink; descends into pelvic cavity around 2 weeks postpartum; **normal size around 6 weeks postpartum**
	   • Rapid uterine contraction may cause abdominal/pelvic cramping

APGAR Scoring System

Sign	0 Points	1 Point	2 Points
Appearance (skin color changes)	Blue-gray, pale	Pink body, blue extremities	Pink all over (no cyanosis)
Pulse	Absent	<100 BPM	≥100 BPM
Grimace (reflex irritability)	Floppy (no response to stimulation)	Minimal response to stimulation	Prompt response to stimulation (pulls away, sneezes, coughs)
Activity (muscle tone)	Absent	Flexed arms and legs	Active movement (flexes arms/legs, resists extension)
Respiration	Absent	Slow, weak, irregular	Vigorous cry

Postpartum Hemorrhage

Etiology & Risk Factors	• **Blood loss of >500mL associated with vaginal delivery or >1,000mL associated with Cesarean delivery and accompanied by signs and symptoms of hypovolemia**
	• Most common cause of maternal death worldwide
	• <u>Etiology</u>: **4 T's**
	  • <u>Tone</u>: **uterine atony is most common cause** (lack of effective contraction of the uterus to stop bleeding)
	  • <u>Tissue</u>: **retained placental tissue**
	  • <u>Trauma</u>: **cervical, perineum or vaginal trauma or lacerations,** uterine rupture
	  • <u>Thrombin</u>: coagulation disorders (hemophilia, von Willebrand disease, idiopathic thrombocytopenic purpura (ITP) or disseminated intravascular coagulation (DIC))
	• <u>Risk Factors</u>: **rapid labor, prolonged labor, uterine overdistention** (multiple gestations, polyhydramnios), **Cesarean,** intra-amniotic infection, anesthesia, **uterine inversion**

Patho-physiology	• Blood vessels of the uterus pass through the myometrium; after labor, the uterine myometrium contracts to provide pressure hemostasis after delivery of the fetus and placenta; failure to contract (uterine atony) prevents this hemostasis to occur leading to hemorrhage
Signs & Symptoms	• **Acute, post-partum vaginal bleeding** • <u>Signs of Hypovolemia</u>: **tachycardia,** tachypnea, **hypotension, weakness,** decreased capillary refill, syncope • <u>Physical Exam</u>: • **Soft, "boggy", non-contracted uterus with dilated cervix**
Diagnosis	• **Clinical Diagnosis** • <u>Labs</u>: **CBC** (hemoglobin, hematocrit, platelets), **coagulation studies** and fibrinogen, type and screen • <u>Ultrasound</u>: may aid it detection of source of bleed or retained placental tissue

Treatment	• **Fluid resuscitation vs blood products for hemodynamic stability** • **Treat Underlying Cause:**		

Tone	Tissue	Trauma	Thrombin

• **Bimanual Uterine Massage is first-line response**
• <u>**Uterotonic Medications**</u> to induce uterine contractions
  • **IV Oxytocin is first-line**
  • Misoprostol, methylergonovine
	• **Suture lacerations** with absorbable sutures	• Detect retained placental tissue with ultrasound
		• Manual removal or curettage
			• Reverse any coagulopathies

Treatment	• **Uterine Inversion:** manually elevate posterior fornix → discontinue uterotonic agents → initiate uterine relaxing agent (nitroglycerin, magnesium sulfate, terbutaline)
Key Words & Most Common	• Blood loss >500mL with vaginal; >1,000mL with C-section • Uterine atony most common cause • Acute vaginal bleeding + tachycardia/hypotension • Resuscitation → bimanual uterine massage + oxytocin

Premature Rupture of Membranes

Etiology & Risk Factors	• **Rupture of amniotic membranes prior to the onset of labor** • Preterm premature rupture of membranes (PPROM) refers to rupture of amniotic membranes prior to the onset of labor prior to 37 weeks' gestation • <u>Etiology</u>: physiologic weakening of membranes, uterine contraction forces • <u>Risk Factors</u>: **short cervical length,** 2nd or 3rd trimester vaginal bleeding, **uterine overdistention (multiple gestations,** polyhydramnios), nutritional deficiencies (copper and vitamin C), low body mass index, low socioeconomic status, **smoking,** sexually transmitted infections (STIs)
Patho-physiology	• Local cytokines, proteinase imbalance, increased collagenase and protease activities result in increased intrauterine pressure and membrane weakening
Signs & Symptoms	• **Leakage or sudden gush of fluid from vagina** • Also known as "water broke" • Fever, foul-smelling vaginal discharge, abdominal pain and fetal tachycardia suggests intra-amniotic infection.

Diagnosis	• **Clinical Diagnosis**
	• **Sterile Speculum Exam: visualization of amniotic fluid passing from cervical canal and pooling in vagina (posterior fornix)**
	  • Cultures, Nitrazine paper test or fern test
	    • <u>**Nitrazine Paper Test**</u>: **detects alkalinity and turns blue if pH>6.5 (normal amniotic fluid pH is 7.1-7.3; vaginal secretion pH is 4.5-6.0)**
	    • <u>Fern Test</u>: amniotic fluid dries in fern pattern (estrogen and amniotic fluid crystallization)
	• <u>Ultrasound</u>: **confirmatory test;** detects oligohydramnios (amniotic fluid volume (AFV) less than the minimum expected for gestational age)
	• *Avoid digital examination to reduce risk of infection*

Treatment	• <u>Expectant Management</u>: admission to hospital for fetal monitoring, activity modifications (modified bedrest), complete pelvic rest, monitor for signs of infection • 90% will go into spontaneous labor within 24 hours • <u>**Antibiotics**</u>: **IV ampicillin + erythromycin *or* azithromycin to prevent infection** (chorioamnionitis or endometritis) • <u>Corticosteroids</u>: **betamethasone; administered to enhance fetal lung maturity; indicated if pregnancy <34 weeks' gestation** • <u>Magnesium Sulfate</u>: consider in pregnancy <32 weeks' gestation to prevent severe neurological dysfunction • <u>Labor Induction</u>: if labor does not occur spontaneously; **prompt delivery if maternal or fetal infection/distress present**
Key Words & Most Common	• Rupture of amniotic membranes prior to onset of labor • Short cervical length, uterine distention (twins), smoking • Leaking or sudden gush of fluid from vagina "water broke" • Clinical diagnosis + sterile speculum exam • Expectant management: admit for monitoring • Antibiotics (ampicillin + erythromycin/azithromycin) to prevent infection

Preterm Labor

Etiology & Risk Factors	• **Labor occurring between 20-36 weeks' gestation**
	   • Labor begins when uterine contractions become strong and regularly spaced at approximately 3 to 5 minutes apart with progressive cervical effacement and dilation
	   • <u>Early Preterm</u>: occurs prior to 33 weeks' gestation
	   • <u>Late Preterm</u>: occurs between 34-36 weeks' gestation
	• <u>Etiology</u>: **stress, infection, cervical insufficiency**, placenta previa or placenta abruption, preterm premature rupture of membranes
	• <u>Risk Factors</u>: inadequate prenatal care, smoking, maternal age <18 or >40 years old, oligohydramnios or polyhydramnios, illicit drug use

Patho-physiology	• Increased cortisol from stress may cause an influx of inflammatory cells into the cervical stroma leading to cytokine and prostaglandin release and stimulating cervical ripening • Inflammatory response syndrome as a result of infection leads to systemic inflammation which triggers parturition pathway to activate
Signs & Symptoms	• **Contractions (abdominal, pelvic, or lower back pain)** • **May experience rupture of membranes** (gush of fluid with leakage of fluid from the vagina) • <u>Physical Exam</u>: • Determine cervical dilation and effacement; **if cervical dilation >2-3cm and >80% effacement, patient is highly likely to deliver**
Diagnosis	• **Clinical Diagnosis** • <u>Infection Workup</u>: urinalysis and urine culture, rectovaginal Group B *Streptococcus* (GBS) culture, STI screen • <u>Ultrasound</u>: determines cervical dilation and effacement; helps distinguish cervical effacement due to cervical insufficiency vs active labor

Treatment	• <u>Conservative</u>: **admit for maternal and fetal monitoring**, if no progressive cervical dilation/effacement and no fetal distress, patient discharged home with restrictions (activity modifications, modified bed rest, complete pelvic rest) if >34 weeks' gestation
	• <u>Corticosteroids</u>: decreases incidence of respiratory distress syndrome and neonatal mortality if <34 weeks' gestation
	   • **Betamethasone given to enhance fetal lung maturity**
	• <u>Tocolytics</u>: used to delay delivery up to 48 hours for corticosteroid administration if <34 weeks' gestation
	   • **Magnesium sulfate exposure demonstrates fetal neuroprotection against severe motor dysfunction**
	• <u>Antibiotics</u>: given as prophylaxis for GBS
	   • **Penicillin G or ampicillin are first-line**; cefazolin, clindamycin or vancomycin as alternatives
	• <u>Progestins</u>: recommended in future pregnancies for women who have a preterm delivery to reduce the risk of recurrence
	   • **17-alpha-hydroxyprogesterone caproate** administered via weekly injection

Key Words & Most Common	• Labor occurring between 20-36 weeks' gestation • Stress, infection, cervical insufficiency • Contractions +/- rupture of membranes • Clinical diagnosis • Corticosteroids (enhance fetal lung maturity) + tocolytic (fetal neuroprotection) + antibiotics (prophylaxis for GBS) if <34 weeks' gestation

Shoulder Dystocia

Etiology & Risk Factors	• **Complication during vaginal delivery in which the baby's anterior shoulder is caught above the mother's pubic bone; considered obstetric emergency** • <u>Etiology</u>: mechanical problem during vaginal delivery • <u>Risk Factors</u>: **fetal macrosomia (diabetes) is greatest risk factor**, post-term pregnancy, **small maternal pelvis or short maternal stature**, multiple gestation, **prolonged second stage of labor**, maternal obesity, advanced maternal age, induction of labor

Patho-physiology	• Mechanical obstruction in which anterior shoulder of baby is unable to traverse the pelvis during delivery of fetal head
	• <u>Fetal Complications</u>: **brachial plexus injuries is most common; clavicular fractures**, long bone fractures, fetal asphyxia, anoxic brain injury, death
	   • <u>Upper Lesions</u>: lateral flexion of head away from affected shoulder
	     • Results in "waiter's tip" palsy (adducted extremity that is internally rotated at shoulder, extended at elbow and pronated at forearm)
	   • <u>Lower Lesions</u>: traction with shoulder in full abduction
	     • Results in "claw hand" palsy (extreme wrist extension, metacarpophalangeal hyperextension and flexion of interphalangeal joints)
	• <u>Maternal Complications</u>: **postpartum hemorrhage**, uterine rupture, perineal/vaginal tearing

Signs & Symptoms	• **Obstructed labor** • <u>Turtle Sign</u>: retraction of baby's head toward the perineum after delivery of fetal head; rare
Diagnosis	• **Clinical Diagnosis** • Head-to-body delivery interval >60seconds

Treatment	• <u>First-Line Maneuvers</u>: *may be combined with extending episiotomy*
	   • **McRoberts Maneuver**: patient's hips are hyperflexed and abducted towards the abdomen to straighten maternal sacrum on lumbar spine
	   • **Suprapubic Pressure**: pressure applied to suprapubic area in downward or rocking motion; attempts to adduct anterior shoulder
	• <u>Second-Line Maneuvers</u>:
	   • Rubin's Maneuver: hand is placed into vagina with pressure to posterior shoulder to attempt fetal shoulder adduction to allow anterior shoulder rotation and delivery
	   • Woods Corkscrew Maneuver: hand placed to anterior aspect of posterior fetal shoulder; shoulder rotated towards back to rotate fetal shoulder 180°
	   • Delivery of Posterior Arm: posterior forearm/wrist of fetus is swept anteriorly across fetal chest to deliver
	   • Gaskin Maneuver: patient on hands and knees (all-fours position), downward traction applied to posterior shoulder
	• <u>Heroic Measures</u>: *last-resort measures when all other maneuvers have failed*
	   • Intentional Clavicle Fracture: fetal clavicle is intentionally fracture to deliver infant; may damage underlying neurovascular structures
	   • Zavanelli Maneuver: fetal head is reduced back into vaginal canal; patient is immediately transported for Cesarean section

Key Words & Most Common	• Complication in which baby's anterior shoulder is mechanically obstructed behind mother's pubic bone • Obstructed labor; turtle sign • Clinical diagnosis • McRoberts maneuver

Breech Presentation

Etiology & Risk Factors	• Breech describes fetal position in which the presenting part is the buttocks or lower extremities • <u>Etiology</u>: **increased or decreased fetal motility** or conditions affecting vertical polarity of uterus (fibroids, placental previa, maternal abdominal wall laxity) • <u>Risk Factors</u>: **prematurity**, **multiple gestations**, congenital anomalies, aneuploidy, fibroids, placental previa
Patho-physiology	• Conditions affecting polarity of uterus inhibit the ability of fetus to turn into vertex position

Signs & Symptoms	• Mother is often asymptomatic
	• 3 Types: frank, complete, incomplete
	  • <u>Frank</u>: both hips are flexed and both knees are extended with feet near fetal face; "pike position" (**most common type**)
	  • <u>Complete</u>: both hips and both knees are flexed; "tuck position"
	  • <u>Incomplete</u>: one or both of the hips are flexed; "footling position"
	• Physical Exam:
	  • <u>Leopold Maneuver</u>: 4 maneuvers to determine estimated fetal weight and presenting position of fetus
	  • Round, hard, mobile structure at fundus and inability to palpate presenting part

Diagnosis	• **Clinical Diagnosis using Leopold maneuver** • **Ultrasound**: fetal lie and presenting part is visualized confirmed
Treatment	• **Immediate OB/GYN consult**: *Zavanelli maneuver may be considered* • <u>Zavanelli Maneuver</u>: fetal head is reduced back into vaginal canal; patient is immediately transported for Cesarean section • **External Cephalic Version**: maneuver to externally rotate fetus into vertex position before labor • <u>Trial of Labor</u>: vaginal breech birth may be attempted if delivery provider is comfortable and mother has low risk of labor or delivery-related complications • **Cesarean Delivery**: C-section significantly decreases perinatal morbidity and mortality versus intended vaginal delivery,
Key Words & Most Common	• Fetal position where presenting part is buttocks or lower extremities • Frank is most common type (hips flexed, knees extended) • Increased/decreased fetal motility or conditions changing vertical polarity of uterus • Leopold maneuver to determine position • Clinical diagnosis + US confirmation • External cephalic version → trial of labor • C-Section

Cesarean Delivery

Etiology & Risk Factors	• **Surgical delivery of fetus by incision into the uterus** • Up to 30% of deliveries in US are Cesarean • **Higher rate of morbidity and mortality than vaginal delivery**
	• **Indicated when safer for mother and/or fetus than vaginal delivery** • <u>Specific Indications</u>: **failure to progress during labor (most common)**, **previous Cesarean delivery**, maternal request, pelvic disproportion, HIV/HSV infection, fetal dystocia, **breech presentation**, **fetal distress** (bradycardia) requiring rapid delivery, **placenta previa**, multiple gestations, maternal hypertension, suspected macrosomia, uterine rupture • *Woman with previous Cesarean delivery is a common indication due to risk of uterine rupture with attempted vaginal delivery after Cesarean section*
Patho-physiology	• Surgeon must traverse all layers between that separate skin from the fetus • Skin → subcutaneous tissue → rectus abdominis fascia → external oblique rectus muscle aponeurosis and transverse abdominis/internal oblique muscle aponeurosis (separates rectus muscles) → parietal peritoneum → uterus → amniotic sac (if present)
Signs & Symptoms	• No true medical contraindications • Ethically, can be contraindicated if mother refuses Cesarean delivery with informed consent
Diagnosis	• Cesarean delivery carries a 20x increased risk of infection • Preoperative prophylactic antibiotics reduce risk of infection by 60-70% • **Single IV dose 1g cephazolin is first-line** • 500mg azithromycin added if Cesarean delivery performed after rupture of membranes or intrapartum due to risk of exposure to vaginal flora • Clindamycin and gentamicin indicated if penicillin-allergic
Treatment	• <u>Mother</u>: **postpartum hemorrhage is greatest risk, infection**, bladder or bowel perforation, reaction to anesthesia, thromboembolism, increased risk during future pregnancies • <u>Fetus</u>: **transient tachypnea, skin lacerations**, clavicle or skull fracture, brachial plexus injury • Long term complications include altered immune development, reduced gut microbiome diversity, increased risk of developing allergies/asthma
Key Words & Most Common	• Mechanical thromboprophylaxis for all women (compression stockings, intermittent pneumatic compression) • Pharmacologic thromboprophylaxis for high-risk women with low molecular weight heparin (LMWH) or unfractionated heparin (UFH) • Held until 6-12 hours postoperatively due to concern of postpartum hemorrhage; continue until mother is ambulatory

Uterine Rupture

Etiology & Risk Factors	• **Complete division of the three layers of the uterus; the endometrium (inner epithelial layer), myometrium (smooth muscle layer), and perimetrium (serosal outer surface)** • Uterine dehiscence is similar condition characterized by incomplete division of the uterus that does not penetrate all layers (peritoneum remains intact) • *Life threatening to both mother and fetus* • Etiology: **healed scar line from prior Cesarean section**; uterine distention, external fetal version, iatrogenic perforation, trauma (motor vehicle accident) Risk Factors: **prior Cesarean section is greatest risk factor**, malpresentation, multiple gestation, polyhydramnios, hypertension, prior myomectomy, use of misoprostol
Patho-physiology	• Previous Cesarean section incision creates weak-point through the three layers of the uterus • Increased pressure within the uterus from contractions, manual pressure, or trauma leads to complete transection at the point of weakness

Signs & Symptoms	• **Acute onset of severe abdominal pain with peritoneal signs**
	   • May be described as "ripping" or "tearing" sensation
	• **Decreased or absent uterine contractions**
	• **Vaginal bleeding**
	• **Fetal bradycardia, reduced variability, late decelerations**
	• Physical Exam:
	   • **Palpable uterine defect**
	   • **Loss of fetal station** (movement of the fetal presenting part towards the abdominal cavity if part of fetus enters the peritoneum)

Diagnosis	• **Clinical Diagnosis** • Labs: CBC (hemoglobin/hematocrit), coagulations studies, type and screen • Ultrasound: may be used to rule out other etiologies of vaginal bleeding including placenta previa, placental abruption or spontaneous abortion • Laparotomy: confirms diagnosis when hemoperitoneum and fetal parts are identified • *Due to emergent nature of uterine rupture, imaging and laboratory tests performed after mother and fetus stabilized*
Treatment	• **Emergent Cesarean Delivery**: immediate delivery of fetus reduces fetal and maternal mortality • **Exploratory Laparotomy**: identifies source of hemorrhage; repair of uterus or **hysterectomy** indicated • **Fluid resuscitation, blood product replacement, airway management**
Key Words & Most Common	• Complete division of 3 layers of uterus • Healed scar line from prior C-section • Acute onset abdominal pain + peritoneal signs • Vaginal bleeding + palpable uterine defect + loss of fetal station • Fetal bradycardia • Clinical diagnosis • Emergent Cesarean delivery + exploratory laparotomy +/- hysterectomy

Umbilical Cord Prolapse

Etiology & Risk Factors	• Umbilical cord exits the cervical os before the presenting part of the fetus; compression results in vasoconstriction and fetal hypoxia • Etiology: **iatrogenic is most common (external cephalic version in setting of ruptured membranes), low-birth weight**, preterm delivery, umbilical cord abnormalities • Risk Factors: **malpresentation**, multiple gestations, preterm rupture of membranes, **intrauterine growth restriction (low-birth weight)**, preterm delivery, polyhydramnios
Patho-physiology	• Presenting part of fetus is not large enough to fill the lower uterus allowing the umbilical cord to present first during labor • Manual compression of the umbilical cord by the descending fetus during delivery leads to fetal hypoxia and bradycardia

Signs & Symptoms	• **Fetal bradycardia**
	   • May be sudden in onset and prolonged
	   • Variable deceleration after previously normal tracing
	• Physical Exam:
	   • **Umbilical cord may be palpable or visualized on vaginal examination; pulsating structure within the vaginal vault**

Diagnosis	• **Clinical Diagnosis**

Treatment	• **Delivery is definitive management**
	   • **Cesarean section is most common delivery method**
	   • Vaginal delivery is option if impending delivery and may be faster
	• **Umbilical Cord Decompression:**
	   • **Manual elevation of fetal presenting part to reduce compression**
	   • Place patient in knee-to-chest position and encourage to not push or cough
	   • Place patient in Trendelenburg to use gravity assist in moving fetus from pelvic floor
	• *Do NOT attempt to reduce umbilical cord*

Key Words & Most Common	• Umbilical cord exits cervical os before fetus leading to compression • Iatrogenic cause is most common • Low-birth weight • Fetal bradycardia • Pulsating structure within vaginal vault • Clinical diagnosis • Delivery via C-section • Cord decompression methods

Spontaneous Abortion

Etiology & Risk Factors	• **Loss of pregnancy prior to 20 weeks of gestation**; often referred to as **"miscarriage"** • <u>Etiology</u>: **fetal chromosomal abnormalities most common, maternal reproductive tract abnormalities** (fibroids, intrauterine adhesions), viral infection (cytomegalovirus, herpesvirus, parvovirus, rubella), autoimmune conditions, trauma, antiphospholipid syndrome, Rh isoimmunization, malnutrition, chronic disease (diabetes, hypertension) • <u>Risk Factors</u>: **advanced maternal age (>35 years old)**, history of spontaneous abortion, drug use (cocaine, alcohol), **cigarette smoking**, poorly controlled chronic disease
Patho-physiology	• Chromosomal abnormalities result in nonviable pregnancy • Multiple types including threatened, inevitable, incomplete, complete, missed, septic
Signs & Symptoms	• **Vaginal bleeding is most common symptom** (with or without pain) • **Crampy abdominal or pelvic pain** • Emotional symptoms such as anxiety, guilt, sadness, feeling of inadequacy may follow
Diagnosis	• <u>**Beta Human Chorionic Gonadotropin (hCG)**</u>: urine and/or blood to diagnose pregnancy • <u>Pelvic Ultrasound</u>: determines location of implantation and embryonic heart rate • Spontaneous abortion criteria include gestational sac 25mm in diameter without yolk sac or embryo or embryo with crown-rump length of 7mm and no cardiac activity • <u>Labs</u>: hemoglobin/hematocrit (acute blood loss anemia), blood type and Rh screen (prepare for blood transfusion or Rh (D)-immune globulin administration), infection workup

Treatment	• <u>Threatened Abortion</u>: observation, close follow-up, bedrest, serial beta-hCG tests
	• <u>Inevitable, Complete, Missed Abortion</u>: uterine evacuation or wait for spontaneous passage of products of conception
	   • <u><12 Weeks</u>: suction curettage or **medical evacuation (misoprostol)**
	   • <u>12-23 Weeks</u>: dilation and evacuation or medical evacuation (misoprostol)
	• <u>Rh (D)-Immune Globulin Administration</u>: if mother is Rh-negative
	• <u>**Emotional Support**</u>: reassurance, formal therapy, support group referral

Key Words & Most Common	• Loss of pregnancy <20 weeks gestation; aka miscarriage • Fetal chromosomal abnormalities most common • Advanced maternal age greatest risk factor • Vaginal bleeding +/- crampy abdominal or pelvic pain • Beta hCG (blood or urine) + pelvic ultrasound • Threatened: observation • Inevitable/complete/missed: uterine evacuation with procedure or medical (misoprostol) • Emotional support

Spontaneous Abortion Types

Classification	Characteristics	Cervical Os	Fetal Tissue Passage	Management
Threatened	• Abdominal pain; vaginal bleeding • <20 weeks gestation	Closed	• No • Products of conception (POC) intact	• <u>Conservative</u>: **observation with close follow-up**; bedrest • **Serial beta-hCG**

Inevitable	• Abdominal pain; vaginal bleeding
	• <20 weeks gestation
		Open	• No
			• Products of conception intact
				• <u>Uterine Evacuation</u>:
				  • Suction curettage if <12 wks
				  • Dilation and evacuation if ≥12 wks
				  • **Medical: misoprostol**

Incomplete	• Abdominal pain; vaginal bleeding
	• <20 weeks gestation
		Open	• **Yes**
			• **Some products of conception expelled from uterus**
				• <u>Expectant</u>: allow POC to pass
				  • Monitor serial beta-hCG and transvaginal ultrasound
				• <u>Uterine Evacuation</u>:
				  • Suction curettage if <12 wks
				  • Dilation and evacuation if ≥12 wks
				  • **Medical: misoprostol**

Complete	• Abdominal pain; vaginal bleeding • <20 weeks gestation	Closed	• **Yes** • **Complete expulsion of products of conception from uterus**	• <u>Rh (D)-Immune Globulin Administration</u>: if indicated • Follow-up beta-hCG

Missed	• Fetal death <20 weeks gestation *without* passage of products of conception for 4 weeks after fetal death	Closed	• No
			• Products of conception intact
				• <u>Uterine Evacuation</u>:
				  • Suction curettage if <12 wks
				  • Dilation and evacuation if ≥12 wks
				  • <u>Medical</u>: **misoprostol**
				• **Can lead to infection**

Septic	• Uterine infection during miscarriage
	• Caused by retained products of conception
	• **Fever** and chills with **foul-smelling, brown discharge; cervical motion tenderness**
		Open or Closed	• No
			• **Often incomplete expulsion of products of conception from uterus**
				• <u>Uterine Evacuation</u>:
				  • Dilation and evacuation to remove POC
				• **Broad-Spectrum Antibiotics**:
				  • **Clindamycin + gentamicin** +/- ampicillin
				  • Regimen modified based on culture results

Elective (Induced) Abortion

Notes	<ul><li>In the United States, about 50% of pregnancies are unintentional</li><li>About 40% of unintentional pregnancies result in induced abortion</li><li>Abortion of previable fetus is regulated by state specific restrictions</li><li>Reasons to pursue elective abortion vary<ul><li>May include **risk to maternal health**, unintended pregnancy, inability to afford child, domestic violence, lack of support, pursuing education or career advancement, unable or unwilling to raise child conceived as result of rape or incest</li></ul></li></ul>
Testing	<ul><li>Confirmation of pregnancy with beta human chorionic gonadotropin (hCG) urine and/or blood</li><li>Gestational age may be determined through ultrasonography or history and physical</li></ul>
Methods	<ul><li>**Instrumental Evacuation**<ul><li>Dilation and Curettage: large diameter suction cannula inserted to uterus<ul><li>Performed at <14 weeks gestation</li></ul></li><li>Manual or Electric Vacuum Aspiration: cannula attached to vacuum source<ul><li>Performed if <9 weeks gestation</li></ul></li><li>Dilation and Evacuation: forceps used to dismember and remove fetus; suction cannula used to aspirate amniotic fluid, placenta, and fetal debris<ul><li>Performed between 14 and 24 weeks</li></ul></li></ul></li><li>**Medical Evacuation**<ul><li>Mifepristone followed by misoprostol 24-48 hours later; safe up to 10 weeks gestation<ul><li>**Mifepristone: progesterone receptor antagonist**; dilates and soften cervix and promotes placental separation from uterine wall</li><li>**Misoprostol: prostaglandin E1 analog**; promotes uterine contractions and dilation</li></ul></li><li>Mifepristone followed by methotrexate 3-7 days later; *less effective and rarely used regimen*<ul><li>Methotrexate: folic acid antagonist; inhibits cellular division and nucleic acid synthesis</li></ul></li><li>Patient should follow-up 1-2 weeks after initial treatment to confirm resolution of pregnancy<ul><li>Ultrasound</li><li>Beta hCG on day of administration and 1 week later</li><li>Urine hCG 5 weeks after administration</li></ul></li></ul></li></ul>
Complications	<ul><li>Hemorrhage (trauma or atonic uterus)</li><li>Infection</li><li>Perforation of uterus or another organ (intestine) by instrument</li><li>Laceration of cervix</li><li>Psychological trauma</li></ul>

Ectopic Pregnancy

Etiology & Risk Factors	<ul><li>**Implantation of an embryo at a site other than the endometrial lining of the uterus (in the fallopian tube, uterine horn, cervix, ovary, or abdominal or pelvic cavity)**</li><li>Location: **ampulla of fallopian tube is most common location (98%)**</li><li>Etiology: **damage to fallopian tubes** (secondary to inflammation, infection, surgery or scarring) **is most common cause**</li><li>Risk Factors: **previous tubal surgery, previous ectopic pregnancy, history of pelvic inflammatory disease**, diethylstilbestrol exposure, smoking, IUD use</li></ul>
Pathophysiology	<ul><li>Tubal damage leads to upregulation of pro-inflammatory cytokines resulting in retention of an oocyte/embryo and promotes invasion and angiogenesis of the fallopian tube</li></ul>
Signs & Symptoms	<ul><li>Triad: (*can also be seen with threatened abortion*)<ul><li>**Unilateral pelvic or lower abdominal pain** (described as dull, sharp, crampy)</li><li>**Vaginal bleeding**</li><li>**Amenorrhea**</li></ul></li><li>Ruptured Ectopic: **severe abdominal pain followed by signs of hemorrhagic shock** (dizziness, **hypotension**, tachycardia, syncope) or peritonitis</li><li>Physical Exam:<ul><li>**Adnexal mass**, unilateral or bilateral adnexal tenderness, **cervical motion tenderness**</li></ul></li></ul>
Diagnosis	<ul><li>**Quantitative Beta Human Chorionic Gonadotropin (hCG)**: confirms pregnancy; serial beta-hCG fails to double or slowly decreases (beta-hCG should double every 48-72h)</li><li>**Transvaginal Ultrasound: identifies location of gestational sac**<ul><li>May identify fetal heartbeat outside of the uterine cavity in ectopic pregnancy</li></ul></li></ul>
Treatment	<ul><li>Administer RhoGAM to Rh-negative women</li><li>**Methotrexate**: inhibits dihydrofolate reductase to block DNA synthesis and destroys trophoblastic tissue<ul><li>**Indicated in hemodynamically stable patients with early gestation (<4cm in diameter), no fetal heart activity, beta-hCG <5,000 and no signs of rupture**</li></ul></li><li>Surgery:<ul><li>**Urgent laparotomy if patient is unstable**</li><li>**Laparoscopic salpingotomy is preferred surgical procedure**; salpingostomy if ruptured or hemorrhage continues after salpingectomy</li></ul></li></ul>
Key Words & Most Common	<ul><li>Implantation of embryo outside the uterus</li><li>Fallopian tube ampulla most common site</li><li>Damage to fallopian tube from previous tubal surgery, ectopic pregnancy or PID most common cause</li><li>Triad: unilateral pelvic/abdominal pain, vaginal bleeding, amenorrhea</li><li>Serial beta-hCG + transvaginal US</li><li>Methotrexate if stable and early</li><li>Surgery if unstable or late</li></ul>

Gestational Trophoblastic Disease

Etiology & Risk Factors	• Neoplasm of placental human chorionic gonadotropin (hCG) producing trophoblast cells • Subdivided into hydatidiform moles (contain villi) and other trophoblastic neoplasms (lack villi) • Etiology: abnormal gametogenesis and/or fertilization • Risk Factors: prior molar pregnancy, extremes of maternal age (<20 or >35 years old), history of spontaneous abortion

Patho-physiology	• Complete Molar Pregnancy: diploid (46XX) resulting from fertilization of single sperm than then duplicates while ovum is absent or inactivated
	  • Abnormal placental tissue (chorionic villi are vesicular and swollen) and fetal tissue does not form
	• Partial Molar Pregnancy: triploid (69XXX or XXY) resulting from fertilization by 2 sperm or a single diploid sperm
	  • Placental tissue contains some vesicular chorionic villi; fetal tissue may be seen but is abnormal and nonviable

Signs & Symptoms	• *Symptoms largely due to elevated levels of hCG* • Vaginal bleeding and abnormal discharge (passage of grape-like vesicle tissue) • Hyperemesis gravidarum (severe nausea and vomiting) • Hyperthyroidism (tachycardia, warm skin, sweating, heat intolerance, and mild tremors) • Early preeclampsia (before 20 weeks' gestation) • Physical Exam: • Uterine size discrepancies (large or smaller than typical gestational age)

Diagnosis	• Quantitative Beta Human Chorionic Gonadotropin (hCG): marked elevation (hCG > 100,000 mIU/mL)
	• Pelvic Ultrasound: gold-standard non-invasive test
	  • Complete Mole: enlarged uterus with central heterogenous mass and multiple interspersed lucent and anechoic areas ("snowstorm" or "bunches of grapes" appearance); absence of fetal tissue and heart tones
	  • Partial Mole: scattered cystic spaces within placenta; may see gestational sac and fetal heart tones
	• Labs: consider thyroid function tests if hCG markedly elevated; CBC if prolonged bleeding

Treatment	• Surgical Uterine Evacuation: dilation and evacuation, suction curettage is mainstay of treatment • Serial Beta hCG: testing every week for 3 weeks then every month for 6 months • Chest X-Ray: look for METS (choriocarcinoma)
Key Words & Most Common	• Neoplasm of abnormal trophoblastic tissue proliferation • Complete mole: vesicular/swollen chorionic villi without fetal tissue • Partial mole: some vesicular chorionic villi; fetal tissue may be seen but nonviable • Vaginal bleeding + grape-like vesicle discharge; hyperemesis gravidarum; early preeclampsia; uterine size discrepancy • Marked elevated beta-hCG + pelvic US • Surgical uterine evacuation

Rh Incompatibility

Etiology & Risk Factors	• Differing pairing of maternal and fetal Rh types • Occurs when Rh(D)-negative women carries a Rh(D)-positive fetus • Etiology: fetomaternal hemorrhage moves significant amounts of RBCs from fetal circulation across placenta to maternal circulation • Mixing of Rh-positive fetal cells with Rh-negative maternal cells causes alloimmunization and anti-Rh(D) IgG antibody production • Risk Factors: exposure to Rh(D) antigen during first pregnancy (during Cesarean section or vaginal delivery, trauma, abruptio placentae, placenta previa, amniocentesis)
Patho-physiology	• Fetal RBCs stimulate maternal antibody production against the Rh antigens resulting in immunogenic pathway activation • Anti-Rh(D) antibodies are produced which may bind to the D antigen on the erythrocyte of the Rh-positive fetus leading to hemolysis of fetal erythrocytes

Signs & Symptoms	• Asymptomatic for mother
	• Detailed history about possible fetal exposure to Rh-positive blood
	  • Delivery (vaginal, Cesarean section), miscarriage, antepartum hemorrhage (abruptio placentae, placenta previa), trauma, invasive procedures (amniocentesis, chorionic villus sampling), ectopic or molar pregnancy
	• Detailed history about possible *non*-fetal exposure to Rh-positive blood
	  • Blood transfusion, bone marrow transplant, needle-stick injury
	• Hemolytic Disease of Neonate (HDN): lethargy, pallor, tachycardia/tachypnea, hypotension, jaundice, scleral icterus

Diagnosis	• Maternal Blood Typing and Rh(D) Antibody Screen: screening at initial prenatal visit to identify if mother is Rh(D)-negative or Rh(D)-positive; repeat at 24-28 weeks' gestation and delivery if Rh(D)-negative
	• Rh(D) Antibody Titer: performed in Rh(D)-negative women
	  • Unsensitized: *no* Rh(D) antibodies present
	  • Sensitized: Rh(D) antibodies are present; if titer is 1:8-1:32 or greater then titer performed every 2-4 weeks; if 1:4, no further testing necessary
	• Study Interpretation:
	  • If Rh(D)-positive: no risk of alloimmunization
	  • If Rh(D)-negative: risk of alloimmunization assessed via antibody screen
	  • If Rh(D)-negative mother is antibody positive: confirmatory study (Coombs test) required to determine management
	  • If Rh(D)-negative mother is antibody negative: paternal Rh testing can be performed

Treatment	• Anti-D Rh Immune Globulin Administration: if mother is Rh-negative and antibody negative • Given at 28 weeks' gestation, within 72 hours of delivery or pregnancy termination, any episode of vaginal bleeding, after amniocentesis or chorionic villus sampling • Intravascular Intrauterine Blood Transfusions: if fetal anemia is likely; given by high-risk pregnancy specialist
Key Words & Most Common	• Occurs when Rh-negative mom carries a Rh-positive fetus • Mixing of Rh-positive fetal cells with Rh-negative maternal cells causes alloimmunization antibody response; can lead to hemolytic disease of neonate • Maternal blood typing and Rh antibody screen → antibody titer if Rh-negative • Anti-D Rh Immune globulin given if mother Rh-negative and antibody negative

Neural Tube Defects

Etiology & Risk Factors	• Birth defects of the central nervous system including the brain, spine or spinal cord
	• Common neural tube defects include spina bifida occulta, spina bifida cystica, myeloschisis, and anencephaly
	   • <u>**Spina Bifida Occulta**</u>: caudal neuropore closure failure; spinal cord, meninges and skin are intact without herniation
	   • <u>**Spina Bifida Cystica**</u>: involves a **meningocele (herniation of meninges only)** and **myelomeningocele (herniation of meninges and neural tissue through vertebral gap)**
	   • <u>Myeloschisis</u>: neural tissue exposure without skin or meningeal covering
	   • <u>**Anencephaly**</u>: rostral neuropore closure; malformation of brain (cerebrum) and cranial vault with normal hindbrain development
	• <u>Etiology</u>: genetic and environmental factors; **folic acid deficiency during pregnancy**
	• <u>Risk Factors</u>: obesity, diabetes, **malnutrition (poor folic acid intake)**, medications (folic acid antagonists, dihydrofolate reductase inhibitors), radiation exposure, stress, low socioeconomic status, hypervitaminosis A, toxoplasmosis exposure, exposure to toxic landfills, rubella

Patho-physiology	• Folic acid synthesizes deoxyribonucleic acid (DNA) and ribonucleic acid (RNA) precursors and promotes cell proliferation as in neurulation • Absence or deficiency of folic acid interrupts neural tissue proliferation and migration during neurulation which contributes to neural tube disorders
Signs & Symptoms	• **Low birth weight** • **Sensory deficits; paralysis or hypotonia** • **Developmental delays** (late ambulation) **and cognitive impairment** • Hydrocephalus • Other congenital abnormalities including cleft palate, undescended testis, omphalocele, cardiac or renal abnormalities
Diagnosis	• <u>**Ultrasound**</u>: identifies and localizes the size and site of neural tube defect; part of prenatal screening • <u>**Serum Alpha-Fetoprotein**</u>: increased level indicates neural tube defect • <u>Serum Acetylcholinesterase</u>: increased level indicates neural tube defect • <u>**Maternal Serum Folic Acid Level**</u>: screening before or during conception helps identify causative factors of neural tube defects
Treatment	• <u>**Folic Acid Supplementation**</u>: **proper nutrition or supplementation necessary for proper neural tube development** • Appropriate intake encouraged 5-6 months prior to conception and immediately upon confirmation of pregnancy • <u>Surgery</u>: fetal postnatal surgery for myelomeningocele to prevent cerebrospinal fluid leakage • <u>Manage Underlying Etiology or Limit Risk Factors</u>: diabetes management, nutrition, medication avoidance, reduced exposures
Key Words & Most Common	• Birth defects of CNS; most common forms include spina bifida and anencephaly • Secondary to folic acid deficiency • Low birth weight, sensory deficits, paralysis, developmental/cognitive delays • Ultrasound + serum alpha-fetoprotein • Folic acid supplementation

Spina Bifida (Open Defect)

Postpartum Depression

Etiology & Risk Factors	• **Depressive symptoms lasting >2 weeks after delivery and meet criteria for major depression** • <u>Etiology</u>: **hormonal, physical, emotional and psychological changes throughout pregnancy** • <u>Risk Factors</u>: **history of depression or anxiety**, reluctance of baby's gender, **risky pregnancy**, **complicated delivery**, victim of sexual or domestic abuse, lifestyle factors
Patho-physiology	• Rapid reproductive hormone changes (estradiol and progesterone) following delivery can be potential stressor in susceptible women • Lower levels of oxytocin implicated in postpartum depression; oxytocin is released during skin-to-skin contact and breastfeeding
Signs & Symptoms	• **Depressive mood or irritability** (subjective or observed) • **Mood swings, crying** • **Loss of interest or mood** (anhedonia) • **Insomnia** or hypersomnia; loss of energy or **fatigue** • **Worthlessness or guilt** (concern if she is a good mother, feeling inadequate) • Change in weight or appetite • **Disinterest in baby** • <u>Severe</u>: **suicidal ideation, thoughts of harming baby, psychotic thoughts or delusions, agitation, unrealistic worries, panic attacks**
Diagnosis	• **Clinical Diagnosis** • <u>Edinburgh Postnatal Depression Scale (EPDS)</u>: 10-item questionnaire filled out by patients to screen for postpartum depression
Treatment	• <u>Conservative</u>: reassurance, support group referral, lactation consultant referral, lifestyle modifications (proper diet and exercise), encouraging bonding with baby • <u>**Cognitive Behavioral Therapy**</u>: **first-line treatment for women with mild to moderate postpartum depression; indicated in all cases of postpartum depression** • <u>**Antidepressants**</u>: **first-line pharmacotherapy** indicated for women with moderate to severe postpartum depression • **Selective serotonin reuptake inhibitors (SSRIs) or serotonin-norepinephrine reuptake inhibitors (SNRIs) initiated and continued for 6-12 months to prevent relapse** • <u>**Admission**</u>: **admit to hospital and remove children to ensure safety if severe postpartum psychosis present and baby is in danger**
Key Words & Most Common	• Depressive symptoms for >2 weeks after delivery • Depressed mood/irritability, mood swings, crying, anhedonia, insomnia, guilt, disinterest in baby • Severe: suicidal ideation, thoughts of harming baby, agitation, panic attacks, psychotic thoughts • Clinical diagnosis • Cognitive behavioral therapy is first-line • Antidepressants (SSRIs or SNRIs) • Admit and remove children for safety if postpartum psychosis present

Abnormal Uterine Bleeding

Etiology & Risk Factors	• Unexplained abnormal bleeding or irregular menstrual cycles present in a nonpregnant female • Normal menstrual cycle has a frequency of 24 to 38 days and lasts 2 to 7 days with an average of 5 to 80 milliliters of blood loss • *Each normal sized tampon or pad holds about 5 milliliters of blood when soaked through; way to quantify blood loss* • <u>Etiology</u>: PALM-COEIN acronym (**Polyp**, <u>A</u>denomyosis, **Leiomyoma**, **Malignancy** and hyperplasia, <u>C</u>oagulopathy, **Ovulatory dysfunction**, <u>E</u>ndometrial disorders, <u>I</u>atrogenic, <u>N</u>ot otherwise classified); *vaginal bleeding before the age of menarche me be result of infection, **trauma** (sexual assault, foreign body), or structural lesions*
Patho-physiology	• **Anovulatory cycle is most common cause**; ovaries produce estrogen, but the corpus luteum does not form; therefore, the normal cyclical secretion of progesterone does not occur leading to unopposed estrogen stimulation of the endometrium; uterine endometrium proliferates and incompletely sloughs causing abnormal bleeding
Signs & Symptoms	• **Vaginal bleeding in a non-pregnant female** • May have cyclic breast tenderness, premenstrual bloating, mood changes, midcycle cramping
Diagnosis	• **No specific test**; should be correlated with menstrual history • <u>Labs</u>: **urine or blood beta-hCG to rule out pregnancy**; consider CBC, ferritin, coagulation studies, thyroid function tests, prolactin, gonadotropins, testosterone and dehydroepiandrosterone sulfate (DHEAS), serum glucose, lipid panel, gonorrhea/chlamydia • <u>Transvaginal Ultrasound</u>: demonstrates uterus size and shape, leiomyomas (fibroids), adenomyosis, endometrial thickness, and ovarian anomalies • <u>**Endometrial Biopsy**</u>: **ordered to rule out endometrial cancer** • Should be performed in women >35 years old with obesity, hypertension or diabetes and **all women with postmenopausal bleeding**

Treatment	• Identify and treat underlying etiology
	• <u>Nonhormonal Management</u>: can be given intermittently when bleeding occurs
	    • <u>Non-Steroidal Anti-Inflammatory Drugs (NSAIDs)</u>: relieve dysmenorrhea by reducing prostaglandin levels
	    • <u>Tranexamic Acid</u>: inhibits plasminogen activation
	• <u>**Hormone Management**</u>: estrogen/progestin contraceptives, progestins, a long-acting progestin-releasing intrauterine device (IUD)
	    • <u>**Combined Estrogen-Progestin Oral Contraceptive Pills**</u>: **first-line medication management**; suppress endometrial development, establishes menstrual patterns
	    • <u>Progesterone</u>: if estrogen therapy is contraindicated; does not control heavy bleeding
	    • <u>Levonorgestrel-Releasing IUD</u>: provides contraception and relieve dysmenorrhea
	• <u>Procedures</u>:
	    • <u>**Hysteroscopy with Dilation and Curettage**</u>: **treatment of choice for severe anovulatory bleeding and refractory to hormonal treatment**; diagnostic and therapeutic
	    • <u>Endometrial Ablation</u>: less invasive than hysteroscopy
	      <u>Hysterectomy</u>: definitive management

Key Words & Most Common	• Polyps, leiomyoma (fibroids), malignancy, ovulatory dysfunction (anovulation is most common cause) • Rule out pregnancy; labs to determine underlying etiology; endometrial biopsy to rule out cancer • Combined OCPs first-line medication management

Dysmenorrhea

Etiology & Risk Factors	• **Uterine pain occurring around time of menses**; may affect normal activities of daily living
	• <u>Etiology</u>: may be primary or secondary; primary is more common
	    • <u>**Primary**</u>: idiopathic and not explained by other gynecologic disorders
	    • <u>**Secondary**</u>: due to pelvic abnormalities (endometriosis is most common cause, uterine adenomyosis, leiomyomas [fibroids], pelvic inflammatory disease)
	• <u>Risk Factors</u>: **early age of menarche**, long/heavy menstrual periods, smoking, family history of dysmenorrhea, **depression/anxiety**, **obesity**, nulliparity

Patho-physiology	• <u>Primary</u>: endometrial cells release prostaglandin F (PGF) at the beginning of endometrial shedding during menstruation; prostaglandins increases uterine tone and causes uterine contractions

Signs & Symptoms	• **Recurrent, crampy abdominal or pelvic pain** (often dull and crampy; can be sharp or throbbing)
	    • **May precede menses by 1-3 days**
	    • **Peaks about 24 hours after onset of menses**
	    • **Subsides after 2-3 days**
	• Pain may radiate to lower back, gluteal area, thighs
	• Headache, nausea, constipation/diarrhea, urinary frequency

Diagnosis	• <u>History</u>: age of symptoms, nature/severity, effect on sexual activity (dyspareunia or infertility), response to NSAIDs, degree of disruption of normal activities • <u>Medical History</u>: identify known causes (endometriosis, fibroids, adenomyosis, method of contraception) • <u>Surgical History</u>: identify procedures that increase risk (cervical conization, endometrial ablation) • <u>Physical Exam</u>: speculum and bimanual examination to evaluate uterine masses and consistency, rectovaginal septum, lesions • <u>Labs</u>: urine or blood beta-hCG to rule out pregnancy; consider gonorrhea/chlamydia testing if PID suspected etiology • <u>**Pelvic Ultrasound**</u>: **highly sensitive to identify pelvic masses** (ovarian cysts, fibroids, endometriosis, uterine adenomyosis) **and can locate abnormally placed IUDs**

Treatment	• <u>Conservative</u>: encourage adequate rest, maintain active lifestyle, **heating pad**, nutritional supplements (omega-3 fatty acids, flaxseed, magnesium, vitamin B, vitamin E, zinc)
	• <u>Medical Therapy</u>:
	    • <u>**Non-Steroidal Anti-Inflammatory Drugs (NSAIDs)**</u>: **first-line medical management**; relieve dysmenorrhea by inhibiting prostaglandins
	    • <u>Hormonal Therapy</u>: combined estrogen-progestin contraceptive pills or progestin-only pills

Key Words & Most Common	• Painful menstruation; may be primary (idiopathic) or secondary (endometriosis or adenomyosis most common) • Recurrent, crampy abdominal/pelvic pain occur around time of menses • History is crucial for accurate diagnosis • Pelvic ultrasound may identify pelvic masses or abnormalities • NSAIDs is first-line treatment

Premenstrual Syndrome (PMS)

Etiology & Risk Factors	• <u>PMS</u>: Luteal-phase disorder characterized physical, behavioral and mood changes occurring 5 days prior to and subsiding within a few hours of the onset of menses • <u>Premenstrual Dysphoric Disorder</u>: **severe PMS with functional impairment;** anger, irritability and tension are prominent symptoms; psychiatric disorder by DSM-5 • <u>Etiology</u>: **unclear etiology; endocrine factors** (hypoglycemia, **estrogen and progesterone fluctuations**, excess aldosterone), genetic predisposition, **serotonin deficiency,** magnesium/calcium deficiency may be contributory • <u>Risk Factors</u>: poor nutrition, high-salt diet, caffeine, alcohol use, poor sleep quality, **stress, perimenopausal**
Patho-physiology	• Progesterone and estrogen fluctuations affect certain neurotransmitters (gamma-aminobutyric acid [GABA], opioids, serotonin, and catecholamine) • Preexisting serotonin deficiency with increased progesterone sensitivity may be implicated • Stress amplifies sympathetic activity and may exacerbate PMS symptoms
Signs & Symptoms	• <u>Physical</u>: **abdominal bloating, fatigue, acne,** breast fullness or pain, **weight gain,** headache, **pelvic pressure,** backache, fluid retention, constipation/diarrhea, palpitations • <u>Emotional</u>: **irritability is most common symptom,** agitation, anger, insomnia, lethargy, depression/anxiety, changes in libido • <u>Behavioral</u>: **food cravings,** lack of concentration, noise sensitivity
Diagnosis	• **Clinical Diagnosis** • Symptoms begin about 5 days prior to menses (luteal phase) and subside a few hours to days after onset of menses • Patient should have at least 1 week of symptom-free days during follicular phase • Symptoms persisting >2 cycles

Treatment	• <u>Lifestyle Modifications</u>: **stress reduction, sleep hygiene, regular aerobic and resistance exercise,** relaxation activities, cognitive behavioral therapy
	• <u>Dietary Modifications</u>: increase protein intake, decreased refined sugar/carbohydrates, consume whole-foods diet, avoid caffeine
	    • Supplementation with vitamin B6, vitamin E, magnesium, calcium, and **chasteberry extract from the agnus castus fruit** have been shown to be beneficial
	• <u>Medication Management</u>:
	    • <u>Non-Steroidal Anti-Inflammatory Drugs (NSAIDs)</u>: relieve aches, pain, and dysmenorrhea
	    • **<u>Combined Oral Contraceptive Pills</u>:** combination of ethinyl estradiol and drospirenone have been shown to decrease symptoms
	    • **<u>Selective Serotonin Reuptake Inhibitors (SSRIs)</u>: first-line medication for treatment of PMS with predominantly emotional symptoms**

Key Words & Most Common	• Physical, behavioral and mood changes occurring 5 days prior to menses and resolving shortly after • Progesterone and estrogen fluctuations and serotonin deficiency may be implicated • Exacerbated by stress • Abdominal bloating, fatigue, acne, weight gain • Irritability, agitation, insomnia, food cravings • Stress reduction + sleep hygiene + dietary modifications • NSAIDs for symptom management • SSRIs first-line for treatment with predominate emotional symptoms

Amenorrhea

Etiology & Risk Factors	• **Absence of menstruation**
	• <u>Primary Amenorrhea</u>: **failure of menses to occur by age 15** (in *presence* of secondary sex characteristics) or **age 13** (in *absence* of secondary sex characteristics)
	    • Gonadal dysgenesis (Turner syndrome, 46,XY), anatomical causes (congenital female reproductive tract anomalies), constitutional delay of puberty
	• <u>Secondary Amenorrhea</u>: **absence of menses for >3 months in a patient with previously normal menstrual cycles OR for ≥6 months in patient with irregular menses**
	    • <u>Physiologic</u>: **pregnancy is the most common cause;** breastfeeding (elevated prolactin and low levels of LH suppresses ovarian hormone secretion)
	    • <u>Thyroid</u>: **hypothyroidism** (increased thyrotropin releasing hormone increases TSH and prolactin; elevated prolactin inhibits LH and FSH necessary for ovulation)
	    • <u>Hypothalamic and Pituitary</u>: prolactin secreting pituitary adenomas (prolactin secretion inhibits FSH and LH release), functional hypothalamic amenorrhea,
	        • **<u>Functional Hypothalamic Amenorrhea</u>: stress, weight loss, or excessive exercise; female athlete triad (amenorrhea, eating disorder, and osteoporosis)**
	    • <u>Ovarian Dysfunction</u>: **polycystic ovarian syndrome (PCOS) (decreased estrogen and increased FSH and LH),** premature ovarian failure
	    • <u>Drug Induced</u>: **progesterone hormonal contraceptives** (medroxyprogesterone acetate) or extended use of combined oral contraceptives, opiates, antipsychotics

Patho-physiology	• During the female menstrual cycle, gonadotropin-releasing hormone (GnRH) is released from the hypothalamus stimulating the pituitary release of follicle-stimulating hormone (FSH) and luteinizing hormone (LH); FSH and LH act on ovaries to activate estrogen and progesterone which carry out the follicular and secretory phase of the menstrual cycle. *Any defect at any level of this normal physiology can cause amenorrhea*
Signs & Symptoms	• **Absence of menstruation** • Physical exam focused on identifying underlying etiology

Diagnosis	• <u>Body Mass Index (BMI)</u>: evaluate for malnutrition, anorexia nervosa, and excessive strenuous exercise
	• <u>Labs</u>:
	    • **<u>Beta-hCG</u>: best initial test to rule out pregnancy**
	    • <u>Prolactin</u>: rule out prolactinoma
	    • <u>Testosterone and DHEAS</u>: rule out hyperandrogenism
	    • <u>Follicle Stimulating Hormone and Luteinizing Hormone</u>: evaluate for hypothalamic amenorrhea
	    • <u>Thyroid Panel</u>: evaluate for thyroid disorder
	• <u>Pelvic Ultrasound</u>: evaluates for congenital anatomic genital tract obstruction

Treatment	• **Treatment directed at underlying disorder** • Patients with stress and eating disorders should undergo behavior modification; SSRIs may be considered
Key Words & Most Common	• Primary: failure of menses by age 15 with secondary sex characteristics or age 13 without secondary sex characteristics; gonadal dysgenesis • Secondary: absence of menses >3 months in patient with previously normal cycles or ≥6 months in patient with irregular menses • Pregnancy is most common cause; breastfeeding, hypothyroidism, prolactinoma, functional hypothalamic amenorrhea (stress, weight loss, exercise), hormonal contraceptives • Beta-HCG is best initial test to rule out pregnancy • Treatment directed at underlying etiology

Leiomyoma (Uterine Fibroids) ♀

Etiology & Risk Factors	• **Benign uterine tumors of smooth muscle origin**; derived from muscle cells of myometrium • <u>Types</u>: **subserosal (under the outer surface of the uterus; most common)**, intramural (in the wall of the uterus), submucosal (under the lining of the uterus) • <u>Etiology</u>: monoclonal cells arising from myometrium; may be related to gene mutations • <u>Risk Factors</u>: **age (>35 years old)**, **African American**, early menarche, **use of oral contraception before the age of 16, high body mass index**
Patho-physiology	• Fibroids have increased expression of estrogen and progesterone receptors compared to normal myometrium; **growth is estrogen dependent** • Ovarian steroids, estradiol, and progesterone may promote growth explaining why fibroid size increases in anovulatory states and pregnancy and decrease after menopause

Signs & Symptoms	• Most are asymptomatic
	• **Abnormal uterine bleeding is most common presenting symptom**
	  • May present as **irregular or heavy menses (menorrhagia)**; *submucosal fibroids may bleed enough to cause anemia*
	• **Lower abdominal/pelvic pain and pressure**
	• **Urinary frequency** or urgency may result from bladder compression
	• **Constipation** may result from intestinal compression
	• <u>Physical Exam</u>:
	  • Normal or may have **palpable, firm, nontender, asymmetric (irregularly shaped) mobile, uterine mass in lower abdomen or pelvis on bimanual exam**

Diagnosis	• <u>Transvaginal Ultrasound</u>: **initial imaging test for suspected fibroids** • **Demonstrates focal heterogenic hypoechoic uterine mass; irregularly shaped uterus** • <u>Magnetic Resonance Imaging (MRI)</u>: may aid in determining vascular extent or degeneration of fibroids

Treatment	• <u>Observation</u>: **first-line as majority of patient do not require treatment**; treatment is determined by symptoms, size and rate of tumor growth and desire to preserve fertility
	• <u>Gonadotropin-Releasing Hormone (GnRH) Agonists</u>: **leuprolide is most effective medical treatment; decreases estrogen production to reduce fibroid size**
	  • Often only given around time of menopause due to long-term side effects or to reduce fibroid size prior to myomectomy or hysterectomy
	• <u>Exogenous Progestins</u>: suppresses estrogen stimulation of fibroid growth; medroxyprogesterone acetate or levonorgestrel-releasing IUD
	• <u>Surgery</u>: reserved for severe cases, rapid growth, recurrent abortions, or refractory to conservative treatment
	  • <u>Myomectomy</u>: **indicated for women wanting to preserve fertility**
	  • <u>Hysterectomy</u>: **definitive treatment**

Key Words & Most Common	• Benign uterine tumor of smooth muscle origin; subserosal most common • Abnormal uterine bleeding, irregular/heavy menses, pelvic pressure • Palpable, irregularly shaped, mobile uterine mass on bimanual exam • Transvaginal ultrasound • Observation → leuprolide or exogenous progestins → surgery

Menopause ♀

Etiology & Risk Factors	• **Physiologic or iatrogenic cessation of menses for >12 consecutive months secondary to loss of ovarian function**; leads to decreased estrogen and progesterone production • Average age of physiologic menopause is 52 years old • <u>Etiology</u>: **physiologic process of aging**; iatrogenic (hysterectomy, oophorectomy, antiestrogen treatment for endometriosis or breast cancer, chemotherapy medication)
Patho-physiology	• As ovaries age, there is a decreased response to the pituitary gonadotropins follicle-stimulating hormone (FSH) and luteinizing hormone (LH) resulting in a shorter follicular phase, fewer ovulations, and decreased progesterone production; resultant decline of estrogen production causes cessation of menstruation
Signs & Symptoms	• <u>Vasomotor Symptoms</u>: **hot flashes (most common perimenopausal symptom), night sweats**, skin flushing, skin/hair/nail changes, increased perspiration • <u>Vaginal Symptoms</u>: **vaginal dryness, dyspareunia (painful intercourse), vulvovaginal atrophy** (causes itching, irritation), urinary urgency, dysuria, frequent UTIs/vaginitis • <u>Neuropsychiatric Symptoms</u>: **irritability, insomnia, fatigue**, anxiety, poor concentration, memory loss, depressive symptoms • <u>Physical Exam</u>: • **Vaginal atrophy with thin mucosa and loss of rugae**; decreased breast size, decreased skin elasticity

Diagnosis	• **Clinical Diagnosis**
	• <u>Labs</u>: follicle stimulating hormone (FSH) level >40mIU/mL is indicative of menopause by ovarian failure
	• <u>Dual-Energy X-ray Absorptiometry (DEXA)</u>: osteoporosis screening recommended to begin at age 65 or sooner if risk factors present (pathologic fracture, medications, fall risk)
	  • Osteopenia: T-score of 1.0 to 2.5
	  • Osteoporosis: T-score >2.5

Treatment	• <u>Lifestyle Modifications</u>: **avoid triggers of hot flashes** (spicy food, bright lights, heavy comforters, etc.), cooling the environment (fans, cooling gel mattress toppers, lowering thermostat), wearing layers that can easily be removed; **exercise, weight loss, proper nutrition; vaginal lubricant**, regular vaginal intercourse or stimulation preserves function
	• <u>Hormone Replacement Therapy</u>: **most effective treatment**; available in various forms (tablets, creams, patches) and different modalities (continuous versus cyclic)
	  • <u>Estrogen only</u>: **recommended only for women without a uterus** (unopposed estrogen may cause uterine hyperplasia and uterine cancer)
	  • <u>Estrogen + Progestin</u>: **recommended for women with an intact uterus** (significantly decreases hot flash severity and frequency; improves urogenital atrophy and sleep disturbances)
	  • <u>Local Estrogen Therapy</u>: enhance blood flow and may reverse vaginal atrophy (vaginal rings, creams, or tablets)
	• <u>Neuroactive Medications</u>: SSRIs, SNRIs, gabapentin have been shown to be moderately effective in reducing hot flushes
	• <u>Complementary Medicine</u>: phytoestrogens (soy, red clover, black cohosh), vitamin E, and omega-3 fatty acids along with proper diet have been shown to reduce symptoms

Key Words & Most Common	• Cessation of menses for >12 consecutive months (physiologic or iatrogenic) • Hot flashes and night sweats; vaginal dryness and atrophy; irritability and insomnia • Clinical diagnosis • Lifestyle modifications • Hormone replacement therapy is most effect treatment (estrogen only indicated for patients without a uterus)

Vulvovaginal Atrophy

Etiology & Risk Factors	• Thinning of the vaginal epithelium and decreased cervical secretions secondary to hypoestrogenic states • <u>Etiology</u>: **hypoestrogenic states such as menopause, postpartum women, lactating women**, progesterone-only contraceptives, hypothalamic amenorrhea, anti-estrogen medication (treatment of uterine fibroids, endometriosis, breast cancer) • <u>Risk Factors</u>: **perimenopausal or menopausal**; bilateral oophorectomy, primary ovarian insufficiency, ovarian failure
Patho-physiology	• Vaginal epithelial cells are stimulated and exfoliated by estrogen which increases glycogen levels that are converted into lactic acid by normal vaginal flora (lactobacilli) • As estrogen levels decrease, the above process is disrupted and vaginal epithelium becomes atrophic and decreased vaginal secretions lead to dryness and reduced lubrication
Signs & Symptoms	• **Vaginal dryness** • **Dyspareunia** (painful intercourse) • Vaginal inflammation • **Recurrent infections (frequent UTIs, vaginitis)** • <u>Physical Exam</u>: • **Vaginal atrophy with thin mucosa and loss of rugae**
Diagnosis	• **Clinical Diagnosis** • Vaginal or urinary cultures, urinalysis if infection suspected
Treatment	• <u>Vaginal Moisturizers</u>: **vaginal lubricants are first-line treatment for short-term relief**(dryness, dyspareunia); do not improve atrophy • <u>Topical Vaginal Estrogen</u>: **safe and effective treatment; enhance blood flow and may reverse vaginal atrophy** (vaginal rings, creams, or tablets) • <u>Systemic Hormonal Replacement Therapy</u>: typically reserved for women experiencing systemic menopausal symptoms in addition to vaginal atrophy
Key Words & Most Common	• Thinning of vaginal epithelium • Secondary to menopause • Vaginal dryness + dyspareunia • Clinical diagnosis • Vaginal moisturizers/lubricants → topical vaginal estrogen

Adenomyosis

Etiology & Risk Factors	• **Presence of ectopic endometrial tissue and stroma within the uterine myometrium** (muscular layer of uterine wall) • <u>Etiology</u>: tissue disruption between the deep endometrium layer (endometrium basalis) and the underlying myometrium • <u>Risk Factors</u>: **age (premenopausal; 35-50 years old), multiparity**, early age of first menarche, short menstrual cycles, high BMI, OCP use, tamoxifen therapy
Patho-physiology	• Estrogen drives endometrial tissue proliferation within the myometrium leading to symptoms • Ectopic adenomyosis foci lead to increased levels of prostaglandins producing dysmenorrhea

Signs & Symptoms	• **Menorrhagia (heavy menstrual bleeding) is most common symptom**
	  • Symptoms of anemia may be present if severe
	• **Dysmenorrhea (painful menstruation)**
	• Chronic pelvic pain/pressure
	• Dyspareunia (painful intercourse)
	• <u>Physical Exam</u>:
	  • **Diffusely enlarged (uniformly shaped), symmetric, "boggy" uterus (may be tender to palpation)**

Diagnosis	• <u>Labs</u>: CBC to rule out anemia; beta-hCG to rule out pregnancy • <u>Transvaginal Ultrasound</u>: **preferred diagnostic imaging modality** • May show echogenic striations and nodules or focal/diffuse myometrial thickening, increased tortuous vessels within the involved myometrium • <u>Magnetic Resonance Imaging (MRI)</u>: may be marginally more sensitive than ultrasound • <u>Histology after Hysterectomy</u>: **definitive diagnosis**

Treatment	• <u>Medical Therapy</u>: aimed to preserve fertility while reducing symptoms
	  • <u>Non-Steroidal Anti-Inflammatory Drugs (NSAIDs)</u>: relieve dysmenorrhea by inhibiting prostaglandins
	  • <u>Hormonal Therapy</u>: combined estrogen-progestin oral contraceptive pills (OCPs), levonorgestrel intrauterine device (IUD), danazol, or aromatase inhibitors
	• <u>Surgery</u>:
	  • <u>Partial Hysterectomy or Myomectomy</u>: invasive procedures that may preserve fertility
	  • <u>Total Hysterectomy</u>: **definitive and most effective treatment**

Key Words & Most Common	• Presence of endometrial tissue within myometrium • Menorrhagia and dysmenorrhea • Diffusely enlarged, symmetric, "boggy" uterus that may be tender • Transvaginal ultrasound preferred imaging modality • Histology after hysterectomy is definitive diagnosis • Total hysterectomy is definitive cure

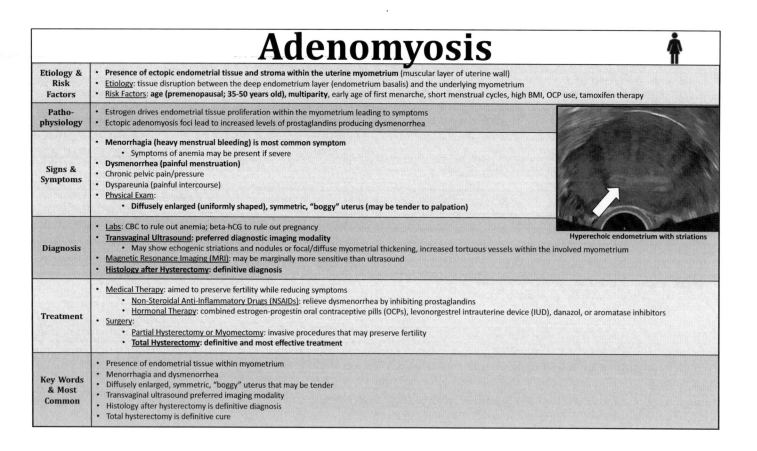
Hyperechoic endometrium with striations

Endometritis

Etiology & Risk Factors	• **Inflammation of the uterine lining, typically caused by ascending bacterial infection from the lower genital or gastrointestinal tract** • Etiology: **postpartum infection secondary to bacteria from vagina and cervix is most common** • **Often polymicrobial**; combination of gram-positive (group B streptococci, *Staphylococcus epidermidis*, and *Enterococcus* spp.), gram-negative (*Gardnerella vaginalis*, *Escherichia coli*, *Klebsiella pneumoniae*, and *Proteus* mirabilis) and anaerobic (*Peptostreptococci*, *Bacteroides* spp., and *Prevotella* spp.) • Risk Factors: **Cesarean section greatest risk factor**; prolonged labor, prolonged rupture of membranes (>24 hours), chorioamnionitis, manual removal of placenta, D&C
Patho-physiology	• Majority of endometritis cases are secondary to childbirth; rupture of amniotic membranes allows translocation of bacteria from the cervix and vagina to ascend and colonize uterine tissue that has been devitalized, bleeding, or damaged (Cesarean section)
Signs & Symptoms	• *Symptoms usually begin within 24-72 hours postpartum* • **Lower abdominal/pelvic pain** • **Fever** • Fatigue, malaise, chills, pallor, tachycardia may also be present Physical Exam: • **Uterine tenderness, vaginal discharge** (may be malodorous and/or bloody), indurated uterus
Diagnosis	• **Clinical Diagnosis** • Labs: urinalysis, urine culture, CBC (leukocytosis of 15000 to 30000 cells/microL is common), blood cultures (if concerned about sepsis) • Pelvic Ultrasound: rule out other diagnoses in postpartum patient (products of conception, infected hematoma, and uterine abscesses)

Treatment	• Antibiotics: broad-spectrum IV antibiotic regimen
	   • **IV clindamycin + gentamicin is first-line**
	   • Ampicillin may be added for enhanced *Enterococcus* coverage
	• Prophylactic Antibiotics: given during Cesarean section to reduce risk
	   • First-generation cephalosporin (cefazolin)

Key Words & Most Common	• Inflammation of uterine lining secondary to infection • Postpartum infection after C-section • Lower abdominal/pelvic pain + fever • Uterine tenderness • Clinical diagnosis • IV clindamycin + gentamicin is first-line

Endometriosis

Etiology & Risk Factors	• **Chronic estrogen-dependent condition characterized by ectopic implantation endometrial tissue (endometrial glands and stroma) outside the uterine cavity** • Location: **ovaries are most common site**; posterior broad ligament, anterior and posterior cul-de-sac and the uterosacral ligament, rectosigmoid colon, bladder • Etiology: retrograde menstruation causes and viable endometrial cells to implant, grow and infiltrate the peritoneal cavity • Risk Factors: **age (peaks at 27 years old), family history of endometriosis**, delayed childbearing or **nulliparity**, early menarche, late menopause, shortened menstrual cycles
Patho-physiology	• Retrograde menstruation causes viable endometrial cells and menstrual fragments to migrate from uterine cavity through the fallopian tube allowing infiltration of the peritoneal cavity where the cells can proliferate and lead to chronic inflammation; ectopic endometrial tissue then responds to cyclical hormone changes

Signs & Symptoms	• Classic Triad:
	   • **Dysmenorrhea** (painful menstruation)
	   • **Dyspareunia** (painful intercourse)
	   • **Infertility**
	• **Cyclical pelvic pain** (pain preceding or during menses)
	• **Dyschezia** (painful defection), dysuria, abnormal bleeding, back pain
	• Physical Exam:
	   • **Often normal**; may have a retroverted and fixed uterus, enlarged/tender ovaries
	   • Fixed ovarian and/or adnexal masses, thickened rectovaginal septum 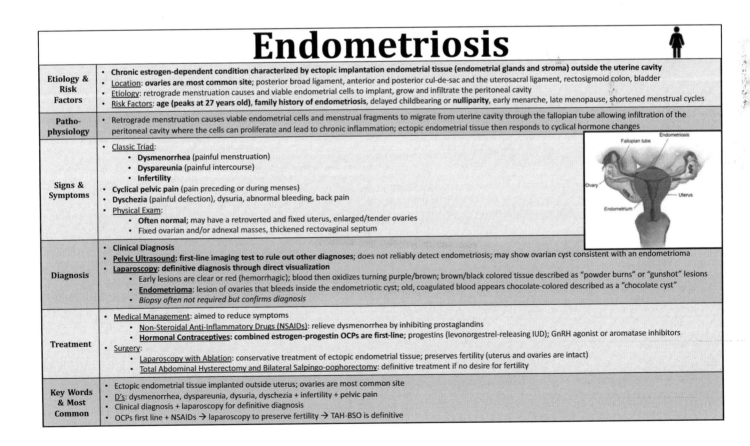

Diagnosis	• **Clinical Diagnosis**
	• **Pelvic Ultrasound: first-line imaging test to rule out other diagnoses**; does not reliably detect endometriosis; may show ovarian cyst consistent with an endometrioma
	• **Laparoscopy: definitive diagnosis through direct visualization**
	   • Early lesions are clear or red (hemorrhagic); blood then oxidizes turning purple/brown; brown/black colored tissue described as "powder burns" or "gunshot" lesions
	   • **Endometrioma**: lesion of ovaries that bleeds inside the endometriotic cyst; old, coagulated blood appears chocolate-colored described as a "chocolate cyst"
	   • *Biopsy often not required but confirms diagnosis*

Treatment	• Medical Management: aimed to reduce symptoms
	   • Non-Steroidal Anti-Inflammatory Drugs (NSAIDs): relieve dysmenorrhea by inhibiting prostaglandins
	   • **Hormonal Contraceptives: combined estrogen-progestin OCPs are first-line**; progestins (levonorgestrel-releasing IUD); GnRH agonist or aromatase inhibitors
	• Surgery:
	   • Laparoscopy with Ablation: conservative treatment of ectopic endometrial tissue; preserves fertility (uterus and ovaries are intact)
	   • Total Abdominal Hysterectomy and Bilateral Salpingo-oophorectomy: definitive treatment if no desire for fertility

Key Words & Most Common	• Ectopic endometrial tissue implanted outside uterus; ovaries are most common site • D's: dysmenorrhea, dyspareunia, dysuria, dyschezia + infertility + pelvic pain • Clinical diagnosis + laparoscopy for definitive diagnosis • OCPs first line + NSAIDs → laparoscopy to preserve fertility → TAH-BSO is definitive

Endometrial Cancer

Etiology & Risk Factors	• Most prevalent gynecologic malignancy in the United States • <u>Types</u>: **adenocarcinoma most common** (>80%), papillary serous; clear cell, adenosquamous, mucinous • <u>Etiology</u>: sporadic mutations secondary to **prolonged unopposed estrogen** (unopposed by progesterone) • <u>Risk Factors</u>: age (postmenopausal women age 50-60 most common), **increased estrogen exposure** (nulliparity, early menarche, late menopause), **polycystic ovarian syndrome, obesity, tamoxifen therapy**, diabetes mellitus, **estrogen-only hormone replacement therapy** • <u>Protective Factors</u>: **combination estrogen-progestin oral contraceptive pills (OCPs) are protective against ovarian and endometrial cancers**
Patho-physiology	• Endogenous or exogenous unopposed estrogen stimulates endometrial proliferation leading to endometrial hyperplasia which progress to invasive cancer • Lymphatic vessels may carry endometrial carcinoma cells to nearby fallopian tubes, cervix and ovaries
Signs & Symptoms	• **Abnormal uterine bleeding** • **Postmenopausal bleeding**, pre- or peri-menopausal bleeding, menorrhagia (heavy menstrual bleeding), metrorrhagia (abnormal uterine bleeding)

Diagnosis	**Staging**
• <u>**Transvaginal Ultrasound**</u>: **screening test; thickened endometrial strip >4mm** • <u>**Endometrial Biopsy**</u>: **definitive diagnosis** • <u>Pelvic MRI</u>: may be indicated to determine origin of tumor and local extension • <u>CT Scan</u>: chest, abdomen, pelvis; indicated in high-grade carcinomas to detect distant metastases	• <u>Stage I</u>: confined to uterine corpus • <u>Stage II</u>: Invasion of the cervical stroma but no extension outside the uterus • <u>Stage III</u>: Local and/or regional spread of the tumor • <u>Stage IV</u>: Involvement of the bladder and/or intestinal mucosa and/or distant metastases

Treatment	• <u>Stage I</u>: **total abdominal hysterectomy with bilateral salpingo-oophorectomy (TAH-BSO)** via laparotomy, laparoscopy or robotic-assisted surgery; may need post-op radiation • <u>Stage II and III</u>: TAH-BSO + sentinel lymph node mapping + pelvic radiation therapy with or without chemotherapy • <u>Stage IV</u>: combination of surgery, radiation therapy and systemic chemotherapy
Key Words & Most Common	• Most prevalent gynecologic malignancy in US • Adenocarcinoma most common • Prolonged unopposed estrogen is greatest risk factor; combined OCPs are protective • Most common >45 years old, increased estrogen exposure, PCOS, obesity, tamoxifen therapy, estrogen-only hormone replacement therapy • Abnormal uterine bleeding (postmenopausal) • Endometrial biopsy definitive diagnosis • TAH-BSO +/- radiation +/- chemotherapy

Pelvic Organ Prolapse

Etiology & Risk Factors	• Herniation of pelvic structures into or beyond the vagina (toward or past the introitus) • <u>Etiology</u>: **pelvic floor muscle weakness**; connective tissue laxity • <u>Risk Factors</u>: **childbirth (especially multiparity or traumatic) leading to pelvic floor weakness, obesity**, repeated heavy lifting, advancing age, connective tissue disorders
Patho-physiology	• Weakening of surrounding pelvic support structures including the uterosacral and cardinal ligament complexes and pelvic floor muscles allow for prolapse of the uterus into the vaginal vault

Signs & Symptoms	

• **Vaginal fullness, heaviness, or "falling out" sensation**
   • Symptoms may be gradual and positional
     • **Worse with prolonged standing or straining** (lifting, bowel movements, coughing, sneezing etc.)
• Lower abdominal or back pain
• <u>Urinary Dysfunction</u>: **urinary urgency and frequency**, sensation of incomplete bladder emptying, **stress incontinence**
• <u>Defecatory Dysfunction</u>: **constipation**, incomplete emptying, fecal urgency or incontinence
• <u>Sexual Dysfunction</u>: **dyspareunia** (painful intercourse), avoidance of sexual activity due to embarrassment
• <u>Physical Exam</u>: **bulging mass visualized on pelvic exam**; performed at rest and with Valsalva maneuver
	• <u>Types</u>:
	   • <u>**Cystocele**</u>: **herniation of anterior vaginal wall + descent of bladder**
	   • <u>**Rectocele**</u>: **herniation of posterior vaginal segment + descent of rectum**
	   • <u>**Enterocele**</u>: **herniation of intestines to or through vaginal wall**
	   • <u>**Uterine/Vaginal Vault Prolapse**</u>: **descent of apex of vagina to lower vagina, hymen, or beyond introitus**
	• <u>Staging</u>: Pelvic Organ Prolapse-Quantification (POP-Q) system
	   • <u>Stage 0</u>: no prolapse
	   • <u>Stage I</u>: most distal prolapse is >1 cm above the hymen
	   • <u>Stage II</u>: most distal prolapse is between 1 cm above and 1 cm below the hymen
	   • <u>Stage III</u>: most distal prolapse is >1 cm below hymen but 2 cm shorter than total vaginal length
	   • <u>Stage IV</u>: complete eversion

Diagnosis	• **Clinical Diagnosis**

Treatment	• <u>Conservative Management</u>:
	   • **Vaginal pessary, pelvic floor muscle training (Kegel exercises)**
	• <u>Surgical Management</u>: techniques may include one or a combination of the following
	   • **Hysterectomy**, pelvic support structure repair (colporrhaphy), uterosacral or sacrospinous ligament fixation suspension, colpocleisis (vagina is suture closed)

Key Words & Most Common	• Pelvic floor weakness secondary to childbirth leads to herniation of structures into/beyond the vagina • Vaginal fullness, heaviness, "falling out" sensation + bulging mass on exam • Urinary, defecatory, sexual dysfunction • Clinical Diagnosis • Vaginal pessary + pelvic floor exercises → surgery

Ovarian Cyst

Etiology & Risk Factors	• Fluid-filled structure within the ovaries; most commonly related to ovulation • <u>Etiology</u>: **physiologic** (follicular or luteal cysts) • <u>Risk Factors</u>: **age (most common during reproductive years)**, infertility treatment (gonadotropins lead to ovarian hyperstimulation), tamoxifen therapy, pregnancy, hypothyroidism, smoking, tubal ligation procedures
Patho-physiology	• <u>Follicular Cysts</u>: **most common**; follicles fail to rupture during ovulation and continue to grow (excessive FSH stimulation or absence of the midcycle LH surge) • <u>Corpus Luteal Cysts</u>: when egg is fertilized, corpus luteum continues to secrete progesterone until 14 weeks' gestation when central hemorrhage dissolves the corpus luteum. If this does not occur, a corpus luteal cyst may form • <u>Theca Lutein Cysts</u>: form as a result of overstimulation in elevated human chorionic gonadotropin (hCG) levels

Signs & Symptoms	• **Often asymptomatic** • **Unilateral dull pelvic pain or pressure** • Dyspareunia (painful intercourse) or bladder pressure may be present • <u>Physical Exam</u>: • Unilateral pelvic tenderness; palpable, mobile cystic adnexal mass	• <u>Ruptured Ovarian Cyst</u>: **sudden onset pelvic pain and tenderness (often during sexual activity or strenuous physical activity); nausea/vomiting; menstrual abnormalities**
Diagnosis	• <u>Transvaginal Ultrasound</u>: **initial imaging test of choice**; evaluates laterality, size, composition, presence of pelvic free fluid, blood flow and vascularity • <u>Follicular</u>: simple, smooth, thin-walled unilocular • <u>Corpus Luteal</u>: complex, thick-walled with peripheral vascularity • <u>Ruptured Ovarian Cyst</u>: adnexal mass + pelvic free fluid • <u>Beta Human Chorionic Gonadotropin (beta-hCG)</u>: rule out pregnancy or ectopic pregnancy • <u>Tumor Markers</u>: CA-125, alpha fetoprotein, beta-hCG if concern for malignancy	
Treatment	• <u>Conservative</u>: **if asymptomatic and small (<5cm) usually resolve spontaneously**; closer observation if 5-8cm • Rest, NSAIDs, serial monitoring with ultrasound after 1-2 menstrual cycles • <u>Surgery</u>: • <u>Laparoscopy or Laparotomy</u>: **indicated for large (>8cm) or characteristics of cancer (solid, nodular, thick septations)** • <u>Oophorectomy</u>: indicated in postmenopausal women with cysts >5cm or large cysts that cannot be removed separate from ovary	• <u>Rupture Ovarian Cyst</u>: observation, analgesics (NSAIDs), rest • May require hospitalization if blood loss, fever, leukocytosis or malignancy suspected • Laparoscopy if hemodynamically unstable

Key Words & Most Common	• Fluid-filled structure within ovaries; often physiologic • Asymptomatic or unilateral dull pelvic pain/pressure • Transvaginal ultrasound • Conservative if small, laparoscopy if large or cancerous

Ovarian Cancer

Etiology & Risk Factors	• Highest mortality rate of all gynecologic cancers; 2nd most prevalent gynecologic cancer (endometrial is 1st) • <u>Etiology</u>: >90% are epithelial in origin; the rest (germ cell tumors, sex-cord stromal tumors) develop from other ovarian cell types • <u>Risk Factors</u>: **family history of ovarian cancer, nulliparity, delayed childbearing, early menarche, late menopause**, Caucasian, **age (>50 years old)**, genetic (BRCA-1 or BRCA-2) • **Risk decreased by combined OCP use**
Patho-physiology	• <u>Type I</u>: arise from atypical proliferative tumors; typically present early stage and are low-grade (except clear-cell), have low proliferative activity and carry good prognosis • <u>Subtypes</u>: low-grade serous carcinoma, endometrioid, clear-cell, and mucinous carcinomas • <u>Type II</u>: high-grade tumors and are usually of advanced stage; high proliferative activity with rapid and aggressive progression • <u>Subtypes</u>: high-grade serous carcinoma, carcinosarcoma, undifferentiated carcinoma
Signs & Symptoms	• **Rarely symptomatic until advanced disease process** (extensive METS) • **Abdominal fullness, bloating and distention**, nausea, early satiety, **constipation** or bowel obstruction, urinary frequency, back pain • **Weight loss** • Increasing abdominal girth • Irregular menses, menorrhagia, postmenopausal bleeding • <u>Physical Exam</u>: • Solid, fixed, irregular, palpable adnexal mass • Ascites, pleural effusion, Sister Mary Joseph's nodule (palpable nodule bulging into the umbilicus) **indicates advanced malignancy**

	Staging
Diagnosis • <u>Pelvic Ultrasound</u>: **initial imaging test of choice**; findings suggesting cancer include a solid component, size >6cm, irregular shape, low vascular resistance and surface growth • <u>Staging Imaging</u>: CT or MRI of chest, abdomen and pelvis may be indicated if advanced metastases suspected • <u>Tumor Markers</u>: **CA-125 (CA 125 is elevated in 80% of advanced epithelial ovarian cancers)**, beta-hCG, lactic dehydrogenase (LDH), alpha-fetoprotein, and inhibin	• <u>Stage I</u>: tumor limited to the ovaries or fallopian tubes • <u>Stage II</u>: tumor involving one or both ovaries or fallopian tubes with pelvic extension or peritoneal cancer • <u>Stage III</u>: tumor involving one or both ovaries or fallopian tubes or peritoneal cancer with microscopically confirmed peritoneal metastases outside the pelvis and/or metastasis to the retroperitoneal lymph nodes • <u>Stage IV</u>: distant metastases excluding peritoneal metastases

Treatment	• <u>Stage I</u>: **total abdominal hysterectomy with bilateral salpingo-oophorectomy (TAH-BSO)** via laparotomy, laparoscopy or robotic-assisted surgery; prognosis generally good • <u>Stage II-IV</u>: **TAH-BSO + lymphadenectomy + adjuvant chemotherapy** (cisplatin or carboplatin and paclitaxel) • <u>Stage IV</u>: combination of surgery, radiation therapy and systemic chemotherapy • <u>CA-125</u>: **levels used to monitor treatment progress** • <u>Prognosis</u>: ovarian cancer is generally detected late in disease course and usually metastatic; often carries a poor prognosis

253

Bartholin Cyst and Abscess 🧍‍♀️

Etiology & Risk Factors	• Obstruction of the Bartholin gland causes a Bartholin cyst which may become infected, forming an abscess • Etiology: idiopathic; **obstruction of Bartholin gland** • Abscesses are generally polymicrobial (*Staphylococcus* spp., *Streptococcus* spp., and *E.coli*; MRSA becoming more common) • Risk Factors: **age (20-30 years old most common), trauma to vagina** (episiotomy, childbirth),
Patho-physiology	• **Bartholin glands (greater vestibular glands) are pair of 0.5cm mucus-secreting glands located at the lower aspect (4 o'clock and 8 o'clock position) of the vaginal introitus** • **Obstruction of the gland leads to collection of mucus and cyst formation that may become infected and form an abscess**

Signs & Symptoms	• Cysts:
	   • **Nontender, unilateral, palpable mass near the vaginal orifice**
	   • Larger cysts (>2cm) may cause discomfort with sexual intercourse and with walking or prolonged sitting
	• Abscess:
	   • **Localized pain and tenderness, unilateral palpable mass near vaginal orifice; may have edema, erythema, or induration**
	   • **May be fluctuant +/- purulent drainage**
	   • Fever, painful intercourse, pain with walking and prolonged sitting, vaginal discharge may be present

Diagnosis	• **Clinical Diagnosis** • Labs: sample of discharge screened for STDs; abscess drainage should be cultured to guide treatment • Biopsy: indicated if atypical presentation in patient >40 years old to rule out vulvar cancer

Treatment	• Conservative: indicated for asymptomatic or mild symptoms;
	   • **Sitz baths**, analgesia (NSAIDs), pelvic rest
	• Incision and Drainage: **indicated for large abscesses**; catheter may be placed for continued drainage
	• Antibiotics: indicated for large abscesses with surrounding cellulitis
	   • **Trimethoprim-sulfamethoxazole OR amoxicillin-clavulanate AND clindamycin**
	• Surgery: indicated for large or recurrent cases
	   • Catheter Insertion: small, balloon-tipped (Word) catheter is inserted, inflated, and left within the cyst for 4-6 weeks; stimulates fibrosis to create a permanent opening
	   • Marsupialization: everted edges of the cyst are sutured to the exterior; performed by gynecologist in operating room
	   • Excision: excision required in recurrent cases

Key Words & Most Common	• Obstruction of Bartholin gland (located at 4 and 8 o'clock position of vaginal introitus) leads to cyst and possible abscess • Cyst: nontender, unilateral, palpable mass • Abscess: localized pain and tenderness + fluctuance + purulence + signs of cellulitis • Clinical Diagnosis • Sitz baths → I&D procedure +/- antibiotics (TMP-SMX or amoxicillin-clavulanate + clindamycin) → surgery

Right Bartholin cyst

Benign Ovarian Mass 🧍‍♀️

Etiology & Risk Factors	• **Non-cancerous, benign neoplasm of the ovaries; also known as "dermoid cyst"** • Most (90%) of ovarian neoplasms in women of reproductive age are benign; risk of malignancy increases with age • Etiology: **no clear etiology** • Risk Factors: late menarche, menstrual irregularities, alcohol abuse, nulliparity, exercise during adolescents (leading to anovulatory state)
Patho-physiology	• **Benign Cystic Teratomas: most common benign ovarian neoplasm; also known as "dermoid cyst"** • Consist mostly of ectodermal issue but do contain tissue from all 3 germ cell layers (sebaceous fluid, hair, teeth) • Fibromas: slow-growing connective tissue tumor • Cystadenomas: serous or mucinous tumors
Signs & Symptoms	• **Often asymptomatic; discovered as incidental finding** • **May lead to adnexal torsion** (especially if mass >4cm) • Vague abdominal/pelvic pain, menstrual irregularities • Physical Exam: • Normal or may have palpable adnexal mass
Diagnosis	• Pelvic Ultrasound: **initial imaging test of choice** • Teratomas: heterogeneous mass with echogenic focus causing shadowing secondary to calcifications, sebum, and hair; fat hair fluid levels are more specific findings • CT Abdomen and Pelvis: most sensitive imaging test; may be used for pre-operative planning

Treatment	• **Surgery: definitive treatment; laparoscopy is gold-standard**
	   • **Surgical removal (simple laparoscopic cystectomy preferred procedure) indicated to reduce risk of adnexal torsion** or malignant transformation of mass
	   • Complete resection with bilateral salpingo-oophorectomy indicated if large (>5cm) mass or distortion of structure or malignant potential

Key Words & Most Common	• Non-cancerous, benign neoplasm of ovaries • Benign cystic teratoma ("dermoid cyst") is most common benign ovarian neoplasm; may contain sebaceous fluid, hair, teeth tissue • Often asymptomatic • Pelvic ultrasound • Surgery; laparoscopy is gold standard

Dermoid cyst on ultrasound

Ovarian Torsion

Etiology & Risk Factors	• Rotation/twisting of the ovary and portion of the fallopian tube on the supporting ligamental structures; also known as adnexal torsion • <u>Etiology</u>: mechanical complication of ovarian cyst of ovarian neoplasm • <u>Risk Factors</u>: **ovarian mass >4cm**, age (**reproductive age**; <50 years old), pregnancy, patient undergoing fertility treatment (ovulation induction)
Patho-physiology	• **Rotation/twisting of the ovary on the supplying vascular pedicle and supporting ligamental structures** (infundibulopelvic ligament, and the utero-ovarian ligament) **interrupting the arterial blood flow leading to ovarian ischemia and subsequent necrosis of the ovary, infarction, hemorrhage, and/or peritonitis** • Torsion most commonly occurs on right ovary (sigmoid colon provides stabilization to the left ovary)

Signs & Symptoms	• **Acute unilateral lower abdominal or pelvic pain**
	   • May be sharp or dull; intermittent (colicky) or constant
	   • Pain may radiate to abdomen, flank or back
	• **Nausea and vomiting**
	• <u>Physical Exam</u>:
	   • **Unilateral, tender, adnexal mass**; may have cervical motion tenderness or peritoneal signs

Diagnosis	• <u>Doppler Ultrasound</u>: **initial imaging test of choice**
	   • **Enlarged ovarian volume and/or ovarian mass**
	   • **Diminished or absent ovarian blood flow** (2/3rd cases have normal blood flow; normal blood flow does *not* exclude torsion)
	• <u>Exploratory Surgery</u>: definitive diagnosis is made by direct visualization of rotated ovary
	• <u>MRI/CT</u>: may be used to rule out other pathology but are not routinely ordered

Treatment	• <u>Surgery</u>: **emergency surgery required to prevent ovarian necrosis**
	   • **Laparoscopic detorsion is first-line procedure**
	   • Cystectomy if benign cyst present to prevent recurrence and preserve ovary
	   • Salpingo-oophorectomy if cyst appears malignant or is necrotic

Key Words & Most Common	• Rotation/twisting of ovary leading to vascular compromise • Acute, unilateral lower abdominal/pelvic pain + nausea and vomiting in reproductive age female • Doppler ultrasound initial test; shows enlarged ovarian volume or ovarian mass +/- diminished blood flow • Laparoscopic detorsion

Polycystic Ovarian Syndrome (PCOS)

Etiology & Risk Factors	• Common hormonal disorder affecting reproductive age females characterized by **irregular menstrual cycles, hyperandrogenism, insulin resistance and bilateral cystic ovaries** • <u>Etiology</u>: environmental and hereditary factors • <u>Risk Factors</u>: **obesity and prepubertal obesity**, insulin resistance, fetal androgen exposure, use of valproic acid
Patho-physiology	• Ovarian hormonal dysregulation secondary to 17-hydroxyprogesterone over response to gonadotropin stimulation alters the gonadotropin-releasing hormone (GnRH) release which leads to an **increase in luteinizing hormone (LH) and decrease in follicle-stimulating hormone (FSH)** biosynthesis and secretion • Luteinizing hormone stimulates ovarian androgen production while decreased FSH prevents aromatase activity within granulosa cells, thus decreasing androgen conversion to estradiol. This self-perpetuating noncyclical hormonal pattern leads to **increased testosterone production, follicular degeneration and bilateral cystic ovaries**
Signs & Symptoms	• <u>Ovulatory Dysfunction</u>: **irregular menses, oligomenorrhea** (infrequent menstruation), **amenorrhea** (absence of menstruation), **infertility** • <u>Hyperandrogenism</u>: **hirsutism** (coarse, dark hair growth in male pattern; face, neck, upper lip, chin, thumbs and toes, around nipples, along lineal alba of lower abdomen) **acne, hair thinning, body odor** • <u>Insulin Resistance</u>: **type II diabetes mellitus, obesity, acanthosis nigricans** (areas of thickened, dark skin of the nape of the neck, axillae, skinfolds, knuckles, elbows) • <u>Other symptoms</u>: fatigue, sleep-related problems (sleep apnea, insomnia), mood swings, depression/anxiety, hypertension, headaches • <u>Physical Exam</u>: • May have bilateral enlarged, smooth, mobile ovaries on bimanual exam; evidence of acanthosis nigricans

Diagnosis	• <u>Rotterdam Criteria</u>: 2 of 3 required for diagnosis
	   • **(1)** ovulatory dysfunction causing menstrual irregularity **(2)** lab or clinical signs of hyperandrogenism **(3)** cystic ovaries on ultrasound
	• <u>Labs</u>: beta-hCG, DHEAs, total testosterone (free testosterone more sensitive), FSH, LH, prolactin, 17-hydroxyprogesterone, lipid panel, fasting insulin, glucose tolerance test
	   • May show **elevated testosterone and increased LH:FSH ratio (≥3:1)**
	• <u>Transvaginal Ultrasound</u>: **imaging test of choice**
	   • Shows enlarged ovaries with >10 follicles per ovary (multiple ovarian cysts) occurring at periphery; resembles a **"string of pearls"**

Treatment	• <u>Lifestyle Modifications</u>: aimed to decrease insulin resistance; **weight loss, regular exercise**, proper diet and nutrition, sleep hygiene • <u>Hormonal Contraceptives</u>: **first-line medical therapy**; intermittent progestin (medroxyprogesterone) or **combination estrogen-progestin contraceptive pills** • <u>Metformin</u>: aims to improve metabolic and glycemic abnormalities to make menstrual cycles more regular; **improves insulin sensitivity, can reduce free testosterone levels** • <u>Spironolactone</u>: anti-androgenic agent that competitively inhibiting dihydrotestosterone at its receptor sites and decreases testosterone levels • <u>Infertility Treatments</u>: **clomiphene** is a selective-estrogen receptor-modulator (SERM) that stimulates ovaries to develop oocyte follicles and reestablish ovulation • <u>Management of Comorbidities</u>: obesity, metabolic syndrome, type II diabetes mellitus, dyslipidemia, endometrial hyperplasia, cardiovascular disease, obstructive sleep apnea
Key Words & Most Common	• Ovulatory dysfunction: irregular or absent menses; infertility • Hyperandrogenism: hirsutism, acne, body odor • Insulin Resistance: T2DM, obesity, acanthosis nigricans • US shows multiple ovarian cysts ("sting of pearls") • Weight loss → OCPs → metformin +/- spironolactone → clomiphene

Vaginal Cancer

Etiology & Risk Factors	• Primary vaginal cancer is quire rare (1% of all gynecologic malignancies); metastases or local extension of malignancies of adjacent structures is more common • <u>Etiology</u>: **squamous cell carcinoma is most common primary tumor (90%)**; secondary tumors are more common overall • <u>Risk Factors</u>: **human papilloma virus (type 16 and 18 most common), age (60-65 years old most common),** vaginal intraepithelial neoplasia, exposure to diethylstilbestrol
Patho-physiology	• HPV is passed through skin-to-skin contact; may be spread through sexual intercourse, hand to genital contact, or oral sex • HPV have oncoproteins that inactivate certain tumor suppressor proteins leading to dysregulation of cell cycle and neoplastic formation of tissue (Cervical intraepithelial neoplasia) and eventually cervical and/or vaginal cancer

Signs & Symptoms	• **Abnormal intermenstrual vaginal bleeding is most common symptom**
	   • **Postcoital** or postmenopausal most common
	• **Watery vaginal discharge**
	• **Dyspareunia** (painful intercourse)
	• <u>Physical Exam</u>:
	   • **Visualized lesion on speculum exam**; may appear as a mass, ulcer, or plaque
	   • Should examine entirety of vagina including anterior and posterior walls; posterior wall of proximal 1/3rd of vagina is most common site

		Staging
Diagnosis	• <u>**Biopsy**</u>: **gold standard for diagnosis** • Colposcopy may be performed to determine biopsy site if no obvious lesion visualized	• <u>Stage I</u>: limited to the vagina • <u>Stage II</u>: invading paravaginal tissue; no pelvic sidewall invasion • <u>Stage III</u>: extension to pelvic wall, lower 1/3rd of the vagina and/or causing hydronephrosis or kidney dysfunction; +/- inguinal lymph node metastases • <u>Stage IV</u>: extension beyond the true pelvis, bladder or rectal involvement and/or distant metastases (lung or bone) +/- lymph node metastases

Treatment	• <u>Local Surgical Excision</u>: may be possible if small (<2cm) lesion and confined to mucosa • <u>Stage I</u>: **radical hysterectomy, upper vaginectomy, and pelvic lymph node dissection** +/- radiation therapy • <u>Stage II-IV</u>: radiation therapy (combination of external beam radiation therapy and brachytherapy) +/- combined chemotherapy
Key Words & Most Common	• Squamous cell carcinoma most common primary tumor • HPV 16 and 18 most common cause • Abnormal vaginal bleeding most common symptom Biopsy is gold standard diagnosis • Local excision if small → hysterectomy, vaginectomy and lymph node dissection (stage I) → radiation +/- chemotherapy if advanced

Vulvar Cancer

Etiology & Risk Factors	• 4th most common gynecologic cancer • <u>Etiology</u>: squamous cell carcinoma most common type (90%); malignant melanoma (5%), transitional cell, adenoid cystic, and adenosquamous carcinomas • <u>Risk Factors</u>: **human papilloma virus (type 16 and 18 most common), increasing age, smoking,** inflammatory vulvar conditions (**lichen sclerosis**, chronic granulomatous disease), prior pelvic radiation, vaginal intraepithelial neoplasia, exposure to diethylstilbestrol
Patho-physiology	• HPV is known to have specific oncoproteins which inactivate the p53 and RB tumor suppressor proteins and leads to unrestricted hyperproliferation and eventually cancer

Signs & Symptoms	• May be asymptomatic
	• **Vulvar pruritus (itching), irritation, pain**
	• **Bleeding, mass lesion, or ulceration** indicates advanced disease
	• <u>Physical Exam</u>:
	   • **Erythematous raised, ulcerative lesion**; scaly patch or plaque
	   • **Labia majora is most common site**; labia minora, clitoris or Bartholin glands may also be affected
	   • *Lesion may mimic sexually transmitted genital ulcers (chancroid), Bartholin gland cyst, condyloma acuminatum (genital warts); consider vulvar cancer in women that develop vulvar lesion with low risk of STIs*

		Staging

Diagnosis	• <u>**Biopsy**</u>: **gold standard for diagnosis**
	   • Dermal punch biopsy is usually diagnostic
	   • Subtle lesions may be delineated by staining the vulva with toluidine blue or using colposcopy
		• <u>Stage I</u>: confined to the vulva
		• <u>Stage II</u>: tumor of any size with adjacent spread (lower 1/3rd of the urethra, lower 1/3rd of the vagina, or anus) with no lymph node metastases
		• <u>Stage III</u>: tumor of any size, with adjacent spread to or presence of nonfixed, nonulcerated lymph nodes
		• <u>Stage IV</u>: tumor of any size with bone or ulcerated lymph node metastases or distance organ metastases

Treatment	• <u>**Surgical Excision**</u>: wide radical excision is standard of care • <u>Stage III-IV</u>: lymph node dissection followed by radiation therapy and chemotherapy (cisplatin or fluorouracil) is performed before surgical excision
Key Words & Most Common	• Squamous cell carcinoma most common • HPV 16 and 18 most common cause • Labia majora most common site • Vulvar pruritus, irritation → bleeding, lesion, ulceration • Biopsy is gold standard • Surgical excision

Pelvic Inflammatory Disease

Etiology & Risk Factors	• Inflammation of the upper female genital tract secondary to infection • <u>Etiology</u>: ascending infection from the vagina and cervix into the endometrium and fallopian tubes • ***Chlamydia trachomatis* (most common)**, ***Neisseria gonorrhoeae****, Gardnerella vaginalis, Mycoplasma genitalium, Haemophilus influenzae, Streptococcus agalactia* • <u>Risk Factors</u>: **history of PID, presence of STI, multiple or new sex partners or a partner who does not use a condom**, non-white ethnicity, low socioeconomic status, **IUD contraceptive**, nulliparity, **age (most common 16-25 years old)**
Patho-physiology	• Inflammation of the upper female genital tract, secondary to infection, leads to scarring, adhesions and partial/total fallopian tube obstruction resulting in loss of ciliated epithelial cells that line the fallopian tubes which impairs ovum transport and increases the risk for infertility and ectopic pregnancy
Signs & Symptoms	• **Lower abdominal or pelvic pain** • **Vaginal discharge (purulent)** • **Dyspareunia** (painful sexual intercourse) • **Vaginal bleeding or postcoital bleeding** • Dysuria, **fever**, malaise, nausea and vomiting • <u>Physical Exam</u>: • **Cervical motion tenderness** (chandelier sign), **adnexal tenderness, mucopurulent cervicitis**, lower abdominal/pelvic tenderness to palpation
Diagnosis	• **Clinical Diagnosis** • Labs: **beta-hCG (rule out ectopic pregnancy), endocervical nucleic acid amplification test (NAAT) for gonorrhea and chlamydia** • <u>Ultrasound/CT</u>: ordered to rule out other pelvic pathology • <u>**Laparoscopy**</u>: **gold-standard for diagnosis** but rarely performed; demonstrates purulent peritoneal material

Treatment	• <u>Antibiotics</u>:
	   • <u>Outpatient</u>: indicated if mild to moderate PID and cervicitis
	      • **IM Ceftriaxone (500mg) + doxycycline** (100mg BID 14 days)
	      • **Metronidazole** (500mg BID 14 days) should be added if there is a concern for trichomonas or recent vaginal instrumentation
	   • <u>Inpatient</u>: indicated if uncertain diagnosis, pregnancy, high fever, tubo-ovarian abscess, inability to tolerate outpatient treatment (vomiting), failed outpatient treatment
	      • **IV Ceftriaxone (1G) + PO/IV doxycycline** (100mg q12h) **+ PO/IV metronidazole** (500mg q12h)
	      • *OR* IV clindamycin + IV gentamicin *OR* IV ampicillin-sulbactam + PO/IV doxycycline
	• <u>Laparoscopy</u>: indicated for tubo-ovarian abscess

Key Words & Most Common	• Ascending infection of female genital tract most commonly caused by C. trachomatis and/or N. gonorrhoeae • Lower abdominal/pelvic pain + purulent vaginal discharge + postcoital bleeding + dyspareunia • Cervical motion tenderness + adnexal tenderness on exam • IM ceftriaxone + doxycycline +/- metronidazole for outpatient treatment

Bacterial Vaginosis

Etiology & Risk Factors	• Condition characterized by overgrowth of normal vaginal flora due to altered microbiome; not considered a sexually transmitted infection • <u>Etiology</u>: **overgrowth of *Gardnerella vaginalis* and decrease in *Lactobacillus acidophilus*** (normal vaginal flora) • <u>Risk Factors</u>: **multiple sexual partners, women who have sex with women** (direct genital contact or shared sexual objects), **douching**, IUD contraceptive, **hygiene products** (some feminine hygiene products, fragrances, lotions, body washes, soaps may disrupt normal vaginal pH), spermicide
Patho-physiology	• *Lactobacilli* spp. is a normal hydrogen peroxide-producing bacteria that maintains vaginal pH and is part of the normal vaginal flora • Disruption of normal vaginal flora leads to overgrowth of *Gardnerella vaginalis* bacteria • Male ejaculate is more alkaline which worsens symptoms (malodourous discharge) after coitus
Signs & Symptoms	• **Vaginal discharge that is malodourous, thin and gray/white** • Described as **"fishy odor"**; becomes stronger when vaginal discharge is more alkaline (after coitus and menses) • **Dyspareunia** • *Vaginal pruritus, irritation, erythema, and edema are not common*

Diagnosis	• <u>**Amsel Criteria**</u>: **3 of 4 criteria met confirms diagnosis**
	   • **Homogenous, thin, gray/white vaginal discharge**
	   • **Positive whiff-amine test** ("fishy odor" when a drop of an alkali solution [10% KOH] is added)
	   • **Vaginal pH >4.5**
	   • **Clue cells on saline wet mount** (bacteria adheres to epithelial cells and obscures their margins)

Treatment	• <u>Conservative</u>: avoid douching, avoid triggers (fragrance, soaps, detergents, etc.), take *Lactobacillus* spp. based probiotic
	• <u>Antibiotics</u>:
	   • <u>**Oral Metronidazole**</u>: **treatment of choice if not pregnant**; oral 500mg BID for 7 days or 2g one time dose
	   • <u>**Intravaginal Metronidazole**</u>: **preferred treatment if pregnant**; 0.75% gel (5g) intravaginally at bedtime for 5 days
	   • <u>**Intravaginal Clindamycin**</u>: 2% cream (5g) intravaginally at bedtime for 7 days
	   • Tinidazole or oral clindamycin are alternatives; secnidazole 2g one time dose if patient compliance is a concern
	• Treatment of asymptomatic sexual partners is unnecessary

Key Words & Most Common	• Overgrowth of *Gardnerella vaginalis* and decreased *Lactobacillus* spp. • Malodourous, thin, gray/white vaginal discharge • Amsel criteria: 1. Homogenous, thin, gray/white discharge 2. Positive whiff test 3. Vaginal pH>4.5 4. Clue cells on saline wet mount • Oral metronidazole is preferred treatment if not pregnant; intravaginal metronidazole if pregnant

Clue Cells

Bacteria adheres to epithelial cell edges

Trichomoniasis

Etiology & Risk Factors	• Sexually transmitted infection caused by a flagellated protozoan that may infect the male or female genital tract • Etiology: *Trichomonas vaginalis*; a flagellated protozoan • Risk Factors: history of STIs, **multiple or new sex partners or a partner who does not use a condom**, contact with infected sexual partner, IV drug abuse,
Patho-physiology	• *Trichomonas vaginalis* is a flagellated protozoan that resides urogenital tract lumen and releases cytotoxic proteins that disrupt the epithelial lining; may increase vaginal pH

Signs & Symptoms	Women	Men

	• **Copious, yellow/green, frothy, malodourous vaginal discharge**
	• **Soreness of vulva or perineum**
	• Dyspareunia, dysuria, urinary frequency
	• Physical Exam:
	   • **Copious yellow/green, frothy malodourous vaginal discharge**, vulvovaginal erythema, **cervical petechiae ("strawberry cervix")**
		• **Mostly asymptomatic**
		• **Urethritis**; epididymitis and prostatitis are rare complications
		• Physical Exam:
		   • Often benign; may have moisture at urethral meatus

Diagnosis	• **Microscopic Examination**: saline wet mount of vaginal secretions demonstrates **trichomonads (motile protozoan with flagella), numerous neutrophils, vaginal pH >4.5** • Nucleic Acid Amplification Test (NAAT): more sensitive than microscopic examination or culture for diagnosis • Urine or Urethral Swab Culture: only validated test for detecting *T. vaginalis* in men

Treatment	• Sexual Education: encourage safe-sex behavior with barrier contraceptives
	• Antibiotics: exposed sexual partners must be treated
	   • **Metronidazole**: treatment of choice; oral 500mg BID for 7 days (women) or 2g one time dose (men or pregnant women)
	   • Tinidazole: 2g one time dose is an alternative
	   • *Topical medications have high failure rates and should not be used*
	• NAAT test of cure recommended for all women treated within three months of treatment

Key Words & Most Common	• *Trichomonas vaginalis* is a flagellated, sexually transmitted protozoan
	• Women: copious, yellow/green, frothy vaginal discharge +/- cervical petechiae ("strawberry cervix")
	• Men: mostly asymptomatic; may develop urethritis
	  Microscopic exam with saline wet mount shows motile flagellated protozoan
	• NAAT is more sensitive; urine/urethral swab culture for men
	• Oral metronidazole is treatment of choice
	   • 500mg BID for 1 days for women
	   • 2g one time dose for men or pregnant women

Vulvovaginal Candiasis

Etiology & Risk Factors	• Inflammation of the vulva and vagina secondary to *Candida* spp. • Etiology: ***Candida albicans* most common** • Risk Factors: **diabetes mellitus, obesity, broad-spectrum antibiotic use, corticosteroid use,** pregnancy, **constrictive undergarments,** immunocompromised, IUD contraceptive
Patho-physiology	• *Candida* spp. superficially penetrate the vaginal mucosal lining and cause an inflammatory response • *Candida* overgrowth secondary to a change in the normal vaginal flora (antibiotic use)

Signs & Symptoms	• **Vulvovaginal pruritus (itching), irritation, burning**
	   • May be worse after coitus or menses
	• **Thick, white, cottage cheese-like vaginal discharge**; may adhere to the vaginal walls
	• Physical Exam:
	   • Vulvovaginal erythema, edema, excoriation
	   • **Thick, white, adherent, vaginal discharge**

Diagnosis	• **Clinical Diagnosis** • **Microscopic Examination: potassium hydroxide (KOH) wet mount demonstrates budding yeast, hyphae, or pseudohyphae; vaginal pH <4.5**

Treatment	• Prevention: keep vulva clean and dry, absorbent 100% cotton underwear to allow air to circulate to reduce moisture, avoid tight-fitting clothing, avoid use of feminine deodorants, bubble baths, fragrant hygiene products
	• Antifungals:
	   • **Oral Fluconazole: first-line medication;** 150mg PO once with a second dose at 72hrs if patient is still symptomatic
	   • **Intravaginal clotrimazole or miconazole are alternatives and first-line for pregnant women**

Key Words & Most Common	• *Candida albicans* infection of vulva and vagina • Diabetes, obesity, recent antibiotic use, constrictive underwear are most common risk factors • Vulvovaginal pruritus + thick, white, cottage cheese-like vaginal discharge • Microscopic exam with KOH prep shows budding yeast, hyphae, pseudohyphae • Oral fluconazole first-line treatment • Intravaginal clotrimazole or miconazole for pregnant women

Pseudohyphae

Cervicitis

Etiology & Risk Factors	• Inflammation of the cervix usually secondary to infection
	• Etiology:
	  • Infectious: **Chlamydia trachomatis (most common)**, *Neisseria gonorrhoeae*, herpes simplex virus (HSV), *Trichomonas vaginalis*, and *Mycoplasma genitalium*
	  • Noninfectious: gynecologic procedure, foreign bodies (pessaries, barrier contraceptives, tampons), chemicals (spermicides, douches, soaps, detergent), allergens (latex)
	• Risk Factors: **multiple or new sex partners or a partner who does not use a condom, age (most common 16-25 years old)**

Patho-physiology	• Infection of the female genitourinary tract by *Chlamydia trachomatis* or *Neisseria gonorrhoeae* allows infiltration of the columnar epithelium of the endocervix leading to inflammation
Signs & Symptoms	• May be asymptomatic • **Mucopurulent vaginal discharge** • **Vaginal bleeding** (after coitus or between menses) • **Dyspareunia, dysuria**, vulvovaginal irritation • Physical Exam: • **Purulent or mucopurulent discharge, cervical friability** (bleeding after touching cervix with swab), **cervical erythema/edema**
Diagnosis	• Clinical Diagnosis • Nucleic Acid Amplification Test (NAAT): most sensitive and specific test; evaluate for gonorrhea, chlamydia, and trichomonas • May be performed on endocervical mucus, vaginal fluid, or urine samples • Saline microscopy, amine whiff test, and vaginal pH to evaluate for bacterial vaginosis

Treatment	• **Empiric treatment recommended for gonorrhea and chlamydia coinfection with IM ceftriaxone (500mg) + oral doxycycline (100mg BID for 14 days)**
	  • Gonorrhea: **IM Ceftriaxone** (500mg)
	    • May give gentamicin + azithromycin OR cefixime if ceftriaxone contraindicated
	  • Chlamydia: oral doxycycline (100mg BID for 14 days); azithromycin (1g as single dose) if pregnant
	• Moxifloxacin indicated if cervicitis persist despite treatment and chlamydia and gonorrhea have been ruled out to cover for *Mycoplasma genitalium* infection

Key Words & Most Common	• Inflammation Of cervix most commonly caused by Chlamydia trachomatis or Neisseria gonorrhoeae • Mucopurulent vaginal discharge + dysuria + dyspareunia • May have cervical friability and purulent discharge on exam • NAAT is most sensitive/specific test • IM ceftriaxone (500mg) + oral doxycycline (100mg BID for 14 days)

Sexual Assault

General Info	• **Any type of sexual activity or contact that a person does not consent to; includes rape and sexual coercion** • May involve force or threats of force; may involve drugs or alcohol • Rape is defined as any vaginal, anal, or oral penetration by another person's sexual organ without consent of the victim • Rape is most commonly an expression of anger or need for psychological power and more violent than it is sexual • People under the age of consent are unable to give consent to any sexual activity with an adult • Female are at greater risk for rape and sexual assault than males; males are less willing to report the crime

Signs & Symptoms	• Rape may result in the following:
	  • Genital injury (lacerations)
	  • Psychological trauma (fear, nightmares, insomnia, anger/embarrassment/guilt, post-traumatic stress disorder, amnesia, anxiety, lack of trust in relationships)
	  • Pregnancy
	  • Sexually transmitted infections (syphilis, gonorrhea, chlamydial infection, trichomoniasis, HPV, hepatitis, HIV)
	  • Additional injuries may occur as a result of the physical violence occurring simultaneously as the assault

Diagnosis	• Collection of Forensic Evidence: if patient chooses to seek counseling prior to medical evaluation, it is recommended to avoid changing clothing, washing or showering, douching, brushing teeth, clipping fingernails or using mouthwash to avoid destroying evidence
	• Physical Exam: privacy must be ensured; each step should be thoroughly explained prior and patient may refuse any part of examination
	  • Description of injuries sustained (including areas of bleeding), description of the attack and the assailant as well as the assailant's behavior
	• Testing: patient has right to refuse testing
	  • Routine Testing: pregnancy test and serologic tests for syphilis, hepatitis B, and HIV; trichomoniasis and bacterial vaginosis testing of vaginal secretions or urine; gonorrheal and chlamydial testing using samples from every penetrated orifice (vaginal, oral, or rectal)
	  • Follow-up tests for pregnancy, untreated STIs, syphilis, hepatitis, and HIV required
	  • Testing for drugs and alcohol is controversial
	• Evidence Collection: can be used to identify assailant
	  • Clothing, smears of buccal, vaginal, rectal mucosa, samples from scalp and pubic hair, fingernail clippings/scrapings, blood and saliva samples, semen samples

Treatment	• Psychological Support: specialist trained in rape crisis intervention should be consulted
	  • Reassurance, nonjudgmental attitude, general support may be provided until specialist can arrive
	• Prevention/Treatment of Infections:
	  • Gonorrhea/Chlamydia: IM ceftriaxone (500mg) + oral doxycycline (100mg BID for 14 days)
	  • Bacterial Vaginosis and Trichomoniasis: metronidazole (500mg BID for 7 days)
	  • Hepatitis B and HPV: vaccination if no documented immunity or is unvaccinated
	  • HIV: post-exposure prophylaxis
	  • Emergency Contraception: levonorgestrel, copper-bearing or levonorgestrel-releasing IUD, ulipristal acetate

References

1. Mastitis in breast.jpg. (2022, December 19). *Wikimedia Commons*. Retrieved 14:29, August 15, 2023 from https://commons.wikimedia.org/w/index.php?title=File:Mastitis_in_breast.jpg&oldid=717754429.
2. Breast Abscess for Incision and Drainage.jpg. (2022, November 15). *Wikimedia Commons*. Retrieved 14:35, August 15, 2023 from https://commons.wikimedia.org/w/index.php?title=File:Breast_Abscess_for_Incision_and_Drainage.jpg&oldid=706323262.
3. Fibrous breast changes.jpg. (2023, March 31). *Wikimedia Commons*. Retrieved 14:37, August 15, 2023 from https://commons.wikimedia.org/w/index.php?title=File:Fibrous_breast_changes.jpg&oldid=745671893.
4. Breast US Fibroadenoma 0531092228218 Nevit.jpg. (2020, August 23). *Wikimedia Commons*. Retrieved 14:39, August 15, 2023 from https://commons.wikimedia.org/w/index.php?title=File:Breast_US_Fibroadenoma_0531092228218_Nevit.jpg&oldid=442315603.
5. GynecomastiaFrontalAsymSevere.jpg. (2022, January 8). *Wikimedia Commons*. Retrieved 14:41, August 15, 2023 from https://commons.wikimedia.org/w/index.php?title=File:GynecomastiaFrontalAsymSevere.jpg&oldid=620136809.
6. MenstrualCycle en.svg. (2023, July 6). *Wikimedia Commons*. Retrieved 15:00, August 15, 2023 from https://commons.wikimedia.org/w/index.php?title=File:MenstrualCycle_en.svg&oldid=780853959.
7. 2906 Placenta Previa-02.jpg. (2023, May 25). *Wikimedia Commons*. Retrieved 16:15, August 15, 2023 from https://commons.wikimedia.org/w/index.php?title=File:2906_Placenta_Previa-_02.jpg&oldid=766922265.
8. Blausen 0737 PlacentalAbruption.png. (2021, May 14). *Wikimedia Commons*. Retrieved 16:18, August 15, 2023 from https://commons.wikimedia.org/w/index.php?title=File:Blausen_0737_PlacentalAbruption.png&oldid=560318145.
9. Spina-bifida.jpg. (2023, March 8). *Wikimedia Commons*. Retrieved 17:59, August 15, 2023 from https://commons.wikimedia.org/w/index.php?title=File:Spina-bifida.jpg&oldid=738801346.
10. Uterine Fibroids.png. (2020, September 25). *Wikimedia Commons*. Retrieved 18:02, August 15, 2023 from https://commons.wikimedia.org/w/index.php?title=File:Uterine_Fibroids.png&oldid=471333286.
11. Linear striations of adenomyosis.jpg. (2020, September 17). *Wikimedia Commons*. Retrieved 18:06, August 15, 2023 from https://commons.wikimedia.org/w/index.php?title=File:Linear_striations_of_adenomyosis.jpg&oldid=462561536.
12. Blausen 0349 Endometriosis.png. (2023, June 28). *Wikimedia Commons*. Retrieved 18:11, August 15, 2023 from https://commons.wikimedia.org/w/index.php?title=File:Blausen_0349_Endometriosis.png&oldid=778038938.
13. Barthonlincyst2011.png. (2022, February 27). *Wikimedia Commons*. Retrieved 18:18, August 15, 2023 from https://commons.wikimedia.org/w/index.php?title=File:Barthonlincyst2011.png&oldid=633338947.
14. Dermoid cyst.jpg. (2023, May 9). *Wikimedia Commons*. Retrieved 18:33, August 15, 2023 from https://commons.wikimedia.org/w/index.php?title=File:Dermoid_cyst.jpg&oldid=761276846.
15. Clue cells - CDC PHIL 3720.jpg. (2020, February 27). *Wikimedia Commons*. Retrieved 18:40, August 15, 2023 from https://commons.wikimedia.org/w/index.php?title=File:Clue_cells_-_CDC_PHIL_3720.jpg&oldid=398879364.
16. Detail of vaginal wet mount in candidal vulvovaginitis.jpg. (2022, October 18). *Wikimedia Commons*. Retrieved 18:47, August 15, 2023 from https://commons.wikimedia.org/w/index.php?title=File:Detail_of_vaginal_wet_mount_in_candidal_vulvovaginitis.jpg&oldid=697286999.

Chapter 7

Endocrine

Primary Adrenal Insufficiency (Addison Disease) 🔄

Etiology & Risk Factors	• Pathology affecting the adrenal gland results in insidious, progressive, hypo-functioning of adrenal cortex • **Primary adrenal insufficiency is characterized by decreased aldosterone and cortisol production secondary to diminished adrenal gland function** • <u>Etiology</u>: **autoimmune destruction of adrenal cortex is most common cause**; destruction of adrenal cortex by infection (tuberculosis, HIV, syphilis, histoplasmosis), thrombosis or hemorrhage of adrenal gland, trauma, metastatic disease, **medications** (ketoconazole, fluconazole, etomidate) **congenital adrenal hyperplasia in children**
Patho-physiology	• **Mineralocorticoid deficiency leads to increased excretion of sodium and decreased excretion of potassium** resulting in hyponatremia and hyperkalemia and may cause severe dehydration, plasma hypertonicity, acidosis, decreased circulatory volume, hypotension, circulatory failure • Glucocorticoid deficiency leads to hypotension, insulin sensitivity and disruption of carbohydrate, fat, and protein metabolism resulting in weakness • **Decreased cortisol leads to increased pituitary adrenocorticotropic hormone (ACTH) production and increased blood beta-lipotropin which has melanocyte-stimulating activity and causes hyperpigmentation of the skin and mucus membranes**

Signs & Symptoms	• **Weakness, fatigue, orthostatic hypotension**
	• Nausea/vomiting/diarrhea, headache, sweating, **cold intolerance**, weight loss, **dehydration**
	• **Salt cravings**
	• Loss of libido, loss of pubic hair, amenorrhea
	• <u>Skin Changes</u>:
	   • **Hyperpigmentation (diffuse tanning of skin especially sun-exposed areas, bony prominences, extensor surfaces, scars, and skin folds)**
	   • **Dark freckles of forehead, face, neck, shoulders**
	   • **Blue/black discolorations of the areolas, lips, mouth, rectum, and vagina**

Diagnosis	• <u>Comprehensive Metabolic Panel (CMP)</u>: ↓sodium, ↑potassium, ↓sodium/potassium ratio (<30:1), ↓glucose, ↓bicarbonate, ↑BUN • <u>Complete Blood Count (CBC)</u>: ↑hematocrit, ↓WBC, ↑eosinophils • <u>Morning Serum Cortisol and Plasma ACTH Levels</u>: ↑plasma ACTH, ↓serum cortisol • <u>ACTH Stimulation Test</u>: **confirms diagnosis; insufficient/absent rise in serum cortisol 30 minutes after ACTH administration (level does not rise above 15-18mcg/dL)** • Normal response is rise of serum cortisol after ACTH administration
Treatment	• <u>Glucocorticoid Replacement</u>: **hydrocortisone (identical to cortisol) is first-line**; prednisone and dexamethasone are alternatives • Total daily dose of hydrocortisone is 15-20 mg; half total given in morning with remaining half split between midday and evening (10mg, 5mg, 5mg) • <u>Mineralocorticoid Replacement</u>: **fludrocortisone is added to replace aldosterone** • <u>Patient Education</u>: stress management education, patients should carry medical alert card and injectable form of cortisol (pre-filled dexamethasone syringe) for emergencies • *Patients may need additional dosing during illness/surgery/fever to recreate the normal "stress" response*
Key Words & Most Common	• Decreased aldosterone and cortisol production due to diminished adrenal gland function (autoimmune destruction is most common cause) • Weakness, fatigue, orthostatic hypotension, salt cravings, cold intolerance, skin hyperpigmentation, dark freckles, blue/black discoloration of mucus membranes and areola • Cosyntropin (ACTH) Stimulation test shows insufficient/absent rise in cortisol • Hydrocortisone + fludrocortisone

Secondary Adrenal Insufficiency 🔄

Etiology & Risk Factors	• Hypo-functioning of the adrenal cortex secondary to inadequate adrenocorticotropic hormone (ACTH) secretion resulting in lack of cortisol • <u>Etiology</u>: **inadequate ACTH secretion** • **Corticosteroid use or stopping long-term corticosteroids (>3months) most common cause**, panhypopituitarism, isolated failure of ACTH secretion
Patho-physiology	• Exogenous corticosteroid use or abrupt discontinuation of corticosteroids without taper results in decreased ACTH stimulation of the adrenal cortex • During periods of metabolic/physiologic stress, adrenals are unable to stimulate corticosteroid release resulting in decreased cortisol levels (does not affect aldosterone levels)
Signs & Symptoms	• **Similar symptoms to Addison disease** • **Hypotension, fatigue, weakness, weight loss, nausea/vomiting**, anorexia, myalgias • Amenorrhea, loss of libido, loss of pubic hair • *Absence of skin manifestations (hyperpigmentation)*
Diagnosis	• <u>Comprehensive Metabolic Panel (CMP)</u>: typically normal electrolyte and BUN levels; **may have hypoglycemia** • <u>Morning Serum Cortisol and Plasma ACTH Levels</u>: ↓plasma ACTH, ↓serum cortisol (*Addison disease has ↑ACTH and ↓serum cortisol*) • <u>ACTH Stimulation Test</u>: normal or subnormal rise in serum cortisol after ACTH administration (*Addison disease has insufficient rise in cortisol*)
Treatment	• <u>Glucocorticoid Replacement</u>: **hydrocortisone (identical to cortisol) is first-line**; prednisone and dexamethasone are alternatives • Total daily dose of hydrocortisone is 15-20 mg; half total given in morning with remaining half split between midday and evening (10mg, 5mg, 5mg) • <u>Mineralocorticoid Replacement</u>: **fludrocortisone is *not* required because the intact adrenals produce aldosterone** • <u>Patient Education</u>: stress management education, patients should carry medical alert card and injectable form of cortisol (pre-filled dexamethasone syringe) for emergencies • *Patients may need additional dosing during illness/surgery/fever to recreate the normal "stress" response*
Key Words & Most Common	• Inadequate ACTH secretion results in lack of cortisol • Corticosteroid use or abruptly stopping corticosteroid use is most common cause • Similar symptoms to Addison disease; hypotension, fatigue, weakness, weight loss, n/v, absence of skin manifestations (hyperpigmentation) • CMP may show hypoglycemia • <u>Morning Cortisol/ACTH</u>: ↓plasma ACTH, ↓serum cortisol (*Addison disease has ↑ACTH and ↓serum cortisol*) • <u>ACTH Stimulation Test</u>: normal or subnormal rise in serum cortisol after ACTH administration (*Addison disease has insufficient rise in cortisol*) • Hydrocortisone

Adrenal Crisis

Etiology & Risk Factors	• Acute, life-threatening presentation of adrenal insufficiency; *can present as complication of primary or secondary adrenal insufficiency* • Etiology: insufficient rise in cortisol during periods of stress to meet demand • Risk Factors: **abruptly stopping corticosteroid therapy (without taper) is most common cause**; "stressful" event (illness [especially GI], infection, pregnancy, surgery, trauma, MI, fever, hypoglycemia), emotional stress, strenuous physical activity, adrenal hemorrhage, patients with Addison disease that did not increase medication dose during illness
Patho-physiology	• The adrenal gland's primary function is to produce mineralocorticoids and glucocorticoids; the pituitary gland produces the adrenocorticotropin hormone (ACTH), which stimulates cortisol release from the adrenal glands • While under stress, hypothalamic-pituitary axis (HPA) stimulation causes an increase in ACTH, which increases the cortisol level; cortisol deficiency causes impaired gluconeogenesis and conversion of norepinephrine into epinephrine leading to hypotension and hypoglycemia

Signs & Symptoms	• Adrenal Crisis:
	  • **Hypotension, tachycardia, abdominal tenderness, fever, confusion/lethargy, hypoglycemia**
	• Primary Adrenal Insufficiency:
	  • Anorexia, weakness/fatigue, hyperpigmentation, hypotension, hyponatremia, hyperkalemia, azotemia, dehydration
	• Secondary Adrenal Insufficiency:
	  • Similar symptoms to primary adrenal insufficiency; no hyperpigmentation, no hyperkalemia, hypotension is less common

Diagnosis	• Complete Blood Count: normocytic normochromic anemia, lymphocytosis, **eosinophilia** • Comprehensive Metabolic Panel (CMP): **hyponatremia, hyperkalemia, hypoglycemia,** may have hypercalcemia, ↑BUN/creatinine • ACTH Stimulation Test: **confirms diagnosis but treatment should not be delayed while diagnostic testing performed**
Treatment	• **Admit to ICU** • Intravenous Fluids: **isotonic fluids (D5NS) to correct hypovolemia and hypoglycemia** • IV Hydrocortisone: **treatment of choice** • Dexamethasone: consider in hemodynamically stable patient if ACTH stimulation test will be performed (does not interfere with cortisol assays)
Key Words & Most Common	• Acute presentation of adrenal insufficiency • Abruptly stopping corticosteroids is most common cause; "stressful" event (especially GI illness) • Hypotension, abdominal tenderness, fever, confusion/lethargy, hypoglycemia • Hyponatremia, hyperkalemia, hypoglycemia • ACTH Stimulation Test confirms diagnosis • Admit to ICU → D5NS fluids → IV hydrocortisone

Cushing Syndrome

Etiology & Risk Factors	• Constellation of nonspecific symptoms related to chronic high levels of excess cortisol or related corticosteroids
	• Etiology: endogenous or exogenous hypercortisolism
	  • Endogenous: **ACTH-secreting pituitary adenomas (Cushing disease) is most common endogenous cause**, ectopic ACTH-secreting tumor (small cell lung carcinoma, medullary thyroid cancer), adrenal hyperplasia or adenoma (excess cortisol secretion)
	  • Exogenous: **iatrogenic (prolonged corticosteroid therapy) is most common cause overall**

Patho-physiology	• Excess cortisol affects transcription and translation of enzyme proteins involved in fat and glycogen metabolism, protein synthesis and the Krebs cycle resulting in an increased rate of gluconeogenesis, glycogenolysis and increased insulin resistance • Protein catabolism causes purple striae of torso, osteoporosis and inhibited wound healing

Signs & Symptoms	• **Weight gain, fatigue, proximal muscle weakness (difficulty brushing hair or standing from seated position)**, headache, **delayed wound healing, easy bruising**, back pain, bone pain, depression, mood swings, erectile dysfunction, mental disturbances, loss of libido, hyperhidrosis, irregular menses, hirsutism
	• Physical Exam:
	  • Cardiovascular: hypertension
	  • Cutaneous: **thin/friable skin**, poor wound healing, easy bruising, **violaceus striae (red/purple, wide, particularly on abdomen)**, acanthosis nigricans
	  • Endocrine: signs of androgen excess (hirsutism, oily skin, **acne**, amenorrhea), glucose intolerance, **obesity**
	  • Metabolic: **fat redistribution; increased truncal fat deposits (central obesity) with thin extremities (slender distal extremities and fingers), back fat deposits ("buffalo hump"); supraclavicular fat pads, "moon facies"** (roundly-shaped, puffy face; earlobes not visualized when viewed from the front)
	  • Musculoskeletal: **proximal muscle atrophy and weakness,**
	  • Ophthalmologic: increased intraocular pressure, cataracts
	  • Psychologic: emotional lability, anxiety

Diagnosis	• Labs: leukocytosis, hyperlipidemia, **hyperglycemia, hypokalemia**, metabolic alkalosis
	• 24-hour Urinary Free Cortisol Measurement: **most specific screening test**; positive if elevated urinary cortisol >120mcg/24 hours
	• 48-hour Low-Dose Dexamethasone Suppression Test: **confirmatory test**; 0.5 mg is given every 6 hours starting at 9am; positive if cortisol level >1.8mg/dL 24 hours later
	• Serum ACTH Tests: differentiate ACTH-independent (↓ACTH level) and ACTH-dependent (↑ACTH or inappropriately normal ACTH) cause of Cushing syndrome
	  • High-Dose Dexamethasone Suppression Test: used if ACTH-dependent (↑ or normal ACTH) to differentiate pituitary ACTH from ectopic source
	    • High-Dose Dexamethasone *will* decrease cortisol by 50% if ACTH source is pituitary adenoma but cortisol *will not* decrease if ACTH secreted by ectopic tumor
	• Pituitary MRI (Cushing disease), unenhanced CT (adrenal adenoma), and chest X-ray/CT (ectopic ACTH-producing lung tumor) are useful to localize the pathology

Treatment	• Corticosteroid Use: **gradual taper of exogenous corticosteroids (prevent adrenal crisis and allow adrenal function to recover)** • ACTH-Secreting Pituitary Tumors: transsphenoidal resection surgery or extirpated with radiation therapy • Corticosteroid-Secreting Adrenocortical Tumors: tumor excision • Ectopic ACTH-Producing Tumors: tumor excision; metyrapone (stimulates the pituitary release of ACTH) or ketoconazole (blocks corticosteroid synthesis) if inoperable

Adrenal Insufficiency Labs

	Potassium	Sodium	BUN	Glucose	ACTH	Cortisol	Aldosterone	Renin	ACTH Stimulation Test
Primary (adrenal)	High	Low	High or Normal	Low or Normal	High	Low	Low	High	Insufficient rise in cortisol
Secondary (pituitary)	Relatively Normal	Relatively Normal	Normal	Low	Low	Low	Normal	Low or Normal	Normal or subnormal rise in cortisol

Cushing Syndrome Labs

	Serum Cortisol 9am	Salivary or Serum Cortisol Midnight	Urinary Free Cortisol	Low-Dose Dexamethasone Suppression Test	High-Dose Dexamethasone Suppression Test	ACTH Level
Normal	Normal	Normal	Normal	Suppression	Suppression	Normal
Cushing Disease (Pituitary)	High or Normal	High	High	No Suppression	Suppression	High
Ectopic ACTH-Producing Tumor	High or Normal	High	High	No Suppression	No Suppression	High
Adrenal Tumor (Cortisol Producing)	High or Normal	High	High	No Suppression	No Suppression	Low

Primary Hyperaldosteronism

Etiology & Risk Factors	• **Renin-independent autonomous production of aldosterone by the adrenal cortex secondary to hyperplasia, adenoma, or carcinoma** • Etiology: **aldosterone-producing adenomas is most common**; aldosterone-producing adrenal carcinoma, ectopic aldosterone secretion from kidneys or ovaries, and bilateral zona glomerulosa hyperplasia, idiopathic
Patho-physiology	• Aldosterone, a potent mineralocorticoid produced by the adrenals, causes **sodium retention and potassium loss** and is regulated by the renin-angiotensin system • Excess aldosterone leads to increased sodium reabsorption leads to hypertension and volume expansion
Signs & Symptoms	• **Triad of hypertension + hypokalemia + metabolic alkalosis** • Hypertension: **diastolic blood pressure tends to be more elevated**; headache or flushing of face • **May present as young patient with multidrug (3+) resistant hypertension** • Hypokalemia: **severe muscle weakness, palpitations**, fatigue, **polyuria/polydipsia** (nephrogenic diabetes insipidus), decreased deep tendon reflexes or **muscle cramps**
Diagnosis	• **Plasma Renin and Aldosterone Levels: elevated plasma aldosterone and low levels of plasma renin activity** (high plasma renin activity indicates secondary etiology) • Ratio of plasma aldosterone to plasma renin activity >20:1 • Labs: **hypokalemia**; metabolic alkalosis • ECG: evidence of hypokalemia (flattening or inversion of T waves → Q-T prolongation → U wave and mild ST depression) • Confirmatory Tests: oral sodium loading test (high urine aldosterone), saline infusion test, fludrocortisone suppression test, captopril challenge test • Imaging: CT or MRI to evaluate for adrenal or extra-adrenal tumor or adrenal hyperplasia

Treatment	• Adenoma: **laparoscopic resection of tumor**
	• Hyperplasia:
	  • **Selective Aldosterone Antagonist: spironolactone is first-line** or eplerenone (does not block androgen receptor which can cause gynecomastia and sexual dysfunction)
	  • Antihypertensives: ACEI, calcium channel blockers, amiloride (sodium channel blocker)

Key Words & Most Common	• Renin-independent autonomous production of aldosterone • Adenoma, hyperplasia, or carcinoma • Aldosterone causes sodium retention and potassium loss • Hypertension: ↑diastolic BP; multidrug resistant HTN • Hypokalemia: severe muscle weakness, palpitations, muscle cramps, polyuria • ↑aldosterone and ↓renin • Adenoma: laparoscopic resection • Hyperplasia: spironolactone

Secondary Hyperaldosteronism

Etiology & Risk Factors	• Reduced renal blood flow stimulates the renin-angiotensin system (RAAS) resulting in increased aldosterone secretion • Etiology: obstructive renal artery disease (renal artery stenosis is most common cause); renal vasoconstriction (hypertension), edematous disorders (CHF, hypovolemia, cirrhosis, nephrotic syndrome)
Patho-physiology	• Aldosterone, a potent mineralocorticoid produced by the adrenals, causes **sodium retention and potassium loss** and is regulated by the renin-angiotensin system • Excess aldosterone leads to increased sodium reabsorption leads to hypertension and volume expansion
Signs & Symptoms	• Triad of hypertension + hypokalemia + metabolic alkalosis • Hypertension: blood pressure tends to be higher than primary hyperaldosteronism; headache or flushing of face • May present as young patient with multidrug (3+) resistant hypertension • Hypokalemia: **severe muscle weakness, palpitations**, fatigue, **polyuria/polydipsia** (nephrogenic diabetes insipidus), decreased deep tendon reflexes or **muscle cramps** • May present with heart failure, cirrhosis, or nephrotic syndrome
Diagnosis	• Plasma Renin and Aldosterone Levels: elevated plasma aldosterone and elevated levels of plasma renin • Labs: hypokalemia; metabolic alkalosis • ECG: evidence of hypokalemia (flattening or inversion of T waves → Q-T prolongation → U wave and mild ST depression) • Imaging: Duplex US, CT or MRI to evaluate for renal artery stenosis
Treatment	• Selective Aldosterone Antagonist: spironolactone is first-line or eplerenone (does not block androgen receptor which can cause gynecomastia and sexual dysfunction) • Antihypertensives: ACEI, calcium channel blockers, amiloride (sodium channel blocker) • Treat Underlying Etiology: surgical revascularization if renal artery stenosis
Key Words & Most Common	• Reduced renal blood flow activates RAAS causing increases aldosterone secretion (aldosterone causes sodium retention and potassium loss) • Renal artery stenosis is most common cause • Hypertension: BP tends to be higher than primary; young patient with multidrug resistant hypertension • Hypokalemia: severe muscle weakness, palpitations, polyuria/polydipsia, muscle cramps • May present with heart failure, cirrhosis, nephrotic syndrome • ↑aldosterone and ↑renin • Spironolactone

	Blood Pressure	Sodium	Potassium	Plasma Renin Activity	Aldosterone
Primary Hyperaldosteronism	↑↑	↑ or normal	↓	↓↓	↑
Secondary Hyperaldosteronism	↑↑↑	↓	↓	↑↑	↑↑

Pheochromocytoma

Etiology & Risk Factors	• Catecholamine-secreting adrenal tumor arising from chromaffin cells
	• Etiology: most are located in the adrenal medulla (90%); paraganglion cells
	   • Most are benign (90%)
	   • Rule of 10's: 10% are malignant, 10% occur bilaterally, 10% occur in children, 10% are extra-adrenal (paraganglioma)
	• Risk Factors: most are sporadic (90%); familial syndromes such as Von Hippel-Lindau syndrome, neurofibromatosis type 1, and multiple endocrine neoplasia syndrome type 2

Patho-physiology	• **Neuroendocrine tumor secretes catecholamines (norepinephrine, epinephrine, dopamine) autonomously and intermittently leading to episodic or continual hypertension** • **Attacks may occur spontaneously or triggered** by lifestyle (physical exertion, stress/anxiety, pain, urination), medications (TCAs, opiates, metoclopramide, glucagon, histamine), foods (cheese, beer, tomatoes, coffee), intraoperative tumor manipulation, intubation, or during anesthetic induction
Signs & Symptoms	• **Hypertension is most prominent**; may be episodic or continual • **Headache (most common symptom), tachycardia, palpitations, diaphoresis**, tachypnea, cold/clammy skin, chest/abdominal pain, weakness, anxiety, weight loss • 5 P's: Pressure (hypertension), Pain (headache), Palpitations, Perspiration, Pallor • Triad: 1. episodic headache 2. diaphoresis 3. tachycardia with hypertension

Diagnosis	• **Plasma Free Metanephrines: most sensitive and specific test (99% sensitive, 89% specific)** demonstrates elevated metanephrine and normetanephrine levels
	• **Urinary Fractionated Metanephrines:** slightly less sensitive and specific than plasma free metanephrines (95% sensitive, 69% specific)
	   • Urinary metabolic products of epinephrine and norepinephrine are metanephrine and normetanephrine, vanillylmandelic acid (VMA), and homovanillic acid (HVA)
	• *Amphetamines, ephedrine, tricyclic antidepressants, and cocaine can affect plasma and urine metanephrine levels*
	• **Imaging: CT or MRI of chest and abdomen with and without contrast used to localize adrenal tumor** after biochemical testing confirms diagnosis
	   • Positron emission tomography (PET) scan is superior to MIBG to evaluate metastatic disease

Treatment	• **Surgical Resection: complete adrenalectomy is gold-standard treatment;** hypertension must be controlled prior to operation (1-2 weeks of medical therapy)
	• **Hypertension Management:** controlled by combination of alpha and beta blockers
	   • **Alpha Blockade: best initial therapy; phenoxybenzamine or phentolamine**
	   • **Beta Blockade: propranolol can be started 2 days to 2 weeks later after adequate alpha blockade has been achieved**
	     • **If beta blockade initiated before alpha blockers, unopposed alpha activity can precipitate hypertensive emergency**
	   • Nitroprusside can be infused for hypertensive crises preoperatively or intraoperatively; phentolamine or nicardipine adjuncts in acute hypertensive crisis

Key Words & Most Common	• Catecholamine-secreting adrenal tumor arising from chromaffin cells • Secretes norepinephrine, epinephrine and dopamine; can be triggered by lifestyle, food, medications, surgery, intubation • 5 P's: Pressure (hypertension), Pain (headache), Palpitations, Perspiration, Pallor; hypertension is most prominent symptom • Plasma free metanephrines + urinary fractionated metanephrines → CT or MRI • Alpha blockade (phenoxybenzamine or phentolamine) → beta blockade (propranolol) → surgical resection (gold standard)

Hypothyroidism

Etiology & Risk Factors	• **State of hypometabolism and deficiency of thyroid hormone**
	• Etiology: primary (caused by the thyroid) or secondary (condition of hypothalamus or pituitary)
	  • Primary: **autoimmune (Hashimoto thyroiditis)**, thyroiditis (may be preceded by hyperthyroidism), post-therapeutic hypothyroidism (radioactive iodine therapy, discontinuation of methimazole/propylthiouracil), iodine deficiency, congenital, **medications (amiodarone**, lithium, iodine) idiopathic
	  • Secondary: insufficient thyrotropin-releasing hormone (TRH) secretion by hypothalamus or insufficiency thyroid stimulating hormone (TSH) by the pituitary
	• Risk Factors: **women, age >60 years old is most common,** family history of thyroid disorders, **other autoimmune diagnoses (adrenal insufficiency,** type 1 diabetes, **pernicious anemia, celiac disease,** premature graying of hair)

Patho-physiology	• Thyrotropin-releasing hormone (TRH) is released by the hypothalamus stimulating the pituitary gland to produce thyroid-stimulating hormone (TSH) which stimulates thyroid gland to produce thyroxine (T4) and triiodothyronine (T3). T4 is converted in peripheral tissue to T3. T3 and T4 levels exert negative feedback on TRH and TSH production. • Disruption of this pathway results in hypothyroidism
Signs & Symptoms	• Constitutional: **weight gain, cold intolerance, lethargy, weakness, fatigue, hoarse voice, slow speech** • Neuropsychiatric: forgetfulness, **paresthesia of hands/feet,** personality changes, anxiety/depression, dull facial expressions, delayed relaxation of deep tendon reflexes • Dermatologic: **facial edema, coarse/dry/thin hair, dry/thick skin, macroglossia, hair loss, non-pitting edema** • Ophthalmic: periorbital swelling, ptosis • Gastrointestinal: **constipation** • Cardiovascular: **bradycardia**
Diagnosis	• Thyroid Function Tests: preferred screening test • Primary hypothyroid profile (increased TSH and decreased free T4) • Thyroid Autoantibodies: **positive antithyroid peroxidase (anti-TPO)** and/or anti-thyroglobulin (anti-Tg) antibodies present in Hashimoto thyroiditis

Treatment	• Thyroid Hormone Replacement: **levothyroxine (synthetic T4) is preferred treatment**
	  • Maintenance dose is 75 to 150mcg QD (dose dependent on age, body mass index, and absorption)
	  • *Most patients require lifelong thyroid hormone replacement*

Key Words & Most Common	• State of hypometabolism and deficiency of thyroid hormone • Autoimmune (Hashimoto thyroiditis) is most common cause in US; iodine deficiency is most common cause worldwide • Weight gain, cold intolerance, lethargy, hoarse voice/slow speech, paresthesia, facial edema, dry/thin skin and hair, hair loss, non-pitting edema, constipation, bradycardia • ↑TSH and ↓T4 • Anti-TPO positive in Hashimoto thyroiditis • Levothyroxine (synthetic T4)

Hashimoto Thyroiditis

Etiology & Risk Factors	• **Autoimmune disease characterized by thyroid cell destruction via cell and antibody-mediated immune processes** • **Most common cause of hypothyroidism in developed countries** (iodine deficiency is most common cause worldwide) • Etiology: **autoimmune; antibody development to thyroid antigens; anti-thyroid peroxidase (anti-TPO) is most common antibody;** anti-thyroglobulin (anti-Tg) and TSH receptor-blocking antibodies (TBII) • Risk Factors: **women age 30-50 is most common;** chromosomal disorders (Down syndrome, Turner syndrome, Klinefelter syndrome), family history of thyroid disorders, **other autoimmune diagnoses (adrenal insufficiency,** type 1 diabetes, **pernicious anemia, celiac disease,** premature graying of hair)
Patho-physiology	• Autoimmune-mediated immune processes lead to the formation of antithyroid antibodies (anti-thyroid peroxidase and anti-thyroglobulin antibodies) causing thyroid cell destruction and progressive fibrosis

Signs & Symptoms	• **Fatigue, cold intolerance,** dry and thickened skin, constipation, **weight gain,** eyelid/facial edema (myxedema), **weakness, lethargy**
	• **Slow hair growth (hair becomes thin, dry, and brittle)**
	• **Decreased muscle strength and increased muscle fatigue**
	• Painless enlargement of thyroid, hoarseness of voice, dyspnea (tracheal compression from goiter)
	• Physical Exam:
	  • **Nontender goiter that is nodular or smooth, firm with a "rubbery" feel**
	  • **Bradycardia, decreased deep tendon reflexes**
	  • **Hair loss, thin/dry/brittle hair, loss of outer 1/3rd of eyebrows**

Diagnosis	• Thyroid Function Tests: preferred screening test
	  • **Primary hypothyroid profile (increased TSH and decreased free T4)**
	• Thyroid Autoantibodies: **positive antithyroid peroxidase (anti-TPO)** and/or anti-thyroglobulin (anti-Tg) antibodies
	• Thyroid Ultrasound: should be performed if palpable nodules or enlarged thyroid
	  • May show heterogeneous, hypoechoic echotexture with septations

Treatment	• Thyroid Hormone Replacement: **levothyroxine (synthetic T4)** • *Most patients require lifelong thyroid hormone replacement*
Key Words & Most Common	• Autoimmune thyroid cell destruction; most common cause of hypothyroidism in developed countries • Women age 30-50 is most common; may have history of autoimmune disease • Fatigue, cold intolerance, weight gain, lethargy, thin/brittle hair • Bradycardia, hair loss, loss of outer 1/3rd of eyebrows • ↑TSH and ↓T4 and + anti-TPO • Levothyroxine

Riedel Thyroiditis

Etiology & Risk Factors	• Rare, chronic, autoimmune thyroiditis characterized by inflammation and dense fibrosis of the thyroid gland and surrounding structures • Etiology: **immunoglobulin G4 (IgG4) related systemic disease**, variant of autoimmune thyroiditis, or systemic fibrosing disorder
Patho-physiology	• Autoimmune mediated replacement of thyroid tissue with dense fibrotic tissue • Fibrosis of extra-thyroidal structures cause mechanical compression of adjacent neck structures (trachea, parathyroid glands, neck muscles, laryngeal nerves, blood vessels)

Signs & Symptoms	• **Compressive Symptoms: dyspnea (tracheal involvement), dysphagia (esophageal involvement),** stridor (laryngeal nerve involvement), venous sinus thrombosis (vascular involvement), neck pain or radicular symptoms (muscular/neurological involvement)
	• **Hard, enlarged, thyroid**
	• Physical Exam:
	  • **Hard, nontender, fixed, rapidly-growing mass of the anterior neck; immobile when swallowing**
	    • "Stone-like, hard-as-wood, rock hard"
	  • *Absence of cervical lymphadenopathy*

Diagnosis	• **Thyroid Function Tests: primary hypothyroid profile (elevated TSH and decreased T4)** in about 70% of patients; euthyroid in 30% • Thyroid Ultrasound: hypoechoic hypovascular mass involving the extra-thyroidal structures • **Open Biopsy: definitive diagnosis; demonstrates dense fibrosis; distinguishes between anaplastic thyroid cancer** • Serum Immunoglobulin G4 (IgG4): may be elevated
Treatment	• Surgery: **subtotal or partial thyroidectomy; indicated to relieve compressive symptoms** • **Corticosteroids: mainstay of medical treatment;** anti-inflammatory and immunosuppressive to reduce further growth
Key Words & Most Common	• Chronic, autoimmune thyroiditis with dense fibrosis of thyroid and surrounding tissue • IgG4 related systemic disease • Compressive Symptoms: dyspnea, dysphagia, stridor, neck pain • Hard, nontender, fixed mass of anterior neck; immobile when swallowing; absence of cervical lymphadenopathy • ↑TSH and ↓T4 • Open biopsy for definitive diagnosis • Thyroidectomy to relieve compressive symptoms • Corticosteroids are mainstay of medical treatment

Subacute Thyroiditis

Etiology & Risk Factors	• **Inflammation of the thyroid gland secondary to viral respiratory tract infection** • *Also known as de Quervain thyroiditis; giant cell thyroiditis; granulomatous thyroiditis* • Etiology: **viral respiratory infection** (coxsackievirus [groups A & B], echovirus, mumps, measles, influenza, SARS-CoV-2) • Risk Factors: **recent viral respiratory infection (viral process precedes symptoms by 2-8 weeks), female, age (25-35 years old most common),** seasonal (fall and summer)
Patho-physiology	• Viral respiratory tract infection causes post-viral inflammation of the thyroid gland causing no new thyroid hormone to be produced and excessive release of triiodothyronine (T3) and thyroxine (T4) which inhibits thyroid stimulating hormone (TSH) release • As no new thyroid hormone is produced, hyperthyroidism is initial presentation followed by euthyroidism then hypothyroidism then return to normal thyroid function

Signs & Symptoms	• *Clinical hyperthyroidism symptoms in acute phase that may progress to hypothyroidism symptoms*
	• **Anterior neck pain**
	  • **Painful thyroid gland worse with head/neck movements and swallowing**
	  • **Pain may radiate to jaw and ears**
	  • May be confused with dental pain, pharyngitis, or otitis
	• **Preceded by upper respiratory infection;** fever, malaise, fatigue, myalgias, pharyngitis, sinus congestion
	• Physical Exam:
	  • **Asymmetrically enlarged, firm, and diffusely tender goiter**

Diagnosis	• **Thyroid Function Tests:**
	  • **Early: hyperthyroid profile (decreased TSH + increased free T4) and negative thyroid antibodies**
	  • **Later (2-8 weeks): euthyroid or transient hypothyroid state** (decrease in free T3 and T4 and rise in TSH) later in the disease course
	• Erythrocyte Sedimentation Rate (ESR): elevated ESR
	• Thyroid Ultrasound: multiple irregular sonolucent areas with reduced blood flow
	• Radioactive Iodine Uptake Scan: confirms diagnosis; shows diffuse, decreased iodine uptake
	• **Fine-Needle Aspiration Biopsy: definitive diagnosis; shows granulomatous inflammation with multinucleated giant cells**

Treatment	• **Supportive: reassurance** • Most cases are self-limiting and return to euthyroid state within 3-4 months • Analgesia: **NSAIDs or aspirin for pain/inflammation** • Oral Corticosteroids: prednisone may be given for severe neck pain refractory to NSAIDs/aspirin; taper over 3-4 week period
Key Words & Most Common	• Inflammation of thyroid gland secondary to viral respiratory tract infection (virus precedes symptoms by 2-8 weeks) • Anterior neck pain worse with head/neck movement and swallowing; pain may radiate to jaw/ears • Asymmetrically enlarged, firm, and diffusely tender goiter • Early: ↓TSH and ↑T4; transient decrease in T3 and rise in TSH later; ↑ESR; biopsy for definitive diagnosis • Supportive care; NSAIDs or aspirin; prednisone taper over 3-4 weeks

Suppurative Thyroiditis

Etiology & Risk Factors	• Bacterial infection of the thyroid gland • <u>Etiology</u>: **gram-positive bacteria (*Staphylococcus*, *Streptococcus*) most common**; mycobacteria or fungus (*Pneumocystis*) possible in immunocompromised • <u>Risk Factors</u>: **extremes of age (primarily affects children)**, chronically ill, **immunocompromised**
Patho-physiology	• Bacterial infection of the thyroid is rare as the organ is encapsulated with rich blood supply and extensive lymphatic drainage • Hematogenous spread or congenital abnormalities (pyriform sinus) are usual source of infection

Signs & Symptoms	• **Acute thyroid pain**
	   • **Worse with hyperextension of the neck**
	   • Pain may radiate to jaw or ears
	• **Superficial erythema of anterior neck**
	• **Fever, chills, pharyngitis**, dysphagia

Diagnosis	• <u>Labs</u>: **leukocytosis, erythrocyte sedimentation rate (ESR) and C-reactive protein (CRP) are significantly elevated**, blood cultures • <u>Thyroid Function Tests</u>: usually within normal limits • <u>Fine Needle Aspiration</u>: **with gram stain and culture** • <u>Thyroid Ultrasound</u>: heterogenous thyroid parenchyma secondary to inflammation; rule out abscess formation
Treatment	• <u>Analgesia</u>: NSAIDs for severe neck pain and inflammation • <u>Antibiotics</u>: **coverage for gram-positive bacteria**; ampicillin, nafcillin/gentamicin, ceftriaxone • Surgery: indicated if fluctuant or abscess demonstrated on ultrasound • *Evaluate for pyriform sinus fistula with barium swallow or endoscopy*
Key Words & Most Common	• Bacterial infection of thyroid gland; gram + (*Staph* or *Strep*) most common • Most common in kids or immunocompromised • Acute thyroid pain + fever • Leukocytosis, ↑ESR/CRP • Antibiotics

Congenital Hypothyroidism

Etiology & Risk Factors	• Thyroid hormone deficiency present at birth • <u>Etiology</u>: **defect in thyroid gland development (thyroid dysgenesis) is most common**; defect of thyroid hormone biosynthesis (dyshormonogenesis) • <u>Risk Factors</u>: **maternal use of anti-thyroid medications** (methimazole or propylthiouracil), maternal thyroid blocking antibodies (mother with autoimmune thyroid disease), **iodine deficiency** (present in developing countries)
Patho-physiology	• Thyroid dysgenesis causes hypofunction of the thyroid gland causing low T4 and T3 levels and elevated TSH levels (hypothalamic and pituitary feedback mechanism) • Thyroid hormone is essential for energy metabolism, growth, and neurodevelopment in child

Signs & Symptoms	• <u>Fetal</u>:
	   • **Growth failure, coarse facial features** (depressed nasal bridge, puffy eyelids, large tongue)
	• <u>Infant</u>:
	   • **Lethargy, hypotonia, large anterior/posterior fontanelles**, jaundice, **weak cry**, constipation, poor feeding, thick/dry/mottled skin, **umbilical hernia**, bradycardia, **macroglossia**
	• <u>Child</u>:
	   • **Mental developmental delays, short stature**, weight gain, weakness, lethargy, decreased metabolic rate, cold intolerance, **goiter symptoms** (hoarseness/dyspnea from tracheal compression), **dry hair, cool/mottled skin**

Diagnosis	• <u>Thyroid Stimulating Hormone (TSH) and Thyroxine (T4) Level</u>: **preferred screening method** • **Demonstrates increased TSH and decreased free T4** • <u>Thyroid Ultrasound</u>: may be indicated to rule out structural thyroid disorders
Treatment	• <u>Thyroid Hormone Replacement</u>: **levothyroxine (synthetic T4)** dosed based on body surface area or age; may require lifelong therapy
Key Words & Most Common	• Thyroid hormone deficiency present at birth • Thyroid dysgenesis is most common cause • <u>Fetal</u>: growth failure, coarse facial features • <u>Infant</u>: lethargy, hypotonia, weak cry, large anterior/posterior fontanelles, umbilical hernia, macroglossia • <u>Child</u>: developmental delays, short stature • ↑TSH and ↓T4 • Levothyroxine

Euthyroid Sick Syndrome

Etiology & Risk Factors	• Nonthyroidal illness syndrome resulting in abnormal thyroid function tests in patients with normal thyroid function • Etiology: **severe critical illness** (sepsis, starvation, myocardial infarction, malignancy, burns/trauma, fracture, major surgery, diabetic ketoacidosis, anorexia nervosa, stress, pneumonia, cardiopulmonary bypass, heart failure, hypothermia, renal failure etc.)
Patho-physiology	• Circulating cytokines (IL1, IL6, TNF-alpha, interferon-beta) secondary to severe critical illness affect the hypothalamus and pituitary glands which inhibit thyroid stimulating hormone (TSH), thyroid releasing hormone (TRH), thyroglobulin, triiodothyronine (T3), and thyroid-binding globulin (TBG) production • **Peripheral conversion of T4 to T3 is inhibited**; decreased clearance of reverse T3 (rT3) generated from T4
Signs & Symptoms	• Specific to etiologic factors; no typical findings of euthyroid sick syndrome
Diagnosis	• <u>Thyroid Stimulating Hormone (TSH)</u>: can be low, normal, or slightly elevated; not as high (<10mIu/L) as primary hypothyroidism • <u>Total Triiodothyronine (T3)</u>: **low T3 is most common abnormality** • <u>Reverse Triiodothyronine (rT3)</u>: **increased rT3** • <u>Thyroxine (T4)</u>: **often normal; low T4 indicates poor prognosis**
Treatment	• **Treat underlying etiology** • Thyroid hormone replacement is not usually indicated
Key Words & Most Common	• Nonthyroidal illness resulting in abnormal thyroid function tests • Secondary to severe critical illness (sepsis, starvation, MI/CHF, malignancy, trauma etc.) • TSH low/normal/slightly elevated • ↓T3 • ↑rT3 • Normal T4 (↓T4 indicates poor prognosis) • Treat underlying etiology

Myxedema Coma

Etiology & Risk Factors	• Rare condition resulting from long-standing hypothyroidism that carries a high mortality rate • Etiology: **disrupted homeostatic mechanism in patient with hypothyroidism** • Risk Factors: **advanced age (>60 years old), females, longstanding hypothyroidism, discontinuation or noncompliance with Levothyroxine therapy** • Precipitating Factors: **infection** (UTI, pneumonia, viral infection, sepsis), bradycardia, trauma/burns, **hypothermia, cold exposure**, hypoglycemia, medications (**amiodarone, lithium**, opioids, anesthetics, beta blockers), GI bleeds, MI, CHF, hypoxemia, cerebrovascular accidents
Patho-physiology	• Thyroid hormone has an effect on many body processes at the genetic and cellular level including **preserving core body temperature**, blood pressure and pulse regulation etc. • Disruption of normal homeostatic mechanisms by an acute precipitating factor in a patient with untreated hypothyroidism leads to severe hypothyroidism
Signs & Symptoms	• **Hypothermia (core body temperature <95.9°F)** • <u>Cardiovascular</u>: **bradycardia, hypotension**, palpitations • <u>Respiratory</u>: hypoventilation, **hypoxia**, hypercapnia • <u>Gastrointestinal</u>: constipation, nausea/vomiting, ileus, abdominal pain • <u>Neurologic</u>: **altered mental status**, psychosis, **obtundation (coma)**
Diagnosis	• <u>Thyroid Function Tests</u>: **increased TSH; decreased free T4 (free T3 and T4 levels may be undetectably low)** • <u>Comprehensive Metabolic Panel (CMP)</u>: **hyponatremia, hypoglycemia** • <u>Complete Blood Count (CBC)</u>: anemia, leukopenia • <u>Arterial Blood Gas (ABG)</u>: **hypoxia**, hypercapnia, and respiratory acidosis • <u>ECG</u>: bradycardia • <u>Other</u>: blood cultures, serum cortisol, CPK,
Treatment	• <u>Resuscitation</u>: **respiratory support** (mechanical ventilation to prevent respiratory collapse and respiratory acidosis), **fluid resuscitation** (be cautious with rapid correction of hyponatremia), **passive warming** (avoid rapid warming) • <u>Thyroid Hormone Replacement</u>: **IV levothyroxine is first-line therapy**; consider T3 replacement (caution in patients with heart disease) • Initial dose of 200-400mcg IV once followed by 75-100mcg IV daily until patient able to tolerate PO medications • <u>Corticosteroids</u>: **IV hydrocortisone given for concomitant adrenal insufficiency**; dexamethasone as alternative
Key Words & Most Common	• Elderly female with longstanding hypothyroidism presenting during winter • May be precipitated by cold exposure, infection, medications • Hypothermia + bradycardia + hypotension + AMS • ↑TSH + ↓T3 and T4; hyponatremia, hypoglycemia • Respiratory and hemodynamic support + passive warming • IV levothyroxine + IV hydrocortisone

Hyperthyroidism

Etiology & Risk Factors	• State of hypermetabolism and elevated serum levels of free thyroid hormones • Etiology: **Graves disease (most common)**, multinodular goiter, thyroiditis, hyperfunctioning "hot" nodule, TSH-secreting pituitary adenoma, iatrogenic • Risk Factors: **medication induced** (inappropriate levothyroxine dose, **amiodarone**, lithium), excess iodine ingestion, other autoimmune conditions
Patho-physiology	• Serum triiodothyronine (T3) increases more than thyroxine (T4) (T4 is converted to T3 in peripheral tissue) which inhibits thyroid stimulating hormone (TSH) release • Enhanced sensitivity to adrenergic hormones causes hypermetabolic features
Signs & Symptoms	• Constitutional: lethargy, **diaphoresis, heat intolerance,** fever, **weakness, weight loss** • Neuropsychiatric: **nervousness, hyperactivity, tremor, irritability,** insomnia, anxiety, depression • Dermatologic: **warm/moist skin,** increased body temperature, hair loss, brittle hair and nails, palmar erythema, onycholysis (separation of the nail from the nail bed) • Ophthalmic: diplopia, stare, eyelid lag, mild conjunctival injection, **ophthalmopathy (exophthalmos [protrusion of eyes anteriorly] is specific to Graves disease)** • Gastrointestinal: **increased appetite, diarrhea** • Cardiovascular: **tachycardia, palpitations,** arrhythmias (atrial fibrillation), dyspnea • Other: menstrual cycle abnormalities, muscle cramps/weakness

Diagnosis	• Thyroid Function Tests: **primary hyperthyroid profile (decreased TSH and increased free T4 and/or T3)**
	  • Secondary (central) hyperthyroid profile (increased TSH and increased free T4) with TSH-secreting pituitary adenoma
	• TSH-Receptor Antibodies: **positive thyroid stimulating immunoglobulin (TSI) is hallmark of Graves disease**
	• Radioactive Iodine Uptake Scan: increased iodine uptake **if due to hormone overproduction;**
	  • Low iodine uptake if due to thyroiditis, iodine ingestion, or overtreatment with thyroid hormones
	  • **Solitary area of increased iodine uptake ("hot nodules") with decreased iodine uptake in surrounding tissue if toxic adenoma**

Treatment	• Radioactive Iodine: **iodine-131 or radioiodine; most common therapy to ablate thyroid**
	  • **Contraindicated in pregnant and breastfeeding women;** may cross placenta/enter breastmilk leading to hypothyroidism of infant
	• Anti-Thyroid Medications: **blocks thyroid peroxidase and decreases the organification of iodide to prevent thyroid hormone biosynthesis**
	  • **Methimazole: preferred medication;** may be used in 2nd/3rd trimester pregnancy or breastfeeding women
	  • **Propylthiouracil (PTU): inhibits peripheral conversion of T4 into T3** (only recommended in 1st trimester pregnancy or thyroid storm due to risk of severe liver failure)
	• Beta Blockers: **may be used to control symptoms** including tremor, hypertension, tachycardia
	  • **Propranolol,** atenolol, metoprolol
	• Thyroidectomy: indicated for patients with large goiter causing anterior neck compressive symptoms, suspicion of thyroid cancer, large thyroid nodules, parathyroid adenoma
	• Trans-Sphenoidal Surgery: definitive and preferred treatment for TSH-secreting pituitary adenoma

Key Words & Most Common	• Graves disease most common cause • Hypermetabolic/increased adrenergic symptoms: diaphoresis, heat intolerance, weakness, tremor, warm/moist skin, weight loss, diarrhea, tachycardia, palpitations • ↓TSH + ↑T3/T4; +TSI with Graves • Radioactive iodine → methimazole/propylthiouracil + propranolol

Graves Disease

Etiology & Risk Factors	• **Autoimmune disease primarily affecting the thyroid gland causing hypermetabolism and increased synthesis and secretion of thyroid hormones** • **Most common cause of hyperthyroidism in the US** • Etiology: **autoimmune; autoantibody against the thyroid receptor for thyroid-stimulating hormone (TSH)** • Risk Factors: **family history, age (20-40 years old most common),** environmental triggers (stress, infection, iodine exposure), **pregnancy (mainly postpartum),** other autoimmune diagnoses (**adrenal insufficiency,** type 1 diabetes, **pernicious anemia, celiac disease,** premature graying of hair)
Patho-physiology	• Thyroid stimulating immunoglobulin (TSI) (also known as thyroid stimulating antibody [TSAb]) is a stimulatory autoantibody against the TSH thyroid receptor resulting in continuous synthesis and secretion of excess T3 and T4 hormones • TSH-receptor autoantibodies in the orbital fibroblasts release of proinflammatory cytokines and activate retroocular fibroblasts and adipocytes leading to infiltrative ophthalmopathy (exophthalmos)

Signs & Symptoms	• Hyperthyroidism: **tachycardia, palpitations, heat intolerance, diaphoresis, fatigue, weight loss,** diarrhea, **tremors, anxiety/nervousness,** insomnia, pruritis, **muscle weakness,** polyuria, loss of libido, neck fullness
	• Ocular Symptoms: **eyelid swelling,** ocular pain, conjunctival erythema, double vision
	• Physical Exam:
	  • **Hypertension, atrial fibrillation, fine tremors, warm and moist skin,** palmar erythema, hair loss, **palpable goiter with thyroid bruit**
	  • **Ophthalmopathy: eyelid retraction, proptosis, exophthalmos (protrusion of eyes anteriorly),** periorbital edema, diplopia
	  • **Pretibial Myxedema:** erythematous patches of legs that subsequently become brawny, associated with non-pitting edema; rare manifestation

Diagnosis	• Thyroid Function Tests: **primary hyperthyroid profile (decreased TSH and increased free T4 and/or T3)** • TSH-Receptor Antibodies: **positive thyroid stimulating immunoglobulin (TSI) is hallmark** • Radioactive Iodine Uptake Scan: increased, diffuse iodine uptake

Treatment	• Radioactive Iodine: **iodine-131 or radioiodine; most common therapy to ablate thyroid**
	  • **Contraindicated in pregnant and breastfeeding women;** may cross placenta/enter breastmilk leading to hypothyroidism of infant
	• Anti-Thyroid Medications: **blocks thyroid peroxidase and decreases the organification of iodide to prevent thyroid hormone biosynthesis**
	  • **Methimazole: preferred medication;** may be used in 2nd/3rd trimester pregnancy or breastfeeding women
	  • **Propylthiouracil (PTU): inhibits peripheral conversion of T4 into T3;** only recommended in 1st trimester pregnancy or thyroid storm due to risk of severe liver failure
	• Beta Blockers: **may be used to control symptoms** including tremor, hypertension, tachycardia, diaphoresis, palpitations, anxiety
	  • **Propranolol,** atenolol, metoprolol
	• Thyroidectomy: indicated for patients with large goiter causing anterior neck compressive symptoms, suspicion of thyroid cancer, large thyroid nodules, parathyroid adenoma
	• Ophthalmopathy: **corticosteroids (prednisone)** indicated with radioactive iodine therapy (initially may exacerbate ophthalmopathy); elevate head of bed; artificial tears
	  • Selenium: cofactor for glutathione peroxidase (major intracellular antioxidant) which removes oxygen free radicals generated during thyroid hormone production
	  • Teprotumumab: insulin-like growth factor 1 (IGF-1) receptor inhibitor that is effective for moderate to severe ophthalmopathy

Plummer Disease

Etiology & Risk Factors	• Hormonally active multinodular goiter with hyperthyroidism; **also known as toxic multinodular goiter** • 2nd most common cause of hyperthyroidism (Graves disease is most common cause) • <u>Etiology</u>: **multiple autonomous functioning nodules of thyroid gland** • <u>Risk Factors</u>: **family history, advanced age, female, smoking, stress,** iodine deficiency leading to hyperplasia, elevated levels of TSH
Patho-physiology	• Hyperplasia of thyroid gland leads to nodule formation and subsequent autonomous activity of the nodules independent of pituitary TSH feedback • Chronic stimuli of thyroid gland induces TSH receptor gene mutations which lead to continuous thyroid activation

Signs & Symptoms	• *Typically fewer signs and symptoms compared to Graves disease*
	• <u>Hyperthyroidism</u>: **tachycardia, palpitations, heat intolerance, diaphoresis, fatigue, weight loss,** diarrhea, **tremors, anxiety/nervousness,** insomnia, pruritis, **muscle weakness,** polyuria, loss of libido, neck fullness
	• <u>Compressive Symptoms</u>: **dyspnea (tracheal involvement), dysphagia (esophageal involvement),** stridor or hoarseness(laryngeal nerve involvement), venous sinus thrombosis (vascular involvement), neck pain or radicular symptoms (muscular/neurological involvement)
	• <u>Physical Exam</u>:
	    • **Multiple soft, smooth, mobile thyroid nodules**
	    • **Palpable goiter**

Diagnosis	• <u>Thyroid Function Tests</u>: **primary hyperthyroid profile (decreased TSH and increased free T4 and/or T3);** may be subclinical • <u>Thyroid Ultrasound</u>: determine quantity, size, and vascularity of nodules • <u>Radioactive Iodine Uptake Scan</u>: **patchy iodine uptake; localized iodine uptake in one or more nodules with decreased uptake of surrounding thyroid tissue** • <u>Fine Needle Aspiration with Biopsy</u>: used to exclude malignancy on "cold" nodules on iodine uptake scan

Treatment	• <u>Surgery</u>: **total, near-total, or subtotal thyroidectomy is mainstay for toxic multinodular goiter;** rapid resolution with low morbidity and mortality
	• <u>Radioactive Iodine</u>: **iodine-131 or radioiodine; most common therapy to ablate thyroid**
	    • **Contraindicated in pregnant and breastfeeding women;** may cross placenta/enter breastmilk leading to hypothyroidism of infant
	• <u>Anti-Thyroid Medications</u>: utilized until radioactive iodine is given and for surgery preparation
	    • **Methimazole: preferred medication;** may be used in 2nd/3rd trimester pregnancy or breastfeeding women
	    • **Propylthiouracil (PTU):** inhibits peripheral conversion of T4 into T3; only recommended in 1st trimester pregnancy or thyroid storm due to risk of severe liver failure

Key Words & Most Common	• Multiple autonomous functioning nodules of thyroid gland • Tachycardia, palpitations, heat intolerance, weight loss, tremors, fatigue, weakness • Multiple soft, smooth, mobile thyroid nodules + palpable goiter • ↓TSH + ↑T3/T4 • <u>RAIU</u>: patchy iodine uptake; localized iodine uptake in nodules with decreased uptake of surrounding tissue • Surgery is mainstay of treatment • RIA vs anti-thyroid medications (methimazole, PTU)

Toxic Adenoma

Etiology & Risk Factors	• Single or multiple nodules of the thyroid gland; usually presents as solitary nodule
	• **May be active or inactive**
	    • <u>Inactive</u>: **most common; asymptomatic as thyroid hormone secretion remains normal**
	    • <u>Active</u>: **referred to as toxic adenomas; symptomatic as thyroid hormone is produced**
	• <u>Etiology</u>: sporadic; may have genetic mutation component (PAX8-PPAR gene rearrangement has strong association)

Patho-physiology	• Monoclonal expansion of thyroid cells, secondary to TSH-receptor gene mutations, lead to nodule formation
Signs & Symptoms	• <u>Hyperthyroidism</u>: **tachycardia, palpitations, heat intolerance, diaphoresis, fatigue, weight loss,** diarrhea, **tremors, anxiety/nervousness,** insomnia, pruritis, **muscle weakness,** polyuria, loss of libido, neck fullness, increased metabolic rate • <u>Compressive Symptoms</u>: **dyspnea (tracheal involvement), dysphagia (esophageal involvement),** stridor or hoarseness (laryngeal nerve involvement), venous sinus thrombosis (vascular involvement), neck pain or radicular symptoms (muscular/neurological involvement) • <u>Physical Exam</u>: • **Solitary, spherical and encapsulated nodule, well demarcated from the surrounding parenchyma, palpable goiter**
Diagnosis	• <u>Thyroid Function Tests</u>: **primary hyperthyroid profile (decreased TSH + increased free T3 or T4)** • <u>Radioactive Iodine Uptake Scan</u>: **solitary area of increased iodine uptake ("hot nodules") with decreased iodine uptake in surrounding tissue** • <u>Thyroid Ultrasound</u>: used to evaluate benign vs malignant lesions (malignant lesions may have hypoechogenicity, microcalcifications, irregular margins) • <u>Fine Needle Aspiration with Biopsy</u>: identifies if lesion has abnormal features or atypia; thyroid adenomas have organized follicular epithelial cells
Treatment	• <u>Observation</u>: if asymptomatic and low concern for malignancy; monitor with serial ultrasounds and/or fine needle aspiration • <u>Radioactive Iodine</u>: **iodine-131 or radioiodine; ablation therapy** • <u>Anti-Thyroid Medications</u>: methimazole or propylthiouracil; blocks thyroid peroxidase and decreases the organification of iodide to prevent thyroid hormone biosynthesis • <u>Surgery</u>: **thyroid lobectomy and isthmusectomy is preferred treatment;** treats compressive symptoms, resolves hyperthyroidism, avoids radiation exposure
Key Words & Most Common	• Single or multiple nodules of thyroid gland • Active nodules produce thyroid hormone; referred to as toxic adenomas • <u>Hyperthyroidism Symptoms</u>: tachycardia, palpitations, heat intolerance, weight loss, tremors • ↓TSH + ↑T3/T4 • Radioactive Iodine Uptake Scan: solitary area of increased iodine uptake • Radioactive iodine to ablate thyroid • Surgery is preferred treatment

272

TSH-Secreting Pituitary Adenoma

Etiology & Risk Factors	• Benign tumor of the anterior pituitary gland that secretes thyroid stimulating hormone (TSH) • Etiology: sporadic; unknown • Most pituitary adenomas are found incidentally on CT scan
Patho-physiology	• Functional tumors are comprised of a cell type that increases secretion of one or more hormones of the anterior pituitary
Signs & Symptoms	• **Hyperthyroidism: tachycardia, palpitations, heat intolerance, diaphoresis, fatigue, weight loss,** diarrhea, **tremors, anxiety/nervousness,** insomnia, pruritis, **muscle weakness,** polyuria, loss of libido, neck fullness, increased metabolic rate • **Compressive Symptoms: bitemporal hemianopsia (impaired peripheral vision of outer visual fields) is most common defect due to compression of optic chiasm;** headache • Physical Exam: • **Hypertension, atrial fibrillation, fine tremors, warm and moist skin,** palmar erythema, hair loss, **palpable goiter**
Diagnosis	• **Thyroid Function Tests: secondary (central) hyperthyroid profile (increased TSH and increased free T4)** • Radioactive Iodine Uptake Scan: increased, diffuse iodine uptake • Pituitary MRI: indicated to distinguish adenoma from aneurysm

Treatment	• **Trans-Sphenoidal Surgery: definitive and preferred treatment** (curative in 50-90% of patients)
	• **Hyperthyroidism Management: necessary prior to surgery to prevent thyroid storm**
	   • Methimazole: prevents thyroid hormone biosynthesis
	   • Somatostatin Analogs (SSA): inhibits TSH secretion

Key Words & Most Common	• Tumor of anterior pituitary gland that secretes TSH • Hyperthyroidism Symptoms: tachycardia, palpitations, heat intolerance, weight loss, tremors • Compressive Symptoms: bitemporal hemianopsia • Secondary (central) hyperthyroid profile ($\uparrow$TSH and $\uparrow$T4) • Pituitary MRI to detect adenoma • Trans-sphenoidal surgery is definitive and preferred treatment

Thyroid Storm

Etiology & Risk Factors	• Acute, life-threatening complication of hyperthyroidism presenting with multi-system involvement, usually after a precipitating event; also known as thyrotoxic crisis • Etiology: **Graves disease most common;** toxic multinodular goiter and toxic thyroid adenoma • Risk Factors: **age (mid 40's most common), females, untreated or undertreated hyperthyroidism** • Precipitating Factors: **abrupt discontinuation of hyperthyroid medications, thyroid surgery, surgery, trauma, infection,** MI, heart failure, **iodine load** (iodinated contrast medium, amiodarone), burns, traumatic brain injury, pregnancy, lithium withdrawal, hyperemesis gravidarum
Patho-physiology	• Rapid increase in thyroid hormone levels in response to a precipitating factor leads to hyperactivity of the sympathetic nervous system, increased catecholamine response, and cytokine release
Signs & Symptoms	• **Hyperthermia: marked fever to 104-106°F** • **Tachycardia:** heart rate out of proportion to fever • **Altered Mental Status: confusion, agitation, delirium,** stupor that may progress to coma or seizure • May also have **palpitations, tremors, hyperhidrosis, ophthalmopathy** (if associated with Graves), **hypotension,** heart failure, atrial fibrillation, dyspnea, wide pulse pressures
Diagnosis	• **Thyroid Function Tests: primary hyperthyroid profile (decreased TSH [TSH may be undetectably low] + increased T3/T4)** • Comprehensive Metabolic Panel (CMP): hypercalcemia, **hyperglycemia** • Complete Blood Count (CBC): **leukocytosis,** thrombocytopenia

Treatment	• **Supportive:**
	   • Fever: **cooling measures** (ice packs, cooling blankets), **acetaminophen** (NSAIDs can displace thyroid hormone off thyroid-binding globulin), **do not aggressively cool** (can cause vasoconstriction)
	   • Dehydration/Hyperglycemia: **IV D5NS**
	   • Agitation: benzodiazepines
	• **Beta Blockers:** treat increased adrenergic tone to **control symptoms** (tremor, hypertension, tachycardia)
	   • **Propranolol,** esmolol (reserpine if BB contraindicated)
	• **Anti-Thyroid Medications: blocks thyroid peroxidase and decreases the organification of iodide to prevent thyroid hormone biosynthesis**
	   • **Propylthiouracil (PTU): preferred medication over methimazole; inhibits peripheral conversion of T4 into T3**
	   • **Potassium Iodide (SSKI): iodine blocks release of thyroid hormone; give 1 hour after PTU to prevent increased hormone production**
	      • *Can substitute radiocontrast dyes, PO Lugol solution, IV sodium iodide as alternative iodine sources*
	   • **Lithium Carbonate: treatment of choice of iodine-induced hyperthyroidism** (contrast load or amiodarone); consider if allergic to iodine
	• **Corticosteroids:** IV hydrocortisone; reduce peripheral conversion of T4 to T3 and treat associated adrenal insufficiency

Key Words & Most Common	• Triad of hyperthermia, tachycardia, altered mental status + hyperthyroid symptoms • $\downarrow$(or undetectable) TSH + $\uparrow$T3/T4 • Cooling measures + acetaminophen + IV D5NS $\rightarrow$ propranolol $\rightarrow$ propylthiouracil (PTU) $\rightarrow$ supersaturated potassium iodide (SSKI) $\rightarrow$ IV hydrocortisone

Hyperthyroidism Disorders

	Graves Disease	Plummer Disease	Toxic Adenoma	TSH-Secreting Pituitary Adenoma
Etiology	• Autoimmune • Triggered by stress, infection, iodine exposure • MCC of hyperthyroidism	• AKA toxic multinodular goiter • Multiple autonomous functioning nodules of thyroid gland • Advanced age	• Solitary autonomously functioning nodule • May have genetic mutation component	• Tumor of anterior pituitary gland that secretes TSH • *Most found incidentally on CT scan*
Patho-physiology	• TSH autoantibodies results in ↑release of thyroid hormones	• Autonomous activity of nodules independent of pituitary TSH feedback	• Expansion of thyroid cells secondary to TSH-receptor gene mutations	• Tumor comprised of cell type that increases TSH secretion
Signs and Symptoms	• Clinical hyperthyroidism • <u>Ophthalmopathy</u>: eyelid retractions, exophthalmos, proptosis • <u>Pretibial Myxedema</u>: pink/brown erythematous patches and non-pitting edema of lower legs	• Clinical hyperthyroidism (*typically less pronounced symptoms than Graves*) • Compressive symptoms (dyspnea, dysphagia, stridor, hoarseness) • *No ophthalmopathy* • Multiple soft, smooth, mobile thyroid nodules	• Clinical hyperthyroidism • Compressive symptoms (dyspnea, dysphagia, stridor, hoarseness) • Solitary, spherical and encapsulated nodule, well demarcated from the surrounding parenchyma; palpable goiter	• Clinical hyperthyroidism • <u>Bitemporal Hemianopsia</u>: impaired peripheral vision of outer visual fields due to compression of optic chiasm • Headache
Diagnosis	• ↓TSH and ↑T3/T4 • + thyroid stimulating immunoglobulin (TSI) • <u>RAIU</u>: ↑ and diffuse iodine uptake	• ↓TSH and ↑T3/T4 • <u>RAIU</u>: patchy areas of iodine uptake; localized uptake at 1+ nodules with surrounding areas of decreased uptake • <u>Ultrasound</u>: evaluate benign vs malignant lesions	• ↓TSH and ↑T3/T4 • <u>RAIU</u>: solitary area of increased iodine uptake ("hot nodule") • <u>Ultrasound</u>: evaluate benign vs malignant lesions	• ↑TSH and ↑T3/T4 (secondary) • <u>RAIU</u>: ↑ and diffuse iodine uptake • <u>Pituitary MRI</u>: adenoma of anterior pituitary
Treatment	• <u>Radioactive Iodine</u>: most common therapy to ablate thyroid • <u>Anti-Thyroids</u>: methimazole or propylthiouracil • <u>Beta Blockers</u>: propranolol for symptoms (tremor, hypertension, tachycardia) • <u>Thyroidectomy</u>: if compressive symptoms or concern for malignancy	• <u>Surgery</u>: total/sub-total thyroidectomy is mainstay • <u>Radioactive Iodine</u>: most common therapy to ablate thyroid • <u>Anti-Thyroids</u>: methimazole or propylthiouracil • <u>Beta Blockers</u>: propranolol for symptoms (tremor, hypertension, tachycardia)	• <u>Observation</u>: if asymptomatic and low concern for malignancy • <u>Radioactive Iodine</u>: most common therapy to ablate thyroid • <u>Anti-Thyroids</u>: methimazole or propylthiouracil • <u>Beta Blockers</u>: propranolol for symptoms (tremor, hypertension, tachycardia) • Surgery: thyroid lobectomy and isthmusectomy is preferred treatment	• <u>Trans-Sphenoidal Surgery</u>: definitive and preferred treatment • <u>Anti-Thyroids</u>: methimazole or propylthiouracil prior to surgery to prevent thyroid storm

Hypothyroidism Disorders

	Hashimoto Thyroiditis	Riedel Thyroiditis	Subacute Thyroiditis	Suppurative Thyroiditis
Etiology	• Autoimmune • Most common cause of hypothyroidism in US • Anti-thyroid peroxidase (anti-TPO) is most common antibody	• Immunoglobulin G4 (IgG4) related systemic disease • Inflammation and dense fibrosis of thyroid	• AKA de Quervain thyroiditis, granulomatous thyroiditis • Viral process precedes symptoms by 2-8 weeks	• Bacterial infection of thyroid gland • Gram + most common (*Staphylococcus, Streptococcus*) • Primarily affects children
Patho-physiology	• Autoimmune antibody development to thyroid antigens	• Autoimmune mediated replacement of thyroid tissue with dense fibrotic tissue	• Inflammation of thyroid gland secondary to viral respiratory tract infection	• Bacterial infection of thyroid; congenital abnormalities (pyriform sinus) may be source

Signs and Symptoms	• Clinical hypothyroidism
	• Nontender goiter that is nodular or smooth, firm with "rubbery" feel
	• Loss of outer 1/3rd of eyebrows
		• Compressive symptoms (dyspnea, dysphagia, stridor, hoarseness)
		• Hard, nontender, fixed mass of anterior neck; immobile when swallowing
		  • "Stone-like, rock hard"
		• *Absence of cervical lymphadenopathy*
			• Clinical hyperthyroidism that may progress to hypothyroidism symptoms
			• Painful thyroid gland worse with head/neck movements and swallowing
			• Asymmetrically enlarged, firm, diffusely tender goiter
				• Fever/chills
				• Painful thyroid
				  • Worse with neck hyperextension of neck
				  • May radiate to jaw/ears
				• Superficial erythema of neck

Diagnosis	• ↑TSH and ↓T3/T4 • + thyroid autoantibodies (antithyroid peroxidase)	• ↑TSH and ↓T3/T4 • <u>Open Biopsy</u>: definitive diagnosis and distinguishes between anaplastic thyroid cancer; shows dense fibrosis	• ↑ ESR (hallmark) • <u>Early</u>: ↓TSH and ↑T3/T4 • <u>Later (2-8 weeks)</u>: ↑TSH and ↓T3/T4 • <u>FNA</u>: definitive diagnosis; shows granulomatous inflammation	• Leukocytosis • ↑↑ ESR/CRP • *Usually euthyroid*
Treatment	• Levothyroxine (synthetic T4)	• <u>Surgery</u>: subtotal or partial thyroidectomy for compressive symptoms • <u>Corticosteroids</u>: mainstay of medical treatment	• <u>Supportive</u>: reassurance; most cases are self-limiting • <u>NSAIDs or ASA</u> for pain/inflammation • <u>Corticosteroids</u>: prednisone for severe neck pain; 3-4 week taper	• NSAIDs for neck pain • Antibiotics (ampicillin, nafcillin/gentamicin, ceftriaxone)

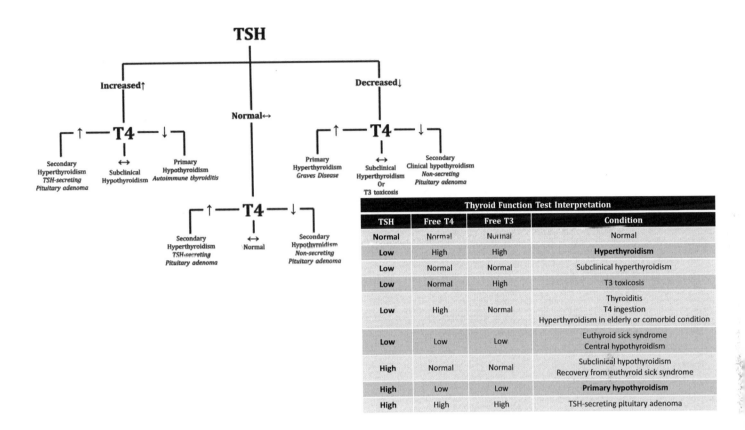

TSH

Increased↑

┌─── ↑ **T4** ↓ ───┐

Secondary Hyperthyroidism
TSH-secreting Pituitary adenoma

Subclinical Hypothyroidism

Primary Hypothyroidism
Autoimmune thyroiditis

Normal↔

┌─── ↑ **T4** ↓ ───┐

Secondary Hyperthyroidism
TSH-secreting Pituitary adenoma

Normal

Secondary Hypothyroidism
Non-secreting Pituitary adenoma

Decreased↓

┌─── ↑ **T4** ↓ ───┐

Primary Hyperthyroidism
Graves Disease

Subclinical Hyperthyroidism
Or
T3 toxicosis

Secondary Clinical hypothyroidism
Non-secreting Pituitary adenoma

Thyroid Function Test Interpretation			
TSH	**Free T4**	**Free T3**	**Condition**
Normal	Normal	Normal	Normal
Low	High	High	**Hyperthyroidism**
Low	Normal	Normal	Subclinical hyperthyroidism
Low	Normal	High	T3 toxicosis
Low	High	Normal	Thyroiditis T4 ingestion Hyperthyroidism in elderly or comorbid condition
Low	Low	Low	Euthyroid sick syndrome Central hypothyroidism
High	Normal	Normal	Subclinical hypothyroidism Recovery from euthyroid sick syndrome
High	Low	Low	**Primary hypothyroidism**
High	High	High	TSH-secreting pituitary adenoma

Papillary Thyroid Carcinoma

Etiology & Risk Factors	• Epithelial malignancy showing evidence of follicular cell differentiation within the thyroid gland • **Most common thyroid cancer (80-90% of all thyroid cancers)** • Etiology: **epithelial malignancy of thyroid gland; ability to invade adjacent structures (lymphatics) is hallmark** • Risk Factors: **radiation exposure** (childhood radiation exposure, medical radiation exposure, **environmental radiation exposure**), **female**, genetics, high iodine intake, **obesity**
Patho-physiology	• Radiation exposure causes chromosomal rearrangements and genetic mutations leading to malignancy • **Local metastases to cervical lymph nodes is most common location**; may metastasize to lungs
Signs & Symptoms	• **Usually asymptomatic** • **Painless thyroid nodule +/- regional (cervical) lymphadenopathy** • Hoarseness and dysphagia may occur secondary to laryngeal nerve involvement • Physical Exam: • **Nontender, firm, fixed nodule (usually <5cm) with irregular border**
Diagnosis	• **Fine Needle Aspiration with Biopsy: initial diagnostic test**; demonstrates change of papillae and nucleus morphology • Thyroid Function Tests: usually normal • Radioactive Iodine Uptake Scan: typically appear as cold (hypo-functioning) nodules
Treatment	• **Surgery: thyroidectomy (total or near-total) followed by postoperative levothyroxine** • **Thyroid Hormone Replacement: levothyroxine (synthetic T4) given postoperatively** to replace normal TSH production and suppress regrowth of tumor • Radioactive Iodine: therapy of choice after thyroidectomy to ablate residual normal thyroid tissue. • *Serum thyroglobulin levels, TSH and neck ultrasound used to monitor for recurrent or persistent disease after treatment*
Key Words & Most Common	• Most common thyroid cancer • Radiation exposure greatest risk factor; female • Painless thyroid nodule +/- cervical lymphadenopathy • Nontender, firm, fixed nodule with irregular border • Fine needle aspiration • Thyroidectomy followed by postoperative levothyroxine

Follicular Thyroid Carcinoma

Etiology & Risk Factors	• Tumor of the follicular cells with both capsular and vascular invasive properties • Second most common type of thyroid cancer (10-15% of all thyroid cancers) • Etiology: follicular malignancy of the thyroid gland • Risk Factors: **radiation exposure** (*less often associated with radiation than papillary*); **iodine deficiency**, elderly, occupational exposures (radiation, pesticides, textiles)
Patho-physiology	• Radiation exposure causes chromosomal rearrangements and genetic mutations leading to malignancy • **More malignant; distal metastases is more common than local metastases (hematogenous spread); lung is most common**; bone, liver, brain
Signs & Symptoms	• **Usually asymptomatic** • **Painless thyroid nodule**
Diagnosis	• <u>Fine Needle Aspiration with Biopsy</u>: may not distinguish between follicular adenoma and carcinoma • <u>Thyroid Ultrasound</u>: solid hypoechoic nodules with micro-calcification, poorly defined margins, vascular patterns • <u>Postsurgical Histology</u>: **definitive diagnosis**
Treatment	• <u>Surgery</u>: **thyroidectomy (total or near-total) followed by postoperative levothyroxine** • <u>Thyroid Hormone Replacement</u>: **levothyroxine (synthetic T4) given postoperatively** to replace normal TSH production and suppress regrowth of tumor • <u>Radioactive Iodine</u>: therapy of choice after thyroidectomy to ablate residual normal thyroid tissue; metastases more reactive to RAI therapy than papillary thyroid cancer • *Serum thyroglobulin levels, TSH and neck ultrasound used to monitor for recurrent or persistent disease after treatment*
Key Words & Most Common	• Tumor of follicular cells; 2nd most common type of thyroid cancer • Radiation exposure, iodine deficiency, elderly, occupational exposure • More malignant than papillary thyroid cancer; distal metastases more common (lung most common METS site) • Painless thyroid nodule • FNA may be insufficient; postsurgical histology for definitive diagnosis • Thyroidectomy followed by postoperative levothyroxine

Medullary Thyroid Carcinoma

Etiology & Risk Factors	• **Tumor arising from the calcitonin-synthesizing parafollicular cells (C-cells) of the thyroid gland** • Constitutes about 5% of all thyroid cancer • Etiology: sporadic (80%); familial (multiple endocrine neoplasia [MEN] 2A, MEN 2B, and familial medullary thyroid cancer [FMTC]), *RET* mutations in neural crest tissue • Risk Factors: **age (50-70 years old most common in sporadic cases; 20-40 years old most common in MEN associated thyroid cancer)**
Patho-physiology	• Tumor arising from the calcitonin-synthesizing parafollicular cells (C-cells) of the thyroid gland and **produces calcitonin (hallmark)** which works to lower calcium in blood • Calcitonin inhibits osteoclast activity and may lower calcium in blood however calcium levels usually normal due to down-regulation of receptors • **More aggressive; local cervical lymph node METS early in disease course** followed by distant METS
Signs & Symptoms	• **Usually asymptomatic** • **Painless thyroid nodule** • **Diarrhea** (secondary to high calcitonin levels) • **Compressive symptoms** (dyspnea, dysphagia, stridor, hoarseness) • Physical Exam: • **Palpable nodule on the superior aspect of the thyroid** (where C-cells are located)
Diagnosis	• <u>Labs</u>: consider carcinoembryonic antigen (CEA) and serum/urinary metanephrine levels (rule out pheochromocytoma prior to surgery [MEN2]) • <u>Serum Calcitonin</u>: **significant elevation of serum calcitonin (hallmark)** • <u>Fine Needle Aspiration</u>: helpful to establish diagnosis but may be nondiagnostic • <u>Thyroid Ultrasound</u>: used to determine lymph node involvement; may show dense, homogenous, conglomerate calcification • <u>Postsurgical Histology</u>: **definitive diagnosis**; shows round or ovoid cells with fibrovascular stroma; characteristic **amyloid deposits that stain with Congo red**
Treatment	• <u>Surgery</u>: **total thyroidectomy + lymph node dissection indicated for all patients** • *Serum calcitonin and CEA levels used to monitor for recurrent or persistent disease after treatment*
Key Words & Most Common	• Tumor arising from calcitonin-synthesizing parafollicular cells • Most are sporadic; may be associated with MEN2 • Painless thyroid nodule + diarrhea + compressive symptoms • Palpable nodule on superior aspect of thyroid • ↑calcitonin • Total thyroidectomy + lymph node dissection

Anaplastic Thyroid Carcinoma

Etiology & Risk Factors	• **Rare, highly aggressive malignant tumor of the thyroid gland** • Constitutes about 2-3% of all thyroid cancers • **Most aggressive of all thyroid cancers and carries poor prognosis** (mortality rate 80% within 1 year of diagnosis); patients often present with metastatic disease • <u>Risk Factors</u>: female **(males carry a worse prognosis), age (>65 years old most common), history of differentiated thyroid cancer**
Patho-physiology	• Progressive accumulation of chromosomal alterations and genetic mutations lead to malignancy • Local invasion aggressively metastasizes to regional lymph nodes and distant sites

Signs & Symptoms	• **Rapid, painful enlargement of thyroid gland**
	• **Compressive symptoms** (dyspnea, dysphagia, stridor, hoarseness)
	• <u>Physical Exam</u>:
	   • **Tender, firm, inferoanterior thyroid mass**
	   • **"Rock hard" thyroid mass; usually fixed to underlying tissue**

Diagnosis	• <u>Thyroid Ultrasound</u>: may show a solid hypoechoic mass with internal calcifications and irregular margins • <u>Fine Needle Aspiration</u>: helpful to establish diagnosis but may be nondiagnostic • <u>Postsurgical Histology</u>: **definitive diagnosis** • <u>CT Scan</u>: useful to define the local extent and detect lymph node metastases
Treatment	• <u>Surgery</u>: debulking surgery is most common procedure to preserve airway; most are not amenable to surgical resection • **Palliative tracheostomy may be performed to preserve airway** • <u>External-Beam Radiation and Chemotherapy</u>: mainly experimental to control local invasion
Key Words & Most Common	• Highly aggressive malignant tumor of thyroid • Carries poor prognosis • Rapid, painful enlargement of thyroid gland + compressive symptoms • Tender, fixed, "rock hard" thyroid mass • Postsurgical histology required for definitive diagnosis • Surgery to preserve airway; most not amenable to resection

Thyroid Nodule

Etiology & Risk Factors	• Benign or malignant discrete lesion within the thyroid gland; may be solitary, multiple, cystic, or solid
	• <u>Etiology</u>: >90% are clinically insignificant, benign lesions
	   • <u>Benign</u>: **Follicular adenoma (hyperplastic colloid goiter) is most common type of nodule**; thyroid cysts, thyroiditis, thyroid adenomas
	   • <u>Malignant</u>: thyroid cancer; **papillary thyroid carcinoma most common malignant cause**
	• <u>Risk Factors</u>:
	   • <u>Benign</u>: **history of ionizing radiation, increasing age, female**, smoking, **obesity**, metabolic syndrome, alcohol use
	   • <u>Malignancy</u>: **history of ionizing radiation, males, age (<20), family history of thyroid cancer or multiple endocrine neoplasia (MEN2)**, solitary nodule, increasing size

Patho-physiology	• Varies depending on etiology of lesion • Radiation may cause somatic mutations of thyroid gland tissue

Signs & Symptoms	• **Most are asymptomatic**
	• <u>Compressive Symptoms</u>: **dyspnea (tracheal involvement), dysphagia (esophageal involvement)**, stridor (laryngeal nerve involvement), venous sinus thrombosis (vascular involvement), neck pain or radicular symptoms (muscular/neurological involvement)
	• **Large, palpable nodule on anterior neck**
	   • May be found incidentally on imaging studies ordered for other reasons
	• <u>Physical Exam</u>:
	   • <u>Benign</u>: **variable**; usually smooth, sharply outline, discrete, painless
	   • <u>Malignant</u>: **solitary, large (>4cm), firm, fixation to adjacent tissue, cervical lymphadenopathy, vocal cord paralysis; no movement with swallowing**

Diagnosis	• <u>Thyroid Function Tests</u>: **initial test performed**;
	   • ↓ **or normal TSH**: radioactive iodine uptake scan indicated (lower malignant potential)
	   • ↑ **TSH**: FNA with biopsy indicated
	• <u>Radioactive Iodine Uptake Scan</u>: performed if TSH is low or subnormal or FNA indeterminant
	   • No or low iodine uptake ("cold nodules") should be biopsied to rule out malignancy
	   • Functional ("hot nodules") have less malignant potential
	• <u>Thyroid Ultrasound</u>: **most sensitive test to detect thyroid lesion**; determines size, vascularity and monitors growth
	   • Malignancy: may have microcalcifications, irregular margins, central vascularity, documented nodule growth, hypoechogenicity, taller-than-wide shape
	• <u>Fine Needle Aspiration</u>: **best test to evaluate nodule**
	   • Indicated in nodules >1cm; or in <1cm if more than one suspicious characteristic on ultrasound, cervical lymphadenopathy or high-risk history.

Treatment	• <u>Observation</u>: observation with follow-up ultrasound every 6-12 months to monitor • <u>Surgery</u>: surgical excision if thyroid cancer is suspected

Type I Diabetes Mellitus

Etiology & Risk Factors	• Autoimmune disease that causes destruction of insulin-producing pancreatic beta cells leading to insulin deficiency • Patients with T1DM require life-long insulin replacement therapy • **Onset usually <30 years old; most commonly presents during childhood (4-6 years old) and early adolescence (10-14 years old)** • <u>Etiology</u>: **autoimmune destruction of the pancreatic islet beta cells** (over months to years) • Risk Factors: **genetic predisposition** (HLA [DR and DQ] alleles), viral infection (*Coxsackievirus* Rubella, EBV or *Enterovirus*), **environmental toxin exposure**, dietary exposures (cow's milk protein exposure, nitrates in drinking water)
Patho-physiology	• Insulin, an anabolic hormone, exercises multiple mechanisms on glucose, lipid, protein, and mineral metabolism • Insulin allows glucose to enter muscle and adipose cells and inhibit breakdown of fat in adipose tissue, stimulates hepatic storage of glucose as glycogen, stimulation amino acid uptake, and stimulates potassium transport into cells • Autoimmune destruction of insulin-producing pancreatic beta cells leads to insulin deficiency

Signs & Symptoms	• **Often asymptomatic until discovery in symptomatic hyperglycemic state or diabetic ketoacidosis**
	• **Symptomatic hyperglycemia is the most common initial presentation**
	  • **Urinary frequency leading to polyuria** (large quantities of urine production), **polydipsia** (excessive thirst), **dehydration**
	  • Dehydration leads to orthostatic hypotension, fatigue, weakness, and mental status changes
	• **Weight loss**, lethargy
	• **Diabetic ketoacidosis is second most common initial presentation**

Diagnosis	• <u>Fasting Plasma Glucose</u>: diagnosis made with elevated fasting glucose measurement (≥126mg/dL) after an 8-12 hour fast on 2 separate occasions • <u>Oral Glucose Tolerance Test (OGTT)</u>: diagnosis made with elevated glucose measurement (≥200mg/dL) 2 hours after ingesting concentrated glucose solution • <u>Glycosylated Hemoglobin A1C (HbA1c)</u>: reflects glycemic control over the previous 2 to 3 months • **≥6.5% indicates diabetes**; 5.7-6.4% indicates prediabetes • <u>Random Plasma Glucose</u>: diagnosis can be made with elevated glucose measurement (≥200mg/dL); should be confirmed with repeat testing

Treatment	• <u>**Insulin Therapy**</u>: **indicated for all type I diabetic patients**
	  • <u>**Basal/Bolus Insulin Therapy**</u>: **preferred therapy to replicate insulin secretion pattern of person without diabetes**
	    • **Longer acting insulin (or a continuous subcutaneous infusion of rapid-acting insulin delivered by a pump) used to simulate basal insulin production**
	    • **Shorter acting insulin used before meals to control postprandial glucose spikes**
	  • <u>Sliding Scale Insulin Therapy</u>: varying doses of rapid-acting insulin administered prior to meals and at bedtime depending on the patient's plasma glucose level

Key Words & Most Common	• Autoimmune destruction of the pancreatic islet beta cells • Onset usually <30 years old; most common during childhood (4-6 years old) and early adolescence (10-14 years old) • Symptomatic hyperglycemia (urinary frequency, polyuria, polydipsia, dehydration), weight loss, fatigue, weakness → diabetic ketoacidosis • Fasting plasma glucose ≥126mg/dL; OGTT ≥200mg/dL; HbA1c >6.5%; Random plasma glucose ≥200mg/dL • Insulin therapy

Type II Diabetes Mellitus

Etiology & Risk Factors	• **Chronic metabolic disorder characterized by persistent hyperglycemia secondary to insulin resistance and relative impairment of insulin secretion** • Accounts for 90% of all cases of diabetes; estimated that 10% of US population is diabetic (estimated 25% of population >65 years old is diabetic) • <u>Etiology</u>: **insulin resistance and impaired insulin secretion** • <u>Risk Factors</u>: **obesity is greatest risk factor, sedentary lifestyle, caloric-dense diet and poor nutrition, age (>45 years old most common)**, family history, hypertension, dyslipidemia, polycystic ovary syndrome, history of gestational diabetes, race/ethnicity (African, Hispanic, Asian American, or American Indian increased risk)
Patho-physiology	• Insulin secretion is inadequate secondary to beta-cell dysfunction and insulin resistance; persistent hyperglycemia develops as insulin secretion cannot compensate • Excess adipose tissue promotes insulin resistance through various inflammatory mechanisms (increased free fatty acid release and adipokine dysregulation)

Signs & Symptoms	• Most are asymptomatic; may be incidental finding
	• **Symptomatic hyperglycemia is the most common initial presentation**
	  • **Urinary frequency leading to polyuria** (large quantities of urine production), **polydipsia** (excessive thirst), **dehydration**
	  • Dehydration leads to orthostatic hypotension, fatigue, weakness, and mental status changes
	• **Poor wound healing, increased infections**
	• Hyperglycemic hyperosmolar state; may present during period of physiologic stress or when glucose metabolism is inhibited (corticosteroid use)

Diagnosis	• <u>Fasting Plasma Glucose</u>: diagnosis made with elevated fasting glucose measurement (≥126mg/dL) after an 8-12 hour fast on 2 separate occasions • <u>Oral Glucose Tolerance Test (OGTT)</u>: diagnosis made with elevated glucose measurement (≥200mg/dL) 2 hours after ingesting concentrated glucose solution • <u>Glycosylated Hemoglobin A1C (HbA1c)</u>: reflects glycemic control over the previous 2 to 3 months • **≥6.5% indicates diabetes**; 5.7-6.4% indicates prediabetes • <u>Random Plasma Glucose</u>: diagnosis can be made with elevated glucose measurement (≥200mg/dL); should be confirmed with repeat testing
Treatment	• <u>Lifestyle Modifications</u>: **weight reduction, aerobic and anaerobic exercise, proper nutrition** (protein prioritized, low-carbohydrate eating plan encouraged), foot care • <u>Biguanides (Metformin)</u>: **first-line therapy**; decreases hepatic glucose production (inhibits gluconeogenesis) and increase peripheral insulin-mediated glucose utilization • <u>Sulfonylureas (Glipizide)</u>: **second-line therapy**; stimulates insulin release from pancreatic cells, decreases hepatic glucose production and increases insulin receptor sensitivity • <u>Thiazolidinediones (Pioglitazone)</u>: **third-line therapy**; increases insulin sensitivity at peripheral receptor sites (adipose, muscle, hepatic cells) to increase glucose utilization • <u>Glucagon-Like Peptide 1 Receptor Agonists (Liraglutide, Semaglutide)</u>: increases glucose-dependent insulin secretion, delays gastric emptying, decreases glucagon secretion • <u>Dipeptidyl Peptidase-4 Inhibitors (DPP4) (Sitagliptin, Linagliptin)</u>: increases glucagon-like peptide 1 which increases insulin release • <u>Sodium Glucose Transport Protein-2 Inhibitor (SGLT-2) (Canagliflozin)</u>: blocks sodium-glucose cotransport at the proximal convoluted tubule decreasing glucose reabsorption • <u>Insulin Therapy</u>: often indicated if patient is uncontrolled with multiple medications
Key Words & Most Common	• Chronic metabolic disorder characterized by persistent hyperglycemia due to impaired insulin secretion and insulin resistance • Obesity is greatest risk factor; sedentary lifestyle, poor diet, increasing age • Often asymptomatic; urinary frequency, polyuria, polydipsia, poor wound healing, increased infections • Fasting plasma glucose ≥126mg/dL; OGTT ≥200mg/dL; HbA1c >6.5%; Random plasma glucose ≥200mg/dL • Lifestyle modifications → metformin → sulfonylureas, DPP-4 inhibitors, GLP-1 agonists, SGLT-2 inhibitors → insulin therapy

Gestational Diabetes

Etiology & Risk Factors	• Glucose intolerance with onset or first recognition during pregnancy; usually subsides postpartum • Etiology: **insulin resistance secondary to placental hormone release, pancreatic beta-cell dysfunction** • Risk Factors: **obesity, sedentary lifestyle**, prior or family history of gestational diabetes, newborn with macrosomia, PCOS, Hgb A1c >5.7, multiple gestations
Patho-physiology	• Placental release of diabetogenic hormones; human placental lactogen provokes and alters insulin receptors which subsequently reduces glucose uptake within the tissue • Maternal hyperglycemia can translate to fetal hyperglycemia and fetal pancreas stimulation; insulin has anabolic properties which promotes fetal tissue growth (macrosomia)

Signs & Symptoms	• Disproportionate weight gain, obesity, elevated BMI
	• Fetal Complications:
	    • **Fetal hyperinsulinemia leads to fetal macrosomia**; macrosomia predisposes to birth injuries (**shoulder dystocia**), preterm labor, delayed fetal lung maturity, **neonatal hypoglycemia**, fetal hyperbilirubinemia, neonatal hypocalcemia and hypomagnesemia
	• Maternal Complications:
	    • >50% chance to develop type 2 diabetes after pregnancy and recurrence of gestational diabetes with subsequent pregnancies
	    • **Preeclampsia**, placental abruption

Diagnosis	• Gestational Diabetes Screen: screening around 24-28 weeks' gestation
	    • One-Hour Glucose Challenge Test: 50g oral glucose solution; patient takes 50g glucose and has lab value drawn one-hour later
	    • Three-Hour Glucose Tolerance Test: 100g oral glucose solution; **indicated if one-hour test is abnormal (≥130 mg/dL); diagnostic gold standard**
	        • *Presence of 2+ abnormal results establishes gestational diabetes diagnosis*
	            • **Fasting glucose >95 mg/dL**
	            • **Glucose at one hour >180 mg/dL**
	            • **Glucose at two hours >155 mg/dL**
	            • **Glucose at three hours >140 mg/dL**

Treatment	• Lifestyle Modifications: **diet modification** (low-carbohydrate), **exercise** (walking), **glucose monitoring** (daily fasting and postprandial glucose measure) • Women with confirmed gestational diabetes diagnosis should be referred to dietician and appropriate support services • Medical Management: indicated when adequate glucose levels (fasting glucose >95mg/dL and postprandial glucose >130-140mg/dL) are unachievable with diet and exercise • **Insulin: first-line medical therapy** (does not cross placenta); goal is fasting glucose <95mg/dL • Oral Hypoglycemic Agents: **metformin or glyburide** are relatively safe if patient is noncompliant or refuses insulin therapy • Labor Induction: occurs at 38-39 weeks in uncontrolled diabetes or evidence of macrosomia; if macrosomia present Cesarean delivery often indicated • *After delivery of placenta, most cases of gestational diabetes resolve* • Antenatal blood glucose monitoring for mother and newborn; newborn can get hypoglycemia during postpartum period

	Mechanism of Action	HbA1c Reduction	Side Effects	Contraindications	Contraindicated in Renal Disease?	Contraindicated in Liver Disease?
Biguanides **Metformin**	↑ peripheral glucose uptake ↓hepatic gluconeogenesis	~↓1.5%	• GI Upset (N/V, Diarrhea) • Lactic Acidosis • ↓B12 (↓ gut absorption) • Weight loss	• Severe renal or hepatic disease, heart failure, alcohol abuse • Iodinated contrast	Yes (↓GFR=↑risk of lactic acidosis)	Yes (hepatotoxic)
Sulfonylureas (Glipizide, Glyburide)	Binds and inhibits ATP-sensitive K⁺ channels in pancreatic beta cells (↑ insulin release)	~↓1.5%	• Hypoglycemic reactions • Weight gain • Disulfiram-like reaction with alcohol	• Type 1 diabetes • Pregnancy or lactation • Renal/hepatic disease • Sulfa allergy	Yes (↓renal excretion = ↑ risk of toxicity)	Yes (↓hepatic metabolism = ↑ risk of toxicity)
Meglitinides (Repaglinide, Nateglinide)	Binds and inhibits ATP-sensitive K⁺ channels in pancreatic beta cells (↑ insulin release)	~↓1.5%	• Hypoglycemic reactions • Weight gain	• Type 1 diabetes • DKA	No (adjust dose only)	No (adjust dose only)
Thiazolidinediones (Pioglitazone, Rosiglitazone)	↑insulin sensitivity at peripheral receptor sites (adipose, muscle, liver cells) ↑glucose utilization and ↓glucose production	~↓1%	• Fluid retention • Weight gain • ↑risk of bladder cancer with pioglitazone	• Heart failure, • History of bladder cancer • Active hepatic disease	No (adjust dose only)	Yes (↓hepatic metabolism = ↑ risk of toxicity)
Sodium Glucose Transport Protein 2 (SGLT-2) Inhibitors (Canagliflozin, Dapagliflozin)	Blocks sodium-glucose cotransport at the proximal convoluted tubule ↓ glucose reabsorption	~↓0.5-1%	• ↑risk of UTIs and candida infections • Hypotension • ↓bone mineral density	• Frequent UTIs or vaginal candidiasis • Osteopenia/porosis • Foot ulcerations • Type 1 diabetes	Yes (diuresis may ↓GFR leading to AKI)	No
Glucagon-Like Peptide 1 (GLP-1) Agonists (Liraglutide, Semaglutide)	↑ glucose-dependent insulin secretion ↓ gastric emptying ↓ glucagon secretion	~↓1-1.5%	• GI Upset (N/V, Diarrhea) • Weight loss • Pancreatitis	• GFR<30 • History of pancreatitis or gastroparesis	Yes	No
Dipeptidyl Peptidase-4 Inhibitors (DPP4) (Sitagliptin, Saxagliiptin)	↑ GLP-1 which ↑ insulin release, ↓hepatic gluconeogenesis and ↑peripheral uptake of glucose	~↓0.5-1%	• Nasopharyngitis • ↑risk of URIs • Pancreatitis	• Active hepatic disease • History of pancreatitis	No (adjust dose only)	Yes
Alpha-Glucosidase Inhibitors (Acarbose, Miglitol)	↓intestinal glucose absorption by inhibiting pancreatic α-amylase and intestinal α-glucosidase hydrolase	~↓0.5-1%	• Malabsorption-related symptoms (flatulence, diarrhea, abdominal pain) • ↑LFTs	• GFR<30 • Relative: history of gastroparesis, IBD	Yes	No

Human Insulin Preparations

Type of Insulin	Onset	Peak	Duration	Insulin Coverage
Rapid-Acting **Lispro** (Humalog) **Aspart** (Novolog) Glulisine	5-15 minutes	45-75 minutes	3-5 hours	• Rapidly absorbed due to amino acid pair reversal to prevent insulin association to dimers and polymers • Most effective at mealtimes to control postprandial glucose spikes • Often used with intermediate or long-acting insulin
Short-Acting Regular	30-60 minutes	2-4 hours	6-8 hours	• Given 30-60 minutes prior to mealtimes • Often used with intermediate or long-acting insulin
Intermediate-Acting **Insulin Isophane (NPH)** **U500 Regular**	2 hours 30 minutes	4-12 hours 4-8 hours	18-26 hours 13-24 hours	• Can cover overnight or about a half of a day • Often used with rapid or short-acting insulin
Long-Acting **Glargine** **U300 Regular** **Detemir** **Degludec**	3-4 hours 6 hours 1-2 hours 1-2 hours	No peak No peak No peak No peak	24 hours 24 hours 14-24 hours >40 hours	• Basal insulin covers for 1 full day • Less hypoglycemic episodes • Often used with rapid or short-acting insulin • Requires 3 days to achieve steady state
Premixed **70% Insulin Isophane (NPH)/30% Regular** 50% Insulin Isophane (NPH)/50% Regular 50% Lispro Protamine/50% Lispro 75% Lispro Protamine/25% Lispro 70% Aspart Protamine/30% Aspart	**30-60 minutes** 30-60 minutes 30-60 minutes 5-15 minutes 5-15 minutes	**Dual (NPH and regular)** 2-12 hours Dual (Lispro protamine and Lispro) Dual (Lispro protamine and Lispro) Dual (Aspart Protamine and Aspart)	**10-16 hours** 10-16 hours 10-16 hours 10-16 hours 10-16 hours	• Often given twice per day at mealtimes

Diagnostic Criteria

Test	Normal	Impaired Glucose Regulation	Diabetes
Fasting Plasma Glucose	<100 mg/dL	100-125 mg/dL	≥126 mg/dL
Oral Glucose Tolerance Test	<140 mg/dL	140-199 mg/dL	≥200 mg/dL
Hemoglobin A1c (HbA1c)	<5.7%	5.8-6.4%	≥6.5%
Random Glucose	<200 mg/dL	-----	≥200 mg/dL

Somogyi Phenomenon

Definition	• Nocturnal hypoglycemia followed by rebound hyperglycemia
Patho-physiology	• Rebound hyperglycemia as a result of counterregulatory growth hormone surge after early morning hypoglycemia
Signs & Symptoms	• Nocturnal hypoglycemic symptoms (nervousness, tachycardia, headache, lightheadedness, dizziness, diaphoresis) **when waking in middle of night** • Rebound symptoms (tachycardia, hypertension)
Diagnosis	• Continuous glucose monitoring device • Frequent blood glucose readings (8-10 times daily)
Treatment	• Preventing hypoglycemia (decrease **nighttime NPH dose** or move NPH does earlier; **high protein snack with a small amount of carbohydrates at night**)

Dawn Phenomenon

Definition	• Periodic hyperglycemia experienced during the morning hours (2am-8am)
Patho-physiology	• Decreased insulin sensitivity and nocturnal rise of counterregulatory cortisol, growth hormones and catecholamines (insulin-antagonists) during the nighttime fast leading to an overall increase in circulating serum glucose
Signs & Symptoms	• Persistent and worsening early morning hyperglycemia
Diagnosis	• Continuous glucose monitoring device • Frequent blood glucose readings (8-10 times daily)
Treatment	• Preventing early morning hyperglycemia (nighttime NPH injection before bed [curbs morning hyperglycemia] or **increase nighttime NPH dose, avoid carbohydrate snack at night**, exercise in evening, increase protein to carbohydrate ratio of evening meal, consume breakfast)

Hypoglycemia

Etiology & Risk Factors	• Low plasma glucose level as a result of sympathetic nervous system stimulation or central nervous system dysfunction • **Defined as a glucose level of ≤70 mg/dL** • <u>Etiology</u>: **complication of diabetes mellitus with oral antihyperglycemic agents (especially sulfonylureas) and insulin, fasting state (too little food), excessive exercise,** alcohol use, adrenal insufficiency, malnutrition, starvation, sepsis, cirrhosis, end-stage renal disease, insulinoma • <u>Risk Factors</u>: poor nutrition, advanced organ failure (especially liver, kidney, or heart failure)
Patho-physiology	• Plasma glucose levels decline causing beta-cell secretion of insulin to also decline leading to a state of increased hepatic and renal gluconeogenesis and hepatic glycogenolysis • As glycogen stores are depleted, glycogenolysis is unable to maintain serum glucose levels; surge in autonomic activity in response to hypoglycemia produces symptoms

Signs & Symptoms	• <u>Neuroglycopenic</u>:
	   • **Altered mental status, lethargy, confusion**
	   • Focal neurological deficits, visual disturbances
	   • Seizure, unresponsiveness
	• <u>Autonomic</u>: *glucose level of ≤55 mg/dL may produce catecholamine surge*
	   • **Anxiety, nervousness**, irritability
	   • Nausea, vomiting
	   • **Palpitations, tremors**, salivation
	   • **Tachycardia** or bradycardia
	   • **Cool, clammy skin; pallor**

Diagnosis	• <u>Blood Glucose Measurement</u>: point-of-care glucose testing
	   • **Glucose level of ≤70 mg/dL**
	   • *Signs and symptoms may not occur until glucose level drops below 55 mg/dL*
	• <u>Whipple's Triad</u>
	   • Symptoms of hypoglycemia + low glucose level (<60mg/dL) at time of symptoms + resolution of symptoms after administration of glucose

Treatment	• <u>Oral Glucose</u>: **first-line; indicated if alert, mild-moderate symptoms, and able to tolerate PO intake**
	   • 15g of fast-acting carbohydrate, fruit juice, hard candy, chewable glucose tablet
	   • <u>Rule of 15's</u>: 15g of glucose/sucrose ingested, recheck glucose 15 minutes later, ingest another 15g of glucose/sucrose if blood glucose not >80mg/dL
	• <u>IV Dextrose or SC/IM Glucagon</u>: **indicated if severe, unconscious, or unable to tolerate PO intake**
	   • IV bolus of D50; subcutaneous or intramuscular glucagon (efficacy of glucagon depends on the size of hepatic glycogen stores; not effective in fasting state)

Key Words & Most Common	• Most common as result of oral antihyperglycemic agents (sulfonylureas) and insulin • AMS, lethargy, confusion, anxiety, nervousness, palpitations, tremors, tachycardia, cool/clammy skin, pallor • Glucose ≤70 mg/dL; symptoms may not be apparent until <55mg/dL • Oral glucose → IV dextrose or SC/IM Glucagon

Diabetic Ketoacidosis (DKA)

Etiology & Risk Factors	• **Acute metabolic complication of diabetes characterized by uncontrolled hyperglycemia, hyperketonemia, and metabolic acidosis; more common in type I diabetes mellitus** • <u>Etiology</u>: **consequence of insulin deficiency and excess counterregulatory hormones** (glucagon, catecholamines, cortisol) • <u>Risk Factors</u>: **uncontrolled or undiagnosed diabetes (especially type 1 diabetes mellitus) or discontinuation/inadequate insulin therapy** • <u>Precipitating Factors</u>: **infection (pneumonia and UTI) is most common**, alcohol abuse, trauma, pulmonary embolism, discontinuation/inadequate insulin therapy, myocardial infarction, **medications (corticosteroids, thiazide diuretics)**, pregnancy, pancreatitis, stroke
Patho-physiology	• <u>Hyperglycemia</u>: Insulin deficiency and excess counterregulatory hormones (glucagon, catecholamines, cortisol) causes increased metabolization of triglycerides and amino acids for energy instead of glucose; hyperglycemia and insulin deficiency leads to osmotic diuresis and depletion of serum electrolytes (sodium, potassium, magnesium, calcium, phosphorus); severe hypokalemia develops due to an extracellular shift of potassium due to metabolic acidosis • <u>Acidosis</u>: insulin deficiency causes lipolysis and accumulation of ketoacids; breakdown of adipose creates first acetoacetate leading to conversion to beta-hydroxybutyrate • <u>Dehydration</u>: dehydration in combination with osmotic diuresis activates RAAS results in further sodium and potassium loss and worsens metabolic acidosis

Signs & Symptoms	• *May be the initial presentation of an undiagnosed T1DM patient*
	• **Symptomatic hyperglycemia is the most common initial presentation**
	   • **Polydipsia (excessive thirst)** and **urinary frequency leading to polyuria** (large quantities of urine production) leading to decreased urine output (volume depleted)
	   • Dehydration leads to orthostatic hypotension, fatigue, weakness, and **mental status changes**
	• **Nausea, vomiting, abdominal pain**
	• Lethargy, somnolence and altered mental status are advanced symptoms
		• <u>Physical Exam</u>:
		   • **Tachycardia, tachypnea**, decreased skin turgor, fruity breath due to exhaled acetone
		   • **Kussmaul respirations (deep, rapid, laborious breaths)**

Diagnosis	• <u>Diagnostic Criteria</u>: **hyperglycemia (glucose >250mg/dL), decreased arterial pH (<7.3), decreased serum bicarbonate (<15mEq/L), and ketones present in urine and serum**
	   • <u>Capillary Blood Glucose</u>: >250mg/dL (blood glucose may be normal or lsightly elevated if impaired gluconeogenesis (liver failure, alcoholism) or SGLT-2 Inhibitor use)
	   • <u>Serum Ketones</u>: beta-hydroxybutyrate elevated
	   • <u>Serum Potassium</u>: **usually elevated initially** (intracellular to extracellular potassium shift due to acidosis and insulin deficiency); may become hypokalemic with insulin
	   • <u>Urinalysis</u>: **ketonuria**; evaluate for UTI as potential precipitating factor
	• *Consider ECG to detect ischemic changes or signs of hypokalemia (low T waves) or hyperkalemia (peaked T waves); CXR to rule out pneumonia as precipitating factor*

Treatment	• <u>Volume Repletion</u>: **critical initial step; volume status should be restored rapidly to raise blood pressure and ensure glomerular perfusion**
	   • **Rapid IV infusion of 0.9% normal saline solution** in the first hour, followed by saline infusions at 250 to 500 mL/hour
	   • 0.45% saline after hypotension and orthostasis resolves if serum sodium level is normal or high
	• <u>Hyperglycemia Correction</u>: **regular insulin infusion** (0.1 unit/kg IV bolus followed by continuous IV infusion of 0.1 unit/kg/hour in 0.9% saline solution)
	   • When plasma glucose <250mg/dL, 5% dextrose can be added to saline infusion (prevents hypoglycemia from insulin therapy)
	• <u>Hypokalemia Prevention</u>: **correction of DKA causes hypokalemia** (insulin shifts potassium intracellularly, causing a decline in serum potassium)
	   • **Goal to maintain a K+ level of 4 to 5 mEq/L**
	   • Potassium replacement held if K+>5.3; 20-30mEq KCl added to each liter of IV fluid if K+ 3.3-5.3; insulin held and KCl given at 40 mEq/hour if K+<3.3

Hyperosmolar Hyperglycemic State (HHS)

Etiology & Risk Factors	• Acute metabolic complication of diabetes mellitus characterized by severe hyperglycemia, dehydration, hyperosmolar plasma and altered consciousness • <u>Etiology</u>: **consequence of insulin deficiency and excess counterregulatory hormones** (glucagon, catecholamines, cortisol) • <u>Risk Factors</u>: **uncontrolled or undiagnosed diabetes (more common with type 2 diabetes mellitus), elderly, obesity**, overconsumption of carbohydrate rich diet/beverages • <u>Precipitating Factors</u>: **infection (respiratory, GI, GU) is most common (50-60% of cases)**, diabetes medication non-adherence, **medications (corticosteroids, beta blockers, diuretics)**, cocaine intoxication, acute coronary syndrome, pancreatitis, stroke
Patho-physiology	• Insulin deficiency leads to hyperglycemia and release of counterregulatory hormones (glucagon, growth hormone, cortisol, catecholamine) which stimulate gluconeogenesis and glycogenolysis; hyperglycemia significantly increases the serum osmolarity causing an osmotic gradient leading to free water, glucose and electrolyte excretion in the urine causing glycosuria and and moderate to severe dehydration • *Not usually associated with severe ketosis or metabolic acidosis as insulin is still produced by the beta cells in the pancreas*
Signs & Symptoms	• **Profound dehydration (hypotension, tachycardia, polydipsia [excessive thirst], dizziness, weakness) is predominant symptom** • **Altered mental status**, confusion, disorientation • Lethargy, seizure, **coma** • <u>Physical Exam</u>: • **Ill-appearing, tachycardia, hypotension**, sunken eyes, decreased skin turgor, **dry mucous membranes, increased capillary refill time**

Diagnosis	• <u>Diagnostic Criteria</u>: **glucose >600mg/dL, serum osmolality >320mOsm/kg, serum bicarbonate >15mEq/L, pH>7.3, serum ketones negative or mildly positive,**
	    • <u>Blood Glucose Level</u>: **marked increase compared to DKA (>600mg/dL)**
	    • <u>Serum Osmolality</u>: **marked elevation (320 to 400mOsm/kg are common)**
	• <u>Comprehensive Metabolic Panel (CMP)</u>: potassium often normal or elevated, hyponatremia (dilutional), marked elevation of BUN and serum creatinine levels
	• *Consider lactate, serum ketones, CBC, UA, lipase, troponin, CXR, ECG*

Treatment	• <u>Volume Repletion</u>: **critical initial step; volume status should be restored rapidly to raise blood pressure and ensure glomerular perfusion**
	    • **Rapid IV infusion of 0.9% normal saline solution** in the first hour, followed by saline infusions at 250 to 500 mL/hour
	    • 0.45% saline after hypotension and orthostasis resolves if serum sodium level is normal or high
	• <u>Hyperglycemia Correction</u>: **regular insulin infusion** (0.1 unit/kg IV bolus followed by continuous IV infusion of 0.1 unit/kg/hour in 0.9% saline solution)
	    • When plasma glucose <250mg/dL, 5% dextrose can be added to saline infusion (prevents hypoglycemia from insulin therapy)
	• <u>Hypokalemia Prevention</u>: **correction of HHS causes hypokalemia** (insulin shifts potassium intracellularly, causing a decline in serum potassium)
	    • **Goal to maintain a K⁺ level of 4 to 5 mEq/L**
	    • Potassium replacement held if K⁺>5.3; 20-30mEq KCl added to each liter of IV fluid if K⁺ 3.3-5.3; insulin held and KCl given at 40 mEq/hour if K⁺<3.3

Key Words & Most Common	• Prototypical patient is elderly with uncontrolled type II diabetes and inadequate access to water; precipitated by infection • Profound dehydration (hypotension, tachycardia, excessive thirst, dizziness) → altered mental status • <u>Diagnostic Criteria</u>: glucose >600mg/dL, serum osmolality >320mOsm/kg, serum bicarbonate >15mEq/L, pH>7.3, serum ketones negative or mildly positive, • Volume repletion (normal saline [0.9%] vs half-normal saline [0.45%]) → D5 + regular insulin infusion → potassium correction

Diabetic Neuropathy

Etiology & Risk Factors	• Broad range of peripheral nervous system dysfunction as a result of diabetes mellitus • <u>Etiology</u>: **diabetes mellitus is most common cause of peripheral neuropathy** • <u>Risk Factors</u>: **poor glycemic control**, advanced age, alcohol use, hypertension, peripheral vascular disease, smoking, dyslipidemia, long duration of diabetes
Patho-physiology	• Exact cause is not well understood; metabolic, neurovascular, and autoimmune pathways have been theorized • Peripheral nervous degradation as a result of oxidative stress

Signs & Symptoms	• <u>Symmetric Polyneuropathy</u>: **most common type of neuropathy**
	    • **Progressive, distal sensory loss occurring in a "stocking-glove" pattern (distal lower extremities and hands)**
	    • Loss of proprioception, light touch, vibratory and temperature sensation; **loss of vibratory sensation is usually first deficit**
	    • Blunted perception of foot trauma from ill-fitting shoes and abnormal weight bearing causes **foot ulceration, infection, fracture**, gait abnormalities, motor dysfunction
	• <u>Autonomic Neuropathy</u>: very common complication affecting the gastrointestinal, cardiovascular, and genitourinary systems
	    • **Orthostatic (postural) hypotension, exercise intolerance, abdominal discomfort, resting tachycardia, nausea, constipation/diarrhea, fecal incontinence**, urinary retention or incontinence, erectile dysfunction, retrograde ejaculation, and decreased vaginal lubrication
	• <u>Radiculopathies</u>: most commonly affect the proximal lumbar (L2-L4) region causing pain, weakness, and lower extremity muscle atrophy; can affect proximal thoracic (T4-T12)
	• <u>Cranial Neuropathy</u>: **most commonly affect CNIII (oculomotor) causing diplopia, ptosis, and anisocoria** (unequal pupil sizes); extraocular muscle palsy with CNIV and CNVI
	• <u>Peripheral Mononeuropathy</u>: **median neuropathy is most common (carpal tunnel syndrome)**; peroneal neuropathy (foot drop)
	• <u>Physical Exam</u>:
	    • Decreased muscle strength, diminished reflexes and sensation (decreased sensation with light touch with a monofilament, vibratory sensation, and proprioception)
	    • Dry/cracked skin suggests autonomic neuropathy; pedal deformities (hammertoes) suggest motor neuropathy

Diagnosis	• **Clinical Diagnosis** • <u>Labs</u>: serum glucose, hemoglobin A1c, complete blood count, erythrocyte sedimentation rate and vitamin B1, B6, and B12 level to rule out other causes of neuropathy • <u>Electromyography and Nerve Conduction Studies</u>: rule out other causes of neuropathy

Treatment	• <u>Glycemic Control</u>: **optimal management of diabetes reduces paresthesia and dysesthesia**
	• <u>Pain Control</u>: indicated when symptoms disrupt sleep or activities of daily living
	    • Antiseizure medication (**pregabalin, gabapentin**), tricyclic antidepressants (**amitriptyline**), or SNRIs (**duloxetine**) can help control symptoms
	    • Topical capsaicin cream, lidocaine patches, alpha-lipoic acid, zinc supplementation are second-line therapies
	• <u>Foot Care</u>: regular, daily self-examination to detect foot trauma or injuries to prevent infection; proper fitting shoe wear

Key Words & Most Common	• Peripheral nervous system dysfunction secondary to diabetes mellitus • Symmetric polyneuropathy is most common; progressive distal sensory loss of lower extremities and hands ("stocking-glove") distribution • Autonomic neuropathy: orthostatic hypotension, exercise intolerance, tachycardia, N/V/C/D • Cranial Neuropathy affecting CNIII causes diplopia, ptosis • Glycemic control + pain control (pregabalin, gabapentin, amitriptyline, duloxetine) + regular foot care

Diabetic Gastroparesis

Etiology & Risk Factors	• Delayed gastric emptying and decreased GI motility without evidence of mechanical obstruction due to dysfunction of autonomic nervous system to sense bowel wall stretch • <u>Etiology</u>: **gastric motor dysfunction and enteric neuropathy** in the setting of long-standing and/or uncontrolled diabetes mellitus • <u>Risk Factors</u>: **poor glycemic control**, advanced age, alcohol use, hypertension, peripheral vascular disease, smoking, dyslipidemia, long duration of diabetes
Patho-physiology	• Chronic hyperglycemia leads to neuronal damage resulting in abnormal myenteric neurotransmission, impaired inhibitory neuronal function, and smooth muscle and pacemaker cell dysfunction causing impaired gastric motor function (autonomic nervous system unable to sense bowel wall stretch to stimulate gastric motility)
Signs & Symptoms	• **Nausea is most common symptom** • Vomiting, **early satiety, post-prandial fullness and bloating** • Upper abdominal discomfort • **Constipation** • <u>Physical Exam</u>: • **Nonspecific**; may have general epigastric distention/tenderness, neuropathy, halitosis (bad breath)
Diagnosis	• <u>Upper Endoscopy</u>: initial test to rule out etiologies (mechanical obstruction, peptic ulcer disease); retained food may be seen with gastroparesis • <u>Nuclear Gastric Emptying Scintigraphy</u>: **gold-standard; shows delayed gastric emptying** without mechanical obstruction

Treatment	• <u>Lifestyle Modifications</u>: **first-line**
	   • <u>Glycemic Control</u>: **optimal management of diabetes reduces the effects of hyperglycemia that cause delayed gastric emptying**
	   • <u>Dietary Modifications</u>: small, frequent meals that are low in fat and carbohydrates and prioritize protein
	   • Alcohol and smoking cessation
	• <u>Antiemetics</u>: initial medical management for symptoms
	   • **Ondansetron**: serotonin (5-HT3) receptor antagonists to reduce nausea as needed
	• <u>Prokinetics</u>: **cornerstone of medical therapy to increase GI motility**
	   • **Metoclopramide**: 5-HT4 receptor activator and dopamine receptor antagonist weak 5-HT3 receptor antagonism promotes GI motility
	   • **Erythromycin**: binds to the motilin receptors responsible for initiating the migrating motor complex at the proximal GI tract
	   • **Domperidone**: dopamine (D2) agonist that does not cross blood-brain-barrier (less extrapyramidal side effects)
	• <u>Surgery</u>: partial gastrectomy with Roux-en-Y gastrojejunostomy and gastric resection is last-resort

Key Words & Most Common	• Enteric neuropathy causes delayed gastric emptying and decreased GI motility • Nausea is most common symptom; early satiety, fullness/bloating, constipation • Upper Endoscopy → nuclear gastric emptying scintigraphy • Glycemic control + dietary modifications • Ondansetron for symptomatic relief • Prokinetics (metoclopramide, erythromycin, domperidone)

Diabetic Nephropathy

Etiology & Risk Factors	• **Renal microvascular complication of diabetes mellitus characterized by persistent albuminuria and progressive decline in glomerular filtration rate** • **Most common cause of end-stage renal disease; 30-40% of patients with diabetes mellitus will develop nephropathy** • Etiology: insulin resistance, genetics, hyperglycemia and autoimmune processes may be related in setting of diabetes mellitus • <u>Risk Factors</u>: **poor glycemic control**, advanced age, alcohol use, **hypertension**, peripheral vascular disease, **smoking, dyslipidemia**, long duration of diabetes
Patho-physiology	• Hyperglycemia leads to the production of reactive oxygen species and activation of multiple inflammatory pathways eventually causing inflammation fibrosis and increased vascular permeability; thickening of glomerular basement membrane and glomerular sclerosis leads to microalbuminuria
Signs & Symptoms	• **Often asymptomatic** • Persistent hypertension • <u>Nephropathy</u>: **fatigue, foamy urine and pedal edema**

Diagnosis	• <u>Diagnostic Criteria</u>: **hypertension, progressive decline in glomerular filtration rate (GFR), persistent albuminuria (>300mg/day) on at least 2 visits, 3-6 months apart**
	• <u>Urine Dipstick</u>: positive proteinuria; *typically a urine dipstick is only positive when protein excretion exceeds 300 to 500 mg/day*
	• <u>24-Hour Urine Collection</u>: **total urinary albumin excretion over 24 hour period**
	   • **Moderate Albuminuria**: excretion of 30 to 300 mg/day; early nephropathy
	   • **Severe Albuminuria**: excretion of >300mg/day; advanced nephropathy
	• <u>Glomerular Filtration Rate (GFR)</u>: monitor progression of disease
	• <u>Renal Biopsy</u>: **definitive diagnosis; Kimmelstiel-Wilson nodules are pathognomonic (nodules of pink hyaline material** in the glomerular capillary loops due to protein leakage), glomerular basement membrane thickening, and glomerular sclerosis, inflammation

Treatment	• <u>Lifestyle Modifications</u>:
	   • <u>Glycemic Control</u>: **optimal management of diabetes to reduce progression**
	   • <u>Dietary Modifications</u>: low-sodium, low-fat, low-carbohydrate diet
	• <u>Angiotensin-Converting Enzyme (ACE) Inhibitor or Angiotensin II Receptor Blocker (ARB)</u>: **indicated at the earliest sign of albuminuria**
	   • **Prevents progression of renal disease by dilating efferent arteriole to lower intraglomerular blood pressure and reduce protein leakage**
	• <u>Renal Replacement</u>: indicated with end-stage renal disease (GFR of 10-15 ml/min); peritoneal or hemodialysis, renal transplant

Key Words & Most Common	• Most common cause of end-stage renal disease characterized by persistent albuminuria and progressive decline in GFR • Often asymptomatic → fatigue, foamy urine, pedal edema • GFR + urine dipstick + 24-hour urine collection for diagnosis • Renal biopsy is definitive; Kimmelstiel-Wilson nodules are pathognomonic • Glycemic control + ACEI/ARB

Diabetic Retinopathy

Etiology & Risk Factors	• Microvascular condition occurring secondary to long-term effects of diabetes mellitus • **Most common cause of new, severe vision loss in working-age adults** • <u>Etiology</u>: **diabetes mellitus** • <u>Risk Factors</u>: **advanced age, poor-glycemic control, hypertension**, obesity, vitamin D deficiency, dyslipidemia
Patho-physiology	• Chronic hyperglycemia and oxidative stress leads cellular and tissue damage • <u>Nonproliferative</u>: increased capillary permeability, microaneurysms, hemorrhage, ischemia and edema leads to retinal thickening secondary to fluid leakage • <u>Proliferative</u>: abnormal neovascularization (new vessel formation) of retina and vitreous cavity leads to vitreous hemorrhage and/or traction retinal detachment
Signs & Symptoms	• **Blurred vision, floaters** (black spots), or **flashing lights** (photopsia) • **Partial or total vision loss (painless)**

Nonproliferative Fundoscopy	Proliferative Fundoscopy

Diagnosis
• **Capillary microaneurysms**
• **Blot and Dot Retinal Hemorrhages**: deep retinal layer hemorrhage
• **Flame-Shaped Hemorrhages**: nerve fiber layer hemorrhage
• **Cotton Wool Spots**: microinfarction of retinal nerve layer
  • **Fuzzy-edged, gray/white spots** that obscure underlying layer
• **Hard Exudates**: suggestive of chronic edema; lipid and lipoprotein deposits
  • **Discrete, yellow spots with sharp margins**
	• **Neovascularization: new, abnormal blood vessel formation**
	  • Visible on optic nerve or retinal surface
	• Vitreous Hemorrhage or tractional retinal detachment
	• Macular edema

Treatment
• **Strict control of blood glucose**
• Focal laser photocoagulation
	• **Strict control of blood glucose and blood pressure**
	• **Intravitreal injection of antivascular endothelial growth factor (anti-VEGF) drugs**
	  • Bevacizumab, ranibizumab, aflibercept
	  • Decreases new vessel formation
	• Focal laser photocoagulation

Key Words & Most Common	• Vision loss secondary to poorly controlled diabetes • Blurred vision, floaters, flashing lights; partial/full vision loss (painless) • Nonproliferative: cotton wool spots, hard exudates, flame-shaped hemorrhage, blot and dot hemorrhage, capillary microaneurysms • Proliferative: neovascularization • Strict blood glucose control → laser photocoagulation; Injected anti-VEGF for proliferative

Syndrome of Inappropriate ADH Secretion (SIADH)

Etiology & Risk Factors	• Inappropriate or continued release of antidiuretic hormone (ADH) from the pituitary gland or ectopic sources
	• <u>Etiology</u>: most commonly occurs secondary to another process
	  • **CNS**: most common etiology; enhanced ADH-release from the pituitary gland due to **hemorrhage (subarachnoid)**, stroke, trauma, tumor, meningitis, hydrocephalus
	  • **Pulmonary**: **small cell lung cancer (SCLC) is the most common tumor that causes ectopic ADH production**, infectious pneumonia (viral, bacterial, tuberculous),
	  • <u>Medications</u>: enhance release/effect of ADH; **carbamazepine, oxcarbazepine, chlorpropamide, cyclophosphamide, and selective serotonin reuptake inhibitors (SSRI)**
	    • **"Ecstasy" (methylenedioxymethamphetamine [MDMA]) is a drug of abuse that is particularly associated with direct release of ADH**
	  • <u>Other</u>: hormone deficiency, hormone administration, hypothyroidism, Human Immunodeficiency Virus (HIV) infection, hereditary SIADH

Patho-physiology	• Inappropriate or continued release of antidiuretic hormone (ADH) from the pituitary gland or ectopic sources (despite normal/increased plasma volume) leads to impaired water excretion (free water retention), hyponatremia and hypo-osmolality as kidneys are unable to dilute the urine and excrete excess water

Signs & Symptoms	• <u>**Hyponatremia Symptoms:**</u>
	  • <u>Mild Hyponatremia</u>: **nausea (without vomiting), malaise, muscle cramping**, difficulty concentrating, cognitive deficits
	  • <u>Moderate Hyponatremia</u>: gait disturbances, falls, **confusion, lethargy**, headache
	  • <u>Severe Hyponatremia</u>: **vomiting (ominous sign)**, cardiopulmonary distress, **somnolence, seizures, coma**
	• <u>Physical Exam</u>: usually no signs of edema

Diagnosis	• <u>**Diagnostic Criteria:**</u>
	  • <u>Serum Osmolality and Serum Sodium</u>: show normovolemic hypotonic hyponatremia (<135mEq/L) with decreased serum osmolality (<275mOsm/kg)
	  • <u>Urine Sodium Concentration and Osmolality</u>: increased urine sodium (>30mEq/L) and increased urine osmolality (>100mOsm/kg); increased specific gravity (>1.015)
	  • <u>Clinical Euvolemia</u>: normal skin turgor, blood pressure within reference range
	  • <u>Absence of Other Causes of Hyponatremia</u>: adrenal insufficiency, hypothyroidism, heart failure, pituitary insufficiency, renal or hepatic disease, drugs that impair renal water excretion
	  • <u>Other</u>: BUN/creatinine values usually normal, serum uric acid is generally low
	• <u>**CXR/CT**</u>: **indicated to evaluate for small cell lung cancer (SCLC)** in patients with long-standing smoking history, weight loss, or pulmonary symptoms
	• *Must rule out hypothyroidism and adrenal insufficiency*

Treatment	• **Treat underlying etiology**
	• <u>Water Restriction</u>: **mainstay of the treatment; goal of <800 mL/day**
	• <u>Sodium Replacement</u>:
	  • **Oral Salt Tablets (NaCl)**: indicated for mild-moderate hyponatremia
	  • **IV Saline + Loop Diuretic (Furosemide)**: loop diuretics inhibit sodium chloride (NaCl) reabsorption in the ascending Loop of Henle resulting in increased urinary sodium and water excretion
	  • **Hypertonic Saline**: reserved for patients with severe hyponatremia and must be used cautiously as **rapid correction risks osmotic demyelination syndrome**
	• <u>Selective Vasopressin Receptor Antagonist</u>: **conivaptan, tolvaptan**; causes water diuresis without significant urinary electrolyte loss
	• <u>Demeclocycline</u>: inhibits ADH-induced water reabsorption in the distal portion of the convoluted tubules; rarely used due to risk of causing acute kidney injury

Diabetes Insipidus

Etiology & Risk Factors	• **Condition that causes deficiency or decreased response to antidiuretic hormone (ADH, also known as vasopressin) leading to inability of kidneys to concentrate urine**
	  <u>Etiology</u>: central or nephrogenic etiologies
	    • <u>Central</u>: most common type; deficient production of ADH; idiopathic is most common cause, autoimmune inflammation of posterior pituitary, trauma, CNS tumor
	    • <u>Nephrogenic</u>: normal ADH secretion but decreased renal sensitivity to ADH; hereditary is most common cause; lithium toxicity, hypokalemia, hypercalcemia

Patho-physiology	• Vasopressin acts to promote water conservation by the kidneys by increasing the distal tubular epithelium permeability to water • **Inadequate or impaired vasopressin secretion or decreased renal sensitivity to ADH causes kidneys to be unable to concentrate urine leading to large production of diluted urine ultimately causing electrolyte imbalances**

Signs & Symptoms	• **Polyuria (large amounts of urine production [3 to 20 L/day]) is hallmark**
	• **Polydipsia** (excessive thirst)
	• **High-volume nocturia** (large amounts of nighttime urine production)
	• **Dehydration may lead to neurologic symptoms of hypernatremia** (confusion, lethargy, neuromuscular excitability, seizures, coma); water intake is less than urinary water loss
	    • *Most common in children or elderly patients with dementia that cannot communicate thirst*
	• <u>Physical Exam</u>:
	    • Signs of dehydration: **tachycardia, hypotension,** sunken eyes, **decreased skin turgor, dry mucous membranes, increased capillary refill time**

Diagnosis	• <u>24-Hour Urine Collection</u>: initial test performed; performed without fluid restriction to test for volume and osmolality
	    • **Decreased urine osmolality (<300mOsm/Kg), decreased urine specific gravity (<1.010)** increased urine volume (>2.5L in adult)
	• <u>Water Deprivation Test</u>: establishes diagnosis; urine volume and osmolality are measured hourly; serum osmolality is measured every 2 hours
	    • <u>Normal Response</u>: progressive urine concentration
	    • <u>Diabetes Insipidus Response</u>: continued production of large amounts of dilute urine (low urine osmolality)
	• <u>Exogenous Vasopressin Stimulation Test</u>: distinguishes central from nephrogenic diabetes insipidus
	    • <u>Central</u>: reduction in urine output + increase in urine osmolality in response to vasopressin (response is indicated by urine osm >800mOsm/L)
	    • <u>Nephrogenic</u>: continued production of large amounts of dilute urine with minimal rise in urine osmolality; no response to exogenous vasopressin

Treatment	• <u>Lifestyle Modifications</u>: **adequate free-water intake, low-solute diet (low salt, low protein)** • <u>Central</u>: **desmopressin is first-line**; desmopressin is a synthetic analog of vasopressin with minimal vasoconstrictive properties • <u>Vasopressin-Releasing Medications</u>: carbamazepine, chlorpropamide are second line • <u>Nephrogenic</u>: correct underlying cause; discontinue the offending agent (lithium) • <u>Thiazide Diuretics</u>: **hydrochlorothiazide**; paradoxically reduce urine output by reducing extracellular fluid volume and increasing proximal tubular resorption • <u>Prostaglandin Inhibitors</u>: **indomethacin**; reduce urine volume by decreasing renal blood flow and glomerular filtration rate (GFR) • <u>Amiloride</u>: indicated for **lithium-induced DI**; inhibits lithium entry through the sodium channel

	Diabetes Insipidus	**SIADH**
Etiology & Risk Factors	• <u>Central</u>: **idiopathic**, autoimmune inflammation of pituitary, trauma, CNS tumor • <u>Nephrogenic</u>: **hereditary**, lithium toxicity, hypokalemia, hypercalcemia, genetic	• Head trauma, CNS tumors, ectopic tumor production (small cell lung cancer), medications, MDMA

Patho-physiology	• **Inadequate ADH**
	    • Central: lack of ADH
	    • Nephrogenic: insensitivity to ADH
		• Excess ADH
		    • Secretion high despite low urine osmolality

Signs & Symptoms	• **Dehydration, polyuria, polydipsia** • **Mental status changes** • **Lethargy, weakness, seizures, coma**	• **Mental status changes** • **Nausea and vomiting, seizures, coma**
Diagnosis	• *HYPER*natremia • ↓urine osmolality • ↓urine specific gravity • ↑urine output	• *HYPO*natremia • ↑urine osmolality • ↑urine specific gravity • ↓urine output
Treatment	• Adequate water intake; **low-sodium** and low-protein diet • <u>Central</u>: desmopressin • <u>Nephrogenic</u>: correct underlying etiology • **HCTZ, indomethacin**	• **Water restriction** • **Sodium replacement** (NaCl tablets, IV NS + furosemide vs hypertonic saline) • **Demeclocycline**

	Serum Na⁺	Serum Osmolality	Urine Osmolality
SIADH	↓	↓	↑
Dehydration	↑	↑	↑
Diabetes Insipidus	↑	↑	↓

Hypercalcemia

Etiology & Risk Factors	• **Elevated serum calcium** (total serum calcium concentration >10.4mg/dL or ionized serum calcium >5.2 mg/dL); normal serum calcium ranges from 8.5 mg/dL-10.5 mg/dL
	• Etiology:
	   • <u>Primary Hyperparathyroidism</u>: **most common cause**; adenoma/hyperplasia of the gland, familial hypocalciuric hypercalcemia, multiple endocrine neoplasia (MEN)
	   • <u>Malignancy</u>: renal carcinomas, leukemias, lymphomas, rhabdomyosarcoma
	   • <u>Hypervitaminosis</u>: **vitamin A or D intoxication**: iatrogenic, excessive milk intake, granulomatous conditions (sarcoidosis, tuberculosis, fungal infections)
	   • <u>Other</u>: **thiazide diuretics, hyperthyroidism, thyrotoxicosis, acute/chronic renal failure, lithium use**, prolonged immobilization

Patho-physiology	• Parathyroid hormone increases serum calcium by increasing intestinal absorption of calcium, mobilizes calcium by enhancing bone resorption, enhancing renal distal nephron calcium reabsorption and stimulating conversion of vitamin D to calcitriol (most active form)

Signs & Symptoms	• *Most patients are asymptomatic*
	• <u>Mnemonic</u>: **Stones, Bones, Groans, Moans, Thrones, Psychic Overtones**
	   • <u>Stones</u>: nephrolithiasis (calcium oxalate and phosphate)
	   • <u>Bones</u>: **bone pain, skeletal muscle weakness**, osteoporosis, osteomalacia, arthritis and pathological fractures
	   • <u>Groans</u>: **abdominal pain, nausea/vomiting, constipation, ileus,** dehydration, pancreatitis
	   • <u>Moans</u>: fatigue, malaise, depression, anxiety, **cognitive dysfunction**
	   • <u>Thrones</u>: polyuria, polydipsia, nocturia
	   • <u>Psychic Overtones</u>: **lethargy, confusion, delirium, psychosis, memory loss,** hallucinations, stupor, coma

Diagnosis	• *Workup includes serum PTH, calcitonin, Vitamin D, ionized calcium, phosphorus, magnesium, alkaline phosphatase levels, renal functions, and urinary calcium-creatinine ratio* • <u>Total Serum and Ionized Calcium Level</u>: **increased serum calcium concentration (>10.4mg/dL) or ionized serum calcium >5.2mg/dL; ionized is more accurate than total** • <u>Intact Parathyroid Hormone (PTH)</u>: differentiates PTH-mediated hypercalcemia (PTH levels are high or high-normal); ordered once hypercalcemia is confirmed • <u>Parathyroid-Related Peptide</u>: ordered if intact PTH is normal or low to rule out malignancy (humoral hypercalcemia of cancer) • <u>Imaging</u>: **CXR** (evaluate for granulomatous disorders, lung cancer, lytic lesions of bone), mammogram (breast cancer), CT, (renal cancer) US/MRI of parathyroid hormones • <u>ECG</u>: **T wave flattening/inversion, shortened QT interval, prolonged PR interval, QRS widening**

Treatment	• <u>Asymptomatic or Ca <12mg/dL</u>: **no immediate treatment required**, avoid aggravating factors (thiazide diuretics, lithium, volume depletion, prolonged inactivity, high Ca diet)
	• <u>Mild Symptoms or Ca 12-14mg/dL</u>: **adequate water intake** (promotes Ca excretion), **oral phosphate** (binds to calcium and prevents absorption)
	• <u>Moderate/Severe</u>:
	   • **IV Fluids + Loop Diuretics: initial management of choice**; isotonic fluids + IV loop diuretics (furosemide) promote calcium excretion; *avoid thiazide diuretics*
	   • **Bisphosphonates: zoledronic acid or pamidronate; inhibit osteoclasts**; drug of choice for cancer-associated hypercalcemia
	   • <u>Calcitonin</u>: adjunct for malignancy-related hypercalcemia; quicker onset of action than bisphosphonates; may be combined with corticosteroids
	   • <u>Denosumab</u>: adjunct for malignancy-related hypercalcemia; monoclonal antibody inhibitor of osteoclastic activity
	   • <u>Corticosteroids</u>: prednisone decreases calcitriol production and intestinal calcium absorption; indicated in vitamin D toxicity and granulomatous conditions (sarcoidosis)

Hypocalcemia

Etiology & Risk Factors	• **Low calcium serum calcium** (total serum calcium concentration <8.8mg/dL or serum ionized calcium concentration <4.7mg/dL) • <u>Fraction</u>: 45% is in free or ionized state (regulated by vitamin D, PTH), 40% bound to plasma proteins (albumin), 15% bound to anions (phosphate, lactate, citrate) • <u>Etiology</u>: **hypoparathyroidism is most common cause overall (autoimmune disorders or accidental removal/damage to parathyroid glands during thyroidectomy), vitamin D deficiency, chronic renal disease** (abnormal renal loss of calcium and decreased renal conversion of vitamin D to active form), **hypomagnesemia,** hyperphosphatemia, hypoalbuminemia, medications (**loop diuretics,** bisphosphonates, phenytoin, phenobarbital, rifampin), pancreatitis
Patho-physiology	• Parathyroid hormone enhances osteoclastic bone resorption and distal tubular reabsorption of calcium, stimulates hydroxylation of 25 hydroxyvitamin D to the active form (1,25-dihydroxy vitamin D); vitamin D stimulates intestinal absorption of calcium, renal absorption of calcium and bone reabsorption; deficiency leads to hypocalcemia

Signs & Symptoms	• *Most patients are asymptomatic*
	• <u>Neurologic</u>: **hypocalcemia decreases excitation threshold and increases neuromuscular excitability**
	   • **Muscle cramps (back and legs most common),** mild encephalopathy (unexplained dementia, depression, psychosis), increased deep tendon reflexes (hyperreflexia), laryngospasm, **bronchospasm, finger or circumoral paresthesia,** tetany, generalized seizures
	   • <u>Chvostek Sign</u>: **involuntary facial muscle spasm elicited with light tapping of facial nerve anterior to the exterior auditory meatus;** indicates latent tetany
	   • <u>Trousseau's Sign</u>: **carpal spasm induced by reduction of blood supply to hand** with tourniquet or blood pressure cuff inflated above systolic blood pressure (forearm)
	• <u>Cardiovascular</u>: congestive heart failure, **arrhythmias (QTc prolongation)**
	• <u>Cutaneous</u>: **dry and scaly skin, brittle nails, coarse hair,** recurrent *Candida* infections
	• <u>Gastrointestinal</u>: diarrhea, abdominal pain/cramping
	• <u>Skeletal</u>: abnormal dentition, osteomalacia, osteodystrophy

Diagnosis	• *Workup includes serum PTH, calcitonin, Vitamin D, ionized calcium, phosphorus, magnesium, alkaline phosphatase levels, renal functions, and urinary calcium-creatinine ratio* • <u>Total Serum and Ionized Calcium Level</u>: **decreased total serum calcium concentration (<8.8 mg/dL) or ionized serum calcium (<4.7 mg/dL); ionized calcium is more accurate** • <u>Serum Albumin Level</u>: ordered to correct the total calcium or directly measure the ionized calcium level • **Corrected Ca = [0.8 x (normal albumin - patient's albumin)] + serum Ca level** • <u>ECG</u>: **prolonged QT interval**
Treatment	• <u>Asymptomatic or Mild</u>: **oral calcium gluconate + vitamin D (calcitriol)** • <u>Symptomatic or Severe</u>: **IV calcium gluconate**; 10mL of 10% solution infused over 10 minutes • <u>Hypomagnesemia</u>: **IV magnesium sulfate** followed by oral magnesium gluconate to correct hypomagnesemia • *Avoid phenothiazine antipsychotics (may precipitate extrapyramidal symptoms); avoid furosemide (worsens hypocalcemia)*
Key Words & Most Common	• Hypoparathyroidism is most common cause • Muscle cramps + finger/oral paresthesia + hyperreflexia + Chvostek sign (facial spasm by tapping facial nerve) + Trousseau's Sign (carpal spasm with inflation of BP cuff) • ↓ total serum calcium or ionized calcium; ECG shows prolonged QT interval • <u>Mild</u>: oral calcium gluconate + vitamin D (calcitriol) • <u>Severe</u>: IV calcium gluconate

Hyperparathyroidism

Etiology & Risk Factors	• **Overactivity of parathyroid gland(s) resulting in elevated serum parathyroid hormone (PTH) levels which leads to hypercalcemia**
	• Etiology:
	    • **PTH Dependent: parathyroid adenoma is most common cause overall (80%)**, parathyroid hyperplasia, hereditary (multiple endocrine neoplasia [MEN] syndromes)
	    • PTH Independent: malignancy, granulomatous, hyperthyroidism, **lithium therapy**, vitamin A or D intoxication, Milk alkali syndrome, adrenal insufficiency
	• Risk Factors: germline and somatic mutations, **chronically low dietary calcium**, obesity and physical inactivity prolonged use of loop diuretics (furosemide), history of neck radiation therapy, **lithium therapy**, hypertension

Patho-physiology	• Parathyroid hormone enhances osteoclastic bone resorption and distal tubular reabsorption of calcium, stimulates hydroxylation of 25 hydroxyvitamin D to the active form (1,25-dihydroxy vitamin D); vitamin D stimulates intestinal absorption of calcium, renal absorption of calcium and bone reabsorption

Signs & Symptoms	• *Most patients are asymptomatic*
	• Mnemonic: **Stones, Bones, Groans, Moans, Thrones, Psychic Overtones for hypercalcemia**
	    • Stones: **nephrolithiasis (calcium oxalate and phosphate)**
	    • Bones: **bone pain, skeletal muscle weakness, osteoporosis,** osteomalacia, arthritis and pathological fractures
	    • Groans: **abdominal pain, nausea/vomiting, constipation, ileus,** dehydration, pancreatitis
	    • Moans: **fatigue, malaise,** depression, anxiety, **cognitive dysfunction**
	    • Thrones: **polyuria, polydipsia, nocturia**
	    • Psychic Overtones: **lethargy, confusion, delirium, psychosis, memory loss,** hallucinations, stupor, coma

Diagnosis	• Triad: **hypercalcemia + increased intact PTH + decreased phosphate** • Total Serum and Ionized Calcium Level: **increased serum calcium concentration (>10.4mg/dL) or ionized serum calcium >5.2mg/dL; ionized is more accurate than total** • Intact Parathyroid Hormone (PTH): **differentiates PTH-mediated hypercalcemia (PTH levels are high or high-normal)** • Phosphate Level: decreased; parathyroid hormone increases urinary phosphate excretion • Parathyroid-Related Peptide: ordered if intact PTH is normal or low to rule out malignancy (humoral hypercalcemia of cancer) • Neck Ultrasound and Parathyroid Nuclear Medicine (Tc-Sestamibi) Scan: standard imaging tests to localize hyperfunctioning parathyroid gland(s); 4D CT or MRI prior to surgery
Treatment	• Surgery: **parathyroidectomy is definitive management;** indicated for symptomatic or progressive hyperparathyroidism • Oral calcium gluconate + vitamin D (calcitriol) may be given post-parathyroidectomy to prevent hypocalcemia • Cinacalcet: calcimimetic agent that increases calcium-sensing receptor sensitivity to extracellular calcium, inhibiting PTH release; **indicated in non-surgical candidates** • **IV Fluids + Loop Diuretics:** indicated for severe hypercalcemia
Key Words & Most Common	• Overactivity of parathyroid gland causing ↑PTH and thus ↑Ca^{2+}; parathyroid adenoma is most common cause, lithium • Mnemonic: Stones, Bones, Groans, Moans, Thrones, Psychic Overtones • Triad: hypercalcemia + ↑ intact PTH + ↓phosphate • Parathyroidectomy is definitive management • Cinacalcet in those unable to undergo surgery

Hypoparathyroidism

Etiology & Risk Factors	• **Deficiency of parathyroid hormone resulting in hypocalcemia, hyperphosphatemia, and increased neuromuscular irritability** • Etiology: **post-operative complications of thyroidectomy, parathyroidectomy or other head/neck surgery is most common;** autoimmune destruction of parathyroid tissue, hypomagnesemia, abnormal development of parathyroid tissue (DiGeorge syndrome), radiation injury, pseudohypoparathyroidism, malignancy • Risk Factors: recent thyroidectomy or head/neck surgery
Patho-physiology	• Parathyroid hormone enhances osteoclastic bone resorption and distal tubular reabsorption of calcium, stimulates hydroxylation of 25 hydroxyvitamin D to the active form (1,25-dihydroxy vitamin D); vitamin D stimulates intestinal absorption of calcium, renal absorption of calcium and bone reabsorption; deficiency of PTH leads to hypocalcemia

Signs & Symptoms	• *Symptoms of hypocalcemia*
	• Neurologic: **hypocalcemia decreases excitation threshold and increases neuromuscular excitability**
	    • **Muscle cramps (back and legs most common),** mild encephalopathy (unexplained dementia, depression, psychosis), increased deep tendon reflexes (hyperreflexia), laryngospasm, **bronchospasm, finger or circumoral paresthesia,** tetany, generalized seizures
	    • Chvostek Sign: **involuntary facial muscle spasm elicited with light tapping of facial nerve anterior to the exterior auditory meatus;** indicates latent tetany
	    • Trousseau's Sign: **carpal spasm induced by reduction of blood supply to hand** with tourniquet or blood pressure cuff inflated above systolic blood pressure (forearm)
	• Cardiovascular: congestive heart failure, **arrhythmias (QTc prolongation)**
	• Cutaneous: **dry and scaly skin, brittle nails, coarse hair,** recurrent *Candida* infections
	• Gastrointestinal: diarrhea, abdominal pain/cramping
	• Skeletal: abnormal dentition, osteomalacia, osteodystrophy

Diagnosis	• Triad: **hypocalcemia + decreased intact PTH + increased phosphate** • Total Serum and Ionized Calcium Level: **decreased total serum calcium concentration (<8.8 mg/dL) or ionized serum calcium (<4.7 mg/dL); ionized calcium is more accurate** • Serum Albumin Level: ordered to correct the total calcium or directly measure the ionized calcium level • **Corrected Ca = [0.8 x (normal albumin - patient's albumin)] + serum Ca level** • Phosphate Level: increased; low parathyroid hormone decreases urinary phosphate excretion • **ECG: prolonged QT interval**
Treatment	• Asymptomatic or Mild: **oral calcium gluconate + vitamin D (calcitriol)** • Symptomatic or Severe: IV calcium gluconate; 10mL of 10% solution infused over 10 minutes • Hypomagnesemia: **IV magnesium sulfate** followed by oral magnesium gluconate to correct hypomagnesemia
Key Words & Most Common	• Deficiency of parathyroid hormone resulting in ↓calcium and ↑phosphate • Muscle cramps + finger/oral paresthesia + hyperreflexia + Chvostek sign (facial spasm by tapping facial nerve) + Trousseau's Sign (carpal spasm with inflation of BP cuff) • ↓ total serum calcium or ionized calcium; ECG shows prolonged QT interval • Mild: oral calcium gluconate + vitamin D (calcitriol) • Severe: IV calcium gluconate

Prolactinoma

Etiology & Risk Factors	• **Prolactin-secreting tumor of the pituitary gland** • **Most common secretory tumor of the pituitary gland** • Etiology: **pituitary adenoma is most common type** • Risk Factors: often sporadic, familial (multiple endocrine neoplasia type 1 *[MEN1]*)
Patho-physiology	• Monoclonal expansion of pituitary lactotrophs that have undergone somatic mutation; prolactin is responsible for lactation, suppression of sex hormones (estrogen in women, testosterone in men), suppression of gonadotropin-releasing hormone leading to decreased follicle stimulating hormone and luteinizing hormone (amenorrhea) • Prolactin inhibits gonadotropin-releasing hormone which causes hypogonadism

Signs & Symptoms	• Compressive Symptoms: headaches, vision changes (visual field defects, blurred vision, decreased visual acuity), cranial nerve palsy, seizures
	• Hyperprolactinemia:
	    • **Males: decreased libido, impotence, erectile dysfunction, oilgozoospermia** (low sperm count; secondary to hypogonadism), **gynecomastia**
	    • **Females: oligomenorrhea** (infrequent menstruation), **amenorrhea** (absence of menstruation), **infertility**, decreased libido, **galactorrhea** (nipple discharge unrelated to normal milk production of breastfeeding)
	• Physical Exam:
	    • **Bitemporal hemianopsia (impaired peripheral vision of outer visual fields) is most common defect due to compression of optic chiasm**, gynecomastia in males

Diagnosis	• Endocrine Studies: **elevated serum prolactin, decreased follicle stimulating hormone (FSH) and decreased luteinizing hormone (LH)** • *If elevated prolactin, workup includes* **thyroid stimulating hormone (TSH),** *comprehensive metabolic panel (CMP),* **pregnancy test,** *growth hormone, ACTH level* • Pituitary MRI with Gadolinium Contrast: most sensitive to identify anatomy; indicated to distinguish adenoma from aneurysm
Treatment	• Observation: indicated asymptomatic; periodic monitoring of labs and imaging • **Dopamine Agonist Therapy: first-line treatment** • **Cabergoline or bromocriptine** are common dopamine agonists to inhibit prolactin; cabergoline is preferred to normalize prolactin level and shrink tumor • Surgery: transsphenoidal resection indicated for prolactinomas refractory to medical management or women with large adenomas (>3cm) wishing to get pregnant
Key Words & Most Common	• Prolactin-secretion tumor of pituitary gland • Pituitary adenoma is most common type • Compressive symptoms: headache, vision change, seizures, bitemporal hemianopsia • Males: ↓libido, impotence, ED, low sperm count • Females: oligomenorrhea, amenorrhea, infertility, galactorrhea • Labs: ↑prolactin, ↓FSH, ↓LH → pituitary MRI • Observation → dopamine agonists (cabergoline or bromocriptine) → transsphenoidal resection

Gigantism and Acromegaly

Etiology & Risk Factors	• **Syndromes of excessive growth hormone (GH) secretion from the anterior pituitary gland resulting in excessive growth of body tissues and metabolic dysfunction** • Etiology: **somatotroph GH-secreting pituitary adenoma is most common cause (95%)**; lymphoma, pancreatic-islet cell tumors, iatrogenic (excessive GH administration) • Risk Factors: mostly sporadic, genetic abnormalities in the X chromosomes
Patho-physiology	• Growth hormone-releasing hormone (GHRH) is the major stimulator while somatostatin is the major inhibitor of the synthesis and release of growth hormone (GH) • Growth hormone stimulates somatic growth, regulates metabolism and controls release of insulin-like growth factor 1 (IGF-1) which controls growth of body tissue

Signs & Symptoms	• Compressive Symptoms: **headaches**, vision changes (visual field defects, blurred vision, decreased visual acuity), cranial nerve palsy, seizures, **bitemporal hemianopsia**
	• **Gigantism: occurs if GH secretion begins before epiphyseal closure in childhood**
	    • Enlargement of skeletal growth and stature with *minimal* bone deformity
	    • Suspected when height is 2-3 standard deviations above normal
	• **Acromegaly: occurs if GH secretion begins after epiphyseal closure**; 20s-40s most common age of diagnosis
	    • **Coarsening of facial features; prominent supraorbital ridge**, broad nose, acne, large lips, tongue enlargement
	    • Elongation of jaw leads to **overbite, teeth malocclusion**, obstructive sleep apnea, TMJ pain, **deepening of voice**
	    • Generalized weakness/lethargy
	    • **Enlargement of extremities; bony expansion and soft tissue swelling of hands and feet**, skull, tongue, forehead and jaw
	        • **Increased ring, shoe, and hat size often appreciated**
	    • **Hyperhidrosis and skin tags**; skin tags are sensitive finding (GH induced epithelial cell hyperproliferation)
	    • **Carpal tunnel syndrome** (swelling of the median nerve)

Diagnosis	• Insulin-Like Growth Factor 1 (IGF-1) Level: **initial test of choice; increased IGF-1 confirms GH excess** • Oral Glucose Tolerance Test (OGTT) with GH Measurement: **confirms diagnosis; increased growth hormone level confirms diagnosis** (normal response is GH suppression) • Pituitary MRI: imaging test of choice; evaluates size, extent of tumor, and degree of optic chiasmal compression

Treatment	• **Surgery: transsphenoidal resection of tumor is first-line treatment of choice**
	• Medical Therapy: indicated as adjunct to surgery or in patients that are not surgical candidates
	    • **Somatostatin Receptor Ligands: octreotide or lanreotide is first-line medical management**; somatostatin inhibits the secretion of growth hormone
	    • Dopamine Agonist Therapy: cabergoline; acts on D2 receptors in somatotrophs to decrease GH secretion; limited efficacy
	    • GH Receptor Antagonist: pegvisomant; decreases IGF-1 levels
	• Radiation Therapy: reserved for primary therapy in surgery is not available

Key Words & Most Common	• Syndrome of excessive GH secretion from somatotroph pituitary adenoma • Gigantism: occurs if GH secretion is before epiphyseal closure in childhood • Acromegaly: occurs if GH secretion begins after epiphyseal closure; coarse facial features, teeth malocclusion, enlargement of hands/feet/skull, skin tags, carpal tunnel • IGF-1 + OGTT with GH measurement → pituitary MRI • Transsphenoidal resection preferred; octreotide if not surgical candidate

Cushing Disease

Etiology & Risk Factors	• Endocrine disorder characterized by excessive adrenocorticotropic hormone (ACTH) production by the pituitary gland leading to excess cortisol release from adrenal gland • <u>Etiology</u>: **ACTH-secreting pituitary adenoma is most common** • ACTH-secreting pituitary adenoma is 2nd most common cause of Cushing syndrome (first is exogenous corticosteroids)
Patho-physiology	• ACTH-secreting adenoma causes an increase in plasma ACTH leading to bilateral adrenal hyperplasia and increased circulating cortisol
Signs & Symptoms	• *Clinical symptoms vary widely among patients* • **Weight gain, proximal muscle weakness, headache** • **Easy bruising**, flushing of the skin, **striae, poor wound healing, hyperpigmentation of skin**, hirsutism, acne • Loss of libido, amenorrhea, erectile dysfunction • Mood and memory changes, mental disturbances (ranging from mild to psychosis)

Diagnosis	• <u>24-hour Urinary Free Cortisol Measurement</u>: **most specific screening test**; positive if elevated urinary cortisol >120mcg/24 hours
	• <u>48 hour Low Dose Dexamethasone Suppression Test</u>: confirmatory test; positive if cortisol level >1.8mg/dL 24 hours later
	• <u>Serum ACTH Tests</u>: increased baseline ACTH
	   • <u>High-Dose Dexamethasone Suppression Test</u>: used if elevated ACTH to differentiate pituitary ACTH from ectopic source
	      • **High-Dose Dexamethasone will *decrease* (suppress) cortisol by 50% if ACTH source is pituitary adenoma**
	• <u>Pituitary MRI</u>: **imaging test of choice**; evaluates size, extent of tumor, and degree of optic chiasmal compression

Treatment	• <u>Surgery</u>: **transsphenoidal resection of tumor is treatment of choice**; extirpation with radiation therapy as adjunct
Key Words & Most Common	• ACTH-secreting pituitary adenoma increases ACTH production leading to excess cortisol • Weight gain + proximal muscle weakness + headache • Striae + poor wound healing • Mental disturbances • ↑ACTH + suppression of cortisol with high-dose dexamethasone suppression test • Pituitary MRI • Transsphenoidal resection surgery

Dwarfism

Etiology & Risk Factors	• **Medical terminology for short-stature** • May be proportionate or disproportionate • <u>Etiology</u>: **familial short stature**, constitutional delay of growth and puberty, idiopathic, **endocrine disorders (growth hormone deficiency), hypopituitarism**, genetic disorders (Down syndrome, Turner syndrome), **achondroplasia**, precocious puberty • <u>Risk Factors</u>: family history, malnutrition
Patho-physiology	• Growth hormone (GH) and insulin-like growth factor 1 (IGF-1) axis is a regulatory pathway for heigh gain • GH, IGF-1, androgens, and thyroid hormones promote chondrogenesis; estrogen stimulates GH and IGF-1 secretion but also promotes chondrocyte deterioration, epiphyseal fusion which ultimately causes a suspension in vertical growth

Signs & Symptoms	• <u>Children</u>: **short stature, growth delays**
	   • Defined as height below 2 standard deviations or in the 3rd percentile for height
	• <u>Adults</u>: central obesity, hypertension, **dyslipidemia**, decreased bone and muscle mass,
	• **Achondroplasia: most common type of disproportionate dwarfism**
	   • Macrocephaly with frontal bossing (**broad forehead**), midface hypoplasia (**small nasal bridge**), rhizomelia (**the proximal portion of the limb is shorter than distal portion**), brachydactyly (**short digits**), **thoracolumbar kyphosis, genu varum** (bowlegs)
	• *Variations of dwarfism depend on underlying genetic disorder*

Diagnosis	• <u>Karyotyping</u>: used to detect genetic disorders (Down syndrome, Turner syndrome) • <u>AP X-Ray of Left Hand/Wrist</u>: may be used to predict bone age and forecast adult height • <u>Pituitary MRI</u>: imaging test to diagnose intracranial masses or developmental anomalies of pituitary • <u>Provocation Tests</u>: utilized to measure the GH reserve; insulin tolerance test,, Arginine HCL test, Glucagon test, physiological stimuli (strenuous exercise, deep sleep, fasting) • No change in growth hormone release indicates hypopituitarism

Treatment	• <u>Hormonal Therapy</u>:
	   • <u>Recombinant Human Growth Hormone Therapy (rhGH)</u>: **effective treatment for growth hormone deficiency**
	   • <u>Gonadotropin-Releasing Hormone (GnRH) Analogs</u>: suppress the release of gonadotropins from the pituitary to slow progression of precocious puberty
	• <u>Surgery</u>: neurosurgery necessary if pituitary mass
	• <u>Psychosocial Support</u>: dwarfism is associated with social stigmatization and extensive mental pressure

Key Words & Most Common	• Endocrine disorders (GH deficiency), hypopituitarism, achondroplasia • Short stature, growth delays • Achondroplasia is most common type of disproportionate dwarfism: broad forehead, small nasal bridge, proximal limb shortening, thoracolumbar kyphosis, genu varum • Hormonal therapy vs surgery; psychosocial support

Hyperprolactinemia

Etiology & Risk Factors	• <u>Etiology</u>: • <u>Pathologic</u>: **pituitary adenoma is most common cause**; hypothyroidism, acromegaly, liver or renal failure, • <u>Physiologic</u>: **pregnancy**, excessive exercise, stress • <u>Pharmacologic</u>: **dopamine antagonists (metoclopramide, promethazine, prochlorperazine), antipsychotics (risperidone, haloperidol)**
Patho-physiology	• Suppression of sex hormones (estrogen in women, testosterone in men) and inhibition of gonadotropin-releasing hormone leads to hypogonadism
Signs & Symptoms	• <u>**Compressive Symptoms**</u>: **present with pituitary adenoma**; headaches, vision changes (visual field defects, blurred vision, decreased visual acuity), cranial nerve palsy, seizures • <u>Hyperprolactinemia</u>: • **Males**: decreased libido, impotence, erectile dysfunction, oilgozoospermia (low sperm count; secondary to hypogonadism), gynecomastia • **Females**: **oligomenorrhea** (infrequent menstruation), **amenorrhea** (absence of menstruation), **infertility**, decreased libido, **galactorrhea** (nipple discharge unrelated to normal milk production of breastfeeding), vaginal dryness • <u>Physical Exam</u>: • **Bitemporal hemianopsia (impaired peripheral vision of outer visual fields) is most common defect due to compression of optic chiasm with pituitary adenoma** • Gynecomastia in males
Diagnosis	• <u>**Endocrine Studies**</u>: **elevated serum prolactin, decreased follicle stimulating hormone (FSH) and decreased luteinizing hormone (LH)** • *If elevated prolactin, workup includes* **thyroid stimulating hormone (TSH)**, *comprehensive metabolic panel (CMP)*, **pregnancy test**, *growth hormone, ACTH level* • <u>**Pituitary MRI with Gadolinium Contrast**</u>: most sensitive to identify anatomy; indicated to distinguish adenoma from aneurysm
Treatment	• *Treatment depends on underlying etiology* • **Discontinue offending medication** • <u>**Dopamine Agonist Therapy**</u>: **first-line treatment** • **Cabergoline or bromocriptine** are common dopamine agonists to inhibit prolactin; cabergoline is preferred to normalize prolactin level and shrink tumor • <u>Surgery</u>: transsphenoidal resection indicated for prolactinomas refractory to medical management or women with large adenomas (>3cm) wishing to get pregnant
Key Words & Most Common	• Prolactin-secretion tumor of pituitary gland • Pituitary adenoma is most common cause • Dopamine antagonists (metoclopramide, promethazine) antipsychotics (risperidone, haloperidol) • <u>Males</u>: ↓libido, impotence, ED, low sperm count • <u>Females</u>: oligomenorrhea, amenorrhea, infertility, galactorrhea • <u>Labs</u>: ↑prolactin, ↓FSH, ↓LH → pituitary MRI • DC offending medication → dopamine agonists (cabergoline or bromocriptine) → transsphenoidal resection

Hypogonadism

Etiology & Risk Factors	• **Congenital or acquired testosterone deficiency with associated decline of spermatozoa production** • <u>Etiology</u>: • <u>Primary</u>: **Klinefelter's syndrome**, anorchia, cryptorchidism (undescended testes), mumps orchitis, hemochromatosis, chemotherapy and age-related • <u>Secondary</u>: idiopathic, Kallman syndrome, Prader-Willi syndrome, **pituitary disorders**, HIV, **obesity**, surgery, trauma, cirrhosis, Cushing syndrome and **stress-induced**
Patho-physiology	• <u>Primary</u>: insufficient synthesis of testosterone by the testicular Leydig cells to inhibit production of follicle-stimulating hormone (FSH) and luteinizing hormone (LH) • <u>Secondary</u>: failure of the hypothalamus to produce gonadotropin-releasing hormone (GnRH); testosterone levels are low and levels of FSH and LH are low or borderline normal
Signs & Symptoms	• <u>Adolescents</u>: • **Delayed puberty** • **Impaired development of secondary sex characteristics** (facial and chest hair, pubic hair, pelvic build (lack of rounded hips), increased muscle mass, voice deepening) • **High-pitched voice, small scrotum, decreased phallic and testicular growth, sparse pubic, body and axillary hair, gynecomastia** • <u>Adults</u>: • **Decreased libido, erectile dysfunction**, mood changes, **sparse body hair, decreased muscle mass**, sleep disorders, **gynecomastia**, decline in cognition, **testicular atrophy**, increased visceral fat
Diagnosis	• **Total and free serum testosterone, serum FSH, and serum LH levels are drawn simultaneously**; FSH and LH used to distinguish primary from secondary • <u>Primary</u>: decreased testosterone + increased FSH/LH • <u>Secondary</u>: decreased testosterone + decreased FSH/LH • <u>**Serum Total and Free Testosterone**</u>: **should be drawn in the morning (before 10:00AM)** • **Decreased total and free serum testosterone diagnoses hypogonadism** (normal total testosterone is 300 to 1000 ng/dL) • **Free testosterone more accurately reflects functional testosterone levels**; sex hormone binding globulin, albumin, and total testosterone may be used to calculate • <u>Semen Analysis</u>: should be included in part of a fertility workup
Treatment	• <u>Lifestyle Modifications</u>: proper nutrition (whole food sources, prioritize protein), weight reduction, increased physical activity (aerobic and resistance exercise) • <u>**Testosterone Replacement Therapy (TRT)**</u>: • **IM injection of testosterone enanthate or cypionate or gel most common**; other forms include lozenges, transdermal patch, nasal spray, subcutaneous implant • *Gel maintains physiologic blood levels more consistently; injections tend to be less expensive* • *Exogenous testosterone impairs spermatogenesis and should be avoided if fertility is a concern* • *Hematocrit (Hct), prostate specific antigen (PSA), and testosterone levels should be monitored quarterly in first year, then semiannually thereafter* • <u>Infertility</u>: • <u>Primary</u>: sperm harvesting with assisted reproductive techniques • <u>Secondary</u>: gonadotropin therapy

Metabolic Syndrome

Etiology & Risk Factors	• **Syndrome of multiple metabolic abnormalities including increased waist circumference (excess abdominal fat), hypertension, insulin resistance and dyslipidemia** • Also known as insulin resistance syndrome or syndrome X • Etiology: **underlying etiology due to poor diet, excess abdominal fat or obesity, lack of physical activity and genetic predisposition** • <u>Risk Factors</u>: **sedentary lifestyle, low muscle-to-fat mass ratio, obesity**, obstructive sleep apnea, chronic kidney/liver disease, polycystic ovarian syndrome, **low-testosterone**
Patho-physiology	• Insulin resistance causes microvascular damage which causes endothelial dysfunction, vascular resistance, hypertension, and inflammation of blood vessels • Endothelial dysfunction and hypertension secondary to metabolic syndrome results in ischemic heart disease
Signs & Symptoms	• **Excess abdominal fat** • **Increased waist circumference** • **Increased waist-to-hip ratio (low muscle-to-fat mass ratio)** • <u>Hypertension</u>: often asymptomatic, may have headaches • <u>Dyslipidemia</u>: arterial bruits, **xanthomas** • <u>Insulin Resistance</u>: peripheral neuropathy, retinopathy, **acanthosis nigricans**

Diagnosis	• <u>Diagnostic Criteria</u>: at least 3 or more of following required to establish diagnosis
	   • **Increased Waist Circumference**: ≥40 inches in men and ≥35 inches in women
	   • **Increased Fasting Glucose**: ≥100 mg/dL
	   • **Increased Blood Pressure**: ≥130/85 mmHg (or medical treatment for hypertension)
	   • **Increased Fasting Triglycerides**: ≥150 mg/dL
	   • **Decreased High-Density Lipoprotein (HDL) Cholesterol**: <40 mg/dL in men and <50 mg/dL in women

Treatment	• <u>Lifestyle Modifications</u>: proper nutrition (whole food sources, prioritize protein), weight reduction, increased physical activity (aerobic and resistance exercise)
	• <u>Weight Loss Medications</u>:
	   • **Orlistat**: inhibits intestinal lipase to decrease fat absorption and improve blood glucose
	   • **Phentermine**: appetite suppressant; short-term use only (<3 months)
	   • <u>Phentermine/Topiramate</u>: combination drug approved for long term use
	   • **GLP-1 Agonists (liraglutide, semaglutide)**: augments glucose-mediated insulin release to induce glycemic control, stimulates satiety to reduces food intake
	   • **Metformin**: inhibits gluconeogenesis and increase peripheral insulin-mediated glucose utilization to promote weight loss
	   • <u>Naltrexone/Bupropion</u>: adjunctive therapy; naltrexone blocks negative feedback on satiety pathways; bupropion induces hypophagia (caloric intake suppression)
	• <u>Surgery</u>: bariatric surgery is most effective single therapy in patients with severe obesity
	• <u>Cardiovascular Risk Factor Management</u>: hypertriglyceridemia management (statin therapy, fibrates, niacin, and omega acids); blood pressure management

Key Words & Most Common	• Metabolic abnormalities due to poor diet, obesity, sedentary lifestyle and genetic predisposition • ↑waist circumference, ↑fasting glucose, ↑blood pressure, ↑fasting triglycerides, ↓HDL cholesterol • Lifestyle modifications → weight loss medications (orlistat, phentermine, GLP-1 agonists, metformin) → bariatric surgery

Multiple Endocrine Neoplasia Type I

Etiology & Risk Factors	• Rare, inherited syndrome characterized by hyperplasia or adenomas of the parathyroid glands, pancreatic islet cell tumors and/or pituitary gland tumors • **3 P's: P**arathyroid, **P**ancreas, **P**ituitary • <u>Etiology</u>: **germline inactivating mutations of the *MEN1* or *menin* gene on chromosome 11** • <u>Risk Factors</u>: family history, age (20-40 years old most common age of diagnosis)
Patho-physiology	• Germline inactivating mutations of the *MEN1* or *menin* gene on chromosome 11 results in hyperplasia or adenomas of parathyroid glands, pancreatic islet cell tumors or pituitary and tumors

Signs & Symptoms	• <u>Parathyroid</u>: **hyperparathyroidism is present in 95% of cases**
	   • **Asymptomatic hypercalcemia or nephrolithiasis is most common presenting manifestation**
	• <u>Pancreas</u>: **pancreatic islet tumors occur in 30-90% of patients**
	   • **Gastrinoma: multiple peptic ulcers**
	   • **Insulinoma: fasting hypoglycemia**
	• <u>Pituitary</u>: **pituitary tumors occur in 15-45% of patients**
	   • **Prolactinoma: most common pituitary tumor**
	• <u>Other</u>: carcinoid tumors, adrenal adenomas, multiple subcutaneous and visceral lipomas, angiofibromas and meningiomas may occur

Diagnosis	• **Workup includes serum calcium, intact parathyroid hormone (PTH), gastrin, and prolactin** • **Genetic Testing: direct DNA sequencing of the *MEN1* gene** • <u>Ultrasonography/CT</u>: utilized to evaluate or localize tumors of the triad

Treatment	• <u>Surgical Excision</u>: **when possible is preferred treatment**
	   • Parathyroidectomy
	   • Transsphenoidal resection of pituitary tumor
	   • Distal subtotal pancreatectomy
	• <u>Medical Management</u>: manage hormone excess
	   • **Octreotide and cinacalcet** to manage hypercalcemia in hyperparathyroidism
	   • **Dopamine agonists** with prolactinoma

Key Words & Most Common	• Inherited syndrome causing overactive endocrine gland tumors of parathyroid, pancreas and pituitary • <u>Parathyroid</u>: hypercalcemia • <u>Pancreas</u>: peptic ulcers or fasting hypoglycemia • <u>Pituitary</u>: prolactinoma most common • Serum Ca^{2+} + intact PTH, + gastrin + prolactin • Surgical excision vs medical management

Multiple Endocrine Neoplasia Type II

Etiology & Risk Factors	• Rare, inherited syndrome characterized by tumors of the adrenal gland, thyroid and parathyroid; further classification to *MEN2A* and *MEN2B* • **MEN2A is more common; comprises of 90%** while *MEN2B* comprises 5% of *MEN2* families • <u>Etiology</u>: **mutations in the *RET* proto-oncogene on chromosome 10** • <u>Risk Factors</u>: family history
Patho-physiology	• Mutations in the *RET* proto-oncogene on chromosome 10 lead to tumor formation of the adrenal, thyroid and parathyroid glands

Signs & Symptoms	• <u>Thyroid</u>: **medullary thyroid cancer (MTC) is the most common manifestation of both *MEN2A* and *MEN2B***
	  • **Solitary thyroid nodule and/or cervical lymphadenopathy is presenting manifestation**
	• <u>Adrenal</u>: **pheochromocytoma of the adrenal glands** occurs in 40-50% of *MEN2A* patients
	  • **Hypertensive crisis is presenting manifestation**
	• <u>Parathyroid</u>: **hyperparathyroidism** occurs in 20% of *MEN2A* patients
	  • **Asymptomatic hypercalcemia or nephrolithiasis is most common presenting manifestation**
	• <u>***MEN2A***</u>: cutaneous lichen amyloidosis (pruritic, pigmented, scaly papules of extremity extensor surfaces and interscapular region)
	• <u>***MEN2B***</u>: marfanoid habitus (decreased upper to lower body ratio, pectus excavatum, scoliosis), mucosal neuromas (red papules) of conjunctiva, lips and tongue and joint laxity

Diagnosis	• **Workup includes serum calcium, intact parathyroid hormone (PTH), plasma free metanephrines, and urinary catecholamine levels** • <u>Genetic Testing</u>: **direct sequencing for *RET* proto-oncogene mutations for both *MEN2A* and *MEN2B*** • <u>Ultrasonography/CT</u>: utilized to evaluate or localize tumors

Treatment	• <u>Surgical Excision</u>: **when possible is preferred treatment**
	  • **Total thyroidectomy and lymph node dissection for medullary thyroid cancer**
	  • Laparoscopic adrenalectomy
	  • Parathyroidectomy

Key Words & Most Common	• Inherited syndrome causing overactive endocrine gland tumors of thyroid, adrenal and parathyroid glands • <u>Thyroid</u>: medullary thyroid cancer • <u>Adrenal</u>: pheochromocytoma • <u>Parathyroid</u>: hyperparathyroidism • <u>Genetic Testing</u>: direct sequencing for *RET* proto-oncogene mutations for both *MEN2A* and *MEN2B* • Surgical excision

Chapter 8
Renal

Nephrotic Syndrome

Etiology & Risk Factors	• Clinical kidney syndrome characterized by proteinuria, hypoalbuminemia, hyperlipidemia, edema and various complications
	• Etiology:
	  • <u>Minimal Change Disease</u>: **most common primary cause in children; cause is unknown**, may occur with viral infections, allergies, medication use (NSAIDs), lymphoma
	  • <u>Focal Segmental Glomerulosclerosis (FSG)</u>: **most common primary cause in adults (African Americans)**; idiopathic, hypertension, drugs (NSAIDs, lithium, heroin), HIV
	  • <u>Membranous Nephropathy</u>: **more common in Caucasians**; medications (NSAIDs, penicillamines), infections, viral hepatitis, autoimmune (SLE), thyroiditis, cancer
	  • <u>Secondary Causes</u>: **diabetic nephropathy is most common secondary cause**, preeclampsia, amyloidosis
	• <u>Risk Factors</u>: **diabetes mellitus**, hypertension, chronic NSAID use, ethnicity (American Indians, African Americans, and Hispanics)

Patho-physiology	• Immunogen and cytokines cause T cell upregulation of circulating permeability factor or downregulation of inhibitor permeability factors cause damage to glomerular cells • Damage to structures that filter serum proteins (capillary endothelial cells, the glomerular basement membrane (GBM), and podocytes) leads to proteinuria

Signs & Symptoms	• Anorexia, malaise
	• **Frothy urine** (high concentration of protein in urine)
	• **Generalized edema worse in the morning**
	  • **Periorbital edema especially present in children**
	  • Dyspnea (pleural effusion, tracheal edema)
	  • Arthralgias (hydrarthrosis)
	  • Abdominal pain (ascites, mesenteric edema)
	• Deep vein thrombosis (DVT)/pulmonary embolism (PE) may be first indication (loss of protein C, S, antithrombin III)

Diagnosis	• <u>Urinalysis</u>: **best initial test; proteinuria of 3+ or 4+ readings on dipstick** or by semiquantitative testing • May demonstrate casts (hyaline, granular, **fatty**, waxy, or epithelial cell casts), lipiduria (**lipids within tubular cells [oval fat bodies], fatty casts**, or free globules) • <u>24-Hour Urine Protein</u>: **confirmatory test; 3g protein in a 24-hour urine collection is diagnostic** • Workup includes **BUN/Cr (elevated), serum albumin (low), total cholesterol and triglyceride levels (elevated)**, HbA1c, glucose, ANA, hepatitis screen, RF, HIV, syphilis • <u>Renal Biopsy</u>: **definitive diagnosis**; not routinely performed
Treatment	• <u>Treat Underlying Etiology</u>: • <u>Minimal Change Disease and FSG</u>: **corticosteroids are first-line**; immunosuppressives (cyclophosphamide, mycophenolate mofetil [MMF], calcineurin inhibitors) • <u>Edema Management</u>: **sodium restriction first-line; IV albumin infusion (correct hypoalbuminemia) followed by loop diuretics (furosemide)** if sodium restriction ineffective • <u>Proteinuria Management</u>: **ACE inhibitors or ARBs**; cause dilation of efferent arteriole to reduce systemic and intraglomerular pressure and proteinuria • <u>Hyperlipidemia Treatment</u>: dietary modifications and statin therapy

Minimal Change Disease

Etiology & Risk Factors	• **Abrupt onset of edema and heavy proteinuria; most common cause of nephrotic syndrome in children** • <u>Etiology</u>: **idiopathic is most common** • May occur secondary to **medications (NSAIDs, lithium antibiotics)**, immunizations, infection, **allergens**, hematologic cancers (especially **Hodgkin lymphoma**) • <u>Risk Factors</u>: **age (most common age 4-8 years old)**, males
Patho-physiology	• Exact pathogenesis is unknown; damage to the glomerular filtration barrier (GFB) increases the renal membrane permeability resulting in urinary loss of protein (primarily albumin)

Signs & Symptoms	• **Periorbital, scrotal, labia, and/or lower extremity edema is most common symptom**
	• **Anorexia, malaise**
	• **Frothy urine** (high concentration of protein in urine)
	• **Generalized edema worse in the morning**
	  • **Periorbital edema especially present in children**
	  • Dyspnea (pleural effusion, tracheal edema)
	  • Arthralgias (hydrarthrosis)
	  • Abdominal pain (ascites, mesenteric edema)
	• *Children may present in setting of severe infections (sepsis, pneumonia, and peritonitis) due to immunoglobulin depletion*

Diagnosis	• Workup includes **BUN/Cr (normal), serum albumin (low), total cholesterol and triglyceride levels (elevated)** • <u>Urinalysis</u>: **best initial test; proteinuria on dipstick** or by semiquantitative testing • Microscopy may demonstrate casts (oval fat bodies and fatty casts) • <u>24-Hour Urine Protein</u>: **confirmatory test; 3g protein in a 24-hour urine collection is diagnostic for nephrotic syndrome** • <u>Renal Biopsy</u>: **definitive diagnosis**; light microscopy often normal; electron microscopy demonstrates diffuse swelling (effacement) of epithelial, immunofluorescent staining is negative
Treatment	• <u>Corticosteroids</u>: **first-line medication**; treatment for 4-6 weeks followed by prolonged taper • <u>Oral Cytotoxic Medications</u>: immunosuppressives (cyclophosphamide or chlorambucil, cyclosporine, mycophenolate mofetil [MMF], rituximab)
Key Words & Most Common	• Idiopathic cause of nephrotic syndrome most commonly seen in children (4-8 years old most common) • Periorbital edema • Frothy urine • Generalized edema, worse in the morning • UA: proteinuria + oval fat bodies and fatty casts on microscopy • 24-Hour Urine: >3g protein in 24-hour urine collection • Renal Biopsy: definitive diagnosis • Corticosteroids

Periorbital Edema

Membranous Nephropathy 👥

Etiology & Risk Factors	• Deposition of immune complexes on the glomerular basement membrane (GBM) with GBM thickening; cause of nephrotic syndrome • **Characterized by proteinuria (>3.5 g/day), peripheral edema, hypertension, frothy urine, and thromboembolic phenomena** • <u>Etiology</u>: **idiopathic is most common; medications (penicillamines, NSAIDs)**, infection (hepatitis B/C, HIV, syphilis), **autoimmune (systemic lupus erythematosus [SLE])**, thyroiditis, parasitic disease (malaria, schistosomiasis), heavy metal poisoning (gold, mercury) • May have underlying cancer (lung, colon, stomach, breast, Hodgkin or non-Hodgkin lymphoma, chronic lymphocytic leukemia, melanoma) • <u>Risk Factors</u>: **most common cause of primary nephrotic syndrome in Caucasian adults**, age (adults most common, **peak incidence between 50-60 years old**), males
Patho-physiology	• Antigen-antibody complexes are deposited between the glomerular basement membrane (GBM) and podocytes; this activates the complement system and generates the membrane attack complex, releasing protease, cytokines and oxidants causing renal tissue damage, loss of membrane anionic charge barrier which causes proteinuria • Loss of protein C, S, antithrombin III may lead to thromboembolic event
Signs & Symptoms	• **Weight gain (generalized fluid retention)** • **Peripheral edema** • **Microscopic hematuria** • **Proteinuria (frothy urine)** • <u>**Thromboembolic Event**</u>: dyspnea (pulmonary embolism), flank pain with hematuria (renal vein thrombosis), calf pain (deep vein thrombosis) and/or heart failure symptoms • <u>Physical Exam</u>: • **Hypertension, peripheral (pedal) edema, anasarca** (generalized accumulation of fluid in interstitial space)

Diagnosis	• Workup includes BUN/Cr (elevated), serum albumin (low), **total cholesterol and triglyceride levels (elevated)**, HbA1c, glucose, ANA, hepatitis screen, RF, HIV, syphilis
	• <u>**Urinalysis**</u>: **best initial test;** proteinuria on dipstick or by semiquantitative testing
	   • May demonstrate casts (cellular casts, fatty casts, and oval fat bodies)
	   • Urinary cholesterol detected by **oval Maltese cross-shaped fat bodies** seen under crossed polarized light microscopy
	• **<u>24-Hour Urine Protein</u>: confirmatory test; 3g protein in a 24-hour urine collection is diagnostic for nephrotic syndrome**
	• <u>**Renal Biopsy**</u>: **definitive diagnosis;** shows diffuse capillary and glomerular basement thickening

Treatment	• ***Treat Underlying Etiology*** • <u>**Edema Management**</u>: **sodium restriction first-line;** IV albumin infusion (correct hypoalbuminemia) followed by loop diuretics (furosemide) if sodium restriction ineffective • <u>**Non-Nephrotic Range Proteinuria**</u>: **ACE inhibitors or ARBs** • <u>**Nephrotic Range Proteinuria**</u>: **immunosuppressive therapy; corticosteroids followed by chlorambucil**
Key Words & Most Common	• Proteinuria, peripheral edema, weight gain, hypertension, frothy urine, thromboembolic phenomena • Most common cause in Caucasian adults • UA: proteinuria + oval Maltese cross-shaped fat bodies on microscopy; Renal biopsy is definitive • Treat underlying etiology + edema management (sodium restriction + loop diuretics) → ACEI/ARB vs immunosuppressive therapy

Focal Segmental Glomerulosclerosis 👥

Etiology & Risk Factors	• Segmental scarring (sclerosis) involving a focal portion of the glomerulus • **Most common idiopathic cause of nephrotic syndrome in adults** • <u>Etiology</u>: **idiopathic most common; drugs (heroin)**, medications (lithium, NSAIDs, interferon alfa, pamidronate), viral infection (hepatitis B/C, HIV, parvovirus, SARS-CoV-2) • <u>Risk Factors</u>: ethnicity (African American most common), males, age (18-45 years old most common)
Patho-physiology	• Idiopathic, viral- or toxin-mediated insult and alteration in intrarenal hemodynamics results in injury and loss of podocytes leading to compensatory podocyte hypertrophy of the remaining podocytes to cover the glomerular capillary surface resulting in effacement and urinary protein loss
Signs & Symptoms	• **Proteinuria (frothy urine)** • **Peripheral edema** • **Hypertension** • **Weight gain (generalized fluid retention)** • May develop over weeks or suddenly (15-20lbs of recent weight gain) • May present with pleural effusion and ascites • Progressive proteinuria → renal failure
Diagnosis	• Workup includes BUN/Cr (elevated), serum albumin (low), **total cholesterol and triglyceride levels (elevated)**, hepatitis screen, RF, ANA, HIV antibody • <u>**Urinalysis**</u>: **best initial test;** proteinuria on dipstick or by semiquantitative testing • **May demonstrate casts (hyaline and broad waxy)** • **<u>24-Hour Urine Protein</u>: confirmatory test; 3g protein in a 24-hour urine collection is diagnostic for nephrotic syndrome** • <u>**Renal Biopsy**</u>: **definitive diagnosis;** shows perihilar or peripheral segmental solidification of the glomeruli
Treatment	• **Treat underlying etiology** • <u>**Corticosteroids**</u>: **first-line medication;** treatment for 4-6 weeks followed by prolonged taper • <u>Oral Cytotoxic Medications</u>: immunosuppressives (cyclophosphamide or chlorambucil, cyclosporine, mycophenolate mofetil [MMF], rituximab)
Key Words & Most Common	• Focal scarring of the glomerulus; most common idiopathic cause of nephrotic syndrome in adults • Proteinuria + edema + hypertension • UA: large amounts of protein; hyaline and broad waxy casts • 24-Hour Urine Protein: confirms diagnosis • Renal Biopsy: definitive diagnosis; perihilar segmental solidification of glomeruli • Corticosteroids

Diabetic Nephropathy

Etiology & Risk Factors	• Renal microvascular complication of diabetes mellitus characterized by persistent albuminuria and progressive decline in glomerular filtration rate • **Most common cause of end-stage renal disease; 30-40% of patients with diabetes mellitus will develop nephropathy** • Etiology: insulin resistance, genetics, hyperglycemia and autoimmune processes may be related in setting of diabetes mellitus • Risk Factors: **poor glycemic control**, advanced age, alcohol use, **hypertension**, peripheral vascular disease, **smoking**, **dyslipidemia**, long duration of diabetes
Patho-physiology	• Hyperglycemia leads to the production of reactive oxygen species and activation of multiple inflammatory pathways eventually causing inflammation fibrosis and increased vascular permeability; thickening of glomerular basement membrane and glomerular sclerosis leads to microalbuminuria
Signs & Symptoms	• **Often asymptomatic** • Persistent hypertension • Nephropathy: fatigue, foamy urine and pedal edema

Diagnosis	• Diagnostic Criteria: hypertension, progressive decline in glomerular filtration rate (GFR), persistent albuminuria (>300mg/day) on at least 2 visits, 3-6 months apart
	• Urine Dipstick: **positive proteinuria**; *typically a urine dipstick is only positive when protein excretion exceeds 300 to 500 mg/day*
	• 24-Hour Urine Collection: total urinary albumin excretion over 24 hour period
	   • Moderate Albuminuria: **excretion of 30 to 300 mg/day**; early nephropathy
	   • Severe Albuminuria: **excretion of >300mg/day**; advanced nephropathy
	• Glomerular Filtration Rate (GFR): **monitor progression of disease**
	• Renal Biopsy: definitive diagnosis; Kimmelstiel Wilson nodules are pathognomonic (**nodules of pink hyaline material** in the glomerular capillary loops due to protein leakage), glomerular basement membrane thickening, and glomerular sclerosis, inflammation

Treatment	• Lifestyle Modifications:
	   • Glycemic Control: **optimal management of diabetes to reduce progression**
	   • Dietary Modifications: low-sodium, low-fat, low-carbohydrate diet
	• Angiotensin-Converting Enzyme (ACE) Inhibitor or Angiotensin II Receptor Blocker (ARB): **indicated at the earliest sign of albuminuria**
	   • **Prevents progression of renal disease by dilating efferent arteriole to lower intraglomerular blood pressure and reduce protein leakage**
	• Renal Replacement: indicated with end-stage renal disease (GFR of 10-15 ml/min); peritoneal or hemodialysis, renal transplant

Key Words & Most Common	• Most common cause of end-stage renal disease characterized by persistent albuminuria and progressive decline in GFR • Often asymptomatic → fatigue, foamy urine, pedal edema • GFR + urine dipstick + 24-hour urine collection for diagnosis • Renal biopsy is definitive; Kimmelstiel-Wilson nodules are pathognomonic • Glycemic control + ACEI/ARB

Nephritic Syndrome

Etiology & Risk Factors	• Manifestation of glomerular inflammation characterized by **hematuria, proteinuria, hypertension, decreased urine output, edema, and dysmorphic red blood cells (RBCs)** • Etiology: poststreptococcal/infectious glomerulonephritis, IgA nephropathy, membranoproliferative, rapidly progressive glomerulonephritis, Goodpasture's, vasculitis, Henoch Schoenlein Purpura
Patho-physiology	• Immune mediated glomerular inflammation leads to structural disruption of glomerular basement membrane which causes increased urinary protein and RBC loss
Signs & Symptoms	• **Periorbital and peripheral (pedal) edema** • **Hematuria (red, cola or tea-colored urine)** • **Proteinuria in non-nephrotic range (frothy urine if protein level high)** • **Hypertension or poorly controlled blood pressure** • **Renal insufficiency characterized by oliguria (reduced urine output)** • May have abdominal or flank pain • *Clinical symptoms may have a variable course depending on underlying etiology* • Physical Exam: • Hypertension, edema (may have signs of fluid overload including JVP distention, pitting edema, and crackles on chest auscultation), pallor,

Diagnosis	• Urinalysis: **initial test performed**
	   • **Hematuria (brownish, tea/cola-colored urine)**, >5 RBCs/HPF
	   • **Non-nephrotic proteinuria** (less than 3.5 g/day)
	   • Acanthocytes, dysmorphic RBCs, and red blood cells (RBCs) casts may be seen
	• *Workup includes BUN/creatinine, ANA, serum C3 and C4 complement levels, ASO titers, ANCA, anti-dsDNA, anti-glomerular basement membrane antibodies, hepatitis screen*

Treatment	• **Mainly supportive treatment** • Antihypertensives: dietary salt and fluid restriction, ACEI/ARBs • Diuretics: loop diuretics may be used to decrease fluid retention; promotes free water and sodium excretion • Corticosteroids: relieve inflammation of the kidney; decrease inflammatory immune response; controversial • Immunomodulators: immunosuppressive medications reduce and inhibit the antigenic effects of the inciting etiology; most useful for rapidly progressive glomerulonephritis • Antibiotics: indicated in certain cases of infectious glomerulonephritis • Dialysis: indicated when disease leads to fulminant renal failure

Immunoglobulin A Nephropathy 🫘

Etiology & Risk Factors	• Nephropathy characterized by IgA immune complex deposition in the glomeruli, progressive hematuria, proteinuria and renal insufficiency • Most common cause of acute glomerulonephritis in adults; also known as Berger's disease • Etiology: autoimmune condition causing antibody-mediated destruction of the glomerular basement membrane; 90% of cases are sporadic • Risk Factors: recent upper respiratory or gastrointestinal infection, male, age (peak onset in adolescent or young adults), Caucasian or Asian
Patho-physiology	• Precipitating factor (infection most common) triggers a dysregulated immune response resulting in IgA overproduction which damages the glomerular basement membrane affecting the filtration of larger molecules causing hematuria; overproduction of cytokines stimulates mesangial cell proliferation
Signs & Symptoms	• Gross hematuria is most common • Described a "cola or tea-colored" urine • Usually begins 1-2 days after febrile mucosal illness (upper respiratory, gastrointestinal) • *Mimics post-infectious glomerulonephritis except symptoms are immediately after or coinciding with illness* • May present as persistent or recurrent macroscopic hematuria or asymptomatic microscopic hematuria • Flank pain, low-grade fever
Diagnosis	• Urinalysis: hematuria, red blood cell casts, dysmorphic red blood cells (acanthocytes), mild proteinuria (usually <1g/day), elevated specific gravity (>1.020) • BUN/Creatinine: serum creatinine usually normal • Renal Biopsy: gold-standard for diagnosis; demonstrates IgA mesangial granular deposits and complement (C3) on immunofluorescent staining
Treatment	• *Usually self-limited and carries a good prognosis* • Hypertension Management: ACE inhibitors or ARBs are first-line (angiotensin inhibition reduces blood pressure, proteinuria and glomerular fibrosis); sodium restriction • Immunosuppression: corticosteroids indicated for persistent or worsening proteinuria or increased serum creatinine • Methylprednisolone + prednisone taper most common regimen • Cyclophosphamide, azathioprine, and cyclosporine are potential steroid-sparing agents • Omega-3 Polyunsaturated Fatty Acids: fish-oil supplements may alter inflammatory cytokine production • Renal Transplant: indicated for patients with end-stage renal disease
Key Words & Most Common	• Nephropathy characterized by IgA immune complexes causing antibody-mediated glomerular basement membrane damage • Most common cause of glomerulonephritis • Gross hematuria • Cola/tea colored • Begins 1-2 days after upper respiratory/GI infection • UA: hematuria, RBC casts, mild proteinuria • Renal biopsy is gold-standard; shows IgA mesangial deposits • ACEI/ARB +/- corticosteroids

Post-Infectious Glomerulonephritis 🫘

Etiology & Risk Factors	• Rapid deterioration of kidney function secondary to a post-infectious inflammatory response • Etiology: Group A *Streptococcus* infection of the skin (impetigo) or throat (pharyngitis) is most common • Viral (hepatitis B/C, HIV, cytomegalovirus, EBV, parvovirus B19), fungal (coccidioidomycosis, histoplasmosis) and parasitic infections (malaria, toxoplasmosis) possible • Risk Factors: age (3-12 years old most common; incidence between 5 to 6 years old), poor hygiene, overcrowding and low socioeconomic status increases risk for outbreaks
Patho-physiology	• *Streptococcal* infection causes immune complexes containing *Streptococcal* antigens and human antibodies to bind to glomerular basement membrane, activating an alternate complement pathway and causing glomerular damage
Signs & Symptoms	• Gross hematuria is most common presenting symptom • Described a "cola or tea-colored" urine • Usually begins 7-14 days after *Streptococcal* pharyngitis or 2-3 weeks after skin infection (impetigo) • *Mimics IgA nephropathy except symptoms are delayed* • Proteinuria (foamy urine), oliguria (low urine output), edema, hypertension and renal insufficiency may be present • Fever indicates persistent infection
Diagnosis	• Urinalysis: hematuria, red blood cell casts, moderate proteinuria (usually 0.5-2g/day), white blood cells; white blood cell, hyaline and cellular casts • Antistreptolysin O Titer: elevated level is most common laboratory finding to indicate *Streptococcus* infection; may be falsely low if patient is/was treated with antibiotics • Serum Complement (C3) Level: low due to complement consumption during acute inflammatory reaction • BUN/Creatinine: elevated in acute phase • Renal Biopsy: not recommended
Treatment	• Supportive: treat volume overload • Loop diuretics (furosemide) + sodium and fluid restriction; ACE inhibitors or calcium channel blockers indicated for hypertension/edema not controlled by diuretics • Antibiotics: antibiotic therapy indicated for active *Streptococcus* infection; *preventive only when initiated in first 36 hours of infection* • Penicillin V, amoxicillin are first-line for *Streptococcal* pharyngitis; cefdinir, cefuroxime, azithromycin, clindamycin are alternatives • Mupirocin 2% ointment is first-line for impetigo • Dialysis: indicated for acute renal failure; manages acid-base imbalance, electrolyte abnormalities and fluid overload
Key Words & Most Common	• Classic patient is 3-12 year-old male 2 weeks s/p *Streptococcus* infection presenting with facial edema and scant amounts of dark urine • Glomerulonephritis secondary to Group A *Streptococcus* infection of the skin (impetigo) or throat (pharyngitis) • Gross hematuria • Cola/tea colored • Begins 10-14 days after *Streptococcal* infection • UA: hematuria, RBC casts, moderate proteinuria; ↑ASO Titer, ↓C3 level • Supportive (loop diuretic + sodium/fluid restriction) +/- antibiotics

Rapidly Progressive Glomerulonephritis (RPGN) 🫘

Etiology & Risk Factors	• Acute nephritic syndrome characterized by microscopic glomerular crescent formation and rapid decline in renal function to end-stage renal disease (weeks/months)
	• <u>Etiology</u>: *any cause of acute glomerulonephritis can present with RPGN*
	   • <u>**Anti-Glomerular Basement Membrane (GBM) Disease**</u>: respiratory exposures (cigarette smoke, viral URI) or other stimulus triggers anticollagen antibodies
	     • <u>**Goodpasture Syndrome**</u>: glomerulonephritis and alveolar hemorrhage in presence of anti-GBM antibodies; antibodies against type IV collagen of GBM
	   • <u>**Granular Immune Complex Disorder**</u>: poststreptococcal glomerulonephritis, collagen vascular disease, visceral abscess, sepsis, lupus nephritis, IgA nephropathy
	   • <u>**Pauci-Immune Disorder**</u>: vasculitis characterized by absence of immune complex or complement deposition and + **antineutrophil cytoplasmic antibodies (ANCA)**
	     • <u>**Microscopic Polyangiitis**</u>: **vasculitis of small renal vessels; + P-ANCA**
	     • <u>**Granulomatosis with Polyangiitis (Wegener's)**</u>: **necrotizing vasculitis; + C-ANCA**

Patho-physiology	• Basement membrane rupture causes extra-capillary fibrin to precipitate followed by parietal cell proliferation to form capsular, crescent-shaped proliferate

Signs & Symptoms	• **Early clinical signs are nonspecific**; weakness, malaise, fatigue, fever, nausea/vomiting, anorexia, arthralgia, abdominal pain
	• **Rapid decline in renal function over weeks to months**
	• **Hematuria and edema**
	• <u>**Anti-GBM Disease**</u>:
	   • **Shortness of breath, cough, hemoptysis due to alveolar hemorrhage**
	• <u>Immune Complex Disorders or ANCA Vasculitis</u>:
	   • Fever, night sweats, weight loss, mucosal ulceration, dyspnea, cough, abdominal pain, palpable purpura

Diagnosis	• <u>**Urinalysis**</u>: **hematuria, red blood cell casts, dysmorphic red blood cells**, proteinuria
	• <u>Complete Blood Count (CBC)</u>: anemia usually present
	• <u>Serologic Testing</u>:
	   • <u>Anti-GBM Antibody Disease</u>: anti-GBM antibodies
	   • <u>Immune Complex RPGN</u>: antistreptolysin O antibodies, anti-DNA antibodies or cryoglobulins
	   • <u>Pauci-Immune RPGN</u>: antineutrophil cytoplasmic antibodies (ANCA) titers
	• <u>**Renal Biopsy: definitive diagnosis**</u>; focal proliferation of glomerular epithelial cells with numerous neutrophils forming a **crescentic cellular mass (crescents)**
	   • <u>Goodpasture Syndrome</u>: linear IgG deposits in glomerular basement membrane

Treatment	• Treatment varies by disease type • <u>**Corticosteroids + Cyclophosphamide or Rituximab**</u>: indicated for immune complex or pauci-immune RPGN • <u>**Plasma Exchange**</u>: indicated for anti-GBM antibody disease • <u>Renal Transplant</u>: effective for all types of RPGN; may recur after graft

Goodpasture Syndrome 🫘

Etiology & Risk Factors	• **Autoimmune syndrome characterized by alveolar hemorrhage and glomerulonephritis caused by circulating anti-glomerular basement membrane (anti-GBM) antibodies** • Also known as anti-GBM disease or Goodpasture's • <u>Etiology</u>: **environmental insult to genetically susceptible individual** • <u>Risk Factors</u>: medications (alemtuzumab), **drug use (smoking, cocaine)**, viral infection (influenza), occupational exposures (metal dust, organic solvents or hydrocarbons), **Caucasian**, age (bimodal distribution 20-30 years and 60-70 years old)
Patho-physiology	• Anti-GBM antibodies are directed against an antigen intrinsic to the glomerular/alveolar basement membrane in response to an inciting stimulus; autoantibodies activate the basement membrane complement resulting in tissue injury

Signs & Symptoms	• **Hemoptysis is predominant symptom**
	• **Cough, dyspnea, fatigue, fever, weight loss**
	• **Hematuria**
	• *Alveolar hemorrhage may precede renal manifestations by weeks to years*
	• <u>Physical Exam</u>:
	   • Clear lungs initially; **crackles and rhonchi auscultated as disease progresses** (alveolar hemorrhage)
	   • Peripheral edema (renal insufficiency)

Diagnosis	• <u>**Serum Anti-GBM Antibodies Test**</u>: **presence of antibodies confirms diagnoses**; methods include indirect immunofluorescence testing or direct enzyme-linked immunosorbent assay (ELISA) • <u>Antineutrophil Cytoplasmic Antibodies (ANCA) Test</u>: only positive in ~25% of patients with Goodpasture syndrome • <u>**Renal Biopsy: definitive diagnosis**</u>; focal segmental necrotizing glomerulonephritis with crescent formation and **linear IgG deposits in glomerular basement membrane** on immunofluorescent staining
Treatment	• <u>Secure Airway</u>: endotracheal intubation and mechanical ventilation indicated for patients with impending respiratory failure due to alveolar hemorrhage • <u>**Plasma Exchange**</u>: exchanges to remove anti-GBM antibodies; performed every other day until antibodies no longer detected • <u>**Corticosteroids + Cyclophosphamide**</u>: **prevents formation of new antibodies**
Key Words & Most Common	• Autoimmune syndrome characterized by alveolar hemorrhage and glomerulonephritis due to anti-GBM antibodies • Smoking most common precipitating factor • Hemoptysis • Hematuria • + anti-GBM antibodies • <u>Renal Biopsy</u>: linear IgG deposits in GBM • Plasma exchange + corticosteroids/cyclophosphamide

ANCA Vasculitis

Etiology & Risk Factors	• Acute nephritic syndrome characterized by microscopic glomerular crescent formation and rapid decline in renal function to end-stage renal disease (weeks/months)
	• <u>Etiology</u>: pauci-immune disorder; vasculitis characterized by absence of immune complex or complement deposition and + **antineutrophil cytoplasmic antibodies (ANCA)**
	  • <u>Granulomatosis with Polyangiitis (Wegener's)</u>: necrotizing vasculitis; + C-ANCA
	  • <u>Microscopic Polyangiitis</u>: vasculitis of small renal vessels; + P-ANCA

Patho-physiology	• Antineutrophilic cytoplasmic antibody (ANCA) antibodies cause small vessel inflammation resulting in necrosis and/or thrombosis of individual loops or larger segments of the glomerulus

Signs & Symptoms	• **Fatigue, fever, and weight loss**
	• <u>**Granulomatosis with Polyangiitis**</u>: involves upper and lower respiratory tracts and kidneys
	  • <u>Upper Respiratory</u>: bloody nasal discharge, **sinusitis**, chronic otitis media, **damage to nasal cartilage**
	  • <u>Lower Respiratory</u>: **alveolar hemorrhage** (cough, hemoptysis, dyspnea)
	  • <u>Renal</u>: **hypertension, oliguria, hematuria, proteinuria**
	• <u>Microscopic Polyangiitis</u>: necrotizing vasculitis of small vessels
	  • **Signs and symptoms of acute renal failure (oliguria, hematuria, abdominal/flank pain, edema)**

Diagnosis	• Antineutrophil Cytoplasmic Antibodies (ANCA) Titers:
	  • <u>**Granulomatosis with Polyangiitis (Wegener's)**</u>: + C-ANCA
	  • <u>**Microscopic Polyangiitis**</u>: + P-ANCA

Treatment	• <u>**Corticosteroids + Cyclophosphamide**</u>: utilized for 6-9 months to achieve remission • <u>Azathioprine</u>: maintenance of remission
Key Words & Most Common	• <u>Granulomatosis with Polyangiitis (Wegener's)</u>: necrotizing vasculitis; + C-ANCA • <u>Microscopic Polyangiitis</u>: vasculitis of small renal vessels; + P-ANCA • Fatigue, fever, weight loss • <u>GP</u>: upper/lower respiratory tract and kidney involvement • <u>MP</u>: necrotizing vasculitis • Corticosteroids + cyclophosphamide

Membranoproliferative Glomerulonephritis

Etiology & Risk Factors	• Immune-mediated disorder characterized by IgG and complements deposited beneath podocytes, glomerular basement membrane thickening and proliferative changes • <u>Etiology</u>: systemic immune complex disorders (**systemic lupus erythematosus, cryoglobulinemia**, Sjögren syndrome), infection (endocarditis, **hepatitis B/C**, HIV), cancer (leukemia, lymphoma, melanoma), sarcoidosis • <u>Risk Factors</u>: **Caucasian, age (30-50 most common), male**
Patho-physiology	• Circulating antibodies bind to intrinsic podocyte antigens causing activation of membrane attack complexes resulting in oxidative damage and DNA damage to podocytes leading to actin cytoskeleton damage resulting in loss of glomerular basement membrane and proteinuria

Signs & Symptoms	• **Presents with mixed nephrotic/nephritic picture**
	• **Signs and symptoms of nephrotic syndrome in 60-80% of patients**
	  • **Anorexia, malaise**
	  • **Frothy urine** (high concentration of protein in urine)
	• **Hematuria**
	• **Hypertension**
	• Renal insufficiency (oliguria)

Diagnosis	• <u>**Urinalysis**</u>: **initial test; demonstrates hematuria and proteinuria** (often in nephrotic range >3.5g/day) • <u>Serum Compliment Profiles</u>: usually decreased C3 and C4 • <u>**Renal Biopsy**</u>: **definitive diagnosis; subendothelial and mesangial immune complex deposits** • *Workup includes HIV, Hepatitis panel, ANA, Anti-DS DNA, ANCA, RF, C3, C4, and serum cholesterol levels to rule out secondary etiologies*

Treatment	• **Treat underlying etiology**
	• <u>**Hypertension Management**</u>: sodium restriction, ACEI/ARB, statins, and loop diuretics
	• <u>**Corticosteroids**</u>: prednisone indicated for children with nephrotic range proteinuria
	  • Treatment course includes prednisone on alternating days for 1+ years
	• <u>**Dipyridamole + Aspirin**</u>: indicated for adults
	  • Treatment course once daily for 1 year

Key Words & Most Common	• Immune-mediated disorder resulting in diffuse proliferative lesions and GBM thickening • Lupus, cryoglobulinemia, hepatitis B/C most common underlying etiology • 30-50 year old Caucasian males most common • Mixed nephrotic/nephritic picture • UA: hematuria, proteinuria (nephrotic range) • Corticosteroids in children • Dipyridamole + aspirin in adults

Henoch Schönlein Purpura

Etiology & Risk Factors	• Acute systemic immunoglobulin A (IgA) mediated small-vessel immune vasculitis of the joints, kidneys, gastrointestinal (GI) tract, skin, CNS and lungs • **Most common vasculitis in children (90% occur in children)** • Etiology: **often preceded by upper respiratory infection (Group A Streptococcus**, Coxsackievirus, parvovirus B19, adenovirus); other environmental or genetic factors • Risk Factors: **age (3-15 years old most common; most present before age 10)**
Patho-physiology	• Antigenic exposure from infection leads to IgA-antibody immune complexes to deposit in the small vessels of the skin, joints, kidneys, and gastrointestinal tract • Influx of pro-inflammatory mediators to specific site leads to clinical manifestations
Signs & Symptoms	• Symptoms may develop over days to weeks • **Rash: palpable purpura**; begins as erythematous/macular/urticarial wheals that progress into ecchymosis and petechiae; most common in lower extremities/buttocks • **Abdominal Pain**: acute pain described as diffuse and colicky; may have GI bleeding • **Arthritis**: migratory arthralgia; typically affects knees and ankles • **Glomerulonephritis**: azotemia (elevated BUN/creatinine), hematuria, proteinuria (frothy urine)
Diagnosis	• **Clinical Diagnosis** • Labs: may have elevated BUN/creatinine; normal PT/PTT and platelets (purpura secondary to vasculitis rather than coagulopathy • Urinalysis: hematuria, proteinuria, RBC casts • **Kidney Biopsy**: definitive diagnosis; shows mesangial IgA deposits and leukoclastic vasculitis; unnecessary if clinical diagnosis is clear
Treatment	• **Supportive: self-limiting disease**; hydration, NSAIDs for pain (if no renal involvement) • **Corticosteroids**: for severe arthralgias, abdominal pain, or renal insufficiency
Key Words & Most Common	• Acute IgA mediated vasculitis most commonly seen in children • Preceded by URI (GAS most common) • Rash (palpable purpura) + Abdominal pain + Arthritis + Glomerulonephritis • Clinical Diagnosis • Kidney biopsy for definitive diagnosis, rarely performed • Supportive care +/- steroids

Acute Kidney Injury

Etiology & Risk Factors	• Characterized by a rapid decline in renal function leading to accumulation of nitrogenous products in the blood (azotemia) with or without oliguria (reduced urine output)
	• Etiology:
	  • **Prerenal: inadequate renal perfusion**
	  • **Intrarenal: intrinsic kidney disease or damage**; may involve renal blood vessels, glomeruli, tubules, or interstitium
	  • **Postrenal: obstruction** in the voiding and/or collecting parts of the urinary system
	• Risk Factors: **radiocontrast agents, atherosclerosis**, chronic hypertension, chronic kidney disease, **NSAID use**, ACE/ARB, sepsis, hypercalcemia

Patho-physiology	• Etiology driven pathogenesis; acute tubular necrosis secondary to renal ischemia, tissue damage, or obstruction leads to effacement of brush border and cell death resulting in tubular cell dysfunction

Signs & Symptoms	• **Often asymptomatic until severe uremia develops**
	  • **Nausea, vomiting, fatigue**, weakness confusion, seizures, coma
	• **Symptoms related to underlying etiology**
	  • **Prerenal: hypotension, thirst, oliguria** (reduced urine output)
	  • **Intrarenal: flank pain, hematuria**, fever, cough, myalgias
	  • **Postrenal: alternating oliguria and polyuria; anuria**

Diagnosis	• **Acute kidney injury suspected with decreased urine output and/or rise in blood urea nitrogen (BUN) and creatinine**
	• Urine: urinalysis, urine sodium, urine creatinine, urine urea, urine protein, urine osmolality and urine sediment microscopy
	• **Basic Metabolic Panel: elevated BUN and creatinine**
	  • **BUN/Creatinine Ratio: >20:1 (prerenal); <12:1 (intrarenal); 12-20:1 (postrenal; normal range)**
	  • May have hyperkalemia, hyponatremia, hyperphosphatemia and hypocalcemia
	• **Renal/Bladder Ultrasound: imaging test of choice**; postvoid residual should be monitored
	• Abdominal CT: determines cause of postrenal failure; *avoid radiocontrast agents*

Treatment	• **Treat underlying etiology** • **Prerenal: IV fluid repletion to restore volume and renal perfusion** • **Intrarenal: varies based on cause** • **Postrenal: removal of obstruction** • **Dialysis: indicated for AEIOU, severe hyponatremia (Na<115mEq/L) or hypernatremia (Na>165mEq/L), creatinine >10 or BUN>100** • **Acidosis, Electrolyte abnormality (hyperkalemia), Ingestions (lithium, ASA, methanol, ethylene glycol), Overload (volume), Uremic pericarditis or encephalopathy**
Key Words & Most Common	• Rapid decline in renal function caused by inadequate renal perfusion (prerenal), intrinsic kidney disease/damage (intrarenal), or obstruction (postrenal) • Often asymptomatic until uremia develops (N/V, fatigue, weakness); symptoms related to underlying etiology • Oliguria + elevated BUN and creatinine • Treat underlying etiology

Prerenal Acute Kidney Injury

Etiology & Risk Factors	• **Prerenal acute kidney injury occurs due to decreased perfusion of nephrons** (*nephron structure still intact*) leading to a decreased glomerular filtration rate (GFR)
	• May lead to intrinsic injury (acute tubular necrosis) if not addressed
	• <u>Etiology</u>: **reduced renal perfusion is most common cause**
	  • <u>**Hypovolemia**</u>: **inadequate oral intake, vomiting/diarrhea**, hemorrhage, **diuretic use**, burns, third space sequestration of fluid
	  • <u>**Hypotension**</u>: sepsis, decreased cardiac output (heart failure, tamponade), **beta blockers, calcium channel blockers**, antihypertensives, valvulopathy
	  • <u>**Renal Artery/Small Vessel Disease**</u>: renal artery embolism or dissection, **renal artery atherosclerosis, efferent arteriole dilation (ACEI/ARBs), afferent arteriole vasoconstriction (NSAIDs, radiocontrast agents)**, microvascular thrombosis, hypercalcemia
	• Typically, does not cause permanent kidney damage unless hypoperfusion is severe and/or prolonged

Patho-physiology	• Renal hypoperfusion causes baroreceptor and heart receptors to increase sympathetic tone to maintain adequate perfusion; Hypoperfusions causes the afferent arteriole to increase renin and antidiuretic hormone secretion; afferent arteriole can maintain adequate perfusion until systolic BP drops to less than 80mmHg • Heart and brain perfusion is maintained resulting in vasoconstriction of renal circulation causing a decrease in glomerular filtration rate (GFR) • Hypoperfusion leads to enhanced reabsorption of sodium and water, resulting in oliguria with high urine osmolality and low urine sodium

Signs & Symptoms	• **Often asymptomatic until severe uremia develops**
	  • **Nausea, vomiting, fatigue**, weakness confusion, seizures, coma
	• **Symptoms related to underlying etiology**
	  • Hypotension, thirst, oliguria (reduced urine output)

Diagnosis	• **Acute kidney injury suspected with decreased urine output and/or rise in blood urea nitrogen (BUN) and creatinine** • <u>**Fractional Excretion of Sodium (FENa)**</u>: **low (<1%)** • <u>**Urine Sodium**</u>: **decreased (<20 mEq/L)** • <u>**Urine Specific Gravity**</u>: **high (>1.020)** • <u>**Urine Osmolality**</u>: **increased (>500 mOsm/kg)** • <u>**Urine Microscopy**</u>: **may show hyaline casts** • <u>**Basic Metabolic Panel**</u>: **elevated BUN and creatinine** • <u>**BUN/Creatinine Ratio**</u>: **>20:1**
Treatment	• **Treat underlying etiology** • **Fluid resuscitation with isotonic IV fluids (restore volume and renal perfusion) is mainstay of treatment**
Key Words & Most Common	• Decreased renal perfusion secondary to hypovolemia, hypotension or renal artery/small vessel disease • Hypotension, thirst, oliguria • FENa <1%; urine Na <20; urine specific gravity >1.020, urine osmolality >500 mOsm/L; BUN/Cr ratio >20:1 • Treat underlying etiology → isotonic fluid repletion

Intrinsic Kidney Injury Interstitial Nephritis

Etiology & Risk Factors	• **Decreased renal function as a result of injury or damage to renal tubules and interstitium characterized by interstitial inflammatory or allergic response**
	• <u>Etiology</u>:
	  • <u>**Medication Hypersensitivity**</u>: **most common cause**; antibiotics (**penicillins**, cephalosporins, fluoroquinolones, sulfonamides), **sulfa-based medications, NSAIDs**, PPIs
	  • <u>Infections</u>: bacteria (*E. coli, Campylobacter, Salmonella*, streptococci), viruses (HIV, EBV, CMV, measles, mumps, HSV), parasites (toxoplasmosis), spirochetes (syphilis)
	  • <u>Systemic Autoimmune Disorders</u>: sarcoidosis, Sjögren's syndrome, cryoglobulinemia, and systemic lupus erythematosus (SLE)
	  • Idiopathic

Patho-physiology	• Interstitial inflammation (nephritis) secondary to immunologic or allergic response within the interstitium results in tubular damage

Signs & Symptoms	• May be asymptomatic or non-specific symptoms (nausea, vomiting, malaise, flank pain)
	• <u>Triad</u>: **fever, rash, eosinophilia**
	  • **Fever (low-grade)**
	  • **Maculopapular skin rash**
	  • **Eosinophilia**

Diagnosis	• <u>Urinalysis</u>: **sterile pyuria and sub-nephrotic range proteinuria are most common findings**; **urine eosinophils** and microscopic hematuria may be present • **WBC casts** • <u>Serum IgE Levels</u>: may be elevated in some patients • <u>Renal Biopsy</u>: **definitive diagnosis**; interstitial edema, interstitial infiltration with lymphocytes, plasma cells, eosinophils and leukocytes; glomeruli are often normal
Treatment	• <u>Discontinuing Offending Medication</u>: spontaneous recover usually within 6-8 weeks after stopping medication • <u>Corticosteroids</u>: may improve renal recovery; T cell-mediated inflammation suppression mitigates fibrosis and renal damage
Key Words & Most Common	• Decreased renal function secondary to renal tubule or interstitium injury characterized by interstitial inflammation or allergic response • Medication hypersensitivity is most common cause; antibiotics, sulfa-based medications, NSAIDs • Triad: fever, maculopapular skin rash, eosinophilia • <u>UA</u>: sterile pyuria (WBC casts) + proteinuria • Discontinue offending medications

Intrinsic Kidney Injury Acute Tubular Necrosis

Etiology & Risk Factors	• Acute kidney injury characterized by acute destruction and necrosis of renal tubular cells of the nephron
	• **Most common type of intrinsic acute kidney injury**
	• Etiology:
	   • <u>Ischemia</u>: **most common cause; hypoperfusion as a result of hypotension or hypovolemia** (vomiting, diarrhea, hemorrhage, dehydration, burns, diuretics)
	   • <u>Nephrotoxins</u>: medications (**aminoglycosides**, amphotericin B, **radiocontrast media**, sulfa drugs, acyclovir, cisplatin, calcineurin inhibitors [cyclosporine], **NSAIDs**)
	   • <u>Sepsis-Induced</u>: systemic hypotension and renal hypoperfusion secondary to vasoconstriction
	• <u>Risk Factors</u>: **most common in hospitalized (ICU patients)**, preexisting chronic kidney disease, diabetes mellitus, preexisting hypovolemia, advanced age

Patho-physiology	• Afferent arteriolar vasoconstriction, backflow of glomerular filtrate, and/or tubular obstruction causes injury to the renal tubular epithelial cells resulting in decreased glomerular filtration rate (GFR) and eventual necrosis of the renal tubular cells of the nephron

Signs & Symptoms	• **Usually asymptomatic**
	• **Oliguria** (decreased urine output)
	• <u>Physical Exam</u>:
	   • Tachycardia, dry mucous membranes, decreased skin turgor, cool extremities, hypotension may indicate volume depletion
	   • **Fever and hypotension may indicate sepsis**

Diagnosis	• *Acute tubular necrosis must be differentiated from prerenal azotemia to guide treatment* • <u>Urinalysis</u>: urine microscopy may show hyaline casts or renal tubular epithelial/granular casts • Renal tubular epithelial cell casts and "muddy brown" granular casts as a result of sloughing of tubular cells into the nephron as a result of ischemia or toxic injury • <u>BUN/Creatinine Ratio</u>: 10-15:1; >20:1 seen in prerenal kidney injury • <u>Fractional Excretion of Sodium (FENa)</u>: **>2%**; <1% seen in prerenal kidney injury • <u>Urine Sodium Concentration</u>: **>40-50 mEq/L indicate acute tubular necrosis**; <20mEq/L seen in prerenal AKI • <u>Urine Osmolality</u>: **<450 mOsm/kg**; >500 mOsm/kg seen in prerenal kidney injury • <u>Urine Specific Gravity</u>: **<1.010**; >1.020 seen in prerenal kidney injury			

Test	ATN	Prerenal
BUN/Cr Ratio	10-15:1	>20:1
Urine Osmolality	<450	>500
Specific Gravity	<1.010	>1.020
Urine Sodium	>40	<20
FENa	>2%	<1%

Treatment	• <u>**Supportive Care**</u>: **remove offending agents and maintaining euvolemia (IV fluids) are first-line** • <u>Diuretics</u>: furosemide; may be utilized to maintain urine output in oliguric state but do not alter the course of kidney injury • <u>N-acetylcysteine</u>: antioxidant agent may be given in contrast-induced ATN; no proven benefit
Key Words & Most Common	• AKI characterized by necrosis of renal tubular cells secondary to ischemia (hypoperfusion), nephrotoxins (radiocontrast dye, NSAIDs, aminoglycosides) or sepsis • Most common in ICU patients • Asymptomatic → oliguria • Renal tubular epithelial cell casts and "muddy brown" granular casts; must differentiate from prerenal azotemia • Remove offending agent + IV fluids

Postrenal Acute Kidney Injury

Etiology & Risk Factors	• Disruption of normal urinary flow secondary to structural or functional obstruction; also known as **obstructive uropathy**
	• Etiology:
	   • **Tubular Precipitation**: medications (acyclovir, sulfonamides, methotrexate), uric acid, calcium oxalate (vitamin C toxicity, ethylene glycol), myoglobin
	   • **Ureteral Obstruction**: nephrolithiasis, ureteral tumors, congenital defects, **tumors**, ureteral trauma, constipation
	   • **Bladder Obstruction**: benign prostatic hypertrophy is most common cause, **prostate cancer**, paraphimosis, phimosis, urethral strictures, anticholinergic medications
	• <u>Risk Factors</u>: **age (>60 years old most common), males**, history of benign prostatic hypertrophy

Patho-physiology	• Obstruction results in increased urine back pressure in the renal collecting ducts leading to an increased glomerular pressure and reduced glomerular filtration rate (GFR) • Obstruction affects renal blood flow; initial increase in glomerular capillary blood flow and blood pressure secondary to reduced afferent arteriolar resistance; renal blood flow is subsequently reduced (after a few hours) due to increased renal vasculature resistance
Signs & Symptoms	• **Alternating oliguria and polyuria is pathognomonic of obstruction** • **Abdominal or flank pain** may be present dependent on level of obstruction • <u>Benign Prostatic Hyperplasia</u>: nocturia, dysuria, urinary urgency or frequency and decreased force of urinary stream • <u>Nephrolithiasis</u>: dull flank pain with sharp radiation to the lower quadrant or groin • <u>Prostate Cancer</u>: unintentional weight loss, night sweats and hematuria; nodular prostate on exam
Diagnosis	• **Acute kidney injury suspected with decreased urine output and/or rise in blood urea nitrogen (BUN) and creatinine** • <u>Basic Metabolic Panel</u>: evaluate blood urea nitrogen (BUN) and creatinine to assess kidney function • **BUN/Creatinine Ratio: 12-20:1 (postrenal; normal range)** • <u>Urinalysis</u>: rule out urinary tract infection; may show hematuria depending on underlying etiology • <u>**Renal and Bladder Ultrasounds**</u>: **initial imaging test to determine level of obstruction and evaluate for hydronephrosis** • CT scan, MRI, cystoscopy, or pyelography may be indicated depending on cause or site of obstruction
Treatment	• **Removal of obstruction is first-line** • <u>**Foley Catheter**</u>: **indicated for bladder obstruction** • Ureteral stents, drains or nephrostomy tube placement indicated for more complex obstruction • <u>Alpha Blockers</u>: tamsulosin, terazosin; indicated in cases of chronic urinary obstructive secondary to BPH (relaxes smooth muscle within the bladder neck and prostate)

Key Words & Most Common	• Disruption of urinary flow secondary to obstruction; benign prostatic hyperplasia is most common cause, nephrolithiasis, prostate cancer, tumors
	  Alternating oliguria and polyuria is pathognomonic
	• BUN/Cr ratio 12-20:1 (normal range)
	• Renal and bladder ultrasound initial imaging test
	   • Removal of obstruction (foley catheter)

Diagnostic Indices in Azotemia

Finding	Prerenal	Intrarenal	Postrenal
BUN (mg/dL)	↑↑	↑	↑
Creatinine (mg/dL)	↑	↑	↑
BUN/Cr Ratio	>20:1	<12:1	12-20:1
Fractional Excretion of Sodium	<1%	>1%	>1%
Urine Osmolality (mOsm/L)	>500	<350	<350
Urine Sodium (mEq/L)	<20	>20	>20
Fractional Urea Excretion	<35%	>50%	n/a
Urine Specific Gravity	>1.020	<1.010	Variable

Acute Kidney Injury Urinalysis

Description	Condition
Red blood cell casts, hematuria, dysmorphic red blood cells	**Acute glomerulonephritis (AGN)**, Vasculitis
"Muddy brown" granular casts or epithelial cell casts	**Acute tubular necrosis (ATN)**
White blood cell casts, pyuria	**Acute interstitial nephritis**, pyelonephritis
Waxy casts (acellular with sharp edges)	Narrow waxy casts: chronic acute tubular necrosis or glomerulonephritis Broad waxy casts: end stage renal disease (tubal dilation)
Fatty casts	**Nephrotic syndrome** (hyperlipidemia), hypothyroidism
Hyaline casts	Non-specific; normal health, fever, exercise, diuretics, renal disease
Normal or near normal urinalysis	Pre- or Post- renal acute kidney injury
Hematuria and pyuria	Urinary tract infection, pyelonephritis
Myoglobin	Rhabdomyolysis

Polycystic Kidney Disease

Etiology & Risk Factors	• **Autosomal dominant disorder** resulting in renal cyst formation which can cause gradual enlargement of both kidneys • **Multisystem progressive disorder resulting in renal cyst formation and enlargement and cysts of other organs** (liver most common, spleen and pancreas) • Etiology: autosomal dominant disorder due to gene *PKD1* (most common) or *PKD2* mutations • Risk Factors: family history, age (20-40 years old most common age of diagnosis)
Patho-physiology	• Polycystin-1 and polycystin-2 are proteins responsible for tubular epithelial cell adhesion and differentiation; mutation causes ciliary and tubular cell flow rate dysfunction • Polycystic kidney disease results in increased levels of cyclic adenosine monophosphate (cAMP) of multiple organs (kidney, liver) which exerts an effect on cellular proliferation
Signs & Symptoms	• Often asymptomatic (50%) • **Abdominal, flank and/or back pain is most common initial symptom** • **Pain due to enlargement of cysts, bleeding within cysts, urinary tract infection, nephrolithiasis** • **Hematuria** • **Hypertension** (increased diastolic blood pressure) • Extrarenal Manifestations: **cerebral aneurysms** (headache, nausea/vomiting, cranial nerve deficits), **hepatic cysts** (RUQ abdominal pain), **valvular disorders** (mitral valve prolapse), **diverticulosis** (LLQ abdominal pain)
Diagnosis	• Urinalysis: mild proteinuria, **microscopic or macroscopic hematuria**; pyuria may be present • Renal Ultrasound: **initial imaging test of choice**; shows cystic changes and enlargement of bilateral kidneys, may have "moth-eaten" appearance due to displaced tissue by cysts • Advanced Imaging: CT scan or MRI are more sensitive; MRI preferred to measure cyst and kidney volume • Genetic Testing: indicated for patients with family history, evidence of PKD and no family history, inconclusive imaging, young patients donating kidney
Treatment	• Supportive: indicated for asymptomatic or mild symptoms; **observation with periodic monitoring with ultrasound** • Flank Pain: must rule out infection, stone, and tumor • Lifestyle modification, avoidance of aggravating activities, cyst aspiration, tricyclic antidepressants (chronic pain syndrome) • Cyst Hemorrhage: self-limiting; modified bedrest, analgesia, **increased fluid intake (fluids inhibit vasopressin release)** • Urinary Tract Infection: trimethoprim-sulfamethoxazole or fluoroquinolone indicated for to prevent retrograde seeding of renal parenchyma • Nephrolithiasis: potassium citrate is the treatment of choice in stone-forming conditions (uric acid, calcium oxalate stones) • Hypertension: **angiotensin-converting enzyme (ACE) inhibitors or angiotensin receptor blockers (ARBs) are antihypertensive of choice** • Surgery: laparoscopic or surgical cyst fenestration if symptoms persist • Hemodialysis, peritoneal dialysis or kidney transplant indicated in patients that develop chronic renal failure
Key Words & Most Common	• Autosomal dominant disorder resulting in renal and multiorgan cyst formation (liver) • Abdominal, flank, back pain + hematuria + hypertension • Renal ultrasound • Symptom-based treatment + ACEI/ARBs indicated for hypertension + increase fluid intake (inhibit vasopressin release)

Chronic Kidney Disease

Etiology & Risk Factors	• Long-standing, progressive deterioration of renal function persisting for ≥3 months • **Defined as estimated glomerular filtration rate (eGFR) <60 mL/min/1.73m² or urinary albumin to creatinine ratio ≥30 mg/g** • <u>Etiology</u>: **diabetes mellitus is most common cause, hypertension is second most common cause**, glomerulonephritis, tubulointerstitial nephritis, cystic renal disease • <u>Risk Factors</u>: **advanced age**, males, **hypertension, diabetes**, obesity, smoking, **insulin resistance**, dyslipidemia, hyperuricemia NSAID use and non-Caucasian ethnicity
Patho-physiology	• Diabetic nephropathy and hypertension related nephrosclerosis causes renal insufficiency which disrupts the kidney's ability to maintain fluid and electrolyte homeostasis • Nephron destruction leads to hypertrophy of remaining nephrons resulting in decreased
Staging	• <u>Stage 0</u>: at-risk patients with normal GFR • <u>Stage 3</u>: GFR 30-59 • <u>Stage 1</u>: kidney damage (proteinuria, abnormal UA, elevated BUN/Cr) with normal GFR • <u>Stage 4</u>: GFR 15-29 • <u>Stage 2</u>: GFR 60-89 • <u>Stage 5</u>: GFR <14 (end-stage renal disease)
Signs & Symptoms	• May be asymptomatic early • **Anorexia, nausea, vomiting, weight loss, stomatitis, and an unpleasant (metallic) taste in the mouth are commonly present** • <u>Mild to Moderate Uremia</u>: **malaise, fatigue, anorexia, decreased mental acuity are early signs** • <u>Severe Uremia</u>: neuromuscular symptoms (muscle spasms and cramps, peripheral sensory/motor neuropathy, hyperreflexia, restless leg syndrome, seizure) • <u>Physical Exam</u>: • **Urea from sweat crystallizes on skin ("uremic frost")**; yellowish/brown, dry skin; dependent edema (renal retention of sodium and water)
Diagnosis	• <u>Basic Metabolic Panel</u>: **elevated BUN and creatinine**; electrolyte abnormalities (hyperkalemia, hyponatremia), hyperphosphatemia • <u>Urinalysis</u>: **proteinuria is best predictor of disease progression**; abnormal sediment; may have RBC/WBC casts, **broad waxy casts seen in end-stage renal disease** • <u>Urine Albumin/Creatinine Ratio (ACR)</u>: assesses degree of proteinuria with early-morning urine sample or 24-hour urine collection; graded A1-A3 • <u>**A1**</u>: ACR<30mg/g; <u>**A2**</u>: ACR 30-300mg/g; <u>**A3**</u>: ACR≥300mg/g • <u>Glomerular Filtration Rate</u>: calculated using CKD-EPI cystatin C equation • <u>Renal Ultrasound</u>: small kidneys with thinned, hyperechoic cortex is classic finding

Treatment	• General Management: address underlying etiology, adjust medication dose for eGFR, moderate dietary protein restriction (controversial)
	• <u>**Hypertension Management**</u>: **blood pressure goal <140/90mmHg; ACE inhibitors or ARBs** decrease the rate of GFR decline in patients with most causes of CKD
	• <u>Diabetes Management</u>: **hemoglobin A1c (HbA1c) goal of <7%**
	• <u>Hyperlipidemia Management</u>: dietary modifications + statin therapy
	• <u>Renal Osteodystrophy</u>: dietary restriction + phosphate binders with calcium containing (calcium acetate; calcium carbonate) or non-calcium containing (lanthanum, sevelamer)
	• <u>**Hypocalcemia and Vitamin D Deficiency**</u>: cholecalciferol (vitamin D_3) or ergocalciferol (vitamin D_2) and calcium supplementation
	• <u>**Dialysis**</u>: indicated with onset of uremic symptoms or inability to control fluid overload, hyperkalemia or acidosis with medications and lifestyle interventions
	  • <u>Non-Diabetics</u>: Indicated when eGFR is ≤10mL/min and/or serum creatinine ≥8mg/dL
	  • <u>Diabetics</u>: dialysis indicated when eGFR is ≤15 mL/min serum creatinine ≥6mg/dL
	• <u>Renal Transplant</u>: indicated when estimated GFR is ≤20mL/min

Renal Osteodystrophy

Etiology & Risk Factors	• Complications of end-stage renal disease that leads to skeletal and extra-skeletal manifestations
	• <u>Etiology</u>: **complication of chronic kidney disease and end-stage renal disease**; further classified into two categories
	  • High bone turnover states (osteitis fibrosa and **hyperparathyroidism**)
	  • Low bone turnover states (adynamic bone disease or heavy metal-induced osteomalacia)

Patho-physiology	• Retention of phosphate due to impaired renal elimination results in hypocalcemia and a compensatory increase in parathyroid hormone (secondary hyperparathyroidism) causing decreased bone mineralization by osteoclast activity • Low activated vitamin D_3 levels result in inability to convert vitamin D3 to its active form, calcitriol, resulting in further hypocalcemia
Signs & Symptoms	• Most are asymptomatic • **Symptoms in the setting of chronic kidney disease or renal failure** • **Bone and joint pain** • **Proximal muscle pain** • **Pathological fractures**

Diagnosis	• <u>Labs</u>:
	  • <u>Early Stage</u>: normal calcium and phosphate levels and increased parathyroid hormone
	  • <u>**Advanced Stage**</u>: decreased calcium, decreased calcitriol (vitamin D), elevated phosphate and elevated intact parathyroid hormone (secondary hyperparathyroidism), elevated alkaline phosphatase
	• <u>X-Ray</u>: **subperiostic bone resorption and periosteal erosions, chondrocalcinosis of the knee joint and pubic symphysis**, osteopenia, **bony cysts** with thin trabecula and cortex, punctate trabecular bone resorption of skull ("salt and pepper appearance")
	• <u>Bone Biopsy</u>: **definitive diagnosis; cystic brown tumors** (bone lesion that arising in setting of excess osteoclast activity)

Treatment	• <u>**Phosphate Binders**</u>: decreases phosphate; goal to maintain serum phosphate **<5.5 mg/dL** to suppress elevated parathyroid hormone levels • **Calcium containing (calcium acetate; calcium carbonate) or non-calcium containing (lanthanum, sevelamer)** • <u>**Vitamin D (Calcitriol) and Calcium Supplementation**</u>: vitamin D causes parathyroid hormone suppression resulting in osteoblast inhibition • <u>**Cinacalcet**</u>: utilized to lower parathyroid hormone levels by improving parathyroid calcium-sensing receptor sensitivity
Key Words & Most Common	• Complication of chronic kidney disease and end-stage renal disease • Bone and proximal muscle pain • ↓calcium, ↓vitamin D, ↑phosphate, ↑PTH, ↑alkaline phosphatase • X-Ray: subperiostic bone resorption, chondrocalcinosis, bony cysts, punctate trabecular bone resorption (skull) • Bone Biopsy: definitive diagnosis; cystic brown tumors • Phosphate binders; Vitamin D/calcium supplementation; cinacalcet

Horseshoe Kidney

Etiology & Risk Factors	• Fusion defect of the kidney characterized by fusion of one pole of each kidney (**lower pole most common**) • <u>Etiology</u>: no clear genetic cause • <u>Risk Factors</u>: **intrauterine exposures** (teratogenic drugs such as thalidomide, alcohol consumption and poor glycemic control), **chromosomal abnormalities** (Edward syndrome, Turner syndrome, Down syndrome); may be associated with other **congenital urologic abnormalities** (**ureteropelvic junction obstruction**, vesicourethral reflux)
Patho-physiology	• Renal parenchyma on both sides of the vertebral column is joined at the corresponding poles (lower pole most common) resulting in isthmus of renal parenchyma or fibrous tissue to join at the midline; ureters remain uncrossed from renal hilum to bladder as they course anteriorly over the isthmus • Obstruction generally occurs secondary to proximal insertion on the renal pelvis • **Complications include increased risk for pyelonephritis, nephrolithiasis and renal cell carcinoma**
Signs & Symptoms	• **Most are asymptomatic** • **Abdominal or flank pain** • **Hematuria** (secondary to urinary tract infection or nephrolithiasis) • **Hydronephrosis** (secondary to vesicourethral reflux or ureteropelvic junction obstruction)
Diagnosis	• <u>**Renal Ultrasound**</u>: imaging test to evaluate kidneys and potential complications • <u>Abdominal CT and MRI</u>: sensitive test to demonstrate anatomy and detect accessory vasculature and surrounding structures • <u>**CT Urography**</u>: best initial test to evaluate anatomy

Treatment	• <u>**Supportive**</u>: majority of cases do not require treatment
	   • Treat complications
	      • <u>Urinary Tract Infection</u>: antibiotics
	      • <u>Nephrolithiasis</u>: extracorporeal shockwave lithotripsy or percutaneous nephrolithotomy
	• **Surgery**: pyeloplasty relieves an uretero-pelvic junction obstruction if residual renal function is adequate

Key Words & Most Common	• Fusion defect of kidney characterized by fusion of one pole of kidney (lower most common) • <u>Complications</u>: pyelonephritis, nephrolithiasis, renal cell carcinoma • Asymptomatic → abdominal/flank pain + hematuria + hydronephrosis • Abdominal imaging (US, MRI, CT, CT Urography) • Supportive (treat complications) → surgery (pyeloplasty)

Hydronephrosis

Etiology & Risk Factors	• Obstruction of urine flow distal to the renal pelvis causing dilation and distention of the collecting system in unilateral or bilateral kidneys
	• <u>Etiology</u>: **urinary tract obstruction due to intrinsic (inside the ureter) or extrinsic compression (outside the ureter)**
	   • <u>Intrinsic</u>: **nephrolithiasis is most common cause, malignancy,** ureteropelvic junction stenosis, ureteral strictures, **benign prostatic hyperplasia**, neurogenic bladder
	   • <u>Extrinsic</u>: **pregnancy**, peripelvic cysts, **malignancy**, trauma, retroperitoneal fibrosis, prostate abscess

Patho-physiology	• Outward flow of urine is obstructed distal to the renal pelvis causes dilation and distention of the collecting system leading to an increase in hydrostatic pressure which can increase the intraglomerular pressure ultimately affecting the glomerular filtration rate
Signs & Symptoms	• **Mostly asymptomatic** • **Dull abdominal or flank pain** (stretching of the renal capsule + genitourinary peristalsis) • **Nausea and vomiting** • Urinary urgency, dysuria, **hematuria** • <u>Physical Exam</u>: • May have costovertebral angle tenderness *Hydronephrosis secondary to kidney stone*
Diagnosis	• <u>Urinalysis</u>: often normal; may show hematuria • <u>Basic Metabolic Panel</u>: used to monitor renal function; may have elevated creatinine • <u>**Renal Ultrasound**</u>: initial imaging test of choice; demonstrates **dilation/distention of collecting system** • <u>**Abdominal CT Scan**</u>: highly sensitive and specific test to evaluate **nephrolithiasis** or evaluate flank pain (able to visualize ureters)
Treatment	• **Treatment varies based on underlying etiology; goal is to remove obstruction** • <u>Urinary Catheter Placement</u>: indicated when lower urinary tract obstruction at the level of the bladder is suspected • <u>**Cystoscopy-Guided Ureteral Stent Placement**</u>: indicated for various intrinsic and extrinsic causes of hydronephrosis at the level of the ureter(s) • <u>Fluoroscopy-Guided Percutaneous Nephrostomy Tube Placement</u>: less invasive procedure performed when ureteral stent is contraindicated • <u>Extracorporeal Shockwave Lithotripsy</u>: indicated for large nephrolithiasis in the renal pelvis • <u>Surgery</u>: indicated for extrinsic compression from pelvic or retroperitoneal tumors and/or aortic aneurysms
Key Words & Most Common	• Urinary tract obstruction distal to renal pelvis; nephrolithiasis is most common cause • Mostly asymptomatic → dull abdominal/flank pain + nausea/vomiting + hematuria • Renal ultrasound • Treatment varies based on underlying etiology • Removal of obstruction

Renal Artery Stenosis

Etiology & Risk Factors	• Diminished blood flow to one or both kidneys as a result of stenosis (partial blockage) or occlusion (complete blockage) of the renal arteries
	• Etiology:
	   • <u>Stenosis</u>: atherosclerosis is most common chronic cause (90%) in elderly; fibromuscular dysplasia (10%) is most common in women 20-50 years old
	   • <u>Occlusion</u>: thromboembolism (atrial fibrillation, myocardial infarction, bacterial endocarditis) is most common acute cause; aortic dissection or renal artery aneurysm
	• <u>Risk Factors</u>: dyslipidemia, smoking, advanced age

Patho-physiology	• Obstruction of renal blood flow causes chronic ischemia leading to adaptive changes within the kidney such as collateral blood vessel formation and renin secretion; this activates the renin-angiotensin-aldosterone system leading to vasoconstriction, and sodium and water retention ultimately causing systemic hypertension

Signs & Symptoms	• <u>Stenosis</u>: may be asymptomatic for years
	   • **Suspect in patient with hypertension beginning at an atypical age (<30 or >50), severe hypertension, or hypertension refractory to multiple (3+) antihypertensives**
	• <u>Occlusion</u>: acute symptoms
	   • **Steady/aching abdominal or flank pain**
	   • Nausea/vomiting
	   • **Oliguria**, hematuria or anuria
	   • Hypertension is less common
	• <u>Physical Exam</u>:
	   • **Abdominal bruit** or signs of atherosclerosis

Diagnosis	• <u>CT Angiography</u>: highly sensitive, noninvasive, fast, widely available; caution with IV contrast (nephrotoxic) • <u>MRA</u>: highly sensitive, noninvasive, safe in patients with GFR>60mL/min • <u>Doppler Ultrasound</u>: highly sensitive, noninvasive; *no risk of contrast-induced nephropathy* • <u>Renal Catheter Arteriography</u>: gold-standard for diagnosis; provides details for surgical procedure but is a more invasive test

Treatment	• Stenosis:
	   • <u>ACE Inhibitor or ARB Therapy</u>: indicated for renovascular hypertension but may be ineffective if patency not restored; **contraindicated if bilateral stenosis or patients with solitary kidney**
	   • <u>Percutaneous Transluminal Angioplasty</u>: with stent placement or surgical bypass of the stenotic segment; indicated if creatinine >4.0, increased creatinine levels with ACE inhibitor therapy or >80% stenosis
	• Occlusion:
	   • <u>Fibrinolytic (Thrombolytic) Therapy</u>: streptokinase, alteplase; indicated if presenting within 3 hours of acute occlusion
	   • <u>Anticoagulation</u>: IV heparin + warfarin or non–vitamin K oral anticoagulants (dabigatran, apixaban, rivaroxaban) indicated in all patients with thromboembolic disorder
	   • <u>Surgical Revascularization</u>: embolectomy; indicated for severe renal failure that does not respond to medical therapy

Pyelonephritis

Etiology & Risk Factors	• Bacterial infection of the renal parenchyma causing inflammation of the kidneys • **Complication of an ascending urinary tract infection (UTI)** spreading from the bladder to the kidney(s) and the collecting systems • <u>Etiology</u>: bacterial infection secondary to fecal flora is most common cause, hematogenous spread, urinary tract obstruction • *Escherichia coli* is most common; *Proteus, Klebsiella,* and *Enterobacter* spp., *S. saprophyticus* • <u>Risk Factors</u>: female (shorter urethra in close proximity to anus), recent catheterization, urinary tract obstruction (tumor, nephrolithiasis), extremes of age, pregnancy
Patho-physiology	• *E. coli* has adhesive molecules (P-fimbriae) allowing the fecal flora to adhere to the urethral mucosal epithelial cells and ascend to the bladder through the urethra and to the kidneys through the ureters; inflammatory cytokines, bacterial toxins and other reactive processes cause pyelonephritis

Signs & Symptoms	• <u>Triad</u>: fever, flank pain, nausea/vomiting
	• <u>Upper Urinary Tract Symptoms</u>: fever and chills, flank pain, colicky abdominal pain, lower back pain/pressure, nausea and vomiting
	• <u>Lower Urinary Tract Symptoms</u>: dysuria, urinary frequency, urgency
	• <u>Physical Exam</u>:
	   • **Costovertebral angle tenderness**
	   • **Fever and tachycardia**

Diagnosis	• <u>Urinalysis</u>: initial test of choice
	   • Pyuria (≥8 WBCs/mcL), positive leukocyte esterase, nitrites (high specificity), hematuria, bacteriuria, cloudy urine
	   • <u>Microscopy</u>: WBC casts (indicate inflammatory reaction)
	• <u>Urine Culture</u>: definitive diagnosis; indicated in pyelonephritis to guide treatment
	   • Complicated cases in pregnancy, postmenopausal, men, children, recent instrumentation or catheterization, immunocompromised, recurrent urinary tract infections
	• <u>Labs</u>: indicated for seriously ill patient or sepsis
	   • CBC (leukocytosis with left shift), BMP (evaluate kidney function and electrolytes), blood cultures

Treatment	• <u>Outpatient Antibiotics</u>:
	   • Ciprofloxacin is first-line; trimethoprim-sulfamethoxazole is second-line; cephalexin, cefdinir, cefixime, levofloxacin are alternatives
	   • *Consider one dose of IV/IM of ceftriaxone or gentamicin if regional susceptibility to ciprofloxacin or TMP-SMX is <80%*
	• <u>Inpatient Antibiotics</u>:
	   • **IV ciprofloxacin, IV ceftriaxone**, IV cefotaxime, piperacillin/tazobactam
	• <u>Pregnancy Antibiotics</u>:
	   • **IV ceftriaxone is preferred antibiotic**, aztreonam if penicillin allergic
	   • Recurrence is common; *consider prophylaxis after resolution with single dose of nitrofurantoin 100mg or cephalexin 250mg at night for remainder of pregnancy*

Renal Cell Carcinoma

Etiology & Risk Factors	• Cancer originating in the **renal cortex (80%)**, **specifically the proximal convoluted renal tubule**, renal pelvis (8%), or parenchymal epithelium • **Most common primary malignant renal tumor (95%); clear cell is most common histological pattern** • <u>Etiology</u>: unknown • <u>Risk Factors</u>: **smoking, hypertension, advanced age**, obesity, chronic renal disease, **dialysis, males**, substance exposures (cadmium, herbicides, asbestos, trichloroethylene)
Patho-physiology	• Proximal renal tubular epithelium is the primary location in which renal cell carcinoma arises as these cells are very metabolically active and have high rate of cellular turnover leading to increased risk of dysplasia
Signs & Symptoms	• Most are asymptomatic until tumor >3cm • <u>Classic Triad</u>: **hematuria + abdominal/flank pain + palpable abdominal mass**; usually only seen in local advanced disease • **Hematuria, abdominal, back or flank pain, palpable flank mass**, fatigue, **weight loss**, anemia, fever, early satiety • **Hypertension**, hypercalcemia often present • <u>Physical Exam</u>: • **Palpable abdominal/flank mass**
Diagnosis	• <u>Urinalysis</u>: **hematuria** • <u>Labs</u>: CBC (**anemia**), serum calcium (**hypercalcemia**), liver function tests • <u>Renal Ultrasound</u>: **initial imaging test**; proceed to CT scan if solid mass or a complex cyst with septations or nodules present on ultrasound • <u>Abdominal CT Scan</u>: **most sensitive imaging test**; indicated if high suspicion or ultrasound negative with unexplained hematuria • Renal mass that is enhanced by radiocontrast strongly suggests renal cell carcinoma
Treatment	• <u>Radical Nephrectomy</u>: **standard treatment for localized renal cell carcinoma** • <u>Nephron-Sparing Surgery (Partial Nephrectomy)</u>: indicated in patients with bilateral involvement, chronic kidney disease, solitary kidney, or in early disease • <u>Systemic Therapies</u>: immune-mediated therapy (interferon alfa-2b, interleukin-2, monoclonal antibody molecular target treatment) are options; minimal long-term efficacy • <u>Palliation</u>: nephrectomy, tumor embolization, external beam radiation therapy and systemic therapy
Key Words & Most Common	• Most commonly originates at the proximal renal tubular epithelium of the renal cortex • Most common primary malignant renal tumor • Clear cell is most common histological pattern • Smoking + advanced age + male + hypertension • Hematuria + abdominal or flank pain/mass + weight loss • Renal ultrasound → abdominal CT scan • Radical nephrectomy is standard treatment

Nephroblastoma (Wilms Tumor)

Etiology & Risk Factors	• Embryonal renal cancer composed of blastemal, stromal, and epithelial elements • **Most commonly seen in children <5 years old**; most common renal malignancy in children and most common cause of abdominal mass in children • <u>Etiology</u>: unknown; genitourinary embryological development dysfunction • <u>Risk Factors</u>: **other congenital abnormalities (genitourinary) including cryptorchidism, hypospadias, horseshoe kidney; age (<5 years old most common)** • **WAGR Syndrome**: <u>W</u>ilms tumor, <u>A</u>niridia, <u>G</u>enitourinary malformations (renal hypoplasia, cystic disease, hypospadias, cryptorchidism) and mental <u>R</u>etardation
Patho-physiology	• Genetic alterations of the normal genitourinary embryological development; chromosomal deletion of *WT1* (a Wilms tumor suppressor gene) may be implicated
Signs & Symptoms	• **Painless, palpable abdominal mass is most common finding** • Abdominal pain, **hematuria, constipation**, nausea/vomiting, anorexia, fever • **Hypertension**
Diagnosis	• <u>Abdominal Ultrasound with Doppler</u>: **best initial imaging study**; determines if mass is cystic or solid and vascular involvement (renal vein or inferior vena cava) • <u>Abdominal CT or MRI</u>: **more sensitive imaging study**; determines tumor extent and spread to regional lymph nodes, contralateral kidney or liver • <u>Chest CT</u>: recommended to detect metastatic pulmonary involvement (lungs is most common metastatic site) • <u>Biopsy</u>: not usually performed due to risk of peritoneal contamination by tumor cells and increasing stage of cancer
Treatment	• <u>Total Nephrectomy followed by Systemic Chemotherapy</u>: treatment with greatest cure rate (80-90%) • <u>Partial Nephrectomy</u>: indicated in bilateral involvement • <u>Postoperative Radiation</u>: may increase overall survival; indicated based on tumor histology and extent of spread
Key Words & Most Common	• Most common in children <5 years old • <u>WAGR Syndrome</u>: Wilms tumor, aniridia, genitourinary malformation, mental retardation • Painless, palpable abdominal mass +/- hematuria, constipation, hypertension • Abdominal Ultrasound → abdominal CT/MRI • Total nephrectomy → systemic chemotherapy

Hyperkalemia

Etiology & Risk Factors	• Defined as a **serum potassium concentration >5.5 mEq/L**
	• Etiology:
	  • **Pseudo-Hyperkalemia**: **most common cause**; caused by hemolysis of RBCs in blood sample, occurs from prolonged application of tourniquet or fist clenching during blood draw, thrombocytosis or leukocytosis
	  • **Diminished Renal Excretion of Potassium**: acute or chronic renal failure inhibits renal potassium excretion
	  • **Reduced Aldosterone Secretion (Hyperaldosteronism)**: **ACE inhibitors/ARBs**, NSAIDs, heparin, antifungals (ketoconazole, fluconazole)
	  • **Aldosterone Inhibition to Mineralocorticoid Receptors**: **spironolactone, eplerenone, potassium sparing diuretics** (amiloride), trimethoprim
	  • Altered Transmembrane Potassium Movement: beta-blockers, digoxin, potassium supplementation, hyperosmolar solutions (mannitol, glucose), salt substitutes
	  • Intracellular Potassium Shifts: **metabolic acidosis (DKA)**, **insulin deficiency**, rhabdomyolysis from a crush injury, burns, excessive exercise, or other hemolytic processes

Patho-physiology	• The majority of potassium is excreted through the urine by the distal convoluted and cortical collecting ducts of the kidneys • Impaired renal function or oliguric states inhibits renal excretion of potassium
Signs & Symptoms	• Potassium levels affect muscle contractility and cardiac conduction; symptoms generally non-specific or asymptomatic until cardiac arrhythmias occur • Neuromuscular: **muscle weakness**, lethargy, **fatigue, paresthesia, paralysis** • Cardiovascular: **palpitations**, chest pain, **cardiac arrhythmias**, dyspnea • Gastrointestinal: abdominal distention, nausea/vomiting, **ileus** (intestinal muscle paralysis)

Diagnosis	• ECG: first test ordered in patient with suspected hyperkalemia; cardiac arrhythmias can be lethal
	  • **5.5-6.5**: **tall, peaked t-waves**
	  • **6.5-7.5**: flattening of p-waves, shortened QT interval
	  • **7-8**: widening of the QRS complex
	  • **8-10**: cardiac arrhythmias, sine wave pattern, asystole
	• Basic Metabolic Panel: **serum potassium >5.5 mEq/L**, evaluate renal function (BUN/creatinine)
	• Evaluate for Underlying Etiology: CBC (leukocytosis or thrombocytosis), glucose (hyperglycemia), bicarbonate (metabolic acidosis), creatinine phosphokinases and urine myoglobin (rhabdomyolysis), renal ultrasound (obstruction)

Treatment	• Mild Hyperkalemia (<6.0 mEq/L and no ECG changes):
	  • Decrease oral potassium intake or discontinue potassium-elevating medications; loop diuretics to increase renal excretion of potassium
	  • Recheck serum potassium level to rule out hemolysis from venipuncture
	• Moderate to Severe Hyperkalemia (>6.0 and/or ECG changes): require prompt attention to stabilize myocardium
	  • **Stabilize Cardiac Membranes**: intravenous **calcium gluconate** or calcium chloride; antagonizes hyperkalemic effect on cardiac muscle
	  • **Shift K+ Intracellular**: intravenous **insulin + glucose** infusion; high-dose **beta-2 agonists (nebulized albuterol)**
	  • **Remove K+**: IV loop diuretic (furosemide) + IV fluids; sodium polystyrene sulfonate (removes K+ via bowel movements; high risk of bowel perforation)
	• **Dialysis: definitive treatment**

Hyperkalemia ECG: V1, V2, V3, Peaked T waves, V4, Small or indiscernible P waves, V5, V6

Hypokalemia

Etiology & Risk Factors	• **Defined as serum potassium concentration <3.5 mEq/L**
	• Etiology:
	  • Decreased Potassium Intake: poor diet
	  • Gastrointestinal Tract Losses: **chronic diarrhea, laxative abuse, vomiting**, bentonite clay ingestion
	  • Intracellular Shift of K+: **insulin administration, metabolic alkalosis** (H+ ions leave cell as K+ enters), hypothermia, caffeine
	  • Renal K+ Loss: Cushing syndrome, hyperaldosteronism (increased mineralocorticoid activity), **hypomagnesemia** (low Mg^{2+} opens Mg^{2+} depending K+ channels), licorice
	  • Medications: **insulin, diuretics** (loop, thiazide, osmotic), amphotericin B, high-dose penicillin, laxatives

Patho-physiology	• Potassium is a predominantly intracellular cation involved in cell regulation and processes; extracellular potassium is in small quantities • Potassium homeostasis is maintained by acute cellular shifts between extracellular and intracellular fluid compartments, renal excretion and gastrointestinal losses • Sodium-potassium ATPase pump requires magnesium to function properly, therefore magnesium deficiency can lead to refractory hypokalemia
Signs & Symptoms	• Potassium levels affect muscle contractility and cardiac conduction; symptoms generally non-specific or asymptomatic • Neuromuscular: **severe muscle weakness**, muscle cramps, **hyporeflexia (decreased deep tendon reflexes), tetany, rhabdomyolysis** • Cardiovascular: **palpitations** (PACs/PVCs), hypotension, bradycardia or atrial/junctional tachycardia, AV block, ventricular tachycardia or fibrillation • Renal: **metabolic alkalosis, polyuria** (causes nephrogenic diabetes insipidus) • Gastrointestinal: nausea/vomiting, **paralytic ileus**
Diagnosis	• ECG: first test ordered in patient with suspected hypokalemia; cardiac arrhythmias can be lethal • **T wave flattening (initial change)**, followed by ST segment depression and an elevated, prominent U wave **(V4-V6)**; premature atrial/ventricle contractions • Basic Metabolic Panel: low serum potassium <3.5 mEq/L is diagnostic • Magnesium Level: hypomagnesemia often occurs with and may worsen hypokalemia; may promoted dysrhythmias such as torsades de pointes

Treatment	• **Potassium Repletion**: oral potassium chloride is first-line and mainstay of treatment
	  • Every 10mEq potassium chloride increases serum potassium by ~0.1mEq/L
	  • IV potassium chloride indicated for severe hypokalemia (<2.5mEq/L) or ECG changes; slow infusion due to risk of peripheral burning, venous sclerosis or phlebitis
	• **Magnesium Repletion**: oral magnesium salts or IV magnesium sulfate indicated for **hypomagnesemia**; difficult to replete potassium if patients are deficient in magnesium
	• Repeat ECG after treatment

Key Words & Most Common	• Serum potassium <3.5 • Chronic diarrhea, laxatives, vomiting, insulin administration, hypomagnesemia, diuretics • Severe muscle weakness and cramps, decreased deep tendon reflexes, palpitations • ECG: T wave flattening → ST depression → prominent U wave • May have concomitant hypomagnesemia • Potassium chloride +/- magnesium

ECG: Prominent U Wave, Depressed ST segment, Biphasic T wave

Hypermagnesemia

Etiology & Risk Factors	• **Defined as serum magnesium concentration >2.5 mEq/L**
	• *Hypermagnesemia is rare in the absence of renal insufficiency*
	• Etiology:
	    • <u>Decreased Renal Excretion</u>: **acute renal insufficiency or chronic kidney disease is most common cause**; hyperparathyroidism (altered calcium metabolism), **lithium**
	    • <u>Increased Intake</u>: iatrogenic (asthma, preeclampsia, torsades de pointes treatment), **excessive laxative or antacid use** (magnesium oxide), milk-alkali syndrome

Patho-physiology	• Magnesium is an effective physiologic extracellular and intracellular calcium channel blocker; intracellular magnesium inhibits several cardiac potassium channels • Most magnesium gets passively reabsorbed in the ascending limb of the loop of Henle; kidney maintains magnesium equilibrium until creatinine clearance is <20mL/min
Signs & Symptoms	• **Mostly asymptomatic** • <u>Mild Hypermagnesemia (<7mEq/L)</u>: **nausea and vomiting,** dizziness, confusion, somnolence • <u>Moderate Hypermagnesemia (7-12mEq/L)</u>: **decreased deep tendon reflexes, muscle weakness,** skin flushing, bladder paralysis, ileus or constipation (GI hypomotility), headache, bradycardia, mild hypotension, **respiratory depression** (diaphragmatic paralysis) • <u>Severe Hypermagnesemia (>12mEq/L)</u>: hypotension, bradycardia (calcium channel blocker-like effects), **conduction defects (heart block), paralysis,** cardiac arrest
Diagnosis	• <u>Serum Magnesium Level</u>: **>2.5mEq/L is diagnostic** • <u>ECG</u>: prolongation of the PR interval, widening of the QRS complex, increased T-wave amplitude

Treatment	• <u>Mild Hypermagnesemia</u>: in presence of normal renal function, discontinue source of magnesium (vitamins, laxatives, antacids)
	• <u>Severe Hypermagnesemia</u>:
	    • <u>Stabilize Cardiac Membranes</u>: **intravenous calcium gluconate** or calcium chloride; antagonizes hyperkalemic effect on cardiac muscle
	    • <u>Remove K$^+$</u>: **IV loop diuretic (furosemide) + IV fluids** promotes renal magnesium excretion
	• **<u>Dialysis</u>: definitive treatment**

Key Words & Most Common	• Serum magnesium >2.5 mEq/L • Acute renal insufficiency or chronic kidney disease is most common cause; lithium, excessive laxative or antacid use • Mostly asymptomatic • N/V → decreased DTR + muscle weakness + respiratory depression → hypotension, bradycardia, heart block, paralysis • ECG: PR prolongation, wide QRS, tall T-wave • Discontinue magnesium source → IV calcium gluconate +/- loop diuretic (furosemide) and IV fluids • Dialysis is definitive treatment

Hypomagnesemia

Etiology & Risk Factors	• **Defined as serum magnesium concentration <1.8 mEq/L**
	• Etiology:
	    • <u>Inadequate Intake</u>: poor diet, malnutrition, starvation, **alcohol use disorder, anorexia nervosa,** critically ill patient (total parenteral nutrition), cancer
	    • <u>Malabsorption</u>: celiac disease, inflammatory bowel disease, **alcohol use disorder** and **chronic diarrhea**
	    • <u>Medications</u>: **thiazide and loop diuretics, chronic proton pump inhibitor use (>1 year), aminoglycoside antibiotics,** amphotericin B, laxative abuse, digitalis
	    • <u>Magnesium Redistribution</u>: **insulin therapy (DKA treatment),** acute pancreatitis, **alcohol withdrawal syndrome,** refeeding syndrome
	    • <u>Increased Renal Loss</u>: alcoholism, **diabetes mellitus,** renal tubular acidosis, hypercalcemia
	    • <u>Endocrine Disorder</u>: hypoparathyroidism (PTH regulates calcium levels), hypocalcemia, hyperaldosteronism

Patho-physiology	• Magnesium affects other electrolytes including sodium, calcium, and potassium; magnesium homeostasis involves the kidney (proximal tubule, thick ascending loop of Henle, and distal tubule), small bowel (jejunum and ileum), and bone; renal and gastrointestinal losses or a particular drug or disease can alter this homeostasis

Signs & Symptoms	• *Neuromuscular hyperexcitation similar to hypocalcemia*
	• <u>Neurologic</u>: hypomagnesemia and hypocalcemia decrease the excitation threshold and increases neuromuscular excitability
	    • **Muscle cramps (back and legs most common),** mild encephalopathy (unexplained dementia, depression, psychosis), **increased deep tendon reflexes (hyperreflexia),** tetany, generalized seizures
	    • <u>Chvostek Sign</u>: **involuntary facial muscle spasm elicited with light tapping of facial nerve anterior to the exterior auditory meatus**; indicates latent tetany
	    • <u>Trousseau's Sign</u>: **carpal spasm induced by reduction of blood supply to hand** with tourniquet or blood pressure cuff inflated above systolic blood pressure (forearm)
	• <u>Cardiovascular</u>: congestive heart failure, **arrhythmias (QTc prolongation)**
	• <u>Gastrointestinal</u>: diarrhea, abdominal pain/cramping

Diagnosis	• <u>ECG</u>: **prolonged QT interval, prolonged PR interval, QRS widening,** peaked T waves (with mild to moderate deficiency), reduced T wave amplitude (with severe deficiency) • <u>Serum Magnesium Level</u>: **<1.8 mEq/L is diagnostic** • <u>Basic Metabolic Panel</u>: frequently occurs with other electrolyte disorders including **hypokalemia, hypocalcemia, and hypophosphatemia**
Treatment	• <u>Mild Hypomagnesemia</u>: **oral magnesium oxide** • <u>Severe Hypomagnesemia</u>: **IV magnesium sulfate** • *Concurrent hypokalemia or hypocalcemia should be addressed; these electrolyte disturbances are difficult to correct until magnesium has been repleted*
Key Words & Most Common	• Serum magnesium <1.8 mEq/L • Poor diet, malnutrition, alcohol use disorder, diarrhea, diuretics, prolonged PPI use, diabetes mellitus • Neuromuscular hyperexcitation similar to hypocalcemia; muscle cramps, increased deep tendon reflexes, weakness, Chvostek sign, Trousseau's sign, arrhythmias • ECG: prolonged QTc, prolonged PR, QRS widening • Frequently occurs with hypokalemia, hypocalcemia, hypophosphatemia • <u>Mild</u> : oral magnesium oxide • <u>Severe</u> : IV magnesium sulfate

Hypernatremia

Etiology & Risk Factors	• **Defined as serum sodium concentration >145 mEq/L**
	• <u>Etiology</u>: can be hypovolemic, euvolemic or hypervolemic
	   • <u>Hypovolemic Hypernatremia</u>: decreased total body water and decreased sodium level
	     • **Gastrointestinal losses (vomiting, diarrhea)**, skin losses (**burns**, perspiration), renal losses (intrinsic renal disease, **loop diuretics**, osmotic diuresis)
	   • <u>Euvolemic Hypernatremia</u>: decreased total body water and near-normal sodium level
	     • Extrarenal losses (tachypnea), skin losses (burns, **excessive perspiration, fever**), **renal losses (diabetes insipidus)**, inadequate water access (infants, elderly)
	   • <u>Hypervolemic Hypernatremia</u>: normal or increased total body water and increased sodium level
	     • **Hypertonic fluid administration (hypertonic saline**, sodium bicarbonate), mineralocorticoid excess (adrenal tumors or adrenal hyperplasia)

Patho-physiology	• Changes in the extracellular volume provides feedback to maintain sodium homeostasis by increasing or decreasing the renal excretion of sodium in the urine • Sodium excretion involves the renin-angiotensin-aldosterone system; when sodium increases, plasma osmolality increases to trigger the thirst response and ADH secretion

Signs & Symptoms	• **Thirst is the most common initial symptom**
	• <u>Central Nervous System Dysfunction</u>: primarily due to cerebral cell shrinkage in the setting of dehydration
	   • **Irritability and agitation**, confusion, disorientation, fatigue, nausea, vomiting, **muscle weakness**, seizures, coma, respiratory arrest
	• **Polyuria, polydipsia (diabetes insipidus)**
	• <u>Physical Exam</u>:
	   • **Doughy or velvety skin** (intracellular water loss), **hypotension, tachycardia**, increased muscle tone with brisk reflexes

Diagnosis	• <u>Serum Sodium Level</u>: **>145 mEq/L is diagnostic**; degree of symptoms vary with level of hypernatremia
	• <u>Urine Volume and Osmolality</u>: may help determine underlying etiology
	   • **Urine osmolality is increased (concentrated) if extrarenal; urine osmolality is decreased (diluted) if diabetes insipidus**
	• <u>Diabetes Insipidus</u>:
	   • <u>24-hour Urine Collection</u>: decreased osmolality, decreased urine specific gravity, increased urine volume
	   • <u>Water Deprivation Test</u>: confirms diagnosis; continued production of large amounts of dilute urine indicated diabetes insipidus

Treatment	• Identify and treat underlying etiology; goal of treatment is replacement of intravascular volume and free water
	• **Oral hydration is preferred initial treatment for hypernatremia**
	• Estimate water deficit necessary to replace with formula: free water deficit (L) = (0.6 x weight in kg) x ((serum Na^+/140) ÷ 1)
	• **Isotonic Fluid Resuscitation: 0.9% normal saline infusion until perfusion deficits corrected followed by 0.45% normal saline until urinary output >0.5 mL/kg/hr**
	   • **Goal is to correct at 0.5mEq/hr**
	   • **Rapid correction (>0.5mEq/hr) can result in cerebral edema caused by excess brain solute)**

Hyponatremia

Etiology & Risk Factors	• **Defined as serum sodium concentration <135 mEq/L**; patients often not symptomatic until <120meq/L
	• <u>Etiology</u>: can be hypovolemic, euvolemic or hypervolemic
	   • <u>Hypovolemic Hyponatremia</u>: decreased total body water and sodium (greater decrease in sodium)
	     • Extrarenal loss (**vomiting, diarrhea**, burns, pancreatitis, rhabdomyolysis, small bowel obstruction), renal loss (**diuretics**, ACE inhibitors, osmotic diuresis)
	   • <u>Euvolemic Hyponatremia</u>: increased total body water and near-normal sodium
	     • Medications (**thiazide diuretics**, NSAIDs, opioids), MDMA (ecstasy), disorders (Addison disease, hypothyroidism, **SIADH**), primary polydipsia, stress, nausea, pain
	   • <u>Hypervolemic Hyponatremia</u>: increased sodium level with greater increased total body water
	     • **Edematous states (congestive heart failure, cirrhosis)**, renal disorders (AKI/CKD, nephrotic syndrome)

Patho-physiology	• Three mechanisms involved in the inability of kidneys to excrete water leading to hyponatremia: high ADH activity (SIADH, cortisol deficiency), low glomerular filtration rate (GFR) impairs the kidney's ability to get rid of water, and low solute intake

Signs & Symptoms	• Patients with mild/moderate hyponatremia (>120 mEq/L) or gradual decrease in sodium (>48 hours) typically have minimal symptoms
	• **Central Nervous System Dysfunction: primarily due to cerebral edema**
	   • <u>Moderate Hyponatremia (>115mEq/L)</u>: **altered mental status, confusion, lethargy, disorientation**, fatigue, gait disturbances, falls, cognitive deficits
	   • <u>Severe Hyponatremia (<115mEq/L)</u>: neuromuscular hyperexcitability, nausea and vomiting, stupor, **hyperreflexia**, seizures, coma, death
	• **Symptoms of rapid correction of sodium may include congestive heart failure and osmotic demyelination syndrome (altered mental status, dysphagia, dysarthria, paresis)**
	   • Severe cerebral edema may occur in premenopausal women with acute hyponatremia (estrogen and progesterone inhibit brain Na^+-K^+-ATPase and decrease solute extrusion from brain cells)

Diagnosis	• **Step 1 – Serum Sodium**: serum sodium concentration <135 mEq/L • **Step 2 - Plasma Osmolality**: differentiates between hypertonic, isotonic, and hypotonic hyponatremia (true hyponatremia is hypotonic; hypotonia proceed to step 3) • **Step 3 - Urine Osmolality**: <100mOsm/kg indicates primary polydipsia; >100mOsm/kg usually indicates a high ADH state (>100mOsm/kg proceed to step 4) • **Step 4 - Volume Status**: hypovolemic vs euvolemic vs hypervolemic (if patient is hypovolemic proceed to step 5) • **Step 5 - Urine Sodium Concentration**: urine sodium <10 mmol/L indicates extrarenal loss of fluid (remote diuretic use and remote vomiting); urine sodium >20 mmol/L indicates renal loss of urine (diuretics, vomiting, cortisol deficiency)
Treatment	• Serum sodium concentration should be corrected no faster than 0.5mEq/L/hour and should not be increased >8mEq/L in first 24 hours • **Rapid correct of sodium causes osmotic demyelination syndrome (central pontine myelinolysis)** • **Hypovolemic Hyponatremia: 0.9% normal saline infusion** + treat underlying etiology • **Euvolemic Hyponatremia: water restriction** + treat underlying etiology • **Hypervolemic Hyponatremia: water restriction + loop diuretics (furosemide) +/- 0.9% normal saline infusion** • **Severe Hyponatremia (<115mEq/L): 3% hypertonic saline infusion +/- desmopressin (prevents overcorrection)**

Hypercalcemia

Etiology & Risk Factors	• **Elevated serum calcium** (total serum calcium concentration >10.4mg/dL or ionized serum calcium >5.2 mg/dL); normal serum calcium ranges from 8.5 mg/dL-10.5 mg/dL • Etiology: • <u>Primary Hyperparathyroidism</u>: **most common cause**; adenoma/hyperplasia of the gland, familial hypocalciuric hypercalcemia, multiple endocrine neoplasia (MEN) • <u>Malignancy</u>: renal carcinomas, leukemias, lymphomas, rhabdomyosarcoma • <u>Hypervitaminosis</u>: **vitamin A or D intoxication**; iatrogenic, excessive milk intake, granulomatous conditions (sarcoidosis, tuberculosis, fungal infections) • <u>Other</u>: thiazide diuretics, hyperthyroidism, thyrotoxicosis, acute/chronic renal failure, **lithium use**, prolonged immobilization
Patho-physiology	• Parathyroid hormone increases serum calcium by increasing intestinal absorption of calcium, mobilizes calcium by enhancing bone resorption, enhancing renal distal nephron calcium reabsorption and stimulating conversion of vitamin D to calcitriol (most active form)
Signs & Symptoms	• *Most patients are asymptomatic* • **Mnemonic: Stones, Bones, Groans, Moans, Thrones, Psychic Overtones** • <u>Stones</u>: nephrolithiasis (calcium oxalate and phosphate) • <u>Bones</u>: **bone pain, skeletal muscle weakness**, osteoporosis, osteomalacia, arthritis and pathological fractures • <u>Groans</u>: **abdominal pain, nausea/vomiting, constipation, ileus**, dehydration, pancreatitis • <u>Moans</u>: fatigue, malaise, depression, anxiety, **cognitive dysfunction** • <u>Thrones</u>: **polyuria, polydipsia, nocturia** • <u>Psychic Overtones</u>: **lethargy, confusion, delirium, psychosis, memory loss**, hallucinations, stupor, coma
Diagnosis	• *Workup includes serum PTH, calcitonin, Vitamin D, ionized calcium, phosphorus, magnesium, alkaline phosphatase levels, renal functions, and urinary calcium-creatinine ratio* • <u>Total Serum and Ionized Calcium Level</u>: **increased serum calcium concentration (>10.4mg/dL) or ionized serum calcium >5.2mg/dL; ionized is more accurate than total** • <u>Intact Parathyroid Hormone (PTH)</u>: differentiates PTH-mediated hypercalcemia (PTH levels are high or high-normal); ordered once hypercalcemia is confirmed • <u>Parathyroid-Related Peptide</u>: ordered if intact PTH is normal or low to rule out malignancy (humoral hypercalcemia of cancer) • <u>Imaging</u>: **CXR** (evaluate for granulomatous disorders, lung cancer, lytic lesions of bone), mammogram (breast cancer), CT, (renal cancer) US/MRI of parathyroid hormones • <u>Electrocardiogram (ECG)</u>: **T wave flattening/inversion, shortened QT interval, prolonged PR interval, QRS widening**
Treatment	• <u>Asymptomatic or Ca <12mg/dL</u>: **no immediate treatment required**, avoid aggravating factors (thiazide diuretics, lithium, volume depletion, prolonged inactivity, high Ca diet) • <u>Mild Symptoms or Ca 12-14mg/dL</u>: **adequate water intake** (promotes Ca excretion), **oral phosphate** (binds to calcium and prevents absorption) • <u>Moderate/Severe</u>: • **IV Fluids + Loop Diuretics: initial management of choice**; isotonic fluids + IV loop diuretics (furosemide) promote calcium excretion; *avoid thiazide diuretics* • **Bisphosphonates: zoledronic acid or pamidronate; inhibit osteoclasts**; drug of choice for cancer-associated hypercalcemia • <u>Calcitonin</u>: adjunct for malignancy-related hypercalcemia; quicker onset of action than bisphosphonates; may be combined with corticosteroids • <u>Denosumab</u>: adjunct for malignancy-related hypercalcemia; monoclonal antibody inhibitor of osteoclastic activity • <u>Corticosteroids</u>: prednisone decreases calcitriol production and intestinal calcium absorption; indicated in vitamin D toxicity and granulomatous conditions (sarcoidosis)

Hypocalcemia

Etiology & Risk Factors	• **Low calcium serum calcium** (total serum calcium concentration <8.8mg/dL or serum ionized calcium concentration <4.7mg/dL) • <u>Fraction</u>: 45% is in free or ionized state (regulated by vitamin D, PTH), 40% bound to plasma proteins (albumin), 15% bound to anions (phosphate, lactate, citrate) • <u>Etiology</u>; **hypoparathyroidism is most common cause overall (autoimmune disorders or accidental removal/damage to parathyroid glands during thyroidectomy), vitamin D deficiency, chronic renal disease** (abnormal renal loss of calcium and decreased renal conversion of vitamin D to active form), **hypomagnesemia**, hyperphosphatemia, hypoalbuminemia, medications (**loop diuretics**, bisphosphonates, phenytoin, phenobarbital, rifampin), pancreatitis
Patho-physiology	• Parathyroid hormone enhances osteoclastic bone resorption and distal tubular reabsorption of calcium, stimulates hydroxylation of 25 hydroxyvitamin D to the active form (1,25-dihydroxy vitamin D); vitamin D stimulates intestinal absorption of calcium, renal absorption of calcium and bone reabsorption; deficiency leads to hypocalcemia
Signs & Symptoms	• *Most patients are asymptomatic* • **Neurologic: hypocalcemia decreases excitation threshold and increases neuromuscular excitability** • **Muscle cramps (back and legs most common)**, mild encephalopathy (unexplained dementia, depression, psychosis), **increased deep tendon reflexes** (hyperreflexia), laryngospasm, **bronchospasm, finger or circumoral paresthesia**, tetany, generalized seizures • **Chvostek Sign: involuntary facial muscle spasm elicited with light tapping of facial nerve anterior to the exterior auditory meatus**; indicates latent tetany • **Trousseau's Sign: carpal spasm induced by reduction of blood supply to hand** with tourniquet or blood pressure cuff inflated above systolic blood pressure (forearm) • <u>Cardiovascular</u>: congestive heart failure, **arrhythmias (QTc prolongation)** • <u>Cutaneous</u>: **dry and scaly skin, brittle nails, coarse hair**, recurrent *Candida* infections • <u>Gastrointestinal</u>: diarrhea, abdominal pain/cramping • <u>Skeletal</u>: abnormal dentition, osteomalacia, osteodystrophy
Diagnosis	• *Workup includes serum PTH, calcitonin, Vitamin D, ionized calcium, phosphorus, magnesium, alkaline phosphatase levels, renal functions, and urinary calcium-creatinine ratio* • <u>Total Serum and Ionized Calcium Level</u>: **decreased total serum calcium concentration (<8.8 mg/dL) or ionized serum calcium (<4.7 mg/dL); ionized calcium is more accurate** • <u>Serum Albumin Level</u>: ordered to correct the total calcium or directly measure the ionized calcium level • **Corrected Ca = [0.8 x (normal albumin - patient's albumin)] + serum Ca level** • <u>Electrocardiogram (ECG)</u>: prolonged QT interval
Treatment	• <u>Asymptomatic or Mild</u>: **oral calcium gluconate + vitamin D (calcitriol)** • <u>Symptomatic or Severe</u>: **IV calcium gluconate**; 10mL of 10% solution infused over 10 minutes • <u>Hypomagnesemia</u>: **IV magnesium sulfate** followed by oral magnesium gluconate to correct hypomagnesemia • *Avoid phenothiazine antipsychotics (may precipitate extrapyramidal symptoms); avoid furosemide (worsens hypocalcemia)*
Key Words & Most Common	• Hypoparathyroidism is most common cause • Muscle cramps + finger/oral paresthesia + hyperreflexia + Chvostek sign (facial spasm by tapping facial nerve) + Trousseau's Sign (carpal spasm with inflation of BP cuff) • ↓ total serum calcium or ionized calcium; ECG shows prolonged QT interval • <u>Mild</u>: oral calcium gluconate + vitamin D (calcitriol) • <u>Severe</u>: IV calcium gluconate

Hyperphosphatemia

Etiology & Risk Factors	• Defined as serum phosphate concentration >4.5mg/dL
	• Etiology:
	  • **Decreased Renal Excretion: severe renal insufficiency or chronic kidney disease is most common cause; hypoparathyroidism** and parathyroid suppression due to hypercalcemia (from excess exogenous vitamin A or D intake)
	  • Transcellular Shifts: tumor lysis syndrome, rhabdomyolysis, crush injuries, diabetic ketoacidosis
	  • Excessive Phosphate Intake: **laxative abuse**, oral consumption

Patho-physiology	• Hyperphosphatemia plays a critical role in the development of secondary hyperparathyroidism and thus increased calcium level which can lead to **calcium precipitation into soft tissues** especially when levels are chronically elevated in the setting of chronic kidney disease • Soft-tissue calcification in the skin is one etiology of excessive pruritis experienced by patients with end-stage renal disease

Signs & Symptoms	• **Most patients are asymptomatic**
	• **Symptomatic hypocalcemia** (due to calcium-phosphate precipitation in the tissues)
	  • **Fatigue**, dyspnea, anorexia, nausea/vomiting, insomnia, muscle weakness, **muscle cramps, tetany, neuromuscular hyperexcitability, hyperreflexia**
	• Prolonged bone demineralization can lead to pathological bone fractures
	• Physical Exam:
	  • **Soft-tissue calcifications** (palpable, hard, subcutaneous nodules often with overlying excoriation from scratching)
	  • Systolic hypertension, widened pulse pressure and left ventricular hypertrophy (vascular calcification and arteriosclerosis)

Diagnosis	• Serum Phosphate Level: >4.5mg/dL is diagnostic • Workup includes basic metabolic panel (BUN/creatinine), vitamin D, serum calcium and magnesium level (hypocalcemia/hypomagnesemia) and PTH level
Treatment	• *Treat underlying etiology* • **Restrict phosphate consumption** (dietary restrictions, discontinue phosphate-containing laxatives) is mainstay of treatment • **IV 0.9% normal saline (if no renal insufficiency)** • **Phosphate Binders: decreases phosphate;** goal to maintain serum phosphate **<5.5 mg/dL** to suppress elevated parathyroid hormone levels • **Calcium containing (calcium acetate; calcium carbonate) or non-calcium containing (sevelamer)** • Dialysis: definitive treatment
Key Words & Most Common	• Serum phosphate >4.5mg/dL • Decreased renal excretion secondary to renal insufficiency or chronic kidney disease most common cause • Asymptomatic → symptomatic hypocalcemia (muscle cramps, neuromuscular hyperexcitability, hyperreflexia) +/- soft tissue calcifications • Phosphate restriction → IV 0/9% normal saline → phosphate binders (calcium acetate/carbonate or sevelamer) → dialysis

Hypophosphatemia

Etiology & Risk Factors	• **Defined as serum phosphate concentration <2.5mg/dL**
	• Etiology:
	  • **Acute: transcellular shifts of phosphate** (superimposed on chronic phosphate depletion) is most common cause
	    • Recovery phase of DKA, **acute alcohol use disorder, refeeding syndrome (after prolonged malnutrition)**, severe burns, severe respiratory alkalosis
	  • **Chronic: decreased renal phosphate reabsorption**
	    • **Hyperparathyroidism**, Cushing syndrome, hypothyroidism, **vitamin D deficiency**, electrolyte disorders (hypokalemia, hypomagnesemia), **diuretic use, antacids**

Patho-physiology	• Hypophosphatemia occurs secondary to inadequate phosphate intake, increased phosphate excretion and shift from extracellular phosphate into the intracellular space • Refeeding syndrome occurs when a malnourished patient has sudden replenishment of carbohydrates, proteins and lipids; insulin and glucose drive phosphate intracellularly • Phosphate provides an energy source for molecular functions with its role in adenosine triphosphate (ATP); **deficiency causes ATP depletion**
Signs & Symptoms	• **Most patients are asymptomatic** • Neuromuscular Dysfunction: **anorexia, muscle weakness, circumoral and fingertip paresthesia, decreased deep tendon reflexes**, decreased mental status, flaccid paralysis • Progressive encephalopathy, seizures, coma, death • Cardiovascular Dysfunction: systolic heart failure (myocytes are less stable), arrhythmias, hypoventilation (decreased diaphragmatic function) • Gastrointestinal Dysfunction: dysphagia, ileus
Diagnosis	• Serum Phosphate Level: **<2.5mg/dL is diagnostic** • 24-hour Urine Collection: determine renal phosphate excretion • Workup includes basic metabolic panel (BUN/creatinine), vitamin D level, serum calcium and magnesium level and PTH level (hyperparathyroidism)

Treatment	• *Treat underlying etiology*
	• **Oral Phosphate Replacement: oral sodium phosphate or potassium phosphate is first-line treatment (may cause diarrhea)**
	  • 1L of milk provides 1g of phosphate and may be more acceptable
	• Intravenous Phosphate Replacement: indicated when phosphate <1.0mg/dL, rhabdomyolysis or CNS symptoms present, or oral replacement contraindicated
	  • IV administration of potassium phosphate

Key Words & Most Common	• Serum phosphate <2.5mg/dL • Acute alcohol disorder, refeeding syndrome, hyperparathyroidism, vitamin D deficiency, antacid and diuretic use • Asymptomatic → neuromuscular dysfunction (anorexia, weakness, paresthesia, decreased DTR) • Oral phosphate replacement (oral sodium phosphate or potassium phosphate)

Acid-Base Approach

1. Check pH (normal pH 7.35-7.45)
   - Acidosis if pH < 7.35
   - Alkalosis if pH >7.45
2. Check pCO_2 (normal pCO_2 35-45)
   - Respiratory if pCO_2 and pH are in the *opposite* direction
   - Compensation if pCO_2 and pH are in the *same* direction
3. Check HCO_3^- (normal HCO_3^- 22-26)
   - Metabolic if HCO_3^- and pH are in the *same* direction
4. If metabolic acidosis present, calculate anion gap
   - Anion Gap (AG) = $Na^+ - (Cl^- + HCO_3^-)$
5. If high anion gap, calculate delta gap to determines if concomitant metabolic alkalosis
   - Delta Gap = (Anion Gap – 12) + HCO_3^- ; concomitant metabolic alkalosis if delta gap > 28
6. <u>Winter's Formula</u>: determines if appropriate respiratory compensation or if a second acid-base disorder is present
   - pCO_2 (expected) = (1.5 x [HCO_3^-] + 8) ± 2
     - If pCO_2 > pCO_2 expected, there is primary respiratory acidosis present
     - If pCO_2 < pCO_2 expected, there is primary respiratory alkalosis present

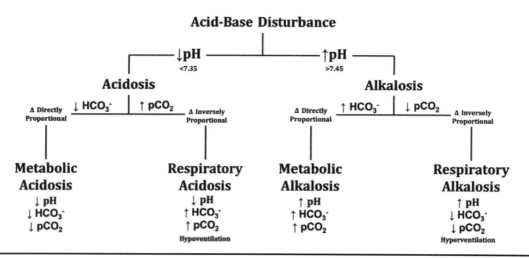

	Acidosis	Alkalosis
Respiratory pCO_2 = 40 (35-45)	↑ pCO_2 >45	↓ pCO_2 <35
Metabolic HCO_3^- = 24 (22-26)	↓ HCO_3^- <22	↑ HCO_3^- >26

↓pH Acidosis
↑pH Alkalosis
then...
Compare pH to pCO_2
<u>ROME</u>
<u>R</u>espiratory = <u>O</u>pposite
<u>ROME</u>
<u>M</u>etabolic = <u>E</u>qual (same direction)

Metabolic Acidosis

Etiology & Risk Factors	• Clinical disturbance defined by a pH <7.35 and a bicarbonate (HCO_3^-) level <24mEq/L
	• <u>Etiology</u>: classification based on the presence or absence of an anion gap; **Anion Gap = Na+ – (Cl^- + HCO_3^-)**; *normal anion gap is 10-12*
	  • <u>Non-Anion Gap</u>: HARDUPS: <u>H</u>yperalimentation, **Acetazolamide**, <u>R</u>enal tubular acidosis, <u>D</u>iarrhea, <u>U</u>retero-pelvic shunt, <u>P</u>ost-hypocapnia, <u>S</u>pironolactone
	    • Gastrointestinal loss (diarrhea), or impaired renal acid secretion (acetazolamide, renal tubular acidosis) are most common causes
	  • <u>Anion Gap</u>: CAT MUDPILERS; <u>C</u>yanide/<u>C</u>arbon monoxide poisoning, <u>A</u>rsenic, <u>T</u>oluene, <u>M</u>ethanol, <u>U</u>remia, **DKA**, **Propylene glycol**, <u>I</u>ron/<u>I</u>soniazid/<u>I</u>nfection, **Lactic acidosis**, <u>E</u>thylene glycol, <u>R</u>habdomyolysis/<u>R</u>enal failure, <u>S</u>alicylates
	    • Ketoacidosis, lactic acidosis, and renal failure are most common causes

Patho-physiology	• Hydrogen ion concentration is determined by acid ingestion, production, excretion, and renal and gastrointestinal bicarbonate losses; bicarbonate minimizes pH alterations • <u>Non-Anion Gap</u>: excessive loss of HCO_3^- replaced by Cl^-; inability to excrete H^+ • <u>Anion Gap</u>: addition of exogenous acids or creation of endogenous acid in pathologic settings (DKA, uremia, lactic acidosis)
Signs & Symptoms	• **Symptoms are primarily those of the underlying disorder** • <u>Mild Acidemia</u>: **often asymptomatic** • <u>Moderate Acidemia</u>: **nausea, vomiting**, malaise, **hyperpnea (long, deep breaths at a normal rate)** due to a compensatory increase in alveolar ventilation (no dyspnea) • <u>Severe Acidemia</u>: **cardiac dysfunction**, impaired cardiac contractility, **arteriolar dilation, venoconstriction (hypotension), ventricular arrhythmias**, shock, coma

Diagnosis	• <u>Step 1 - Arterial Blood Gas</u>:
	  • **Metabolic Acidosis when pH <7.35 and bicarbonate (HCO_3^-) level <24mEq/L**
	• <u>Step 2 - Anion Gap Calculation</u>: **determine if anion gap**
	  • Anion Gap = Na+ – (Cl^- + HCO_3^-)
	• <u>Step 3 - Delta Gap</u>: **determines if concomitant metabolic alkalosis**
	  • Delta Gap = (Anion Gap – 12) + HCO_3^-; concomitant metabolic alkalosis if delta gap > 28
	• <u>Step 4 - Winter's Formula</u>: **determines if appropriate respiratory compensation or if a second acid-base disorder is present**
	  • pCO₂ (expected) = (1.5 x [HCO_3^-] + 8) ± 2 ; *in an acute setting pCO₂ should decrease by 1 mmHg for every 1 mEq decrease in HCO_3^-*
	    • **If pCO₂ > pCO₂ expected, there is primary respiratory acidosis present**
	    • **If pCO₂ < pCO₂ expected, there is primary respiratory alkalosis present**
	• <u>Basic Metabolic Panel</u>: evaluate electrolytes

Treatment	• **Treatment is directed at underlying disorder** • <u>Hemodialysis</u>: indicated for renal failure and some cases of ethylene glycol, methanol and salicylate intoxication • <u>Sodium Bicarbonate</u>: consider when HCO_3^- <4mEq/L, pH<7.2 with shock or cardiac dysfunction, severe hyperchloremic acidemia • Controversial due to assumed risks

Metabolic Alkalosis

Etiology & Risk Factors	• **Clinical disturbance defined by a pH >7.45 and a bicarbonate (HCO_3^-) level >24mEq/L**
	• <u>Etiology</u>:
	  • <u>Excess Loss of H^+</u>: **gastric losses (vomit, nasogastric suction, chronic diarrhea)**
	  • <u>Increased Bicarbonate</u>: excess enteral bicarbonate or alkali intake (milk-alkali syndrome) or increased parenteral citrate or acetate intake; increased renal absorption
	    • Severe hypokalemia, primary hyperaldosteronism, Cushing syndrome, toxic ingestion of licorice
	  • <u>Diuretic Induced</u>: **loop and thiazide diuretics** block sodium and chloride reabsorption leading to increased bicarbonate absorption at the proximal tubule
	  • <u>CLEVER PD</u>: <u>C</u>ontraction, <u>L</u>icorice, <u>E</u>ndo (Conn/Cushing), <u>V</u>omiting, <u>E</u>xcess alkali, <u>R</u>efeeding alkalosis, <u>P</u>ost-hypercapnia, <u>D</u>iuretics

Patho-physiology	• Intracellular shift, gastrointestinal loss or excessive renal loss of H^+ or retention/addition of bicarbonate ions leads to the net increase in bicarbonate levels in the blood • Large volume gastric loss (vomiting, NG suction) correlates with a loss of hydrogen chloride (acid) leading to a relative increased bicarbonate level in the blood, driving alkalosis • Thiazide and loop diuretics induce secondary hyperaldosteronism by increasing sodium and fluid load to distal nephron, activating the renin-angiotensin-aldosterone system

Signs & Symptoms	• **Symptoms are primarily those of the underlying disorder**
	• **Symptoms often vague and nonspecific and usually result from contaminant hypocalcemia and hypokalemia**
	• <u>Hypocalcemia Symptoms</u>: severe alkalemia increases protein binding of ionized calcium (Ca^{2+})
	  • Fatigue, headache, dyspnea, anorexia, nausea/vomiting, insomnia, muscle weakness, **muscle cramps, tetany, neuromuscular hyperexcitability, hyperreflexia**, seizures
	• <u>Hypokalemia Symptoms</u>: hypovolemia can lead to potassium depletion
	  • Muscle weakness and cramps, decreased deep tendon reflexes, palpitations

Diagnosis	• <u>Step 1 - Arterial Blood Gas</u>:
	  • **Metabolic Alkalosis when pH >7.45 and bicarbonate (HCO_3^-) level >24mEq/L**
	• <u>Step 2 - Anion Gap Calculation</u>: **determine if anion gap**
	  • Anion Gap = Na+ – (Cl^- + HCO_3^-)
	• <u>Step 3- Winter's Formula</u>: **determines if appropriate respiratory compensation or if a second acid-base disorder is present**
	  • pCO₂ (expected) = (1.5 x [HCO_3^-] + 8) ± 2
	    • **If pCO₂ > pCO₂ expected, there is primary respiratory acidosis present**
	    • **If pCO₂ < pCO₂ expected, there is primary respiratory alkalosis present**
	• <u>Labs</u>: basic metabolic panel (evaluate electrolytes); tests directed at suspected etiology

Treatment	• **Treatment is directed at underlying disorder** • <u>Volume Repletion</u>: **0.9% normal saline**; repletion of extracellular volume decreases Na^+ reabsorption; Cl^- delivery to distal tubule increases Cl^-/bicarbonate exchange • <u>Potassium Repletion</u>: **potassium chloride**; K^+ moves H^+ out of cells (acidosis) and inhibits hypokalemia • <u>Acetazolamide</u>: carbonic anhydrase inhibitor; increases HCO_3^- excretion but increase urinary losses of K^+ and phosphate (PO_4^-) • <u>Spironolactone</u>: aldosterone antagonists indicated to correct mineralocorticoid excess if indicated • <u>Hemodialysis</u>: indicated for renal failure, severe electrolyte abnormalities or volume overload

Respiratory Acidosis

Etiology & Risk Factors	• Clinical disturbance defined as an increase in carbon dioxide partial pressure (pCO_2) +/- compensatory bicarbonate (HCO_3^-) increase; **pH is usually low, may be near normal**
	  • pH <7.4, pCO_2 >45
	• <u>Etiology</u>: ventilation failure (hypoventilation) causes carbon dioxide (CO_2) accumulation
	  • <u>Acute</u>: **CNS depression (opioids**, sedatives, trauma), cardiopulmonary arrest, pneumonia, cerebrovascular accident (CVA)
	  • <u>Chronic</u>: **chronic obstructive pulmonary disease (COPD)**, obesity, **sleep apnea**, neuromuscular disorders (Guillan-Barre syndrome, myasthenia gravis)
	  • <u>CHAMPP</u>: **C**NS depression (drugs [opioids], Guillan-Barre, CVA), **H**emo/pneumothorax, **A**irway obstruction (COPD), **M**yopathy, **P**neumonia, **Pulmonary edema**

Pathophysiology	• In a hypoventilation state, more CO_2 is produced than can be eliminated leading to a net increase in CO_2 leading to an increase in hydrogen (H^+) ions (acidemia) and a slight increase in bicarbonate (HCO_3^-) which acts as a buffer

Signs & Symptoms	• **Symptoms are primarily those of the underlying disorder**
	• **Headache, dyspnea**, anxiety, **wheezing**, sleep disturbances (drowsiness), confusion
	• **Altered mental status**, myoclonus, seizures
	• <u>Physical Exam</u>:
	  • **Cyanosis due to hypoxemia**; pursed-lip breathing
	  • Gait disturbances, **tremor**, decreased deep tendon reflexes, papilledema, obtundation

Diagnosis	• <u>Arterial Blood Gas</u>:
	  • **Respiratory Acidosis when pH <7.4 and pCO_2 >45mmHg**
	  • **If HCO_3^- is in the *opposite* direction as the pH, there is partial metabolic compensation (full compensation if normal range pH level)**
	• <u>Labs</u>: basic metabolic panel (evaluate electrolytes); tests directed at suspected etiology

Treatment	• **Treatment is directed at underlying disorder**
	• <u>**Adequate Alveolar Ventilation**</u>:
	  • <u>**Bronchodilators**</u>: **beta-agonists**, anticholinergic drugs, and methylxanthines indicated for COPD
	  • <u>**Naloxone**</u>: **indicated in opioid overdose**
	  • <u>**Noninvasive Positive Pressure Ventilation**</u>: **CPAP indicated for COPD**
	  • <u>**Endotracheal Intubation**</u>: **indicated for severe acidemia (pH<7.25)**

Key Words & Most Common	• Hypoventilation: opioid overdose, COPD, sleep apnea most common
	• Symptoms of underlying disorder; may have dyspnea, headache, wheezes, AMS, cyanosis
	• <u>ABG</u>: pH<7.4, pCO_2>45; if CO_3^- is in opposite direction as pH there is partial metabolic compensation (full compensation if normal pH)
	• Treat underlying disorder
	  • <u>COPD</u>: beta-agonists, anticholinergics, CPAP
	  • <u>Opioid Overdose</u>: naloxone
	  • <u>Severe</u>: intubation

Respiratory Alkalosis

Etiology & Risk Factors	• **Clinical disturbance defined as a decrease in carbon dioxide partial pressure (pCO_2)** +/- compensatory bicarbonate (HCO_3^-) decrease; **pH is usually high or near normal**
	• **Most common acid-base abnormality**
	• <u>Etiology</u>: **ventilation increase in rate or volume (hyperventilation) causes carbon dioxide (CO_2) to be exhaled away**
	  • **Psychogenic hyperventilation (anxiety/stress/panic attack)**, hypoxia (**severe asthma**, pneumonia, pulmonary embolism, **high altitude**), CHF/pulmonary edema, infection (sepsis or fever), increased intracranial pressure (head trauma, CVA, CNS tumor), **salicylate (aspirin) overdose**, **excessive mechanical ventilation**, pregnancy
	  • <u>CHAMPPS</u>: **C**NS disease, **H**ypoxia, **A**nxiety, **M**echanical ventilation, **P**rogesterone/**P**regnancy, **S**alicylates/**S**epsis

Pathophysiology	• Hypoxic stimulation causes hyperventilation in response to correct the hypoxia at the expense of a CO2 loss • Acute respiratory alkalosis is associated with a higher bicarbonate level as there is insufficient time to lower the HCO_3^- levels to compensate for the alkalemia; chronic respiratory alkalosis is associated with a low or near-normal HCO_3^- level

Signs & Symptoms	• <u>**Acute**</u>: **symptoms are primarily those of the underlying disorder**
	  • Light-headedness, **anxiety**, peripheral or circumoral paresthesia, muscle cramps, headache, syncope
	• <u>Chronic</u>: usually asymptomatic
	• <u>Physical Exam</u>:
	  • **Hyperventilation; tachypnea or hyperpnea may be only sign**

Diagnosis	• <u>Arterial Blood Gas</u>:
	  • **Respiratory Acidosis when pH >7.4 and pCO_2 <35mmHg**
	  • **If HCO_3^- is in the *opposite* direction as the pH, there is partial metabolic compensation (full compensation if normal range pH level)**
	• <u>Labs</u>: basic metabolic panel (evaluate electrolytes); tests directed at suspected etiology
	• <u>Imaging</u>: x-ray or CT may be necessary to identify anatomical or infectious cause

Treatment	• **Treatment is directed at underlying disorder** • <u>Anxiolytics</u>: **benzodiazepines** (alprazolam, diazepam, lorazepam) **indicated for acute anxiety** • <u>Mechanical Ventilation</u>: may be indicated if severe alkalosis or respiratory compromise
Key Words & Most Common	• Most common acid-base abnormality • Hyperventilation causes CO_2 to be exhaled away • Anxiety, stress, panic attack, hypoxia (asthma, high altitude), salicylate overdose • Hyperventilation, tachypnea, hyperpnea, anxiety • <u>ABG</u>: pH>7.4 and pCO_2 <35; if CO_3^- is in opposite direction as pH there is partial metabolic compensation (full compensation if normal pH) • Treat underlying disorder • <u>Anxiolytics</u>: benzodiazepines

References

1. Nephrotic eyes.JPG. (2020, October 30). *Wikimedia Commons*. Retrieved 19:35, August 15, 2023 from https://commons.wikimedia.org/w/index.php?title=File:Nephrotic_eyes.JPG&oldid=507901732.
2. Hydro.jpg. (2020, September 12). *Wikimedia Commons*. Retrieved 19:40, August 15, 2023 from https://commons.wikimedia.org/w/index.php?title=File:Hydro.jpg&oldid=456162228.
3. Type3FMD.jpg. (2020, October 19). *Wikimedia Commons*. Retrieved 20:01, August 15, 2023 from https://commons.wikimedia.org/w/index.php?title=File:Type3FMD.jpg&oldid=494841054.
4. ECG in hyperkalemia.svg. (2020, September 21). *Wikimedia Commons*. Retrieved 20:04, August 15, 2023 from https://commons.wikimedia.org/w/index.php?title=File:ECG_in_hyperkalemia.svg&oldid=467195626.
5. ECG Pattern Of Hypokalemia.png. (2023, January 8). *Wikimedia Commons*. Retrieved 20:05, August 15, 2023 from https://commons.wikimedia.org/w/index.php?title=File:ECG_Pattern_Of_Hypokalemia.png&oldid=723689193.

Chapter 9
Genitourinary

Urge Incontinence

Etiology & Risk Factors	• Characterized by a sudden urge to urinate and results in involuntary leakage of urine • <u>Etiology</u>: **overactivity of the detrusor muscle**, poor detrusor muscle compliance and bladder hypersensitivity • <u>Risk Factors</u>: **advanced age, female, obesity, previous hysterectomy or pelvic surgery, parity,** pulmonary disease, diabetes mellitus, dementia, prolonged catheterization
Patho-physiology	• <u>Detrusor Muscle Overactivity</u>: **uninhibited (involuntary) contractions of the smooth muscle during bladder filling** (idiopathic or neurological disorder) • <u>Poor Detrusor Muscle Compliance</u>: failure of the bladder to stretch leads to an increase in bladder pressure (pelvic radiotherapy or prolonged catheterization) • <u>Bladder Hypersensitivity</u>: urothelial inflammation/infection may lead to overactive bladder; imbalance of urinary microbiota alters function and sensation (cystitis)
Signs & Symptoms	• **Leakage of urine accompanied by or immediately preceded by urgency** • **Increased urinary urgency and frequency** (>7 micturition episodes per day) • **Pain with a full bladder** • **Nocturia** • **Increased urinary retention**, weak flow rate, small volume voids
Diagnosis	• **Clinical Diagnosis** • <u>Urinalysis</u>: rule out other pathology • <u>**Postvoid Residual Volume**</u>: **volume >50mL**

Treatment	• <u>Bladder Training</u>: **first-line treatment**; demonstrates improvement in 75% of patients
	  • **Lifestyle modifications,** voiding diary, **timed frequent voiding,** altered fluid intake, **avoid bladder irritants** (caffeine, smoking, spicy food, citrus), **pelvic floor training**
	• <u>Medication</u>: second-line treatment
	  • <u>**Antimuscarinic Agents**</u>: **first-line medical therapy; Oxybutynin is most effective;** tolterodine may have less side effects; **promotes smooth muscle relaxation**
	  • <u>**Beta-3 Agonists**</u>: **mirabegron;** causes direct relaxation of detrusor muscles
	  • <u>Tricyclic Antidepressants</u>: **imipramine;** has central and peripheral anticholinergic activity and alpha-adrenergic agonist effects
	• Percutaneous stimulation of tibial nerve (PTNS), temporary chemical denervation of the bladder detrusor muscle, and sacral neuromodulation are third-line treatments

Key Words & Most Common	• Sudden urge to urinate resulting in involuntary leakage of urine • Detrusor muscle overactivity is most common • Urinary urgency and frequency + pain with full bladder + nocturia + urinary retention • Clinical diagnosis → postvoid residual volume >50mL • Bladder training is first-line • <u>Medications</u>: antimuscarinics (oxybutynin, tolterodine), beta-3 agonists (mirabegron), tricyclic antidepressants (imipramine)

Overflow Incontinence

Etiology & Risk Factors	• **Involuntary leakage of urine due to an overdistended bladder; secondary to urinary retention or incomplete bladder emptying**
	• <u>Etiology</u>: **overly full bladder**
	  • <u>**Neurologic Disorders or Autonomic Dysfunction**</u>: **most common cause;** spinal cord injuries, multiple sclerosis, diabetes mellitus, peripheral neuropathy, **spinal stenosis**
	  • <u>Bladder Outlet Obstruction</u>: **benign prostatic hypertrophy**, pelvic organ prolapse, abdominal or pelvic mass (uterine fibroids, tumors, prostate cancer)

Patho-physiology	• Bladder outlet obstruction or neurologic disorder leads to a chronically overdistended bladder, resulting in the inability to contract (**detrusor muscle underactivity**) • Overflow of urine results as the bladder is not able to empty completely
Signs & Symptoms	• **Involuntary leakage of urine without warning (urge) or triggers (stress)** • Common during change in positions • **Weak or intermittent urinary stream, hesitancy, frequency** • **Sensation of incomplete bladder emptying** • **Nocturia**
Diagnosis	• **Clinical Diagnosis** • <u>Urinalysis</u>: rule out other pathology • <u>**Postvoid Residual Volume**</u>: **volume >200mL**
Treatment	• <u>Clean Intermittent Catheterization or Indwelling Urethral Catheter</u>: **first-line treatment** • <u>Relief of Obstruction</u>: surgical removal of abdominal or pelvic mass • <u>**Alpha-Adrenergic Antagonists**</u>: **tamsulosin, terazosin;** relieve symptoms of outlet obstruction, reduces postvoid residual and outlet resistance, increases urinary flow rate • **Indicated in management of bladder outlet obstruction or benign prostatic hypertrophy** • <u>5-Alpha-Reductase Inhibitors</u>: finasteride, dutasteride; reduce prostate size and obstructive symptoms in benign prostatic hypertrophy • <u>Cholinergics</u>: bethanechol; may increase detrusor muscle activity but generally ineffective
Key Words & Most Common	• Involuntary leakage of urine due to an overly full bladder • Neurologic or autonomic; bladder outlet obstruction (BPH) • Urine leakage without warning or trigger • Weak/intermittent urine stream, hesitancy, frequency, nocturia • Clinical diagnosis → postvoid residual volume >200mL • Clean intermittent catheterization or indwelling urethral catheter + relief of obstruction • Alpha-adrenergic antagonists (tamsulosin)

Stress Incontinence

Etiology & Risk Factors	• Involuntary leakage of urine that occurs with increases in intraabdominal pressure (exertion, coughing, sneezing, laughing, straining, jumping)
	• Etiology:
	  • **Increased Intraabdominal Pressure**: exertion, coughing, sneezing, laughing, straining, jumping
	  • **Pelvic Floor Weakness**: childbirth, surgery, atrophic vaginitis (postmenopausal estrogen loss)
	  • **Urethral Hypermobility**: insufficient pelvic floor muscle support of the vaginal connective tissue to urethra and bladder neck
	• Risk Factors: **female**, age (**most common type of incontinence in younger women**; peak incidence 45-50 years old), pregnancy

Patho-physiology	• Pressure in the urethra falls below that of the bladder when intraabdominal pressure is raised and resistance to urine flow is impeded, leading to involuntary leakage of urine
Signs & Symptoms	• **Involuntary urine leakage occurring with increases in intraabdominal pressure** • **No urge to urinate prior to leakage**
Diagnosis	• **Clinical Diagnosis** • Urinalysis: rule out other pathology • Urinary Stress Test: patient's bladder must be full; patient sits upright or close to upright with the legs spread, relaxes the perineal area, and coughs vigorously once; leakage of urine indicates positive test • Cotton Swab Test: lubricated cotton swab is placed into the female urethra and patient is asked to Valsalva; positive result if angle change is >30°
Treatment	• **Pelvic Floor Muscle Strengthening: Kegel exercises are initial treatment**; the pelvic muscles (pubococcygeus and paravaginal) are contracted and held to strengthen • Pelvic floor physical therapy • Lifestyle Modifications: protective pads, weight loss, controlling fluid intake, prompted (timed) voiding, constipation management, smoking cessation, avoidance of caffeine • Mechanical Devices: cones, **pessaries**, urethral plugs; considered if refractory to pelvic floor muscle strengthening and lifestyle modifications • Surgery: definitive treatment; **bladder neck suspension (urethral hypermobility)**, periurethral injections of bulking agents, **urethral/bladder sling procedures**, urethropexy • Alpha-Adrenergic Agonists: pseudoephedrine, phenylpropolamine; stimulates urethral smooth muscle contraction
Key Words & Most Common	• Involuntary leakage of urine during increased intraabdominal pressure • Exertion, coughing, sneezing, laughing, straining, jumping • Clinical diagnosis • Urinary stress test • Pelvic floor muscle strengthening + lifestyle modifications → mechanical devices (pessaries) → surgery (urethral/bladder sling procedures)

Pelvic Organ Prolapse

Etiology & Risk Factors	• Herniation of pelvic structures into or beyond the vagina (toward or past the introitus) • Etiology: **pelvic floor muscle weakness**; connective tissue laxity • Risk Factors: **childbirth (especially multiparity or traumatic) leading to pelvic floor weakness, obesity**, repeated heavy lifting, advancing age, connective tissue disorders		
Patho-physiology	• Weakening of surrounding pelvic support structures including the uterosacral and cardinal ligament complexes and pelvic floor muscles allow for prolapse of the uterus into the vaginal vault		

Signs & Symptoms	• **Vaginal fullness, heaviness, or "falling out" sensation**
	  • Symptoms may be gradual and positional
	    • **Worse with prolonged standing or straining** (lifting, bowel movements, coughing, sneezing etc.)
	• Lower abdominal or back pain
	• Urinary Dysfunction: **urinary urgency and frequency**, sensation of incomplete bladder emptying, **stress incontinence**
	• Defecatory Dysfunction: **constipation**, incomplete emptying, fecal urgency or incontinence
	• Sexual Dysfunction: **dyspareunia** (painful intercourse), avoidance of sexual activity due to embarrassment
	• Physical Exam: **bulging mass visualized on pelvic exam**; performed at rest and with Valsalva maneuver
		• Types:
		  • **Cystocele: herniation of anterior vaginal wall + descent of bladder**
		  • **Rectocele: herniation of posterior vaginal segment + descent of rectum**
		  • **Enterocele: herniation of intestines to or through vaginal wall**
		  • **Uterine/Vaginal Vault Prolapse: descent of apex of vagina to lower vagina, hymen, or beyond introitus**
		• Staging: Pelvic Organ Prolapse-Quantification (POP-Q) system
		  • Stage 0: no prolapse
		  • Stage I: most distal prolapse is >1 cm above the hymen
		  • Stage II: most distal prolapse is between 1 cm above and 1 cm below the hymen
		  • Stage III: most distal prolapse is >1 cm below hymen but 2 cm shorter than total vaginal length
		  • Stage IV: complete eversion	

Diagnosis	• **Clinical Diagnosis**		

Treatment	• Conservative Management:
	  • **Vaginal pessary, pelvic floor muscle training (Kegel exercises), topical estrogen for atrophic vaginitis**
	• Surgical Management: techniques may include one or a combination of the following
	  • **Hysterectomy**, pelvic support structure repair (colporrhaphy), uterosacral or sacrospinous ligament fixation suspension, colpocleisis (vagina is suture closed)		

Key Words & Most Common	• Pelvic floor weakness secondary to childbirth leads to herniation of structures into/beyond the vagina • Vaginal fullness, heaviness, "falling out" sensation + bulging mass on exam • Urinary, defecatory, sexual dysfunction • Clinical Diagnosis • Vaginal pessary + pelvic floor exercises → surgery		

Peyronie Disease

Etiology & Risk Factors	• **Fibrosis/scarring of the tunica albuginea leads to contracture of the fascia causing an abnormal penile curvature/deviation and may cause painful erections** • <u>Etiology</u>: fibrosis of the tunica albuginea • <u>Risk Factors</u>: **penile trauma (vigorous sexual intercourse, certain sports)**, connective tissue disorders, family history, hypogonadism, diabetes mellitus, alcohol/smoking use
Patho-physiology	• Tunica albuginea is comprised of type 1 collagen fibers; fibrous plaque forms if the penis is abnormally bent or squeezed causing contracture/scarring of the collagen fibers and alters the elastic properties of the tunica albuginea leading to penile curvature and painful erection
Signs & Symptoms	• **Penile curvature towards affected side** • **Penile pain/curvature with erection** • Severe curvatures can prevent penetration • Penile shortening • **Erectile dysfunction**
Diagnosis	• **Clinical Diagnosis** • <u>Penile Ultrasound</u>: identifies areas of fibrosis or calcifications
Treatment	• <u>Observation</u>: **indicated for mild curvature (<30°) and no sexual dysfunction**; resolution may occur spontaneously or over several months • <u>Medical Management</u>: **indicated for curvature >30° but <90° and no sexual dysfunction; vitamin E**, tamoxifen, procarbazine, omega-3 fatty acids, vitamin E with L-carnitine • Intralesional injection with collagenase *Clostridium hystolyticum*, interferon-a-2b, and verapamil if present for >3 months • <u>Surgical Management</u>: indicated for curvature impairing satisfactory sexual relations, stable deformity without pain >3 months, extensive plaque, failed conservative treatment
Key Words & Most Common	• Fibrosis/scarring of the tunica albuginea leads to contracture of the fascia causing an abnormal penile curvature/deviation and may cause painful erections • Penile curvature and pain with erection • Erectile dysfunction • Clinical diagnosis • Observation → medical management → surgical management

Vesicoureteral Reflux

Etiology & Risk Factors	• **Retrograde urine flow from the bladder into the upper urinary tract** • <u>Etiology</u>: **congenital anomalies of the ureterovesical junction is most common cause**
Patho-physiology	• Inadequate closure or incompetent ureterovesicular junction causes failure of the normal flap valve mechanism which permits urine reflux from the bladder into the ureter and renal pelvis
Signs & Symptoms	• <u>Prenatal</u>: **hydronephrosis on prenatal ultrasound** • <u>Postnatal</u>: **febrile urinary tract infection** • Fever, abdominal/flank pain, dysuria, frequency, urgency, inability to hold urine
Diagnosis	• <u>Kidney, Ureter, Bladder Ultrasound</u>: **initial imaging test**; evaluates kidney size, evidence of hydronephrosis or scarring • Postnatal ultrasound performed on all patients with prenatal hydronephrosis • <u>Voiding Cystourethrogram (VCUG)</u>: **gold-standard for diagnosis**; urinary bladder filled with water-soluble contrast to allow visualization of the bladder under fluoroscopy

Treatment	• <u>Observation</u>: indicated in mild to moderate cases; most resolve spontaneously over months to years
	• <u>Antibiotic Prophylaxis</u>: indicated in children with mild to moderate vesicoureteral reflux
	  • Trimethoprim-sulfamethoxazole, nitrofurantoin or cephalexin
	• <u>Anticholinergic Medications</u>: oxybutynin or solifenacin indicated in severe cases; promotes smooth muscle relaxation
	• <u>Surgery</u>: **indicated for recurrent infections, impaired renal growth, renal scarring or bladder dysfunction**
	  • Endoscopic injection of a bulking agent or ureteral reimplantation
	
	VCUG demonstrating bilateral vesicoureteral reflux

Key Words & Most Common	• Retrograde urine flow from bladder into upper urinary tract • Congenital anomalies is most common cause • Hydronephrosis on prenatal ultrasound → febrile UTI • <u>KUB US</u>: initial imaging test • <u>Voiding Cystourethrogram</u>: gold-standard • Observation + antibiotic prophylaxis → surgery

Acute Cystitis

Etiology & Risk Factors	• **Urinary tract infection (UTI) confined to the bladder** • Etiology: *Escherichia coli* (86%) is most common cause, *Staphylococcus saprophyticus*, *Klebsiella* spp., *Proteus* spp., *Enterobacter* spp., *Citrobacter* spp., or *Enterococcus* spp. • Risk Factors: **women** (shorter urethra in close proximity to anus), **sexual intercourse**, **pregnancy** (progesterone and estrogen cause ureter dilation and inhibits peristalsis), spermicidal use, **age (elderly)**, **postmenopausal**, **diabetes mellitus**, indwelling catheter use, recent instrumentation or surgery of urinary tract, fecal incontinence
Patho-physiology	• *E. coli* has adhesive molecules (P-fimbriae) allowing the fecal flora to adhere to the urethral mucosal epithelial cells and ascend to the bladder through the urethra • Complicated UTIs: children, elderly, pregnancy, anatomic abnormality, diabetes mellitus, immunocompromised, chronic kidney disease, indwelling catheter, males
Signs & Symptoms	• **Urinary frequency** (using bathroom <2 hours apart) • **Urinary urgency** • **Dysuria** (burning or stinging sensation when passing urine) • **Suprapubic or lower back pain** • **Cloudy urine, foul-smelling urine or hematuria** • Complicated: altered mental status, fever, abdominal pain, weakness (may be only symptom in elderly)
Diagnosis	• Urinalysis: initial test of choice • Pyuria (≥8 WBCs/mcL), positive leukocyte esterase, nitrites (high specificity), hematuria, bacteriuria, cloudy urine • Urine Culture: definitive diagnosis; indicated in complicated cases to guide treatment

	Uncomplicated	Complicated	Pregnant

Treatment	• First-Line Antibiotics:
	  • **Nitrofurantoin**: 5-7 days
	  • **Trimethoprim-Sulfamethoxazole**: 3 days
	  • Fosfomycin: 1 time dose
	• Second-Line Antibiotics:
	  • Cephalexin, amoxicillin-clavulanate, ciprofloxacin (avoid in uncomplicated UTIs)
	• Adjunct: **phenazopyridine** (bladder analgesic); should only be used for 48 hours due to side effects (methemoglobinemia, hemolytic anemia) and risk of masking symptoms
		• **Ciprofloxacin**: 7-10 or 14 days
		• Cefpodoxime: 10-14 days
		• Trimethoprim-Sulfamethoxazole: 7-10 days
		• Nitrofurantoin: 7 days
		• *Consider one dose of IV/IM of ceftriaxone or gentamicin if regional susceptibility to ciprofloxacin or TMP-SMX is <80%*
		• *May require inpatient treatment if altered mental status, fever, weakness, or indwelling catheter/recent hospitalization*
			• **Amoxicillin-Clavulanate**: 7 days
			• **Cephalexin**: 3-5 days
			• **Nitrofurantoin**: 7 days
			• Cefpodoxime: 5-7 days

Pyelonephritis

Etiology & Risk Factors	• Bacterial infection of the renal parenchyma causing inflammation of the kidneys • **Complication of an ascending urinary tract infection (UTI)** spreading from the bladder to the kidney(s) and the collecting systems • Etiology: **bacterial infection secondary to fecal flora is most common cause**, hematogenous spread, urinary tract obstruction • *Escherichia coli* is most common; *Proteus, Klebsiella,* and *Enterobacter* spp., *S. saprophyticus* • Risk Factors: **female** (shorter urethra in close proximity to anus), **recent catheterization**, **urinary tract obstruction** (tumor, nephrolithiasis), extremes of age, **pregnancy**
Patho-physiology	• *E. coli* has adhesive molecules (P-fimbriae) allowing the fecal flora to adhere to the urethral mucosal epithelial cells and ascend to the bladder through the urethra and to the kidneys through the ureters; inflammatory cytokines, bacterial toxins and other reactive processes cause pyelonephritis

Signs & Symptoms	• Triad: fever, flank pain, nausea/vomiting
	• Upper Urinary Tract Symptoms: **fever and chills, flank pain**, colicky abdominal pain, lower back pain/pressure, **nausea and vomiting**
	• Lower Urinary Tract Symptoms: dysuria, urinary frequency, urgency
	• Physical Exam:
	  • **Costovertebral angle tenderness**
	  • **Fever and tachycardia**

Diagnosis	• Urinalysis: initial test of choice
	  • Pyuria (≥8 WBCs/mcL), positive leukocyte esterase, nitrites (high specificity), hematuria, bacteriuria, cloudy urine
	  • Microscopy: WBC casts (indicate inflammatory reaction)
	• Urine Culture: definitive diagnosis; indicated in pyelonephritis to guide treatment
	  • Complicated cases in pregnancy, postmenopausal, men, children, recent instrumentation or catheterization, immunocompromised, recurrent urinary tract infections
	• Labs: indicated for seriously ill patient or sepsis
	  • CBC (leukocytosis with left shift), BMP (evaluate kidney function and electrolytes), blood cultures

Treatment	• Outpatient Antibiotics:
	  • **Ciprofloxacin is first-line; trimethoprim-sulfamethoxazole is second-line**; cephalexin, cefdinir, cefixime, levofloxacin are alternatives
	  • *Consider one dose of IV/IM of ceftriaxone or gentamicin if regional susceptibility to ciprofloxacin or TMP-SMX is <80%*
	• Inpatient Antibiotics:
	  • **IV ciprofloxacin, IV ceftriaxone**, IV cefotaxime, piperacillin/tazobactam
	• Pregnancy Antibiotics:
	  • **IV ceftriaxone is preferred antibiotic**, aztreonam if penicillin allergic
	  • *Recurrence is common; consider prophylaxis after resolution with single dose of nitrofurantoin 100mg or cephalexin 250mg at night for remainder of pregnancy*

Urethritis

Etiology & Risk Factors	• Lower urinary tract infection causing inflammation of the urethra
	• Etiology:
	    • ___Chlamydia trachomatis___: **most common cause**; 5-8 day incubation period
	    • ___Neisseria gonorrhea___: abrupt onset; 3-4 day incubation period
	    • Other Infectious: *Trichomonas vaginalis, Ureaplasma urealyticum, Mycoplasma genitalium*, Herpes Simplex virus, *Treponema pallidum, Candida*
	    • Other Non-Infectious: trauma, irritation (friction from clothing or sex, physical activity such as biking, soaps, detergents, lotions)
	• Risk Factors: male, young age, unprotected sexual intercourse, and multiple sexual partners

Patho-physiology	• Bacterial infection of the lower urinary tract causes inflammation of the urethra; most commonly transmitted via unprotected sexual intercourse

Signs & Symptoms	• **Commonly asymptomatic**
	• **Urethral discharge**
	    • ___Chlamydia trachomatis___: tends to be more mucoid or thin/watery discharge; 5-8 day incubation period
	    • ___Neisseria gonorrhea___: purulent or mucopurulent discharge; 3-4 day incubation period
	• **Dysuria**
	• **Penile or vaginal pruritus**

Diagnosis	• **Clinical Diagnosis**
	• **Nucleic Acid Amplification Test: most sensitive and specific test**; first-catch urine or urethral swab
	• Gram Stain Test: >2 WBC/hpf on gram stain
	    • ___Chlamydia trachomatis___: no organisms generally seen on Gram stain (organism is a small, gram-negative obligate intracellular parasitic bacteria)
	    • ___Neisseria gonorrhea___: **gram-negative diplococci** bacteria on Gram stain
	• Urinalysis: suspect with positive leukocyte esterase or >10 WBCs/hpf (pyuria) on microscopy
	    • Suspect *Chlamydia* in a young, sexually active female patient with pyuria and no bacteriuria

Treatment	• **Coinfection of *Gonorrhea* and *Chlamydia* is common; empiric treatment of <u>both</u> is recommended if one entity suspected and/or test results are not available**
	• ___Chlamydia trachomatis___: **doxycycline 100mg BID for 7 days**
	    • Azithromycin 1g oral (single dose) if pregnant
	• ___Neisseria gonorrhea___: **ceftriaxone 500mg IM**; (1g if weight >150kg)
	    • Gentamicin 240mg IM + Azithromycin 2g oral (single dose) if ceftriaxone contraindicated (anaphylaxis to penicillins or cephalosporin allergy)

Key Words & Most Common	• *Chlamydia trachomatis* is most common cause; *Neisseria gonorrhea* is second most common cause • Asymptomatic → urethral discharge + dysuria in sexually active patient • NAAT is most sensitive and specific test • Empiric treatment with doxycycline 100mg BID for 7 days (*Chlamydia*) and ceftriaxone 500mg IM (*Gonorrhea*)

Prostatitis

Etiology & Risk Factors	• Inflammation of the prostate gland; may be acute or chronic (symptoms for >3 months)
	• Etiology:
	    • Bacterial: ***Escherichia coli* is most common cause;** *Chlamydia trachomatis, Neisseria gonorrhea* **is most common in young, sexually active males <35;** *Proteus, Klebsiella, Enterobacter, Serratia* and *Pseudomonas*
	    • Non-Bacterial: structural or functional abnormality, trauma, repetitive activities (sports, bike riding)
	• Risk Factors: **urinary tract obstruction**, phimosis, **unprotected vaginal or anal sex, indwelling catheter**, transurethral biopsy/surgery, sexual abuse

Patho-physiology	• Bacterial: Secondary to ascending bacterial infection from urethritis, cystitis, and/or epididymitis or secondary to direct inoculation from prostate biopsy or manipulation • Non-Bacterial: Impaired urinary sphincter relaxation and dyssynergic voiding results in elevated urinary pressure causing reflux of urine into the prostate triggering an inflammatory response; chronic trauma causes transient inflammation

Signs & Symptoms	• Irritative Symptoms: **dysuria, urinary frequency, urinary urgency**
	• Obstructive Symptoms: **hesitancy, weak or interrupted stream, incomplete voiding**
	• Acute: **fever**/chills, myalgias, **malaise, perineal pain or fullness**, lower back/pelvic pain
	• Chronic: more subtle symptoms; **recurrent UTIs**
	• Physical Exam:
	    • Acute: rectal exam reveals **exquisitely tender and boggy prostate**
	    • Chronic: rectal exam often unremarkable; may have nontender, boggy prostate

Diagnosis	• **Clinical Diagnosis** • Urinalysis: **pyuria and bacteriuria** • *Prostate massage may be performed prior to providing sample in chronic cases; prostate massage should be avoiding in acute prostatitis due to risk of bacteremia* • Urine Culture: **definitive diagnosis; indicated to guide treatment** • Transrectal Ultrasonography or Cystoscopy: may be necessary to identify suspected prostatic abscess if patient fails initial antibiotic therapy

Treatment	• Antibiotics: guided based on suspected or identified organism
	    • Acute:
	        • **Fluoroquinolones (ciprofloxacin or levofloxacin) or trimethoprim-sulfamethoxazole for 28 days if not associated with STDs**
	        • **500mg IM ceftriaxone + doxycycline 100mg BID for 14 days if concern for** *Chlamydia trachomatis, Neisseria gonorrhea* **as primary organism**
	    • Chronic:
	        • **Fluoroquinolones (ciprofloxacin or levofloxacin) or trimethoprim-sulfamethoxazole for 6-12 weeks**
	        • Alpha-adrenergic blockers (tamsulosin) or muscle relaxers (cyclobenzaprine) may provide symptomatic relief
	• Perineal or Transrectal Aspiration: indicated if prostatic abscess present

Epididymitis

Etiology & Risk Factors	• Infection or inflammation of the epididymis (the tubular structure located on the posterosuperior aspect of the testicle)
	• Etiology:
	   • Bacteria: most common cause
	     • *Chlamydia trachomatis* (**most common cause**) and/or *Neisseria gonorrhea* is most common in men <35 years old; *Ureaplasma, E. coli, Trichomonas*
	     • *Escherichia coli* **is most common cause in men >35 years old;** *Klebsiella, Proteus, Pseudomonas*
	   • Other: chemical (exercising or having sexual intercourse with a full bladder), drug-induced (amiodarone), viral infections (cytomegalovirus, mumps), trauma
	• Risk Factors: male, young age, unprotected sexual intercourse, and multiple sexual partners

Patho-physiology	• Bacteria of the lower urinary tract ascends through the genitourinary tract and causes inflammation/infection of the epididymis • Retrograde flow or stagnation of urine results in infection of the epididymis

Signs & Symptoms	• **Gradual onset of localized testicular pain and swelling**
	   • Usually **unilateral**
	   • May start as flank pain that migrates to the scrotum
	• **Urinary Symptoms: dysuria, urinary frequency, urgency or urinary incontinence**
	• **Urethral discharge (if associated with STDs)**
	• Physical Exam:
	   • Scrotal edema and tenderness; skin overlying the scrotum may appear warm, erythematous, inflamed and indurated
	   • **Tenderness to palpation of the epididymis along the posterior and superior aspect of the testicle**
	   • **Positive Prehn Sign: relief of pain with elevation of testicle**
	   • **Intact Cremasteric Reflex:** stroking of the skin of the inner thigh causes the cremaster muscle to contract and pull ipsilateral testicle toward the inguinal canal

Diagnosis	• **Clinical Diagnosis** • **Scrotal Ultrasound: best initial test; demonstrates enlarged epididymis and increased testicular blood flow; used to rule out testicular torsion** • Urinalysis: may show pyuria or bacteriuria • **Nucleic Acid Amplification Test: most sensitive and specific test to identify** *Chlamydia trachomatis* or *Neisseria gonorrhea*

Treatment	• **Supportive**: scrotal elevation (jockstrap when upright) to provide support, analgesics (NSAIDs), scrotal cool compresses
	• Antibiotics: guided based on suspected or identified organism
	   • **Fluoroquinolones (ciprofloxacin or levofloxacin) or trimethoprim-sulfamethoxazole for 10 days if not associated with STDs**
	   • **500mg IM ceftriaxone + doxycycline 100mg BID for 10 days if concern for** *Chlamydia trachomatis, Neisseria gonorrhea* as primary organism

Key Words & Most Common	• *Chlamydia trachomatis* and/or *Neisseria gonorrhea* is most common cause in men <35 years old • Gradual onset of unilateral testicular pain/swelling; + Prehn sign; + cremasteric reflex • Clinical diagnosis + UA → ultrasound • Supportive → antibiotics (fluoroquinolones [ciprofloxacin or levofloxacin] vs ceftriaxone + doxycycline if chlamydia or gonorrhea suspected)

Orchitis

Etiology & Risk Factors	• Inflammation of the testis
	• Etiology:
	   • **Viral: mumps and rubella are the most common viral causes;** coxsackievirus, varicella, echovirus, and cytomegalovirus
	   • Bacterial: *Escherichia coli, Klebsiella pneumoniae, Pseudomonas aeruginosa,* and *Staphylococcus* and *Streptococcus* spp.
	     • *Neisseria gonorrhoeae, Chlamydia trachomatis* and *Treponema pallidum* in most common in sexually active males
	• Risk Factors: **lack of immunization with MMR vaccination,** history of epididymitis, unprotected vaginal or anal sex, multiple sexual partners, long-term use of foley catheter, bladder outlet obstruction, anatomic abnormality

Patho-physiology	• Mumps orchitis is caused by parenchymal edema, congestion of the seminiferous tubules, and perivascular infiltration by lymphocytes

Signs & Symptoms	• **Scrotal pain and swelling**
	   • **Usually unilateral**
	   • **Occurs 4-7 days after onset of parotitis (mumps)**
	• Physical Exam:
	   • **Tenderness, enlargement, and induration of the testis**
	   • Erythema and edema of the skin overlying the scrotum
	   • **Intact Cremasteric Reflex:** stroking of the skin of the inner thigh causes the cremaster muscle to contract and pull ipsilateral testicle toward the inguinal canal

Diagnosis	• **Clinical Diagnosis** • **Scrotal Doppler Ultrasound:** ordered to rule out testicular torsion; shows inflammation of testicle • **Serum Immunofluorescence Antibody Testing: confirms diagnosis of mumps orchitis** • Urinalysis: rule out urinary tract infection • Nucleic Acid Amplification Test: rule out *Chlamydia trachomatis* or *Neisseria gonorrhea* as infectious cause

Treatment	• **Supportive:** scrotal elevation (jockstrap when upright) to provide support, bedrest, analgesics (NSAIDs), scrotal cool compresses
	• Antibiotics: indicated enteric or sexually transmitted bacteria is suspected etiology
	   • Fluoroquinolones (ciprofloxacin, ofloxacin or levofloxacin) for 10-14 days if not associated with STDs
	   • 500mg IM ceftriaxone + doxycycline 100mg BID for 14 days if concern for *Chlamydia trachomatis, Neisseria gonorrhea* as primary organism

Key Words & Most Common	• Inflammation of the testis • Mumps is most common cause • Scrotal pain/swelling occurs 4-7 days after onset of parotitis (mumps) • Tenderness + enlargement of testis • Clinical diagnosis + doppler ultrasound; serum immunofluorescence antibody testing to confirm • Supportive care

Testicular Torsion

Etiology & Risk Factors	• Urologic emergency caused by rotation of the testis • <u>Etiology</u>: **twisting of the spermatic cord causes strangulation of testicular blood supply** • <u>Risk Factors</u>: **age (10-20 years old and neonates at greatest risk)**, cryptorchidism (undescended testicle), trauma
Patho-physiology	• Abnormal development of the tunica vaginalis and spermatic cord leads to insufficient fixation of the lower pole of the testis to the tunica vaginalis (bell-clapper deformity) leading to increased testicular mobility; testicle may twist around the spermatic cord causing strangulation of blood supply leading to ischemia of the testicle

Signs & Symptoms	• **Abrupt onset of unilateral testicular pain, inguinal or lower abdominal pain**
	• **Nausea and vomiting**
	• <u>Physical Exam</u>:
	  • **Swollen and tender testicle**
	  • **Transverse (horizontal) lie and in a retracted (high-riding) position**
	  • <u>**Negative Prehn Sign**</u>: no relief of pain with testicle elevation; not reliable for predicting torsion
	  • <u>**Absent Cremasteric Reflex**</u>: no elevation of testicle with stroking of the inner thigh

Diagnosis	• <u>**Clinical Diagnosis**</u>: do not delay urologic consultation for workup • <u>**Scrotal Doppler Ultrasound**</u>: **most common initial test**; indicated for equivocal cases • Demonstrates decreased or absent blood flow to the testicle • <u>Urinalysis</u>: included as part of workup • <u>**Surgical Exploration**</u>: **definitive diagnosis**; direct visualization of rotation of testicle

Treatment	• <u>**Immediate Urological Consultation**</u>: **for detorsion and orchiopexy** (permanent fixation of a testicle into the scrotum)
	  • **Salvage rate drops significantly after 6 hours of pain onset**
	• <u>**Manual Detorsion**</u>: **may be attempted by experienced provider if surgical intervention is not immediately available**
	  • Detorsion of testis by rotating in an outward/lateral direction, repeat 2-3 times; pain relief guides procedure

Key Words & Most Common	• Urologic emergency caused by rotation of the testis on the spermatic cord causing testicular ischemia • Most common in adolescent males and neonates • Abrupt onset of unilateral testicular pain + nausea/vomiting • Transverse (horizontal) lie and high-riding position • Negative Prehn sign + absent cremasteric reflex • Clinical diagnosis → doppler ultrasound → surgical exploration • Immediate urological consult for detorsion and orchiopexy

TWIST Score

Finding	Points
Testicular Swelling	2
Firm Testicle	2
Absent Cremasteric Reflex	1
Nausea or Vomiting	1
High-Riding Testicle	1

Positive Predictive Value 100% >5 points
Negative Predictive Value 100% <2 points
Score 2-5 require ultrasound evaluation

Cryptorchidism

Etiology & Risk Factors	• **Failure of one or both testes to descend into the scrotum by 4 months of age**
	  • Can occur on either side or both; **right is most common**
	• **Most common congenital defect of the male genitalia**
	• **Most (80%) cryptorchid testes descend by 3 months old**
	• <u>Etiology</u>: exact etiology unknown
	• <u>Risk Factors</u>: **prematurity is greatest risk factor**, small for gestational age, **maternal obesity and/or diabetes**, family history, congenital malformation syndromes
	  • <u>In Utero Exposures</u>: chemical endocrine disruptors, pesticides, alcohol, cigarette smoke

Patho-physiology	• Transient hormone deficiency may contribute to a lack of testicular descent and impaired spermatogenic tissue development • Impaired Sertoli cell and Leydig cell function may cause infertility due to poor semen quality in adults
Signs & Symptoms	• **No palpable testicle within the scrotum** • **Minimal scrotal rugae** • **May have inguinal hernia or fullness** (if testicle located in the inguinal canal)
Diagnosis	• **Clinical Diagnosis** • <u>Ultrasound</u>: non-contributory in routine use
Treatment	• <u>**Observation**</u>: **recommended if infant is <6 months old** (most [80%] testicles descend by 3 months old); reevaluation at 6 months of age • <u>**Surgical Orchiopexy**</u>: **recommended for congenital undescended testes between the ages of 6 and 18 months**; may be performed as early as 4 months old • <u>Hormone Treatment</u>: human chorionic gonadotropin (hCG) stimulates testosterone; indicated only in cases of undescended testis associated with Prader-Willi Syndrome • <u>Complications</u>: • Increased risk of testicular cancer (reduced 2-3x if orchiopexy performed before puberty), infertility, increased risk of testicular torsion, psychological consequence
Key Words & Most Common	• Failure of one or both testes to descend into the scrotum by 4 months old; most descend spontaneously by 3 months old • Prematurity is greatest risk factor • No palpable testicle in scrotum + minimal scrotal rugae • Clinical diagnosis • <u>Observation</u>: <6 months old • <u>Orchiopexy</u>: 6-18 months old

Testicular Cancer

Etiology & Risk Factors	• Most common solid tumor malignancy in men aged 15 to 35 years old • <u>Etiology</u>: genetic and environmental factors • <u>Risk Factors</u>: **cryptorchidism (2.5-20x increased risk) is greatest risk factor**; family history, infection (HPV, EBV, CMV), testicular trauma, high maternal estrogen levels

Patho-physiology	• <u>**Germinal Cell Tumors**</u>**: most common type (95%)**
	  • <u>**Nonseminomas**</u>: mixed types (teratomas, choriocarcinomas, yolk sac tumors); increased serum alpha-fetoprotein and beta-hCG and resistant to radiation
	  • <u>**Seminomas**</u>: transformed germ cells that are blocked in their differentiation; no increase in serum alpha-fetoprotein and sensitive to radiation
	• <u>Sex Cord Stromal Tumor</u>: (5%)
	  • <u>Leydig or Sertoli Cell Tumors</u>: may be benign and may secrete hormones (androgens, estrogens) leading to precocious puberty in children

Signs & Symptoms	• **Nontender testicular mass is most common symptom** • **May have dull testicular pain or heaviness** • Secondary hydrocele possible • May have endocrine abnormalities from elevated hCG levels (gynecomastia, hyperthyroid profile); rare manifestation • <u>Physical Exam</u>: • Firm, fixed testicular mass that does not transilluminate
Diagnosis	• <u>Scrotal Ultrasound</u>: initial imaging test of choice; cancer suspected with hypoechoic, solid, vascularized intratesticular lesion visualized • <u>Serum Tumor Markers</u>: **alpha-fetoprotein (elevated in nonseminomas)**, beta-HCG, and lactate dehydrogenase (LDH) • <u>Abdominal, Pelvic, and Chest CT</u>: necessary for staging using standard TNM (tumor, node, metastasis) system

Treatment	• <u>**Radical Inguinal Orchiectomy**</u>**: mainstay of management**; therapeutic and provides tissue for histopathological diagnosis
	  • <u>Retroperitoneal Lymph Node Dissection</u>: standard treatment for nonseminoma
	  • <u>Cosmetic Testicular Prosthesis</u>: may be placed at time of orchiectomy
	• <u>Radiation Therapy</u>: indicated in management of seminoma (no role for radiation therapy in nonseminoma)
	• <u>Chemotherapy</u>: platinum-based combination chemotherapy indicated for nodal masses >5 cm, lymph node metastases above the diaphragm or visceral metastases
	• <u>Prognosis</u>: generally excellent (5-year survival rate >95% with seminoma or nonseminoma localized to the testis)

Key Words & Most Common	• Most common solid tumor in men age 15-35 years old
	• Cryptorchidism is greatest risk factor
	• Germinal cell tumors most common
	  • <u>Nonseminomas</u>: ↑AFP and beta-hCG and resistant to radiation
	  • <u>Seminomas</u>: ↔AFP and sensitive to radiation
	• Nontender testicular mass +/- dull testicular pain or heaviness
	• Scrotal ultrasound + serum tumor markers → abdominal/pelvic/chest CT
	• Radical Inguinal orchiectomy +/- retroperitoneal lymph node dissection

Hydrocele

Etiology & Risk Factors	• **Collection of serous fluid between the parietal and visceral layers of the tunica vaginalis of the scrotum** • Most common cause of painless scrotal swelling • <u>Etiology</u>: **idiopathic is most common**; congenital patency of processus vaginalis, reactive hydrocele secondary to inflammatory conditions (epididymitis, orchitis, tumor) • <u>Risk Factors</u>: breech presentation, low birth weight, gestational progestin use, residing in warm climate
Patho-physiology	• <u>**Communicating**</u>**: patent processes vaginalis (congenital) causes connection with peritoneal cavity** • <u>Noncommunicating</u>: excessive production of serous fluid (secondary hydrocele), defective absorption of serous fluid, impaired lymphatic drainage of scrotal structures

Signs & Symptoms	• **Painless scrotal swelling**
	  • **Swelling may increase throughout the day**
	• May experience dull ache or heaviness sensation of scrotum with increasing size
	• <u>Physical Exam</u>:
	  • **Transillumination of scrotum**
	  • Fluid collection primarily located anterolateral to the testis
	  • Swelling may worsen with Valsalva if communicating 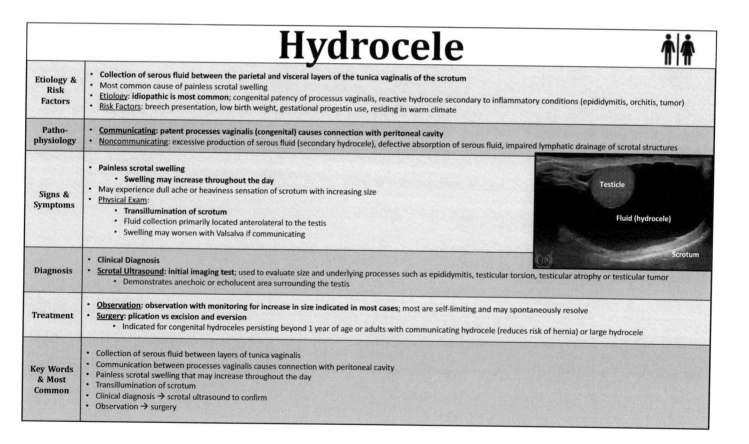

Diagnosis	• **Clinical Diagnosis** • <u>Scrotal Ultrasound</u>: **initial imaging test**; used to evaluate size and underlying processes such as epididymitis, testicular torsion, testicular atrophy or testicular tumor • Demonstrates anechoic or echolucent area surrounding the testis
Treatment	• <u>**Observation**</u>: observation with monitoring for increase in size indicated in most cases; most are self-limiting and may spontaneously resolve • <u>Surgery</u>: plication vs excision and eversion • Indicated for congenital hydroceles persisting beyond 1 year of age or adults with communicating hydrocele (reduces risk of hernia) or large hydrocele
Key Words & Most Common	• Collection of serous fluid between layers of tunica vaginalis • Communication between processes vaginalis causes connection with peritoneal cavity • Painless scrotal swelling that may increase throughout the day • Transillumination of scrotum • Clinical diagnosis → scrotal ultrasound to confirm • Observation → surgery

Image labels: Testicle, Fluid (hydrocele), Scrotum

Spermatocele

Etiology & Risk Factors	• **Fluid filled cyst that develops on the epididymis and contains sperm** • Also known as epididymal cyst • <u>Etiology</u>: unknown • <u>Risk Factors</u>: scarring of epididymis secondary to inflammation or trauma
Patho-physiology	• Scarring of seminiferous tubules on the head of the epididymis may cause diverticulum that gradually accumulates sperm forming a fluid filled cyst

Signs & Symptoms	• **Painless, cystic testicular mass**
	  • **Described as "small, pea-sized mass"**
	• <u>Physical Exam</u>:
	  • **Round, soft (fluid-filled), mobile mass of the epididymis occurring at the superior, posterior aspect of the epididymis and separate from the testicle**
	  • **Transillumination of mass**

Diagnosis	• <u>Scrotal Ultrasound</u>: definitive diagnosis and most accurate imaging test; confirms fluid filled cyst of the epididymis
Treatment	• <u>Observation</u>: no treatment necessary; monitor size and symptoms • <u>Surgery</u>: surgical excision indicated for chronic pain but rarely performed
Key Words & Most Common	• Fluid filled cyst of the epididymis that contains sperm • Painless, cystic mass of testicle • "Small, pea-sized mass" • Round, soft, fluid-filled, mobile mass of the epididymis • + transillumination of cyst • Scrotal ultrasound • Observation

Varicocele

Etiology & Risk Factors	• **Abnormal dilation and enlargement of the scrotal venous pampiniform plexus; varicose veins** • Can impair sperm production/function leading to infertility • <u>Etiology</u>: unknown; anatomical cause • **Left-side most common; increased angle (near 90°) of the left internal spermatic vein as it joins the left renal vein**
Patho-physiology	• Increased angle of the left internal spermatic vein as it joins the left renal vein causes vascular congestion which damage sperm production and function secondary to excess heat from the increased blood flow and oxidative stress, reduced oxygenation, hydrostatic pressure, toxin formation, and hypoxia • Isolated right-sided varicocele may indicate right renal cell carcinoma due to vena cava obstruction

Signs & Symptoms	• **Mostly asymptomatic**
	• **May have dull scrotal pain or heaviness**
	• May cause testicular atrophy
	• <u>Physical Exam</u>:
	  • **Nontender, soft scrotal mass superior to the testicle; described as a "bag of worms"**
	  • **Increased dilation with standing or with Valsalva**
	  • Decreased dilation when supine

Diagnosis	• **Clinical Diagnosis** • <u>Scrotal Ultrasound</u>: **initial imaging test of choice**; used to monitor of size and testicular atrophy • Demonstrates dilation of pampiniform plexus >3mm in diameter • <u>Abdominal CT</u>: indicated in isolated right-sided varicocele to evaluate for right renal cell carcinoma

Treatment	• <u>Supportive</u>: scrotal elevation (jockstrap when upright) to provide support, analgesics (NSAIDs), scrotal cool compresses
	• <u>Observation</u>: indicated for most cases; ultrasound to monitor for testicular atrophy
	• <u>Semen Analysis</u>: indicated as part of infertility workup or to determine if surgery is indicated
	• <u>Surgery</u>: percutaneous venous embolization, spermatic vein ligation, or laparoscopic varicocelectomy
	  • **Indicated for pain, infertility or abnormal semen parameters, testicular atrophy or delayed testicular growth and development in adolescence**
	  • Improved semen parameters in 80% of patients and improved conception rates in 40-60% of patients after surgery

Key Words & Most Common	• Abnormal dilation of scrotal venous pampiniform plexus; "varicose veins" • Left is more common due to increased angle of left internal spermatic vein and left renal vein junction • Asymptomatic → dull scrotal pain/heaviness • Nontender, soft scrotal mass; "bag of worms" • Clinical diagnosis + scrotal ultrasound • Supportive + observation → semen analysis → surgery

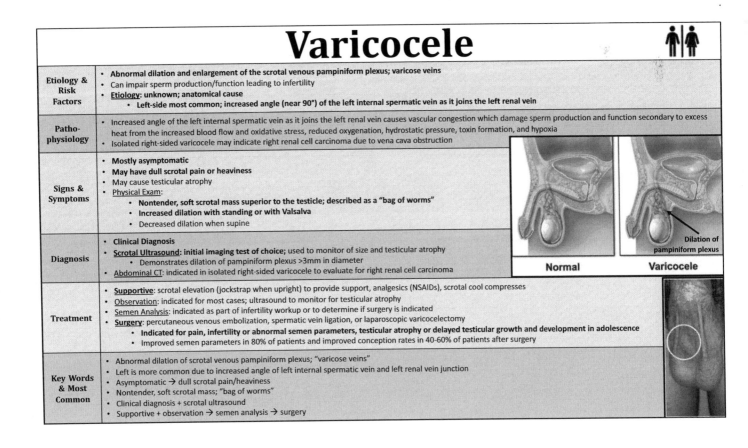

Normal   Varicocele

Dilation of pampiniform plexus

Urethral Strictures

Etiology & Risk Factors	• Narrowing of the urethral lumen causing obstructive symptoms
	• Etiology:
	   • **Idiopathic**: may be secondary to repetitive microtrauma to perineum
	   • **Iatrogenic: trans-urethral resection (TUR) procedure is most common iatrogenic cause; prolonged catheterization**, cystoscopy
	   • **Trauma**: saddle injuries or penile fracture; injury sustained during sexual intercourse
	   • **Inflammatory: post-infectious inflammation** (gonococcal urethritis is most common cause)

Patho-physiology	• Inflammation and fibrous changes of the corpus spongiosum causes contraction compression of the urethral lumen leading to compressive symptoms

Signs & Symptoms	• **Chronic obstructive voiding symptoms**
	   • **Weak urinary stream**
	   • **Hesitancy**
	   • **Incomplete bladder emptying**
	• **Double urine stream or spraying of urine**
	• Dysuria; recurrent UTIs (including prostatitis)
	• Sexual dysfunction
	• Physical Exam:
	   • May have palpable fibrosis of urethra

Diagnosis	• **Cystoscopy: helps to determine the location of the stricture;** may not be able to visualize beyond initial stricture if significant obstruction present • **Retrograde Urethrography: confirms diagnosis;** allows visualization of the entire urethra up to the bladder
Treatment	• Transurethral Procedures: urethral dilation or internal urethrotomy • **Urethral dilation is typically the standard and initial treatment modality** • Surgical Procedures: stricture resection and anastomosis, urethroplasty, and perineal urethrostomy
Key Words & Most Common	• Narrowing of urethral lumen leading to obstructive symptoms • Idiopathic, iatrogenic, trauma, inflammatory • Chronic obstructive voiding symptoms (weak stream, hesitancy, incomplete bladder emptying) • Double urine stream or spraying of urine • Cystoscopy vs retrograde urethrography • Urethral dilation is typically first-line treatment

Bladder Cancer

Etiology & Risk Factors	• Neoplasm that arises from the urinary bladder • **Most common malignancy of genitourinary system** • Etiology: **urothelial (transitional cell) carcinoma is most common type (90%)**; squamous cell carcinoma, adenocarcinoma, sarcoma, small cell carcinoma Risk Factors: **smoking is greatest risk factor**, medications (**cyclophosphamide**, pioglitazone), age (>40 years old), **Caucasian, male**, chronic irritation (urolithiasis, catheter use) • **Occupational exposure to hydrocarbons or industrial chemicals used in dyes, rubber**, electric, **leather**, cable, **paint**, and textile industries
Patho-physiology	• Transitional cell carcinomas is most common type of bladder cancer; papillary carcinomas is most common subtype which usually arises from hyperplasia or dysplasia
Signs & Symptoms	• **Painless gross or microscopic hematuria is most common presenting symptom** • Usually intermittent • Irritative Voiding Symptoms: **dysuria, urgency, frequency** • Pelvic pain or pelvic mass with advanced cancer 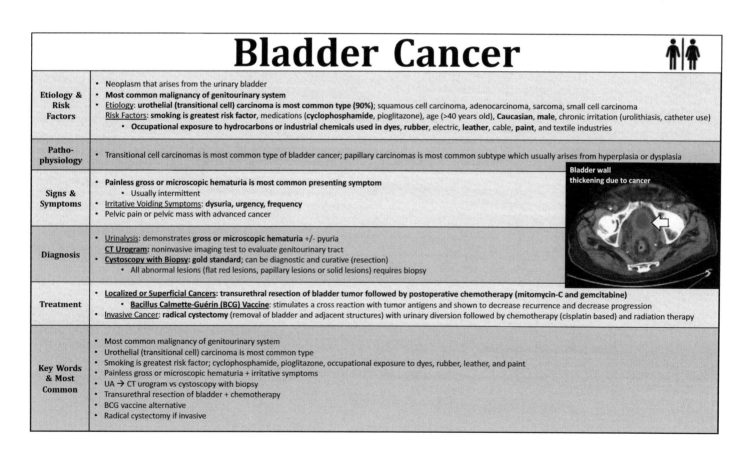
Diagnosis	• Urinalysis: demonstrates **gross or microscopic hematuria** +/- pyuria **CT Urogram:** noninvasive imaging test to evaluate genitourinary tract • **Cystoscopy with Biopsy: gold standard**; can be diagnostic and curative (resection) • All abnormal lesions (flat red lesions, papillary lesions or solid lesions) requires biopsy
Treatment	• **Localized or Superficial Cancers:** transurethral resection of bladder tumor followed by postoperative chemotherapy (mitomycin-C and gemcitabine) • **Bacillus Calmette-Guérin (BCG) Vaccine:** stimulates a cross reaction with tumor antigens and shown to decrease recurrence and decrease progression • **Invasive Cancer: radical cystectomy** (removal of bladder and adjacent structures) with urinary diversion followed by chemotherapy (cisplatin based) and radiation therapy
Key Words & Most Common	• Most common malignancy of genitourinary system • Urothelial (transitional cell) carcinoma is most common type • Smoking is greatest risk factor; cyclophosphamide, pioglitazone, occupational exposure to dyes, rubber, leather, and paint • Painless gross or microscopic hematuria + irritative symptoms • UA → CT urogram vs cystoscopy with biopsy • Transurethral resection of bladder + chemotherapy • BCG vaccine alternative • Radical cystectomy if invasive

Bladder wall thickening due to cancer

Phimosis

Etiology & Risk Factors	• **Describes difficulty or inability to retract the foreskin over the glans**
	• Not a urological emergency (unless urinary retention results)
	• <u>Etiology</u>:
	   • **Physiologic**: prepuce is non-retractile at birth and may remain so for months to years; **most cases resolve by 5 years old**
	   • **Pathologic**: scarring of the preputial opening secondary to balanitis xerotica obliterans (BXO), trauma, inflammation, or infection

Patho-physiology	• <u>Physiologic</u>: epithelial lining of the glans and prepuce are contiguous with the preputial adhesions being part of the normal developmental process • <u>Pathologic</u>: balanitis xerotica obliterans (BXO) causes a sclerotic constricting band of tissue 1-2 cm proximal to the distal end of the penis, prohibiting retraction of the foreskin
Signs & Symptoms	• **Inability to retract the foreskin over the glans** • Acute urinary retention or nocturnal enuresis secondary to urinary outflow obstruction is rare but possible complication
Diagnosis	• **Clinical Diagnosis** • Ensure patient is able to urinate and no evidence of urinary retention
Treatment	• **Supportive**: reassurance and education on proper hygiene; no treatment required in physiologic phimosis • Manual stretching exercises of the foreskin is often effective • <u>Topical Corticosteroids</u>: betamethasone 0.5% 2-3x per day for 4-8 weeks; inhibits collagen deposition and scar formation • <u>Surgery</u>: circumcision is definitive management
Key Words & Most Common	• Difficulty or inability to retract foreskin over the glans • May be physiologic or pathologic • Most physiologic cases resolve by 5 years old • Clinical diagnosis • Supportive care if physiologic • Topical corticosteroids (betamethasone) • Circumcision is definitive

Inability to retract foreskin over the glans

Paraphimosis

Etiology & Risk Factors	• **Urologic emergency occurs when the retracted foreskin is unable to be reduced to the normal position**
	• <u>Etiology</u>:
	   • **Iatrogenic**: foreskin is retracted for cleaning, placement of a urinary catheter, cystoscopy procedure or penile examination and not promptly reduced
	   • Penile coital trauma, balanoposthitis (inflammation of glans penis secondary to poor hygiene, infections, allergies, STDs), self-inflicted injury
	• <u>Risk Factors</u>: most common in uncircumcised adolescent male

Patho-physiology	• Retracted foreskin becomes trapped behind the corona of the glans, forming a tight constricting of penile tissues that functions as a tourniquet and can cause impairment of distal venous and lymphatic drainage and decrease arterial blood flow to the glans eventually causing ischemia and necrosis

Signs & Symptoms	• **Severe pain, and swelling of the distal penis**
	• May have obstructive urinary symptoms
	• <u>Physical Exam</u>:
	   • **Enlarged, tender, and erythematous glans**
	   • **Constricting band of foreskin tissue behind the glans**
	   • **Flaccid penile shaft**

Diagnosis	• **Clinical Diagnosis**

Treatment	• **Manual Reduction**: initial management
	   • Apply and maintain circumferential pressure for several minutes to reduce edema
	   • Release pressure and advance foreskin over glans
	   • May use cool compresses or compressive bandages to aid in reduction
	• <u>Adjunctive Therapy</u>: indicated if manual reduction unsuccessful
	   • Apply granulated sugar to exposed glans (acts as osmotic agent to reduce swelling), hyaluronidase injection to reduce edema, Babcock clamps applied to foreskin
	• **Dorsal Slit Procedure**: definitive management; incision made into foreskin to aid in reduction; indicated if impaired perfusion and urology consult unavailable

Key Words & Most Common	• Retracted foreskin is unable to be reduced over the glans penis • Urologic emergency • Iatrogenic is common cause; foreskin is retracted for cleaning, catheter, cystoscopy, examination and not promptly reduced • Severe pain + swelling of glans and foreskin • Constricting band of foreskin tissue behind the glans • Clinical diagnosis • Manual reduction → apply granulated sugar or hyaluronidase injection → dorsal slit procedure

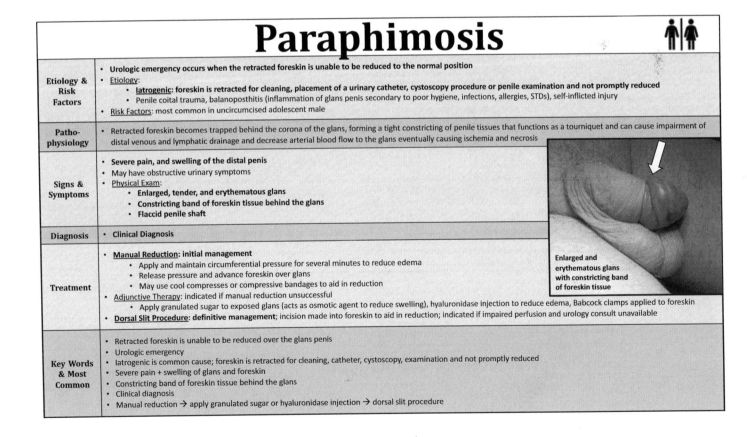

Enlarged and erythematous glans with constricting band of foreskin tissue

Benign Prostatic Hyperplasia (BPH) 🧍🧍

Etiology & Risk Factors	• Benign, nonmalignant growth or hyperplasia of the periurethral prostate gland; may lead to bladder outlet obstruction • <u>Etiology</u>: part of normal aging process; hormonally depending on dihydrotestosterone (DHT) production • <u>Risk Factors</u>: age (>50 years old most common) is greatest risk factor, metabolic syndrome, obesity, family history
Patho-physiology	• Dihydrotestosterone (DHT) has direct effects on the stromal and epithelial tissue of the prostate gland which has paracrine and endocrine effects that influence cellular proliferation and apoptosis leading to hyperplasia • Hyperplasia causes progressive narrowing of the prostatic urethra lumen causing urine outflow obstruction
Signs & Symptoms	• May be asymptomatic • <u>Irritative Symptoms</u>: urinary frequency, nocturia, urgency • <u>Obstructive Symptoms</u>: hesitancy, weak or intermittent stream, incomplete voiding, dribbling of urine at end of stream • <u>Acute Urinary Retention</u>: marked abdominal or pelvic discomfort, overflow incontinence • Symptoms may be worse with anesthetics, anticholinergics, sympathomimetics, opioids, or alcohol • <u>Physical Exam</u>: • **Digital Rectal Exam (DRE): uniformly enlarged and nontender prostate with rubbery consistency**
Diagnosis	• <u>Urinalysis</u>: may have microscopic hematuria; used to rule out other diagnoses • <u>Ultrasound</u>: aids to determine hydronephrosis secondary to obstruction and post-void residual volume • <u>Prostate Specific Antigen (PSA)</u>: correlated with prostate size and degree of obstruction to determine risk of prostatic cancer • **>1.5ng/mL indicates enlarged prostate; >4.0ng/mL warrants further testing or biopsy; >5.0ng/mL indicates high risk of prostate cancer** • <u>Transrectal Ultrasound-Guided Needle Biopsy</u>: indicated if suspicious for prostate cancer

Treatment	• <u>Observation</u>: prostate specific antigen level monitored annually
	• <u>Lifestyle Modifications</u>: weight loss, limiting caffeine and nighttime fluid intake, avoiding constipation, limiting diuretics, timed voiding, pelvic floor exercises
	• Medical Therapy:
	   • <u>Alpha-Blockers</u>: tamsulosin, alfuzosin; **best initial therapy; promotes stromal smooth muscle relaxation** and improves urinary flow but *does not* reduce prostate size
	   • <u>5-Alpha Reductase Inhibitors</u>: finasteride, dutasteride; **block conversion of testosterone to DHT to reduce prostate size over time** (6-12 months)
	• <u>Surgery</u>: transurethral resection of the prostate (TURP) is the standard procedure; removes excess prostate tissue and relieve obstruction
	   • Indicated for recurrent UTIs or urinary retention, renal insufficiency, high-pressure urinary retention, increased post-void residual volume, urolithiasis

Key Words & Most Common	• Benign growth or hyperplasia of prostate gland • Irritative and obstructive symptoms → urinary retention • DRE: uniformly enlarged and nontender prostate with rubbery consistency • PSA to determine risk → transrectal biopsy • Observation + lifestyle modifications → medical therapy (alpha blockers [tamsulosin]; 5-alpha reductase inhibitors [finasteride]) → surgery (TURP)

Prostate Cancer 🧍🧍

Etiology & Risk Factors	• Most common non-dermatologic cancer in men > 50 in the US • <u>Etiology</u>: **adenocarcinoma is most common type** (95%) • <u>Risk Factors</u>: **increasing age is greatest risk factor, positive family history**, increased height, **obesity**, hypertension, **sedentary lifestyle**, persistently elevated testosterone levels, Agent Orange exposure, and **ethnicity (African-Americans have higher incidence)**
Patho-physiology	• Cancer begins with a cellular mutation within the normal prostate glandular tissue (beginning with the peripheral basal cells) and may spread to the immediate surrounding prostate tissue to form a tumor nodule

Signs & Symptoms	• **Usually asymptomatic**
	• **Symptoms similar to benign prostatic hyperplasia**
	   • **Urinary frequency, nocturia, urgency, hesitancy, weak or intermittent stream, incomplete voiding, dribbling of urine at end of stream, urinary retention**
	• **Mass effect can cause spinal cord compression** leading to paresthesia, leg weakness, pain, paralysis, and urinary and fecal incontinence
	• Metastatic disease can cause **significant bone pain** (back [vertebrae], pelvis, hip, rib pain)
	• <u>Physical Exam</u>:
	   • **Digital Rectal Exam (DRE): firm, indurated, nodular, asymmetrically enlarged prostate**

Diagnosis	• <u>Prostate Specific Antigen (PSA)</u>: **>4.0ng/mL warrants further testing or biopsy; >5.0ng/mL indicates high risk of prostate cancer; >10ng/mL indicates high risk for METS** • <u>Transrectal Ultrasound-Guided Needle Biopsy</u>: **most accurate test**; indicated if PSA >4ng/mL in patients with palpable nodular mass on DRE • <u>Multiparametric MRI</u>: may help define the local extent of the tumor in patients with locally advanced prostate cancer • <u>Gleason Grading System</u>: used to stage prostate cancer by determining malignant potential; based on the the microscopic arrangement, architecture and pattern of the cells
Treatment	• <u>Active Surveillance</u>: indicated for very low-risk patients, clinically localized prostate cancer or if life-limiting disorders coexist (<10-year life expectancy) • Includes periodic DRE, PSA measurement, and close monitoring of symptoms • <u>Radical Prostatectomy</u>: surgical removal of prostate with seminal vesicles and regional lymph nodes; indicated for patients < 75 years old with confined prostate tumor • <u>External Beam Radiation Therapy</u>: indicated for localized or advanced cancer; fewer side effects with very similar overall survival as radical prostatectomy for localized cancer • <u>Hormonal Therapy</u>: **androgen deprivation therapy;** bilateral orchiectomy or LHRH agonists (leuprolide, goserelin) + antiandrogens (flutamide) +/- radiation therapy • <u>Chemotherapy</u>: indicated in progressive cancer despite a testosterone level consistent with castration
Key Words & Most Common	• Adenocarcinoma is most common type • Age is greatest risk factor; family history, obesity, African-American • Symptoms similar to BPH • DRE: firm, indurated, nodular, asymmetrically enlarged prostate • PSA: >4.0ng/mL → transrectal US guided biopsy • Active surveillance → radial prostatectomy vs external beam radiation

Urolithiasis

Etiology & Risk Factors	• Solid particles within the urinary system; **nephrolithiasis** (renal calculi), **ureterolithiasis** (calculi within the ureter), and **cystolithiasis** (calculi within the urinary bladder)
	• Etiology: 4 major types
	   • **Calcium: calcium oxalate is most common type** (70%); calcium phosphate (15%); secondary to **hypercalciuria, hyperparathyroidism**, renal tube acidosis
	   • **Uric Acid:** second most common type (10%); secondary to elevated uric acid levels from high protein food, **gout**, chemotherapy, hyperuricosuria, or urine pH<5.5
	   • **Struvite:** composed of **magnesium ammonium phosphate; forms staghorn calculi due to UTI** caused by urea-splitting bacteria (**Proteus, Pseudomonas, Klebsiella**)
	   • **Cystine:** cystinuria; secondary to rare congenital defect in reabsorption of cysteine
	• Risk Factors: **poor oral fluid intake**, high animal protein intake, high oxalate intake (beans, beer, berries, coffee, chocolate, nuts, teas, soda, spinach, potatoes), high salt intake

Patho-physiology	• High concentration of the underlying composition begins to collect and crystallize within the renal parenchyma and forms a renal calculi; the crystals continue to aggregate and enlarge; **stone may then migrate into the ureter which increases luminal tension, hydronephrosis, and prostaglandin release leading to symptoms** • **Most common location for a stone to obstruct is the ureteropelvic junction (UPJ)** due to the narrow diameter

Signs & Symptoms	• **Sudden onset of sharp/crampy back or flank pain**
	   • **May radiate to the groin or to anterior abdomen**
	   • Pain may be intermittent or "colicky"
	   • **Patient may be unable to find a comfortable position**
	• **Nausea/vomiting + hematuria**
	• Physical Exam:
	   • **Pain depends on location of stone; flank pain** (upper ureter), anterior abdominal pain (mid ureter), groin pain (distal ureter), UTI-symptoms (ureterovesical junction)
	   • Costovertebral angle tenderness to percussion if located at the ureteropelvic junction

Diagnosis	• **Urinalysis:** microscopic or gross hematuria most common; acidic urine (pH<5.5) associate with uric acid and cystine stones; alkaline urine (pH>7.2) associated with struvite • Urine Culture: consider for all patients or those at greater risk for infection • Labs: **CBC** (if concern for infection), **BMP (renal function)**, urine beta-hCG (guides imaging choice) • Kidney Ureter Bladder (KUB) X-Ray: **only calcium and struvite stones are radiopaque;** lacks sensitivity for small stones • **Renal Ultrasound: initial imaging test** in children or pregnant patient; detects location of stone and complications (hydronephrosis) • **Non-Contrast CT Abdomen and Pelvis: imaging test of choice;** determines size and location of stone

Treatment	• **Analgesia: oral (ibuprofen) and IV (ketorolac) NSAIDs are first-line treatment for pain;** opioids reserved for refractory or severe pain; IV lidocaine
	• Antiemetics: **ondansetron**, metoclopramide, promethazine
	• Expulsive Therapy:
	   • **Alpha-Blockers: tamsulosin;** facilitates calculus passage by promoting smooth muscle relaxation and improves urinary flow
	   • Increased Oral or IV Fluids: traditionally recommended; *increased fluid administration has not been shown to speed the passage of calculi*
	• **Flexible Ureteroscopy: most common method;** allows for visualization and removal of stone or stent placement to provide immediate relief to obstructed or at-risk kidney
	• Extracorporeal Shockwave Lithotripsy: breaks up larger stones to facilitate passage
	• Percutaneous Nephrolithotomy: most invasive procedure; **reserved for large stones (>10mm), struvite stones**, or when other modalities have failed

Stone Size	Passage Rate
1-4 mm	78%
4-7 mm	60%
≥8 mm	39%

Penile Cancer

Etiology & Risk Factors	• Uncommon malignancy; patients often delay seeking medical attention due to embarrassment, guilt, fear, and denial of the condition
	• Etiology:
	   • **Squamous Cell Carcinoma: most common type;** associated with HIV, HPV 16 and 18
	   • Other Malignant Neoplasms: basal cell carcinoma, melanoma, sarcomas, and adenosquamous carcinoma
	   • Bowen' Disease: carcinoma in situ of the penile shaft that carries a 5-10% risk of progressing to SCC; associated with HPV 16
	• Risk Factors: **age (>60 years old** most common), **balanitis, lack of circumcision**, sexually transmitted infections (**HIV and HPV**), **poor hygiene**, smoking, phimosis, penile trauma

Patho-physiology	• Most commonly begin as small, erythematous lesion on the glans or prepuce that may grow to become fungating and exophytic or ulcerative and infiltrative cancer

Signs & Symptoms	• **Skin lesion or palpable nodule on the penis**
	   • **Most common on the glans, the coronal sulcus or the prepuce**
	   • May present with a **sore or ulcer that has not healed**
	• Physical Exam:
	   • **Inguinal lymphadenopathy**
	   • Painless skin lesion, palpable nodule or ulcer with subtle induration of skin

Diagnosis	• **Biopsy: punch, incisional, or excisional required for diagnosis** • If positive, **lymph node evaluation required;** initially spreads to the inguinal lymph nodes then the pelvic and retroperitoneal nodes • CT or MRI: aids in staging localized cancer and evaluating lymph nodes
Treatment	• Small, Superficial Lesions: **topical treatment with 5-fluorourcil or imiquimod and laser ablation** • Invasive and High-Grade Lesions: **radical resection;** partial vs total penectomy depending on extent of lesion • Bilateral ilioinguinal lymphadenectomy indicated in invasive cancer
Key Words & Most Common	• Squamous cell carcinoma most common; associated with HPV 16 and 18 • Skin lesion or palpable nodule on penis • May present as a nonhealing sore/ulcer • Inguinal lymphadenopathy • Biopsy • Topical treatment with 5-fluorourcil or imiquimod → radical resection

Erectile Dysfunction

Etiology & Risk Factors	• Defined as the consistent or recurrent inability to achieve or maintain an erection suitable for satisfactory sexual intercourse; also known as impotence
	• Etiology:
	  • <u>Vascular</u>: **most common cause**; **atherosclerosis**, diabetes, smoking, obesity, dyslipidemia, hypertension
	  • <u>Neurologic</u>: diabetic neuropathy, stroke, seizures, multiple sclerosis, peripheral and autonomic neuropathies, **spinal cord injuries**, **spinal stenosis**, surgical injury
	  • <u>Psychogenic</u>: stress, **general anxiety**, depression, guilt, fear of intimacy, **performance anxiety**; may be situational (involving a particular partner or place)
	  • <u>Hypogonadism</u>: decreased testosterone level
	  • <u>Medications</u>: **beta-blockers**, thiazide diuretics, **spironolactone**, calcium channel blockers, **SSRIs**, TCAs; **alcohol can cause temporary erectile dysfunction**

Patho-physiology	• Atherosclerosis of the cavernous arteries of the penis decreases the arterial blood vessel dilation capacity and smooth muscle relaxation which inhibits the amount of blood that is able to enter the penis; endothelial dysfunction, mediated by low levels of nitric oxide secondary to smoking, diabetes, or low testosterone levels, reduces the vasodilation ability of small arterioles, inhibiting blood flow to the penis
Signs & Symptoms	• **Inability to achieve or maintain an erection** • May have physical exam findings or symptoms consistent with underlying etiology
Diagnosis	• **Clinical Diagnosis** • <u>**Depression Screen**</u>: **vital to screen as may not always be apparent** • <u>Labs</u>: consider **testosterone**, prolactin, luteinizing hormone, hemoglobin A1C, lipid panel, cortisol level • <u>Nocturnal Penile Tumescence</u>: used to evaluate erections during sleep; may help differentiate between organic and psychogenic etiology • <u>Penile Duplex Ultrasound</u>: evaluates penile blood flow
Treatment	• **Treat underlying etiology** • <u>**Phosphodiesterase-5 (PDE5) Inhibitors**</u>: **first-line therapy; sildenafil, tadalafil, vardenafil** • Inhibits hydrolysis of cGMP to promote cGMP-dependent smooth muscle relaxation leading to ability to generate and maintain an erection • <u>Intracavernosal Injection Therapy</u>: prostaglandin E1 (alprostadil); may be compounded with papaverine and phentolamine for increased efficacy • <u>Mechanical Devices</u>: elastic ring placed at the base of the erect penis, vacuum pump (draws blood into the penis via suction) • <u>Penile Prosthesis</u>: semi-rigid silicone rod or saline-filled inflatable device is implanted within the penis to instantly produce an erection
Key Words & Most Common	• Inability to achieve of maintain an erection • Vascular is most common cause (atherosclerosis), neurologic, psychogenic, hypogonadism, medications (beta-blockers, spironolactone, SSRIs), alcohol • Clinical diagnosis • Treat underlying etiology • Phosphodiesterase-5 inhibitors (sildenafil, tadalafil) is first-line therapy

Hypospadias

Etiology & Risk Factors	• **Anatomical congenital malformation of the male external genitalia resulting in abnormal <u>ventral</u> (downward) position of the urethral opening** • May be associated with penile curvature and abnormal foreskin development • <u>Etiology</u>: **genetic, endocrine and environmental factors** • In-utero exposure to estrogens found in pesticides (fruits and vegetables) and plastic linings (water bottles, food containers, etc.)
Patho-physiology	• Failure of tubularization and fusion of the urethral groove during embryonal development resulting in abnormal urethral fold and ventral position of the urethral opening

Signs & Symptoms	• **Downward deflection of urinary stream**
	• **Erectile dysfunction**
	• **Penile curvature**
	• Increased risk of UTIs
	• <u>Physical Exam</u>:
	  • **Ventral (downward) position of the urethral meatus**
	  • Glandular groove and dorsal hood of the foreskin; prepuce is incomplete ventrally
	  • Abnormal penile curvature (chordee)

Diagnosis	• **Clinical Diagnosis**

Treatment	• <u>Surgery</u>: **urethroplasty** involves construction of the urethra using skin from the penile shaft or foreskin
	  • **Neonatal circumcision contraindicated** (foreskin is used to repair the defect)
	  • **Usually performed between 6-18 months of age**

Key Words & Most Common	• Congenital anomaly resulting in a ventrally located urethral opening • Downward deflection of urinary stream + penile curvature • Ventrally located urethra • Clinical diagnosis • Urethroplasty • Circumcision contraindicated

Ventral (downward) position of urethral meatus

Epispadias

Etiology & Risk Factors	• Anatomical congenital malformation of the male external genitalia resulting in abnormal <u>dorsal</u> (upward) position of the urethral opening • <u>Etiology</u>: usually seen as a component in the spectrum of **bladder exstrophy-epispadias-complex (BEEC)** • **Isolated epispadias is rare**
Patho-physiology	• Failure of midline penile fusion resulting in the urethra to tubularize on the dorsal aspect of the penis

Signs & Symptoms	• **Upward deflection of urinary stream**
	• **Urinary incontinence**
	• Increased risk of UTIs
	• <u>Physical Exam</u>:
	   • **Dorsal (upward) position of the urethral meatus**
	   • Absent dorsal foreskin
	   • Abnormal penile curvature (chordee)

Diagnosis	• **Clinical Diagnosis** • Associated bladder exstrophy usually diagnosed via prenatal ultrasound
Treatment	• <u>Surgery</u>: surgical reconstruction of the penis with bladder outlet reconstruction required to preserve continence
Key Words & Most Common	• Congenital anomaly resulting in a dorsally located urethral opening • Upward deflection of urinary stream + Urinary incontinence • Dorsally located urethra • Clinical diagnosis • Surgical reconstruction of the penis and bladder outlet

Urethral Trauma

Etiology & Risk Factors	• Trauma to urethra characterized by crush, bruising, laceration, or transection injuries
	• **More common in men**
	• <u>Etiology</u>:
	   • <u>Blunt Trauma</u>: **most common cause**; anterior urethral injury (**straddle-type falls** or direct impact) or posterior urethral injury (**pelvic fracture**, motor vehicle accidents)
	   • <u>Iatrogenic</u>: improper urethral catheterization and transurethral instrumentation
	   • <u>Other</u>: confused, disoriented or agitated patients pull out indwelling catheters; inserting objects into the urethra during sexual activity, **penile fractures**

Patho-physiology	• Trauma to urethra can cause scar tissue formation leading to fibrosis, stenosis, and/or stricture formation within the urethra resulting in urinary retention

Signs & Symptoms	• **Gross hematuria**
	• **Urinary retention**
	• **Pain or inability to void**
	• Sudden onset of pain during intercourse
	• <u>Physical Exam</u>:
	   • **Blood at the urethral meatus**
	   • **Scrotal swelling; "butterfly" pattern of ecchymosis of the perineum**
	   • **Distended urinary bladder**
	   • **High-riding prostate**

Diagnosis	• <u>Retrograde Urethrogram</u>: **gold-standard diagnostic test; must per performed prior to transurethral catheterization as it may potentiate urethral disruption** • <u>Urinalysis</u>: hematuria
Treatment	• <u>Urethral Catheterization</u>: indicated in urethral contusions • <u>Suprapubic Cystotomy</u>: indicated in partial or complete urethral disruption prior to surgical repair • <u>Surgery</u>: urethroplasty often required for severe injuries
Key Words & Most Common	• More common in men • Blunt trauma is most common cause (straddle injuries, pelvic fracture, MVA), improper catheterization, penile fractures • Grosse hematuria + inability to void + urinary retention • Blood at the urethral meatus + distended bladder • Retrograde urethrogram is gold-standard • Catheterization vs suprapubic cystotomy

Priapism

	Low-Flow (Ischemic)	High-Flow (Non-Ischemic)

Etiology & Risk Factors	• Painful, prolonged, persistent erection unaccompanied by sexual desire or excitation or any erection lasting >4 hours
	• Etiology:
	  • Idiopathic is most common, sickle cell disease, medications (SSRIs, trazodone, antipsychotics, PDE5 inhibitors [sildenafil]), drugs (cocaine)
		• Prolonged, persistent erection unaccompanied by sexual desire or excitation or any erection lasting >4 hours
		• Etiology:
		  • Arterio-cavernosal shunt due to groin or straddle injury/trauma, high spinal injury, head trauma

Patho-physiology	• Most common type; decreased venous outflow causes increased intracorporal pressure that results in a compartment syndrome situation with tissue ischemia and hypoxia of the cavernous tissue, cavernosal acidosis and penile pain	• Increased arterial inflow; perineal or penile injury or trauma results in fistula formation between the cavernosal artery and the corpus cavernosum
Signs & Symptoms	• Painful erection • Rigid penile shaft (corpus cavernosum) with flaccid penile glans and spongiosum	• Usually painless • Partially rigid shaft with rigid penile glans
Diagnosis	• Clinical Diagnosis • Cavernosal Blood Gas: hypoglycemia, hypoxemia, hypercarbia, and acidemia • Penile Doppler Ultrasound: minimal or absent cavernosal blood flow	• Clinical Diagnosis • Cavernosal Blood Gas: similar to ABG and normal glucose • Penile Doppler Ultrasound: normal to high cavernosal blood flow

Treatment	• Aspiration and Saline Irrigation: initial therapy
	  • Aspiration of blood from the base of the corpora cavernosa followed by saline irrigation
	• Intracavernosal Injection: phenylephrine is first-line medication
	  • Alpha agonists lead to contraction of cavernous smooth muscle resulting in increased venous outflow
	• Surgical Shunt: indicated if unsuccessful with aspiration and injection or if priapism present for >48 hours
		• Observation: most resolve within hours to days
		• Conservative: ice packs and analgesia
		• Selective Embolization or Surgical Ligation: indicated if refractory to conservative measures

Key Words & Most Common	• Idiopathic, sickle cell disease, medications (trazodone, sildenafil), cocaine • Decreased venous outflow • Painful erection • Cavernosal Blood Gas: hypoglycemia, hypoxemia, hypercarbia, acidemia • Penile Doppler US: minimal/absent cavernosal blood flow • Aspiration and saline irrigation → phenylephrine injection → surgical shunt	• Arterio-cavernosal shunt secondary to groin/straddle trauma • Increased arterial inflow • Painless erection • Cavernosal Blood Gas: similar to ABG, normal glucose • Penile Doppler US: normal to high cavernosal blood flow • Observation → ice packs/analgesia → embolization or surgical ligation

Urinary Incontinence in Children

Etiology & Risk Factors	• Distinct episodes of urinary incontinence occurring ≥2 times per month in children >5 years of age
	  • Diurnal Incontinence: daytime urinary incontinence
	  • Enuresis (Bed-Wetting): nocturnal urinary incontinence
	• Etiology:
	  • Diurnal Incontinence: bladder irritability (UTI), detrusor muscle weakness, constipation, incorrect position when voiding (females), structural abnormalities
	  • Enuresis (Bed-Wetting): maturation delay, incomplete toilet training, increased nighttime urine volume, difficulty arousing from sleep
	• Risk Factors: unusual stress (low socioeconomic status, parental divorce, birth of a sibling), family history of urinary incontinence as a child

Patho-physiology	• Abnormalities in either the storage phase (bladder size and compliance) or voiding phase (bladder contraction and external urinary sphincter synchronization) of urination can lead to urinary incontinence
Signs & Symptoms	• Daytime or nocturnal urinary incontinence

Diagnosis	• DSM-5 Diagnostic Criteria:
	  1. Involuntary or intentional voiding of urine into bed or clothes
	  2. Clinically significant distress or functional impairment from urinary incontinence
	  3. 5 years-old or developmental level of a 5 year-old
	  4. Behavior not attributed to another medical condition
	• Primary: continence was never established; child never achieved urinary continence for ≥6 months
	• Secondary: continence was achieved then lost; incontinence episode occurring after period of >6 months of urinary control
	• Testing to rule out alternative causes such as urinary tract infection, constipation, seizure, diabetes, or sleep apnea.

Treatment	• Behavioral: first-line therapy
	  • Motivational therapy, education, reassurance
	  • Bladder training, regular voiding schedule, timed voiding prior to sleep, fluid restriction at night, planned nighttime waking to urinate
	• Enuresis Alarm: most effective treatment; sensor is placed on bed pad or undergarments and alarm goes off when wet; continue until 21-28 consecutive dry nights
	• Medication: rarely indicated if a child is <7 years-old
	  • Desmopressin: anti-diuretic hormone; given 1 hour prior to bedtime to reduce urine production; indicated only for short-term use
	  • Imipramine: tricyclic antidepressant; anticholinergic effects cause detrusor muscle relaxation leading to decreased bladder contractility and decreased enuresis

Key Words & Most Common	• Urinary incontinence episodes occurring ≥2 times per month in children >5 years of age • Diurnal: daytime incontinence; bladder irritability (UTI) • Enuresis: nocturnal incontinence; maturation delay, difficulty arousing from sleep • Unusual stress (parental divorce, birth of a sibling) is greatest risk factor • Behavioral therapy → enuresis alarm → medications (desmopressin)

References

1. Peyronie's disease.jpg. (2023, February 25). *Wikimedia Commons*. Retrieved 21:49, August 15, 2023 from https://commons.wikimedia.org/w/index.php?title=File:Peyronie%27s_disease.jpg&oldid=735699528.
2. Vesicoureteral-reflux-004.jpg. (2020, September 13). *Wikimedia Commons*. Retrieved 21:52, August 15, 2023 from https://commons.wikimedia.org/w/index.php?title=File:Vesicoureteral-reflux-004.jpg&oldid=457495510.
3. Ultrasonography of hydrocele.jpg. (2022, October 12). *Wikimedia Commons*. Retrieved 21:57, August 15, 2023 from https://commons.wikimedia.org/w/index.php?title=File:Ultrasonography_of_hydrocele.jpg&oldid=695881704.
4. Spermatocele.JPG. (2020, October 4). *Wikimedia Commons*. Retrieved 21:58, August 15, 2023 from https://commons.wikimedia.org/w/index.php?title=File:Spermatocele.JPG&oldid=480298507.
5. Varicocele.png. (2022, September 22). *Wikimedia Commons*. Retrieved 22:06, August 15, 2023 from https://commons.wikimedia.org/w/index.php?title=File:Varicocele.png&oldid=690780531.
6. Photo légendé d'une Varicocèle.jpg. (2021, May 25). *Wikimedia Commons*. Retrieved 22:08, August 15, 2023 from https://commons.wikimedia.org/w/index.php?title=File:Photo_l%C3%A9gend%C3%A9_d%27une_Varicoc%C3%A8le.jpg&oldid=564293305.
7. BladderwallthickeningduetoCaMark.png. (2022, March 12). *Wikimedia Commons*. Retrieved 22:11, August 15, 2023 from https://commons.wikimedia.org/w/index.php?title=File:BladderwallthickeningduetoCaMark.png&oldid=637752085.
8. Phimosis.jpg. (2023, February 1). *Wikimedia Commons*. Retrieved 22:12, August 15, 2023 from https://commons.wikimedia.org/w/index.php?title=File:Phimosis.jpg&oldid=729441100.
9. Paraphimosis.jpg. (2023, January 18). *Wikimedia Commons*. Retrieved 22:15, August 15, 2023 from https://commons.wikimedia.org/w/index.php?title=File:Paraphimosis.jpg&oldid=725881277.
10. Benign Prostatic Hyperplasia nci-vol-7137-300.jpg. (2020, September 27). *Wikimedia Commons*. Retrieved 22:16, August 15, 2023 from https://commons.wikimedia.org/w/index.php?title=File:Benign_Prostatic_Hyperplasia_nci-vol-7137-300.jpg&oldid=473429685.
11. Penis with Hypospadias. 01.jpg. (2023, July 28). *Wikimedia Commons*. Retrieved 22:21, August 15, 2023 from https://commons.wikimedia.org/w/index.php?title=File:Penis_with_Hypospadias._01.jpg&oldid=787552753.

Chapter 10
Neurologic

Traumatic Brain Injury (TBI)

Etiology & Risk Factors	• Mechanical injury to brain tissue that temporarily or permanently impairs brain function; may result in cognitive, physical, social, emotional, or behavioral symptoms • Etiology: falls (especially in elderly and children) is most common cause, motor vehicle accidents or other transportation-related causes (bicycle crashes, collision with pedestrian, etc.), physical assault, sports activities (football, hockey, boxing, rugby), penetration
Patho-physiology	• Primary injury leads to bruising of brain parenchyma (contusions), intra- and extra-parenchymal hemorrhages (hematomas), or diffuse axonal injury • Secondary injury results as increased intracranial pressure occurs compressive and restricting perfusion of the brain leading to ischemia, brain herniation, and cellular death
Signs & Symptoms	• *Range of symptoms ranges from mild to severe and vary based on specific type of TBI* • **Physical injuries secondary to trauma** • **Loss of consciousness** (usually seconds to minutes) • <u>Cognitive Function Impairment</u>: confusion or amnesia (retrograde), **difficulty concentrating**, impaired processing time, impaired calculation and executive function • <u>Physical Impairment</u>: **headache, dizziness,** insomnia, **nausea/vomiting,** uneven gait, blurred vision, seizure • <u>Behavioral Impairment</u>: anxiety, irritability, depression, **sleep disturbances, emotional lability,** loss of initiative • <u>Cushing Reflex</u>: hypertension, bradycardia, irregular respirations

Diagnosis	• <u>Glasgow Coma Scale</u>: classifies severity of injury
	   • <u>Mild</u>: score >13
	   • <u>Moderate</u>: score of 9-12
	   • <u>Severe</u>: score of <8
	• <u>Non-contrast Head CT</u>: **best initial imaging test to evaluate acute head injuries**
	   • **Use validated decision rule to determine need to neuroimaging** (Canadian CT Head Rule)
	• <u>MRI Head</u>: indicated later in course to detect subtle contusions, diffuse axonal injury and brain stem injury
	• <u>CT Angiography</u>: indicated if vascular injury is suspected

Treatment	• *Treatment based on severity of TBI and extent of underlying trauma*
	• <u>Mild TBI</u>: **discharge home with close observation and strict return precautions,** cognitive and physical rest, avoid strenuous exercise
	• <u>Moderate TBI</u>: **admit for observation** with frequent clinical and neurological assessments
	• <u>Severe TBI</u>: admit to intensive care unit (ICU)
	   • <u>Airway</u>: **early endotracheal intubation;** avoid hypoxia
	   • <u>Breathing</u>: avoid hyperventilation in first 24-48 hours (hypocapnia induces cerebral vasoconstriction)
	   • <u>Circulation</u>: avoid hypotension; **fluid resuscitation with isotonic saline + vasopressors (phenylephrine) if refractory**
	   • <u>Reduction of Intracranial Pressure</u>:
	      • **Elevate Head of Bed: 30 degrees or reverse Trendelenburg;** keep head and neck in neutral position (improves cerebral venous drainage)
	      • <u>Osmotherapy</u>: **hypertonic saline is standard of care;** mannitol (increased tonicity draws water out of the brain parenchyma and into the intravascular space)
	   • <u>Seizure Control</u>: benzodiazepines (levetiracetam) and antiepileptic drugs (phenytoin or fosphenytoin)
	   • <u>Neurosurgery Intervention</u>: **indicated with abnormal CT scan;** surgical evacuation of hematoma, decompressive craniectomy, skull fracture care

Cerebral contusions

Validated Decision Rule

Canadian CT Head Rule for Minor Head Injury

Inclusion Criteria

Blunt head trauma causing loss of consciousness, amnesia, disorientation

Glasgow Coma Scale 13-15

Age ≥16 years old

No coagulopathy or use of anti-coagulant medication

No seizure

Head CT indicated if one or more of the following present

High Risk

Age ≥65 years old

Vomiting >2 episodes

Suspected open or depress skull fracture

Signs suggesting basilar skull fracture
(hemotympanum, racoon eyes, CSF otorrhea or rhinorrhea, Battle's sign)

Glasgow Coma Scale <15 at 2 hours post-injury

Medium Risk

Retrograde amnesia >30 minutes

Dangerous Mechanism
(pedestrian struck by vehicle, ejection from motor vehicle, fall from elevation >3 feet or 5 stairs)

Minor Head Injury: defined as a witnessed loss of consciousness, definite amnesia, or witnessed disorientation in patients with GCS of 13-15. Not applicable if warfarin use, bleeding disorder, or patient suffering seizure prior to arrival to ED.

Classification of Severity

Glasgow Coma Scale

Eye Opening	Score	Verbal Response	Score	Motor Response	Score
Spontaneously	4	Oriented	5	Obeys Commands	6
Verbal Command	3	Disoriented, able to answer questions	4	Localization Response to Pain	5
Response to pain	2	Inappropriate answer to questions	3	Withdrawal Response to Pain	4
No Eye Opening	1	Incomprehensible Speech	2	Abnormal Flexion Response to Pain	3
		No Verbal Response	1	Abnormal (Rigid) Extension Response to Pain	2
				No Motor Response	1

<u>Mild TBI</u>: score of 13 or higher
<u>Moderate TBI</u>: score of 9-12
<u>Severe TBI</u>: score of 8 or less

Concussion

Etiology & Risk Factors	• Form of mild traumatic brain injury leading to altered mental status with or without loss of consciousness
	• Etiology: blunt force trauma or acceleration/deceleration head injury
	  • Falls (especially in elderly and children) is most common cause, motor vehicle accidents or other transportation-related causes (bicycle crashes, collision with pedestrian, etc.), physical assault, sports activities (football, hockey, boxing, rugby), penetration
	• Risk Factors:
	  • Repeat Injury: patient that has suffered one concussion is 2-4x more likely to suffer another concussion
	  • Second-Impact Syndrome: acute, often fatal brain swelling occurs with second sustained concussion before complete recovery from a previous concussion

Patho-physiology	• Acceleration, deceleration or head rotation result in acute axonal injury via neurofilament organization disruption; ion channel depolarization releases electrolytes and neurotransmitters resulting in neurologic dysfunction; alterations in glucose metabolism cause reduced cerebral blood flow resulting in mitochondrial dysfunction • Brain dysfunction secondary to excitotoxicity (neuronal damage caused by excessive excitatory neurotransmitter [glutamate] release)
Signs & Symptoms	• May have loss of consciousness • Confusion: dazed or stunned, blank expression, blunted affect • Amnesia: retrograde (pre-traumatic) or antegrade (post-traumatic); may not recall plays or assignment if sports-related • Vision Disturbance: double vision, photophobia • Physical Impairment: headache, dizziness, nausea, uneven gait, tinnitus • Post-Concussion Syndrome: may be present days or weeks after initial injury • Chronic headaches, impaired short-term memory, difficulty concentrating, fatigue, disrupted sleep, personality changes (irritability, mood lability), photo/phono-phobia • Signs of Increased Intracranial Pressure: vomiting, worsening headache, increased disorientation, changing levels of consciousness, seizure

Diagnosis	• Clinical Diagnosis
	• Glasgow Coma Scale: classifies severity of injury
	  • Mild TBI: score >13
	• Non-Contrast Head CT: best initial imaging test to evaluate acute head injuries
	  • Use validated decision rule to determine need to neuroimaging (Canadian CT Head Rule)
	• MRI Head: indicated later in course to detect subtle contusions, diffuse axonal injury and brain stem injury; indicated for symptoms lasting >7-14 days or worsening symptoms
	• CT Angiography: indicated if vascular injury is suspected

Treatment	• Removal from Contest or Activity: second-impact syndrome can be life-threatening • Observation: family members encouraged to monitor for signs of deterioration (decreased consciousness, focal neurologic deficits, vomiting, worsening headache, seizure) • Analgesia: acetaminophen or NSAIDs indicated for headache based on severity of injury • Cognitive and Physical Rest: mainstay of management • School and work activities, driving, alcohol, excessive brain stimulation (computers, television, video games, bright/flashing lights), physical exertion should be avoided • Return to Play Protocol: symptomatic patients should refrain from activity until asymptomatic for at least 1 week then follow a graduated approach to return to play

Epidural Hematoma

Etiology & Risk Factors	• Extra-axial collection of blood between the outer layer of the dura mater and the inner skull, confined by the lateral sutures (coronal sutures) where the dura inserts • Life-threatening condition • Etiology: acute head trauma; often associated with temporal skull fracture • Risk Factors: motor vehicle accidents, physical assaults, accidental falls
Patho-physiology	• Blunt trauma to temporal or temporoparietal region results in rupture of the middle meningeal artery results in bleeding between the outer layer of the dura mater and the inner skull, confined by the coronal sutures (where the dura inserts)

Signs & Symptoms	• 3 Classic Phases: loss of consciousness → lucid interval → neurologic deterioration
	  • Loss of Consciousness: initial loss of consciousness following acute head trauma
	  • Complete Transient Recovery: also known as a "lucid interval"; patient regains consciousness and seems fine
	  • Rapid Neurological Deterioration: mental status changes, headache, vomiting, focal neurologic deficits (hemiparesis), decreased level of consciousness, seizure
	• Elevated Intracranial Pressure: ipsilateral pupil dilation (secondary to uncal herniation and oculomotor nerve compression), elevated blood pressure, bradycardia, and irregular breathing

Diagnosis	• Non-contrast Head CT: initial imaging test of choice
	  • Demonstrates a biconvex (lens-shaped, lemon-shaped) hyperdense lesion with sharp margins in the temporoparietal region
	  • Does not cross coronal suture lines (differentiates epidural form subdural hematoma)
	• Brain MRI: more sensitive than CT scan; rarely performed in acute setting

Treatment	• Craniotomy and Hematoma Evacuation: treatment of choice for acute and symptomatic epidural hematomas
	• Observation: indicated if small and patient is stable
	• Reduction of Intracranial Pressure:
	  • Elevate Head of Bed: 30 degrees or reverse Trendelenburg
	    • Keep head and neck in neutral position (improves cerebral venous drainage)
	  • Intubation and Mechanical Ventilation: preserve airway; consider short-term hyperventilation
	  • Osmotherapy: hypertonic saline is standard of care
	    • Mannitol (increased tonicity draws water out of the brain parenchyma and into the intravascular space)

Key Words & Most Common	• Collection of blood between dura mater and skull; confined by lateral sutures • Often associated with temporal skull fracture • 3 Classic Phases: loss of consciousness → lucid interval → neurologic deterioration • Non-contrast head CT shows biconvex (lens-shaped) hyperdense lesion with sharp margins • Craniotomy and hematoma evacuation

Biconvex (lens-shaped) hyperdense lesion

Subdural Hematoma

Etiology & Risk Factors	• Abnormal collection of blood between the dura mater and arachnoid membranes • <u>Etiology</u>: **sudden acceleration-deceleration of the brain**, blunt head trauma • **Resultant shearing of the cortical bridging veins** • <u>Risk Factors</u>: **elderly and alcoholics** (increased brain atrophy), **children <2 years old** (accidental or intentional trauma, also known as "shaken baby syndrome")
Patho-physiology	• Sudden acceleration-deceleration injury as a result of violent, repeated movements or blunt head trauma causes shearing of the cortical bridging veins resulting in collection of blood between the dura mater and arachnoid membranes

Signs & Symptoms	• <u>Adults</u>: variable presentation; often secondary to trauma
	   • **Gradual increase in generalized neurologic symptoms** (headache, dizziness, nausea/vomiting) **and/or focal neurologic symptoms**
	   • **Altered mental status** (irritability, lethargy), alterations in orientation, level of arousal and/or cognition
	   • May have **loss of consciousness**
	• <u>Infants</u>: injuries often contradicts the history given by the caretaker
	   • **Abnormal breathing patterns, apneic episodes**
	   • **Abnormal feeding or refusal to feed, changes in behavior,** vomiting, abnormal movements or seizures
	   • May have other signs of abusive trauma **(bruising, limb deformities)**
	   • **Retinal hemorrhages**
	• <u>Elevated Intracranial Pressure</u>: ipsilateral pupil dilation, elevated blood pressure, bradycardia, and irregular breathing

Diagnosis	• <u>Non-Contrast Head CT</u>: initial imaging test of choice
	   • **Demonstrates concave (crescent-shaped) opacity overlying brain tissue that can cross suture lines**
	   • **Large hematomas may cause midline shift**
	   • Acute hematomas appear hyperdense; chronic hematomas appear hypodense

Treatment	• <u>Observation</u>: indicated if stable with small hematoma and no signs of brain herniation and no signs of increased intracranial pressure • <u>Surgical Evacuation</u>: indicated if hematoma >10mm, midline shift >5mm, or signs of increased intracranial pressure • Craniotomy, decompressive craniectomy, burr hole trephination (only indicated if extended time to assessment by neurosurgeon) • **Report abuse to the appropriate state child protection authority if concern for non-accidental trauma**
Key Words & Most Common	• Bleeding between dura mater and arachnoid membranes • Sudden acceleration-deceleration of brain or trauma shears cortical bridge veins • Most common in elderly and alcoholics or children <2 (child abuse possible) • <u>Adults</u>: gradual increase in general neurologic symptoms • <u>Infants</u>: abnormal breathing patterns, abnormal feeding, changes in behavior, retinal hemorrhages • Non-contrast head CT shows concave (crescent-shaped) opacity overlying brain tissue that can cross suture lines • Observation vs surgical evacuation → report suspected abuse

Concave (crescent-shaped) opacity that crosses suture lines

Intracerebral Hemorrhage

Etiology & Risk Factors	• **Focal bleeding from a blood vessel within the brain parenchyma**
	• **Also known as hemorrhagic stroke**
	• <u>Etiology</u>:
	   • <u>Primary</u>: **hypertension is most common cause overall**; cerebral amyloid angiopathy is most common cause in elderly
	   • <u>Secondary</u>: **arteriovenous malformation**, coagulopathy (iatrogenic, congenital, acquired), neoplasm, drug abuse
	• <u>Risk Factors</u>: **hypertension, advanced age, alcohol abuse, anticoagulant (warfarin) use, drug use (cocaine)**, poor diet, smoking

Patho-physiology	• Chronic arterial hypertension leads to weakening of arteriosclerotic small arteries which eventually rupture causing extravasation of blood into the brain parenchyma • Blood accumulates as a mass that compresses the adjacent brain tissue leading to neuronal dysfunction

Signs & Symptoms	• *Often clinically indistinguishable from ischemic stroke and subarachnoid hemorrhage*
	• **Neurologic symptom progression over minutes to hours**
	• **Headache, nausea/vomiting, altered mental status** often precede neurologic deficits
	• <u>Focal Neurologic Deficits</u>: hemiplegia, hemiparesis, seizure, unilateral weakness, paresthesias
	• <u>Increased Intracranial Pressure</u>: due to obstructive hydrocephalus
	   • **Elevated blood pressure** (diastolic >110mmHg), postural headache, **papilledema, vomiting, diplopia**
	   • Confusion, loss of consciousness, seizure

Diagnosis	• <u>Non-Contrast Head CT</u>: initial imaging test of choice; helps distinguish between ischemic stroke and subarachnoid hemorrhage • **Demonstrates an area of hyperdensity within the parenchyma and surrounding hypodensity (perivascular edema)**

Treatment	• <u>Supportive</u>: measures to prevent increased intracranial pressure
	   • Elevate head of bed (30°), limit IV fluids, pain control, stool softeners, sedation, consider intubation
	• <u>Discontinue/Reverse Anticoagulation</u>: fresh frozen plasma, prothrombin complex concentrate, tranexamic acid, vitamin K or platelet transfusions as indicated
	• <u>Blood Pressure Management</u>: aggressive reduction indicated if systolic BP >100mmHg or mean arterial pressure >150mmHg
	   • **IV nicardipine or IV labetalol preferred**
	• <u>Surgery</u>: early evacuation of large lobar cerebral hematomas

Key Words & Most Common	• Bleeding within the brain parenchyma; most common secondary to hypertension • Neurologic symptoms progress over minutes to hours • Headache, nausea/vomiting, altered mental status → focal neurologic deficits → increased intracranial pressure • Non-contrast head CT shows hyperdense area within the parenchyma • Supportive + discontinue/reverse anticoagulation • Aggressive BP management (nicardipine or labetalol) • Surgical evacuation

Hyperdensity within parenchyma and surrounding hypodensity

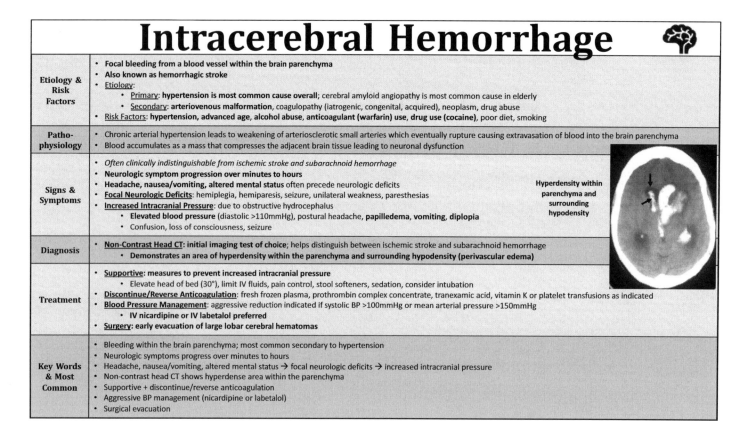

Cerebral Aneurysm

Etiology & Risk Factors	• Focal dilations that occur at weak points along the cerebral arterial circulation • Most common location is in anterior circulation, usually at junctions or bifurcations along the circle of Willis • <u>Etiology</u>: most are acquired; genetic predisposition • <u>Risk Factors</u>: **advanced age, hypertension, smoking, alcohol abuse, atherosclerosis are greatest risk factors**; **cocaine use**, tumors, trauma, family history, **connective tissue disorder** (autosomal dominant polycystic kidney disease, Ehlers-Danlos or Marfan syndrome)
Patho-physiology	• Hemodynamic stress from hypertension or turbulent blood flow on the internal elastic lamina causes structural fatigue and tissue breakdown over time • Eventually, vascular wall histologic changes lead to aneurysmal formation and growth • <u>3 Types</u>: saccular (berry) is most common, fusiform (circumferential), myotic (infectious)
Signs & Symptoms	• **Most are asymptomatic** • **Large aneurysms may cause compression of adjacent structures** • Ocular palsies, diplopia, squint, orbital pain • Rupture of cerebral aneurysm leads to subarachnoid hemorrhage
Diagnosis	• **Most cerebral aneurysms are diagnosed incidentally or in the setting of subarachnoid hemorrhage** • <u>Neuroimaging</u>: indicated in high-risk patients • Brain MRI, CT angiography (CTA), or conventional angiography (digital subtraction angiography)
Treatment	• <u>Observation</u>: serial imaging and reduction of risk factors indicated for small, asymptomatic aneurysms • <u>Management of Risk Factors</u>: combination of diet, exercise, statin and antihypertensive therapy, diabetes control • <u>Endovascular Coiling</u>: indicated in large or symptomatic aneurysms or aneurysm located in posterior circulation
Key Words & Most Common	• Focal dilations occurring at weak points along cerebral arterial circulation • Age, hypertension, smoking, alcohol use, atherosclerosis greatest risk factors • Most asymptomatic; may cause compression if large • Neuroimaging to diagnose; most are diagnosed incidentally • Observation + management of risk factors if small or asymptomatic • Endovascular coiling if large or symptomatic

C

Digital subtraction angiography demonstrates aneurysm at anterior cerebral artery

Subarachnoid Hemorrhage

Etiology & Risk Factors	• **Abnormal collection of blood between the arachnoid membranes and pia mater** • <u>Etiology</u>: **ruptured cerebral aneurysm (congenital intracranial saccular or berry aneurysm is most common)**, head trauma, arteriovenous malformation, bleeding disorders • <u>Risk Factors</u>: **hypertension and smoking are greatest risk factors, family history, atherosclerosis**, age (40-60 years old most common) alcohol abuse, drug use (cocaine, amphetamines), connective tissue disease (Ehlers-Danlos or Marfan syndrome), family history of polycystic kidney disease, estrogen deficiency
Patho-physiology	• Hemorrhage secondary to a ruptured cerebral aneurysm causes blood to collect between the arachnoid membranes and pia mater • Bleeding in the subarachnoid space causes an aseptic chemical meningitis that can increase intracranial pressure

Signs & Symptoms	• **Sudden, severe "thunderclap" headache**
	  • **Reaches maximal intensity within seconds to minutes**
	  • Usually unilateral (often in occipital area)
	  • **Described as "worst headache of my life"**
	• May be associated with syncope, delirium, **nausea/vomiting**, seizures, **meningeal symptoms (photophobia, neck stiffness)**
	• May have history of mild headache for 1-3 weeks prior (sentinel leak occurs in 30-50% of patients)
	• <u>Physical Exam</u>:
	  • <u>Meningeal Signs</u>: nuchal rigidity, positive Brudzinski and Kernig signs and jolt test
	  • Bilateral extensor plantar responses (Babinski sign)
	  • **Retinal hemorrhages**

Diagnosis	• <u>Non-Contrast Head CT</u>: **initial imaging test of choice; demonstrates subarachnoid hemorrhage** and may aid in diagnosis of cerebral aneurysm • <u>Lumbar Puncture</u>: indicated if initial CT negative, no concern for increased intracranial pressure and subarachnoid hemorrhage is clinically suspected • **Increased opening pressure, numerous RBCs, xanthochromia** (yellow to pink CSF from RBC lysis causing release of breakdown products [bilirubin and oxyhemoglobin]) • <u>CT Angiogram</u>: all 4 arteries (2 carotid and 2 vertebral arteries) should be evaluated to identify source of bleeding and confirm location of intracerebral aneurysms

Treatment	• <u>Supportive</u>: bed rest, elevate head of bed, pain control, discontinue/reverse all anticoagulation, stool softeners (prevent increased intracranial pressure with Valsalva)
	• <u>Blood Pressure Management</u>: indicated if mean arterial pressure is > 130 mm Hg; euvolemia should be maintained
	  • Labetalol, **nicardipine**, enalapril are preferred antihypertensives
	• <u>Vasospasm Prevention</u>:
	  • <u>Nimodipine</u>: calcium channel blocker to reduce cerebral vasospasms
	  • <u>Magnesium Sulfate</u>: controversial treatment; prevents vasospasm acting as NMDA antagonist and a calcium channel blocker
	• <u>Surgery</u>: **endovascular coiling or surgical clipping; indicated to prevent rebleeding within the first 24 hours**

Key Words & Most Common	• Collection of blood between arachnoid membranes and pia mater due to ruptured cerebral (saccular or berry) aneurysm • Sudden, severe "thunderclap" headache reaching maximal intensity within seconds to minutes • Non-contrast head CT initial imaging test of choice • BP management → vasospasm prevention (nimodipine) → surgery (endovascular coiling or surgical clipping)

Subarachnoid hemorrhage extending into bilateral sulci

Tension Headache

Etiology & Risk Factors	• **Headache characterized by mild, generalized (vise-like) pain** without incapacitation, nausea, or photo/phonophobia • Also known as muscle contraction headache, stress headache or psychomyogenic headache • <u>Etiology</u>: various factors; nutritional, muscular, environmental and genetics • **Stress, poor posture (excessive neck flexion)**, eye strain, TMJ dysfunction, **sleep disturbance**, vitamin B12 deficiency, vitamin D deficiency, poor electrolyte intake, **dehydration, overexertion**
Patho-physiology	• Exact pathophysiology unknown; myofascial trigger points, excessive pericranial muscle contractions, tightening of the suboccipital and the upper neck musculature (leads to "pulling" of the dural matter), autonomic dysfunction have been implicated

Signs & Symptoms	• **Bilateral headache**
	   • **Described as pressure, tight, "band-like" or "vice-like"**
	   • **Non-throbbing (non-pulsatile)**
	   • **Steady or aching headache** (worsens throughout the day)
	• Headache *worsened* by stress, fatigue, noise, light glare
	• Headache *not worsened* with routine activity and not associated with pulsating, nausea, vomiting, photo/phonophobia, or focal neurologic symptoms (visual aura) or deficits
	• <u>Physical Exam</u>:
	   • **Usually benign exam**; may have **pericranial muscle tenderness** (head, neck, shoulder tenderness)

Diagnosis	• **Clinical Diagnosis**
	• <u>Definition</u>:
	   • Headache lasting 30 minutes to 7 days
	   • 2 or more of the following: bilateral location, pressure/tight (non-pulsatile), mild-to-moderate intensity, not aggravated by routine activity (walking, bending over)
	   • No nausea or vomiting; no photophobia or phonophobia
	   • Not attributed to another disorder

Treatment	• <u>**Supportive**</u>: adequate hydration, trigger avoidance, **local heat, trigger point massage, relaxation, exercise programs, improvement of posture**, acupuncture, physical therapy
	• <u>**Analgesia**</u>: **NSAIDs are mainstay of treatment**; acetaminophen alternative for those than cannot tolerate NSAIDs
	   • Ibuprofen, naproxen, aspirin, acetaminophen, ketoprofen, diclofenac, ketorolac
	   • **400mg ibuprofen and 1,000mg of acetaminophen is considered best pharmacologic treatment**
	• <u>Chronic Medical Management</u>: **tricyclic antidepressants (amitriptyline)** can help prevent chronic tension-type headaches

Key Words & Most Common	• Triggered by stress, poor posture, eye strain, sleep deprivation, overexertion, dehydration • Bilateral headache + pressure/tight/"band-like"/"vice-like"; non-throbbing • Clinical diagnosis • Supportive care + analgesia (NSAIDs)

Migraine Headache

Etiology & Risk Factors	• **Episodic, primary headache disorder characterized by unilateral, throbbing pain, worse with exertion, and accompanied by nausea, photophobia and/or phonophobia** • <u>Etiology</u>: combination of genetic and environmental factors • <u>Risk Factors</u>: **female, family history**, age (presents initially during puberty, continues through 40 years old), **oral contraceptives**, hormone therapy • <u>Precipitating Factors</u>: **stress is most common trigger, hormonal changes** (menstruation, ovulation, pregnancy), skipped meals, **weather changes**, insufficient sleep, odors (fragrances, gasoline, cologne, perfume), **neck pain, bright light exposure**, alcohol, smoking, late sleeping, heat or cold exposure, certain foods
Patho-physiology	• Neurovascular pain syndrome characterized by altered central neuronal processing (brain stem nuclei activation, cortical hyperexcitability) and trigeminovascular system involvement which initiates a neuropeptide release causing acute cranial nerve and dura mater inflammation and parasympathetic dilation of intracranial arteries

Signs & Symptoms	• <u>**Prodrome**</u>: premonitory symptoms including yawning, mood changes, neck pain, food cravings, loss of appetite, nausea, sound sensitivity, sweating, increased thirst
	• <u>**Aura**</u>: focal neurological symptom lasting <60 minutes (5-20 minutes most common) that accompany or follow the headache
	   • **Visual aura is most common type; flashes of bright light**, "foggy" vision, zigzag lines, and **scintillating scotoma** (multi-colored, arc-shaped, wavy, visual phenomena)
	   • Auditory, somatosensory, loss of function (aphasia, hearing loss) aura also possible
	• <u>**Headache Attack**</u>: may last hours to day (average 4-72 hours)
	   • **Unilateral, pulsatile (throbbing) headache of moderate-to-severe pain intensity**
	   • **Aggravated by routine physical activity** (walking, bending over, coughing)
	   • Accompanied by **nausea/vomiting, photophobia and/or phonophobia**
	• <u>Physical Exam</u>: usually normal; may have aphasia, dysarthria, paresthesia, weakness

Diagnosis	• **Clinical Diagnosis** • <u>*Red Flags*</u>: *pain reaching peak intensity within seconds to minutes, onset after age 50, increasing headache intensity, history of cancer, fever, AMS, papilledema, focal deficits*

Treatment	• <u>**Lifestyle Modifications**</u>: **relaxation techniques, avoidance of triggers, good sleep hygiene**, regular exercise, cognitive behavioral therapy, **stress reduction, yoga**, dark room
	   • Butterbur, magnesium, melatonin supplements may reduce frequency
	• <u>**Acute (Abortive) Treatment**</u>: *consider parenteral medications if nausea and vomiting*
	   • <u>**NSAIDs**</u>: **first-line for mild attacks**; ibuprofen, naproxen, aspirin, acetaminophen, ketoprofen, diclofenac, ketorolac; acetaminophen as alternative
	   • <u>**Triptans**</u>: **sumatriptan**, zolmitriptan; indicated in moderate-to-severe attacks or refractory to NSAIDs
	   • <u>**Antiemetics**</u>: **metoclopramide**, chlorpromazine, prochlorperazine; indicated as adjunctive therapy with NSAIDs/triptans to decrease nausea/vomiting
	     • <u>**Antihistamines**</u>: diphenhydramine may be added to prevent or treat dystonic reactions associated with metoclopramide
	   • <u>**Ergots**</u>: **ergotamine, dihydroergotamine**; indicated in moderate-to-severe attacks or refractory to other treatments (more side effects)
	   • *IV fluids and placing patient in a dark and quit room helpful in combination with acute treatments*
	• <u>**Prophylactic (Preventative) Treatment**</u>: indicated in frequent or long-lasting headaches, associated with disability, and/or affecting quality of life
	   • <u>**Beta-Blockers**</u>: **propranolol**, metoprolol; especially effective in hypertensive and non-smoker patients
	   • <u>**Calcium Channel Blockers**</u>: **verapamil**, flunarizine; especially effective in women of childbearing age or patients with Raynaud's phenomenon
	   • <u>**Antidepressants**</u>: **amitriptyline** (TCA), venlafaxine (SNRI); especially effective in patients with depression, anxiety disorders and/or insomnia
	   • <u>Anticonvulsants</u>: valproate, topiramate; especially effective in patients with epilepsy

Cluster Headache

Etiology & Risk Factors	• **Short-lasting unilateral headache with one or more autonomic symptom ipsilateral to the headache** (lacrimation, nasal congestion, conjunctival injection, or ear fullness) • <u>Etiology</u>: exact etiology is unclear • <u>Risk Factors</u>: **male (10x greater risk than female), age (>40 most common), alcohol, stress, family history**, prior brain surgery, head trauma • <u>Precipitating Factors</u>: **alcohol**, stress, ingestion of certain foods, **usually worse at nighttime**, watching television, hot weather, sexual activity
Patho-physiology	• Exact pathophysiology is unknown; circadian periodicity suggests hypothalamic dysfunction

Signs & Symptoms	• **Severe, unilateral headache**
	  • **Localized to periorbital or temporal region**
	  • Described as **sharp, lancinating** (piercing or stabbing sensation)
	  • Attacks typically last <2 hours with spontaneous remission
	  • **Attacks occur several times per day and around the same time everyday** (may awaken from sleep)
	• <u>Physical Exam</u>:
	  • <u>Ipsilateral Autonomic Features</u>: **conjunctival injection or lacrimation, nasal congestion, rhinorrhea**, eyelid or forehead edema, miosis, ptosis, **facial flushing**
	    • <u>Horner's Syndrome</u>: ptosis, miosis, anhidrosis
	  • **Patients are often agitated and restless** (pacing the floor, hitting head)

Diagnosis	• **Clinical Diagnosis** • <u>Neuroimaging</u>: consider CT/MRI to rule out structural etiology

Treatment	• <u>**Acute Treatment**</u>:
	  • <u>Oxygen Therapy</u>: **high-flow 100% oxygen is first-line and most effective therapy**
	  • <u>Triptans</u>: **sumatriptan**, zolmitriptan; subcutaneous or intranasal formulary indicated in moderate-to-severe attacks
	  • <u>Other</u>: intranasal lidocaine (4%), octreotide, ergotamine, dihydroergotamine
	• <u>**Preventative Treatment**</u>:
	  • **Verapamil is first-line** for initial preventative therapy
	  • Suboccipital blockade, corticosteroids, lithium, valproic acid, melatonin, and intranasal capsaicin are alternatives for prevention

Key Words & Most Common	• Middle aged male + alcohol or stress • Worse at night • Severe unilateral periorbital/temporal headache described as sharp/piercing/stabbing • Autonomic Symptoms: conjunctival injection, tearing, nasal congestion, rhinorrhea, facial flushing • Clinical Diagnosis • High-flow 100% Oxygen fist-line for initial treatment → triptans • Verapamil is first-line for prevention

Trigeminal Neuralgia

Etiology & Risk Factors	• **Severe paroxysmal, lancinating facial pain secondary to 5th cranial nerve (trigeminal nerve) disorder** • <u>Etiology</u>: **compression of the trigeminal nerve root by an aberrant loop of an intracranial artery** (anterior inferior cerebellar artery, basilar artery) **is most common cause** • Idiopathic, mass effect (tumor, aneurysm), arteriovenous malformation, multiple sclerosis plaque • <u>Risk Factors</u>: **most common in middle-aged women**
Patho-physiology	• Trigeminal nerve compression causes local demyelination at the compression site; ectopic nerve impulse generation (ephaptic transmission) and spinal trigeminal nucleus central pain pathway disinhibition leads to symptoms

Signs & Symptoms	• **Paroxysmal, severe, unilateral headache**
	  • **Pain follows trigeminal nerve distribution (maxillary distribution most common)**
	  • **Pain lasts seconds**, up to 2 minutes; can occur many times per day
	  • **Pain described as lancinating, excruciating, incapacitating; described as a "lightning bolt" strike or stabbing sensation**
	  • **May be triggered by light stimulus** (light touch, shaving, brushing teeth, washing face, chewing, smoking, talking, cold air exposure, gentle breeze)
	• <u>Physical Exam</u>:
	  • Often normal neurological exam; light palpation of "trigger zones" may initiate severe pain or facial muscle spasms

Diagnosis	• **Clinical Diagnosis** • <u>Neuroimaging</u>: consider CT/MRI to rule out structural etiology • *Development of trigeminal neuralgia in a young patient should raise concern for multiple sclerosis*

Treatment	• <u>**Medical Management**</u>:
	  • **Carbamazepine: first-line agent; decreases neuronal response to peripheral stimulation**
	  • **Oxcarbazepine**, baclofen, lamotrigine, gabapentin, phenytoin, amitriptyline are alternative, second-line agents
	• <u>Surgical Management</u>:
	  • Posterior fossa microvascular decompressive surgery indicated for severe or refractory cases

Key Words & Most Common	• Severe, paroxysmal, lancinating facial pain due to CNV (trigeminal) compression • Most common in middle-aged women • Severe, unilateral headache + pan following CNV distribution (maxillary) • Triggered by light stimulus • Clinical diagnosis • Cabamazepine is first-line

Trigeminal Nerve

Idiopathic Intracranial Hypertension 🧠

Etiology & Risk Factors	• Condition characterized by idiopathic increased intracranial pressure (ICP) in the setting of normal imaging and cerebrospinal fluid (CSF) studies • Also known as **pseudotumor cerebri** • <u>Etiology</u>: **idiopathic** • <u>Risk Factors</u>: **obese women of childbearing age is most common**; associated with obesity, weight gain, pregnancy, vitamin A toxicity, thyroid disorders • <u>Medications</u>: cyclosporine, tetracycline, amiodarone, sulfa antibiotics, lithium, corticosteroid withdrawal, thyroid hormone replacement, oral contraceptives
Patho-physiology	• Idiopathic accumulation of CSF through decreased absorption or increased production leads in increased intracranial pressure • Proposed mechanisms involve the vascular, hormonal, and cellular systems.

Signs & Symptoms	• <u>Headache</u>: **pulsatile in quality and worse in morning, changes in posture or with Valsalva**
	   • Pain may be bilateral, frontal or retrobulbar (worse with eye movements)
	• <u>Transient Vision Loss</u>: may be monocular or binocular, partial or complete and lasts seconds at a time (due to optic disc edema and temporary optic nerve ischemia)
	• <u>Diplopia</u>: binocular and horizontal diplopia (due to CNVI [abducens] palsy)
	• <u>Pulsatile Tinnitus</u>: described as heartbeat or "whooshing" sound
	• <u>Photopsia</u>: may have flashing lights
	• <u>Physical Exam</u>:
	   • <u>Fundoscopic Exam</u>: **papilledema** (usually bilateral and symmetric)
	   • <u>CNVI (abducens) Palsy</u>: esotropia and horizontal diplopia
	   • <u>Visual Field Loss</u>: increased blind spot and loss of inferonasal vision

Diagnosis	• <u>Neuroimaging</u>: performed prior to lumbar puncture to rule out intracranial mass
	   • **Magnetic Resonance Imaging (MRI) with Venography (MRV): preferred imaging study**; normal parenchyma and ventricles, may have transverse sinus stenosis
	   • <u>CT Scan</u>: performed if MRI contraindicated; less sensitive and specific
	• **Lumbar Puncture: CSF opening pressure >25cmH$_2$O**; normal CSF analysis

Treatment	• <u>**Carbonic Anhydrase Inhibitors**</u>: **acetazolamide is first-line**; decreases CSF production and functions as a diuretic • <u>Topiramate</u>: weak carbonic anhydrase activity and may lead to weight loss • <u>Diuretics</u>: furosemide, chlorthalidone; adjunct therapy as less effective than carbonic anhydrase inhibitors • <u>Repeat Lumbar Puncture</u>: may transiently relieve symptoms or lead to a complete resolution by decreasing CSF pressure • <u>Weight Loss</u>: weight loss of 5 to 10% of total body weight may achieve complete resolution • <u>Surgery</u>: optic nerve sheath fenestration or CSF shunt (ventriculoperitoneal or lumboperitoneal) indicated in cases refractory to medical treatment
Key Words & Most Common	• Idiopathic increased ICP in setting of normal neuroimaging and CSF studies (lumbar puncture) Obese women of childbearing age is most common presentation • Headache + transient vision changes (vision loss, diplopia, flashing lights) + pulsatile tinnitus + papilledema • Acetazolamide is first-line

Normal Pressure Hydrocephalus 🧠

Etiology & Risk Factors	• **Dilation of cerebral ventricles characterized by gait disturbance, urinary incontinence, dementia, and normal or slightly elevated cerebrospinal fluid (CSF) opening pressure**
	• <u>Etiology</u>:
	   • <u>Primary</u>: **idiopathic with no identifiable cause**
	   • <u>Secondary</u>: **develops as complication of another disorder** (subarachnoid hemorrhage, meningitis, tumor, traumatic brain injury, radiation)
	• <u>Risk Factors</u>: **age (>70 years old most common)**

Patho-physiology	• Exact pathophysiology is unknown; may be result of defect in cerebrospinal fluid (CSF) resorption leading to buildup within the ventricles that leads to an increased intracranial pressure

Signs & Symptoms	• <u>Triad</u>: **gait disturbances, dementia/cognitive dysfunction and urinary incontinence**
	   • <u>Gait Disturbance</u>: **most common and earliest finding**; **"magnetic gait" with feet stuck to floor; wide-based, shuffling gait, taking small steps and difficulty turning**
	   • <u>Dementia</u>: **impaired executive function, difficulty concentrating, memory loss**, psychomotor depression, apathy
	   • <u>Urinary Incontinence</u>: **presents as urinary urgency early in course and progresses to urinary incontinence**
	• <u>Other</u>: weakness, malaise, rigidity, lethargy, hyperreflexia
	• *Usually do not have symptoms of elevated ICP such as headache, nausea/vomiting, vision changes*

Diagnosis	• <u>Neuroimaging</u>: **MRI is more sensitive than CT scan**
	   • **MRI: preferred imaging study**; demonstrates ventricular enlargement disproportionate to cortical atrophy, compressed sulci, dilated Sylvian fissures
	• **Lumbar Puncture: normal CSF opening pressure**
	   • Removal of 30-50mL of CSF may improve neurologic symptoms and support diagnosis

Treatment	• <u>**Surgery**</u>: **ventriculoperitoneal shunt is treatment of choice** • Marked improvement with removal of CSF during lumbar puncture may predict response to shunting procedure
Key Words & Most Common	• Dilation of cerebral ventricles with normal CSF opening pressure • <u>Gait Disturbance</u>: "magnetic gait" with feet stuck to floor; wide-based and shuffling gait, small steps, difficulty turning • <u>Dementia</u>: impaired executive function and difficulty concentrating → memory loss • <u>Urinary Incontinence</u>: urinary urgency → incontinence • <u>MRI</u>: preferred imaging study • <u>LP</u>: normal CSF opening pressure • Ventriculoperitoneal shunt

Bacterial Meningitis

Etiology & Risk Factors	• **Bacterial infection of the meninges leading to acute inflammation**
	• Etiology: bacteremia or direct extension from local infection (otitis media, sinusitis, mastoiditis)
	  • *Streptococcus pneumoniae*: **most common cause in adults and children** (ages 3 months to 10 years old)
	  • **Group B *Streptococcus*: most common cause in infants** (<2 months old); due to exposure to vaginal and perineal flora during vaginal delivery
	  • *Neisseria meningitidis*: **most common cause in adolescents** (ages 11-17 years old)
	  • *Listeria monocytogenes*: increased incidents in neonates, immunocompromised and adults >50 years old
	  • Other: *Haemophilus influenzae, Escherichia coli, Staphylococcus aureus, Staphylococcus albus*, and gram-negative bacilli
	• Risk Factors: **recent otitis media or sinusitis**, immunocompromised, alcoholism, pneumonia, age (pediatric), **close contact with others (military barracks, college dormitories)**

Patho-physiology	• Bacteremia results in bacteria crossing the blood-brain barrier and access the meninges • Congenital abnormality or trauma results in an abnormal communication between the nasopharynx and subarachnoid space allow local infection to enter CSF

Signs & Symptoms	• **Triad: fever, headache, neck stiffness**
	• **Fever, headache, neck stiffness, lethargy, obtundation**
	• Tachycardia, **photophobia**, seizures, vomiting, prodromal URI, rash (meningococcemia)
	• Physical Exam:
	  • **Nuchal Rigidity**: rigidity of neck muscles with flexion
	  • **Kernig's Sign**: pain with hip flexed at 90° and knee extension
	  • **Brudzinski Sign**: involuntary lifting of legs with passive flexion of the neck
	  • **Jolt Test: most sensitive test**; exacerbation of pre-existing headache with horizontal rotation of the head at frequency of 2 rotations/second
	  • **Purpura Fulminans**: purpuric lesions with jagged edges indicate meningococcemia

Diagnosis	• **Lumbar Puncture (LP) and CSF Analysis: definitive diagnosis and best initial test**; analyzed for Gram stain, culture, complete cell count (CBC), glucose and protein levels • **Decreased glucose, increased neutrophils, increased protein levels, increased opening pressure and positive bacteria on Gram stain or culture** • Head CT Scan: indicated prior to LP to rule out mass effect if papilledema, seizures, focal neurological deficits, known CNS lesion, stroke, or focal CNS infection present • *Workup includes CBC, BMP, blood culture; elevated CRP and procalcitonin levels suggest bacterial etiology*

Treatment	• **Antibiotics**: empiric treatment should be started as quickly as possible
	  • **Neonates (<1 month old): ampicillin + cefotaxime OR gentamicin**
	  • **Infants/Children (>1 month old): ceftriaxone + vancomycin**
	  • **Adults (<50 years old): ceftriaxone + vancomycin**
	  • **Adults (>50 years old or immunocompromised):** ceftriaxone + vancomycin + ampicillin
	• **Dexamethasone**: used to decrease cerebral and cranial nerve inflammation and edema; best-established for patients with pneumococcal meningitis
	• *Neisseria meningitidis* Post-Exposure Prophylaxis: indicated for direct contacts within home, school or daycare, direct exposure to secretions, intubation without facemask
	  • Rifampin (600mg BID x 2 days); Ciprofloxacin (500mg one time dose); Ceftriaxone (250mg IM one time dose)
	• Other Measures: elevation of head of bed to 30°, hyperventilation to a pCO_2 of 27-30mmHg (causes intracranial vasoconstriction), IV mannitol (osmotic diuresis)

Aseptic Meningitis

Etiology & Risk Factors	• **Inflammation of the meninges with negative cerebrospinal fluid (CSF) bacterial cultures**
	• Etiology:
	  • **Viral: most common cause; Enterovirus (Coxsackievirus and Echovirus) are most common**; HSV2, varicella-zoster virus, Epstein-Barr virus, MMR, HIV, West Nile
	  • Fungal: *Candida, Cryptococcus neoformans, Histoplasma capsulatum, Coccidioides immitis,* and *Blastomyces dermatitides*
	  • Parasitic: *Toxoplasma gondii*, naegleria, neurocysticercosis, trichinosis, and *Hartmannella*
	  • Non-infectious: sarcoidosis, Sjögren's syndrome, SLE and granulomatosis with polyangiitis; medications (NSAIDs, antibiotics), neoplastic (metastasis or leukemia)
	• Risk Factors: **age (children aged 4-7 years old most common)**, male, immunocompromised

Patho-physiology	• Hematogenous spread or reactivation of latent viral infection • Infiltration of brain parenchyma is spared therefore delirium, confusion, seizures, and focal or global neurologic deficits are absent

Signs & Symptoms	• *Manifestations resemble bacterial meningitis but are typically less severe*
	• Prodrome of viral infection (fever, myalgias, gastrointestinal or respiratory symptoms) **followed by signs and symptoms of meningitis**
	• **Triad: fever, headache, neck stiffness**
	• **Fever, headache, neck stiffness, no focal neurological deficits**
	• Physical Exam:
	  • **Nuchal Rigidity**: rigidity of neck muscles with flexion
	  • **Kernig's Sign**: pain with hip flexed at 90° and knee extension
	  • **Brudzinski Sign**: involuntary lifting of the legs with passive flexion of the neck
	  • **Jolt Test: most sensitive test**; exacerbation of pre-existing headache with horizontal rotation of the head at frequency of 2 rotations/second

Diagnosis	• *Must rule out bacterial meningitis* • **Lumbar Puncture (LP) and CSF Analysis: definitive diagnosis and best initial test**; analyzed for Gram stain, culture, complete cell count (CBC), glucose and protein levels • **Normal glucose, lymphocytic predominance, mildly increased protein levels, increased opening pressure and *negative* bacteria on Gram stain or culture** • Viral serologic tests, **PCR**, or culture of CSF or other sources (blood, throat, nasopharyngeal, stool) may aid in identifying causative virus
Treatment	• *Empiric antibiotics may be initiated until bacterial meningitis is ruled out based on suspicion* • **Supportive**: antipyretics/analgesics (NSAIDs, acetaminophen), IV fluids, discontinue offending medication • **Antivirals: IV acyclovir indicated with HSV meningitis or varicella-zoster virus meningitis** • **Dexamethasone**: adjunct used to decrease cerebral and cranial nerve inflammation and edema
Key Words & Most Common	• Enterovirus (coxsackievirus and echovirus) most common • Symptoms similar to bacterial meningitis but typically less severe • Viral infection prodrome → fever, headache, neck stiffness • LP: normal glucose, lymphocytic predominance, mildly increased protein, negative bacteria • Supportive +/- IV acyclovir +/- dexamethasone

Encephalitis

Etiology & Risk Factors	• Infection of brain parenchyma of the temporal and inferior frontal lobes causing distinct neurologic abnormalities
	• Etiology:
	   • **Herpes simplex virus (HSV) most common cause in US**
	   • Varicella zoster virus, Epstein-Barr virus, enteroviruses (coxsackievirus and echovirus), MMR, cytomegalovirus (CMV), dengue virus, rabies virus
	   • Arboviruses (eastern equine, western equine, St. Louis, Venezuelan equine, Zika and West Nile) is common cause worldwide
	• Risk Factors: age (bimodal distribution of **young and elderly**), immunocompromised, **epidemiologic factors** (time of the year, geography, animal or insect exposure)

Patho-physiology	• Viral invasion of brain parenchyma causes an inflammatory response which disrupts normal neural cell function; untreated cases can cause hemorrhagic necrosis and death • Gray matter is predominantly affected causing distinct neurologic abnormalities (cognitive/psychiatric signs, lethargy, seizure)

Signs & Symptoms	• **Prodrome of viral infection** (fever, myalgias, gastrointestinal or respiratory symptoms) **may precede neurological symptoms**
	• **Fever, headache, seizures, altered mental status**
	   • **Altered Mental Status: behavioral and personality changes, hallucinations, cognitive decline, speech and movement disturbances**
	• **Olfactory seizures may manifest as a foul smell aura (rotten eggs, burnt meat) indicate temporal lobe involvement and suggest HSV etiology**
	• Physical Exam:
	   • **Focal neurologic deficits** (hemiparesis, sensory deficits, cranial nerve palsies)

Diagnosis	• Neuroimaging:
	   • **Head CT Scan**: performed prior to LP to rule out space-occupying lesion; may show edema and petechial hemorrhages, low-density lesions in the temporal lobes (HSV)
	   • **MRI: most sensitive imaging modality**; may show edema in the orbitofrontal and temporal areas
	• **Lumbar Puncture**: analyzed for opening pressure, complete cell count, glucose, protein, **polymerase chain reaction (PCR) testing for HSV-1, HSV-2, and enteroviruses**
	   • **Normal glucose, moderate lymphocytosis, moderately increased protein**

Treatment	• **Supportive: antipyretics/analgesics (NSAIDs, acetaminophen), IV fluids** • **Antivirals: IV acyclovir**; early empiric treatment has been shown to significantly decrease morbidity/mortality and limit long-term behavioral/cognitive impairment severity • *Seizures may require valproic acid or phenytoin; status epilepticus may require benzodiazepines*
Key Words & Most Common	• Infection of brain parenchyma most commonly caused by herpes simplex virus (HSV) • Prodrome of viral infection → fever, headache, seizures, altered mental status • Focal neurologic deficits • MRI is most sensitive imaging modality • LP: normal glucose, moderate lymphocytosis, moderately increased protein; viral PCR testing should be performed • IV acyclovir

Huntington Disease

Etiology & Risk Factors	• **Autosomal dominant neurodegenerative disorder characterized by chorea, neuropsychiatric symptoms, and progressive cognitive deterioration** • Etiology: cytosine, adenine, and guanine (CAG) trinucleotide repeats on the short arm of chromosome 4p16.3 in the *Huntingtin* (*HTT*) gene • Risk Factors: **age (30-50 years old most common age of presentation), family history**
Patho-physiology	• Mutation resulting in CAG trinucleotide repeat on the Huntingtin (HTT) gene on chromosome 4 leads to neurodegeneration and neurotoxicity, as well as degeneration and atrophy of the neurons in the putamen, caudate nucleus and cerebral cortex

Signs & Symptoms	• Signs and symptoms develop insidiously **starting around age 35-40**
	• **Behavioral Changes: psychiatric disturbances, depression, apathy, irritability, anhedonia**, antisocial behavior, bipolar or schizophreniform disorder
	• **Abnormal Movements:**
	   • **Chorea: rapid, nonrhythmic, jerky, non-suppressible involuntary movement of distal muscles and face, worsened with voluntary, semi-purposeful movements**
	   • **Athetosis: slow, nonrhythmic, writhing movements of the distal muscles**; often present with altering proximal limb posture
	   • **Myoclonic jerks**, pseudo-tics, **"puppet-like" gait, facial grimacing**, inability to move eyes without blinking/head thrusting (oculomotor apraxia), inability to sustain motor act (tongue protrusion, grasping)
	• **Dementia: cognitive decline** (specific executive functions and organizing, multitasking, planning)

Diagnosis	• **Clinical Diagnosis + positive family history** • Genetic Testing: **confirmatory test**; genetic test measures number of CAG repeats to determine penetrance • Neuroimaging: CT/MRI shows caudate and frontal-predominant cortical atrophy
Treatment	• **Supportive Care: progressive disease that is usually fatal within 15-20 years after presentation; end-of-life care should be discussed** • Antipsychotics: chlorpromazine, haloperidol, risperidone, olanzapine; may partially suppress chorea and agitation • Vesicular Monoamine Transporter Type 2 (VMAT-2) Inhibitor: **tetrabenazine; depletes dopamine to lessen chorea and dyskinesias** • Benzodiazepines: may be used intermittently to treat chorea and sleep disturbances
Key Words & Most Common	• Autosomal dominant neurodegenerative disorder • 30-50 years old most common age of presentation • Behavioral Changes: depression, psychiatric disturbances, irritability, anhedonia • Abnormal Movements: chorea, athetosis, myoclonic jerks • Dementia: cognitive decline • Clinical diagnosis + family history + genetic testing • Supportive care + tetrabenazine to treat chorea and dyskinesias

Essential Tremor

Etiology & Risk Factors	• Involuntary rhythmic and oscillatory movement of antagonistic muscle groups with a relatively constant frequency and variable amplitude • <u>Etiology</u>: autosomal dominant inherited disorder of unknown etiology • <u>Risk Factors</u>: family history, monozygotic twins
Patho-physiology	• Neuropathology within the brainstem (locus coeruleus) and cerebellum causes alternating contractions of antagonistic muscles producing the tremor

Signs & Symptoms	• <u>Intentional Tremor</u>: postural, bilateral action tremor
	  • **Most commonly affects the upper extremity (bilateral arms and hands), head, neck and/or voice** (tremor of the lower extremity is uncommon with essential tremor)
	  • **Maximal tremor with voluntary/intentional movement or adrenergic activity** (emotional stress or anxiety)
	  • **Tremor may be relieved by small amounts of alcohol**
	• <u>Physical Exam</u>:
	  • **Tremor increases at the end of goal-directed movements (drinking from a glass or finger-to-nose testing)**
	  • Tremor reproduced with arms suspended against gravity in a fixed posture

Diagnosis	• **Clinical Diagnosis; diagnosis of exclusion** • <u>Neuroimaging</u>: CT/MRI to rule out structural etiology (trauma, stroke, mass lesion, Wilson disease) otherwise not routinely indicated • <u>Labs</u>: consider thyroid function, copper, ceruloplasmin, heavy metal screen

Treatment	• <u>Supportive</u>:
	  • **Limb weights** (wrist weights) may be used to dampen tremor and improve symptoms
	  • Avoidance of precipitating or aggravating factors (caffeine, alcohol, medications, exercise, fatigue, sleep deprivation or stress)
	  • **Relaxation techniques**, good sleep hygiene, regular exercise, biofeedback, **stress reduction, yoga**
	• <u>Medical Therapy</u>:
	  • **Propranolol is first-line for severe or situational symptoms**
	  • **Primidone (barbiturate)** indicated if refractory to propranolol; may be used in combination with propranolol
	  • Alprazolam (benzodiazepine) indicated for tremor and chronic anxiety; continuous use should be avoided
	• <u>Interventional Therapy</u>:
	  • Deep brain stimulation (DBS), focused ultrasound, or radio-surgical gamma knife thalamotomy indicated to treat persistently disabling limb tremor

Key Words & Most Common	• Involuntary rhythmic and oscillatory movements with autosomal dominant pattern • Intentional tremor most commonly affects upper extremities, head, neck, voice • Tremor increases at end of goal-directed movement (finger-to-nose testing); may decrease with alcohol consumption • Clinical diagnosis of exclusion • Avoid triggers + stress reduction → propranolol +/- primidone

Parkinson Disease

Etiology & Risk Factors	• **Slowly progressive, neurodegenerative movement disorder characterized by resting tremor, rigidity, bradykinesia, and gait and/or postural instability** • <u>Etiology</u>: **idiopathic loss of dopaminergic neurons in the substantia nigra of the basal ganglia** • <u>Risk Factors</u>: **age (45-65 years old most common age of onset)**, family history, exposure to pesticides, herbicides, or industrial plant pollution
Patho-physiology	• Dopamine is inhibitory while acetylcholine is an excitatory central nervous system (CNS) neurotransmitter • Degeneration and loss of dopaminergic neurons of the substantia nigra cause dopamine depletion of the putamen (part of basal ganglia) and acetylcholine inhibition failure, resulting in the characteristic motor manifestations

Signs & Symptoms	• <u>Triad</u>: **resting tremor, bradykinesia, muscle rigidity**
	• <u>Resting Tremor</u>: **often initial symptom**
	  • Slow and coarse tremor often involving hands and/or feet; thumb moving against index finger ("pill-rolling" tremor)
	  • **Worse at rest** and with emotional stress
	  • **Improves with voluntary activity and intentional movement; *absent during sleep***
	• <u>Bradykinesia</u>: **voluntary movement slowness and decreased automatic movements**
	  • Repetitive motor activity results in a progressive or sustained decrease in amplitude of movement (hypokinesia), movement becomes hard to initiate (akinesia)
	  • Manifests as shuffling gait or lack of swinging of arms while walking
	• <u>Muscle Rigidity</u>: **increased resistance to passive movement;** semirhythmic jerks occur with attempts to move a rigid joint, producing a ratchet-like effect (**cogwheel rigidity**)
	• <u>Facial Involvement</u>: **masklike facies** (hypomimia) **with open mouth and reduced blinking**, widened palpebral fissure
	  • <u>Myerson's Sign</u>: glabellar tap reflex; repetitively tapping nasal bridge produces a sustained blink response
	• <u>Postural Instability</u>: **develops later in disease course**; stooped posture, difficulty initiating walking, turning, and stopping
	  • Displacing patient's center of gravity causes patient to fall forward (propulsion) or backward (retropulsion) due to loss of postural reflexes
	  • <u>Festination</u>: inadvertently quickening of gait with progressive shortening of stride length; precursor to freezing of gait
	• **Normal deep tendon reflexes** and no muscle weakness; **dementia, depression, sleep disorders are common**

Diagnosis	• **Clinical Diagnosis;** *must differentiate from corticospinal tract lesions (paresis, hyperreflexia, extensor plantar response [Babinski reflex])* • <u>Post-Mortem Histology</u>: loss of dopamine pigment in the substantia nigra and synuclein-filled Lewy bodies in the nigrostriatal system

Treatment	• <u>Levodopa/Carbidopa</u>: **most effective and first-line treatment**
	  • **Levodopa**: metabolic precursor of dopamine; crosses the blood-brain barrier into the basal ganglia where a decarboxylation reaction converts it to active dopamine
	  • **Carbidopa**: reduces peripheral conversion of levodopa into dopamine which lowers required dose and adverse effects of levodopa
	• <u>Dopamine Agonists</u>: pramipexole, ropinirole, rotigotine; actively stimulates dopamine receptors in the basal ganglia
	• <u>NMDA-Receptor Antagonist</u>: **amantadine**; increases presynaptic dopamine release and inhibit dopamine reuptake; may slow progression of Parkinson disease and dyskinesias
	• <u>Selective MAO-B Inhibitors</u>: selegiline, rasagiline; inhibits enzymatic break down of dopamine in the brain to prolong levodopa action
	• <u>Anticholinergics</u>: benztropine, trihexyphenidyl; inhibits excitatory effects of acetylcholine
	• <u>Catechol *O*-methyltransferase (COMT) Inhibitors</u>: entacapone, tolcapone; inhibits the breakdown of levodopa and dopamine
	• <u>Surgery</u>: deep brain stimulation is effective treatment for patients with levodopa-induced dyskinesias or significant motor fluctuations

Amyotrophic Lateral Sclerosis (ALS) 🧠

Etiology & Risk Factors	• **Neurodegenerative disease of the upper and lower motor neurons resulting in progressive motor degeneration** • Also known as Lou Gehrig's disease • <u>Etiology</u>: **unknown**; most cases (90-95%) are sporadic • <u>Risk Factors</u>: male, age **(>40 years old most common)**
Patho-physiology	• Degeneration and gliosis of axons within the anterior and lateral columns of the spinal cord lead to progressive deterioration of the corticospinal tracts, anterior horn cells, and/or bulbar motor nuclei resulting in progressive motor dysfunction

Signs & Symptoms	• **Asymmetric limb weakness is most common presenting symptom**
	   • **Random unilateral cramping, weakness, and muscle atrophy of the hands (most commonly) or feet**
	   • **Muscle weakness progresses** to the forearms, shoulders, and lower limbs
	   • Inability to initiate and control motor movements especially fine motor movements (buttoning a shirt)
	• <u>Bulbar Palsy</u>: **dysphagia, voice hoarseness, slurred or nasally speech; difficulty handling salivary secretions and choking on liquids (secondary to dysphagia)**
	• <u>Pseudobulbar Affect</u>: **inappropriate, involuntary, and uncontrollable excesses of laughter or crying**
	• *Sensation, consciousness, cognition, voluntary eye movements, sphincter function (bowel and bladder) and sexual function usually are spared*
	• <u>Physical Exam</u>: **mixed upper and lower motor neuron signs and symptoms**
	   • <u>Upper Motor Neuron</u>: spasticity, stiffness of movement, hyperreflexia, weakness
	   • <u>Lower Motor Neurons</u>: progressive bilateral muscle fasciculations, muscle atrophy, hyporeflexia, weakness
	   • Difficulty controlling facial expression and tongue movements

Diagnosis	• Clinical Diagnosis • Electromyography: further supports diagnosis; demonstrates findings of acute denervation, chronic denervation and chronic reinnervation

Treatment	• <u>Supportive Care</u>: 50% of patients die within 3 years of onset (respiratory failure secondary to progressive diaphragmatic and intercostal muscle weakness)
	   • CPAP, BiPAP and ventilator may be necessary for respiratory support as the disease advances
	   • Diet modifications (progressive muscle weakness causes impaired mastication and dysphagia)
	• <u>Riluzole</u>: modulates the actions of glutamate and reduces glutamate-induced excitotoxicity; improves survival (by 2-6 months)

Key Words & Most Common	• Neurodegenerative disease of upper and lower motor neurons • Asymmetric limb weakness + cramping + muscle atrophy of distal extremities (hands/feet) • <u>Bulbar Palsy</u>: dysphagia, hoarse voice, change in speech • <u>Pseudobulbar Affect</u>: uncontrollable excess laughter/crying • Clinical diagnosis + electromyography to support diagnosis • Supportive care • Riluzole may improve survival

Tourette Syndrome 🧠

Etiology & Risk Factors	• **Neurodevelopmental disorder characterized by multiple motor and vocal tics beginning in childhood** • <u>Etiology</u>: **idiopathic**; combination of genetic and environmental factors • <u>Risk Factors</u>: **male, family history**, monozygotic twins • **Onset usually in early childhood (4-6 years old most common) with peak severity at middle childhood (10-12 years old)**
Patho-physiology	• Abnormal dopamine pathways at the presynaptic, intrasynaptic, and postsynaptic levels disrupt the excitatory and inhibitory pathways of the basal ganglia • GABA (gamma-aminobutyric acid) disruption may cause cortico-basal ganglia dysfunction

Signs & Symptoms	• <u>Simple Tics</u>: **brief movement or vocalization**, usually without social meaning
	   • **Motor**: blinking, grimacing, head jerking or thrusting, **shrugging of shoulders**
	   • **Verbal**: grunting or barking, nasal sniffling or snorting, **throat clearing**
	• <u>Complex Tics</u>: **longer lasting movement or vocalizations that may involve a combination of simple tics**, usually with social meaning (recognizable speech, gestures or words)
	   • **Motor**: combination of simple tics (head thrusting + shoulder shrugging), sexual or obscene gestures (copropraxia), **imitating other's movements** (echopraxia)
	   • **Verbal**: saying socially inappropriate words such as obscenities or ethnic slurs (coprolalia), **imitating other's phrases or words** (echolalia)
	• Tics are often exacerbated by stress and fatigue; tics are most prominent when patient is relaxed (watching television, sitting still) and lessen with engaging in activity

Diagnosis	• **Clinical Diagnosis** • <u>DSM5 Diagnostic Criteria</u>: multiple motor and vocal tics present for >1 year with onset prior to 18 years old and not caused by effects of a substance or medical condition

Treatment	• <u>Supportive</u>: reassurance, education on coping strategies, prognosis, and treatment options; school programs and support
	   • Having an educated and supportive teacher at school is one of most significant influential factor
	• <u>Comprehensive Behavioral Intervention for Tics (CBIT)</u>: **behavioral therapy and habit reversal therapy is first-line**
	• <u>Medical Management</u>:
	   • <u>Alpha-Adrenergic Agonists</u>: **clonidine, guanfacine**; indicated for mild symptoms that do not respond to behavioral/habit reversal therapy
	   • <u>Antipsychotics</u>: risperidone, haloperidol, pimozide; indicated for more severe or uncontrollable symptoms

Key Words & Most Common	• Neurodevelopmental disorder of childhood characterized by motor and vocal tics for >1 year • Onset 4-6 years old; peaks at 10-12 years old • Simple Motor: blinking, shrugging shoulders, head thrusting • Simple Verbal: grunting, barking, throat clearing • Complex Motor: head thrusting + shoulder shrugging, sexual or obscene gestures, imitation of actions • Complex Verbal: saying obscenities or ethnic slurs, imitation of phrases or words • Clinical • Supportive → behavioral and habit reversal therapy → medications

Cerebral Palsy

Etiology & Risk Factors	• Group of permanent central nervous system (CNS) disorders characterized by impaired voluntary movement or posture
	• Etiology: **prenatal developmental malformations or perinatal or postnatal CNS damage**
	   • Prenatal: **congenital brain malformations**, intrauterine infections, **intrauterine stroke**, chromosomal abnormalities
	   • Perinatal: **perinatal asphyxia, stroke, CNS** infections, kernicterus
	   • Postnatal: **accidental or non-accidental trauma, stroke,** CNS infection, **anoxic insult**
	• Risk Factors: **prematurity is greatest risk factor**, multiple gestation, intrauterine growth restriction, preeclampsia, abnormal placental pathology, maternal substance abuse, meconium aspiration, perinatal hypoglycemia

Patho-physiology	• Damage to the fetal or infant's brain as a result of trauma, hypoxic or anoxic insult or other CNS damage results in abnormal CNS development

Signs & Symptoms	• **Symptoms usually manifest by 2 years old**
	• **Spasticity: hallmark of disorder**
	   • **Characterized by a state of resistance to passive range of motion**
	   • Upper Limb Spasticity: **flexed elbow, clenched fist, flexed wrist, pronated forearm**, thumb flexed into palm
	   • Lower Limb Spasticity: **plantar flexed foot/ankle, flexed toes**, equinovarus foot (foot points down and inward)
	• May result in hemiplegia, quadriplegia, diplegia, or paraplegia
	• May have intellectual or learning disabilities or developmental abnormalities
	• Physical Exam:
	   • **Hyperreflexia, hypertonic muscles**, joint contractures, limb-length discrepancies, weak and poorly coordinated voluntary movements
	   • Scissor Gait: hypertonia and flexion of the legs, hips and pelvis with extreme adduction leads to knees and thighs cross or touch

Diagnosis	• **Clinical Diagnosis** • Brain MRI: **preferred imaging test to evaluate for abnormal neuroanatomy in the motor areas of the brain** • *Workup may include screening for associated conditions*
Treatment	• **Multidisciplinary team approach** • **Physical and Occupational Therapy: first-line**; directed at stretching, strengthening, and facilitating proper movement patterns • Orthotics, bracing, constraint therapy may be added • Botulinum Toxin Injection: injection to muscle to inhibit hypertonia and prevent fixed contractures • Spasticity Management: benzodiazepines, baclofen, dantrolene, tizanidine, cyclobenzaprine • Analgesia: anti-inflammatories for pain control; gabapentin • Antidepressants: depression and anxiety common • Surgery: baclofen pump placement, tendon releases, limb rotation/derotation surgery, spinal fusion, strabismus repair, deep brain stimulation

Restless Leg Syndrome

Etiology & Risk Factors	• **Chronic movement disorder characterized by an irresistible urge to move the legs**
	• Etiology:
	   • Primary: **idiopathic**; may be familial
	   • Secondary: **iron deficiency, pregnancy**, peripheral neuropathy, **alcohol abuse**, end-stage renal disease, diabetes mellitus, **folate or magnesium deficiency**, fibromyalgia
	• Risk Factors: psychiatric factors, **pregnancy**, stress, fatigue, medications (neuroleptics, TCAs, SSRI/SNRI, lithium, beta-blockers), **alcohol, caffeine, drug withdrawal**

Patho-physiology	• Not fully understood Dysfunction of the dopaminergic system and diminished iron stores in the brain; high estrogen levels may play a role in pregnancy

Signs & Symptoms	• **Strong, perceived need to move the legs at rest**
	   • **Urge is relieved with initiation of leg movement**
	   • May be **uncomfortable and unpleasant sensation** (creeping or crawling sensation, itching, burning, paresthesia, throbbing) **localized to deep structures** (not skin level)
	• **Symptoms worse at night or with prolonged periods of inactivity or rest** (sitting in movie theater, waiting room etc.)
	   • May disturb sleep
	   • Involuntary, forceful dorsiflexion of the foot or leg twitching during sleep
	• Physical Exam:
	   • Often normal

Diagnosis	• **Clinical Diagnosis** • Polysomnography: quantifies leg movement frequency and characterizes sleep patterns • Labs: CBC, BMP, thyroid panel, iron studies (serum iron, transferrin, ferritin, total iron-binding capacity), magnesium, vitamin B12, folate to determine underlying etiology
Treatment	• Lifestyle Modifications: sleep hygiene, proper nutrition, exercise, warm or cool baths, massage, avoidance of alcohol and caffeine • **Dopamine Agonists: pramipexole, ropinirole, rotigotine**; actively stimulates dopamine receptors in the basal ganglia • **Alpha2-Delta Calcium-Channel Ligands: gabapentin**, pregabalin; indicated with severe sleep disturbances, comorbid insomnia, anxiety, pain • **Iron Supplementation**: indicated in patients with serum ferritin <75mcg/L; ferrous sulfate 325 mg + vitamin C 250 mg on empty stomach • Benzodiazepines: clonazepam; may improve sleep continuity but does not reduce leg movement
Key Words & Most Common	• Idiopathic, iron deficiency, pregnancy, alcohol abuse, caffeine, drug withdrawal • Irresistible urge to move the legs • Urge relieved with initiating leg movement • Creeping/crawling sensation, itching, burning localized to dep structures • Worse at night or prolonged inactivity • Clinical diagnosis • Lifestyle modifications → dopamine agonists (pramipexole, ropinirole) → gabapentin, pregabalin +/- iron supplementation

Bell's Palsy

Etiology & Risk Factors	• Idiopathic, unilateral peripheral cranial nerve VII (facial nerve) palsy characterized by hemifacial weakness and paresis of the upper and lower face • Etiology: • **Idiopathic is most common**, viral implication (**herpes simplex virus,** varicella-zoster virus, and Epstein-Barr virus) or in setting of known associations (Ramsay-Hunt syndrome and Lyme disease [bilateral Bell's palsy], sarcoidosis, diabetes mellitus) • Risk Factors: **diabetes, pregnancy (3rd trimester),** recent URI, dental nerve block, preeclampsia, obesity, hypertension
Patho-physiology	• Facial muscles are innervated peripherally by the ipsilateral cranial nerve VII and centrally by the contralateral cerebral cortex; central innervation tends to be bilateral for the upper face (forehead muscles) and unilateral for the lower face, therefore both central and peripheral lesions may paralyze the lower portion of the face • A peripheral lesion will cause compression of cranial nerve VII that will affect the upper face (forehead) more than a central lesion (stroke)

Signs & Symptoms	• **Sudden onset of unilateral increased sound sensitivity** (hyperacusis) **and retroauricular pain** (precedes facial symptoms by 24-72 hours)
	• Numb or heavy sensation of the face
	• Taste disturbance (anterior 2/3rd of the tongue)
	• Changes in eye tearing or salivation
	• Physical Exam:
	  • **Unilateral facial weakness or paralysis** <u>involving the forehead</u>
	    • **Inability to wrinkle forehead, raise eyebrow, blink, smile or grimace on affected side**
	    • **Loss of nasolabial fold, drooping of corner of mouth**
	    • **Incomplete closure of eyelid on affected side**
	  • *Weakness and paralysis only affects the face and does not involve the extremities*
	
	Inability to wrinkle forehead/raise eyebrow
	Drooping of corner of mouth

Diagnosis	• **Clinical Diagnosis**; diagnosis of exclusion
	  • **Must distinguish from a central lesion (hemispheric stroke or tumor)**
	  • **Patients with central lesion are able to wrinkle their forehead, furrow their brow and close their eyes tightly; may have unilateral extremity weakness**
	• MRI: indicated if gradual or other neurologic deficits are present; detect facial nerve inflammation and can rule out schwannoma, hemangioma or a space-occupying lesion

Treatment	• Supportive: **artificial tears to replace lacrimation;** intermittent use of tape or eye patch to keep eye closed (especially during sleep) to prevent corneal ulceration/keratitis • Corticosteroids: **initiation within the first 48-72 hours of symptom onset results in a faster and more complete recovery** • **Prednisone 60mg for 1 week followed by gradual taper** • Antivirals: valacyclovir, acyclovir may be effective if herpes simplex virus or varicella-zoster virus; *recent data suggest that antiviral drugs provide no benefit* • *Consider empiric doxycycline if high index of suspicion for Lyme disease based on clinical presentation or lab results*
Key Words & Most Common	• Unilateral facial weakness or paralysis involving the forehead (inability to wrinkle forehead, raise eyebrow, blink, smile on affected side) • Loss of nasolabial fold + drooping corner of mouth + NO unilateral extremity weakness or paralysis • Clinical diagnosis • Supportive (artificial tears, eye protection) + corticosteroids (prednisone)

Guillain-Barré Syndrome

Etiology & Risk Factors	• **Acute polyneuropathy due to immune-mediated peripheral nerve myelin sheath destruction** • Etiology: autoimmune reaction secondary to infectious disorder, surgery, or immunization • Infection: ***Campylobacter jejuni* infection is most common**; enteric viruses, herpesviruses (cytomegalovirus and Epstein-Barr virus), *Mycoplasma pneumoniae* infection
Patho-physiology	• Infection or immune system stimulus results in an autoimmune responds in which autoantibodies mistakenly attack the myelin sheath of peripheral nerves leading to demyelination and nerve damage resulting in inhibition of nerve impulses

Signs & Symptoms	• **Ascending, symmetric weakness and paresthesias**
	  • **Usually starts in distal lower extremities** then progresses to the arms; **progressive weakness**
	  • May progress to **weakness of diaphragm and intercostal muscles** leading to respiratory compromise
	  • Weakness of facial and bulbar (oropharyngeal) muscles leading to **dysphagia,** dehydration and malnutrition
	• Physical Exam:
	  • **Decreased or absent deep tendon reflexes, flaccid paralysis, weakness**
	  • Sphincter tone usually remains intact
	  • Autonomic Dysfunction: fluctuation of blood pressure, cardiac arrhythmias, tachycardia, **respiratory failure,** constipation, urinary retention, pupillary changes

Diagnosis	• **Clinical Diagnosis** • Electrodiagnostic Testing: nerve conduction studies and electromyography; show **slowed motor nerve conduction velocities and evidence of segmental demyelination** • Lumbar Puncture with CSF Analysis: shows **albumin-cytologic dissociation (increased protein but low or normal white blood cell count)** • Pulmonary Function Test: indicated to assess peak inspiratory pressure and forced vital capacity to determine need for intubation and mechanical ventilation • Spinal MRI: used to rule out other etiologies; may show selective enhancement of the anterior spinal nerve roots (inflammatory breakdown of the blood-nerve barrier)
Treatment	• Admit for Observation: admission to ICU for monitoring and vital support • Intubation and Mechanical Ventilation: indicated with progressive dyspnea or dysphagia, hypoxia, aspiration, reduced forced vital capacity, negative inspiratory force • Intravenous Immunoglobulin (IVIG): **first-line treatment of choice**; act by its immune-modulating action; preferred over plasmapheresis due to convenience and availability • Plasmapheresis: indicated if IVIG is ineffective; act by removing pathogenic antibodies and complement proteins but is associated with greater hemodynamic instability • Corticosteroids: **not indicated**; do not improve and may worsen the outcome
Key Words & Most Common	• Autoimmune reaction secondary to infectious disorder, surgery, immunization • *Campylobacter jejuni* most common • Ascending, symmetric weakness and paresthesias starting in distal extremities • Decreased or absent DTR • Clinical diagnosis + electrodiagnostic testing + LP with CSF analysis (↑protein, ↓WBC) + PFT • Admit +/- intubation → IVIG/plasmapheresis

Myasthenia Gravis

Etiology & Risk Factors	• Autoimmune peripheral nerve disorder due to autoantibody degradation, dysfunction, and blockade of acetylcholine receptor at the neuromuscular junction (NMJ) • <u>Etiology</u>: **autoantibody- and cell-mediated destruction of acetylcholine receptors** • **Abnormal thymus gland** (thymic hyperplasia or thymoma) in 75% of cases • <u>Risk Factors</u>: **female (20 to 40 years old) and males (50 to 80 years old)**; history of other autoimmune condition (autoimmune hyperthyroidism, RA, SLE, pernicious anemia) • <u>Precipitating Factors</u>: infection, surgery, medications (aminoglycosides, quinines, magnesium sulfate, procainamide, calcium channel blockers)
Patho-physiology	• Autoantibodies against acetylcholine receptors (AChRs) bind to the postsynaptic membrane at the neuromuscular junction and interrupt neuromuscular transmission

Signs & Symptoms	• <u>Ocular Weakness</u>:
	   • **Ptosis and diplopia usually initial symptoms**
	   • May have cranial nerve III, IV, VI weakness
	   • **Pupils are spared**
	• <u>Muscle Weakness</u>:
	   • **Progressive weakness with prolonged/repetitive use of affected muscle; weakness resolves with rest**
	   • **Bulbar (Oropharyngeal) Weakness**: weakness with prolonged mastication, **dysphagia**, dysphonia (voice hoarseness), dysarthria (altered voice)
	   • **Proximal muscle weakness, weak hand grip, expressionless face** and weak neck muscle (dropped-head syndrome)
	   • **Weakness of diaphragm and intercostal muscles** leads to respiratory compromise (myasthenic crisis)
	• <u>Physical Exam</u>:
	   • **Sensation and deep tendon reflexes are normal**
	
	Strabismus and ptosis

Diagnosis	• <u>Anticholinesterase Test</u>: edrophonium temporarily improves symptoms; no longer used in the US • <u>Ice Pack Test</u>: full or partial resolution of ptosis after applying icepack to closed eye for 2 minutes indicates a positive test • <u>Prolonged Upward Gaze Test</u>: developing of ptosis or diplopia with prolonged, fixed, upward gaze held for 30 seconds indicates a positive test • <u>**Serum Acetylcholine Receptor Antibody Level**</u>: **initial test of choice**; positive antibodies present in 80 to 90% of patients • <u>**Electromyography**</u>: **most accurate test**; repetitive nerve stimulation shows a decrease in amplitude of the compound muscle action potential response • <u>Imaging</u>: chest x-ray, CT, or MRI should be performed to evaluate for thymic hyperplasia and/or thymoma
Treatment	• <u>**Anticholinesterase Inhibitors**</u>: **pyridostigmine, neostigmine first-line**; prevents acetylcholine destruction by cholinesterase and allow transmission of impulse across the NMJ • <u>**Corticosteroids**</u>: prednisone; indicated if symptoms continue despite pyridostigmine use; azathioprine or cyclosporine are alternatives to steroids • <u>**Intravenous Immunoglobulin (IVIG) or Plasmapheresis**</u>: **indicated if severe symptoms or myasthenic crisis** • <u>**Thymectomy**</u>: indicated for patients with generalized myasthenia and <80 years old or any patient with thymic hyperplasia or thymoma; removes source of antibodies

Lambert-Eaton Myasthenic Syndrome

Etiology & Risk Factors	• **Immune-mediated, myasthenia-like syndrome characterized by limb muscle weakness limbs and sparing of the ocular and bulbar muscles** • <u>Etiology</u>: **autoantibodies against the voltage-gated calcium channels at the neuromuscular junction (NMJ)** • <u>Risk Factors</u>: advanced age, males, intrathoracic tumors (**small or oat cell lung carcinoma**), malignancy • **Characteristic patient is an elderly male with history of cigarette smoking and lung cancer**
Patho-physiology	• Antibodies against the presynaptic voltage-gated calcium channels prevent acetylcholine release from the nerve terminals into the neuromuscular junction space leading to muscle weakness

Signs & Symptoms	• **Proximal muscle weakness that improves with repeated muscle use** (myasthenia gravis worsens with repeated muscle use)
	   • **Especially affects proximal leg muscles causing alteration in gait, difficulty rising from a chair, or climbing stairs**
	• Myalgias, muscle stiffness (hips and shoulders), paresthesias
	• <u>**Autonomic Symptoms**</u>: **dry mouth is most common**, postural hypotension, erectile dysfunction
	• <u>Physical Exam</u>:
	   • **Hyporeflexia, ptosis, sluggish pupillary response**
	   • Unaffected eye movement, no muscle atrophy, no sensory dysfunction
	   • <u>Lambert Sign</u>: grip strength increases on repeated evaluation with handshake

Diagnosis	• <u>Voltage-Gated Calcium Channel Antibody Assay</u>: positive antibodies confirms diagnosis • <u>Electrophysiologic Testing</u>: increased response to repetitive nerve stimulation and increased amplitude of the compound muscle action potential • <u>Imaging</u>: CT or MRI to evaluate for underlying malignancy
Treatment	• **Treatment of underlying malignancy** • <u>**Anticholinesterase Inhibitors**</u>: **pyridostigmine is first-line**; prevents acetylcholine destruction by cholinesterase and allow transmission of impulse across the NMJ • <u>Cholinergic Agonists</u>: guanidine; enhances acetylcholine release and slows depolarization and repolarization rate of muscle cell membranes • <u>Potassium Channel Blockers</u>: amifampridine; prolongs presynaptic nerve terminal depolarization and increases acetylcholine release • Corticosteroids, intravenous immunoglobulin (IVIG) or plasmapheresis are alternatives
Key Words & Most Common	• Characteristic patient is an elderly male with history of cigarette smoking and lung cancer • Proximal muscle weakness that improves with repeated muscle use • Alteration in gait, difficulty rising from a chair or climbing stairs • Hyporeflexia • Treat underlying malignancy • Pyridostigmine is first-line

Multiple Sclerosis (MS)

Etiology & Risk Factors	• Autoimmune disease of the central nervous system (CNS) characterized by chronic inflammation and nerve demyelination with a relapsing-remitting or progressive course • <u>Types</u>: **relapsing-remitting** (episodic exacerbations lasting 24-48 hours), **primary progressive** (gradual deterioration acute acute exacerbations), **secondary progressive** (relapsing-remitting pattern that becomes progressive) • <u>Etiology</u>: unknown; combination of immune, environmental, and genetic factors • <u>Risk Factors</u>: **age (20-40 years old most common age of onset), female**, vitamin D deficiency, latent viral infection (Epstein-Barr virus), HLA-DR2 allotype
Patho-physiology	• Immune-mediated attack on myelin causes focal inflammation resulting in plaques and blood-brain barrier damage eventually causing myelin destruction and axonal injury • Fibrous scarring of injured glial cells (gliosis) occurs which impedes transmission of nerve impulses

Signs & Symptoms	• <u>**Muscle/Sensory Deficits**</u>: **most common presenting symptoms**
	  • **Paresthesias of one or more extremities, trunk or one side of the face**
	  • **Lower extremity weakness** worse than upper extremity; **clumsiness, stiffness or unusual limb fatigue**
	  • Decreased proprioception, pain, or temperature sensation; **difficulty with gait and balance**
	  • <u>Upper Motor Neuron Signs</u>: **hyperreflexia, positive (upward) Babinski sign**, spasticity, muscle rigidity
	  • <u>**Uhthoff Phenomenon**</u>: **acute exacerbation of symptoms with heat exposure** (warm weather, exercise, hot showers, hot tubs, fever)
	  • <u>Lhermitte's Sign</u>: neck flexion causes acute, shock-like pain that radiates from spine down the leg
	• <u>**Visual Disturbances**</u>: **result of optic neuritis**
	  • **Unilateral partial vision loss;** preceded by retrobulbar pain
	  • Blurred vision, **diplopia**, scotomas, nystagmus, diplopia
	  • <u>**Afferent Pupillary Defect**</u>: **abnormal reaction to light stimuli**; light shined into normal eye causes pupil constriction in both eyes and rapidly swinging light from unaffected to affected eye causes pupil dilation in both eyes **when light stimulus (Marcus-Gunn pupil)**
	• <u>Internuclear Ophthalmoplegia</u>: inability to adduct affected eye with horizontal nystagmus of the contralateral eye; convergence ("cross eyed") is preserved
	• <u>Dysautonomia</u>: bladder or bowel dysfunction or incontinence, urinary retention, constipation, erectile dysfunction
	• <u>Cerebellar Symptoms</u>: Charcot's neurologic triad (intentional tremor, scanning/staccato speech, nystagmus), ataxia, slurred speech
	• <u>**Cognitive Dysfunction**</u>: **depression**, apathy, poor judgement, inattention, emotional lability,

Diagnosis	• **Clinical Diagnosis** • <u>**Brain MRI with Gadolinium**</u>: **initial and most accurate test; multiple hyperintense white matter plaques**; contrast differentiates active (inflamed) vs older plaques • <u>**Lumbar Puncture with CSF Analysis**</u>: indicated if MRI nondiagnostic; **shows elevated protein, increased total IgG, increased free kappa light chains, oligoclonal bands** • Oligoclonal IgG bands on electrophoresis indicate inflammatory cells have penetrated the blood-brain barrier
Treatment	• <u>**High-Dose Corticosteroids**</u>: **IV methylprednisolone and/or oral prednisone first-line treatment**; shortens acute exacerbations, slows progression and improves MRI measures • <u>**Plasmapheresis**</u>: plasma exchange indicated if corticosteroids are ineffective; useful for relapsing types, not used for primary progressive types • <u>**Immunomodulator Therapy**</u>: **beta-interferon or glatiramer first-line for prevention of relapse and progression**; decreases acute exacerbation frequency and delays disability • <u>Anti-alpha-4 Integrin Antibody</u>: natalizumab; monthly infusion to inhibits leukocyte passage across the blood-brain barrier; risk of progressive multifocal leukoencephalopathy • <u>Symptom Control</u>: amantadine (fatigue) antidepressants (depression), stool softeners/laxatives (constipation), gabapentin (paresthesias), baclofen (spasticity)

White matter plaque

Astrocytoma

Etiology & Risk Factors	• **Central nervous system (CNS) tumor that develops from astrocytes (star-shaped glial cell that form a large portion of the brain parenchyma)** • **Most common CNS tumor of childhood** (most cases occur between 5-9 years old) • <u>Etiology</u>: unknown • <u>Risk Factors</u>: **exposure to ionizing radiation**
Patho-physiology	• <u>**Pilocytic Astrocytoma (Grade I)**</u>: benign in nature, cystic consistency, **typically infratentorial, classically presents in childhood** • <u>**Diffuse Astrocytoma (Grade II)**</u>: more common in adults; tend to invade surrounding tissue but develop relatively slowly; may progress to glioblastoma • <u>**Anaplastic Astrocytoma (Grade III)**</u>: more common in adults; lack of endothelial proliferation, more aggressive type • <u>**Glioblastoma (Grade IV)**</u>: most common primary CNS tumor, peak age is 65 years old; **very poor prognosis**
Signs & Symptoms	• <u>General Symptoms</u>: **early morning headaches (may wake patient up at night), nausea/vomiting**, cognitive difficulties, personality changes, **gait disturbances** • <u>Focal Symptoms</u>: **seizures, aphasia, visual field defects or vision changes, cranial nerve deficits** • <u>Increased Intracranial Pressure</u>: headache, nausea/vomiting, papilledema, ataxia, drowsiness, stupor secondary to mass effect • <u>Physical Exam</u>: • **Localizing features based on neurological deficits**
Diagnosis	• <u>**Brain MRI with Gadolinium Contrast**</u>: **imaging test of choice**; determines disease extent and helps detect recurrence; grade I/II are non-enhancing, grade III/IV are enhancing • <u>Brain Biopsy</u>: guided by imaging studies; required to determine tumor type and grade

Treatment	• <u>**Low-Grade Astrocytoma**</u>:
	  • <u>**Surgical Resection**</u>: **primary treatment**
	  • <u>Chemotherapy</u>: indicated in children with unresectable tumor or inability to fully excise tumor or tumor that progresses or recurs after surgery
	  • <u>Radiation Therapy</u>: rarely used in children due to risk of long-term cognitive impairment
	• <u>**High-Grade Astrocytoma**</u>:
	  • **Combination of surgery, chemotherapy and radiation therapy**
	  • **Very poor prognosis**; overall survival at 3 years is only 20 to 30%

Key Words & Most Common	• CNS tumor developing from astrocytes • May be related to ionizing radiation exposure • Early morning headache + N/V + gait disturbances • Seizures, visual field defects, vision changes, CN deficits • Contrast enhanced brain MRI → brain biopsy • Surgical resection +/- chemotherapy +/- radiation therapy

Low grade astrocytoma of midbrain

Glioblastoma Multiforme

Etiology & Risk Factors	• Grade IV astrocytoma
	• Most common and most aggressive primary malignant central nervous system tumor in adults
	• <u>Etiology</u>: unknown; combination of environmental and genetic factors
	• <u>Risk Factors</u>: **age (>50 years old most common), males, neurofibromatosis, exposure to ionizing radiation**, HHV-6 or cytomegalovirus infections, occupational exposures (pesticides, petroleum refining, rubber manufacturing)
	• <u>Types</u>:
	    • <u>Primary</u>: **most common (90%) and most aggressive type**, more common in older adults (mean age of 62 years old); arises de novo (not from lower-grade tumor)
	    • <u>Secondary</u>: more common in younger adults (mean age of 45 years old); arises from lower-grade astrocytoma or oligodendroglioma

Patho-physiology	• Genetic alterations and epigenetic mutations lead to increase expression and suppression of genes and cellular and extracellular matrix changes • Primary tumors arise from neural stem cell precursors; secondary tumors arise from mature neural cell (astrocyte) mutations
Signs & Symptoms	• **Rapidly progressive neurological symptoms over days to weeks** • <u>General Symptoms</u>: **early morning headaches (may wake patient up at night), nausea/vomiting**, cognitive difficulties, personality changes, **gait disturbances** • <u>Focal Symptoms</u>: **seizures**, aphasia, **visual field defects or vision changes, cranial nerve deficits** • <u>Increased Intracranial Pressure</u>: headache, nausea/vomiting, papilledema, ataxia, drowsiness, stupor secondary to mass effect • <u>Physical Exam</u>: • **Localizing features based on neurological deficits**
Diagnosis	• <u>Brain MRI with Gadolinium Contrast</u>: initial imaging test of choice; shows **tumor involving the corpus callosum that extends into occipital and temporal lobes resulting in a butterfly wing pattern ("butterfly" glioma)**, lesion has **variable rings of enhancement with central necrosis and irregular (serpiginous) margins** • <u>Post-Surgical Histopathology</u>: definitive diagnosis; malignant astrocytes and necrotic regions surrounded by pseudo palisading (tumor cells lining the necrotic regions)
Treatment	• **Maximal surgical excision followed by chemoradiotherapy is recommended treatment** • **Very poor prognosis**; overall survival at 3 years is only 20 to 30%
Key Words & Most Common	• Most common and most aggressive primary malignant CNS tumor • Rapidly progressive neurological symptoms over days to weeks • Early morning or nocturnal headaches +N/V + gait disturbances + neurological deficits + visual disturbances • Brain MRI with gadolinium contrast • Maximal surgical excision followed by chemoradiotherapy

Meningioma

Etiology & Risk Factors	• **Benign, slow-growing central nervous system (CNS) tumor commonly arising from the arachnoid meningothelial cells of the brain and spinal cord meninges** • <u>Etiology</u>: sporadic; neurofibromatosis type 2 • <u>Risk Factors</u>: **female, obesity**, alcoholism, **ionizing radiation exposure, exogenous hormone use, hormone replacement therapy, use of oral contraceptive pills**, breast cancer
Patho-physiology	• Meningiomas express progesterone, estrogen, and androgen receptors on their membranes resulting in changes in size during pregnancy and the luteal phase of the menstrual cycle • Can develop wherever there is dura; most commonly develops over the cerebral convexities, along the base of the skull, and in the posterior fossa; rarely within ventricles
Signs & Symptoms	• Often asymptomatic • **Symptoms or focal neurologic signs are due to compression and brain displacement (do not invade brain parenchyma) and depend tumor location** • <u>Upper Motor Neuron Symptoms</u>: **hypertonia** or clonus, **hyperreflexia**, positive Babinski sign, **paresis**, paralysis • <u>General Symptoms</u>: anosmia, **headaches, dizziness, visual impairments, seizures**, papilledema, and **behavioral changes** • <u>Spinal Meningioma</u>: pain, weakness, hypotonia, hyporeflexia, **paresthesias**
Diagnosis	• <u>Brain MRI with Gadolinium Contrast</u>: preferred imaging test; homogenous, dense, enhanced dural-based lesions with or without brain edema • <u>Histology</u>: spindle-cells arranged in a "whorled" pattern; meningothelial cells eventually mineralize to form psammoma bodies (round, concentric calcifications)
Treatment	• <u>Observation</u>: indicated if small and asymptomatic; annual or biennially imaging with brain MRI • <u>Surgery</u>: **surgical resection** (if possible) indicated for symptomatic lesions or lesions with accelerated growth • Radiation or chemotherapy may be used if not surgical candidate or as adjuvant treatment
Key Words & Most Common	• Benign, slow-growing CNS tumor arising from meninges of brain/spinal cord • Female, OCP use, ionizing radiation exposure, hormone replacement therapy greatest risk factors • Signs and symptoms due to compression and brain displacement and depend on tumor location • Brain MRI with contrast • Observation vs surgical resection

355

Primary Brain Lymphoma

Etiology & Risk Factors	• Extranodal non-Hodgkin lymphoma involving the brain, spinal cord, cerebrospinal fluid (CSF), leptomeninges, and eyes with no evidence of any disease outside the CNS • <u>Etiology</u>: unknown; **may be related to an acquired or congenital immunodeficiency** • <u>Risk Factors</u>: **advanced age, history of Epstein-Barr virus**, history of autoimmune disease (RA, SLE, sarcoidosis), immunosuppression (AIDS, post-transplant, chemotherapy)
Patho-physiology	• Recurrent *MYD88* and *CD79B* gene mutations affect the B-cell signaling pathways • Origin of lymphoma cells unclear

Signs & Symptoms	• <u>Focal Deficits</u>: **depend on location of lesion**
	   • Change in personality, **seizures, confusion**, lethargy, increased intracranial pressure symptoms (headaches, nausea, vomiting, papilledema)
	• <u>Intraocular Involvement</u>: present in about 20-30% of cases
	   • Vision floaters, **blurry vision, diminished visual acuity and vision fields**

Diagnosis	• <u>Brain MRI with Gadolinium Contrast</u>: **preferred imaging test**; isodense or hypodense ring-enhancing lesion of the deep white matter (similar to cerebral toxoplasmosis) • <u>Lumbar Puncture with CSF Analysis</u>: indicated if focal enhancement on MRI • <u>Brain Biopsy</u>: **definitive diagnosis**; *corticosteroids are lymphocytotoxic and can obscure pathologic diagnosis* • Workup includes slit lamp examination of the eyes, chest, abdomen, pelvis CT scan, bone marrow biopsy, CBC, CMP, HIV, hepatitis B, and C serology, lactate dehydrogenase
Treatment	• <u>Corticosteroids</u>: **rapid improvement initially but typically recur** <u>Chemotherapy</u>: **high-dose IV methotrexate is most effective therapy** • *Whole-brain radiation can cause clinically significant leukoencephalopathy*
Key Words & Most Common	• Lymphoma of brain, spinal cord, CSF, leptomeninges, eyes • Focal deficits include seizures, confusion, headaches, n/v • Intraocular involvement includes blurry vision, floaters, diminished visual acuity • Brain MRI with contrast • Corticosteroids → high-dose IV methotrexate

Oligodendroglioma

Etiology & Risk Factors	• **Diffusely infiltrating glioma often involving the cortical gray matter; resembles oligodendrocytes** • <u>Oligodendrocytes</u>: myelin generating cells of the central nervous system (CNS) • **Slow-growing glioma most commonly seen in frontal lobes** • <u>Etiology</u>: unknown • <u>Risk Factors</u>: age (50-60 years old most common), male
Patho-physiology	• Tumor found predominantly in the white matter of the cerebral hemisphere, most commonly in the frontal lobes; temporal and parietal lobe involvement is possible • Characterized by deletion of the p arm of chromosome 1 and the q arm of chromosome 19 (1p/19q codeletion)
Signs & Symptoms	• **Often asymptomatic**; slow-growing tumor • **Headache and seizures are most common presenting symptoms** • Focal neurological deficits based on tumor location

Diagnosis	• <u>Neuroimaging</u>:
	   • <u>Head CT Scan</u>: initial imaging test; hypodense or isodense peripheral mass that is cortically based with a gyriform pattern of cortical calcification
	   • <u>**Brain MRI**</u>: **more accurate imaging test**; helps define the true extent and infiltration of the tumor
	• <u>Brain Biopsy</u>: **definitive diagnosis**; gelatinous gray mass, with cystic areas and small focal hemorrhages
	• <u>Genetic Marker Testing</u>: deletion of the p arm of chromosome 1 and the q arm of chromosome 19 (1p/19q codeletion)

Treatment	• **Combination of surgery, chemotherapy and radiation therapy**
Key Words & Most Common	• Glioma resembling oligodendrocytes • Slow-growing and most common in frontal lobes • Asymptomatic → headache and seizures + focal neurological deficits • Brain MRI + brain biopsy → genetic marker testing • Surgery, chemotherapy, radiation therapy

Ependymoma

Etiology & Risk Factors	• **Glial cell tumors arising from ependymal cells that line the ventricular system and parts of the the spinal column** • <u>Etiology</u>: unknown • <u>Risk Factors</u>: **most common in children (5 years old is mean age of diagnosis)**
Patho-physiology	• Based on genetic mutations and variations • Most commonly seen in the 4th ventricle, spinal cord, and medulla
Signs & Symptoms	• **Nausea/vomiting, headache** (due to increased intracranial pressure) • Irritability, sleeplessness in infants
Diagnosis	• <u>**Neuroimaging**</u>: **CT/MRI**; demonstrates non-enhancing and well-demarcated intraventricular lesion (isodense on CT and isointense on MRI T1 images) • <u>Brain Biopsy</u>: definitive diagnosis; perivascular pseudo rosettes (tumor cells arranged radially around a central vessel)
Treatment	• **Surgical resection followed by adjuvant radiation therapy** • Insufficient evidence to support the chemotherapy use
Key Words & Most Common	• Glial cell tumors arising from ependymal cells of the ventricular system • Most common in children (around age 5) • Nausea/vomiting + headache • Neuroimaging → brain biopsy Surgical resection → adjuvant radiation therapy

Ependymoma of 4th ventricle

Alzheimer Disease

Etiology & Risk Factors	• **Neurodegenerative disease that causes progressive behavior and cognitive impairment including memory, comprehension, language, attention, reasoning, and judgment** • **Most common type of dementia** • <u>Etiology</u>: unknown; progressive neuronal cell death • <u>Risk Factors</u>: **increasing age is greatest risk factor;** history of traumatic head injury, depression, **vascular disease**, smoking, **family history**, increased homocysteine levels • <u>Protective Factors</u>: **higher education**, estrogen therapy, NSAID use, **stimulating activities (reading, playing musical instruments, puzzles)**, healthy diet, **regular exercise**
Patho-physiology	• Accumulation of abnormal neuritic plaques and neurofibrillary tangles • Extracellular amyloid-beta protein deposition (neuritic plaques) occurs around meningeal and cerebral vessels and gray matter and are neurotoxic • Neurofibrillary tangles are hyperphosphorylated Tau protein aggregates that form twisted helical filament pairs which destabilize axonal microtubules
Signs & Symptoms	• *It is important to interview family members or caregivers as patients with cognitive decline rarely have insight into their cognitive and functional limitations* • Gradual progression of signs and symptoms • <u>**Loss of Short-Term Memory**</u>: most common initial symptom • **Asking the same question repeatedly, frequently misplacing objects**, forgetting appointments, **increasing reliance on memory aids** (reminder notes or lists) • <u>**Impaired Reasoning**</u>: poor or inappropriate social interactions, wearing inappropriate clothes for the current weather) • <u>**Difficulty Handling Complex Tasks**</u>: increased reliance on family members for help) • <u>**Poor Judgement**</u>: inability manage bank account, making poor financial decisions, paying less attention to hygiene) • <u>**Language or Visuospatial Dysfunction**</u>: difficulty recalling common words, speaking or writing errors, inability to recognize faces or common objects) • <u>**Behavioral Changes**</u>: wandering, confusion, increased agitation, yelling, persecutory ideation
Diagnosis	• **Clinical Diagnosis** • <u>Brain MRI</u>: **cerebral atrophy (specifically atrophy of the medial temporal lobe)**, widened third ventricle, reduced hippocampal volume, white matter lesions • <u>Cerebrospinal Fluid Analysis</u>: low beta-amyloid 42 and elevated Tau protein

Treatment	• <u>**Supportive**</u>: fostering supportive and familiar environment, orientation reinforcement, providing security objects, safety measures, cognitive stimulation
	• <u>**Cholinesterase Inhibitors**</u>: donepezil, rivastigmine, galantamine; moderately improves cognitive and memory function in some patients
	  • Inhibits acetylcholinesterase (AChE) to improve the availability of acetylcholine
	• <u>***N*-methyl-d-aspartate (NMDA) Receptor Antagonist**</u>: memantine; indicated in moderate to severe disease to improve cognition and functional capacity
	  • Blocks NMDA receptor to slows intracellular calcium accumulation and reduce glutamate excitotoxicity
	• <u>Anti-Amyloid Monoclonal Antibody</u>: aducanumab; monthly infusion of human IgG1 anti-amyloid monoclonal antibody is a disease-modifying treatment

Key Words & Most Common	• Neurodegenerative disease causing progressive behavioral and cognitive impairment • Increasing age and family history are greatest risk factors • Loss of short-term memory, impaired reasoning, difficulty handling complex tasks, poor judgement, language dysfunction, behavioral changes • Clinical diagnosis; brain MRI shows cerebral atrophy • Supportive +/- cholinesterase inhibitors (donepezil, rivastigmine, galantamine) +/- NMDA receptor antagonists (memantine

357

Vascular Dementia

Etiology & Risk Factors	• Chronic progressive cognitive decline resulting in functional impairment due to cerebrovascular disease • <u>Etiology</u>: diffuse or focal cerebral infarction (lacunar infarcts) • <u>Risk Factors</u>: **hypertension is greatest risk factor; advancing age (>70 years old)**, male, hyperlipidemia, diabetes mellitus, tobacco use, history of CVA, atrial fibrillation
Patho-physiology	• Atherosclerosis, thrombosis, or vasculopathy causes acute and chronic cerebral tissue ischemia, gliosis and demyelination leading to cognitive decline and neurological deficits

Signs & Symptoms	• **Similar cognitive impairment to other dementias** (memory loss, impaired reasoning, difficulty handling tasks, poor judgement, language dysfunction, behavioral changes)
	• <u>**Cognitive Deficits**</u>: **depends on the area affected**
	  • <u>Medial Frontal</u>: impaired executive function, apathy (lack of interest or concern), abulia (inability to act decisively)
	  • <u>Left Parietal</u>: apraxia (inability to perform tasks or movements), aphasia (inability to understand or express speech), agnosia (inability to process sensory information)
	  • <u>Right Parietal</u>: hemineglect (unawareness or unresponsiveness to objects, people, and other stimuli), confusion, visuospatial abnormalities
	• **Typically causes memory loss *later* and affects reasoning and executive function *earlier* than Alzheimer dementia**
	• **Abrupt functional decline and/or stepwise progression of symptoms**
	  • Infarct initiates abrupt onset of functional decline followed by subtle recovery; multiple-infarcts causing decline to progress in discrete steps
	• <u>**Focal Neurological Deficits**</u>: **depends on the area affected**
	  • Exaggeration of deep tendon reflexes, extensor plantar response, gait abnormalities, extremity weakness, urinary difficulty, hemiplegia, pseudobulbar palsy, aphasia

Diagnosis	• **Clinical Diagnosis** • Rule out other causes of symptoms (CBC, CMP, thyroid-stimulating hormone level, rapid plasma regain (RPR), vitamin B12, folate, PHQ9 depression screen, ECG, lipid panel) • <u>**Brain MRI**</u>: **multiple cortical or subcortical infarcts, multiple lacunar infarcts, periventricular white matter lesions**
Treatment	• <u>**Supportive**</u>: **fostering supportive and familiar environment**, orientation reinforcement, providing security objects, safety measures, cognitive stimulation • <u>**Manage Vascular Risk Factors**</u>: strict blood pressure control, cholesterol-lowering therapy, blood glucose regulation, smoking cessation
Key Words & Most Common	• Chronic progressive cognitive decline due to cerebrovascular disease • Diffuse or focal cerebral infarction • Hypertension and advance age is greatest risk factor • Similar cognitive impairment to other dementias (memory loss, impaired reasoning, difficulty handling tasks, poor judgement, language dysfunction, behavioral changes) • Typically causes memory loss later than Alzheimer dementia • Abrupt functional decline or stepwise progression of symptoms • Clinical diagnosis + brain MRI • Supportive + managing vascular risk factors

Differences Between Vascular Dementia and Alzheimer Disease

Clinical Evaluation	Vascular Dementia	Alzheimer Disease
History of Present Illness	• **Abrupt or stepwise progression in cognitive decline after multiple infarcts**	• **Slow, gradual deterioration of cognition**
Past Medical/Family History	• Cerebrovascular risk factors (hypertension, hyperlipidemia, diabetes mellitus, tobacco use) • History of coronary artery disease or peripheral artery disease	• Family history of Alzheimer disease
Mental Status	• **Variable mental status based on area of brain affected** • Subtle executive function and reasoning decline secondary to subcortical ischemic vascular disease	• **Memory impairment more prominent**
Neurological Findings	• **Focal deficits, gait disturbances**	• **Impaired mental status**
Cardiovascular Findings	• May have signs of cardiovascular risk factors (skin changes related to peripheral artery disease, lower extremity edema related to heart failure, hypertension, irregular heart rate)	• Usually normal
Neuroimaging (MRI/CT)	• **Multiple cortical or subcortical infarcts, multiple lacunar infarcts, periventricular white matter lesions**	• **Cerebral atrophy (specifically atrophy of the medial temporal lobe)**, widened third ventricle, reduced hippocampal volume, white matter lesions

Frontotemporal Dementia

Etiology & Risk Factors	• **Irreversible deterioration of cognition sporadic and hereditary disorders that cause localized frontal and temporal lobe degeneration** • <u>Etiology</u>: **sporadic or familial** (mutation of chromosome 17q21-22) • <u>Risk Factors</u>: **male, age (58 years old most common age at presentation)**; age of onset earlier than Alzheimer disease
Patho-physiology	• Abnormal protein aggregate deposition in the frontal and temporal lobes results in neuronal degeneration, microvacuoles formation, and astrocytosis

Signs & Symptoms	• Generally causes marked change in personality, social behavior, and language function (syntax and fluency) with less memory changes than Alzheimer disease
	• <u>**Behavioral Variant**</u>: **altered personality and behavioral changes**
	  • **Disinhibition, social inappropriate behaviors, apathy** (loss of sympathy and empathy for others), impaired abstract thinking, gradual worsening of executive function
	• <u>**Semantic Variant**</u>: **language function changes**; speech is fluid but may not make sense
	  • **Impaired word finding or loss of vocabulary** (paraphasia), **impaired comprehension**, impaired retrieval of information, disorganized responses
	• <u>Physical Exam</u>:
	  • Preserved memory, visuospatial and constructional skills
	  • Preserved orientation and general motor skills

Diagnosis	• **Clinical Diagnosis** • <u>Brain MRI</u>: nonspecific atrophy and hypoperfusion in the frontal and temporal lobes

Treatment	• <u>**Supportive**</u>: **ensuring safety is important**
	  • **Fostering supportive and familiar environment**, reinforce orientation, provide security objects, **safety measures**
	  • Cognitive stimulation (reading, board games, social interaction, puzzles)
	• Symptoms treated as needed

Key Words & Most Common	• Irreversible deterioration of cognition due to degeneration of the frontal and temporal lobe degeneration • Familial; age of onset earlier than Alzheimer disease (mean age of 58 years old) • Behavioral variant has altered personality and behavioral changes • Semantic variant has language function changes • Preserved memory, visuospatial, orientation and motor skills • Clinical diagnosis + brain MRI (atrophy of frontal and temporal lobes) • Supportive measures

White matter atrophy of the frontal lobes

Lewy Body Dementia

Etiology & Risk Factors	• **Chronic, progressive cognitive deterioration characterized by diffuse presence of abnormal protein inclusions (Lewy bodies) in the cytoplasm of cortical neurons** • <u>Etiology</u>: unknown; **various genetics, environmental, and age-related factors** • <u>Risk Factors</u>: **history of Parkinson disease** (40% of patients will develop dementia); **age (>70 years old most common)**
Patho-physiology	• Decreased acetylcholine levels in the temporal and parietal cortex result in visual hallucinations; increased regulation of muscarinic M1 receptors in the temporal lobe result in delusions characteristic of Lewy body dementia
Signs & Symptoms	• <u>**Extrapyramidal Symptoms**</u>: **parkinsonism; rigidity, bradykinesia, unstable gait, repeated falls** (tremor does not occur early; deficits usually symmetric) • <u>**Cognitive Fluctuations**</u>: **attention span variations**; periods of being alert, oriented and coherent alternate with episodes of drowsiness, delirium and confusion • <u>**Progressive Dementia**</u>: impaired attention and executive function; memory loss occurs later in disease course • <u>**Visual Hallucinations**</u>: recurrent and complex/detailed hallucinations • <u>**Autonomic Dysfunction**</u>: orthostatic hypotension and unexplained syncope; extreme sensitivity to antipsychotics • <u>**Sleep Dysfunction**</u>: vivid dreams without the usual physiologic paralysis of skeletal muscles during REM sleep results in patient acting out dream
Diagnosis	• **Clinical Diagnosis** • **Diagnosis considered probable with 2 of the 4 following core features:** • Cognitive fluctuations, visual hallucinations, REM sleep dysfunction, parkinsonism • Rule out other causes of symptoms (CBC, CMP, thyroid-stimulating hormone level, rapid plasma regain (RPR), vitamin B12, folate, PHQ9 depression screen, ECG, lipid panel)
Treatment	• <u>**Supportive**</u>: **fostering supportive and familiar environment**, orientation reinforcement, providing security objects, **safety measures** • <u>**Cholinesterase Inhibitors**</u>: **donepezil, rivastigmine, galantamine**; moderately improves cognitive function in some patients • Inhibits acetylcholinesterase (AChE) to improve the availability of acetylcholine • <u>**Levodopa/Carbidopa**</u>: **effective treatment for extrapyramidal symptoms but may worsen psychiatric symptoms** • <u>**Palliative Measures**</u>: may be more appropriate than highly aggressive interventions or hospital care in advanced cases
Key Words & Most Common	• Chronic, progressive cognitive deterioration characterized by presence of Lewy bodies • Cognitive fluctuations + visual hallucinations + sleep dysfunction + extrapyramidal symptoms (parkinsonism) • Clinical diagnosis • Supportive +/- cholinesterase inhibitors (rivastigmine, galantamine) +/- levodopa/carbidopa (may worsen psychiatric symptoms) → palliation

Focal (Partial) Seizure

Etiology & Risk Factors	• Abnormal neuronal discharge of electrical impulse from one focal section of one hemisphere
	• <u>Two Classifications</u>: simple or complex partial seizure
	   • <u>Simple Partial Seizures</u>: focal aware seizure; without impairment of consciousness
	   • <u>Complex Partial Seizures</u>: focal impaired-awareness seizure; with impairment of consciousness
	• <u>Etiology</u>: multiple genetic, structural, metabolic, autoimmune, infectious, or unknown factors
	• <u>Risk Factors</u>: male, age (bimodal distribution of young and elderly), blood vessel pathology, congenital developmental abnormality, traumatic brain injury

Patho-physiology	• Gamma-aminobutyric acid (GABA) is an inhibitory neurotransmitter; when GABA is released, the glutamate receptor initiations and ensuing uninhibited, unsynchronized neuronal action that causes a focal discharge of electrical impulse resulting in seizure activity
Signs & Symptoms	• **Focal autonomic, motor, and/or sensory dysfunction depending on lobe affected** • <u>Autonomic Dysfunction</u>: GI sensations (pain, nausea, vomiting, hunger), **flushing**, sexual arousal, piloerection, blood pressure changes, **palpitations** • <u>Motor Dysfunction</u>: rhythmic, jerking movements, muscle tightening or rigidity; may spread to other parts of the affected limb or body (**Jacksonian march**) • <u>Sensory Dysfunction</u>: paresthesias, **hot or cold sensation**, sensation of movement and visual, olfactory, auditory, or gustatory sensations • <u>Behavioral Arrest</u>: cessation of movement and unresponsiveness • <u>Automatisms</u>: repetitive behaviors (facial grimacing, clenching jaw, picking/patting, repeating words or phrases, lip smacking, staring into space, rapid eye movement, patting, hand rubbing) may accompany complex seizures • <u>Cognitive Dysfunction</u>: language impairment, hallucinations, distorted perceptions, déjà vu • <u>Emotional Dysfunction</u>: anxiety, intense fear, joy or other affect without subjective emotion • *Complex partial seizures may present with aura sensation in which patient claims to feel, see, hear, taste, or smell a not-present sensation*

Diagnosis	• <u>Neuroimaging</u>: CT/MRI to rule out structural causes
	• <u>Labs</u>: complete blood count, comprehensive metabolic panel, drug screen, blood alcohol level, toxin screen, and thyroid panel to rule out reversible causes
	• <u>Electroencephalogram (EEG)</u>: aids in detection of origin of seizure activity; helps predict if seizure will be controlled or uncontrolled
	   • <u>Simple Partial</u>: focal discharge at onset of seizure
	   • <u>Complex Partial</u>: interictal spike or slow waves at a focal site

Treatment	• <u>Supportive</u>: elimination of cause, avoidance or use of safety measures in situations when loss of consciousness could be life threatening (driving, swimming, climbing, bathing)
	• <u>Antiseizure Medications</u>: no drug of choice; can be treated with multiple types of medications
	   • <u>Carbamazepine</u>: first-line medication; blocks use-dependent sodium channels which inhibits sustained, repetitive neuronal firing
	   • <u>Lamotrigine</u>: first-line medication; blocks voltage-gated sodium channels which stabilizes neuronal membranes
	   • Second-line medications include valproate, topiramate, oxcarbazepine, or gabapentin

Key Words & Most Common	• <u>Simple Partial</u>: no impairment of consciousness with motor, sensory, autonomic, psychic symptoms • <u>Complex Partial</u>: with impairment of consciousness + simple partial seizure symptoms; may be accompanied by automatisms

Absence Seizure

Etiology & Risk Factors	• **Generalized seizure (involving both hemispheres) during which the patient is unresponsive** • <u>Etiology</u>: genetic predisposition (multifactorial inheritance) and altered neurotransmitter function • <u>Risk Factors</u>: **most commonly seen in childhood; age of onset typically between 4-10 years old (peak between 5-7 years old)** • <u>Precipitating Factors</u>: **hyperventilation**, heightened state of arousal, sleep deprivation, medication use
Patho-physiology	• Neurons from the thalamocortical network can synchronously discharge in an oscillatory or single spike pattern pattern resulting in brief impairment of consciousness and absence of motor activity followed by an abrupt return to baseline

Signs & Symptoms	• **"Blank Stare" Episodes: sudden, marked impairment of consciousness without loss of body tone**
	   • Brief (5-10 seconds) pause/staring episodes associated with loss of awareness, unresponsiveness, and behavioral arrest
	   • Automatisms (eyelid twitching and lip smacking) **may occur if episode lasts >10 seconds**
	   • May occur 10-30+ times per day
	   • No postictal phase and not preceded by aura
	• <u>Physical Exam</u>:
	   • May be provoked by hyperventilation
	   • Patient may be asked to blow pinwheel or piece of paper for 2 minutes to provoke seizure that may be seen clinically or on EEG

Diagnosis	• <u>Electroencephalogram (EEG)</u>: **primary diagnostic tool; demonstrates bilateral, synchronous and symmetrical 3-Hertz spike-and-wave activity that starts and ends abruptly**

Treatment	• <u>Supportive</u>: adequate sleep, stress reduction, avoiding triggers, breathing exercises, ketogenic or a medium-chain triglyceride diet may be beneficial
	• <u>Medication Management</u>:
	   • **Ethosuximide: first-line medication**; suppresses the paroxysmal 3 cycle/second spike-and-wave activity associated with lapses of consciousness
	   • **Valproic Acid: second-line medication**; increases effects of GABA and may inhibit glutamate/NMDA receptor-mediated neuronal excitation; avoid in pregnancy
	   • <u>Lamotrigine</u>: third-line medication; blocks voltage-gated sodium channels which stabilizes neuronal membranes
	   • *Some sodium channel blockers (phenytoin, carbamazepine, gabapentin, pregabalin, and vigabatrin) can worsen absence seizures*

Key Words & Most Common	• Most common in children aged 4-10 years old (peak 5-7 years old) • "Blank Stare" Episodes: sudden impairment of consciousness lasting 4-10 seconds without loss of body tone • May be provoked by hyperventilation • <u>EEG</u>: bilateral symmetric 3-Hertz spike-and-wave activity • Ethosuximide is first-line • Valproic acid is second-line

Generalized Tonic-Clonic Seizure 🧠

Etiology & Risk Factors	• Simultaneous neuronal discharge of both hemispheres (diffuse brain involvement) characterized by a seizure that has a tonic phase followed by clonic muscle contractions • Also known as a grand mal seizure • <u>Etiology</u>: **genetic predisposition**, structural brain abnormalities, or metabolic disturbances • <u>Risk Factors</u>: **family history of epilepsy, traumatic brain injury**, stroke, brain tumors, **developmental disorders**, infectious diseases, **drug or alcohol abuse**, sleep deprivation • <u>Precipitating Factors</u>: fever, menstrual period, **sleep deprivation, stress, strong emotions**, strenuous exercise, loud music, **flashing lights, drug use** (cocaine, amphetamines)
Patho-physiology	• Imbalance between excitatory and inhibitory neurotransmitters causes abnormal synaptic connectivity resulting in synchronous and simultaneous neuronal discharge in both hemispheres of the brain

Signs & Symptoms	• **Tonic-Clonic Seizures**:
	  • **Loss of Consciousness**: abrupt loss of consciousness without aura followed by tonic phase
	  • **Tonic Phase**: may start with a scream and **generalized stiffening (contraction and rigidity) of the body with or without respiratory arrest** followed by clonic phase
	  • **Clonic Phase**: clonic jerking (repetitive, rhythmic, symmetric jerking motion) usually lasting <3 minutes followed by postictal phase
	  • **Postictal Phase**: postictal sleepiness, **confusion**, agitation, somnolence, headache, personality and mood changes
	• Physical Exam:
	  • **Evidence of trauma sustained during seizure; tongue bites**, cracked teeth, bruises and scrapes, fracture from fall, posterior shoulder dislocation

Diagnosis	• <u>Neuroimaging</u>: CT/MRI to rule out structural causes • <u>Labs</u>: complete blood count, comprehensive metabolic panel, drug screen, blood alcohol level, toxin screen, and thyroid panel to rule out reversible causes • <u>Electroencephalogram (EEG)</u>: shows generalized, bilateral, symmetric bursts of high-amplitude (4-7/Hz) rapid spiking during active episodes

Treatment	• **Treat underlying cause if identified**
	• **Supportive**: roll onto side to decrease the risk of asphyxiation and aspiration during active seizure or postictal phase, pad/pillows on guard rails of bed, bite guard to prevent oral/dental trauma, avoidance or use of safety measures in situations when loss of consciousness could be life threatening (driving, swimming, climbing, bathing)
	• **Prophylactic/Long-Term Therapy**:
	  • **Valproate: first-line monotherapy**; increases effects of GABA and may inhibit glutamate/NMDA receptor-mediated neuronal excitation; avoid in pregnancy
	  • **Lamotrigine**: second-line medication; blocks voltage-gated sodium channels which stabilizes neuronal membranes
	  • **Levetiracetam**: alternative second-line medication; binds to specific synaptic vesicle proteins in the brain which regulates neurotransmitter release
	  • **Topiramate**: alternative second-line medication; blocks voltage-gated sodium channels, enhances GABA activity and blocks glutamate activity
	• **Acute Therapy**:
	  • **Benzodiazepines: lorazepam, midazolam; initial therapy to control active seizure**; potentiates GABA-mediated CNS inhibition and block cortical and limbic arousal

Key Words & Most Common	• Loss of consciousness → tonic phase (generalized stiffening of body) → clonic phase (repetitive, rhythmic jerking motion) → postictal phase (confusion, agitation) • EEG: generalized, symmetric bursts of high-amplitude spiking during episodes • Valproate first-line; lamotrigine, levetiracetam, topiramate are alternatives • Benzodiazepines (lorazepam, midazolam) for acute seizure

Status Epilepticus 🧠

Etiology & Risk Factors	• **Neurological emergency defined as a single, continuous seizure lasting >5 minutes or continuous/recurrent seizure activity without recovery between seizures** • <u>Etiology</u>: CNS infections, metabolic abnormalities, CVA, **head trauma, drug toxicity or drug withdrawal syndrome**, hypoxia, hypertensive emergency, structural abnormalities • <u>Risk Factors</u>: **history of epilepsy**, age (bimodal distribution in infants and elderly)
Patho-physiology	• Breakdown in the normal mechanisms that regulate the balance between excitatory neurotransmitters (glutamate, aspartate, acetylcholine), inhibitory neurotransmitters (gamma-aminobutyric acid [GABA]) and inhibitory mechanisms (calcium ion-dependent potassium ion current and magnesium blockade of NMDA) lead to excessive neuronal excitation and sustained and persistent seizures
Signs & Symptoms	• **Single, continuous seizure lasting >5 minutes or continuous/recurrent seizure activity without recovery between seizures** • Convulsive status epilepticus characterized by generalized tonic-clonic movements of the extremities and impaired mental status • Non-convulsive status epilepticus may have impaired mental status with or without subtle motor signs (tonic eye deviation)
Diagnosis	• **Clinical Diagnosis** • **Head CT**: often indicated to determine if intracranial mass or hemorrhage is present • <u>Labs</u>: blood glucose level, electrolytes (Ca, Na, Mg), complete blood count, lumbar puncture with CSF analysis, toxicology screen, CK, lactate, anti-seizure medication levels
Treatment	• **Supportive**: protect patient from injury (roll onto side to decrease the risk of asphyxiation and aspiration, pad/pillows on guard rails of bed, jaw thrust to prevent oral trauma) • **Benzodiazepines: first-line agent to rapidly control seizure**; potentiates GABA-mediated CNS inhibition and block cortical and limbic arousal • **IV lorazepam preferred**; IV diazepam; IM midazolam alternative if unable to obtain IV access • **Phenytoin or Fosphenytoin: second-line agent** indicated if no response to benzodiazepines; blocks voltage-gated sodium channels to stabilize neuronal membranes • **Valproate**: alternative second-line agent indicated if no response to benzodiazepines; increases GABA effects, inhibits glutamate/NMDA receptor-mediated neuronal excitation • **Levetiracetam**: alternative second-line agent preferred in pregnancy; binds to specific synaptic vesicle proteins in the brain which regulates neurotransmitter release • **Phenobarbital**: third-line agent if refractory to phenytoin; binds to GABA receptors and potentiates GABA-mediated CNS inhibition • General Anesthetics: propofol, midazolam, ketamine, lacosamide indicated if refractory
Key Words & Most Common	• Single, continuous seizure lasting >5 minutes or continuous/recurrent seizure activity without recovery between seizures • Clinical diagnosis + head CT to rule out mass or hemorrhage • Benzodiazepines (lorazepam) → phenytoin or fosphenytoin → valproate, levetiracetam → phenobarbital

Lacunar Infarct

Etiology & Risk Factors	• **Type of ischemic stroke characterized by occlusion of small deep penetrating branches of the cerebral arteries in the pons and basal ganglia** • Etiology: **occlusion of vascular supply to a focal part of the brain**; may have embolic fragments from a cardiac or large vessel disease origin • Risk Factors: **hypertension and diabetes mellitus are greatest risk factors**; smoking, hyperlipidemia, carotid artery atherosclerosis, PAD, history of TIA
Patho-physiology	• Cerebral arteries from the circle of Willis, including branches from the middle cerebral artery, anterior cerebral artery, posterior cerebral artery, and/or basilar artery supply blood to the cerebrum, cerebellum, and brainstem; occlusion or blockage of these small deep penetrating arteries causes lacunar infarct
Signs & Symptoms	• **Pure Motor Hemiparesis: most common presentation; contralateral hemiparesis or weakness of the face, arm, and leg** • *Cortical signs (aphasia, cognitive deficit, visual symptoms) are always absent* • **Ataxic Hemiparesis**: contralateral face and leg hemiparesis and contralateral limb ataxia (impaired balance or coordination) • **Pure Sensory Deficits**: absent or abnormal sensation (pain, touch, pressure, vision, hearing, taste, temperature) of the contralateral face, arm, and leg • **Sensorimotor**: combination of contralateral sensory and motor loss • **Dysarthria**: "clumsy hand syndrome"; tongue, larynx, facial muscle weakness, dysphagia, dysarthria; contralateral clumsiness of upper extremity
Diagnosis	• **Head CT: initial imaging test; demonstrates small, ill-defined hypodensities usually within the central and noncortical aspects (pons and basal ganglia)** • **CT Angiogram**: may demonstrate filling defect secondary to occlusion of vessel by thrombus, arterial narrowing and/or extensive vessel disease • **Brain MRI: most accurate imaging test** • Carotid Ultrasound: may aid in diagnosis of atherosclerosis and carotid artery stenosis

Treatment	• **Tissue Plasminogen Activator (TPA): indicated if presenting within 4.5 hours of symptom onset**
	• **Dual Antiplatelet Therapy (DAPT): aspirin and clopidogrel indicated if outside TPA window**
	  • Treatment initiated within 24 hours of symptom onset and continued for 21 days
	• **Management of Risk Factors**:
	  • Hypertension: allowing for permissive hypertension unless the marked blood pressure elevation (>220/120mmHg)
	  • Diabetes: goal to lower blood glucose levels to 60-180 mg/dL
	• Good Prognosis: partial or complete resolution within hours to weeks after insult

Key Words & Most Common	• Type of stroke characterized by occlusion of small deep penetrating branches of cerebral arteries • Hypertension and diabetes mellitus are greatest risk factors • 5 Classic Presentations: pure motor hemiparesis, ataxic hemiparesis, pure sensory deficits, sensorimotor, dysarthria • Head CT is initial imaging test • TPA vs DAPT as indicated • Manage underlying risk factors

Transient Ischemic Attack (TIA)

Etiology & Risk Factors	• **Transient episode of neurologic dysfunction secondary to focal brain, spinal cord or retinal ischemia without acute infarction or tissue injury** • Etiology: emboli is most common etiology • Risk Factors: **diabetes mellitus, hypertension, advanced age, dyslipidemia, smoking, obesity, sedentary lifestyle**, alcoholism, poor diet, psychosocial stress
Patho-physiology	• Cryptogenic: the most common classification characterized by cortical pattern of ischemia with no clear identifiable cardioembolic, lacunar, or atherosclerotic source • Cardioembolic: blood clot within the left atrium secondary to atrial fibrillation • Lacunar Infarcts: small vessel arteriolosclerosis • Large-Vessel Atherosclerosis: lack of blood flow distal to arterial stenosis or arterial embolism (emboli from carotid or vertebral arteries most common)

Signs & Symptoms	• **Symptoms last for a few minutes with complete resolution within 1 hour**; often resolve by time of presentation
	• **Focal, unilateral weakness, paralysis or paresis of the face, arm, or leg**
	• **Dysarthria** (slurred speech), **dysphagia** (difficulty swallowing), **aphagia** (inability to swallow)
	• **Vision changes** (visual field defects, diplopia, vision loss)
	  • **Amaurosis Fugax**: transient monocular vision loss; described as "shade pulled down over one eye"
	• Physical Exam:
	  • Cranial Nerve Deficits: monocular vision loss, disconjugate gaze, facial droop, hemianopia, diplopia, abnormal tongue movement
	  • Motor Deficits: difficulty with balance and coordination, unilateral weakness in the upper or lower extremities
	  • Cardiac Exam: carotid bruit or irregular irregular rhythm may be heard
		ABCD2 Stroke Risk Score
		
		Age >60 years old (1 point)
		
		BP >140/90 (1 point)
		
		Clinical Symptoms:
		Slurred speech (1 point)
		Unilateral weakness (2 points)
		
		Duration:
		>10 minutes (1 point)
		>60 minutes (2 points)
		
		Diabetes mellitus (1 point)
		
		0-3 points = 3.1% 90-day risk
		4-5 points = 9.8% 90-day risk
		6-7 points = 17.8% 90-day risk

Diagnosis	• **Labs**: point of care glucose, CBC, CMP, coagulation tests, troponin, pregnancy test, drug screen, lipid panel, infection workup • **Head CT**: initial study to rule out hemorrhage, mass lesion, or infarct (may not identify infarcts for >24 hours) • **CT Angiography**: recommended if an MRI cannot be performed; evaluates for large vessel occlusion or carotid stenosis • **Diffusion Weighted MRI**: most accurate imaging test to rule out an infarct • **Conventional Angiography**: definitive diagnosis; invasive procedure that is rarely performed • Carotid Doppler Ultrasound: evaluate for carotid artery stenosis • Ancillary Testing: rule out cardioembolic source, ECG, echocardiogram)	

Treatment	• **Antiplatelet Therapy: aspirin and/or clopidogrel indicated as first-line medical management**
	  • Aspirin: indicated for ABCD2 score <4 points
	  • Aspirin + Clopidogrel: indicated for ABCD2 score ≥4 points
	• **Carotid Endarterectomy**: indicated in internal carotid artery stenosis >50%; arterial angioplasty plus stenting alternative
	• **Management of Risk Factors**:
	  • Combination of diet, exercise, antiplatelet, statin, antihypertensive therapy, diabetes control has been shown to reduce subsequent stroke risk by 80-90%	

Ischemic Stroke

Etiology & Risk Factors	• Acute onset of neurological impairment secondary to vascular injury that reduces cerebral blood flow to specific region of brain; also know as cerebrovascular accident
	• Etiology: **hypoperfusion secondary to thrombotic or embolic cause**
	   • **Thrombotic: most common cause (80%); atherosclerosis,** vasculitis, **vertebral and carotid artery dissection,** hypercoagulable state, drug use (cocaine, amphetamine)
	   • **Embolic:** valvular vegetations, atrial fibrillation, valvular disease, patent foramen ovale, fat emboli
	• Risk Factors: **hypertension is greatest risk factor: dyslipidemia, diabetes mellitus,** atrial fibrillation, smoking, obesity, sedentary lifestyle, poor diet, drug use

Patho-physiology	• Hypoperfusion of the brain secondary to thrombosis or embolisms leads to oxygen and nutrient deprivation resulting in brain cell dysfunction, injury, and death • Extent and location of damage depends on size and location of affected artery and duration of ischemia

Signs & Symptoms	• **Signs and symptoms of ischemic stroke depend on the part of brain affected**
	• General Symptoms:
	   • **Focal, unilateral weakness, paralysis or paresis of the face, arm, or leg**
	   • **Dysarthria** (slurred speech), **dysphagia** (difficulty swallowing), **aphagia** (inability to swallow)
	   • **Vision changes** (visual field defects, diplopia, vision loss)
	   • **Dizziness,** headache, loss of balance/coordination, **confusion, altered mental status**

Diagnosis	• **Clinical Diagnosis** • Labs: point of care glucose, CBC, CMP, coagulation tests, troponin, pregnancy test, drug screen, lipid panel • ECG: stroke often associated with coronary artery disease • **Non-Contrast: best initial test,** indicated to rule out hemorrhagic stroke; may be normal within first 6-24 hours • **Diffusion Weighted MRI: most accurate imaging test** to rule out an infarct

Treatment	• **Tissue Plasminogen Activator (tPA): alteplase; indicated within 3 hours of symptom onset for diagnosed ischemic stroke with measurable neurological deficit**
	   • Contraindications: BP >185/110, active internal or intracranial hemorrhage, recent bleeding, bleeding disorder, recent head trauma, recent intracranial surgery
	   • *May be used within 4.5 hours in patients <80 years old, NIH stroke scale <25, no history of diabetes, no history of ischemic stroke*
	• **Mechanical Thrombectomy: consider in all patients, even if those who received fibrinolytic therapy**
	   • **Can be performed within 24 hours of symptom onset (6-16 hours recommended) for patients with large arterial occlusion of the proximal anterior circulation**
	   • Improved reperfusion, early neurological recovery and improved functional outcome compared to alteplase alone
	• **Blood Pressure Management: labetalol,** nicardipine, clevidipine, hydralazine
	   • Indicated if >180/110mmHg if thrombolytics are to be used
	   • Indicated if >180/105mmHg for the first 24 hours after IV alteplase OR
	   • Indicated if >220/120 if no plan to use thrombolytics
	• **Antiplatelet Therapy: aspirin, clopidogrel;** indicated for secondary prevention for subsequent non-cardioembolic strokes; dual therapy indicated for TIA or minor stroke
	• **Anticoagulant Therapy:** dabigatran, apixaban, rivaroxaban; indicated for secondary prevention of cardioembolic strokes (warfarin nonvalvular or valvular atrial fibrillation)
	• **Statin Therapy:** atorvastatin; indicated for all patients with evidence of atherosclerotic stroke and low-density lipoprotein (LDL) cholesterol ≥100 mg/dL

Middle Cerebral Artery Infarct

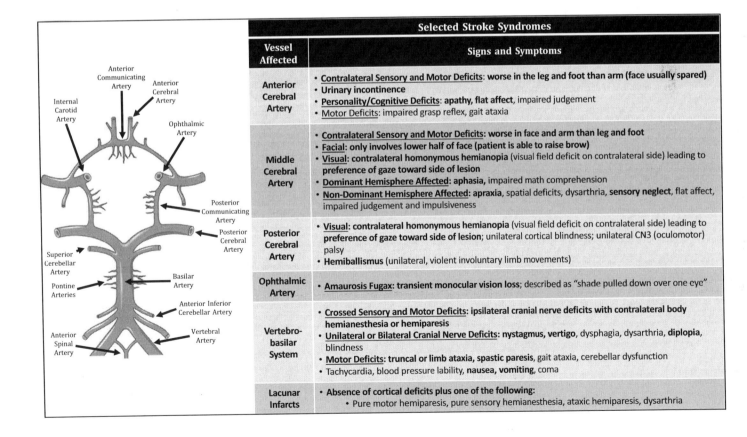

Selected Stroke Syndromes

Vessel Affected	Signs and Symptoms
Anterior Cerebral Artery	• **Contralateral Sensory and Motor Deficits: worse in the leg and foot than arm (face usually spared)** • **Urinary incontinence** • **Personality/Cognitive Deficits: apathy, flat affect,** impaired judgement • Motor Deficits: impaired grasp reflex, gait ataxia
Middle Cerebral Artery	• **Contralateral Sensory and Motor Deficits: worse in face and arm than leg and foot** • **Facial: only involves lower half of face (patient is able to raise brow)** • **Visual:** contralateral homonymous hemianopia (visual field deficit on contralateral side) leading to preference of gaze toward side of lesion • **Dominant Hemisphere Affected: aphasia,** impaired math comprehension • **Non-Dominant Hemisphere Affected: apraxia,** spatial deficits, dysarthria, **sensory neglect,** flat affect, impaired judgement and impulsiveness
Posterior Cerebral Artery	• **Visual:** contralateral homonymous hemianopia (visual field deficit on contralateral side) leading to preference of gaze toward side of lesion; unilateral cortical blindness; unilateral CN3 (oculomotor) palsy • **Hemiballismus** (unilateral, violent involuntary limb movements)
Ophthalmic Artery	• **Amaurosis Fugax: transient monocular vision loss;** described as "shade pulled down over one eye"
Vertebro-basilar System	• **Crossed Sensory and Motor Deficits: ipsilateral cranial nerve deficits with contralateral body hemianesthesia or hemiparesis** • **Unilateral or Bilateral Cranial Nerve Deficits: nystagmus, vertigo,** dysphagia, dysarthria, **diplopia,** blindness • **Motor Deficits: truncal or limb ataxia, spastic paresis,** gait ataxia, cerebellar dysfunction • Tachycardia, blood pressure lability, **nausea, vomiting,** coma
Lacunar Infarcts	• **Absence of cortical deficits plus one of the following:** • Pure motor hemiparesis, pure sensory hemianesthesia, ataxic hemiparesis, dysarthria

Arteriovenous Malformation

Etiology & Risk Factors	• Abnormal fistulas between cerebral arteries and veins • **Most commonly occurs at the junction of cerebral arteries** (parenchyma of the frontal-parietal region, frontal lobe, lateral cerebellum, or overlying occipital lobe) • Etiology: **sporadic** or due to genetic syndromes (Osler-Weber-Rendu syndrome, Cobb syndrome) • <u>Risk Factors</u>: **history of genetic syndrome**, male, history of head trauma, hypertension, smoking, drug use, pregnancy (hormone change)
Patho-physiology	• Altered flow dynamics or structural vascular abnormalities cause increased arterial flow directly into venous structures predisposes the venous wall to disruption and hemorrhage
Signs & Symptoms	• **Often asymptomatic** • **Symptomatic presentation with spontaneous intracranial hemorrhage** • **Headache and seizure most common presenting symptoms** • Cranial bruit
Diagnosis	• **Most cerebral aneurysms are diagnosed incidentally or in the setting of acute hemorrhage** • <u>**Neuroimaging**</u>**:** • **Contrast or non-contrast head CT, brain MRI, CT angiography (CTA), or conventional angiography**
Treatment	• <u>Observation</u>: serial imaging and reduction of risk factors considered if low risk of rupture • <u>Surgery</u>: **surgical resection, endovascular embolization, stereotactic radiosurgery or combination is primary treatment**
Key Words & Most Common	• Abnormal fistula between cerebral arteries and veins • Altered flow dynamics leads to increased arterial flow into venous structure increasing risk of rupture and hemorrhage • Often asymptomatic until hemorrhage occurs • Headache and seizure most common symptoms • Neuroimaging to diagnose • Surgical resection, endovascular embolization, stereotactic radiosurgery primary treatment

Basilar Skull Fracture

Etiology & Risk Factors	• **Fracture of one of the bones that compose the base of the skull** • **Most commonly involves the temporal bone**; may involve occipital, sphenoid, ethmoid, and/or orbital plate of the frontal bone • <u>Etiology</u>: **high-velocity blunt force trauma (motor vehicle accidents, motorcycle accidents, pedestrian injuries, falls, assault)**
Patho-physiology	• Blunt trauma causes fracture of the bones that compose the base of the skull; skull fractures are often associated with other central nervous systems (CNS) pathologies including epidural hematoma secondary to temporal bone weakness and the proximity of the middle meningeal artery
Signs & Symptoms	• **Cranial nerve deficits, headache, loss of consciousness, altered mental status, nausea/vomiting**, dizziness, tinnitus, nystagmus, **loss of smell and hearing** • <u>**Periorbital Ecchymosis (Raccoon Eyes)**</u>: pooling of blood surrounding the eyes; presentation may be delayed 1-3 days • <u>**Retroauricular or Mastoid Ecchymosis (Battle's Sign)**</u>: pooling of blood behind the ears in the mastoid region; presentation may be delayed 1-3 days • <u>**Hemotympanum**</u>: pooling of blood behind the tympanic membrane; earliest clinical finding with presentation within minutes to hours • <u>**Cerebrospinal Fluid (CSF) Rhinorrhea or Otorrhea**</u>: CSF leak from ear or nose; presentation may be delayed hours to days • **"Halo" Sign**: drop of fluid placed on tissue paper, rapidly expanding ring of clear fluid around red blood defines positive test
Diagnosis	• **Clinical Diagnosis** • <u>**Non-Contrast Head CT**</u>: **first-line imaging test**; linear or non-displaced fractures may be difficult to detect • Multidetector CT (MDCT) thin-slice scanning of face and skull base may aid in the detection of subtle fractures
Treatment	• **Emergent neurosurgery evaluation** • Prophylactic antibiotics and tetanus immunization often indicated • **Nasogastric tubes and nasotracheal intubation are absolutely contraindicated**
Key Words & Most Common	• Fracture of temporal bone most common • High-velocity blunt force trauma (MVA, assault, motorcycle accidents, falls) • Periorbital ecchymosis (raccoon eyes) • Retroauricular/mastoid ecchymosis (Battle's sign) • Hemotympanum • CSF rhinorrhea/otorrhea • Non-contrast head CT • Emergent neurosurgery evaluation

Basilar skull fracture

C1 Burst (Jefferson) Fracture

Etiology & Risk Factors	• **Fracture of the anterior arch and posterior arch of the C1 (atlas) vertebrae** • Etiology: **dive into shallow water, football tackle**, motor vehicle collision • Mechanism of Injury: **axial loading mechanism** (combined with flexion/extension or rotation) or **hyperextension of the neck** • Risk Factors: low-energy trauma in elderly patients; high-impact trauma in young patients
Patho-physiology	• C1 articulates with C2 and condyles of the occipital bone, joining the skull with the cervical spine • C1 does not contain a vertebral body and is comprised of thin anterior and posterior arches; axial loading transmits force through occipital condyles to the lateral structures

Signs & Symptoms	• **Proximal neck pain following traumatic mechanism**
	• Physical Exam:
	  • **Decreased neck range of motion**
	   Usually no neurologic symptoms

Diagnosis	• **Lateral Cervical X-Ray: increase in the predental space between C1 and odontoid (dens)**; atlantodens interval >3mm in adults and >5mm in children • **Odontoid (Open-Mouth) X-Ray: lateral step-off mass of C1**; lateral mass displacement >7mm indicates transverse ligament rupture • Cervical Spine CT Scan: indicated if positive fracture on x-ray or polytrauma (often associated with other cervical fractures

Treatment	• **Non-Operative Management: indicated for stable fractures** (nondisplaced with intact transverse ligament)
	  • **External Immobilization: rigid cervical orthosis ("C-collar") or halo for 6-12 weeks**
	• **Operative Management: indicated for unstable fractures** (displaced or disruption of transverse ligament)
	  • **Posterior C1-C2 fusion vs occipitocervical fusion**

Key Words & Most Common	• Fracture of anterior and posterior arch of C1 (atlas) • Axial loading mechanism +/- hyperextension of neck (dive into shallow water, football tackle Proximal neck pain + decreased ROM • Lateral cervical x-ray shows increased predental space between C1 and odontoid • Odontoid x-ray shows lateral step-off mass of C1 • External immobilization for stable fractures • Operative management for unstable fractures

Fracture of anterior and posterior arch of C1

Odontoid Fractures

Etiology & Risk Factors	• **Fracture of the odontoid process (dens) of the C2 vertebrae (axis)** • Etiology: **dive into shallow water, football tackle**, motor vehicle collision, **fall from standing position, fall downstairs** • Mechanism of Injury: **hyperextension or hyperflexion of the cervical spine** • Risk Factors: bimodal age distribution (early adults and elderly)
Patho-physiology	• Type I (Stable): oblique avulsion fracture of the tip of odontoid; avulsion of alar ligament (stable) • **Type II (Unstable): most common type**; fracture at base of odontoid (dens) where it attaches to the C2 body; high associate with nonunion due to blood supply interruption • Type III (Unstable): extension of the fracture through upper portion of C2 body (unstable)

Signs & Symptoms	• **Proximal neck pain following traumatic mechanism**
	  • **Worse with motion**
	• May have dysphagia if retropharyngeal hematoma present
	• Physical Exam:
	  • **Decreased neck range of motion**
	   Usually no neurologic symptoms

Diagnosis	• Cervical X-Ray: performed if CT unavailable; lower sensitivity and specificity • **Odontoid (open mouth) view allows greatest visualization** • **Cervical Spine CT Scan: imaging test of choice to identify fracture pattern**

Treatment	• Observation: indicated with os odontoideum (odontoid aplasia or hypoplasia)
	• **External Immobilization:**
	  • **Rigid Cervical Orthosis ("C-collar"): indicated for type I and type III fractures for 6-12 weeks**
	  • **Halo Fixation: indicated for type II in young patients without risk factors for nonunion or if not surgical candidate**
	• **Surgery: anterior odontoid screw fixation indicated for type II fractures**

Key Words & Most Common	• Fracture of the odontoid process (dens) of the C2 vertebrae (axis) • Dive into shallow water, football tackle, fall from standing position or downstairs • Type II is unstable and most common type • Proximal neck pain following traumatic mechanism • Cervical x-ray (odontoid [open mouth] view) • Cervical CT is imaging test of choice • Type I and III: external immobilization (rigid cervical orthosis or halo fixation) • Type II: surgery vs halo fixation

Fracture of odontoid process of C2 vertebrae

Hangman's Fracture

Etiology & Risk Factors	• Traumatic bilateral fracture of the pedicles or pars interarticularis of the C2 vertebrae with an associated traumatic subluxation (spondylolisthesis) of C2 on C3 • Unstable fracture also known as **traumatic spondylolisthesis of the axis** • Etiology: **motor vehicle accidents** (chin hitting steering wheel), **diving injuries, contact sports**; judicial hanging • Mechanism of Injury: **extreme hyperextension and axial loading** or extreme hyperextension and distraction • Risk Factors: bimodal age distribution (early adults and elderly), osteoporosis, metastatic burden, vitamin D deficiency
Patho-physiology	• Hyperextension and axial compression of C2 pedicle between adjoining articular processes of C1 and C3 leads to bilateral fracture of the pedicles or pars interarticularis

Signs & Symptoms	• **Posterior neck pain**
	• **Cervical radiculopathy**
	• Physical Exam:
	   • **Decreased neck range of motion**
	   Usually no neurologic symptoms (diameter of neural canal is greatest at C2)

Diagnosis	• **Cervical X-Ray**: lateral, anteroposterior (AP), and open-mouth odontoid views necessary; demonstrates subluxation of C2 on C3 • **Cervical CT Scan**: imaging test of choice to identify fracture pattern • Cervical MRI: preferred test to evaluate ligamentous construct, disc space, spinal cord, nerve roots, and other soft tissue injuries

Treatment	• **External Immobilization:**
	   • **Rigid Cervical Orthosis**: indicated for fractures with <3mm horizontal displacement
	   • **Closed Reduction and Halo Fixation**: indicated for fractures with 3-5mm of horizontal displacement
	• **Surgery**: internal fixation indicated for fractures with >5mm displacement with severe angulation

Key Words & Most Common	• Traumatic bilateral fracture of the pedicles or pars interarticularis of C2 vertebrae + traumatic subluxation of C2 on C3 • MVA, diving injuries, contact sports • Extreme hyperextension and axial loading is most common mechanism • Posterior neck pain + radiculopathy • Cervical x-ray vs cervical CT scan • Rigid cervical orthosis in fractures <3mm displacement • Halo fixation in fractures 3-5mm of displacement • Surgery in fractures >5mm displacement

C1
C2
C3
C4
Spondylolisthesis of C2 on C3

Cervical Spinous Process Fracture

Etiology & Risk Factors	• Isolated avulsion fracture of the spinous processes of the lower cervical (C7 most common) or upper thoracic (C6-T3) vertebrae • Also known as a **"clay-shoveler's fracture"** • Etiology: **motor vehicle accident** most common • Mechanism of Injury: **quick deceleration resulting in hyperflexion of the neck**; considered a "stable" fracture
Patho-physiology	• Quick deceleration injury (MVA) results in hyperflexion of the neck causing the muscles to pull on the supraspinous ligament leading to an avulsion fracture of the spinous process

Signs & Symptoms	• **Lower neck or upper back pain**
	   • **"Pain between the shoulder blades"**
	• Physical Exam:
	   • **Focal midline tenderness to palpitation**
	   • **Reduced or painful range of motion of the neck**
	   • Usually no neurologic deficits

Diagnosis	• **Cervical X-Ray**: initial imaging test performed; lateral, anteroposterior (AP), and open-mouth odontoid views necessary • **Lateral View**: most sensitive view; avulsion fracture of the spinous process • **Cervical CT Scan**: imaging test of choice to identify fracture pattern

Treatment	• **Conservative**: nonoperative management is first-line
	   • **Pain control (NSAIDs)**
	   • **Rigid Cervical Orthosis ("C-collar")**: high rates of union with immobilization
	• Surgery: surgical excision indicated for nonunion or refractory pain

Key Words & Most Common	• Isolated avulsion fracture of the spinous process of the lower cervical (C7) or upper thoracic (C6-T3) vertebrae • MVA; quick deceleration results in hyperflexion of the neck • Lower neck or upper back pain + focal midline tenderness to palpation • Cervical x-ray → cervical CT scan • Conservative treatment (NSAID + C-collar)

Vertebral Burst Fractures

Etiology & Risk Factors	• Acute vertebral fracture • Etiology: **fall from height**, trauma • Mechanism of Injury: **axial load with flexion compromises the anterior and middle column causing bone expansion in all directions** • Risk Factors: **osteoporosis is greatest risk factor**; trauma, cancer, chemotherapy, infection, long-term steroid use, hyperthyroidism, radiation therapy, smoking, alcohol abuse, **low estrogen levels**, anorexia
Patho-physiology	• Axial loading injury causes compression of the vertebral body resulting in retropulsion of the bone fragments leading to spinal canal damage and neurological deficits secondary to spinal cord compression • Stable: ligaments are intact and no posterior displacement of fracture segment • Unstable: >50% compression of spinal cord, >50% loss of vertebral heigh, >20° of angulation or evidence of neurologic deficits
Signs & Symptoms	• **Focal spine pain** following axial load injury • Complete or incomplete spinal cord injury is common
Diagnosis	• Spinal X-Ray: initial imaging test: demonstrates comminuted vertebral body and loss of vertebral height • Spinal CT Scan: **most sensitive imaging modality**; visualizes the spin in three planes to properly grade the extent of the injury
Treatment	• Conservative: **stabilization prior to orthopedic or neurosurgery consult** • Pain control (NSAIDs), rigid cervical orthosis ("c-collar") • Surgery: **vertebroplasty or kyphoplasty often indicated**
Key Words & Most Common	• Acute vertebral fracture sustained by fall from heigh • Axial load with flexion Osteoporosis is greatest risk factor • Focal pain • Spinal x-ray → CT • Conservative vs surgery

Complex Regional Pain Syndrome

Etiology & Risk Factors	• Neuropathic pain disorder characterized by ongoing pain disproportionate to degree of bone or soft tissue injury (trauma, surgery, fracture)
	  • **Sensory, motor, and autonomic dysfunction**
	• Etiology: **fracture (most common)**, trauma, surgery, sprains, contusions, crush injuries, procedure sites, amputation
	  • **Upper extremity most common**
	• Risk factors: **female, age (60-70yo most common)**, asthma, ACEI use, menopause, osteoporosis, migraine, smoking	

Patho-physiology	• Unclear pathophysiology • Central sympathetic sensitization, peripheral nociceptor sensitization and neuropeptide release leads to ongoing pain and inflammation	
Signs & Symptoms	• Sensory: **regional pain (burning/aching) is hallmark symptom**; hyperalgesia (extreme sensitivity to pain), **allodynia** (pain to stimulus that does not usually provoke pain) • Cutaneous Changes: **edema, dry or hyperhidrotic skin**, red/mottled skin, increased/decreased temperature • Trophic Changes: shiny, atrophic skin; cracking or excessive growth of nails, hair loss • Motor Abnormalities: **decreased range of motion, weakness**, tremors, spasms • Psychologic Stress: depression, anxiety, anger (often secondary to frustration of unclear cause or prolonged course)	

Diagnosis	• **Clinical Diagnosis**
	• X-Ray: may show bone demineralization
	• Bone Scintigraphy: increased uptake/activity
		• Budapest Criteria (1 symptom in three of the four categories)
		  • Sensory: hyperalgesia or allodynia
		  • Vasomotor: temperature or skin color asymmetry to contralateral side
		  • Sudomotor/Edema: sweating changes, sweating asymmetry, edema
		  • Motor/Trophic: trophic changes to hair/skin/nails; ↓ ROM, motor dysfunction (weakness, tremor, dystonia)

Treatment	• Conservative: analgesia (**NSAIDs**), physical/occupational therapy, desensitization therapy, transcutaneous electrical nerve stimulation, acupuncture
	  • Vitamin C prophylaxis has been hypothesized to lower risk of CRPS after fractures
	  • Behavioral therapy for psychologic stress
	• Medications: oral corticosteroids, tricyclic antidepressants, antiseizure medications may be attempted
	  • Gabapentin often has greatest benefit
	  • Ketamine infusion may aid in acute flare	

Key Words & Most Common	• Sensory, motor, and autonomic dysfunction most common after fracture • Hyperalgesia/allodynia, temperature/skin color asymmetry; sweating asymmetry or edema; changes to hair/skin/nails and motor dysfunction • Clinical diagnosis • NSIADs + physical therapy • Gabapentin vs TCAs	

Carpal Tunnel Syndrome

Etiology & Risk Factors	• Entrapment neuropathy caused by compression of the median nerve as it travels through the carpal tunnel in the wrist • <u>Etiology</u>: **repetitive wrist flexion/extension** (drawing, typing, video games), trauma, edema • <u>Risk Factors</u>: **females**, **age (40-60yo most common)**, **diabetes**, **pregnancy**, hypothyroidism, occupations with repetitive wrist flexion/extension, obesity, autoimmune disorders
Patho-physiology	• Increased pressure, local edema, or tendinous inflammation leads to compression of the median nerve as it travels through the carpal tunnel causing entrapment neuropathy

Signs & Symptoms	• **Burning/aching pain and paresthesia in median nerve distribution**
	  • Palmar aspect of thumb, index, middle and radial aspect of ring finger
	• **Waking at night** (patient may shake hand to restore sensation)
	• **Thenar atrophy** and weakness occurs in advanced cases
	• <u>Physical Exam</u>:
	  • **Tinel Sign**: paresthesia is reproduced by tapping the volar aspect of wrist
	  • **Phalen Sign**: paresthesia is reproduced by holding flexion of both wrists for 30-60 seconds
	  • <u>Carpal Compression Test</u>: paresthesia is reproduced by applying direct, firm pressure to carpal tunnel of the wrist in neutral position

Diagnosis	• **Clinical Diagnosis** • <u>Electrophysiologic Testing</u>: **gold standard**; often not required for diagnosis

Treatment	• <u>Conservative</u>: **activity modifications, proper hand ergonomics** (keyboard at proper height), physical therapy, analgesia (NSAIDs)
	  • <u>Immobilization</u>: **volar splint is initial management; especially beneficial at night**
	• <u>Corticosteroid Injection</u>: injection if refractory to conservative treatment
	• <u>Surgery</u>: carpal tunnel release if severe or refractory to all other conservative treatments
	           Bilateral thenar atrophy

Key Words & Most Common	• Median nerve entrapment as it travels through the carpal tunnel • Repetitive wrist use • Female, middle age, pregnancy, occupation • Burning/aching pain + paresthesia • Night symptoms • + Tinel; + Phalen sign • Clinical diagnosis • Wrist splint + activity/ergonomic modifications → steroid injection → surgery

Syncope

Etiology & Risk Factors	• **Sudden, brief loss of consciousness with loss of postural tone followed by spontaneous recovery**
	• <u>Etiology</u>: **cerebral hypoperfusion**
	  • <u>Benign</u>: **vasovagal is most common cause**, volume depletion, orthostatic hypotension, medication-related
	  • <u>Pathologic</u>: cardiac arrhythmias, carotid sinus syncope, valvular abnormalities, psychogenic
	• <u>Risk Factors</u>: vary based on underlying etiology

Patho-physiology	• Vasovagal is most common cause and often precipitated by prolonged standing, crowded places, hot environment, severe pain, extreme fatigue or exposure to stressful situation (sight of blood, injury, needles) leading to vasodilatation and bradycardia resulting in cerebral hypoperfusion

Signs & Symptoms	• <u>Vasovagal</u>: **more common in standing or seated position**
	  • **Prodrome of blurred vision, diaphoresis, nausea, dizziness, weakness**
	  • **Followed by bradycardia, hypotension, and loss of consciousness**
	  • **Spontaneous recovery within seconds to minutes**
	  • **General pallor, diaphoresis, and headache common with regain of consciousness**
	• <u>Neurocardiac</u>: more commonly occurs while in lying position
	• <u>Physical Exam</u>:
	  • Vital signs are essential; bradycardia and hypotension often present; weak pulse
	  • Orthostatic vital signs should be performed

Diagnosis	• **Clinical Diagnosis; vasovagal syncope is diagnosis of exclusion** • <u>Labs</u>: CBC (hemoglobin), BMP (electrolytes), point of care glucose • <u>Cardiovascular Workup</u>: **ECG for all patients**; consider echocardiogram, cardiac enzymes, continuous cardiac monitoring, Holter monitor • <u>Cerebrovascular Workup</u>: consider CT head, carotid doppler ultrasound, MRI brain or MRA, EEG
Treatment	• <u>Conservative</u>: **indicated for benign etiology** • **Adequate hydration and electrolyte intake, avoid stimuli that precipitated event,** discontinue offending medication, gradual change in posture • Referral to specialist for non-benign related etiology
Key Words & Most Common	• Transient loss of consciousness associated with loss of postural tone followed by spontaneous recovery • Vasovagal most common cause • Prodrome of blurred vision, diaphoresis, nausea, dizziness → bradycardia, hypotension, loss of consciousness → spontaneous recovery within seconds to mintures • Clinical diagnosis of exclusion; ECG should be performed for all patients • Conservative vs referral based on etiology

Spinal Cord Injury

Etiology & Risk Factors	• Disruption of nerve function leading to loss of motor and sensory function **below the level of injury** that can cause significant morbidity and permanent disability • Etiology: major trauma is most common (**penetrating trauma, burst fracture, MVA, violence/assault, hyperextension/hyperflexion**), spinal stenosis, tumor, aortic dissection • Risk Factors: **male**, bimodal distribution (young adults or elderly), history of osteoporosis
Patho-physiology	• Direct trauma causes damage the vertebrae, ligaments and/or disks of the spinal column causing damage of spinal cord tissue and nerve function; motor and sensory function is lost below the injury. Ischemia, hematoma, spinal cord edema may develop due to secondary vascular injury causing further damage • Neuronal damage mediated by excessive neurotransmitter release from damaged cells, cytokine inflammatory immune response, apoptosis and free radical accumulation

	Complete Transection Syndrome	Anterior Cord Syndrome	Central Cord Syndrome	Brown-Séquard syndrome

Signs & Symptoms	• **Immediate, complete, flaccid paralysis**
	• **Autonomic dysfunction** below level of injury
	• **Loss of anal sphincter tone, priapism**
	• **Loss of all sensation and reflex activity** below level of injury
		• Motor Deficits: **paraplegia below the level of the lesion (corticospinal)**
		• Sensory Deficits: **loss of pain and temperature sensation worse in lower than upper extremity (lateral spinothalamic)**
		  • May develop autonomic dysfunction, orthostasis, bowel/bladder/sexual dysfunction
		• Preserved: **vibration and pressure sensation, proprioception, light touch (2-point) discrimination preserved** (dorsal column spared)
			• Motor Deficits: **quadriparesis (worse in upper than lower extremities)**
			• Sensory Deficits: **loss of pain and temperature sensation worse in upper than lower extremities**
			  • +/- bladder dysfunction or urinary retention
			• Preserved: **"sacral sparing" intact toe flexion, normal rectal tone, intact perianal sensation; proprioception and vibratory sensation preserved** (dorsal column spared)
				• **Unilateral hemisection of the spinal cord**
				• Ipsilateral Deficits: **spastic paralysis and loss of position sense below the lesion**
				• Contralateral Deficits: **loss of pain and temperature sensation below the injury**

Diagnosis	• Non-Contrast Spinal CT Scan: initial imaging test indicated in all cases of suspected spinal cord injury to determine fracture; poor sensitivity for soft tissue injury • MRI: indicated to assess the level of injury and extent of soft tissue injury
Treatment	• **Neurogenic shock management + intubation** • **Pain control/sedation** • Surgery: indicated for **unstable spine fractures or progressive neurological deficits** • *Steroids are no longer recommended*

References

1. Brain trauma CT.jpg. (2023, February 6). *Wikimedia Commons*. Retrieved 22:26, August 15, 2023 from https://commons.wikimedia.org/w/index.php?title=File:Brain_trauma_CT.jpg&oldid=730409110.
2. Trigeminal Nerve.png. (2020, October 13). *Wikimedia Commons*. Retrieved 22:35, August 15, 2023 from https://commons.wikimedia.org/w/index.php?title=File:Trigeminal_Nerve.png&oldid=488547416.
3. Bells palsy diagram.svg. (2023, July 10). *Wikimedia Commons*. Retrieved 22:40, August 15, 2023 from https://commons.wikimedia.org/w/index.php?title=File:Bells_palsy_diagram.svg&oldid=781993115.
4. MSMRIMark.png. (2020, November 15). *Wikimedia Commons*. Retrieved 22:45, August 15, 2023 from https://commons.wikimedia.org/w/index.php?title=File:MSMRIMark.png&oldid=512767565.
5. Astrozytom.jpg. (2022, June 3). *Wikimedia Commons*. Retrieved 22:47, August 15, 2023 from https://commons.wikimedia.org/w/index.php?title=File:Astrozytom.jpg&oldid=661129356.
6. Glioblastoma - MR sagittal with contrast.jpg. (2021, April 16). *Wikimedia Commons*. Retrieved 22:49, August 15, 2023 from https://commons.wikimedia.org/w/index.php?title=File:Glioblastoma_-_MR_sagittal_with_contrast.jpg&oldid=553314166.
7. MRIMeningioma.png. (2020, October 6). *Wikimedia Commons*. Retrieved 22:50, August 15, 2023 from https://commons.wikimedia.org/w/index.php?title=File:MRIMeningioma.png&oldid=482386573.
8. OligodendrogliomaMRI.png. (2020, October 19). *Wikimedia Commons*. Retrieved 22:52, August 15, 2023 from https://commons.wikimedia.org/w/index.php?title=File:OligodendrogliomaMRI.png&oldid=494802217.
9. Ependymom sag FLAIR.jpg. (2022, March 31). *Wikimedia Commons*. Retrieved 22:53, August 15, 2023 from https://commons.wikimedia.org/w/index.php?title=File:Ependymom_sag_FLAIR.jpg&oldid=645451026.
10. Pick's disease.png. (2020, October 14). *Wikimedia Commons*. Retrieved 22:58, August 15, 2023 from https://commons.wikimedia.org/w/index.php?title=File:Pick%27s_disease.png&oldid=489163660.
11. CT of lacunar strokes.jpg. (2022, November 25). *Wikimedia Commons*. Retrieved 23:00, August 15, 2023 from https://commons.wikimedia.org/w/index.php?title=File:CT_of_lacunar_strokes.jpg&oldid=709323447.
12. MCA Territory Infarct.svg. (2022, January 23). *Wikimedia Commons*. Retrieved 23:03, August 15, 2023 from https://commons.wikimedia.org/w/index.php?title=File:MCA_Territory_Infarct.svg&oldid=623823753.
13. "File:Cardiovascular system - Circle of Willis -- Smart-Servier.png." *Wikimedia Commons*. 22 Jan 2023, 12:25 UTC. 5 Apr 2023, 14:54
14. EpiduralHematoma.jpg. (2020, October 30). *Wikimedia Commons*. Retrieved 23:05, August 15, 2023 from https://commons.wikimedia.org/w/index.php?title=File:EpiduralHematoma.jpg&oldid=507021295.
15. Subduralandherniation.PNG. (2021, June 21). *Wikimedia Commons*. Retrieved 23:08, August 15, 2023 from https://commons.wikimedia.org/w/index.php?title=File:Subduralandherniation.PNG&oldid=570299938.
16. Takayasu.PNG. (2020, September 19). *Wikimedia Commons*. Retrieved 23:11, August 15, 2023 from https://commons.wikimedia.org/w/index.php?title=File:Takayasu.PNG&oldid=464566982.
17. SubarachnoidP.png. (2023, July 18). *Wikimedia Commons*. Retrieved 23:13, August 15, 2023 from https://commons.wikimedia.org/w/index.php?title=File:SubarachnoidP.png&oldid=784568480.
18. Intracerebral hemorrhage 2.jpg. (2020, September 20). *Wikimedia Commons*. Retrieved 23:17, August 15, 2023 from https://commons.wikimedia.org/w/index.php?title=File:Intracerebral_hemorrhage_2.jpg&oldid=465887735.
19. BasSkullFracMark.png. (2022, June 2). *Wikimedia Commons*. Retrieved 23:20, August 15, 2023 from https://commons.wikimedia.org/w/index.php?title=File:BasSkullFracMark.png&oldid=660917485.
20. Jeffersonfraktur - 84jm- CT axial - 001.jpg. (2022, March 30). *Wikimedia Commons*. Retrieved 23:22, August 15, 2023 from https://commons.wikimedia.org/w/index.php?title=File:Jeffersonfraktur_-_84jm-CT_axial_-_001.jpg&oldid=645420038.
21. OdontoidType3Mark.png. (2020, October 14). *Wikimedia Commons*. Retrieved 23:24, August 15, 2023 from https://commons.wikimedia.org/w/index.php?title=File:OdontoidType3Mark.png&oldid=489754142.
22. Hangman's fracture.JPG. (2020, September 4). *Wikimedia Commons*. Retrieved 23:27, August 15, 2023 from https://commons.wikimedia.org/w/index.php?title=File:Hangman%27s_fracture.JPG&oldid=447861762.
23. BurstCoL4LCT.png. (2020, July 12). *Wikimedia Commons*. Retrieved 23:30, August 15, 2023 from https://commons.wikimedia.org/w/index.php?title=File:BurstCoL4LCT.png&oldid=432679130.
24. Untreated Carpal Tunnel Syndrome.JPG. (2020, September 25). *Wikimedia Commons*. Retrieved 23:32, August 15, 2023 from https://commons.wikimedia.org/w/index.php?title=File:Untreated_Carpal_Tunnel_Syndrome.JPG&oldid=470760641.

Chapter 11
Psychiatry & Behavioral Science

Child Abuse

Etiology & Risk Factors	• Defined as actions (abuse) or inactions (neglect) by an individual's caregiver or parent which inflicts physical, sexual, or emotional harm on the individual
	• Etiology: **parent or caregiver responsible for the care are the most common perpetrator**
	  • Abuse: **poor impulse control of caregiver,** inadequate self-esteem or emotional maturity of caregiver, caregiver history of abuse as a child
	  • Neglect: **poor stress-coping skills,** unsupportive family systems, stressful life circumstances, financial and environmental stressors
	• Risk Factors: **poor socioeconomic status,** domestic violence (direct or indirect), **drug and alcohol abuse, unwanted or unplanned pregnancy,** gender-based discrimination, **child with special needs, disability or difficult behaviors,** untreated mental health disorder o caregiver

Additional Information	• **Physical:** evidence of hitting, slapping, kicking, punching, hair pulling, pushing, twisting of any extremity • **Sexual:** any type of sexual activity or contact that a person does not consent to including unwanted touching, grabbing, kissing, or rape • **Psychological:** abusive language, social isolation, financial control • **Neglect:** failure to provide food, clothing, shelter or supervision; failure to provide affection, love or emotional support; failure to enroll in school; inadequate medical care

Signs & Symptoms	• History provided is often inconsistent with the evidence of injury, changes to caregiver report, delays in care, injuries in various stages of healing
	• **Skin Lesions: most common finding;** may be subtle or severe
	  • Bruising: **injuries to face, cheeks, buttocks, ears, torso, neck in an immobile child** (<6 months of age)
	  • Burns: intentional immersion injuries of extremities, buttocks or perineum; cigarette burns
	• **Retinal Hemorrhages:** present in abusive head trauma ("shaken baby syndrome")
	• Fractures: **metaphyseal fractures** (caused by shaking child), rib fractures, spinous process fractures
	• Sexual Abuse: may show physical or behavioral signs
	  • Physical: incontinence, difficulty walking or sitting, bruising or lacerations of mouth, anus or genitals, vaginal discharge or bleeding, pregnancy in minor
	  • Behavioral: **child may exhibit sexual knowledge, initiation of sexual acts with peers, behavioral or personality changes, sexting or posting nude photos**
	• Emotional Abuse: **anxiety/depression, low self-esteem,** superficial in interpersonal relationships, passive, people-pleasing behavior, lack of privacy, **fearful and sensitive affect**
	• Neglect: **poor hygiene, malnutrition,** fatigue, **lack of appropriate clothing,** failure to thrive, stunted growth, failure to meet developmental milestones

Diagnosis	• **Clinical Diagnosis** • Workup: consider x-ray imaging, neuroimaging, ophthalmic examination, forensic evidence collection in setting of sexual assault as indicated
Treatment	• **Treatment of Injuries: repeat of lacerations, burn wound treatment, fracture care, STI treatment, emergency contraception if indicated** • **Reporting to Appropriate Agency:** healthcare professionals are mandatory reporters; child protective agencies and social workers will evaluate and help determine plan • **Ensure Safety of Child:** create safety plan; options include protective hospitalization, placement with relative or temporary housing, temporary foster care • **Counseling and Support Services:** offer counseling or psychotherapy to victim and family members to prevent long-lasting effects on development and sexual adaptation • Follow-Up: follow-up plan should be implemented with aid of social services to evaluate child's well being (weight checks if malnourished, random physical evaluation, etc.)
Key Words & Most Common	• Parent or caregiver responsible for care is most common perpetrator • Abuse includes physical, sexual, psychological and neglect • Treatment of injuries + report to appropriate agency + ensure safety of child

Domestic Violence

Etiology & Risk Factors	• **Physical, sexual, and/or psychologic abuse between people who live together (sex partners, parents or guardians and children, children, grandparents, siblings)** • Etiology: typically stems from **behavioral dysfunction of the abuser** • **Anger management issues, jealousy,** low self-esteem, feeling inferior, cultural beliefs, **personality or psychological disorder, alcohol/drug use,** learned behavior • Risk Factors: **low education level, low socioeconomic status,** childhood abuse, growing up in a family where domestic violence was accepted, alcohol/drug use, **pregnancy**
Additional Information	• 1 in 4 women and 1 in 7 men will experience physical violence; 1 in 3 women and 1 in 6 men will experience sexual violence • A woman who leaves an abusive partner has a 70% greater risk of being murdered by the abuser compared to staying • The average reported prevalence of abuse during pregnancy is approximately 30% emotional abuse, 15% physical abuse, and 8% sexual abuse • 80-90% of domestic violence victims abuse or neglect their children

Signs & Symptoms	• Abuse can be sexual, physical or psychological
	• **Physical:** hitting, slapping, kicking, punching, pulling hair, pushing, twisting of any extremity
	  • **Contusions (often in central pattern [head, face, neck, thorax, abdomen]),** musculoskeletal injuries, "accidental" injuries, burns, injuries inconsistent with history
	• **Sexual:** any type of sexual activity or contact that a person does not consent to including unwanted touching, grabbing, kissing, or rape
	  • **Contusions or lacerations around breasts, genitals or mouth,** injuries consistent with rape, genital lacerations, **pain or pruritus of anogenital area,** pregnancy, difficulty walking or sitting, vaginal discharge, bleeding or evidence of STI
	• **Psychological:** abusive language, social isolation, financial control
	  • **Anxiety and depression, low self-esteem,** insecurity, superficial in interpersonal relationships, passive or people-pleasing behavior, **fearful and sensitive affect**

Diagnosis	• **Clinical Diagnosis** • Workup: consider x-ray imaging, neuroimaging, forensic evidence collection in setting of sexual assault, toxicology screen, urinalysis, pregnancy test, STI testing
Treatment	• **Treatment of Injuries: treat injuries, provide reassurance, evaluate emotional/mental status** • **Ensure Safety of Victim: determine if legal intervention is needed** • **Counseling and Support Services:** offer shelter options, legal services, and counseling for victim however *it is the patient's right to accept or refuse help*
Key Words & Most Common	• Physical, sexual, and/or psychologic abuse between people who live together • Low education level, low socioeconomic status, pregnancy are greatest risk factors • Abuse can be physical, sexual, or psychological • Clinical diagnosis • Treat injuries → ensure safety → provide counseling and support services

Elder Abuse

Etiology & Risk Factors	• Includes any physical, psychological, sexual abuse, financial exploitation and/or neglect of an elder
	• <u>Etiology</u>: **caregiver responsible is the most common perpetrator**; may also be family member
	• <u>Risk Factors</u>:
	   • <u>Caregiver</u>: **caregiver burnout is greatest risk factor**, substance abuse, financial dependence on the victim, undiagnosed/untreated mental illness, personality disorders
	   • <u>Victim</u>: **chronic health challenges** (incontinence, dementia, functional/cognitive impairment), **progressive mental and behavioral changes**, shared living arrangements

Additional Information	• <u>Physical Abuse</u>: intentional physical force to inflict pain or cause impairment of the victim
	   • **Hitting, inappropriate use of restraints**, hair pulling, forcibly feeding a person, pinching, pushing, pulling
	• <u>Psychological Abuse</u>: **threats of harm or institutionalization**, harassment, intimidation, **yelling**, isolation, infantilization (**treating the elder like a child**)
	   • May cause anxiety, depression, social withdrawal, despair, hopelessness of the victim
	• <u>Sexual Abuse</u>: any nonconsensual sexual act in which the victim is forced into or are incapable of understanding/consenting to the sexual act
	   • Rape, **unwanted touching, forced nudity**, explicit photography, **inappropriately exposing of oneself to the victim**
	• <u>Financial Exploitation</u>: withholding or misuse of the resources (money, property, other assets) to the detriment of the victim or benefit of the perpetrator
	   • **Stealing assets, forging the victim's signature on documents or checks**, inappropriate changing of a will, overpaying for products or services
	• <u>Neglect</u>: intentional or unintentional failure to provide necessary care to the elder
	   • **Withholding food or water, inappropriate clothing for weather**, failure to give or refill medications, failure to provide assistive devices (hearing aids, glasses, walkers)

Signs & Symptoms	• **Unexplained or frequent injuries, delay of care following the onset of illness or injury**, noncompliance with the medical regimen, missing follow-up appointments
	• <u>Physical Exam</u>:
	   • <u>Abuse</u>: **Patterned or linear bruising, bruising in various stages of healing**, subconjunctival hemorrhages, oral injuries, bruising in suspicious regions (wrists, the ulnar aspect of the forearms, face, neck, ears, back, abdomen), anogenital trauma
	   • <u>Neglect</u>: **malnutrition or dehydration, wearing dirty or inappropriate clothing, lack of personal hygiene** (long hair, toenails or fingernails), **presence of pressure ulcers**

Diagnosis	• **Clinical Diagnosis** • <u>Workup</u>: consider x-ray imaging, neuroimaging, forensic evidence collection in setting of sexual assault, STI testing
Treatment	• <u>**Treatment of Injuries**</u>: **treat injuries, evaluate emotional/mental status** • <u>**Reporting to Appropriate Agency**</u>: report to Adult Protective Services to investigate the abuse • <u>**Ensure Safety of Victim**</u>: may require contacting law enforcement or hospital security, social work, hospital legal team, and possibly applying for emergency guardianship • <u>**Counseling and Support Services**</u>: **offer shelter options, legal services, and counseling for victim** • Coordination of home health services, meal delivery, transportation, or referral to senior care centers
Key Words & Most Common	• Caregiver burnout + chronic health challenges and progressive mental/behavioral changes of the victim is greatest risk factor • Physical, psychological, sexual abuse, financial exploitation, and/or neglect • Unexplained bruising in various stages of healing, malnutrition, dehydration, dirty clothing, lack of personal hygiene, present of pressure ulcers • Treat injuries → report to Adult Protective Services → ensure safety → provide support services

Sexual Assault

Etiology & Risk Factors	• **Any type of sexual activity or contact that a person does not consent to; includes rape and sexual coercion** • May involve force or threats of force; may involve drugs or alcohol • **Rape is defined as any vaginal, anal, or oral penetration by another person's sexual organ without consent of the victim** • *Rape is most commonly an expression of anger or need for psychological power and more violent than it is sexual* • People under the age of consent are unable to give consent to any sexual activity with an adult • **Female are at greater risk for rape and sexual assault** than males; males are less willing to report the crime

Signs & Symptoms	• **Rape may result in the following:**
	   • Genital injury (lacerations)
	   • Psychological trauma (fear, nightmares, insomnia, anger/embarrassment/guilt, post-traumatic stress disorder, amnesia, anxiety, lack of trust in relationships)
	   • Pregnancy
	   • Sexually transmitted infections (syphilis, gonorrhea, chlamydial infection, trichomoniasis, HPV, hepatitis, HIV)
	   • Additional injuries may occur as a result of the physical violence occurring simultaneously as the assault

Diagnosis	• <u>**Collection of Forensic Evidence**</u>: if patient chooses to seek counseling prior to medical evaluation, it is recommended to avoid changing clothing, washing or showering, douching, brushing teeth, clipping fingernails or using mouthwash to avoid destroying evidence
	• <u>**Physical Exam**</u>: privacy must be ensured; each step should be thoroughly explained prior and patient may refuse any part of examination
	   • Description of injuries sustained (including areas of bleeding), description of the attack and the assailant as well as the assailant's behavior
	• <u>**Lab Testing**</u>: patient has right to refuse testing
	   • Pregnancy test and serologic tests for syphilis, hepatitis B, and HIV; trichomoniasis and bacterial vaginosis testing of vaginal secretions or urine; gonorrheal and chlamydial testing using samples from every penetrated orifice (vaginal, oral, or rectal)
	   • Follow-up tests for pregnancy, untreated STIs, syphilis, hepatitis, and HIV required
	   • Testing for drugs and alcohol is controversial
	• <u>**Evidence Collection**</u>: can be used to identify assailant
	   • Clothing, smears of buccal, vaginal, rectal mucosa, samples from scalp and pubic hair, fingernail clippings/scrapings, blood and saliva samples, semen samples

Treatment	• <u>**Psychological Support**</u>: specialist trained in rape crisis intervention should be consulted
	   • Reassurance, nonjudgmental attitude, general support may be provided until specialist can arrive
	• <u>**Prevention/Treatment of Infections**</u>:
	   • <u>Gonorrhea/Chlamydia</u>: IM ceftriaxone (500mg) + oral doxycycline (100mg BID for 14 days)
	   • <u>Bacterial Vaginosis and Trichomoniasis</u>: metronidazole (500mg BID for 7 days)
	   • <u>Hepatitis B and HPV</u>: vaccination if no documented immunity or is unvaccinated
	   • <u>HIV</u>: post-exposure prophylaxis
	   • <u>Emergency Contraception</u>: levonorgestrel, copper-bearing or levonorgestrel-releasing IUD, ulipristal acetate

Panic Disorder

Etiology & Risk Factors	• Recurrent unexpected panic attacks • <u>Etiology</u>: **chemical imbalance** (abnormalities in gamma-aminobutyric acid [GABA], cortisol, serotonin), genetic and environmental factors • <u>Risk Factors</u>: **family history, female, age (20-30 years old), major depression**, OCD, social phobias, asthma, COPD, IBS, hypertension, mitral valve prolapse
Additional Information	• Alterations in several neurotransmitters, including serotonin (regulation of mood, anxiety, and sleep), norepinephrine (stress response), and gamma-aminobutyric acid (GABA) (inhibitory neurotransmitter that regulates anxiety and stress responses) • Abnormalities in several brain regions, including the amygdala (involved in fear and anxiety generation), hippocampus (involved in memory and contextual processing), and prefrontal cortex (involved in cognitive control, decision making and fear response)
Signs & Symptoms	• <u>Panic Attack</u>: **sense of intense fear or discomfort (impending doom) followed by 4 or more of the following symptoms of sympathetic system overdrive** • <u>Cognitive</u>: **fear of dying, fear of going crazy or losing control**, feelings of unreality (derealization), or **detachment from the self** (depersonalization) • <u>Somatic</u>: **chest pain/discomfort, dizziness, choking feeling,** chills or hot flashes, nausea/abdominal distress, paresthesias, **palpitations or tachycardia, shortness of breath, sweating, trembling or shaking** • Panic attacks may occur in situations tied to a specific phobia or trigger • Frequently seek medical care due to worry about heart, lung, or brain disorders • Many patients also have symptoms of major depression
Diagnostic Criteria	• **Recurrent panic attacks associated with 1 or more of the following for ≥1 month** • **Panic attack followed by persistent concern about future attacks** (anticipatory anxiety) • **Persistent worrying about the implications of the attacks** (losing control, going crazy) • **Maladaptive behavioral response to the panic attacks** (avoiding activities, exercise or social situations to try to prevent further attacks) • Symptoms are not related to substance abuse, medical condition (thyroid or cardiac disorder, hypoglycemia), or other psychiatric disorder
Treatment	• <u>Supportive</u>: reassurance and patient education • <u>Cognitive Behavioral Therapy (CBT)</u>: treatment to focus on thinking and behavioral techniques (relaxation, desensitization, examining behavior consequences) • <u>Benzodiazepines</u>: **alprazolam, lorazepam, diazepam are first-line medical management indicated for panic attacks**; long term use may lead to physical dependence or abuse • <u>Antidepressants</u>: indicated for long-term medical management of panic disorder • <u>Selective Serotonin Reuptake Inhibitors (SSRIs)</u>: **sertraline, citalopram, fluoxetine are first-line for long-term medical management** • <u>Selective Norepinephrine Reuptake Inhibitors (SNRIs)</u>: venlafaxine • <u>Tricyclic Antidepressants (TCAs)</u>: adjunct if SSRIs/SNRIs are ineffective
Key Words & Most Common	• <u>Panic Attack</u>: fear of dying, fear of going crazy or losing control, feelings of unreality (derealization), or detachment from the self (depersonalization), chest pain/discomfort, dizziness, choking feeling, chills or hot flashes, nausea/abdominal distress, paresthesias, palpitations or tachycardia, shortness of breath, sweating, trembling or shaking • <u>Panic Disorder</u>: recurrent panic attacks + anticipatory anxiety OR persistent worrying about implication of the attacks OR maladaptive behavioral response to the attacks • Supportive + CBT is first line for mild-cases • Antidepressants (SSRIs) for long-term management; benzodiazepines (alprazolam) for panic attacks

Agoraphobia

Etiology & Risk Factors	• **Anxiety that occurs when one is in a public or crowded place in which a potential escape or obtaining help is difficult** • <u>Etiology</u>: **temperamental, environmental and genetic factors** • <u>Risk Factors</u>: **parental overprotectiveness, presence of childhood fears** or night terrors, grief or bereavement experienced early in life, unhappy or traumatic childhoods
Additional Information	• <u>Temperamental</u>: neuroticism, anxiety disorders, OCD, dependent personality • <u>Environmental</u>: negative or traumatic events in childhood, reduced warmth or overprotectiveness in childhood, traumatic childhood, early grief or bereavement • <u>Genetic and Physiological Predisposition</u>: family history of agoraphobia, concomitant panic disorder
Signs & Symptoms	• **Fear and anxiety out of proportion to potential danger of situation** • Severe cases can lead to the people becoming homebound
Diagnostic Criteria	• **Marked, persistent (≥6 months) fear or anxiety involving 2 or more of the following situations** • **Using public transportation (automobiles, buses, trains, airplanes)** • **Being in open spaces (marketplaces, parking lots, bridges)** • **Being in enclosed spaces (theaters or malls)** • **Standing in lines or crowds** • **Being outside of the home alone** • Patients actively avoid the situation, and the associated fear, anxiety, or avoidance of the situation leads to significant distress or impairment of social or occupational function
Treatment	• <u>Cognitive Behavioral Therapy (CBT)</u>: **most effective treatment;** patients are taught to recognize and control their thinking and beliefs of the situation • <u>Exposure Therapy</u>: patients are encouraged to seek out, confront, and remain in contact with an uncomfortable situation until their fear/anxiety is relieved • <u>Antidepressants</u>: SSRIs are generally first-line for medical management; SNRIs and TCAs are alternative therapies
Key Words & Most Common	• Anxiety surrounding a public or crowded situation in which a potential escape or obtaining help may be difficult • Fear and anxiety out of proportion to danger of situation such as using public transport, being in open or enclosed spaces, standing in lines or crowds, being outside of home • CBT + exposure therapy +/- antidepressant medications

Generalized Anxiety Disorder

Etiology & Risk Factors	• Mental health disorder characterized by excessive, persistent, and unrealistic fear, worry, or feeling of being overwhelmed • <u>Etiology</u>: **combination of environmental, genetic, neurobiological and childhood factors** • <u>Risk Factors</u>: **female, stress** (occupational, financial, relationship), **family history**, comorbid conditions (major depression), physical conditions (diabetes), **history of childhood abuse or neglect, substance abuse disorder**, unmarried, poor general health, **low education level, sedentary lifestyle**
Patho-physiology	• Alterations in neurotransmitter signaling, brain circuitry, and stress response systems within the amygdala and prefrontal cortex regions of the brain responsible for emotional regulation and cognitive processing • Abnormalities of low serotonin and elevated noradrenergic system activity and alteration of the GABA system leads to signs and symptoms of general anxiety

Signs & Symptoms	• **Multiple fears, worries, or feelings of being overwhelmed not focal to a specific situation**
	   • Precipitation factors include work and family responsibilities, finances, health, safety, chores
	• <u>Somatic Symptoms</u>: **vague or nonspecific complaints are most common**
	   • **Shortness of breath, palpitations, chest pain, nausea, fatigue, headache, dizziness, restlessness, sweating, trembling**
	• <u>Psychiatric Symptoms</u>: **excessive and nonspecific anxiety and/or worry**, emotional lability, difficulty concentrating, **insomnia**

Diagnostic Criteria	• **Excessive fear, anxiety, or worry, occurring the majority of days for more than 6 months and are associated with 3 or more of the following:** • **Restlessness or on-edge feeling, easily fatigued, difficulty concentrating, muscle tension, disturbed sleep** • Symptoms are not related to substance abuse, medical condition (thyroid or cardiac disorder, hypoglycemia), or other psychiatric disorder

Treatment	• <u>Lifestyle Modifications</u>: regular exercise, stress-reduction techniques (meditation or deep breathing exercises) limiting caffeine and alcohol intake, maintaining a healthy diet, sleep hygiene, and engaging in social support and hobbies/activities
	• <u>Cognitive Behavioral Therapy (CBT)</u>: psychoeducation, altering maladaptive thought patterns, exposure therapy to anxiety-provoking situations
	• <u>Medical Management</u>: indicated for patients that fail lifestyle modifications and CBT
	   • <u>Antidepressants</u>: **generally, first-line for medical management; SSRIs** (sertraline, escitalopram, fluoxetine) or SNRIs (venlafaxine)
	   • <u>Benzodiazepines</u>: **anxiolytics (alprazolam, lorazepam) indicated for short-term use while long-term therapy takes effect;** may lead to physical dependence or abuse
	   • <u>Buspirone</u>: adjunct medication to SSRIs; does not cause sedation but has a therapeutic lag in the efficacy of 2-3 weeks

Key Words & Most Common	• Mental health disorder characterized by excessive, persistent, unrealistic fear or worry • Somatic: shortness of breath, palpitations, nausea, fatigue, headache, dizziness, restless • Psychiatric: anxiety, worry, emotional lability, difficulty concentrating, insomnia • Excessive fear, anxiety, or worry, for > 6 months associated with 3+ of the following: • Restlessness or on-edge feeling, easily fatigued, difficulty concentrating, muscle tension, disturbed sleep • Not focal to specific situation • Lifestyle modifications + CBT are first-line • SSRIs/SNRIs +/- benzodiazepines

Social Anxiety Disorder

Etiology & Risk Factors	• **Marked fear or anxiety of one or more social situations in which the individual is exposed to scrutiny of others** • <u>Etiology</u>: genetic and **environmental factors** • <u>Risk Factors</u>: **female, overly controlling or intrusive parent**, negative or traumatic life-events, **childhood trauma or neglect**, chronic stress, **low self-esteem**
Patho-physiology	• Limbic system dysregulation (particularly the amygdala) results in impaired processing of emotional and social information leading to a heightened fear response • Neurotransmitter system abnormalities involving serotonin, dopamine, and glutamate have been implicated
Signs & Symptoms	• **Excessive fear of embarrassment, humiliation, or rejection by others** • Sweating, flushing, nausea/vomiting, trembling (quavering voice), tachycardia or difficult thought processing or inability to find words • **Situational anxiety surrounding specific situations** • Public speaking, acting in a theatrical performance, playing a musical instrument, meeting new people. eating with others, having a conversation with someone new, signing a document before witnesses, using a public restroom

Diagnostic Criteria	• **Marked, persistent (≥6 months) fear or anxiety about a social or performance situation in which the individual may be scrutinized by others**
	   • **Fear of humiliation, embarrassment, rejection or offending others**
	• All of following present:
	   • Exposure to social situations almost always triggers fear, anxiety, or expected panic attacks
	   • Active avoidance of the situation
	   • Fear or anxiety is out of proportion to the actual threat or danger
	   • Fear, anxiety, and/or avoidance cause significant distress or significantly impair social or occupational functioning

Treatment	• <u>Cognitive Behavioral Therapy (CBT)</u>: psychoeducation, teaching patients to recognize and control distorted thinking, exposure therapy to anxiety-provoking situations
	• <u>Medical Management</u>: indicated for patients that fail lifestyle modifications and CBT
	   • <u>Antidepressants</u>: **generally, first-line for medical management; SSRIs** (sertraline, escitalopram, fluoxetine) or SNRIs (venlafaxine)
	   • <u>Benzodiazepines</u>: anxiolytics (alprazolam, lorazepam) may be used situationally or in the short-term; may lead to physical dependence or abuse
	   • <u>Beta Blockers</u>: **propranolol, atenolol; reduce symptoms (tachycardia, trembling, and sweating) related to performance anxiety and public speaking**

Key Words & Most Common	• Marked fear or anxiety in social situations that may involve scrutiny by others • Excessive fear of embarrassment, humiliation, reception or offending others • Public speaking, performance, playing an instrument, meeting new people, eating in public, using a public restroom • CBT +/- antidepressants (SSRIs) • Propranolol may be used to reduce symptoms related to performance anxiety

Major Depressive Disorder

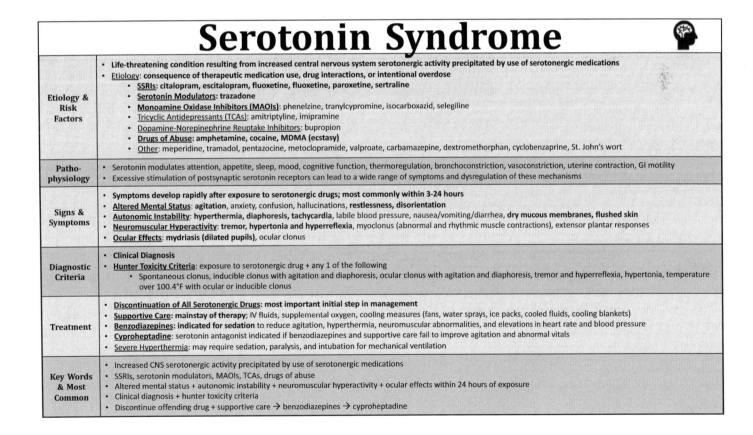

Etiology & Risk Factors	• Persistently depressed mood or anhedonia causing social or occupational impairment • <u>Etiology</u>: multiple biological, genetic, environmental, and psychosocial factors • <u>Risk Factors</u>: **family history, female, traumatic or stressful life events** (loss of a loved one, a relationship breakup or divorce, financial difficulties), **medical conditions** (chronic pain, thyroid disorders, heart disease), **substance abuse** (drugs, alcohol), **personality traits** (pessimism, low self-esteem, and a tendency to worry)
Patho-physiology	• Imbalance and abnormal regulation of cholinergic, catecholaminergic (noradrenergic or dopaminergic), glutamatergic, and serotonergic neurotransmission • Neuroendocrine dysregulation of the hypothalamic-pituitary-adrenal, hypothalamic-pituitary-thyroid, and/or hypothalamic-pituitary-growth hormone axis • Abnormalities in brain structure and function, including decreased activity in the prefrontal cortex and hyperactivity in the amygdala
Signs & Symptoms	• **Tearful eyes, furrowed brows, frowning, poor posture, poor eye contact, lack of facial expression, minimal body movement, speech changes** (soft voice, short responses) • **Neglect of personal hygiene** (unkept hair or facial hair, long fingernails and toenails, body odor, poor dentition)
Diagnosis	• 5 or more of the following symptoms present almost every day for at least 2 weeks; one symptom must be depressed mood or loss of interest or pleasure (anhedonia) • **Depressive mood, anhedonia, fatigue, insomnia or hypersomnia, significant weight loss or weight gain or increased appetite, psychomotor agitation or retardation (restlessness or slowness), feelings of worthlessness or inappropriate guilt, decreased concentration or indecisiveness, recurrent thoughts of death or suicide** • Symptoms must cause significant distress or significantly impair social or occupational functioning • Symptoms are not related to substance abuse, medical condition (thyroid or cardiac disorder, hypoglycemia), or other psychiatric disorder

Treatment	• <u>Lifestyle Modifications</u>: regular exercise, stress-reduction techniques (meditation or deep breathing exercises) limiting caffeine and alcohol intake, maintaining a healthy diet, sleep hygiene, and engaging in social support and hobbies/activities
	• <u>Psychological Support</u>: weekly or biweekly follow-up, reassurance, encouragement, referral to support groups
	• **Psychotherapy**: cognitive behavioral therapy (CBT), interpersonal therapy, supportive therapy, psychoeducation
	• <u>Antidepressants</u>: indicated for patients that fail lifestyle modifications and CBT
	  • <u>SSRIs</u>: sertraline, escitalopram, citalopram, fluoxetine are first-line treatment options and most commonly prescribed medication
	  • <u>SNRIs</u>: venlafaxine, duloxetine; may be used in patients with depression and chronic pain disorder
	  • <u>Serotonin Modulators</u>: trazodone
	  • <u>Atypical Antidepressants</u>: bupropion and mirtazapine; may be used in patients that experience sexual-related side effects of SSRIs/SNRIs
	  • <u>Tricyclic Antidepressants (TCAs)</u>: amitriptyline, imipramine; not commonly prescribed due to side effects
	  • <u>Monoamine oxidase inhibitors (MAOIs)</u>: tranylcypromine, phenelzine; not commonly prescribed due to side effects
	• <u>**Electroconvulsive Therapy (ECT)**</u>: indicated in patients unresponsive to medical therapy or in cases of rapid reduction of symptoms (suicidality, psychosis, refusal to eat/drink)
	• <u>Other</u>: phototherapy (seasonal depression), psychostimulants, vagus nerve stimulation, medicinal herbs (St. John's wort), deep brain stimulation

Key Words & Most Common	• Persistently depressed mood or anhedonia almost every day for at least 2 weeks + 5 or more of: • Depressive mood, anhedonia, fatigue, insomnia or hypersomnia, significant weight loss or weight gain or increased appetite, psychomotor agitation or retardation (restlessness or slowness), feelings of worthlessness or inappropriate guilt, decreased concentration or indecisiveness, recurrent thoughts of death or suicide • Lifestyle modifications + psychological support → psychotherapy → antidepressants (SSRIs first-line)

Serotonin Syndrome

Etiology & Risk Factors	• **Life-threatening condition resulting from increased central nervous system serotonergic activity precipitated by use of serotonergic medications**
	• <u>Etiology</u>: **consequence of therapeutic medication use, drug interactions, or intentional overdose**
	  • <u>**SSRIs**</u>: **citalopram, escitalopram, fluoxetine, fluoxetine, paroxetine, sertraline**
	  • <u>**Serotonin Modulators**</u>: **trazadone**
	  • <u>**Monoamine Oxidase Inhibitors (MAOIs)**</u>: phenelzine, tranylcypromine, isocarboxazid, selegiline
	  • <u>Tricyclic Antidepressants (TCAs)</u>: amitriptyline, imipramine
	  • <u>Dopamine-Norepinephrine Reuptake Inhibitors</u>: bupropion
	  • <u>**Drugs of Abuse**</u>: **amphetamine, cocaine, MDMA (ecstasy)**
	  • <u>Other</u>: meperidine, tramadol, pentazocine, metoclopramide, valproate, carbamazepine, dextromethorphan, cyclobenzaprine, St. John's wort

Patho-physiology	• Serotonin modulates attention, appetite, sleep, mood, cognitive function, thermoregulation, bronchoconstriction, vasoconstriction, uterine contraction, GI motility • Excessive stimulation of postsynaptic serotonin receptors can lead to a wide range of symptoms and dysregulation of these mechanisms
Signs & Symptoms	• **Symptoms develop rapidly after exposure to serotonergic drugs; most commonly within 3-24 hours** • <u>**Altered Mental Status**</u>: **agitation**, anxiety, confusion, hallucinations, **restlessness, disorientation** • <u>**Autonomic Instability**</u>: **hyperthermia, diaphoresis, tachycardia**, labile blood pressure, nausea/vomiting/diarrhea, **dry mucous membranes, flushed skin** • <u>**Neuromuscular Hyperactivity**</u>: **tremor, hypertonia and hyperreflexia**, myoclonus (abnormal and rhythmic muscle contractions), extensor plantar responses • <u>**Ocular Effects**</u>: **mydriasis (dilated pupils)**, ocular clonus
Diagnostic Criteria	• **Clinical Diagnosis** • <u>**Hunter Toxicity Criteria**</u>: exposure to serotonergic drug + any 1 of the following • Spontaneous clonus, inducible clonus with agitation and diaphoresis, ocular clonus with agitation and diaphoresis, tremor and hyperreflexia, hypertonia, temperature over 100.4°F with ocular or inducible clonus
Treatment	• <u>**Discontinuation of All Serotonergic Drugs**</u>: **most important initial step in management** • <u>**Supportive Care**</u>: **mainstay of therapy**; IV fluids, supplemental oxygen, cooling measures (fans, water sprays, ice packs, cooled fluids, cooling blankets) • <u>**Benzodiazepines**</u>: **indicated for sedation** to reduce agitation, hyperthermia, neuromuscular abnormalities, and elevations in heart rate and blood pressure • <u>**Cyproheptadine**</u>: serotonin antagonist indicated if benzodiazepines and supportive care fail to improve agitation and abnormal vitals • <u>Severe Hyperthermia</u>: may require sedation, paralysis, and intubation for mechanical ventilation
Key Words & Most Common	• Increased CNS serotonergic activity precipitated by use of serotonergic medications • SSRIs, serotonin modulators, MAOIs, TCAs, drugs of abuse • Altered mental status + autonomic instability + neuromuscular hyperactivity + ocular effects within 24 hours of exposure • Clinical diagnosis + hunter toxicity criteria • Discontinue offending drug + supportive care → benzodiazepines → cyproheptadine

Neuroleptic Malignant Syndrome

Etiology & Risk Factors	• Life threatening neurologic emergency associated with the use of neuroleptic agents • <u>Etiology</u>: **first-generation (typical) antipsychotics (haloperidol) are most common**, second-generation antipsychotics (**risperidone, olanzapine**), antiemetics (**metoclopramide, promethazine**), withdrawal of anti-Parkinson medication (levodopa, amantadine) • <u>Risk Factors</u>: **male, age (less than 40 years old most common), high-dose or rapid increase in dose of antipsychotic medication**, sensitivity to neuroleptic agents, dehydration
Patho-physiology	• Excessive dopamine receptor blockade in the basal ganglia causes dopamine and acetylcholine dysregulation, leading to altered thermoregulation, muscle rigidity, autonomic dysfunction, and altered mental status
Signs & Symptoms	• Most commonly occurs within the first 2 weeks of treatment with neuroleptic drugs • <u>Altered Mental Status</u>: **earliest symptom; agitated delirium**, lethargy, unresponsiveness (encephalopathy) • <u>Motor Abnormalities</u>: **generalized, severe muscle rigidity (lead-pipe rigidity)**, dystonia, chorea, tremor, **hyporeflexia** • <u>Autonomic Hyperactivity</u>: **tachycardia**, arrhythmias, tachypnea, **hypertension, hypersalivation, diaphoresis, incontinence, regular-sized pupils** • <u>Hyperthermia</u>: **temperature often >104°F; most common presenting symptom**
Diagnostic Criteria	• **Clinical Diagnosis** • <u>Labs</u>: CBC (WBC>10k), electrolyte studies (hypocalcemia, hypomagnesemia, hyperkalemia, metabolic acidosis), total CK (>1000), LFTs (transaminitis)
Treatment	• <u>Discontinuation of Causative Medication</u>: **most important initial step in management** • <u>Supportive Care</u>: **mainstay of therapy**; IV fluids, supplemental oxygen, cooling measures (fans, water sprays, ice packs, cooled fluids, cooling blankets) • <u>Benzodiazepines</u>: **indicated for sedation** to reduce agitation, hyperthermia, neuromuscular abnormalities, and elevations in heart rate and blood pressure • <u>Dopamine Agonists</u>: bromocriptine or amantadine; may help restore dopaminergic activity • <u>Dantrolene</u>: skeletal muscle relaxant only indicated to treat severe hyperthermia and rigidity
Key Words & Most Common	• Neurologic emergency caused by neuroleptic agents • First-generation antipsychotics (haloperidol) most common cause • Seen with high-dose or rapid increase in dose of antipsychotics or withdrawal of dopamine agonist medication • AMS + motor abnormalities (lead-pipe rigidity and hyporeflexia) + autonomic hyperactivity (tachycardia, hypertension, diaphoresis) + hyperthermia • Discontinue causative medication + supportive therapy • Dopamine agonists or benzodiazepines as indicated

	Serotonin Syndrome	Neuroleptic Malignant Syndrome
Onset	Abrupt	Gradual
Course	Rapidly Resolving	Prolonged
Neuromuscular Findings	Myoclonus and Tremors	Diffuse Rigidity
Reflexes	Increased	Decreased
Pupils	Mydriasis	Normal

Bipolar Disorder

Etiology & Risk Factors	• Mental health disorder characterized by chronically occurring episodes of elevated moods (mania or hypomania) alternating with periods of depression • <u>Etiology</u>: combination of genetic, epigenetic, neurochemical, and environmental factors • <u>Risk Factors</u>: **family history is greatest risk factor, childhood abuse and neglect, stressful events** (childbirth, divorce, unemployment, disability, and early parental loss) • <u>Precipitating Factors</u>: alcohol use, sympathomimetic drugs (cocaine, amphetamine), antidepressant use (tricyclics, noradrenergic reuptake inhibitors)
Patho-physiology	• Dysregulation of monoaminergic neurotransmitters (dopamine and serotonin) and intracellular signaling systems that regulate mood as well as structural and functional abnormalities in brain regions involved in emotion regulation and cognitive control (prefrontal cortex and amygdala) • <u>**Bipolar I Disorder**</u>: **presence of at least one manic episode and cycles with occasional depressive episodes** • <u>**Bipolar II Disorder**</u>: **presence of major depressive episodes with at least one hypomanic episode** (current or previous manic episode indicates a bipolar I disorder diagnosis)

Signs & Symptoms	• <u>Mania</u>: abnormal and persistently elevated, expansive, or irritable mood for *at least* 1 week with marked social or occupational impairment 3+ of the following symptoms
	  • **Inflated self-esteem or grandiosity, decreased need for sleep**, more talkative or pressured speech, **flight of ideas** or racing thoughts, easily distracted, increased goal directed activity, **excessive involvement in high-risk activities** (spending sprees, gambling, dangerous sports, promiscuous sexual activity, unwise investments)
	  • <u>**Manic Psychosis**</u>: extreme grandiose or persecutory delusions (being Jesus or being followed), hallucinations, marked increase in activity (screaming, swearing, singing)
	• <u>Hypomania</u>: less extreme variant of mania involving an abnormal and persistently elevated, expansive, or irritable mood for *less than* 1 week
	  • Symptoms similar to mania but do not cause marked social or occupational impairment and not associated with psychotic episodes
	• <u>Depressive Episode</u>: symptoms similar to major depressive disorder
	  • **Depressive mood, anhedonia, fatigue, insomnia or hypersomnia, significant weight loss or weight gain or increased appetite, psychomotor agitation or retardation (restlessness or slowness), feelings of worthlessness or inappropriate guilt, decreased concentration or indecisiveness, recurrent thoughts of death or suicide**

Diagnostic Criteria	• <u>**Bipolar I Disorder**</u>: **presence of at least one manic episode and cycles with occasional depressive episodes** • <u>**Bipolar II Disorder**</u>: **presence one hypomanic episode and major depressive episodes** • *Consider workup for alternative diagnosis including point of care glucose, CBC, CMP, toxicology screen, thyroid panel, EtOH, urinalysis, aspirin or acetaminophen level*

Treatment	• <u>Supportive</u>: lifestyle modifications, education, sleep hygiene, information about conjugal consequences (divorce) and increased risk of infection with sexual promiscuity
	• <u>Psychotherapy</u>: **cognitive, behavioral and interpersonal therapy**
	• <u>Mood Stabilizers</u>: **first-line for medical therapy**
	  • **Lithium: first-line medication indicated for acute mania and long-term management; commonly used monotherapy**
	  • **Valproic Acid or Carbamazepine: alternative first-line medication; indicated for rapid cycling or mixed features**
	• <u>Second-Generation (Atypical) Antipsychotics</u>: **aripiprazole, olanzapine, quetiapine, risperidone, ziprasidone; monotherapy or adjunctive therapy to mood stabilizers**
	• <u>Antidepressants</u>: therapy may be used as adjunct in bipolar II but **antidepressant monotherapy may precipitate manic episode**
	• <u>Other</u>: electroconvulsive therapy for refractory or acute mania with suicidal ideation; phototherapy (seasonal depression/mania), transcranial magnetic stimulation

Persistent Depressive Disorder

Etiology & Risk Factors	• **Depressive symptoms that persist for 2 or more years without remission**; also known as **dysthymia** or chronic major depression • <u>Etiology</u>: combination of biological, social, and psychological factors • <u>Risk Factors</u>: **female, family history, childhood trauma** (abuse or neglect), **chronic stress**, substance abuse, chronic medical conditions, chronic pain
Patho-physiology	• Similar neurochemical (dopamine, epinephrine, norepinephrine, GABA, and glutamate) imbalance and neuroendocrine abnormalities as major depressive disorder • Abnormalities in brain structure and function, including decreased activity in the prefrontal cortex and hyperactivity in the amygdala

Signs & Symptoms	• **Chronic, depressed mood for at least 2 years in adults (or at least 1 year in children/adolescents)**
	• <u>Physical Exam</u>:
	  • **Tearful eyes, furrowed brows, frowning, poor posture and eye contact, lack of facial expression, minimal body movement, speech changes** (soft voice, short answer)
	  • **Neglect of personal hygiene** (unkept hair or facial hair, long fingernails and toenails, body odor, poor dentition)
	• May have major depressive episodes or meet criteria for major depressive disorder on a continuous basis

Diagnostic Criteria	• **Chronic, depressed mood for at least 2 years in adults (or at least 1 year in children/adolescents) lasting most of the day and most days of the week not symptom free for 2 or more months at a time plus at least 2 of the following symptoms:** • **Decreased appetite or overeating, insomnia or hypersomnia, fatigue, low self-esteem, poor concentration or indecisiveness, feelings of hopelessness**
Treatment	• <u>Lifestyle Modifications</u>: regular exercise, stress-reduction techniques (meditation or deep breathing exercises) limiting caffeine and alcohol intake, maintaining a healthy diet, sleep hygiene, and engaging in social support and hobbies/activities • <u>Psychological Support</u>: weekly or biweekly follow-up, reassurance, encouragement, referral to support groups • <u>Psychotherapy</u>: cognitive behavioral therapy (CBT), interpersonal therapy, supportive therapy, psychoeducation • <u>Antidepressants</u>: **indicated for patients that fail lifestyle modifications and CBT** • **SSRIs (first-line medication), SNRIs, TCAs, MAO inhibitors** • <u>Other</u>: phototherapy (seasonal depression), psychostimulants, vagus nerve stimulation, medicinal herbs (St. John's wort), deep brain stimulation
Key Words & Most Common	• Chronic, depressed mood for at least 2 years in adults (or at least 1 year in children/adolescents) lasting most of the day and most days of the week not symptom free for 2 or more months at a time plus at least 2 of the following symptoms: • Decreased appetite or overeating, insomnia or hypersomnia, fatigue, low self-esteem, poor concentration or indecisiveness, feelings of hopelessness • Lifestyle modifications + psychological support → psychotherapy → antidepressants (SSRIs first-line)

Cyclothymic Disorder

Etiology & Risk Factors	• Characterized by hypomanic and mini-depressive periods lasting for a few days, follow an irregular course, and are less severe than those in bipolar disorder • Similar to bipolar II disorder but less severe • <u>Etiology</u>: combination of genetic susceptibility, neurotransmitter dysregulation, and environmental factors • <u>Risk Factors</u>: **family history, childhood trauma** (abuse or neglect), **chronic stress**, substance abuse, chronic medical conditions, chronic pain, **hormone imbalance**
Patho-physiology	• Abnormalities in the regulation of certain neurotransmitters, including dopamine, serotonin, and norepinephrine
Signs & Symptoms	• **Alternations between euphoric and depressive dispositions** • <u>Depressive Symptoms</u>: depressed mood, irritability, hopelessness, helplessness, insomnia, fatigue, anhedonia, negative affect, headaches, suicidal ideation • <u>Hypomanic Symptoms</u>: impulsiveness, grandiosity or racing thoughts, increased sociability, excessive physical activity, pressured speech, minimal sleep • <u>Interpersonal and Social Consequences</u>: employment instability (changing jobs frequently), impulsive and frequent changes of residence, repeated breakups, episodic alcohol and/or drug abuse
Diagnostic Criteria	• **At least 2 years of mild manic, hypomanic, and depressive episodes that do not meet the full diagnostic criteria for full manic, hypomanic, or major depressive episodes** • **Symptom-free periods are not longer than 2 months**

Treatment	• <u>Supportive</u>: lifestyle modifications, education, sleep hygiene, information about conjugal consequences (divorce) and increased risk of infection with sexual promiscuity
	• <u>Psychotherapy</u>: **cognitive, behavioral and interpersonal therapy**
	• <u>Mood Stabilizers</u>: **first-line for medical therapy**
	   • <u>Lithium</u>: **first-line medication indicated for acute mania and long-term management; commonly used monotherapy**
	   • <u>Valproic Acid or Carbamazepine</u>: **alternative first-line medication; indicated for rapid cycling or mixed features**
	• <u>Second-Generation (Atypical) Antipsychotics</u>: **aripiprazole, olanzapine, quetiapine, risperidone, ziprasidone; monotherapy or adjunctive therapy to mood stabilizers**
	• <u>Antidepressants</u>: therapy may be used as adjunct in bipolar II but **antidepressant monotherapy may precipitate manic episode**
	• <u>Other</u>: electroconvulsive therapy for refractory or acute mania with suicidal ideation; phototherapy (seasonal depression/mania), transcranial magnetic stimulation

Key Words & Most Common	• Hypomanic and mini-depressive episodes lasting few a few days, irregular, and less severe than bipolar disorder • Alteration between hypomanic and depressive symptoms without meeting full diagnostic criteria for manic, hypomanic or major depressive episodes • Supportive care + psychotherapy • Mood stabilizers (lithium vs valproic acid vs carbamazepine) +/- antipsychotics

Premenstrual Syndrome (PMS)

Etiology & Risk Factors	• <u>PMS</u>: **Luteal-phase disorder characterized physical, behavioral and mood changes occurring 5 days prior to and subsiding within a few hours of the onset of menses** • <u>Premenstrual Dysphoric Disorder</u>: **severe PMS with functional impairment;** anger, irritability and tension are prominent symptoms; psychiatric disorder by DSM-5 • <u>Etiology</u>: **unclear etiology; endocrine factors** (hypoglycemia, **estrogen and progesterone fluctuations**, excess aldosterone), genetic predisposition, **serotonin deficiency**, magnesium/calcium deficiency may be contributory • <u>Risk Factors</u>: poor nutrition, high-salt diet, caffeine, alcohol use, poor sleep quality, **stress, perimenopausal**
Patho-physiology	• Progesterone and estrogen fluctuations affect certain neurotransmitters (gamma-aminobutyric acid [GABA], opioids, serotonin, and catecholamine) • Preexisting serotonin deficiency with increased progesterone sensitivity may be implicated • Stress amplifies sympathetic activity and may exacerbate PMS symptoms
Signs & Symptoms	• <u>Physical</u>: **abdominal bloating, fatigue, acne**, breast fullness or pain, **weight gain**, headache, **pelvic pressure**, backache, fluid retention, constipation/diarrhea, palpitations • <u>Emotional</u>: **irritability is most common symptom**, agitation, anger, insomnia, lethargy, depression/anxiety, changes in libido • <u>Behavioral</u>: **food cravings**, lack of concentration, noise sensitivity
Diagnostic Criteria	• **Clinical Diagnosis** • Symptoms begin about 5 days prior to menses (luteal phase) and subside a few hours to days after onset of menses • Patient should have at least 1 week of symptom-free days during follicular phase • Symptoms persisting >2 cycles

Treatment	• <u>Lifestyle Modifications</u>: **stress reduction, sleep hygiene, regular aerobic and resistance exercise**, relaxation activities, cognitive behavioral therapy
	• <u>Dietary Modifications</u>: increase protein intake, decreased refined sugar/carbohydrates, consume whole-foods diet, avoid caffeine
	   • Supplementation with vitamin B6, vitamin E, magnesium, calcium, and **chasteberry extract from the agnus castus fruit** have been shown to be beneficial
	• <u>Medication Management</u>:
	   • <u>Non-Steroidal Anti-Inflammatory Drugs (NSAIDs)</u>: relieve aches, pain, and dysmenorrhea
	   • <u>**Combined Oral Contraceptive Pills**</u>: combination of ethinyl estradiol and drospirenone have been shown to decrease symptoms
	   • <u>**Selective Serotonin Reuptake Inhibitors (SSRIs)**</u>: **first-line medication for treatment of PMS with predominantly emotional symptoms**

Key Words & Most Common	• Physical, behavioral and mood changes occurring 5 days prior to menses and resolving shortly after • Progesterone and estrogen fluctuations and serotonin deficiency may be implicated • Exacerbated by stress • Abdominal bloating, fatigue, acne, weight gain • Irritability, agitation, insomnia, food cravings • Stress reduction + sleep hygiene + dietary modifications • NSAIDs for symptom management • SSRIs first-line for treatment with predominate emotional symptoms

Suicide

Etiology & Risk Factors	• <u>Suicide</u>: death caused by an intentional act of self-harm that is intended to be lethal • <u>Suicidal Behavior</u>: suicide attempts and preparatory behaviors to completed suicide • <u>Suicidal Ideation</u>: process of thought about, considering, and/or planning suicide • <u>Etiology</u>: combination of genetic, environmental, and psychologic/behavioral factors • <u>Risk Factors</u>: **depression is greatest risk factor, increased age, gender (females attempt suicide more often, men more often complete suicide), access to firearms, mental illness, previous suicide attempt**, substance abuse, marital status (single, never married greatest risk), childhood trauma, chronic medical conditions, **chronic stress** • <u>Precipitating Factors</u>: relationship disruption (**divorce**), occupational disruptions (**unemployment**), death of family or friend, financial stress, **bullying** (cyberbullying, social rejection, discrimination, humiliation)
Patho-physiology	• Abnormalities in the regulation of certain neurotransmitters, including dopamine, serotonin, and norepinephrine combined with risk factors increases likelihood of suicide behavior
Signs & Symptoms	• **Depressed mood and anhedonia** • <u>**Activities Associated With Suicidal Behavior**</u>: making a will, excessive cleaning and organizing living space, inexplicably visiting friends or family members, purchasing a firearm, writing a suicide note, frequent visits to primary care physician • <u>**Suicide-Related Characteristics**</u>: preoccupation with death, sense of isolation or social withdrawal, emotional distance (lives alone, never married, no intimate relationships), distraction or lack of humor (appears "in their own world"), dwelling in the past, feelings of hopelessness or helplessness
Diagnostic Criteria	• Clinical Diagnosis • Must assess suicide risk including suicidal behavior and ideation; SAD PERSONS score may aid in determining need for admission

Treatment	• <u>Intervention</u>: **first-step in management is assuring the patient's safety and preventing patient from committing suicide**
	   • Patient must not be left alone, remove all potentially dangerous objects (cords, IV tubing, scalpels etc.), continuous monitoring with sitter or video
	• <u>Admission</u>: suicide risk patients often require admission for observation and psychiatric evaluation
	• <u>Mental Health Management</u>: **safety planning**, offering crisis resources, counseling on removal or storage of lethal weapons, frequent contact (telemedicine, follow-ups)
	   • **Psychotherapy** (cognitive-behavioral therapy, dialectical behavior therapy, collaborative assessment and management of suicidality [CAMS], family therapy)
	• **Treatment of underlying disorder**

Key Words & Most Common	• Depression is greatest risk factor; access to firearms, underlying mental illness, previous suicide attempt, recent change in circumstance (job loss, divorce) • Depressed mood and anhedonia • Clinical diagnosis • Intervention → admission → mental health management (safety planning and psychotherapy) → treat underlying disorder

Suicide Prevention

Assess	1. Inquire about past and present suicide ideation and behavior 2. Identify risk factors 3. Implement and maintain safety measures
Intervene	1. Develop a safety plan for maintaining continued safety measures and restricting lethal means 2. Initiate coping strategies and support 3. Develop plan for underlying mental health disorder
Monitor	1. Increase availability and access to provider or mental health resources 2. Increased monitoring during periods of high-risk 3. Involve family and social support

SAD PERSONS Score

Sex = Male	1 point
Age <19 or >45	1 point
Depressed symptoms	2 points
Psychiatric history or past suicide attempt	1 point
EtOH/drug use history	1 point
Rational thought loss	2 points
Separated/divorced/widowed or sickness with 3 or more prescription medications	1 point
Organized plan or serious attempt	2 points
No social support	1 point
Stated attempt	2 points
<6 points: may discharge home if caregiver available and safety and crisis plan developed **6-8 points**: consult psychiatry to determine admission plan **>8 points**: admit for psychiatric evaluation and treatment	

Oppositional Defiant Disorder (ODD)

Etiology & Risk Factors	• Childhood disruptive behavior disorder involving problems with the self-control of emotions and behaviors characterized by persistent angry or irritable mood, argumentative or defiant behavior, or vindictiveness toward others • Etiology: combination of genetic, environmental and psychosocial factors • Risk Factors: adults that engage in loud, argumentative, interpersonal conflicts in front of child is greatest risk factor; family history, male, age (5-10 years old most common age), childhood trauma, low socioeconomic status, low education level
Additional Information	• Genetics: heritability is around 50%; may have concomitant underlying ADHD or depression • Environmental: childhood trauma and/or harsh, inconsistent parenting • Psychosocial: general temperament (irritability, impulsivity, poor frustration, emotional reactivity)
Signs & Symptoms	• Defiant towards authority but *not* associated with physical aggression, violating other's basic rights or breaking law (unlike conduct disorder) • Frequently loses temper, negative, angry or irritable mood, easily annoyed • Argumentative and defiance towards adults • Defiant behavior with intentional vindictiveness or spitefulness; refusal to follow rules • Deliberately annoying towards others • Many children lack basic social skills

Diagnostic Criteria	• Diagnosed in child with at least 4 of the following symptoms present for 6 or more months; symptoms must be severe and disruptive
	  • Angry or Irritable Mood: often loses temper, angry and resentful, touchy or irritable mood
	  • Argumentative or Defiant Behavior: argues with authority figures, actively refuses or defies to comply with authority figures or rules,
	  • Vindictiveness: blames others for misbehaviors and negative attitude, child has been spiteful or vindictive 2 or more times within the past 6 months
	• Severity: mild (symptoms confined to only 1 setting), moderate (present in 2 settings) and severe (present in 3+ settings)

Treatment	• Behavior Modification Therapy: rewards-based behavior-modification program is treatment of choice; problem-solving skills and conflict management training, parental management training for proper discipline, enforcing rules, setting limits and maintaining a reward system • Medical Management: indicated if comorbid condition • Stimulants and non-stimulants (ADHD), antidepressants (depression), mood stabilizers (aggression, mood dysregulation, bipolar disorder)
Key Words & Most Common	• Childhood disruptive behavior involving problems with self-control of emotions and behavior, angry or irritable move, argumentation or defiant behavior and vindictiveness • Adults in family that engage in loud, argumentative, interpersonal conflicts in front of child is greatest risk factor • Defiant towards authority but *not* associated with physical aggression, violating other's basic rights or breaking law (unlike conduct disorder) • Behavior modification therapy focusing on rewards-based behavior modification is treatment of choice

Conduct Disorder

Etiology & Risk Factors	• Persistent pattern of behavior that violates the rights of others (or animals) and deviates sharply from age-appropriate societal norms or rules • Etiology: multiple biological, psychosocial neurological, environmental factors • Risk Factors: family history, male, childhood trauma, low socioeconomic status, low education level, lack of social support, social isolation, comorbid mental health disorders (ADHD, depression, oppositional defiance disorder), substance abuse
Additional Information	• May progress to antisocial personality disorder • Biological Factors: insensitivity to punishment, antisocial behavior, aggressive temperament, low levels of plasma dopamine beta-hydroxylase, high testosterone levels • Psychosocial Factors: frequent marital conflict among parents, harsh parenting, exposure to domestic violence, parent with alcohol abuse, lack of adequate parenting, low socioeconomic status without parental support • Neurological Factors: developmental delays (lead to poor social skills, learning disabilities and below-average intellectual capacity), traumatic brain injury, seizures • Environmental Factors: school (large classroom sizes, lack of positive feedback, lack of counseling), exposure to gang violence in community, no positive role model, lack of affectionate parenting, poor living conditions
Signs & Symptoms	• Engagement in physical and/or sexual violence • Lack of empathy for victims and lack of remorse for committing crimes • Symptoms of comorbid mental health condition

Diagnostic Criteria	• Exhibits pattern of behavior that violates the rights of others or animals and disregards age-appropriate societal norms
	  • Aggression Towards People and/or Animals: bullying, initiating fights, using weapons, threatening behavior, abusive or cruel to animals or people
	  • Destruction of Property: deliberately causing damage to property including acts of arson or vandalism
	  • Deceitfulness or Theft: lies to obtain goods or favors, breaks into cars or homes, shoplifting, acts of forgery; lack of remorse for actions
	  • Serious Violation of Rules: stays out late at night, frequent running away from home, school truancy

Treatment	• Psychosocial Management:
	  • Parental management training for proper discipline, enforcing rules, setting limits and maintaining a reward system
	  • Anger management training and behavioral modification
	  • Multisystemic therapy with community and family involvement to improve family dynamics and academic function
	  • Psychotherapy directed at problem-solving skills and resolving personal conflict
	• Medical Management: indicated if comorbid condition
	  • Stimulants and non-stimulants (ADHD), antidepressants (depression), mood stabilizers (aggression, mood dysregulation, bipolar disorder)

Key Words & Most Common	• Patterns of behavior that violate the rights of others or animals and disregards age-appropriate societal norms • Aggression towards people/animals, destruction of property, deceitfulness or theft, serious violation of rules • Psychosocial management is first-line; parental management training, anger management training, behavioral modification, psychotherapy

Dissociative Identity Disorder

Etiology & Risk Factors	• **Dissociative disorder characterized by 2 or more identities or personality states that alternate** • Also known as **multiple personality disorder** • Etiology: combination of environmental, genetic, and neurobiological factors • Risk Factors: **severe trauma, stress or abuse experienced during childhood is greatest risk factor**; early loss (death of a parent), medical illness, overly stressful events
Patho-physiology	• Traumatic experiences result in alterations in neural circuitry as well as brain structure/function leading to dissociation of memories, emotions, and sense of self maintained across behavioral states as a means of coping with the severe trauma, stress, or abuse

Signs & Symptoms	• <u>Multiple Identities</u>:
	  • **Possession Form**: patient speaks and acts in an obvious different manner that may seem as though another person or a spirit (demon or God) has taken over
	  • **Non-Possession Form**: patients experience feelings of depersonalization such as detachment from physical and mental processes or experience sudden thoughts, impulses, emotions that are not their own
	  • **Disruption of identity may be observed by others** (rapid change in attitude, preferences, or opinions that suddenly revert)
	• <u>Amnesia</u>:
	  • **Gaps in memory of traumatic personal events** (inability to recall childhood memories or periods of time in which the trauma was experienced)
	  • **Lapses in dependable memory**; discovery of things done or said without recollection of doing so
	  • Inability to recall everyday events, important personal information and/or traumatic or overly stressful events
	• May have visual, tactile, olfactory and/or gustatory hallucinations

Diagnostic Criteria	• **Patients experience 2 or more personality states or identities with substantial discontinuity of sense of self and sense of agency** • **Patients experience gaps in everyday memory, important personal information, and traumatic events** • **Symptoms result in significant distress or impairment of social or occupational function**

Treatment	• <u>Ensure Safety</u>: ensure safety of patient (commonly experience suicidal ideation and self-injurious behavior)
	• <u>Psychotherapy</u>: directed at evaluation of the traumatic experiences and discussing the problematic identities and rational of dissociations
	  • Reassessment of memories with different personalities to aid in tolerating, processing, and integrating the past trauma among personalities
	  • Focus on returning the patient's relationship to self as a whole and to the rest of the world
	• <u>Hypnosis</u>: accessing alternate identities to facilitate communication, stabilization and interpretation among them in attempt to integrate the various personality states
	• <u>Medication Management</u>: not indicated as primary treatment; may be used to treat certain underlying symptoms or comorbid conditions

Key Words & Most Common	• Dissociative disorder characterized by 2+ identities or personality states • Severe trauma, stress, or abuse (especially sexual abuse) experienced during childhood • Multiple identities + amnesia • Patients experience 2+ personality states or identities with discontinuity of sense of self, experience gaps in everyday memory, important personal information, and traumatic events and symptoms result in significant distress or impairment of social/occupational function • Ensure safety → pharmacotherapy → hypnosis

Depersonalization/Derealization Disorder

Etiology & Risk Factors	• **Dissociative disorder characterized by the persistent or recurrent feelings of being detached (dissociated) from one's body or mental processes**
	  • **Depersonalization**: feeling of being an outside observer of one's life; "out of body feeling"
	  • **Derealization**: feelings of being detached from one's surrounding environment
	• <u>Etiology</u>: combination of environmental, genetic, and neurobiological factor
	• <u>Risk Factors</u>: **childhood abuse or neglect is greatest risk factor**; childhood domestic violence, impaired or mentally ill parent, unexpected death of friend of family member
	• <u>Precipitating Factors</u>: personal, financial or occupational stress, depression, use of illicit drugs,

Patho-physiology	• Dysregulation of the brain's emotional processing centers such as an overactive or hypersensitive amygdala (area responsible for processing of emotional stimuli) leading to disconnection between emotional and sensory experiences • Alteration of neural circuitry as a result of experienced trauma leads to abnormalities of self-awareness and sensory information processing

Signs & Symptoms	• <u>Depersonalization</u>: **feeling of detachment from one's body, mind, feelings, and/or sensations**
	  • Patients describe feeling "unreal, robot-like, or automated" in terms of emotions
	  • **Emotionally numb** ("emotional flat-line")
	  • Disconnection from memories or unclear recollection of events
	• <u>Derealization</u>: **feeling of detachment from one's surrounding environment**
	  • "Dream-like" or "fog-like" state that separates the patient from experiencing his/her surroundings
	  • Distorted perception of objects, sound, or time

Diagnostic Criteria	• **Patients experience persistent or recurrent episodes of depersonalization and/or derealization** • **Patients understand their dissociative experiences are not real (intact sense of self and reality)** • **Symptoms cause significant distress or impairment of social/occupational function**

Treatment	• <u>Psychotherapy</u>: **most effective treatment; various approaches may be required**
	  • <u>Cognitive Techniques</u>: blocking of obsessive thoughts about the "unreal" state of living
	  • <u>Behavioral Techniques</u>: engaging patient in various tasks to distract them from feelings of depersonalization/derealization
	  • <u>Grounding Techniques</u>: engaging the 5 sense to have patient feel more intact with surroundings (standing barefoot on grass, holding ice cube in hand, loud music)
	  • <u>Psychodynamic Therapy</u>: coping techniques to manage negative feelings or experiencing and underlying conflicts

Key Words & Most Common	• <u>Depersonalization</u>: feeling of being an outside observer of one's life, detachment from one's body, mid, feelings, and/or sensations • <u>Derealization</u>: feelings of detachment from one's surrounding environment • Childhood abuse or neglect is greatest risk factor • Psychotherapy is most effective treatment

Dissociative Amnesia

Etiology & Risk Factors	• Dissociative disorder involving the inability to recall important personal information • Etiology: combination of environmental, genetic, and neurobiological factors • Risk Factors: **severe traumatic experience** (physical or **sexual abuse, rape**, genocide, **natural disasters**, death of a close friend or family member, **armed combat**)
Patho-physiology	• Alterations in neural pathways and circuits related to the stress response and memory processing retrieval systems within the brain • Changes within the brain are initiated by experiencing traumatic events that result in a temporary or persistent inability to recall certain memories

Signs & Symptoms	• **Memory loss inconsistent with normal forgetfulness**
	• **Localized Amnesia: inability to recall a specific event during a specific period of time (usually during periods of stress or trauma)**
	   • Inability to recall events during period of time of being abused as a child, time spent in intense combat
	   • Woman who was raped in a stairwell refuses to enter a stairwell even though she cannot recall the events or location surrounding the rape
	• **Selective Amnesia**: inability to recall some of the specifics surrounding an event or time period
	• **Systematized Amnesia**: forgetting specific categorical information (forgetting all information about a specific family member)
	• **Continuous Amnesia**: forgetting each new event as it occurs
	• **Dissociative Fugue**: abrupt travel away from home and bewildered wandering associated with loss of identity or inability to recall the past

Diagnostic Criteria	• **Patients are unable to recall important personal information (typically stress- or trauma-related) that is inconsistent with normal forgetfulness** • **Symptoms cause significant distress or impairment of social/occupational function**
Treatment	• **Supportive: creation of a safe and supportive environment**, reassurance, education • **Psychotherapy: most effective treatment** • May be combined with hypnosis or drug-facilitated interviews to restore memory
Key Words & Most Common	• Dissociative disorder involving the inability to recall important personal information • Most often associated with severe trauma (sexual assault, sexual abuse, rape) • Memory loss inconsistent with normal forgetfulness • May be localized, selective, systematized, continuous amnesia • Patients are unable to recall important personal information (typically stress- or trauma-related) that is inconsistent with normal forgetfulness • Symptoms cause significant distress or impairment of social/occupational function • Supportive + psychotherapy

Pica

Etiology & Risk Factors	• **Persistent eating of non-nutritive, non-food material over a period of at least 1 month** • Etiology: multiple psychological, cultural and behavioral factors, **iron-deficiency anemia** • Risk Factors: **stress, underlying mental health disorder, nutritional deficiency**, child neglect, pregnancy, low socioeconomic status, mental retardation
Patho-physiology	• Impaired oxygen-carrying capacity of the blood results in the release of neurochemicals that trigger the craving for ice; chewing ice may provide temporary relief for oral inflammation, a common symptom of iron deficiency anemia • Thought by patient in vulnerable stages of human cell replication and embryogenesis (childhood, pregnancy) that non-nutritive substances offers protection from harmful toxins through binding of toxins and impairing absorption with undigestible material
Signs & Symptoms	• **Ingestion of nutritive, non-food material** • **Dirt**, raw starches, **ice, paint**, charcoal, **chalk**, paper, ash, **hair**, clothing, baby powder, **soap**, coffee grounds, eggshells • Complications: **intestinal obstruction** (impaction of undigestible material), **lead intoxication** (eating paint), bowel perforation, parasitic infection (eating dirt)

Diagnostic Criteria	• **Persistent eating of non-nutritive, non-food material for at least 1 month**
	   • **Ingestion of the material is inappropriate for the patient's developmental level**
	   • **Ingestion of these materials is not related to cultural tradition**
	• Labs: evaluate for nutritional deficiencies (folate, iron/ferritin, zinc), **toxicity testing (lead level),** stool test (parasitic infection)
	• Imaging: abdominal x-ray, barium studies, endoscopy; indicated with abdominal symptoms to evaluate for obstruction and ensure passage of material

Treatment	• **Reduce Access**: reducing access to items (removal and repainting of non-lead-based paint), provide appropriate substitute with similar texture • **Behavioral Modifications**: addressing underlying mental health disorder • **Nutritional Supplementation**: indicated for identified nutritional deficiencies
Key Words & Most Common	• Persistent eating of non-nutritive, non-food material for at least 1 month • Dirt, ice, paint, chalk, hair, soap most common items • Reduce access + behavioral modifications • Nutritional supplementation as indicated

Binge-Eating Disorder

Etiology & Risk Factors	• Recurrent episodes of consuming large amounts of food in a short period of time time occurring every week over 3 or more months • Etiology: multiple psychological, social, cultural, and biological factors • Risk Factors: **childhood obesity, lack of controlled eating in childhood**, perfectionism, parental psychopathology, **family weight concerns and projection, distorted body image**, low self-esteem, substance abuse, **childhood abuse**
Patho-physiology	• Emotional or environmental stressors result in dysregulation of the brain's reward centers, including the dopamine and opioid systems, leading to a maladaptive coping mechanism that results in overeating and loss of control
Signs & Symptoms	• **Eating a larger amount of food than most people would eat under similar circumstances** • **Severe distress after binge eating**; sense of losing control
Diagnostic Criteria	• **Recurrent episodes of binge-eating occurring at least once per week for 3 months and 3 or more of the following** • **Eating rapidly, eating until feeling uncomfortably full, eating large amounts of food when not physically hungry, eating alone (because of embarrassment), feeling disgusted or guilty from over-eating** • **Patient has a sense of lack of control over-eating** • **Binge eating is not followed by purging** (self-induced vomiting, misuse of laxatives or enemas), **excessive exercise or fasting** • **Does not involve constant overeating ("grazing")**

Treatment	• Supportive: diet and exercise plan, education regarding disorder, reassurance, weight loss plan
	• Psychotherapy: **cognitive behavioral therapy or interpersonal psychotherapy is first-line in management**
	• Medical Management: indicated if patient does not have access or is non-compliant with psychotherapy
	  • Antidepressants: **SSRIs** may have short-term effectiveness to eliminate binge-eating
	  • Stimulants: **lisdexamfetamine** is approved for the treatment of moderate to severe binge eating disorder
	  • Antiepileptics: **topiramate** has been associated with appetite-suppression and weight loss

Key Words & Most Common	• Recurrent episodes of binge-eating occurring at least once per week for 3 months and 3 or more of the following • Eating rapidly, eating until feeling uncomfortably full, eating large amounts of food when not physically hungry, eating alone (because of embarrassment), feeling disgusted or guilty from over-eating • Patient has a sense of lack of control over-eating • Binge eating is not followed by purging, excessive exercise or fasting • Does not involve constant overeating • Supportive + psychotherapy → medication (SSRIs, lisdexamfetamine, topiramate)

Bulimia Nervosa

Etiology & Risk Factors	• **Eating disorder characterized by recurrent episodes of binge eating followed by inappropriate compensatory behavior to prevent weight gain** • Etiology: multiple psychological, social, cultural, and biological factors • Risk Factors: **female, lack of controlled eating in childhood**, perfectionism, parental psychopathology, **family weight concerns and projection, distorted body image**, low self-esteem, substance abuse, **childhood abuse**
Patho-physiology	• Neurotransmitter dysregulation of serotonin and dopamine, which are involved in the regulation of appetite, mood, and reward processing • Abnormalities in brain structure and function, particularly in areas of the brain involved in impulse control and emotion regulation

Signs & Symptoms	• Binge-Purge Behavior: rapid consumption of large amounts of food followed by inappropriate compensatory behavior
	  • **Binge Behavior**: consuming sweet, high-fat foods ice cream, cake, chips, cookies) during episode is common; often triggered by psychosocial stress
	  • **Compensatory Behavior**: self-induced vomiting, use of laxatives, excessive exercise, prolonged fasting; behavior is ego-dystonic (troublesome to the patient)
	• **Usually maintains a normal weight or may be overweight**
	• Physical Exam:
	  • **Erosion of dental enamel of the front teeth** (damage from stomach acid exposure secondary to vomiting)
	  • Russell's Sign: **scars or calluses on the dorsum of the hand from self-induced vomiting** (back of hand rubs against teeth while attempting to trigger gag reflex)
	  • **Painless parotid (salivary) gland swelling**

Diagnostic Criteria	• **Recurrent binge eating episodes characterized by the uncontrolled consumption of large amounts of food occurring once per week for 3 or more months**
	  • **Accompanied by a sense of loss of control**
	  • **Inappropriate compensatory behavior to influence body weight**
	  • **Perception of self-worth is unduly influenced by body shape and weight concerns**
	• Labs: may show **hypokalemia**, hypomagnesemia, **elevated amylase**, metabolic alkalosis

Treatment	• Psychotherapy: **cognitive behavioral therapy is first-line and treatment of choice**; interpersonal therapy to help identify and alter current interpersonal problems • Medication Management: • Antidepressants: **fluoxetine** (SSRI) is only FDA-approved medication show to reduce the binge-purge behavior cycle
Key Words & Most Common	• Binge eating episodes followed by self-induced vomiting, laxative abuse, excessive exercise or prolonged fasting • Behavior is troublesome to the patient • Patient usually normal or overweight • Erosion of teeth enamel, scars on dorsum of the hand, parotid gland swelling • Cognitive behavioral therapy is most effective treatment

Anorexia Nervosa

Etiology & Risk Factors	• Eating disorder characterized by a relentless pursuit of maintaining a thin body habitus, fear of obesity, distorted body image, and nutrient intake restriction, leading to a significantly low body weight • Etiology: multiple psychological, social, cultural, and biological factors • Risk Factors: **childhood obesity, female**, mood disorders, **personality traits** (perfectionism, meticulous, compulsive), **childhood abuse**, weight-related concerns from family or peers, **athletics requiring thin physique** (dancers, long-distance running), low self-esteem, **middle-to-upper socioeconomic status**
Patho-physiology	• Abnormalities in the hypothalamus-pituitary-adrenal axis, alterations in neurotransmitter systems (dopamine [eating behavior and reward] and serotonin [impulse control and neuroticism]), and changes in brain structure and function combined with one or more of the above risk factors results in development of eating disorder • Malnutrition can result in endocrine abnormalities (hypogonadotropic hypogonadism, hypothyroidism, increased cortisol), hypokalemia, metabolic alkalosis • **Binge Eating/Purging Type**: binge eating episodes followed by compensatory behavior such as self-induced vomiting laxative abuse, diuretics, or enemas • **Restricting Type**: strict, reduced food intake, dieting, fasting, vigorous or excessive exercise, stimulant medication abuse

Signs & Symptoms	• Preoccupation and anxiety surrounding maintain a low body weight or certain body image
	  • Behaviors include excessive water intake, food-related obsession (hoarding, concealing, wasting), studying of diets, calories and nutrition labels
	  • Behavior is ego-syntonic (behavior is acceptable and in harmony with self-image goals)
	• Common symptoms include **amenorrhea, cold intolerance**, constipation, extremity edema, **fatigue**, irritability, dehydration, **bloating, abdominal distress, constipation**
	• Physical Exam:
	  • **Greatly reduced body fat** (thin, emaciated appearance), **bradycardia, hypotension**, hypothermia, **lanugo hair** (soft, fine hair usually only found on neonates), arrhythmia, salivary gland hypertrophy, edema
	  • **Russell's Sign**: scars or calluses on the dorsum of the hand from self-induced vomiting (back of hand rubs against teeth while attempting to trigger gag reflex)

Diagnostic Criteria	• **Restriction of food intake resulting in a significantly low body weight** • **Intense ear of excessive weight gain or obesity or persistent behavior to prevent weight gain** • **Distorted body image** (misperception of body weight and appearance) **or denial of the seriousness of illness despite being underweight** • **Low body weight defined as a body mass index (BMI) of less than 17kg/m² or a body weight <85% of ideal weight** • Labs: **hypokalemia** (secondary to GI loss), **increased BUN/Cr** (dehydration), **hyperchloremic metabolic alkalosis** (secondary to vomiting), **hypogonadotropic hypogonadism** (low estrogen or low testosterone), **hypothyroidism**

Treatment	• **Life-Saving Measures**: hospitalization indicated for patients <75% expected body weight, rapid and severe weight loss, metabolic complications, or medically unstable
	• **Nutritional Supplementation**: oral feedings with solid foods preferred, liquid supplements are alternative; nasogastric tube feeding required in severe cases
	  • **Refeeding Syndrome**: most common complication after prolonged starvation; glucose is used to produce ATP and increased insulin leads to hypophosphatemia and hypokalemia which may result in cardiac and respiratory compromise
	• **Psychotherapy**: cornerstone of long-term treatment; cognitive behavioral therapy, supervised meals, normalized eating and weight gain
	• Medical Management:
	  • Antidepressants: SSRIs indicated if underlying depression and may help with weight gain
	  • Atypical Anti-Psychotics: olanzapine may help with weight gain

Body Dysmorphic Disorder

Etiology & Risk Factors	• Condition characterized by a preoccupation with a perceived defect or flaw in one's physical appearance that is either not observable or only slightly observed by others • Etiology: multiple biological, cultural, psychosocial, and neuropsychological factors • Risk Factors: **childhood abuse or neglect is greatest risk factor; female**, age (adolescence is most common), comorbid mental health condition (anxiety or depression)
Patho-physiology	• Alterations in the frontostriatal and limbic circuits (anterior cingulate cortex, orbitofrontal cortex, and basal ganglia), which are responsible for processing sensory information and emotional regulation, may play a role in the development and maintenance of body dysmorphia

Signs & Symptoms	• **Concern or fixation on a perceived defect in physical appearance**
	  • Hair thinning, acne, wrinkles, scars, vascular markings, complexion, skin color (tanning) or excessive facial or body hair
	  • **Focus on specific body parts**; shape or size of the nose, ears, eyes, mouth, breasts, buttocks, legs
	  • **Muscle dysmorphia** is the preoccupation that one's body is not sufficiently lean and muscular; more common in men
	  • **May commit repetitive acts in response to preoccupation** (mirror checking, observing or photographing specific body parts, seeking reassurance, skin picking)
	• May have history of multiple cosmetic procedures and/or unnecessary surgical interventions (multiple rhinoplasties or breast augmentations most common)

Diagnostic Criteria	• **Preoccupation with 1 or more perceived appearance flaws that are not observable or only slightly observed by others** • **Repetitive behaviors performed in response to the appearance concerns** • **Preoccupation causes significant distress or impairment of social or occupational function**

Treatment	• Medical Therapy:
	  • Antidepressants: **SSRIs** (fluoxetine, sertraline, citalopram) are first-line medications
	  • Tricyclic Antidepressants: **clomipramine** has potent and specific serotonergic effects
	• **Psychotherapy: cognitive behavioral therapy (CBT)** and/or cognitive restructuring utilized as prevention
	  • Awareness training, stimulus control, avoidance of triggers, competing response training

Key Words & Most Common	• Concern or fixation on a perceived defect in physical appearance • Focus on specific body parts or appearance aspects (hair thinning, acne, skin color, body hair etc.) • Clinical Criteria: preoccupation with 1 or more perceived appearance flaws that are not observable or only slightly observed by others, repetitive behaviors performed in response to the appearance concerns, preoccupation causes significant distress or impairment of social or occupational function • SSRIs +/- clomipramine • Psychotherapy (CBT)

Obsessive-Compulsive Disorder (OCD)

Etiology & Risk Factors	• Disorder characterized by intrusive thoughts with or without compensatory actions to alleviate the stress brought on by these thoughts • <u>Etiology</u>: combination of genetic and environmental factors • <u>Risk Factors</u>: **comorbid mental health disorder (anxiety is most common, depression)**, family history, childhood abuse, severe traumatic experiences, stressful life events
Patho-physiology	• Dysfunction in the activity of the cortico-striato-thalamo-cortical (CSTC) circuit; abnormal communication of the orbitofrontal cortex, anterior cingulate cortex, basal ganglia • Overactive dopaminergic and glutamatergic neurotransmission in the frontostriatal pathways and diminished activity of serotonergic and GABAnergic neurotransmission in the frontolimbic systems

Signs & Symptoms	• <u>Obsessions</u>: **recurrent or intrusive thoughts, images, or urges**
	  • Thoughts may be related to reducing harm or risk to self or others, fear of contamination, pathologic doubt (forgetting to turn off stove to avoid danger), symmetry or precision (ordering or counting), or aggression
	  • Typically, unwanted and unpleasant, causing significant anxiety or distress; patient may ignore or suppress the obsession or neutralize by performing a compulsion
	• <u>Compulsions</u>: **the drive to perform repetitive behaviors, rituals or mental acts to reduce the anxiety or prevent harm**; usually time consuming or cause distress
	  • <u>Washing</u>: excessive cleaning, hand washing, showering
	  • <u>Checking</u>: ensuring stove is off, doors are locked, electronic devices unplugged
	  • <u>Counting</u>: repeating a behavior a certain number of times, television volume must be on even/odd number, counting objects (stairs, steps, tiles)
	  • <u>Ordering</u>: arranging tableware or workplace items in a specific pattern, arranging clothes by color, arranging books by alphabetical order; obsession with symmetry

Diagnostic Criteria	• Presence of obsessions, compulsions or both • Obsessions or compulsions must be time-consuming (> 1 hour per day) and/or cause significant distress or functional impairment

Treatment	• <u>Combination Therapy</u>: **medical therapy (SSRIs) and cognitive behavioral therapy (CBT) with exposure and response prevention (ERP) is most effective treatment**
	  • **<u>Cognitive Behavioral Therapy (CBT)</u>**: cognitive restructuring may be useful identify and manage behaviors; focus on altering malicious and harmful thoughts
	  • **<u>Exposure and Response Prevention (ERP)</u>**: exposure to a specific fear enables the patient to resist the urge to perform a compulsion with a goal to restructure and alter the habituation created by the compulsion
	• <u>Medical Therapy</u>:
	  • <u>Antidepressants</u>: **SSRIs (fluoxetine, sertraline, citalopram) are first-line medications; higher-dose may be required**
	  • <u>Tricyclic Antidepressants</u>: **clomipramine** has potent and specific serotonergic effects
	    Other: memantine, lamotrigine, N-acetylcysteine, ketamine, topiramate, and glycine may be included as adjunctive medications

Key Words & Most Common	• Disorder characterized by intrusive thoughts with or without compensatory actions to alleviate the stress brought on by these thoughts • <u>Obsessions</u>: recurrent or intrusive thoughts, images, or urges • <u>Compulsions</u>: the drive to perform repetitive behaviors, rituals or mental acts to reduce the anxiety or prevent harm • Combination of CBT and ERP and medical therapy (SSRIs) is most effective treatment

Trichotillomania

Etiology & Risk Factors	• Disorder characterized by recurrent pulling out of one's hair resulting in hair loss • <u>Etiology</u>: multiple neuropsychiatric and cognitive components • <u>Risk Factors</u>: **female (90%), comorbid mental health condition (anxiety, stress, OCD and depression most common)**, traumatic or stressful life experiences, childhood abuse
Patho-physiology	• Neurotransmitter system abnormalities (serotonin) and alterations in the brain regions that involve impulse control, emotion regulation, and motor planning may play a role

Signs & Symptoms	• **Chronic pulling of the hair**
	  • Usually with hands, fingers or tweezers
	  • Most commonly involves the scalp, eyebrows, and eyelashes but can involve any body hair (beard, arm or leg hairs)
	  • Some may show ritualistic behavior; patient may inspect the hair, roll the hair between their fingers, pull the strands between their teeth, or chew/swallow their hair
	• <u>Physical Exam</u>:
	  • **Signs range from thinning hair, eyebrows or eyelashes to complete alopecia or fully missing eyelashes and/or eyebrows**
	  • May wear wigs, hates or scarves to hide areas of hair loss

Diagnostic Criteria	• **Patient actively removes hair from a body region, involving a concentrated or diffuse area that results in bald spots or thinning of the hair** • **Patient has made repeated attempts to decrease or stop the hair pulling** • **Patient experiences significant distress or impairment in functioning from the the hair-pulling** • **Hair loss is not caused by another medical condition (alopecia areata, tinea capitis)**

Treatment	• <u>Psychotherapy</u>: **cognitive behavior therapy with a focus on habit reversal therapy is most effect management**
	  • Utilizes awareness training, stimulus control and competing response training to identify cognitive distortions and develop stress-management techniques
	• <u>Medical Therapy</u>:
	  • <u>Antidepressants</u>: **SSRIs (fluoxetine, sertraline, citalopram)** show modest benefits
	  • N-acetylcysteine (a partial glutamatergic agonist) has shown some efficacy

Key Words & Most Common	• Disorder characterized by recurrent pulling out of one's hair resulting in hair loss • Female, comorbid anxiety, stress, OCD and/or depression most common risk factors • May have thinning of hair to complete alopecia or fully missing eyelashes/eyebrows • Cognitive behavior therapy focusing on habit reversal therapy

Hoarding Disorder

Etiology & Risk Factors	• Disorder characterized by a persistent difficulty to discard or part with possessions, regardless of their actual value resulting in accumulation of large number of possessions that may clutter living spaces to the point they may become unusable • <u>Etiology</u>: combination of genetic, environmental, and psychological factors • <u>Risk Factors</u>: **elderly, comorbid mental health condition (anxiety, stress, and depression most common)**, traumatic life experiences (death of a friend or family member),
Patho-physiology	• May be related to abnormal activity in certain brain regions, such as the anterior cingulate cortex and insula • Abnormalities in the serotonin system, which plays a role in regulating mood and anxiety • Underlying information-processing deficits, emotional attachment issues, behavioral avoidance, and inconsistent beliefs about the value or nature of possessions

Signs & Symptoms	• Strong desire to save or refusal to discard possessions regardless of value
	  • **Results in large accumulation of possessions that congest and clutter living space** (may become unusable)
	  • **Significant distress surrounding parting with the items** or contemplating parting with them
	  • **Inconsistent beliefs about the value of the possessions**
	• Results in significant social or occupational impairment (patient may restrict access to home and refuse family members, friends, handymen to enter due to embarrassment)
	• <u>Animal Hoarding</u>: accumulation of many animals without adequate nutrition, sanitation, and veterinary care despite deterioration in the health of the animals (weight loss, sickness) or environment (overcrowding, lack of sanitation)

Diagnostic Criteria	• Patients have persistent difficulty discarding or parting with possessions, regardless of their actual value • Difficulty discarding possessions is due to the perceived need to save the items and to the distress associated with parting The accumulated possessions congest and clutter active living areas resulting in compromised ability to use that space • Hoarding results in significant distress or impairment social, occupational or other areas of function

Treatment	• **Psychotherapy: cognitive behavioral therapy is most effective treatment**; difficult to address
	  • Focuses on helping the patient discard possessions, understand inherent value of the possessions, refrain from acquiring new possessions and improve their decision-making skills
	• <u>Medication Management</u>:
	  • <u>Antidepressants</u>: **SSRIs** (fluoxetine, sertraline, citalopram) show modest benefits if concurrent obsessive-compulsive disorder is present

Key Words & Most Common	• Disorder characterized by a persistent difficulty to discard or part with possessions, regardless of their actual value • Results in accumulation of large number of possessions that clutter living spaces to the point they are unusable • Results in significant social or occupational impairment • Cognitive behavioral therapy is most effective treatment

Excoriation (Skin-Picking) Disorder

Etiology & Risk Factors	• Disorder characterized by recurrent picking of one's skin resulting in skin lesions • <u>Etiology</u>: combination of genetic, environmental, and psychological factors • <u>Risk Factors</u>: **comorbid mental health condition (anxiety, body dysmorphic disorder), female, chronic stress**, personality traits (perfectionism), **substance abuse (stimulants)**
Patho-physiology	• Dysregulation of neurotransmitters, specifically dopamine and serotonin, in the brain's reward and impulse control center

Signs & Symptoms	• **Recurrent picking of one's skin**
	  • **May pick normal skin or minor lesions** (calluses, pimples, or scabs)
	  • **May be triggered by intrusive thoughts** (removal of a lesion that they perceive as unattractive or cancerous)
	• Patient may avoid social situations out of embarrassment
	• <u>Physical Exam</u>:
	  • **Multiple areas of self-inflicted skin trauma in various stages of healing**
	  • May result in scarring, infections, excessive bleeding
	  • May wear long sleeves, pants, gloves or makeup to cover skin lesions

Diagnostic Criteria	• **Visible skin lesions as a result of picking** • **Patient has made repeated attempts to decrease or stop the skin-picking** • **Patient experiences significant distress or impairment in functioning from the the skin-picking**

Treatment	• **Psychotherapy: cognitive behavioral therapy is most effective treatment**
	  • Focus on identification of triggers for skin picking, learn coping strategies to manage those triggers, and develop new, healthier behaviors to replace the skin picking
	• <u>Medical Therapy</u>:
	  • <u>Antidepressants</u>: **SSRIs** (fluoxetine, sertraline, citalopram) show modest benefits
	  • N-acetylcysteine (a partial glutamatergic agonist) has shown some efficacy

Key Words & Most Common	• Recurrent picking of one's skin • Visible skin lesions as a result of picking • Patient has made repeated attempts to decrease or stop the skin-picking • Patient experiences significant distress or impairment in functioning from the the skin-picking • Cognitive behavioral therapy is first-line treatment

Attention-Deficit/Hyperactivity (ADD/ADHD) Disorder

Etiology & Risk Factors	• **Neurodevelopmental disorder characterized by inattention, hyperactivity, and impulsivity that is not age-appropriate** • Etiology: combination of genetic, environmental, sensorimotor, physiologic, behavioral, and neurobiological factors • Risk Factors: **family history, male**, age (onset 4-12 years old), low birth weight, head trauma, iron deficiency, obstructive sleep apnea, lead exposure, prenatal exposure to alcohol, tobacco, or illicit drugs, **poor nutrition (diet high in sugar and processed foods and low in micronutrients), comorbid conduct and oppositional defiant disorders**
Patho-physiology	• Abnormalities in the anterior cingulate gyrus and dorsolateral prefrontal cortex which are involved in regulating attention, working memory, and impulse control • Imbalance of certain neurotransmitters, particularly dopamine and norepinephrine, which are responsible for regulating attention, motivation, and reward • Certain genes are related to dopamine signaling and neurotransmitter pathways identifying a familial component

Signs & Symptoms	• **Inattention**: signs appear with tasks that require mental vigilance, rapid reaction time, visual and perceptual recollection, and sustained listening
	• **Impulsivity: hasty actions that have the potential for a negative outcome** (running across street, suddenly quitting school or a job)
	• **Hyperactivity**: excessive activity; difficulty sitting still when it is appropriate (at church or school); **fidgeting, talkative, or restless behavior**
	• Physical Exam:
	   • **Difficulty sitting still on exam table** (frequently getting up and down, playing with table paper, grabbing at medical equipment)
	   • Motor incoordination or clumsiness, perceptual-motor dysfunction

Diagnostic Criteria

At least 6 signs of inattentiveness and/or 6 signs of hyperactivity/impulsivity and present for 6 or more months, not age-appropriate, occur in at least 2 settings (home and school), present before 12 years old, and interfere with function

Inattention	Hyperactivity and Impulsivity
• 1. Misses details or makes careless mistakes • 2. Difficulty sustaining attention on tasks • 3. Does not seem to listen when spoken to directly • 4. Does not follow directions or complete tasks • 5. Difficulty organizing tasks/activities • 6. Avoids or is reluctant to engage in tasks that require sustained mental effort • 7. Often loses things needed to complete activities and tasks • 8. Easily distracted • 9. Forgetful in daily activity	• 1. Fidgets and squirms in their seat • 2. Constantly in motion (often leaves seat) • 3. Runs or climbs when activity is inappropriate • 4. Difficulty playing quietly • 5. always on the go, touching or playing with everything • 6. Talks excessively • 7. Blurts out appropriate or inappropriate comments • 8. Difficulty waiting turn • 9. Interrupts or intrudes on others

Treatment	• **Lifestyle Modification**: regular exercise, adequate nutrition, sleep hygiene • **Behavioral Therapy: social skills training, classroom modifications and parent education;** strategies to improve organization, time management, and communication skills • **Stimulant Medications: methylphenidate, amphetamine/dextroamphetamine, dexmethylphenidate are first-line medical treatments** • Inhibits reuptake and increases availability of dopamine and norepinephrine in the extra-neuronal space to improve attention and reduce impulsivity/hyperactivity • **Non-Stimulant Medications: atomoxetine** (selective norepinephrine reuptake inhibitor), **guanfacine** (alpha-2 agonist), bupropion or venlafaxine (SNRIs) • Alternative Treatments: elimination diets, vitamin or nutritional supplementation, antioxidants, biochemical interventions have shown to be helpful in some cases

Autism Spectrum Disorder

Etiology & Risk Factors	• **Neurodevelopmental disorder characterized by impaired social interaction and communication, repetitive and stereotyped behavior, and uneven intellectual development** • Etiology: combination of genetic, environmental, sensorimotor, physiologic, behavioral, and neurobiological factors • Risk Factors: **male, family history**, advanced maternal/paternal age, **prematurity or low birth weight**, prenatal toxin exposure (pesticides, pollution), comorbid neurological conditions (epilepsy or tuberous sclerosis), **prenatal or perinatal complications** (hypoxia, infection, fetal distress)
Patho-physiology	• Not fully understood; may be related to abnormal neural connectivity, differences in the structure and function of the brain's reward system, and an imbalance in excitatory and inhibitory signaling

Signs & Symptoms	• **Social Communication and Interaction Deficits**:
	   • **Social/Emotional Reciprocity Deficits**: difficulty initiating or responding to social interactions or conversation, no sharing of emotions, no response to affection; difficulty understanding what is not explicitly stated (metaphors, humor, jokes)
	   • **Nonverbal Social Communication Deficits**: difficulty interpreting body language, gestures, facial expressions; avoiding eye contact, avoids social situations
	   • **Difficulty Developing and Maintaining Relationships**: difficulty making friends or adjusting behavior for different social situations
	• **Restricted, Repetitive, Stereotyped Behaviors, Interests and/or Activities**:
	   • **Repetitive Movements or Stereotyped Speech**: repeated hand flapping or finger flicking, repeating phrases or imitated speech, lining up toys
	   • **Strict Adherence to Routines and Rituals**: distress with changes in clothing, meals, or daily routines
	   • **Highly Restricted, Abnormally Intense, Fixated Interests**: engrossed with the vacuum cleaner
	   • **Extreme Reaction to Sensory Input**: abnormal sensitivity to visual, auditory or olfactory stimuli; unusual attachment to ordinary objects

Diagnostic Criteria	• Evidence of social interaction and communication impairment and 2 or more of the restricted, repetitive, stereotyped behaviors or interests described above

Treatment	• **Applied Behavioral Analysis: approach to therapy that includes specific cognitive, social, or behavioral skills that are taught in a stepwise fashion**
	   • Goal to improve, change, or develop specific behaviors (social, language and communication skills, reading, academics, hygiene, punctuality, and occupational skills)
	• **Speech and Language Therapy:** strategies are implemented to help compensate for focal deficits in motor function, motor planning, and sensory processing
	• Medication Management: indicated for more severe cases
	   • Atypical Antipsychotics: risperidone, aripiprazole; may treat behavioral problems (ritualistic, self-inflicted injuries, aggressive behavior)
	   • Selective Serotonin Reuptake Inhibitors (SSRIs): may help treat ritualistic behavior
	   • Mood Stabilizers: valproate; may treat self-inflicted injury and outburst behavior
	   • ADHD Medication: stimulant and non-stimulant medication for inattention, impulsivity and hyperactivity
	• Alternative Therapies: mixed efficacy
	   • Gluten-free diet, diet low in processed sugar/carbohydrates, vitamin supplementation (B6, B12, D); chelation, auditory integration and hyperbaric oxygen therapies

Cluster A	**Schizoid Personality Disorder**	
Etiology & Risk Factors	• Disorder is characterized by a pervasive pattern of voluntary social withdrawal, detachment, and general disinterest in social relationships and anhedonia introversion • Described as aloof, blunted affect, isolated, disengaged, and distant with a limited range of emotions in interpersonal relationships • <u>Etiology</u>: combination of genetic, environmental and neurobiological factors • <u>Risk Factors</u>: **childhood experiences (neglect, emotional abuse, and a lack of nurturing, socialization, or affection), male**, early life stressors, family history, social isolation	
Patho-physiology	• Not well understood; may be related to abnormal brain activity, specifically in the areas of the brain responsible for emotional processing and social interaction	
Signs & Symptoms	• <u>Social Withdrawal</u>: **isolation is predominant feature; little or no desire for close relationships** (no close friends, rarely date and seldom marry, little interest in sexual activity) • <u>Social Detachment</u>: **socially inept, aloof, disengaged, self-absorbed, distant, blunted affect with limited range of emotions**; do not react appropriately to major life events • <u>Significant Introversion</u>: prefers solitary activities (computer gaming), quiet, loner "hermit-like" behavior • <u>Anhedonia</u> : little pleasure in activities, rarely react or show emotion in social situations, lack response to praise or criticism	

Diagnostic Criteria	• Patients show detachment from and general disinterest in social relationships with limited expression of emotions in interpersonal interactions and ≥4 of the following:
	    • **No desire for or enjoyment of close relationships** (including family, friends, or intimate partners)
	    • **Strong preference of solitary activities**
	    • **Little interest in sexual relationships or intimacy**
	    • **Anhedonia** or general lack of enjoyment in any activity
	    • **No close friends or confidants**
	    • General indifference to praise or criticism by others
	    • Emotionally distant and disengaged with blunted affect	

Treatment	• **Psychotherapy: cognitive behavioral therapy with focus on acquiring social skills and developing general interests** • **Encouragement to share interests in topics (possessions, collections, hobbies, gaming) that may appeal to others with solitary preferences to establish a relationship and facilitate a therapeutic friendship** • <u>Medication Management</u>: short-term low-dose antipsychotics, antidepressants or psychostimulants have little efficacious studies • Prognosis is generally poor with little improvement over time	
Key Words & Most Common	• Disorder is characterized by a pervasive pattern of voluntary social withdrawal, detachment, and general disinterest in social relationships and anhedonia introversion • Family history of mental illness, childhood abuse/neglect, social isolation • Preference of solitary activities, lack of interest in close relationships, limited emotional and sexual expression, lack of enjoyment in activities • Psychotherapy to acquire social skills to facilitate therapeutic friendships	

Cluster A	**Schizotypal Personality Disorder**	
Etiology & Risk Factors	• Disorder characterized by pervasive pattern of discomfort and reduced capacity for personal relationships, distorted cognition, bizarre perceptions, and eccentric behavior • Similar to schizophrenia without psychosis (no hallucinations or delusions) • <u>Etiology</u>: combination of genetic, environmental and neurobiological factors • <u>Risk Factors</u>: **childhood abuse or neglect, social isolation**, prenatal and perinatal complications, family history of psychotic disorders, substance abuse	
Patho-physiology	• Not fully understood; may involve abnormalities in brain structure and function, including reduced gray matter volume and altered connectivity in regions associated with perception, language, and social cognition; dysregulation of dopaminergic and glutamatergic systems may contribute to the development of schizotypal features	
Signs & Symptoms	• Social isolation and discomfort, **peculiar behavior, unusual beliefs or magical thinking, odd speech or language**, and perceptual or cognitive distortions • Excessive social anxiety that does not diminish with familiarity, **odd beliefs or superstitions** • **Unusual perceptual experiences**, distorted cognition and reasoning • **Restricted range of emotions, inappropriate or flat affect**, have difficulty understanding and interpreting social cues	

Diagnostic Criteria	• Persistent pattern of intense discomfort and decreased capacity for close relationships, cognitive or perceptual distortions and eccentric behavior and ≥5 of the following:
	    • **Ideas of reference** (idea that everyday occurrences/items have a special significance) *without* delusions of reference (similar ideas held with more conviction)
	    • **Odd beliefs or magical thinking** (belief in clairvoyance, telepathy, superstition, having a sixth sense, preoccupation with paranormal phenomena, fantasies)
	    • **Unusual perceptual experiences**
	    • **Odd thoughts, speech and/or language** (excessively elaborate or metaphorical)
	    • Suspicious or paranoid thoughts
	    • Incongruous or restricted affect
	    • **Peculiar, eccentric behavior and appearance**
	    • No close friends or confidants
	    • Excessive social anxiety that does not diminish with familiarity	

Treatment	• <u>Psychotherapy</u>: **first-line treatment; combination of cognitive behavioral, individual and/or group therapy**
	    • **Goal is to reduce subjective stress, enable patient to understand internal problems, decrease abnormal behavior, and modify specific problematic traits/behaviors**
	    • Increase awareness how behavior may be perceived by others
	• <u>Medication Management</u>: atypical antipsychotics indicated for psychotic episodes or suspiciousness; antidepressants indicated to alleviate comorbid anxiety	

Key Words & Most Common	• Disorder characterized by pervasive pattern of discomfort and reduced capacity for personal relationships, distorted cognition, bizarre perceptions, and eccentric behavior • Childhood abuse or neglect, social isolation are greatest risk factors • Ideas of reference without delusions, odd beliefs or magical thinking, unusual perceptual experiences, odd thoughts/speech/language, peculiar or eccentric behavior • Psychotherapy is first-line	

Cluster A	# Paranoid Personality Disorder 🧠
Etiology & Risk Factors	• Disorder characterized by a pervasive pattern of unwarranted distrust and suspicion of others that involves interpreting other's motives as malicious behavior • Etiology: combination of genetic, environmental and neurobiological factors • Risk Factors: **childhood abuse or neglect, male, family history of psychotic disorders, history of interpersonal conflict or violence**, history of repeated betrayals experienced by others, **certain personality traits** (suspiciousness, hostility, and rigidity), substance abuse
Patho-physiology	• Not fully understood; may be related to abnormalities in brain regions related to processing emotions, leading to heightened vigilance and mistrust of others
Signs & Symptoms	• **Pervasive distrust and suspicion that others are planning to harm, deceive, or exploit them** • Secondary to distrust in others, they may feel a need to be in control and autonomous over situations • Unjustified feeling they may be attacked • **Reluctance to confide in others** due to a fear that the information will be used against them • **Hypervigilant about potential insults, threats, and disloyalty** • **Reading into hidden meanings of innocent remarks or events and holding grudges for perceived slights** • **Jealousy in intimate relationships**

Diagnostic Criteria	• **Persistent distrust and suspiciousness of others with 4 or more of the following:**
	  • Unjustified suspicion that others are planning to harm, deceive, or exploit them
	  • Preoccupation with unjustified doubts about the reliability of others
	  • Reluctance to confide in others due to fear that information will be used against them
	  • Misinterpretation of innocent remarks or events as having hidden hostile or threatening meaning
	  • Holding of grudges, does not easily forgive others
	  • Perception of attacks on his or her character or reputation and may react angrily or counterattack
	  • Unjustified suspicions that their spouse or partner is unfaithful

Treatment	• **Psychotherapy: first-line treatment; combination of cognitive behavioral, individual and/or group therapy** • **Goal is to reduce subjective stress, enable patient to understand internal problems, decrease abnormal behavior, and modify specific problematic traits/behaviors** • Medication Management: atypical antipsychotics indicated for excessive suspiciousness; antidepressants indicated to alleviate comorbid anxiety
Key Words & Most Common	• Pervasive distrust and suspicion that others are planning to harm, deceive, or exploit them; reluctance to confide in others, hypervigilance about insults or threates, reading into hidden meanings of innocent actions, jealousy and holding of grudges • Childhood abuse or neglect, family history, history of interpersonal conflict/violence or repeated betrayals are greatest risk factors • Psychotherapy is first-line

Cluster B	# Antisocial Personality Disorder 🧠
Etiology & Risk Factors	• Disorder characterized by a pervasive pattern of disregard for consequences and for the rights of others with behaviors that deviate sharply from the norms of society • Etiology: combination of genetic, environmental, and social factors • Risk Factors: **childhood abuse, neglect or trauma, male,** family history, low-socioeconomic status, **lack of parental supervision as child, association with delinquent peers during adolescence,** history of comorbid mental health disorder, **substance abuse**
Patho-physiology	• Not fully understood; impulsive aggression may be related to abnormal serotonin transporter functioning; patients may have structural and functional abnormalities in certain areas of the brain, particularly those involved in decision-making and empathy
Signs & Symptoms	• **Behavior that deviates sharply from the norms, values and laws of society** • **May demonstrate disregard for others and the law by destroying property, hostility towards others, or criminal acts (stealing)** • **May seemingly be nice and charismatic to those that do not know their history** • **Impulsivity;** does not have ample thought or consideration of consequences or safety of self or others (binge drinking, taking large amounts of drugs, drunk driving) • **Socially and financially irresponsible** (frequently changes jobs, homes, relationships; failure to pay bills) • **Easily provoked with aggression towards others** (getting into fights, assaults, road rage etc.)

Diagnostic Criteria	• **Persistent disregard for the rights of others, be at least 18 years old with a history of conduct disorder by 15 years old and 3 or more of the following:**
	  • Failure to comply with social norms and disregard and violation of the rights of others and committing unlawful acts
	  • Deceitful; frequently lying, using of aliases, or exploiting others for personal pleasure or gain
	  • Impulsive behavior
	  • Easily provoked or aggressive towards others
	  • Recklessness and disregard for the safety of self or others
	  • Consistently acting irresponsible
	  • Lack of remorse for actions

Treatment	• **Psychotherapy: first-line treatment; cognitive behavioral therapy** • **Goal is to establish limits, modify specific problematic traits/behaviors, and avoiding actions that have legal consequences** • Medication Management: mood stabilizers, antidepressants, antipsychotics may be indicated based on symptoms; avoid medications with abusive potential
Key Words & Most Common	• Pervasive pattern of disregard for consequences and for the rights of others with behaviors that deviate sharply from the norms of society • Childhood abuse, neglect or trauma is greatest risk factor • Stealing, binge drinking, drunk driving, impulsivity, assaults, road rage, frequently changes jobs/relationships, financially irresponsible • Psychotherapy is first-line

Cluster B	Borderline Personality Disorder
Etiology & Risk Factors	• Disorder characterized by a pervasive pattern of unstable/unpredictable mood and affect that causes instability in relationships, self-image, and mood • Etiology: combination of genetic, environmental, and social factors • Risk Factors: **childhood abuse, neglect or trauma, female**, family history, history of unstable or chaotic relationships or repeated betrayals or interpersonal conflicts, history of comorbid mental health disorder, **certain personality traits** (emotional instability, impulsivity, and a tendency to experience intense emotions)
Patho-physiology	• Not fully understood; abnormalities in several areas of the brain, including the limbic system and prefrontal cortex, which are involved in regulating emotions and behavior; dysfunction in the neurotransmitter systems, including serotonin and dopamine
Signs & Symptoms	• **Feeling of abandonment or neglect associated with an intense fear or anger** • **Changing views of others abruptly and dramatically**; "black-and-white thinking" (thinking in polarizing extremes of good and bad, splitting) • May idealize relationship early and then suddenly feels that the other person does not care enough then becomes disillusioned and belittles/becomes angry with them • **Difficulty controlling anger**; often becomes inappropriate and intensely angry • **Changes in mood** (dysphoria, irritability, anxiety) • **Self-sabotaging behavior** (dropping out of school early, preemptively ending a promising relationship); fear of abandonment • **Impulsivity leading to self-damaging behaviors** (substance abuse, reckless driving, binge eating, spending, self-mutilation) • May have dissociative episodes, paranoid thoughts

Diagnostic Criteria	• **Persistent pattern of unstable relationships, self-image, and emotions (emotional dysregulation) and pronounced impulsivity and 5 or more of the following:**
	   • Desperate efforts to avoid abandonment
	   • Unstable and intense relationships that alternate between idealizing and devaluing the other person
	   • Unstable self-image
	   • Impulsivity in self-damage behaviors
	   • Repeated suicidal behavior and/or gestures or threats
	   • Persistent feelings of emptiness
	   • Rapid changes in mood
	   • Inappropriately intense anger or problems controlling anger
	   • Temporary paranoid thoughts or severe dissociative symptoms exacerbated by stress

Treatment	• **Psychotherapy: first-line treatment; cognitive behavioral therapy** with focus on emotional dysregulation social skills; dialectical behavioral therapy • Goal is to teach skills to manage emotions, set goals, manage negative expectations, identify support network • Medication Management: mood stabilizers, antidepressants, antipsychotics may be indicated based on symptoms; avoid medications with abusive potential
Key Words & Most Common	• Mental health disorder characterized by instability in emotions, relationships and self-image • Intense and unstable emotions, impulsivity, fear of abandonment, self-har, suicidal behavior • Psychotherapy is first-line

Cluster B	Histrionic Personality Disorder
Etiology & Risk Factors	• Disorder is characterized by a pervasive pattern of excessive emotionality and attention seeking behavior • Etiology: combination of genetic, environmental, and social factors • Risk Factors: **childhood abuse, neglect or trauma, female**, family history, **negative childhood experiences (lack of attention or validation)**, history of comorbid mental health disorder, history of unstable or chaotic relationships, **certain personality traits** (emotional instability, impulsivity, and tendency to seek out attention/validation from others)
Patho-physiology	• Not fully understood; genetic predisposition and environmental factors (childhood trauma or neglect) contribute to the formation of maladaptive personality traits that may lead to the development of histrionic personality disorder
Signs & Symptoms	• **Attention-seeking behavior;** demand to be the center of attention • **Lively, dramatic, overly emotional, seductive, enthusiastic, flirtatious behavior** • **Inappropriate clothing, seductive and sexually provocative behavior** • **Emotional expression is often dramatic and exaggerated** • **Seeks reassurance and praise;** easily influenced by others and trends • **Hyperinflated relationships;** may believe relationships are closer than they really are

Diagnostic Criteria	• **Persistent pattern of excessive emotionality and attention seeking behavior with 5 or more of the following:**
	   • Desire to be center of attention
	   • Inappropriately sexually seductive or provocative interaction with others
	   • Shallow emotional expression
	   • Consistent use of physical appearance to gain attention
	   • Impressionistic and vague speech
	   • Self-dramatization, theatricality, and extravagant emotional expression
	   • Easily influenced by others or situations
	   • Belief that relationships are more intimate than they are

Treatment	• **Psychotherapy: first-line treatment; cognitive behavioral therapy** with focus on underlying internal conflicts • Goal is to substitute speech for behavior, teach communications skills to be less dramatic and help patient understand their behavior is a maladaptive way to attract attention and manage their self-esteem; help patient understand and manage emotions and behaviors • Medication Management: mood stabilizers, antidepressants, antipsychotics may be indicated based on symptoms; avoid medications with abusive potential
Key Words & Most Common	• Characterized by a pervasive pattern of excessive emotionality and attention seeking behavior • Need for attention, exaggerated emotions, inappropriate seductiveness, overly dramatic behavior • Seeks reassurance and praise, inappropriate clothing and sexually provocative behavior • Psychotherapy is first-line

Cluster B	# Narcissistic Personality Disorder	
Etiology & Risk Factors	• **Disorder characterized by a pervasive pattern of grandiosity, excessive sense of self-importance, superiority, need for admiration and lack of empathy** • Etiology: combination of genetic, environmental, cultural and social factors • Risk Factors: **childhood abuse or trauma, childhood experiences** (lack of empathy and validation), **history of overvaluation and overindulgence** (excessively praised and overvalued by their parents or caregivers), cultural factors (emphasis on individualism and success), **certain personality traits** (grandiose sense of self-importance, a lack of empathy, sense of entitlement)	
Patho-physiology	• Not fully understood; may be associated with abnormalities in brain regions involved in empathy, self-reflection, and emotional regulation. These abnormalities may result in the characteristic traits such as grandiosity, lack of empathy, and a sense of entitlement	
Signs & Symptoms	• **Overestimation of their abilities** • **Exaggerate of their achievements** (may imply an underestimation of the worth and achievements of others) • **Fantasy of great achievements** (desire to be admired for their intelligence, beauty, prestige, accomplishments, success, and influence) • **Inflated self-image** (belief that they are special, entitled, and may feel as though they should only associate with others that are as special or talented) • **Fragile self-esteem** (sensitive and bothered by criticism, loss of power; may feel humiliated with defeat or failure) • **Lack of empathy** (may react to situations with rage)	

Diagnostic Criteria	• **Persistent pattern of grandiosity, need for admiration, and lack of empathy with 5 or more of the following:**
	  • An exaggerated, unfounded sense of their own importance and talents (grandiosity)
	  • Preoccupation with fantasies of unlimited achievements, money, influence, power, intelligence, beauty, or perfect relationship
	  • Belief that they are special and unique and should only associate with people of the highest caliber
	  • Desire to be unconditionally admired
	  • Sense of entitlement
	  • Lack of empathy
	  • Envy of others with a belief that others envy them
	  • Arrogance and haughtiness	

Treatment	• Psychotherapy: first-line treatment; cognitive behavioral therapy with focus on underlying internal conflicts • Goal is to increase self awareness, develop empathy, improve interpersonal relationships and address underlying emotional issues • Medication Management: mood stabilizers, antidepressants, antipsychotics may be indicated based on symptoms; avoid medications with abusive potential	
Key Words & Most Common	• **Disorder characterized by a pervasive pattern of grandiosity, excessive sense of self-importance, superiority, need for admiration and lack of empathy** • Childhood abuse/trauma/experiences, history of overvaluation and overindulgence • Exaggerated sense of achievements, inflated self-image, fragile self-esteem, lack of empathy • Psychotherapy is first-line	

Cluster C	# Avoidant Personality Disorder	
Etiology & Risk Factors	• **Disorder characterized by the avoidance of social situations or interactions due to an intense fear of rejection, criticism, or humiliation** • Etiology: combination of genetic, environmental, cultural and social factors • Risk Factors: **childhood abuse or trauma, childhood experiences** (repeated rejection or criticism from parents or peers), **lack of social support or positive reinforcement**, cultural factors (emphasis on conformity and fitting in), **certain personality traits** (shyness, social anxiety, and low self-esteem)	
Patho-physiology	• Not fully understood; some studies implicate an overactive amygdala, which may contribute to excessive fear and avoidance of social situations or reduced activity in the prefrontal cortex, which may lead to difficulties in regulating emotions and social behavior	
Signs & Symptoms	• **Social inhibition** (avoiding social interaction; may refuse promotion out of fear coworkers will criticize them, avoid parties, avoid making new friends) • **Timid or shy behavior with a lack of confidence** • **Low self-esteem and a sense of inadequacy** • **Relative isolation** • **Emotional sensitivity** (sensitive to criticism, rejection, insults, jokes)	

Diagnostic Criteria	• **Persistent pattern of avoiding social interaction, feeling inadequate, and being hypersensitive to criticism and rejection with 4 or more of the following:**
	  • Avoidance of occupation-related activities involving social contact due to fear of criticism, rejection or disapproval
	  • Unwillingness to interact with people unless they are certain of being liked
	  • Cautious of close relationships due to fear of ridiculed or humiliation
	  • Preoccupation with being criticized or rejected in social situations
	  • Inferiority or inadequacy complex
	  • Self-assessment as socially incompetent, unappealing, or inferior to others
	  • Reluctance to take new risks or participate in new activities out of fear of embarrassment	

Treatment	• Psychotherapy: first-line treatment; cognitive behavioral therapy with focus on social skills • Goal is to increase self-esteem, develop coping skills, build social skills, and address underlying emotional issues • Medication Management: antidepressants, anxiolytics may be indicated based on symptoms; avoid medications with abusive potential	
Key Words & Most Common	• Disorder characterized by the avoidance of social situations or interactions due to an intense fear of rejection, criticism, or humiliation • Social inhibitions, timid or shy behavior, lack of confidence, low self-esteem, emotional sensitivity • Psychotherapy is first-line	

Cluster C	**Dependent Personality Disorder** 🧠
Etiology & Risk Factors	• Disorder characterized by a pervasive, excessive need to be taken care of, leading to submissive and clinging behaviors • <u>Etiology</u>: combination of genetic, environmental, cultural and social factors • <u>Risk Factors</u>: **childhood abuse or trauma, childhood experiences** (overprotective or controlling parenting results in persistent fear of abandonment and an excessive need for approval and support), **lack of social support or positive reinforcement** (results in reliance on others for decision-making), cultural factors (gender-role stereotypes), **certain personality traits** (low self-esteem, anxiousness, and passivity)
Pathophysiology	• Not fully understood; may have abnormalities in the brain regions (amygdala, hypothalamus, prefrontal cortex, insula, cingulate cortex) associated with stress, anxiety, and fear as a result of early life trauma or adverse experiences
Signs & Symptoms	• **Submissive behavior** (do not think they can care for themselves; use submissive behavior to get others to care for them) • **Need for reassurance and advice when making decisions** (may let others make decisions in all aspects of life) • **Inferiority complex** (take criticism or disapproval as proof of incompetence) • **Lack of independence** (difficulty initiating new tasks or working by themselves) • **Approval seeking behavior** (goes to great lengths to obtain approval) • **Dependent relationships** (immediately try to find new relationship when one ends)

Diagnostic Criteria	• **Persistent, excessive need to be taken of, resulting in submissiveness and clinging and 5 or more of the following:**
	  • Difficulty making decisions without an advice and reassurance from others
	  • Need to hold others responsible for most important aspects of their life
	  • Difficulty expressing disagreement with others due to fear or disapproval
	  • Difficulty initiating projects or tasks independently because they are not confident in their judgment and/or abilities
	  • Going to great lengths to obtain approval and support of others
	  • Feelings of intense discomfort or helplessness when alone due to fear of being unable to care for themselves
	  • Urgent need to establish a new relationship with someone who will care for and support when a close relationship ends
	  • Unrealistic preoccupation with fears of being left to take care of themselves

Treatment	• <u>Psychotherapy</u>: **first-line treatment; cognitive behavioral therapy** with focus on examining fears of independence and difficulties with assertiveness • Goal is to increase self-esteem, develop coping skills, build self-reliance, and address underlying emotional issues • <u>Medication Management</u>: antidepressants, anxiolytics may be indicated based on symptoms; avoid medications with abusive potential
Key Words & Most Common	• **Disorder characterized by a pervasive, excessive need to be taken care of, leading to submissive and clinging behaviors** • Childhood abuse/trauma/experiences, lack of social support or positive reinforcement are greatest risk factors • Submissive behavior, need for reassurance and advance for decision making, inferiority complex, lack of independence, approval seeking behavior, dependent relationships • Psychotherapy is first-line

Cluster C	**Obsessive-Compulsive Personality Disorder** 🧠
Etiology & Risk Factors	• Disorder characterized by a pervasive preoccupation with orderliness, perfectionism, and control without obsessions or compulsions • <u>Etiology</u>: combination of genetic, environmental, cultural and social factors • <u>Risk Factors</u>: **childhood abuse or trauma, male, childhood experiences** (parental criticism or over-control,), **high stress or traumatic experiences** (results in developing rigid coping mechanisms), cultural factors (emphasis on achievement and success), **certain personality traits** (perfectionism, rigidity, and excessive conscientiousness)
Pathophysiology	• Not fully understood; may be related to alterations in brain circuits involved in reward, motivation, and decision-making; dysfunction in the cortico-striatal-thalamo-cortical (CSTC) circuitry, which regulates repetitive behaviors and cognitive flexibility
Signs & Symptoms	• **Preoccupation with order, perfectionism and control of situations**; interferes with flexibility and effectiveness • **Rigid and stubborn** (insist that everything be done in a certain, specific way; results in difficulty delegating tasks) • **Intense focus on rules, details, procedures, schedules and lists in order to maintain control**; often plan far in advance • **Preoccupation with details** (may result in incomplete or delayed work completion) • **Tightly controlled affection** (may relate to others in a formal, stiff or serious manner)

Diagnostic Criteria	• **Persistent pattern of preoccupation with order, perfectionism, and control of self, others and/or situations with 4 or more of the following:**
	  • Preoccupation with order, details, rules, schedules, organization and lists
	  • Drive and desire for perfection interferes with completion of the task
	  • Excessive devotion to work and productivity results in neglect of leisure activities and social interaction
	  • Excessive conscientiousness, fastidiousness and inflexibility regarding ethical and moral issues and values
	  • Unwillingness to discard worn-out or worthless objects (even with no inherent or sentimental value)
	  • Reluctance to delegate or work with others and insists upon having things be done in a certain, specific way
	  • A miserly approach to spending for themselves and others because they see money as something to be saved for future endeavors
	  • Rigid, stubborn, serious or restricted affect

Treatment	• <u>Psychotherapy</u>: **first-line treatment; cognitive behavioral therapy** with focus on developing a greater sense of self-awareness, flexibility, and emotional resilience
	  • Goal is to increase self-awareness, develop coping skills, increasing flexibility and address underlying emotional issue
	  • *Therapy may be difficult due to patient's rigidity, stubbornness and need for control*
	• <u>Medication Management</u>: antidepressants, anxiolytics may be indicated based on symptoms; avoid medications with abusive potential

Key Words & Most Common	• Disorder characterized by a pervasive preoccupation with orderliness, perfectionism, and control without obsessions or compulsions • Preoccupation with order, perfectionism and control of situations; rigid and stubborn behavior, intense focus on rules, details, lists, procedures, preoccupation with details, tightly controlled affection • Psychotherapy is first-line

Delusional Disorder

Etiology & Risk Factors	• Disorder characterized by firmly held false beliefs (delusions) persisting for at least 1 month, *without* other symptoms of psychosis • <u>Etiology</u>: combination of genetic, environmental, and psychological factors • <u>Risk Factors</u>: **family history, substance abuse, traumatic life events** (physical or sexual abuse), **high levels of stress**, cultural factors (belief in supernatural or paranormal experiences), **pre-existing mental illness**
Patho-physiology	• Not fully understood; may be related to abnormalities in the brain's processing of information and its perception of reality; certain brain regions (prefrontal cortex and limbic system) may be involved in the development of delusional beliefs; abnormalities in neurotransmitters such as dopamine, serotonin, and glutamate have been implicated • <u>Nonbizarre Delusion</u>: involving situations that could occur (being followed, poisoned, infected, stalked, or deceived by partner) • <u>Bizarre Delusion</u>: involve implausible situations (believing that someone removed their internal organs)

Signs & Symptoms	• **Feeling of being exploited**
	• **Preoccupation with trustworthiness or loyalty of acquaintances**
	• **Perceived threats from benign remarks or events**
	• **Persistent bearing of grudges with a readiness to respond to perceived slights**
	• <u>Several Subtypes:</u>
	   • **Erotomania**: belief that another person is in love with them
	   • **Grandiose**: belief that they have a grandiose talent or have made an important discovery
	   • **Jealous**: belief that their spouse, partner or lover is unfaithful
	   • **Persecutory**: belief that they are being plotted against, spied on, maligned or harassed
	   • **Somatic**: delusion related to a bodily function (physical deformity, odor, disease, syndrome or parasite)

Diagnostic Criteria	• **At least 1 delusion lasting for 1 or more months without other psychotic symptoms and no significant impairment in function** • **Behavior is not obviously bizarre or odd** • Does not meet criteria for schizophrenia • Symptoms are not related to substance abuse, medical condition or other psychiatric disorder
Treatment	• <u>Atypical Antipsychotics</u>: **risperidone or olanzapine are first-line medical management**; indicated to reduce the intensity of the delusions and associated symptoms • <u>Psychotherapy</u>: **cognitive-behavioral therapy (CBT)** with focus on identifying and challenging the delusions and developing a more realistic and adaptive thought process • <u>Hospitalization</u>: may be necessary to ensure the individual's safety; delusions may cause them to engage in dangerous behaviors
Key Words & Most Common	• **Disorder characterized by firmly held false beliefs (delusions) persisting for at least 1 month, *without* other symptoms of psychosis** • Feeling exploited, untrustworthy of others, perceived threats from benign remarks or events, persistent bearing of grudges • Erotomania, grandiose, jealousy, persecutory, somatic subtypes • Atypical antipsychotics (risperidone or olanzapine) is first-line + psychotherapy

Schizophrenia

Etiology & Risk Factors	• **Psychotic disorder characterized by hallucinations, delusions and abnormal/disturbed thought, perception, behavior and emotion** • <u>Etiology</u>: combination of genetic, environmental, and neurological factors • <u>Risk Factors</u>: **family history (strong genetic predisposition), substance abuse** (nicotine, alcohol, cannabis, cocaine), **childhood trauma, abuse, or neglect**, prenatal and perinatal exposures (exposure to viral infections, malnutrition, complications during pregnancy or delivery), urban living, **social isolation**
Patho-physiology	• Dysregulation of several neurotransmitters, including dopamine, glutamate, and GABA; may be related to excess dopamine in the mesolimbic and mesocortical pathways • Abnormalities in brain structure and function (enlarged cerebral ventricles, thinning of the cortex, decreased size of the anterior hippocampus and other brain regions)

Signs & Symptoms	• <u>**Positive Symptoms**</u>: symptoms are "added to" normal behavior
	   • **Hallucinations**: sensory perceptions that are not perceived by anyone else; may be auditory (most common), visual, olfactory, gustatory or tactile
	   • **Delusions**: false beliefs that are held and maintained despite clear contradictory evidence; may be persecutory, grandiose, reference, control, jealousy, nihilism
	   • **Disorganized Speech**: thoughts are disconnected and tangentially rambling
	• <u>**Negative (Deficit) Symptoms**</u>: symptoms "take away" from normal behavior
	   • **Cognitive Deficits**: impaired attention, processing speed, working memory, abstract thinking, executive function, problem solving, understanding social interaction
	   • **Blunted Affect**: poor eye contact, lack of spontaneous movement, lack of vocal inflections, lack of facial expression, flat affect
	   • **Alogia**: poverty of speech (speaks sparingly), increased latency of response
	   • **Avolition**: decreased initiative, failure of appropriate role responsibilities, poor hygiene and grooming, lack of motivation, inability to set goals
	   • **Anhedonia**: lack of interest in activities, intimacy, or sex
	   • **Asociality**: socially withdrawn, little interest in relationships and failure to engage with others socially

Diagnostic Criteria	• **2 or more of the characteristic symptoms (delusions, hallucinations, disorganized speech, disorganized behavior, negative symptoms) for at least 6 months** • Prodromal or attenuated signs of illness with social, occupational or self-care impairments evident for at least 6 months including 1 month of active symptoms • Symptoms cause significant impairment of social or occupational functioning • Symptoms are not related to substance abuse, medical condition or other psychiatric disorder • <u>Neuroimaging</u>: CT scan may demonstrate ventricular enlargement (lateral and third), decreased cortical volume and grey matter, abnormal white mater • *Consider toxicology screen, CBC, CMP, ECG, fasting glucose as part of acute psychosis workup*

Treatment	• <u>**Second-Generation (Atypical) Antipsychotics**</u>: **risperidone, quetiapine or olanzapine are first-line medical management**
	   • Lower risk of extrapyramidal side effects but carry increased risk of metabolic syndrome development
	• <u>**First-Generation (Typical) Antipsychotics**</u>: **haloperidol, droperidol, fluphenazine**
	   • More effective for positive symptoms and minimally effective on negative symptoms
	   • Increased risk of extrapyramidal symptoms, tardive dyskinesia and neuroleptic malignant syndrome
	• <u>Psychotherapy</u>: **cognitive-behavioral therapy (CBT)**, psychosocial skill training and vocational rehabilitation programs, skills training, individual, family and group therapy
	• <u>Acute Psychosis</u>: hospitalization may be necessary to ensure the individual's safety; agitation and hallucinations may cause them to engage in dangerous behaviors
	   • **Haloperidol**, risperidone, olanzapine indicated in extremely agitated psychosis

Post-Traumatic Stress Disorder (PTSD) 🧠

Etiology & Risk Factors	• Disorder characterized by recurring, intrusive recollections of an overwhelming traumatic event
	• <u>Etiology</u>: **exposure to actual or threatened death, serious injury or sexual violence**
	   • <u>**Direct Experience**</u>: serious injury or the threat of death of self
	   • <u>**Indirect Experience**</u>: witnessing others being seriously injured, killed, or threatened with death; learning of events that occurred to close family members or friends
	• <u>Risk Factors</u>: **exposure to trauma (combat, sexual assault, natural disaster or serious injury), childhood abuse, trauma, or neglect,** history of mental health condition, lack of social support, substance abuse, social isolation

Patho-physiology	• Dysregulation of the hypothalamic-pituitary-adrenal (HPA) axis, which controls the body's stress response, leads to a prolonged and exaggerated stress response • Altered neurotransmitter function (GABA, glutamate, serotonin, neuropeptide Y, and endogenous opioids) have been implicated
Signs & Symptoms	• <u>**Intrusive Thoughts**</u>: **recurrent, unwanted, and distressing memories of the traumatic event;** flashbacks/nightmares in which the person feels/acts as if the event is recurring • <u>**Avoidance**</u>: **avoiding stimuli associated with the traumatic event** such as places, people, situations including feelings or thoughts that trigger memories related to the event • <u>**Negative Alterations in Mood and Cognition**</u>: **negative changes in beliefs or feelings about oneself or others**; distorted feelings of blame or guilt, persistent negative emotions, inability to remember important aspects of the traumatic event • <u>**Hyperarousal**</u>: **hypervigilance, irritability, and exaggerated startle response resulting in difficulty concentrating or sleeping and feeling constantly on edge**

Diagnostic Criteria	• **Direct or indirect exposure to a traumatic event and have symptoms from each of the following categories for more than 1 month**
	   • <u>**Intrusion Symptoms**</u>: recurrent, involuntary, intrusive, disturbing memories or dreams ranging from flashbacks to losing awareness of the present surroundings
	   • <u>**Avoidance Symptoms**</u>: avoiding thoughts, feelings, memories, activities, places, conversations, or people associated with the event
	   • <u>**Negative Effects on Cognition and Mood**</u>: dissociative amnesia, inability to remember important aspects of the event, negative feelings of self, world or others, anhedonia, negative emotions (horror, anger, shame/guilt), feeling detached
	   • <u>**Altered Arousal and Reactivity**</u>: difficulty sleeping, irritability or angry, reckless or self-destructive behavior, difficulty concentrating, hypervigilance

Treatment	• <u>**Psychotherapy**</u>: **cognitive behavioral therapy (CBT), prolonged exposure therapy, and eye movement desensitization and reprocessing (EMDR)**
	   • Goal is to help the individual process and overcome their traumatic memories; help modify critical and punitive attitude associated with survivor guilt
	• <u>Medical Management</u>:
	   • **SSRIs are first line medical treatment**
	   • **Prazosin** may be used for nightmares and hypervigilance
	   • **Trazodone** may be used for insomnia
	   • TCAs, MAO inhibitors and atypical antipsychotics may be considered based on symptoms

Key Words & Most Common	• **Disorder characterized by recurring, intrusive recollections of an overwhelming traumatic event** • Exposure to trauma, childhood abuse/neglect, mental health history, lack of social support, substance abuse, and social isolation are greatest risk factors • Dysregulation of the hypothalamic-pituitary-adrenal (HPA) axis and altered neurotransmitter function • Intrusive thoughts, avoidance, negative mood and cognition, and hyperarousal • Treatment options include psychotherapy (CBT, prolonged exposure therapy, EMDR) and medical management (SSRIs, prazosin for nightmares, trazodone for insomnia)

Adjustment Disorder 🧠

Etiology & Risk Factors	• **Disorder characterized by maladaptive emotional and/or behavioral symptoms/reaction caused by an identifiable stressor** • <u>Etiology</u>: combination of biological, psychological and environmental factors • <u>Risk Factors</u>: **exposure to a stressful or traumatic event (loss of a loved one, relationship issues, financial difficulties, job loss, moving, starting college, changing jobs),** pre-existing mental health conditions, **lack of social support,** certain personality traits (neuroticism or low emotional stability), chronic stress, low socioeconomic status
Patho-physiology	• Abnormal stress response resulting in inappropriate release of cortisol, epinephrine and norepinephrine, leading to emotional and behavioral symptoms • Alterations in the hypothalamic-pituitary-adrenal (HPA) axis and sympathetic nervous system function have been implicated
Signs & Symptoms	• **Depressed mood** (feeling sad, crying episodes) • **Anxiety or nervousness** • **Misconduct** (feeling overwhelmed, difficulty concentrating, social withdrawal) • **Behavioral Symptoms** (sleeping too much or too little, changes in appetite, anhedonia)

Diagnostic Criteria	• **Emotional or behavioral symptoms within 3 months of exposure to a stressor and 1 or more of the following:**
	   • **Marked distress that is out of proportion to the stressor**
	   • **Symptoms significantly impair social or occupational functioning**

Treatment	• <u>**Lifestyle Modification**</u>: **stress management and relaxation techniques, mindfulness,** physical exercise, adequate nutrition, sleep hygiene, avoiding drugs, alcohol and tobacco • <u>**Psychotherapy**</u>: **brief psychotherapy, cognitive behavioral therapy, and/or supportive psychotherapy is initial management of choice** • Goal to explore emotions, identify sources of stress and develop coping strategies • *Medications only used in selected cases but do not have clear evidence supporting use*
Key Words & Most Common	• Characterized by maladaptive emotional and/or behavioral symptoms/reaction caused by an identifiable stressor • Depressed mood, anxiety or nervousness, misconduct, and emotional or behavioral symptoms • Lifestyle modification such as stress management, relaxation techniques, and physical exercise can help manage symptoms • Psychotherapy, including brief psychotherapy and cognitive-behavioral therapy, is the initial management of choice; medications are only used in selected cases

Illness Anxiety Disorder

Etiology & Risk Factors	• Disorder characterized by preoccupation with having or acquiring a serious medical illness or disorder • Also known as **hypochondriasis** • <u>Etiology</u>: combination of biological, psychological, and environmental factors • <u>Risk Factors</u>: **family history, childhood trauma or abuse, history of a serious medical illness or disorder, major life stressor** (divorce, loss of job), certain personality traits (poor coping skills, difficulty managing stress, perfectionism), health-related anxiety, social isolation, lack of social support
Patho-physiology	• Not fully understood; may be related to altered response to stress and illness-related cues in the brain including misinterpretation of non-pathologic physical symptoms or normal bodily functions
Signs & Symptoms	• **High level of concern and excessive worry, fear and anxiety about their health** • **Misinterpreting bodily sensations or mild symptoms as signs of a serious illness** (gas pains, abdominal bloating, sweating, etc.) • **Frequently checking for physical signs of illness or disease** (looking at their throat in a mirror, checking their skin for lesions) • **Care seeking** (frequently seeking reassurance from medical professionals, family members or friends about their health status ["doctor shopping"]) • **Undergoing unnecessary medical procedures** • **Constantly researching about various illnesses and disease and their symptoms**
Diagnostic Criteria	• Patient is preoccupied with having or acquiring a serious illness with no or minimal somatic symptoms • Patient is highly anxious about health and easily alarmed about personal health issues • Patient frequently evaluates health status or maladaptively avoids healthcare • Symptoms are not related to substance abuse, medical condition or other psychiatric disorder
Treatment	• <u>Reassurance</u>: regularly-scheduled appointments for continued education and reassurance that their symptoms are not indicative of a serious illness • <u>Psychotherapy</u>: **cognitive-behavioral therapy (CBT) is the most effective form of psychotherapy** • Goal to help patients understand their irrational thoughts and behaviors and help them develop realistic beliefs and coping strategies • <u>Medical Management</u>: antidepressants may be indicated based on symptoms • *Provider must carefully interpret signs and symptoms the patient is demonstrating and correlate as to not miss a potential diagnosis*
Key Words & Most Common	• Disorder characterized by preoccupation with having or acquiring a serious medical illness or disorder • Excessive worry, fear, and anxiety about their health and misinterpret bodily sensations as signs of serious illness • Reassurance, cognitive-behavioral therapy, and medical management if indicated

Functional Neurological Symptom Disorder

Etiology & Risk Factors	• **Disorder characterized by neurologic symptoms or deficits that develop unconsciously and usually involve motor or sensory function** • Formerly known as **conversion disorder** (patients "convert" their psychological beliefs into neurological symptoms) • <u>Etiology</u>: combination of biological, psychological, and social factors • <u>Risk Factors</u>: **female, history of physical or emotional trauma, childhood abuse or neglect, stressful life events, comorbid mental health condition**, chronic pain or serious illness/injury, history of illness or disability in the family
Patho-physiology	• Not fully understood; may be related to abnormal nervous system function secondary to psychological factors, such as emotional distress or trauma
Signs & Symptoms	• **Abrupt onset of symptoms following a traumatic or stressful event** • <u>Motor Symptoms</u>: weakness, tremors,, abnormal gait, abnormal movements or postures, difficulty swallowing, globus sensation (lump in the throat) • <u>Sensory Symptoms</u>: paresthesia, pain, paralysis of an arm or leg, loss of sensation, blindness, double vision, urinary retention, hearing difficulty • *Episodes are often brief but can occasionally become chronic*
Diagnostic Criteria	• **Presence of 1 or more symptoms of neurological dysfunction (voluntary motor or sensory) that cannot be explained clinically by another medical or psychiatric condition** • **Symptoms are *not* intentionally produced or feigned** • Symptoms cause significant distress or impairment of social or occupational function
Treatment	• <u>Supportive</u>: **education and reassurance**, physical therapy (if difficulty with mobility or motor function), occupational therapy (if functional impairment present) • <u>Psychotherapy</u>: **cognitive behavioral therapy** focusing on identifying and changing negative thought patterns and behaviors that contribute to the patient's symptoms • <u>Hypnotherapy</u>: treatment that induces a relaxed state in which the patient is more receptive to positive suggestions • <u>Medication Management</u>: antidepressants and anxiolytics can be used to treat coexisting anxiety or depressive disorders that may be contribuotry
Key Words & Most Common	• Disorder characterized by neurologic symptoms or deficits that develop unconsciously and usually involve motor or sensory function • Also known as conversion disorder • Abrupt onset of motor or sensory symptoms following a traumatic or stressful event • Presence of 1 or more symptoms of neurological dysfunction (voluntary motor or sensory) that cannot be explained clinically by another medical or psychiatric condition • Symptoms are *not* intentionally produced or feigned • Supportive + psychotherapy and/or hypnotherapy

Factitious Disorder

Etiology & Risk Factors	• Disorder characterized by intentional falsification or exaggeration of physical or psychologic symptoms without an obvious external incentive; the motivation for this behavior is to assume the sick role • Previously known as **Munchausen syndrome** • <u>Etiology</u>: combination of biological, psychological, environmental and social factors • <u>Risk Factors</u>: **childhood trauma, abuse or neglect, comorbid mental health condition, stressful life events**, learned behavior (faking symptoms gains attention or sympathy from others), **certain personality traits** (impulsivity, attention-seeking behavior, or a need for control)
Patho-physiology	• Not fully understood; may be related to abnormalities in brain structure and function in areas that are involved in emotional processing and self-awareness (prefrontal cortex, insula, amygdala, and anterior cingulate cortex)

Signs & Symptoms	• <u>Factitious Disorder Imposed on Self</u>: patient presents themselves as injured, impaired or ill
	  <u>Factitious Disorder Imposed on Another</u>: presents another person as injured, impaired, or ill (child, elder, or mentally disabled family member)
	• **Intentional creation or exaggeration of symptoms of illness or disorder**
	  • Complain of specific (abdominal/chest) pain suggesting a more serious diagnosis, mimic symptoms (limping, refusal to use extremity), alteration of diagnostic testing
	• **Simulation of physical exam findings consistent with an illness or disorder**
	  • Pricking finger to add blood to a urine sample, inoculating wound with bacteria to get an infection, inject or purposefully consume toxins, intentionally hurt/injure themselves to bring on symptoms
	• **Extensive knowledge of medical terminology**
	  • Knowing that pain from a myocardial infarction may radiate to shoulder or jaw
	• **Increased willingness or eager to undergo diagnostic testing or surgery** to gain sympathy
	• **Peregrination** (moving from one medical provider or hospital to another)

Diagnostic Criteria	• **Intentional falsification or exaggeration of physical or psychologic symptoms for primary gain** (to assume sick role to obtain sympathy) • **Deceptive behavior without external incentives** (time off work, financial compensation, etc.); **malingering involves falsification of symptoms for secondary gain** • Presentation of illness imposed on another • Symptoms are not related to substance abuse, medical condition or other psychiatric disorder

Treatment	• **No clearly effective treatment**
	  • **Early psychiatric consult may be necessary early if suspected** to avoid unnecessary use of medication, invasive procedures, or exploratory surgeries
	  • **Confrontation should be made in a non-threatening manner** to avoid leaving against medical advice
	• <u>Psychotherapy</u>: cognitive-behavioral therapy (CBT) with a focus on identifying and changing negative thought patterns and behaviors
	  • Goal to improve coping skills and address any underlying emotional issues
	• <u>Reporting to Appropriate Agency</u>: reporting to child or adult protective service may be necessary if imposed on another

Somatic Symptom Disorder

Etiology & Risk Factors	• Disorder characterized by multiple persistent physical symptoms that are associated with excessive and maladaptive thoughts, feelings, and behaviors related to the symptoms with no physical cause identified during diagnostic workup • Previously known as **somatization disorder** • <u>Etiology</u>: combination of biological, psychological, and social factors • <u>Risk Factors</u>: **female, age (<30 years old most common), childhood trauma or abuse**, family history, **history of medical illness or hospitalization, chronic stress, certain personality traits** (neuroticism, introversion, or a tendency to catastrophize symptoms or health concerns), social isolation, low socioeconomic status
Patho-physiology	• Not fully understood; alterations in pain perception, immune function, and other physiological systems in combination with psychological factors such as emotional distress, anxiety, and depression lead to development of the disorder
Signs & Symptoms	• **Recurring and vague physical symptoms that are not explained by a physical or medical cause** • **Shortness of breath, fatigue, gastrointestinal distress, headaches, dysmenorrhea, dysuria, dysphagia, amnesia, vomiting, general pain are most common complaints** • **Excessive worry about symptoms causing significant impairment of daily life** (may miss work or social activities) • Frequently seeks medical evaluations and treatments (laboratory tests, imaging studies, specialist referrals) often with little or no relief of symptoms • Obsessive focus on physical symptoms (frequent internet searches, excessive self-examination)

Diagnostic Criteria	• **Symptoms must be distressing or or result in disruption of daily life for 6 or more months with 1 or more of the following:**
	  • Disproportionate and persistent thoughts about the seriousness of the symptoms
	  • Persistently high anxiety about health or the symptoms
	  • Excessive time and energy spent on the symptoms or health concerns
	• *A thorough workup is necessary to rule out any underlying medical causes of the symptoms*

Treatment	• <u>Reassurance</u>: regularly-scheduled appointments for continued education and reassurance • <u>Psychotherapy</u>: **cognitive-behavioral therapy (CBT) is the most effective form of psychotherapy** • Goal to help patients understand their irrational thoughts and behaviors and help them develop realistic beliefs and coping strategies • <u>Medical Management</u>: antidepressants may be indicated based on symptoms • *Provider must carefully interpret signs and symptoms the patient is demonstrating and correlate as to not miss a potential diagnosis*
Key Words & Most Common	• Disorder characterized by multiple persistent physical symptoms that are associated with excessive and maladaptive thoughts, feelings, and behaviors • Recurring/vague symptoms (SOB, fatigue, GI distress, headaches, dysmenorrhea, dysuria, dysphagia, general pain) • Excessive worry about symptoms causing significant occupational or social impairment • No physical cause identified during diagnostic workup • Reassurance + psychotherapy is most effective

Tobacco Use/Dependence

Etiology & Risk Factors	• Major individual and public health problem and most important modifiable risk factor for preventable pulmonary, cardiac and cancer-related deaths • Etiology: combination of biological, psychological, behavioral and social factors • Risk Factors: **early initiation** (younger use leads to a more severe addiction and greater difficulty quitting), **family history, male, peer pressure, comorbid mental health condition, substance abuse**, exposure to secondhand smoke, **exposure to media propaganda, advertising and marketing**, low education level, low socioeconomic status
Patho-physiology	• Nicotine, the addictive substance in tobacco, binds to nicotinic acetylcholine receptors in the brain, causing the release of dopamine, a neurotransmitter associated with reward and pleasure; nicotine use can lead to changes in brain circuitry that reinforce drug-seeking behavior and addiction • Tar byproducts from tobacco smoke induce metabolizing enzymes in the liver (primarily CYP2A6), leading to multiple drug interactions • Increased risk of developing coronary artery disease, COPD, lung and other cancers, asthma, upper respiratory infections, erectile dysfunction, peptic ulcer disease, osteoporosis, pneumonia, periodontitis, GERD, macular degeneration, diabetes, rheumatoid arthritis
Signs & Symptoms	• **Nicotine increases heart rate, blood pressure, and respiratory rate** • **Smoking may cause user to feel increased energy and arousal, increased ability to concentrate, decreased tension or anxiety and a sense of pleasure** • Mild Nicotine Toxicity: nausea, vomiting, headache, and weakness • Severe Nicotine Toxicity: cholinergic toxidrome with nausea, vomiting, salivation, lacrimation, diarrhea, urination, muscle fasciculations and weakness • **Nicotine Withdrawal: nicotine cravings, restlessness, anxiety, irritability, sleep disturbances, headaches,** increased appetite, difficulty concentrating, weight gain
Diagnostic Criteria	• **Clinical Diagnosis**

Treatment	• Supportive Care: indicated for nicotine toxicity
	• Tobacco Cessation:
	  • **Therapy: counseling and support therapy, cognitive behavioral therapy**
	  • **Encouragement:** encouraging temporary abstinence and reduction in consumption even if patient relapses after periods of abstinence; establish a quite date
	  • **Nicotine Tapering:** nicotine gum, nasal sprays, transdermal patches, lozenges, inhaler; **combination therapy (long-acting patch + short-acting gum) more effective**
	  • **Bupropion: antidepressant medication indicated to aid in smoking cessation when used with nicotine tapering therapy**
	    • Increases release of dopamine and norepinephrine to reduce nicotine craving and withdrawal symptoms
	  • **Varenicline: most effective monotherapy available for smoking cessation**
	    • **Partial antagonism at the nicotine receptors to reduce nicotine activity and partial agonism to block effects of nicotine**
	    • Mitigates nicotine withdrawal symptoms and decreases the pleasurable effects of smoking if the patient relapses

Key Words & Most Common	• Nicotine is addictive and causes changes in brain circuitry that reinforce drug-seeking behavior and addiction. • Smoking increases the risk of various health problems, including cancer, heart disease, and respiratory issues. • Tobacco cessation options include therapy, nicotine tapering, bupropion, and varenicline

Opioid Dependency

Etiology & Risk Factors	• **Disorder characterized by compulsive, long-term self-administration of opioids for nonmedical purposes** • Types of Opioids: natural (**morphine, codeine**), semi-synthetic (**oxycodone, hydrocodone, hydromorphone**), fully-synthetic (**fentanyl, tramadol, methadone**) • Etiology: combination of biological, psychological, behavioral and social factors • Risk Factors: **family history, chronic stress, trauma, childhood abuse or trauma,** low socioeconomic status, comorbid mental health condition, **history of substance abuse, recent surgery receiving opioid pain medication, chronic pain**
Patho-physiology	• Opioids interact with specific opioid receptors in the central nervous system (particularly areas and tracts associated with pain perception) and on receptors of sensory nerves, mast cells, and gastrointestinal tract cells to reduce the perception of pain and increase feelings of pleasure • Prolonged opioid use can lead to changes in the brain's reward and pleasure centers, resulting in dependence, tolerance, withdrawal symptoms, and increased risk of overdose

Signs & Symptoms	• Opioid Intoxication:
	  • **Drowsiness, impaired social functioning, impaired memory, slow or slurred speech, nausea/vomiting, constipation**
	  • **Pupillary constriction (miosis),** altered mental status, respiratory depression, bradycardia, hypotension
	• Opioid Withdrawal:
	  • **Lacrimation,** hypertension, **pruritus, tachycardia, nausea/vomiting,** abdominal cramping, diarrhea, **diaphoresis,** yawning, **piloerections, pupillary dilation (mydriasis),** flu-like symptoms, rhinorrhea, myalgia

Diagnostic Criteria	• **Pattern of opioid use causes clinically significant impairment or distress with 2 or more of the following over a 12-month period:** • Taking opioids in large amounts or for a longer time than intended, persistent desire or unsuccessful attempt to decrease use, spending a great deal of time obtaining, using, or recovering from opioids, craving opioids, failing to meet obligations at work, home or school, recurrent social or occupational distress as a result of opioid use, developed tolerance to opioids, having opioid withdrawal symptoms

Treatment	• Long-Term Maintenance: oral opioid receptor agonists are an alternative to opioid substitution with tapering
	  • **Methadone: potent, long-acting opioid receptor agonist**
	    • Indicated to suppress withdrawal symptoms and dependency without providing a significant high or oversedation
	  • **Buprenorphine: mixed, partial opioid receptor agonist-antagonist**
	    • Indicated to manage withdrawal symptoms and cravings in opioid dependency, treat chronic pain and aid in detoxification from opioids
	    • Blocks receptors, which inhibits concomitant illicit use of heroin or other opioids
	  • **Naltrexone: competitive opioid antagonist**
	    • Indicated for patients with less severe or early-stage opioid dependency with a strong motivation to remain abstinent

Key Words & Most Common	• Disorder characterized by compulsive, long-term self-administration of opioids for nonmedical purposes • Intoxication: drowsiness, impaired social functioning, impaired memory, slow or slurred speech, nausea/vomiting, constipation, pupillary constriction • Withdrawal: lacrimation, pruritus, tachycardia, nausea/vomiting, diaphoresis, piloerections, pupillary dilation, flu-like symptoms • Long-term maintenance includes methadone, buprenorphine, naltrexone

Opioid Toxicity

Etiology & Risk Factors	• Symptoms that can result from the use of opioid drugs, which include both prescription painkillers and illegal opioids • <u>Types of Opioids</u>: natural (**morphine, codeine**), semi-synthetic (**oxycodone, hydrocodone, hydromorphone**), fully-synthetic (**fentanyl, tramadol, methadone**) • <u>Etiology</u>: combination of biological, psychological, behavioral and social factors • <u>Risk Factors</u>: **opioid tolerance, combining opioids with other drugs (alcohol, benzodiazepines), high opioid doses, misuse or abuse of opioids** (taking without a prescription or taking them in a way that is different from the prescribed method), low socioeconomic status, **comorbid mental health condition, history of substance abuse, chronic pain**
Patho-physiology	• Opioids interact with specific opioid receptors in the central nervous system (particularly areas and tracts associated with pain perception) and on receptors of sensory nerves, mast cells, and gastrointestinal tract cells to reduce the perception of pain, increase feelings of pleasure and may cause significant respiratory depression • Prolonged opioid use can lead to changes in the brain's reward and pleasure centers, resulting in dependence, tolerance, withdrawal symptoms, and increased risk of overdose
Signs & Symptoms	• **Euphoria, drowsiness, impaired social functioning, impaired memory, slow or slurred speech, nausea/vomiting, constipation** • **Delirium, hypotension, bradycardia, hypothermia, urinary retention, altered mental status, pupillary constriction (miosis)** • **Respiratory depression** • Seizures, coma, death
Diagnosis	• **Clinical Diagnosis** • Urine drug toxicology screen confirms diagnosis

Treatment	• <u>Supportive</u>:
	  • <u>Secure Airway</u>: airway management and respiratory support is the first priority; endotracheal intubation may be indicated
	  • <u>Fluid Replacement</u>: IV fluids and electrolyte replacement
	  • <u>Psychosocial Support</u>: counseling or referral to addiction treatment programs, to address underlying issues and prevent relapse
	  • <u>Safety</u>: soft physical restraints may be indicated prior to naloxone administration as it precipitates acute withdrawal
	• <u>Medication Management</u>:
	  • <u>Naloxone</u>: opioid antagonist
	    • Indicated in acute intoxication or overdose to acutely reverse the effects of opioids; respiratory depression is most common indication
	    • **IV administration preferred**; IM, subcutaneously, or intranasal administration is also effective
	  • <u>Clonidine</u>: centrally acting adrenergic (alpha-2-agonist) drug indicated to suppress sympathetic/autonomic symptoms and signs of opioid withdrawal

Key Words & Most Common	• **Opioid tolerance, combining opioids with other drugs (alcohol, benzodiazepines), high opioid doses, misuse or abuse of opioids are greatest risk factors** • **Euphoria, drowsiness, impaired social functioning, impaired memory, slow or slurred speech, nausea/vomiting, constipation** • **Delirium, hypotension, bradycardia, hypothermia, urinary retention, altered mental status, pupillary constriction (miosis)** • **Respiratory depression** • Clinical diagnosis + drug toxicology screen • Secure airway → naloxone

Alcohol Dependency

Etiology & Risk Factors	• **Disorder characterized by a pattern of alcohol use that includes cravings and manifestations of tolerance and/or withdrawal symptoms** • <u>Etiology</u>: combination of genetic, environmental, and psychological factors • <u>Risk Factors</u>: **family history (children of alcoholics)**, early initiation, **peer pressure or social influences, comorbid mental health condition**, increased tolerance to alcohol, **chronic stress, childhood trauma/abuse/neglect**, chronic pain, availability (ease of access), **certain personality traits** (social isolation, dependency, self-destructive impulsivity)
Patho-physiology	• Chronic alcohol use changes in the brain neurotransmitter systems of the brain, specifically those related to the reward (dopamine) and stress (cortisol) pathways, leading to the development of tolerance and withdrawal symptoms • Positive-effect regulation results in alcohol use for a positive reward (euphoria); negative-effect regulation is seen when patients consume alcohol to cope with negative feelings including depression, anxiety, isolation, or feeling worthless • Chronic alcohol consumption leads to damage of the liver, brain, and pancreas
Signs & Symptoms	• **Slurred speech and difficulty articulating words clearly, impaired judgment and decision-making ability** • **Loss of coordination and balance, nausea and vomiting, impotence, gynecomastia** • **Headache, dizziness, blurred or double vision, memory impairment or blackouts, emotional instability** • Impairment of social and occupational function, injuries sustained while intoxicated • <u>Physical Exam</u>: • **Tachycardia, hypertension, flushed skin**, elevated body temperature, nystagmus, gynecomastia, male pattern baldness, testicular atrophy, telangiectasias
Diagnostic Criteria	• **Clinically significant impairment or distress as with 2 or more of the following symptoms over a 12-month period:** • Consuming alcohol in large quantities or for an extended period of time, persistent desire or unsuccessful attempt to decrease use, craving alcohol, spending an extended amount of time obtaining, consuming or recovering, failure to meet obligations at home, work, or school because of alcohol use, failure to stop drinking alcohol because of problems associated with alcohol use, using alcohol in hazardous situations, continuing to consume alcohol with a physical disorder (liver disease) or mental disorder (depression) caused or exacerbated by alcohol, having a tolerance to alcohol, experiencing alcohol withdrawal symptoms

Treatment	• <u>Supportive</u>: psychotherapy, individual or group therapy, inpatient and residential rehabilitation programs
	  • Goal is to enhance motivation and teach patients to avoid circumstances that precipitate drinking and encourage social support of abstinence
	  • Alcoholics Anonymous (AA) is the most common self-help group
	• <u>Medication Management</u>: used with counseling rather than monotherapy
	  • <u>Disulfiram</u>: interferes with the hepatic metabolism of acetaldehyde (an intermediary product in the oxidation of alcohol) so that acetaldehyde accumulates
	    • Deters alcohol use by producing unpleasant symptoms are produced including hypotension, palpitations, skin flushing, dizziness, nausea, vomiting, headache
	  • <u>Naltrexone</u>: competitive opioid antagonist; indicated to decrease the relapse rate and number of drinking days, reduce alcohol craving and alcohol-induced euphoria
	  • <u>Clonidine</u>: centrally acting adrenergic (alpha-2-agonist) drug indicated to suppress sympathetic/autonomic symptoms and signs of alcohol withdrawal

Alcohol Withdrawal

Etiology & Risk Factors	• Range of symptoms that occur when a person who is dependent on alcohol abruptly stops or reduces their alcohol consumption • Etiology: dysregulation of neurotransmitter systems and hyperexcitability of the central nervous system as a result of abruptly stopping or reducing alcohol consumption • Risk Factors: **abruptly stopping or reducing alcohol consumption, heavy alcohol use, previous episodes of alcohol withdrawal**, comorbid medical or psychiatric conditions, older age, family history of alcoholism
Patho-physiology	• Chronic alcohol use leads to neuroadaptation and changes in the brain's neurotransmitter systems, particularly gamma-aminobutyric acid (GABA) and glutamate • Abrupt cessation of alcohol results in an unopposed glutamate activity and reduced GABA activity leading to increased neuronal excitation and hyperactivity of the autonomic nervous system causing withdrawal symptoms • Chronic alcohol use can lead to pancreatitis, gastritis, hepatitis, cardiomyopathy, peripheral neuropathy, brain damage, malnutrition, cancer

Signs & Symptoms	• **Acute Intoxication**: tranquility, mild sedation, decreased motor coordination, impaired judgement, unsteady gait, nystagmus, slurred speech, memory impairment, loss of behavioral inhibitions, delirium, lethargy, obtundation
	• **Mild Withdrawal Syndrome**: symptoms usually begin 6-48 hours after last consumption of alcohol
	  • **Tremor, weakness, headache, diaphoresis, hyperreflexia, gastrointestinal symptoms** (nausea/vomiting/diarrhea)
	• **Alcohol Hallucinosis**: symptoms usually begin 12-48 hours after last consumption of alcohol
	  • **Visual (most common), auditory and/or tactile hallucination; patient has clear consciousness and normal vital signs**
	• **Delirium Tremens**: symptoms usually begin 48-72 hours after alcohol withdrawal
	  • Delirium (altered consciousness), hallucinations, agitation, confusion, disorientation, anxiety, diaphoresis, abnormal vital signs (tachycardia, hypertension, fever)

Diagnosis	• **Clinical Diagnosis** • Labs: blood alcohol content (BAC), point of care glucose test, CBC, magnesium, CMP (liver enzymes), coagulation studies, serum ammonia, serum, alubmin

Treatment	• Supportive:
	  • **Secure Airway: airway management and respiratory support is the first priority; endotracheal intubation may be indicated**
	  • **Fluid Replacement: IV fluids, oral rehydration**
	  • **Psychosocial Support**: counseling or referral to addiction treatment programs, to address underlying issues and prevent relapse
	  • Safety: soft physical restraints may be indicated if patient becomes combative or aggressive
	• Medication Management:
	  • **Electrolyte Replacement and Vitamin Supplementation: IV thiamine (B1) prevents Wernicke encephalopathy, multivitamins (B12 and folate), magnesium**
	  • **Benzodiazepines: diazepam, lorazepam, oxazepam are mainstays of therapy;** potentiates GABA mediated CNS inhibition (alcohol mimics GABA at receptor sites)
	    • **Lorazepam and oxazepam are preferred in patients with severe liver disorder** (advanced cirrhosis or alcoholic hepatitis)
	  • Phenobarbital: used as an alternative or in conjunction with benzodiazepines if benzodiazepines are ineffective alone

Wernicke-Korsakoff Syndrome

Etiology & Risk Factors	• **Neurological disorder characterized by confusion, nystagmus, partial ophthalmoplegia and ataxia secondary to a thiamine (vitamin B1) deficiency**
	  • **Wernicke Encephalopathy: acute neurological symptoms caused by a thiamine deficiency**
	  • **Korsakoff Psychosis: chronic neurological symptoms caused by a thiamine deficiency**
	  • **Wernicke-Korsakoff Syndrome: presence of Wernicke encephalopathy and Korsakoff psychosis simultaneously**
	• Etiology: chronic alcohol abuse or malnutrition
	• Risk Factors: **alcoholism, chronic malnutrition or malabsorption**, gastrointestinal surgery or disease, **prolonged vomiting**, increased metabolic requirements (cancer)

Patho-physiology	• Excessive alcohol intake interferes with thiamine absorption within the gastrointestinal tract and hepatic storage of thiamin • Thiamine is essential for normal brain function; deficiency leads to lactic acidosis, altered brain metabolism and alterations in myelination

	Wernicke Encephalopathy	**Korsakoff Psychosis**
Signs & Symptoms	• **Oculomotor Abnormalities: horizontal and vertical nystagmus; ophthalmoplegia** (weakness or paralysis of the eye muscles) resulting in diplopia and ptosis • **Vestibular Dysfunction: vertigo, ataxia (lack of coordination),** difficulty with balance, **gait abnormalities (wide-based and slow gait with short-spaced steps)** • **Confusion: profound disorientation,** inattention, **drowsiness, stupor** • **Autonomic Dysfunction: sympathetic hyperactivity** (tremor, agitation) **or hypoactivity** (hypotension, hypothermia, syncope)	• **Retrograde Amnesia:** inability to recall past events or memories • **Anterograde Amnesia:** inability to form new memories (past memories maintained) • **Personality Changes:** disorientation, emotional changes (apathy, euphoria, flat affect), decreased initiative • **Confabulation:** striking feature; imaginary fabrication or confusion surrounding events they are unable to recall • Occurs in 80% of untreated patients with Wernicke encephalopathy

Diagnosis	• **Clinical Diagnosis**

Treatment	• **Supportive:** oral and IV rehydration, correction of electrolyte abnormalities, general nutritional therapy
	• **Alcohol Cessation: mandatory to prevent progression**
	• **Parenteral Thiamine:** replenishing thiamine necessary to prevent further morbidity/mortality
	  • **IV or IM thiamine should be administered immediately** and continued once per day for 3-5 days
	• **Parenteral Magnesium:** hypomagnesemic state may be resistant to thiamine therapy (magnesium is a necessary cofactor in thiamin-dependent metabolism)
	  • **IV or IM magnesium sulfate** should be administered with thiamine

Key Words & Most Common	• Wernicke Encephalopathy: oculomotor abnormalities + vestibular and autonomic dysfunction + confusion • Korsakoff Psychosis: retrograde/anterograde amnesia + personality changes + confabulation • Due to thiamine (vitamin B1) deficiency • Chronic alcohol abuse or malnutrition is most common cause • Clinical diagnosis • Supportive + alcohol cessation • Parenteral thiamine + magnesium

Cocaine Intoxication

Etiology & Risk Factors	• Includes the range of physical, psychological, and behavioral changes that occur when someone uses cocaine • <u>Etiology</u>: ingestion, inhalation, injection or insufflation of cocaine • <u>Risk Factors</u>: **male, age** (adolescent and young adults most common), **increased frequency and duration of use, comorbid mental health condition, peer pressure or social influences, comorbid mental health condition, certain personality traits** (social isolation, dependency, self-destructive impulsivity), ease of access
Patho-physiology	• Cocaine enhances serotonin, dopamine and norepinephrine activity in the central and peripheral nervous systems by inhibiting the reuptake of biogenic amines resulting in euphoria, increased energy, and enhanced focus and motivation; dopamine activity enhancement plays largest role in symptoms and reinforcement leading to dependency
Signs & Symptoms	• **Elevated or euphoric mood** • **Hyperstimulation, heightened sensory perception and alertness** • **Psychomotor agitation, increased sense of energy**, restlessness, **agitation**, irritability, **pressured speech** • **Impaired judgement and decision making**, anxiety, paranoia • Nausea, vomiting, diarrhea, seizures • <u>Physical Exam</u>: • **Sympathomimetic Toxidrome**: tremor, flushing, diaphoresis, **pupillary dilation (mydriasis), hypertension, tachycardia, hyperthermia** • <u>Complications</u>: **myocardial ischemia and infarction** ("cocaine chest pain"), arrythmia, acute psychosis, rhabdomyolysis, stroke, intracranial hemorrhage, aortic dissection • <u>Withdrawal</u>: post-intoxication depression, anhedonia, hypersomnia, dysphoria, difficulty concentrating, **somnolence** ("cocaine washout syndrome"), increased appetite
Diagnosis	• **Clinical Diagnosis** • Urine drug toxicology screen confirms diagnosis • Workup to monitor complications; CMP, troponin, CK, coagulation studies, ECG

Treatment	• <u>Supportive</u>: IV fluids, cooling blankets/ice packs for hyperthermia, nasal irrigation of nares, reassurance (cocaine is short-acting), do not use restraints (risk of rhabdomyolysis)
	• <u>Medication Management</u>:
	  • **Sedation: benzodiazepines (lorazepam or diazepam) are first-line medication for sedation**
	    • Avoid haloperidol for sedation if abnormal vital signs as it may lead to seizures, dysrhythmias, hyperthermia
	  • **Hypertension: phentolamine (alpha-adrenergic antagonist) is first-line for hypertension**
	    • **Beta-blockers are contraindicated** as may lead to paradoxical hypertension

Key Words & Most Common	• Elevated or euphoric mood, hyperstimulation, increased energy, agitation, pressured speech, impaired judgement • Tremor, flushing, hyperthermia, pupillary dilation (mydriasis), hypertension, tachycardia, diaphoresis • Clinical diagnosis • Supportive → sedation (benzodiazepines) • Phentolamine is first-line antihypertensive • Beta-blockers contraindicated

Ketamine and Phencyclidine (PCP) Intoxication

Etiology & Risk Factors	• **Ketamine and phencyclidine (PCP) are N-methyl-D-aspartate receptor antagonists and dissociative anesthetic and hallucinogenic drugs that can cause intoxication** • <u>Etiology</u>: ingestion, inhalation, or injection of PCP or ketamine; ketamine may be used illicitly or therapeutically for sedation, pain control and depression • <u>Risk Factors</u>: **male, age** (adolescents/young adults more likely to experiment with illicit drugs), **increased frequency and duration of use, comorbid mental health condition, peer pressure or social influences, comorbid mental health condition, certain personality traits** (social isolation, dependency, self-destructive impulsivity), ease of access
Patho-physiology	• N-methyl-D-aspartate (NMDA) receptors play a critical role in many important physiological processes, such as synaptic plasticity, learning, and memory • NMDA receptor antagonism causes a release of dopamine, serotonin, and norepinephrine, leading to stimulation and increased activity in the brain; sigma receptors binding inhibits the reuptake of dopamine, contributing to the euphoric effects and potential for addiction
Signs & Symptoms	• Mix of cholinergic, anticholinergic and sympathomimetic symptoms • **Euphoria followed by anxiety and mood lability** • **Dissociation, hallucinations**, delirium, psychomotor agitation • **Impulsivity, rage**, homicidal ideation, **feelings of strength and invulnerability** • <u>Physical Exam</u>: • Tachycardia, hyperthermia, **combativeness, ataxia**, dysarthria, **muscular hypertonicity, multidirectional (vertical, horizontal, rotary) nystagmus**, hyperreflexia, myoclonic jerks, hypertension, erythematous/dry skin
Diagnosis	• **Clinical Diagnosis** • Urine immunoassay may detect PCP

Treatment	• <u>Supportive</u>: observation with frequent monitoring
	  • **Secure Airway: airway management and respiratory support is the first priority; endotracheal intubation may be indicated**
	  • <u>Safety</u>: soft physical restraints may be indicated if patient becomes combative or aggressive; place in a quiet, calming, low-stimulus environment
	  • <u>Hyperthermia Management</u>: cooling blankets/ice packs
	  • <u>Rehydration</u>: IV fluids
	• <u>Medication Management</u>:
	  • **Sedation: benzodiazepines (lorazepam or diazepam) are first-line medication for sedation** if acutely agitated

Key Words & Most Common	• NMDA receptor antagonists and dissociative anesthetic and hallucinogenic drugs • Euphoria followed by anxiety and mood lability • Dissociation, hallucinations, impulsivity, rage, feeling of strength/invulnerability • Hypertonicity, ataxia, multidirectional nystagmus • Clinical diagnosis • Supportive +/- benzodiazepines for sedation

Marijuana Intoxication

Etiology & Risk Factors	• Under the influence of cannabis or marijuana • Etiology: ingestion, inhalation of cannabis or marijuana • Risk Factors: **male, age** (adolescents/young adults more likely to experiment with illicit drugs), **increased frequency and duration of use, comorbid mental health condition, peer pressure or social influences, comorbid mental health condition, certain personality traits** (social isolation, dependency, self-destructive impulsivity), ease of access
Patho-physiology	• The active chemical compound in the marijuana plant is THC (delta-9-tetrahydrocannabinol) which binds to cannabinoid receptors in the brain and body which alters the normal functioning of the endocannabinoid system and produces a range of physiological and psychological effects
Signs & Symptoms	• **Euphoria, giddiness, dreamy state of consciousness, relaxation, intensification of sensory experiences, lethargy** • **Anxiety**, disinhibition, depression, fear, paranoia, **panic reactions** (may be related to the setting in which the drug was taken) • **Increased appetite, dry mouth** • **Impaired concentration, coordination**, sense of time, depth perception, and reaction time may occur for up to 24 hours • **Conjunctival injection** • Decreased fertility and reduced sperm count with chronic use • <u>Cannabinoid Hyperemesis Syndrome</u>: **cyclic episodes of nausea and vomiting in patients that frequently use cannabis and has relief with hot baths/showers**
Diagnosis	• **Clinical Diagnosis** • Urine drug toxicology screen confirms diagnosis

Treatment	• <u>Supportive</u>: treatment not usually required; symptomatic management
	   • Chronic abuse requires behavioral therapy in a drug treatment program
	• <u>**Cannabinoid Hyperemesis Syndrome**</u>:
	   • **Cessation of Marijuana Use: definitive management**
	   • <u>Antiemetics</u>: **ondansetron**, metoclopramide, diphenhydramine
	   • <u>Sedation</u>: benzodiazepines (lorazepam or diazepam) or antipsychotics (haloperidol) if patient experiencing anxiety, panic, paranoia
	   • **Thermoregulation: hot shower, capsaicin cream applied to abdomen/arms/back**

Key Words & Most Common	• Euphoria, dream-like state, relaxation, intense sensorium, lethargy • Anxiety, panic reactions, impaired concentration and coordination • Increased appetite, dry mouth, conjunctival injection • <u>Cannabinoid Hyperemesis Syndrome</u>: cyclic episodes of nausea and vomiting in patients that frequently use cannabis and has relief with hot baths/showers • Clinical diagnosis • Supportive → cessation of use + antiemetics + hot shower or capsaicin cream for cannabinoid hyperemesis syndrome

Grief Reaction

Etiology & Risk Factors	• **Describes the normal psychological and emotional response to the loss of a loved one, or to any other significant life change that results in a sense of loss or separation** • Also known as **bereavement or mourning** • Etiology: **death of a pet, friend or family member, job loss is most common**, relationship breakup, divorce, catastrophic damage to home or other possession, disability • Risk Factors: **nature and circumstance of death (sudden, unexpected or traumatic deaths or deaths of children/young adults), close or dependent relationship with the deceased**, history of trauma or loss, comorbid mental health condition, **lack of social support, lack of coping skills**, other life stressors (financial or relationship problems)
Patho-physiology	• Elevated level of cortisol causes alterations in the levels of certain neurotransmitters such as serotonin, norepinephrine and dopamine and changes in hypothalamic-pituitary-adrenal (HPA) axis activity resulting in psychological and physical symptoms
Signs & Symptoms	• <u>5 Stages</u>: denial, anger, bargaining, depression and acceptance • <u>**Feelings**</u>: **shock, emotional numbness, sadness**, helplessness, depression, yearning, denial, **anger**, guilt, apathy • <u>**Thoughts**</u>: disbelief, confusion, **difficulty concentrating** • <u>**Physical Sensations**</u>: **tightness or heaviness in the chest**, globus sensation ("lump in the throat"), **loss of appetite**, nausea, headache, paresthesias, muscle weakness, fatigue • <u>**Behavior**</u>: insomnia or hypersomnia, anhedonia, **mood lability** (irritation, aggression) • <u>**Somatic Symptoms**</u>: chest pain, dysphagia, **dyspnea, gastrointestinal distress (nausea, vomiting, diarrhea)**, weakness
Diagnosis	• **Clinical Diagnosis**
Treatment	• <u>Normal Grief</u>: usually resolves within 6 months to 1 year • <u>Complicated Grief</u>: **complicated grief therapy, cognitive-behavioral therapy (CBT)** • <u>Benzodiazepines</u>: short-duration use may be indicated for insomnia in specific patients
Key Words & Most Common	• Psychological and emotional response to the loss of a loved one, or to any other significant life change that results in a sense of loss or separation • Shock, numbness, sadness, anger, disbelief, difficulty concentrating • Tightness or heaviness in the chest, globus sensation, loss of appetite, weakness, fatigue • Insomnia or hypersomnia, mood lability • Chest pain, dyspnea, GI distress • Clinical diagnosis • Usually resolves within 6 months to 1 year; grief therapy for complicated cases

Narcolepsy

Etiology & Risk Factors	• Disorder characterized by chronic excessive daytime sleepiness, often with sudden onset of rapid eye movement sleep and frequent uncontrollable sleep attacks • Etiology: combination of genetic and environmental factors • Risk Factors: **family history, human leukocyte antigen (HLA) haplotypes**, age (adolescents and young adults most common), **autoimmune disorders**, traumatic brain injury, infection (*Streptococcal* infections or H1N1 flu), **hypocretin deficiency**, obstructive sleep apnea
Patho-physiology	• Autoimmune destruction of hypocretin-producing neurons in the hypothalamus leads to hypocretin deficiency (also known as orexin) which is a neurotransmitter that regulates sleep-wake cycles and promotes wakefulness

Signs & Symptoms	• **Excessive Daytime Sleepiness: primary symptom; falling asleep throughout the day**, sleep attacks (rapidly sleeping without warning) at inappropriate times or during times of monotonous activity (reading, watching television, attending meetings)
	  • May result in low productivity, disruption of relationships, poor concentration, low motivation, depression, reduced quality of life, potential for physical injury (motor vehicle accidents)
	• **Cataplexy: transient episodes of muscular weakness or paralysis evoked by sudden emotions** (excitement, joy, laughter, anger, surprise); may resemble loss of muscle tone
	  • Weakness often begins in the face (ptosis, jaw may droop, hypotonic face, nodding head) and lower extremities (limbs become limp, weakness, paralysis)
	• **Hypnagogic and Hypnopompic Hallucinations: vivid auditory or visual hallucinations** occurring as the patient is falling asleep (hypnagogic) or upon waking (hypnopompic)
	• **Sleep Paralysis**: complete inability to move for 1-2 minutes immediately after waking or before falling asleep
	• **Disturbed Nocturnal Sleep**: disturbed sleep due to increased level of arousal

Diagnosis	• **Nocturnal Polysomnography**: diagnosis and excludes alternative/coexisting causes of daytime sleepiness
	  • Narcolepsy diagnosed with spontaneous awakenings, mild reduced sleep efficiency, increased non-REM sleep, REM sleep within 15 minutes after onset of sleep
	• **Multiple Sleep Latency Testing (MSLT)**: identifies onset of sleep onset rapid eye movement (REM) and measures mean sleep latency
	  • Narcolepsy diagnosed if patient falls asleep within 8 minutes (normal patients within 10-15 minutes) and include sleep onset rapid eye movements

Treatment	• **Modafinil: first-line in medical management; indicated in narcoleptic patients *with* cataplexy** to improve control of sleepiness and promote evening wakefulness
	  • May promote wakefulness by increasing the release of wake-promoting neurotransmitters in the brain, such as dopamine, norepinephrine, and histamine
	  • **Armodafinil** is an *R*-enantiomer of modafinil with similar benefits but is longer-acting
	• **Solriamfetol: alternative first-line medication; indicated in excessive daytime sleepiness patients *without* cataplexy**
	  • Dopamine and norepinephrine reuptake inhibitor that increases extracellular levels of these neurotransmitters, leading to increased wakefulness and alertness
	• **Pitolisant**: histamine-3 receptor inverse agonist; indicated for treatment of excessive daytime sleepiness and cataplexy
	• **Sodium Oxybate**: indicated for treatment of cataplexy and excessive daytime sleepiness associated with narcolepsy
	• **Stimulants**: methylphenidate, dextroamphetamine; only indicated if patients do not respond to or cannot tolerate wake-promoting medications

Key Words & Most Common	• Excessive daytime sleepiness, cataplexy, hallucinations, sleep paralysis, disturbed nocturnal sleep • Nocturnal polysomnography followed by multiple sleep latency testing for diagnosis • Modafinil is first-line medication; indicated if cataplexy present • Solriamfetol is alternative first-line medication; indicated if cataplexy not present

Insomnia

Etiology & Risk Factors	• Sleep disorder characterized by difficulty falling asleep, staying asleep, or waking early and not being able to fall back asleep, leading to problems of daytime functioning
	• Etiology:
	  • **Medical Conditions**: chronic pain, asthma, heartburn, restless legs syndrome
	  • **Psychiatric Conditions**: depression, anxiety
	  • **Substance Use**: alcohol, caffeine, nicotine
	  • **Medications**: antidepressants, stimulants
	  • **Poor Sleep Hygiene**: irregular sleep schedule, exposure to screens before bedtime, excessive naps, exercise or excitement (watching thrilling TV show) late in evening
	  • **Acute Emotional Stressors**: job loss, hospitalization, a death in the family
	• Risk Factors: **female, medical conditions** (chronic pain, respiratory disorders, psychiatric disorders), substance use, **stressful life events, shift work**

Patho-physiology	• Variety of factors that can disrupt the normal sleep-wake cycle resulting in poor sleep quality and daytime fatigue, which can worsen the condition leading to a chronic sleep disorder
Signs & Symptoms	• **Difficulty falling asleep, staying asleep or both** • **Fatigue, irritability, difficulty concentrating, decreased performance in work, school or daily activities** • **Waking earlier than desired with trouble falling back asleep** • Anxiety, depression
Diagnosis	• **Presence of 1 or more of following symptoms occur at least 3 nights per week for at least 3 months:** • **Difficulty falling asleep, difficulty staying asleep, waking up too early or poor sleep quality** • Polysomnography or Actigraphy: objective measures of sleep quality

Treatment	• **Lifestyle Modifications**: proper nutrition, adequate daytime exercise, stress reduction, cessation of alcohol, tobacco and caffeine
	• **Sleep Hygiene: first-line and most effective**
	  • Limiting daytime naps, cool dark room, regular sleep schedule, avoiding screens or bright lights within 2 hours of bedtime
	• Psychotherapy: **cognitive-behavioral therapy**
	• **Relaxation Therapy**: meditation, breathing exercises, yoga
	• Medication Management:
	  • **Benzodiazepines**: temazepam, lorazepam, and triazolam; may be used short-term
	  • **Benzodiazepine Receptor Agonists**: zolpidem, zopiclone, and zaleplon; preferred for chronic management
	    • More selective action at the GABA-A receptor subtype responsible for sedation resulting in lower risk of dependence and withdrawal symptoms
	  • **Off-Label: antidepressants** (trazodone, mirtazapine, amitriptyline), typical antipsychotics (olanzapine, quetiapine), anticonvulsants (gabapentin)
	• Alternative Therapy: **melatonin**, valerian root, chamomile, passionflower, L-glycine, lemon balm and magnesium

Chapter 12
Dermatologic

Acne Vulgaris

Etiology & Risk Factors	• Skin condition characterized by comedones, papules, pustules, nodules, and/or cysts • Etiology: obstruction and inflammation of pilosebaceous units • Risk Factors: **hormonal changes (increased androgen levels during puberty, pregnancy or hormonal imbalance)**, family history, **skin type** (oily skin), medications (corticosteroids, androgens, lithium, OCPs), **diet (processed carbohydrate and sugars, dairy products, trans fats)**, increased stress, occupational exposure, humidity, sweating
Patho-physiology	• **4 Major Factors**: excess sebum production, follicular plugging with sebum and keratinocytes (follicular hyperkeratinization), colonization of follicles by *Cutibacterium acnes* (formerly *Propionibacterium acnes*), inflammatory response • **Non-Inflammatory Acne**: comedones are sebaceous plugs impacted within follicles • **Inflammatory Acne**: papules and pustules develop with *C. acnes* colonization of closed comedones which breaks sebum down into free fatty acids that cause follicular epithelial irritation, eliciting an inflammatory response by neutrophils and lymphocytes

Signs & Symptoms	• Commonly seen in areas with increased sebaceous glands such as the **face, back, chest, shoulders, proximal arms**
	• **Comedones**: small, non-inflammatory bumps that form on the skin when hair follicles become clogged with excess oil (sebum) and dead skin cells
	   • **Open Comedones (Blackheads)**: incomplete blockage; exposure to air causes oxidation of melanin in the sebum and keratin that are clogging the pore
	   • **Closed Comedones (Whiteheads)**: complete blockage; closure prevents the oxidation of the trapped sebum and keratin within the follicle
	• **Papules**: small, raised, solid 2-5mm lesions appearing on the skin surface; relatively deep compared to pustules
	• **Pustules**: small, raised, solid 2-5mm suppurative (pus-filled) lesions appearing on the skin surface; relatively superficial compared to papules
	• **Nodules**: larger, deeper, more inflamed and painful lesions than papules; lack cystic structure
	• **Cysts**: suppurative (pus-filled) nodule; chronic cystic acne may result in small and deep pits, larger pits, shallow depressions, hypertrophic scarring, keloids

Diagnosis	• **Clinical Diagnosis** • **Mild**: <20 comedones or <15 inflammatory lesions • **Moderate**: 20-100 comedones or 15-50 inflammatory lesions • **Severe**: >5 cysts, >100 comedones or >50 inflammatory lesions

Treatment	• **Lifestyle Modifications**: clean affected area twice daily with mild soap, dietary change (low glycemic diet; elimination of dairy products), short exposure to direct sunlight
	• **Topical Medications**:
	   • **Retinoids: tretinoin**; vitamin A derivatives indicated to unclog pores and prevent the formation of new comedones
	   • **Benzoyl Peroxide**: gel, cream, wash; kills bacteria that cause acne and reduces inflammation
	   • **Topical Antibiotics: clindamycin, erythromycin**; kills bacteria that cause acne and reduces inflammation
	   • **Salicylic Acid**: helps to unclog pores and prevent the formation of new comedones; has some anti-inflammatory properties
	• **Oral Medications**:
	   • **Oral Antibiotics: doxycycline and minocycline are first-line**; erythromycin, tetracycline and azithromycin are adjuncts
	   • **Oral Contraceptives**: may help regulate hormonal imbalances that can lead to acne; *may exacerbate acne in some cases*
	   • **Spironolactone**: aldosterone antagonist works by blocking the effects of androgen hormones on the skin
	   • **Oral Isotretinoin: most effective therapy; indicated for severe/refractory acne**; vitamin A derivative that decreases inflammation, sebum production and keratinization

Rosacea

Etiology & Risk Factors	• Chronic inflammatory acneiform skin condition characterized by facial flushing, telangiectasias, erythema, papules, pustules, and rhinophyma • Etiology: **unknown**; combination of genetic and environmental factors such as abnormalities in blood vessels, immune system dysfunction, and microbial infections • Risk Factors: **age (30-50 years old most common), fair complexion**, family history, **increased or prolonged sun exposure, certain foods and drinks (spicy foods, alcohol, hot beverages), stress**, hormonal changes, medications (corticosteroids, blood pressure medications, amiodarone), **hot or cold weather, hot showers/baths, wind exposure**
Patho-physiology	• Not fully understood; may be related to abnormal vasomotor control, impaired facial venous drainage, increased follicular mites (*Demodex folliculorum*), increased angiogenesis, ferritin expression, and reactive oxygen species, capillary vasodilation, abnormal pilosebaceous activity
Signs & Symptoms	• **Pre-Rosacea Phase**: centrofacial erythema, flushing and blushing of skin with burning and stinging; persists through other phases • **Vascular Phase**: facial erythema and edema with multiple telangiectasis (persistent vasomotor instability) • **Inflammatory Phase**: papulopustular formation (acne-like rash) • **Late Phase**: coarse tissue hyperplasia of the cheeks and nose (**rhinophyma**) as a result of tissue inflammation, collagen deposition and sebaceous gland hyperplasia • **Ocular Rosacea**: may accompany facial; represents blepharoconjunctivitis, iritis, scleritis, or keratitis, leading to pruritus, foreign body sensation, edema, erythema of the eye • Physical Exam: • **Absence of comedones (distinguishes from acne vulgaris)**; rhinophyma (erythematous, hyperplastic nose), cutaneous edema
Diagnosis	• **Clinical Diagnosis**

Treatment	• **Avoidance of Triggers**: use of sunscreen or protective garments, dietary modification, stress reduction, discontinue offending medication, temperature-controlled environment
	• **Topical Management**: indicated for mild-moderate cases
	   • **Metronidazole cream (first-line for papulopustules), topical azelaic acid, or topical ivermectin**
	   • Benzoyl peroxide may be added for improved control
	   • Sodium sulfacetamide, clindamycin, and erythromycin are less-effective options
	   • **Topical brimonidine** (alpha-2-selective adrenergic agonist) **or topical oxymetazoline hydrochloride** indicated for persistent facial erythema or flushing
	• **Oral Management**: indicated for moderate to severe cases in combination with topical therapy
	   • **Oral Antibiotics: doxycycline, minocycline**, tetracycline, erythromycin, azithromycin
	   • **Oral Isotretinoin: indicated for severe/refractory acne**
	• Rhinophyma Treatment Techniques: dermabrasion, laser ablation, tissue excision
	• Telangiectasia Treatment Techniques: laser and electrocautery

Key Words & Most Common	• Centrofacial erythema, flushing, blushing of skin • Erythema and edema with telangiectasis • Papulopustular formation (acne-like rash without comedones); coarse tissue hyperplasia of cheeks/nose • Avoidance of triggers → topical medications (metronidazole, azelaic acid, ivermectin) → oral antibiotics (doxycycline, minocycline) → oral isotretinoin

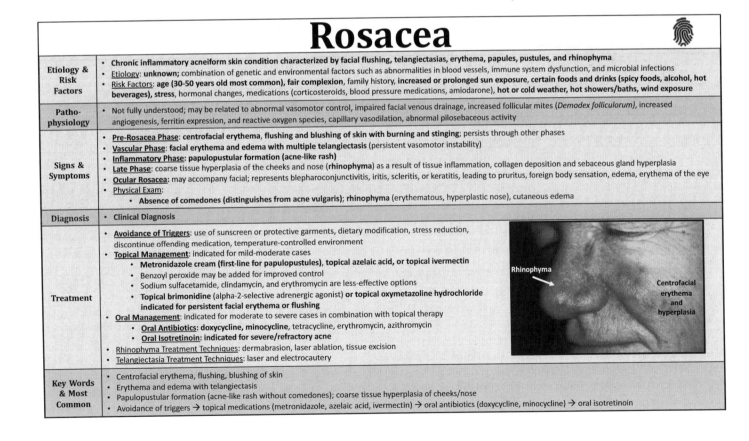

Rhinophyma

Centrofacial erythema and hyperplasia

Folliculitis

Etiology & Risk Factors	• Inflammation or infection of 1 or more hair follicles • <u>Etiology</u>: **bacterial** (*Staphylococcus aureus* most common; *Pseudomonas aeruginosa* implicated in hot tub folliculitis), fungal, viral or parasitic • <u>Risk Factors</u>: **immunocompromised, friction (tight clothing, shaving, sweating)**, certain skin conditions (acne, eczema), **exposure to hot tubs or pools, exposure to contaminated items (towels, razors, clothing)**, occupations requiring tight clothing (athletes, firefighters, healthcare workers), use of topical corticosteroids
Patho-physiology	• Perspiration, friction, occlusion, and/or trauma may potentiate infection of the hair follicle
Signs & Symptoms	• **Mild pain, pruritus, irritation of affected area** • **Superficial, singular or cluster of perifollicular papules, pustules, or inflammatory nodules** • Infected hairs fall out or are easily removed
Diagnosis	• **Clinical Diagnosis**
Treatment	• <u>Supportive</u>: avoid tight clothing when possible, only use clean towels/razors, wash with antibacterial soap after exposure to contaminated items, hot tubs or pools • <u>Topical Management</u>: • **Topical Clindamycin 1%: first-line medication**; most folliculitis are caused by *S. aureus* • **Topical Mupirocin 2%: alternative first-line medication** • **Benzoyl Peroxide 5%**: may be added while showering as an alternative or in addition to topical clindamycin; indicated for hot tube folliculitis • <u>Oral Management</u>: indicated for extensive cutaneous involvement • **Oral Cephalexin: first-line oral medication**; 250-500mg 3-4x per day • <u>Oral Dicloxacillin</u>: alternative oral medication • *Gram stain and culture (rule out gram-negative or MRSA etiology) or potassium hydroxide wet mount (rule out fungal etiology) indicated if resistant or refractory to treatment*
Key Words & Most Common	• Inflammation/infection of 1 or more hair follicles • *S. aureus* is most common cause; *P. aeruginosa* most common in hot tub folliculitis • Friction, tight clothing, shaving, sweating, exposure to hot tubs/pools, use of contaminated towels/razors • Mild pain + pruritus + irritation • Superficial perifollicular papules/pustules • Clinical diagnosis • Supportive (most cases resolve without treatment → topical clindamycin/mupirocin → cephalexin/dicloxacillin if extensive

Erythema Multiforme

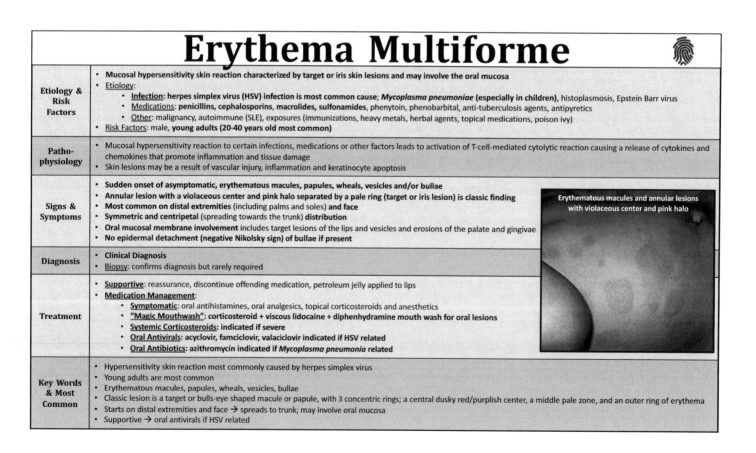

Etiology & Risk Factors	• **Mucosal hypersensitivity skin reaction characterized by target or iris skin lesions and may involve the oral mucosa** • <u>Etiology</u>: • <u>Infection</u>: **herpes simplex virus (HSV) infection is most common cause**; *Mycoplasma pneumoniae* **(especially in children)**, histoplasmosis, Epstein Barr virus • <u>Medications</u>: **penicillins, cephalosporins, macrolides, sulfonamides**, phenytoin, phenobarbital, anti-tuberculosis agents, antipyretics • <u>Other</u>: malignancy, autoimmune (SLE), exposures (immunizations, heavy metals, herbal agents, topical medications, poison ivy) • <u>Risk Factors</u>: male, **young adults (20-40 years old most common)**
Patho-physiology	• Mucosal hypersensitivity reaction to certain infections, medications or other factors leads to activation of T-cell-mediated cytolytic reaction causing a release of cytokines and chemokines that promote inflammation and tissue damage • Skin lesions may be a result of vascular injury, inflammation and keratinocyte apoptosis
Signs & Symptoms	• **Sudden onset of asymptomatic, erythematous macules, papules, wheals, vesicles and/or bullae** • **Annular lesion with a violaceous center and pink halo separated by a pale ring (target or iris lesion) is classic finding** • **Most common on distal extremities** (including palms and soles) **and face** • **Symmetric and centripetal** (spreading towards the trunk) **distribution** • **Oral mucosal membrane involvement** includes target lesions of the lips and vesicles and erosions of the palate and gingivae • **No epidermal detachment (negative Nikolsky sign) of bullae if present**
Diagnosis	• **Clinical Diagnosis** • <u>Biopsy</u>: confirms diagnosis but rarely required
Treatment	• <u>Supportive</u>: reassurance, discontinue offending medication, petroleum jelly applied to lips • <u>Medication Management</u>: • <u>Symptomatic</u>: oral antihistamines, oral analgesics, topical corticosteroids and anesthetics • **"Magic Mouthwash": corticosteroid + viscous lidocaine + diphenhydramine mouth wash for oral lesions** • <u>Systemic Corticosteroids</u>: indicated if severe • <u>Oral Antivirals</u>: acyclovir, famciclovir, valaciclovir indicated if HSV related • <u>Oral Antibiotics</u>: azithromycin indicated if *Mycoplasma pneumonia* related
Key Words & Most Common	• Hypersensitivity skin reaction most commonly caused by herpes simplex virus • Young adults are most common • Erythematous macules, papules, wheals, vesicles, bullae • Classic lesion is a target or bulls-eye shaped macule or papule, with 3 concentric rings; a central dusky red/purplish center, a middle pale zone, and an outer ring of erythema • Starts on distal extremities and face → spreads to trunk; may involve oral mucosa • Supportive → oral antivirals if HSV related

Erythematous macules and annular lesions with violaceous center and pink halo

Stevens-Johnson Syndrome (SJS) and Toxic Epidermal Necrolysis (TEN) 👆

Etiology & Risk Factors	• Severe mucocutaneous hypersensitivity reactions characterized by detachment of the epidermis and extensive skin necrosis
	• <u>Stevens-Johnson Syndrome</u>: involves <10% of skin body surface area
	• <u>Toxic Epidermal Necrolysis</u>: involves >30% of the skin body surface area
	• <u>Etiology</u>:
	  • <u>Medication</u>: **most common cause overall; sulfa drugs most common, antibiotics** (ampicillin, amoxicillin, fluoroquinolones, cephalosporins), **antiepileptics** (phenytoin, carbamazepine, phenobarbital, valproic acid), **NSAIDs** (meloxicam, ibuprofen), miscellaneous (allopurinol)
	  • <u>Infection</u>: *Mycoplasma pneumoniae*, HIV, HSV
	  • <u>Other</u>: malignancy, immunization, graft-vs-host disease, idiopathic

Patho-physiology	• Altered drug metabolism leads to an accumulation of reactive drug metabolites which may trigger a T-cell-mediated cytotoxic reaction to the drug antigens in keratinocytes • Immune system reaction in which the body's immune cells attack and destroy the skin and mucous membranes

Signs & Symptoms	• Prodrome of general malaise, fever, URI symptoms, and keratoconjunctivitis that begins 1-3 weeks after starting the offending medication
	• Erythematous macules with purpuric center (target configuration) appear suddenly
	  • Most common on face, neck, and upper trunk but can appear anywhere
	• Macules coalesce into widespread, large, flaccid bullae that slough over 1-3 days
	• Involves mucosal membranes (ocular and oral involvement can be severe)
	  • Painful oral crusts, keratoconjunctivitis, genital involvement (urethritis, phimosis)
	• Skin sloughs with lateral pressure revealing weepy, painful and erythematous underlying skin (positive Nikolsky sign)

Diagnosis	• **Clinical Diagnosis** • <u>Biopsy</u>: confirms diagnosis; demonstrates full-thickness necrotic epithelium
Treatment	• **Discontinue inciting medication if identified** • <u>**Supportive**</u>: **fluid and electrolyte replacement**, pain management, airway management • <u>**Burn Unit Admission**</u>: indicated for severe cases, prompt treatment of secondary bacterial infections; daily wound care following burn protocols
Key Words & Most Common	• Severe hypersensitivity reaction characterized by detachment of epidermis and extensive skin necrosis • <u>Stevens-Johnson Syndrome</u>: involves <10% of skin body surface area • <u>Toxic Epidermal Necrolysis</u>: involves >30% of the skin body surface area • Sulfa medication is most common offending agent • Prodrome of fever + URI symptoms → erythematous macules with purpuric center that coalesce to flaccid bullae • Involve mucosal membranes • Skin sloughing (+ Nikolsky sign) • Discontinue offending agent + supportive care → burn unit admission

Erythematous macules with purpuric center and oral crusts

Alopecia Areata 👆

Etiology & Risk Factors	• **Condition characterized by sudden, patchy, nonscarring hair loss** • <u>Etiology</u>: **autoimmune disorder** • <u>Risk Factors</u>: **other autoimmune disorder (thyroiditis, vitiligo, SLE, Addison's disease)**, family history, **history of atopic dermatitis, emotional or physical stress**, immunization
Patho-physiology	• T-cell mediated autoimmune attack on hair follicle matrix epithelium, leading to the miniaturization and eventual dormancy of the hair follicle

Signs & Symptoms	• <u>Hair Abnormalities</u>: occurs over weeks, non-painful, non-pruritic
	  • **Discrete, circular patches of hair loss**
	  • **Short, broken hairs that taper near the proximal hair shaft (resemble exclamation points)** located at the patch margins
	  • Scalp and facial hair are most common areas affected; can occur anywhere
	• <u>Nail Abnormalities</u>: **fine pitting of the nails**, trachyonychia (roughness of the nail), nail fissuring

Diagnosis	• **Clinical Diagnosis** • <u>Biopsy</u>: definitive diagnosis; demonstrates lymphocytic inflammatory infiltrates surrounding the bulbar region of the hair follicles

Treatment	• <u>**Corticosteroids**</u>: **most effective treatment**
	  • <u>**Intralesional Corticosteroids**</u>: **first-line treatment**; triamcinolone acetonide injected every 2-6 weeks shows improvement of localized hair regrowth
	  • <u>**Topical Corticosteroids**</u>: **alternative first-line**; clobetasol propionate indicated in patients unable to tolerate injections or **extensive involvement**; *may induce folliculitis*
	  • <u>**Oral Corticosteroids**</u>: effective treatment however relapse is common after cessation of therapy
	• <u>Topical Anthralin</u>: used to stimulate a mild irritant reaction
	• <u>Topical Minoxidil</u>: adjuvant to corticosteroid or anthralin treatment

Key Words & Most Common	• Sudden, patchy, nonscarring hair loss • Most common secondary to autoimmune disorder • Autoimmune disorder (autoimmune thyroiditis, SLE most common), atopic dermatitis, stress greatest risk factors • Discrete, circular patches of hair loss • Short, broken hairs that taper near scalp (resemble exclamation points) • Nail pitting and fissuring • Clinical diagnosis • Intralesional corticosteroids injection first-line

Circular patches of hair loss

Androgenetic Alopecia

Etiology & Risk Factors	• **Progressive hair loss that occurs when the hair follicles shrink over time due to the influence of androgen hormones** • Follows a characteristic distribution (**male-pattern or female-pattern hair loss**) • <u>Etiology</u>: **genetic predisposition and hormonal influences** • <u>Risk Factors</u>: **increasing age, male, family history**, certain medical conditions (autoimmune disorders), **sedentary lifestyle, poor nutrition**, medications, **stress**
Patho-physiology	• DHT is a potent androgen hormone produced by testosterone by the enzyme 5-alpha reductase • Scalp hair follicles have greater number of androgen receptors increasing the sensitivity to DHT causing hair follicles to prematurely enter that catagen phase of hair growth leading to hair follicle miniaturization and hair loss
Signs & Symptoms	• Varying degrees of hair thinning and nonscarring hair loss • Gradual in onset and usually occurs after puberty • <u>Males</u>: **bitemporal thinning or hair loss of frontotemporal regions progressing to involve the vertex** • <u>Females</u>: **diffuse hair thinning or hair loss of the vertex (crown and top of head) that spares the frontal hairline** • Usually demonstrated as a wider hair part or a visible scalp
Diagnosis	• **Clinical Diagnosis** • <u>Dermoscopy</u>: demonstrates miniaturized hair and brown perihilar casts

Treatment	• <u>Topical Minoxidil</u>: **first-line treatment for new onset alopecia involving a smaller area**
	    • Dilates blood vessels allowing oxygen and nutrient flow to promote and lengthen the anagen (growth phase) and promotes growth in hair follicle diameter and length
	    • Hair regrowth usually takes 8-12 months and use is continued indefinitely (hair loss resumes if therapy is stopped)
	• <u>Oral Finasteride</u>: **5-alpha reductase inhibitor to inhibit the conversion of testosterone to dihydrotestosterone**
	• <u>Hormonal Modulators</u>: oral contraceptives or spironolactone may be useful for female-pattern hair loss
	• <u>Alternative Therapies</u>: low-level laser light therapy, autologous platelet-rich plasma injections may promote follicular growth
	• <u>Surgery</u>: follicle transplant, scalp flaps

Key Words & Most Common	• Progressive hair loss secondary to androgen hormone influence • Male, family history, sedentary lifestyle, poor nutrition, chronic stress are greatest risk factors • <u>**Males**</u>: **bitemporal thinning or hair loss of frontotemporal regions progressing to involve the vertex** • <u>**Females**</u>: **diffuse hair thinning or hair loss of the vertex (crown and top of head) that spares the frontal hairline** • Clinical Diagnosis • Topical minoxidil or oral finasteride is often first-line treatment

Onychomycosis

Etiology & Risk Factors	• **Fungal infection of the nail plate and/or nail bed** • <u>Etiology</u>: **dermatophyte infection is most common (*Trichophyton rubrum*)**; nondermatophyte molds (*Aspergillus, Scopulariopsis, Fusarium*); *Candida albicans* • <u>Risk Factors</u>: **increasing age, tinea pedis, males**, preexisting nail dystrophy (psoriasis), **exposure to tinea pedis or onychomycosis (public showers, pool decks, hotel carpet)**, diabetes, peripheral vascular disease, immunocompromised state
Patho-physiology	• Dermatophyte, yeast, or mold infection of the nail plate, nail bed or both, leading to an inflammatory reaction that results in dystrophic changes characterized by thickening, discoloration and deformity of the nail

Signs & Symptoms	• Most common on the **great toe**
	• **Opaque, thickened, and or cracked nails**
	• Patches of white or yellow discoloration and deformity of the nails
	• 3 Characteristic Patterns:
	    • <u>Distal Subungual</u>: nail thickening and yellowing with keratin and debris accumulation underneath and distally causing nail separation from the nail bed
	    • <u>Proximal Subungual</u>: nail changes begin proximally; indicates immunosuppression
	    • <u>White Superficial</u>: chalky white scale spreads beneath the nail surface

Diagnosis	• <u>Dermoscopy</u>: aids in clinical diagnosis; presence of subungual short spikes and longitudinal striae • <u>Potassium Hydroxide (KOH) Wet Mount Examination</u>: easily accessible rapid test; proximal nail scrapings are sampled and examined for hyphae; only 60% sensitive • <u>Periodic Acid-Schiff (PAS) Test</u>: **most sensitive rapid test**; performed on nail clippings • <u>Fungal Culture or PCR</u>: most specific test but lacks sensitivity; test but takes several weeks to result

Treatment	• *Confirmation of fungal infection is essential prior to initiating treatment as only 50% of dystrophic nails are secondary to fungal infection*
	• <u>Supportive</u>: keep nails short, keep feet clean and dry, wear absorbent socks (cotton or wool), use of antifungal foot powder, avoid wearing old or wet shoes
	• <u>Oral Antifungals</u>: **most effective treatment**
	    • <u>Terbinafine</u>: **first-line and most effective medication**; 250 mg once a day for 12 weeks
	    • <u>Itraconazole</u>: indicated for both dermatophytes and *Candida albicans*; 200 mg 2 times per day 1 week a month for 3 months
	    • *Baseline liver function studies should be drawn and trended during treatment due to risk of hepatotoxicity*
	• <u>Topical Antifungals</u>:
	    • <u>Efinaconazole or Tavaborole</u>: indicated if contraindication to oral antifungals or side effects not worth risk to patient

Key Words & Most Common	• Fungal infection of nail plate and/or nail bed • Dermatophyte (Trichophyton rubrum) most common cause • Exposure to public showers, pool decks, hotel carpet is most common risk factor • Opaque, thickened, and or cracked nails with patches of white or yellow discoloration • KOH or PAS rapid test + fungal culture • Oral antifungals (terbinafine) are most effective

Thickened, opaque/discoloration of nails

Paronychia

Etiology & Risk Factors	• Inflammation or infection of the proximal and/or lateral nail folds • <u>Etiology:</u> bacterial infection most common cause (*Staphylococcus aureus* most common; *Streptococcal pyogenes, Pseudomonas pyocyanea* and Proteus vulgaris) • <u>Risk Factors:</u> **female, trauma (biting/picking nailbed, finger sucking, ingrown toenail, manicures)**, chronic irritation (water submersion, detergent or chemical exposure), immunosuppression
Patho-physiology	• Trauma to the nail and nail fold leads to disruption of the protective barrier which allows organisms to enter and causing an acute infection
Signs & Symptoms	• **Pain, warmth, erythema and edema along the nail margin (lateral and/or proximal nail fold)** • **Purulence may accumulate** along the nail margin or beneath the nail (fluctuance on exam)
Diagnosis	• Clinical Diagnosis

Treatment	• <u>Supportive:</u> **warm water or warm saline soaks**, hand hygiene, avoid inciting factors (manicures, biting nails, irritations)
	• <u>Topical Antibiotic Ointment:</u> mupirocin 2% or triple antibiotic ointment indicated if mild or after incision and drainage
	• <u>Oral Antibiotics:</u> indicated for mild to moderate cases
	  • **Cephalexin or dicloxacillin are first-line**
	  • **Amoxicillin-clavulanic acid or clindamycin** if associated with nail biting
	  • Trimethoprim-sulfamethoxazole, clindamycin or doxycycline indicated if concern for MRSA
	• <u>Incision and Drainage:</u> **indicated if purulence or fluctuance present**
	  • Consider digital block for anesthesia
	  • Incise area of greatest fluctuance parallel to nail (do not incise perpendicular to nail) with #11 scalpel or iris scissors

Key Words & Most Common	• Inflammation/infection of proximal and/or lateral nail folds • Most commonly caused by *S. aureus* • Common with nail biting/picking, finger sucking, manicures • Pain, warmth, erythema and edema along along the nail margin +/- purulence • Clinical diagnosis • Warm water/saline soaks + oral antibiotics (cephalexin, amoxicillin-clavulanic acid or TMP-SMX) • I&D if purulent or fluctuant

Erythema and edema along the nail margin (proximal/lateral nail fold)

Felon

Etiology & Risk Factors	• **Subcutaneous pyogenic infection of the pulp space compartments of the distal finger** • <u>Etiology:</u> **bacterial infection most common cause** (*Staphylococcus aureus* most common; *Streptococcal pyogenes*); paronychia can progress to a felon • Risk Factors: **female, trauma (biting/picking nailbed, finger sucking, ingrown toenail, manicures), foreign body penetration (splinter, animal bite)**, chronic irritation (water submersion, detergent or chemical exposure), immunosuppression, **history of paronychia**
Patho-physiology	• Penetrating skin trauma introduction of bacteria into the fingertip pulp leading to infection and inflammation. The inflammatory response leads to increased pressure within the closed compartment of the fingertip, resulting in severe pain, swelling and abscess formation • Delayed treatment may allow infection spread to adjacent tissues, leading to more serious complications such as osteomyelitis, flexor tenosynovitis, sepsis, amputation

Signs & Symptoms	• **Severely painful, erythematous, edematous distal finger**
	  • **May have fluctuance** with abscess formation
	  • Necrotic appearing distal tissue secondary to increased pressure in pulp space may be present

Diagnosis	• **Clinical Diagnosis** • Consider x-ray to rule out radiopaque foreign body

Treatment	• <u>Supportive:</u> **warm water or warm saline soaks**, hand hygiene, elevation, removal of foreign body
	• <u>Incision and Drainage:</u> **indicated if purulence or fluctuance present**
	  • Digital block
	  • Incision should be made along the **ulnar aspect of the index, middle, and ring fingers** and along the **radial aspects of the thumb and little finger**
	  • Incision should be from 5 mm distal to flexor DIP crease to 5 mm proximal to nail plate border
	• <u>Oral Antibiotics:</u> indicated for associated cellulitis
	  • **Cephalexin or dicloxacillin are first-line**
	  • **Amoxicillin-clavulanic acid or clindamycin** if associated with nail biting
	  • **Trimethoprim-sulfamethoxazole**, clindamycin or doxycycline indicated if concern for MRSA

Key Words & Most Common	• Subcutaneous infection of pulp space of distal finger • S. aureus is most common cause • Penetrating trauma (splinter, animal bite, manicure, nailbed biting) is greatest risk factor • Severely painful, erythematous, edematous distal finger +/- fluctuance • Clinical diagnosis • I&D if fluctuant/purulent +oral antibiotics (cephalexin, amoxicillin-clavulanic acid or TMP-SMX)

Onychocryptosis

Etiology & Risk Factors	• **Incurvation or impingement of a toenail border into its adjacent nail fold** • <u>Etiology</u>: toenail growing into the skin of the toe • <u>Risk Factors</u>: **improper or excessive trimming of toenails, tight-fitting shoes or socks**, toe injury, family history, **curved or irregularly shaped toenails**, poor foot hygiene, **abnormal gait** (toe-walking), congenital variations in nail contour, bulbous toe shape
Patho-physiology	• Improper or excessive trimming of toenail or tight-fitting shows or socks cause the toenail plate to grow into the adjacent skin causing irritation and inflammation
Signs & Symptoms	• **Pain and swelling at the distal corner of the toenail fold** • **May involve entire lateral margin** • Pain may be gradual and may be mild or only noted with certain footwear
Diagnosis	• **Clinical Diagnosis**
Treatment	• <u>**Supportive**</u>: **larger toe box footwear,** warm water soaks, elevation, proper nail trimming techniques • <u>**Toenail Lifting**</u>: toenail is lifted and cotton is inserted between the ingrown nail plate and painful fold • Using a thin toothpick; prevents from growing into adjacent skin • <u>**Partial Toenail Excision**</u>: indicated in severe cases especially if concomitant paronychia present
Key Words & Most Common	• Toenail growing into skin of toe • Most common due to improper trimming of toenails or tight-fitting shoes/socks • Pain and swelling of distal corner of toenail fold • Clinical diagnosis • Supportive → toenail lifting → toenail excision

Edema at distal corner of toenail fold

Herpetic Whitlow

Etiology & Risk Factors	• **Cutaneous infection of the distal aspect of the finger caused by herpes simplex virus (HSV)** • <u>Etiology</u>: **contact with oral herpes or autoinoculation from genital herpes** • <u>Risk Factors</u>: **history of or exposure to HSV-1 (most common) or HSV-2**, immunocompromised, **poor hand hygiene, nail-biting**, finger-sucking, skin trauma, sharing personal items (towels, razors, or other personal care items that may have come into contact with the virus)
Patho-physiology	• Exposure to herpes simplex virus type 1 or type 2 results in viral invasion through break in skin barrier and subsequent viral replication within the epidermal and dermal cells that travels along nerve fibers to the sensory nerve ganglion. • HSV then becomes dormant in the ganglion until it reactivates and travels back along the nerve to the skin surface, causing recurrent outbreaks of the infection

Signs & Symptoms	• Infection usually occurs 2 to 20 days following exposure
	• **Intense pain, erythema and edema of finger**
	  • Pain may be burning or pruritic sensation
	• **Vesicular bullae develop on the volar or dorsal distal phalanx usually around the nail;** occurs 2-3 days after pain begins
	  • **Vesicles then coalesce into large, honeycomb-like bullae** in 5 to 6 days
	• Distal finger may be indurated and tender (not as tense as a felon)

Diagnosis	• **Clinical Diagnosis** • <u>Viral Culture</u>: most specific test; unroofing of vesicles and swabbing of fluid • <u>Polymerase chain reaction (PCR) by Immunofluorescence</u>: most sensitive test to confirm diagnosis and differentiate herpes simplex virus type 1 from type 2

Treatment	• <u>**Supportive**</u>: hand hygiene, avoid trauma (manicures, biting nails, irritants), elevation, pain control, keep vesicles covered to avoid autoinoculation and transmission
	• <u>**Antivirals**</u>: may shorten the duration of symptoms
	  • <u>**Topical Acyclovir 5%**</u>: shortens duration and viral shedding in primary infection
	  • <u>**Oral Acyclovir**</u>: 800mg twice daily may prevent recurrences if given immediately after onset of symptoms
	• <u>**Incision and Drainage: contraindicated**</u> as there is no symptomatic relief, may lead to transmission to others and/or cause viremia or bacterial superinfection

Key Words & Most Common	• Infection of distal aspect of finger caused by HSV • HSV 1 is most common • Intense pain, erythema, edema of finger • Vesicles at distal phalanx around nail that coalesce into large bullae • Clinical diagnosis • Antivirals (topical acyclovir shortens duration; oral acyclovir prevents recurrence) • I&D is contraindicated

Vesicular bullae at dorsal distal phalanx

Brown Recluse Spider Bite

Etiology & Risk Factors	• **Local tissue injury, inflammation and infection secondary to envenomation by a brown recluse spider**
	• <u>Etiology</u>: brown recluse spider (*Loxosceles reclusa*) which have a **violin pattern** on the anterior cephalothorax
	• <u>Risk Factors</u>:
	    • **Most common in the southwestern and midwestern US**
	    • Usually found in **woodpiles**, sheds, closets, **garages, basements**, and other places that are dry and undisturbed; **most commonly inhabit rotting wood or cardboard**

Patho-physiology	• Venom contains sphingomyelinase D which is the protein component that is cytotoxic and hemolytic; the procoagulant enzymes may cause thrombosis and ischemia leading to local necrosis

Signs & Symptoms	• <u>Systemic Reaction</u>:
	    • Malaise, fever and chills, nausea/vomiting, generalized morbilliform rash are initial symptoms
	• <u>Local Reaction</u>:
	    • **Initial bite is usually painless** followed by increasing pain over the subsequent 2-8 hours
	    • Bite site may have **2 small puncture wounds** with surrounding erythema and burning/pruritic pain
	    • **Center of bite will blanch and become paler as the outer edge becomes more erythematous and edematous** ("red halo"; indicates local vasospasm) over 3-4 hours
	    • **Hemorrhagic bullae then develops with ecchymotic center; may ruptures revealing an ulcer that undergoes eschar formation and can become necrotic**
	    • "Red, white and blue" sign (erythema, blanching, ecchymosis)
	    • Skin sloughing may occur

Diagnosis	• **Clinical Diagnosis**

Treatment	• <u>Supportive</u>: elevation of extremity, tetanus prophylaxis, **pain control** (NSAIDs, opioids if severe)
	• **<u>Local Wound Care</u>**:
	    • **Clean daily with soap and water, wound debridement** as indicated
	    • **Local application of ice** (sphingomyelinase D is temperature dependent and may slow necrosis process)
	    • Topical antibiotic ointment (polymyxin/bacitracin/neomycin; mupirocin) may be used
	• <u>Oral Antibiotics</u>: indicated if secondary infection develops (cellulitis)

Key Words & Most Common	• Local tissue injury/infection secondary to brown recluse spider bite • Most common in southwestern and midwestern US • Found in woodpiles, garages, basements, rotting wood or cardboard • Painless bite → 2 small puncture wounds + surrounding erythema + burning pain • Hemorrhagic blister forms surrounded by blanched skin (vasoconstriction) → ecchymosis → ruptures revealing ulcer that undergoes eschar formation and becomes necrotic • Clinical diagnosis • Pain control + local wound care +/- antibiotics

Ulcer with eschar formation

Black Widow Spider Bite

Etiology & Risk Factors	• **Local tissue injury, inflammation and infection secondary to envenomation by a black widow spider**
	• <u>Etiology</u>: black widow spider (*Latrodectus spp.*) which has a **shiny black body and red hourglass shape on the abdomen**
	• <u>Risk Factors</u>:
	    • **Present throughout the US**
	    • Occupational or recreational exposure to **woodpiles, rubble, garages, abandoned buildings**, or engaging in activities such as **gardening, hiking, camping**

Patho-physiology	• Venom has a combination of biologically active proteins, peptides and proteases; neurotoxic component includes alpha-latrotoxin which affects neuromuscular transmission and results in massive release of neurotransmitters (acetylcholine, dopamine, norepinephrine, glutamate) which causes muscle cramps, tachycardia, hypertension

Signs & Symptoms	• <u>Local Reaction</u>:
	    • **Initial painful** ("pinprick" sensation), **erythematous and edematous bite site** (blanched circular patch with surrounding erythematous perimeter)
	    • Followed by the **development of a central punctum** (central, dark comedone opening)
	    • Bite site may have **2 small puncture wounds**
	    • **Isolated diaphoresis and piloerection around bite site**
	• <u>Systemic Reaction</u>:
	    • Headache, nausea/vomiting, diaphoresis, photophobia, dyspnea
	    • **Neuromuscular symptoms (severe muscle pain, spasms and cramping are most prominent features)**
	    • Increased autonomic function (**tachycardia, tachypnea, hypertension**)
	• **<u>Latrodectism</u>: systemic syndrome caused by neurotoxic venom components of widow spider bites**
	    • **Diffuse muscle rigidity and cramping**, tenderness and burning around at the bite site, truncal and abdominal tenderness, nausea, and vomiting,
	    • Restlessness, anxiety, diaphoresis, dizziness, headache
	    • Diffuse erythematous rash, pruritus, extremity edema, increased skin temperature over affected area

Diagnosis	• **Clinical Diagnosis**

Treatment	• <u>Supportive</u>: elevation of extremity, tetanus prophylaxis, **pain control** (NSAIDs, opioids if severe)
	• **<u>Local Wound Care</u>**:
	    • **Clean daily with soap and water, wound debridement** as indicated
	    • **Local application of ice** (pain control)
	    • Topical antibiotic ointment (polymyxin/bacitracin/neomycin; mupirocin) may be used
	• <u>Oral Antibiotics</u>: indicated if secondary infection develops (cellulitis)
	• **<u>Black Widow Spider Antivenom</u>: safe and highly effective; usually only indicated for elderly patients or patients with significant comorbidities**
	• Benzodiazepines or muscle relaxants may be indicated for severe muscle spasms

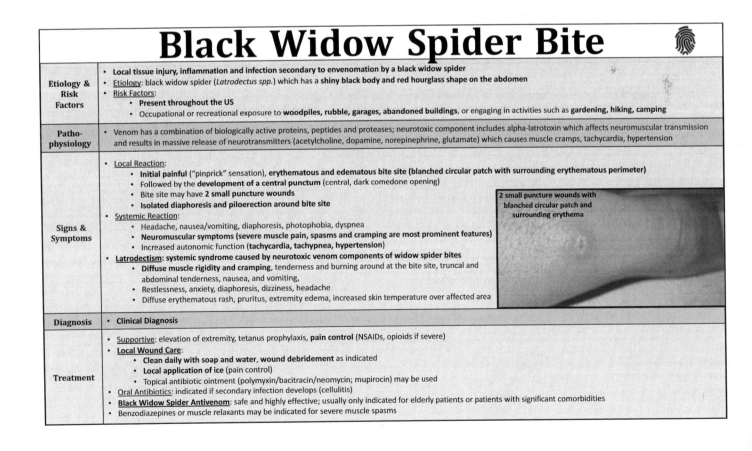

2 small puncture wounds with blanched circular patch and surrounding erythema

Hymenoptera Stings

Etiology & Risk Factors	• Local or systemic reaction due to venomous material injected by an insect, including bees, wasps, hornets, yellow jackets, and fire ants • Etiology: Apids (honeybees, bumblebees), Vespids (wasps, yellow jackets, hornets), Formicids (nonwinged fire ants) • Risk Factors: outdoor activities that increase exposure to insects (hiking, gardening, picnicking, camping) wearing brightly colored or floral-patterned clothing
Patho-physiology	• Apids: usually do not sting unless provoked; single sting results in dislodging of a barbed stinger into the wound; melittin is the main pain-inducing component of the venom • Vespid: stingers do not stay in the skin which allows the insect to sting multiple times; allergenic venom contains phospholipase, hyaluronidases and antigen 5 protein • Formicids: fire ants anchor to the person and repeatedly stings and rotates body in an arc; venom is hemolytic, cytolytic, antimicrobial and insecticidal

Signs & Symptoms	• Immediate burning, pain and pruritus at sting site
	  • May develop urticarial wheal at sting site
	  • May have stinger present if apid sting
	• Erythema, edema and induration develops surrounding the sting site minutes to hours after sting (usually peaks 48 hours after sting)
	  • Often misdiagnosed as secondary bacterial cellulitis
	• Allergic reactions may present with diffuse urticaria, angioedema, bronchospasm (wheezing, shortness of breath), refractory hypotension

Diagnosis	• Clinical Diagnosis • Secondary bacterial cellulitis may be considered if erythema and edema appear 1-2 days after the sting (rather than immediately), have systemic symptoms (fever/chills) or increasing pain level
Treatment	• Supportive: cool compresses, tetanus prophylaxis, pain control (NSAIDs, opioids if severe) • Immediate Removal of Stinger: most important initial step if present; methods include scraping with a thin, dull edge (edge of a credit card, dull side of scalpel) • Oral Antihistamines: H1 blockers (diphenhydramine) initial medication management indicated for mild or local reactions • Topical Treatment: topical antihistamines, lidocaine patches or cream, intradermal injection of 1% lidocaine, and topical mid-potency corticosteroids (triamcinolone 0.1%) • Parenteral Treatment: consider IM corticosteroids if mild to moderate symptoms without signs of anaphylaxis • Anaphylaxis: parenteral epinephrine, IV fluids and vasopressors if necessary
Key Words & Most Common	• Immediate burning, pain, pruritus + urticarial wheal at sting site • Surrounding erythema, edema, induration develops minutes to hours later (peaks 48 hours after) • May have evidence of anaphylaxis • Clinical diagnosis • Immediate removal of stinger → pain control → oral antihistamines • Anaphylaxis management if present

Urticarial wheal with surrounding erythema

Erythema Infectiosum

Etiology & Risk Factors	• Viral infection also known as fifth disease • Etiology: parvovirus B19 • Risk Factors: seasonal (most common in spring), age (most common among children 5-7 years old), high risk exposures (daycare or school settings)
Patho-physiology	• Transmission: respiratory droplets; 4-14 day incubation period • Parvovirus B19 infects and destroys reticulocytes resulting in a transient suppression of erythropoiesis (leading to aplastic crisis in patients with sickle cell disease) • Transplacental transmission possible in pregnant females without immunity; can result in stillbirth or severe fetal anemia with widespread edema (hydrops fetalis)
Signs & Symptoms	• Nonspecific flu-like symptoms (low-grade fever, malaise, coryza, pharyngitis) initially • Erythematous malar rash appears over the cheeks ("slapped-cheek" appearance) and circumoral pallor for 2-4 days • Symmetric, reticular or lacy, maculopapular rash appears on the extremities (especially upper) and/or trunk; usually spares the palms and soles usually lasting for 5-10 days • Rash may recur for several weeks, exacerbated by sunlight, exercise, heat, fever and/or emotional stress • Arthralgias may be present in older children and adults
Diagnosis	• Clinical Diagnosis • Serologies: Parvovirus B19 specific IgM-antibody confirms diagnosis

Treatment	• Supportive: mainstay of treatment; self-limited disease
	  • Analgesia/antipyretics (acetaminophen and/or NSAIDs)
	  • Oral hydration
	• IV Immunoglobulin: indicated for immunocompromised children
	• Pregnancy: regular fetal monitoring and close follow-up with obstetrician

Key Words & Most Common	• AKA fifth disease • Viral infection caused by parvovirus B19 • Most common in spring and in children • 4-14 day incubation period • Nonspecific flu-like symptoms → erythematous malar rash over cheeks → reticular/lacy maculopapular rash of extremities and trunk • Clinical diagnosis • Supportive treatment

Erythematous malar rash with a "slapped-cheek" appearance

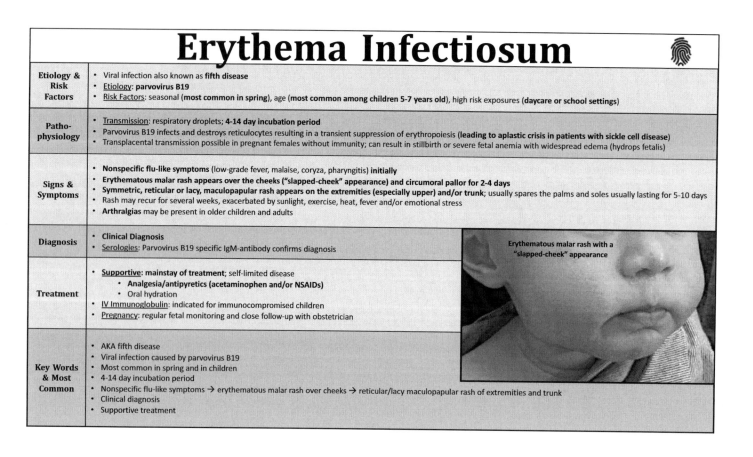

Measles (Rubeola)

Etiology & Risk Factors	• Highly contagious RNA virus that primarily affects the respiratory system • Etiology: **measles virus, part of the Paramyxovirus family** • Risk Factors: **lack of immunization, international travel to areas with outbreaks, exposure to international terminal at airports or interaction with foreign visitors** (U.S. tourist attractions), **crowded areas** (schools, dorms, military barracks, daycare centers, public transportation), **immunocompromised**
Patho-physiology	• Transmission: respiratory droplets; **7-14 day incubation period** • Virus enters the respiratory tract (nasopharynx) and infects the mucous membranes, then spreads throughout the body via the bloodstream, causing a systemic infection; viral replication initially occurs in immune cells of the lymphatic system and may also infect and damage the respiratory epithelium and skin, leading to characteristic rashes

Signs & Symptoms	• **Prodrome:**
	  • **Fever, coryza, cough and conjunctivitis** followed by Koplik spots
	• **Koplik Spots: pathognomonic enanthem**
	  • **Small 1-3mm pale white papules with erythematous base on the buccal mucosa**; precedes rash by about 24-48 hours
	  • **Most commonly on oral mucosa opposite the 1st and 2nd upper molars**; may be extensive
	  • Spots resemble "grains of white sand surrounded by red base"
	• **Generalized Exanthem:** appears 3-5 days after symptom onset; 1-2 days after Koplik spots appear
	  • **Morbilliform (maculopapular), erythematous rash beginning on face at the hairline and behind the ears**
	  • **Descending rash spreads to trunk and extremities (including palms and soles) as the lesions fade on the face**
	  • Rash usually lasts 3-5 days and may fade rapidly, leaving a darkened, coppery-brown discoloration followed by desquamation

Diagnosis	• **Clinical Diagnosis** • **Viral Detection via Polymerase Chain Reaction (PCR): preferred testing method to confirm diagnosis** • Measles IgM Serology: frequent false positives; no longer recommended

Treatment	• **Supportive: mainstay of treatment**; self-limited disease
	  • **Analgesia/antipyretics (acetaminophen and/or NSAIDs)**
	  • Oral hydration
	• **Vitamin A Supplementation:** reduces morbidity and mortality
	  • Dose is once per day for 2 days
	    • **≥1 Year:** 200,000 international units (IU)
	    • **6-11 Months:** 100,000 IU
	    • **≤6 Months:** 50,000 IU
	• Prevention: live-attenuated virus vaccine containing measles, mumps, and rubella
	  • First dose recommended at 12-15 months; second dose recommended at 4-6 years old

Morbilliform Rash

Koplik Spots

Hand-Foot-and-Mouth Disease

Etiology & Risk Factors	• Etiology: **coxsackievirus A16 most common cause**; enterovirus 72 or other enteroviruses • Risk Factors: seasonal (**most common in summer and early fall**), age (**most common among children <5 years old**), high risk exposures (**daycare or school settings**)
Patho-physiology	• Transmission: **fecal-oral or oral-oral** • Virus invasion through oral ingestion (GI or upper respiratory tract) and then replicates in the lymphoid tissue of the lower intestine and the pharynx with subsequent spread to the regional lymph nodes

Signs & Symptoms	• **Prodrome:**
	  • Mild fever, reduced appetite, URI symptoms, sore mouth or mouth pain, general malaise
	• **Oral Enanthem:** occurs 1-2 days later
	  • **Painful vesicles surrounded by a thin, erythematous halo**
	  • **Eventually ulcerate with a grey-yellow base and erythematous rim**
	  • **Found on buccal mucosa, tongue, soft palate and gingiva**
	• **Exanthem:** follows oral enanthem; lasts about 10 days
	  • **Erythematous macular, maculopapular or vesicular greyish-yellow, 2-6mm lesions that involve the distal extremities (including palms and soles)**
	    • **Red papules that change to grey vesicles on the hands and feet most common**
	  • Usually not painful or pruritic

Diagnosis	• **Clinical Diagnosis** • Viral Detection via Polymerase Chain Reaction (PCR): preferred testing method to confirm diagnosis

Treatment	• **Supportive: mainstay of treatment**; self-limited disease
	  • **Analgesia/antipyretics (acetaminophen and/or NSAIDs)**
	  • Oral hydration
	• **Dietary Modifications:** soft diet, avoid acidic or excessively salty foods
	• **Oral Lesions:** mixture of viscous lidocaine, liquid ibuprofen and liquid diphenhydramine can be used to swish and spit or gargle to coat oral ulcers
	  • ***Lidocaine is contraindicated in infants (due to risk of lidocaine toxicity and FDA block box warning)***

Key Words & Most Common	• Coxsackievirus A16 most common cause • Most common in summer/fall and in children <5 years old • Prodrome: fever + URI symptoms • Oral Enanthem: painful, erythematous oral vesicles that ulcerate • Exanthem: erythematous maculopapular rash that changes to grey vesicles on hands and feet • Supportive treatment

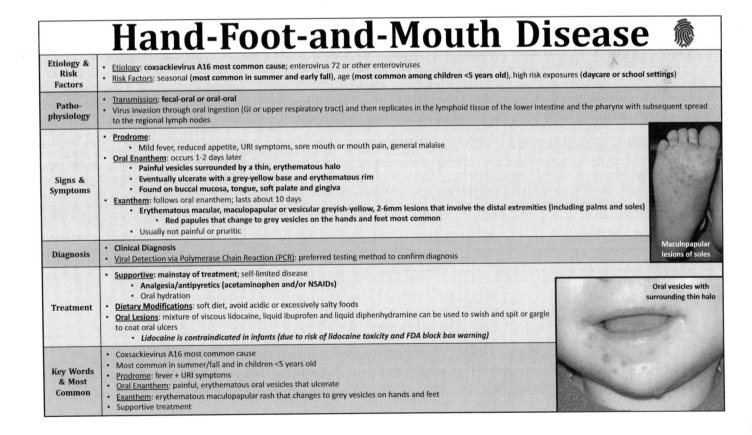

Maculopapular lesions of soles

Oral vesicles with surrounding thin halo

Herpangina

Etiology & Risk Factors	• <u>Etiology</u>: **coxsackievirus type A most common**; coxsackievirus type B, other enteroviruses • <u>Risk Factors</u>: seasonal (**most common in summer and early fall**), age (**most common among children 3-10 years old**), high risk exposures (**daycare or school settings**)
Patho-physiology	• Virus invasion through oral ingestion and infects the cells lining the upper GI or upper respiratory tract, leading to inflammation and the formation of small, painful ulcers or blisters in the mouth and throat

Signs & Symptoms	• <u>Prodrome</u>:
	  • **Sudden onset of high fever, sore throat, malaise**
	• <u>Oral Enanthem</u>: occurs 24-48 hours after prodrome
	  • **Small, painful, yellow-white or grayish papules that become vesicles with an erythematous rim**
	  • **Lesions then become shallow ulcers before healing**; usually heal in 1-7 days
	  • **Most common on posterior pharynx** (soft palate, tonsillar pillars, uvula)
	• <u>Other</u>: decreased appetite (secondary to oral pain), pharyngitis, odynophagia, malaise, headache, nausea

Diagnosis	• **Clinical Diagnosis** • <u>Viral Detection via Polymerase Chain Reaction (PCR)</u>: preferred testing method to confirm diagnosis

Treatment	• **Supportive: mainstay of treatment**; self-limited disease
	  • **Analgesia/antipyretics (acetaminophen and/or NSAIDs)**
	  • Oral hydration
	  • Oral hygiene (using a soft toothbrush and salt-water rinses)
	• <u>Dietary Modifications</u>: soft diet, avoid acidic or excessively salty foods
	• <u>Oral Lesions</u>: mixture of viscous lidocaine, liquid ibuprofen and liquid diphenhydramine can be used to swish and spit or gargle to coat oral ulcers
	  • *Lidocaine is contraindicated in infants (due to risk of lidocaine toxicity and FDA block box warning)*

Key Words & Most Common	• Coxsackievirus A16 most common cause
	• Most common in summer/fall and in children 3-10 years old
	• <u>Prodrome</u>: sudden onset high fever + sore throat + malaise
	• <u>Oral Enanthem</u>: Small, painful, grayish papules that become vesicles with erythematous rim
	  • Become shallow ulcers before healing
	  • Most common on posterior pharynx
	• Supportive treatment

Oral herpangitic lesions

Cellulitis

Etiology & Risk Factors	• **Acute bacterial infection of the skin and subcutaneous tissue** • <u>Etiology</u>: **group A beta-hemolytic streptococci (*Streptococcus pyogenes*) most common cause**; *Staphylococcus aureus*, MRSA, *S. agalactiae*, gram-negative bacilli • <u>Risk Factors</u>: **skin conditions resulting in breaks in the skin** (eczema, psoriasis, tinea), **skin injuries** (lacerations, abrasions, punctures, burns), **immunocompromised**. IV drug use, **obesity, chronic venous insufficiency or lymphedema**, history of cellulitis
Patho-physiology	• Bacteria breaches the epidermis resulting in a cytokine and neutrophilic response leading production of antimicrobial peptides and keratinocyte proliferation resulting in an epidermal inflammatory response • *Streptococci* infection results in diffuse, rapidly spreading infection as specific enzymes (streptokinase, DNase, hyaluronidase) disrupt the cellular components that usually contain and localize the inflammation

Signs & Symptoms	• **Most common in lower extremities and unilateral** (stasis dermatitis mimics cellulitis but is typically bilateral)
	• <u>Local Symptoms</u>:
	  • **Localized macular erythema, edema, warmth and tenderness**
	  • **Indistinct margins** that are tender and indurated (firm)
	• <u>Systemic Symptoms</u>:
	  • **Fever**, chills, **regional lymphadenopathy**, malaise, myalgias, **lymphangitis (streaking)**, tachycardia

Diagnosis	• **Clinical Diagnosis** • <u>Wound Culture</u>: may be indicated if no response to initial antibiotic regimen • *Suspect MRSA if purulent, penetrating trauma, surgical wound, recent hospitalization, IV drug use, implanted medical device, history of MRSA, nasal colonization of MRSA*

Treatment	• **Supportive**: immobilization and elevation of the affected area to reduce edema, analgesia (acetaminophen, NSAIDs), cool, wet dressings to relieve local discomfort
	• **Antibiotics**:
	  • <u>Mild/Moderate Infection</u>: **dicloxacillin or cephalexin is first-line**; clindamycin, clarithromycin or azithromycin alternatives if penicillin allergic
	    • Consider single IM injection of ceftriaxone in outpatient setting based on extent
	  • <u>MRSA Infection</u>:
	    • <u>Oral</u>: **trimethoprim-sulfamethoxazole, clindamycin, doxycycline**
	    • <u>IV</u>: **vancomycin is first-line**; linezolid, daptomycin
	  • <u>Mammalian Bite Infection</u>: **amoxicillin-clavulanate is first-line (covers for Pasteurella multicide)**; clindamycin *plus* either ciprofloxacin *or* trimethoprim-sulfamethoxazole if penicillin allergic
	  • <u>Saltwater-Related Infection</u>: PO/IV doxycycline plus IV cefepime (covers for *Vibrio vulnificus*); PO/IV ciprofloxacin alternative
	  • <u>Freshwater-Related infection</u>: PO/IV ciprofloxacin (covers for *Aeromonas spp.*); PO trimethoprim-sulfamethoxazole, IV ceftriaxone

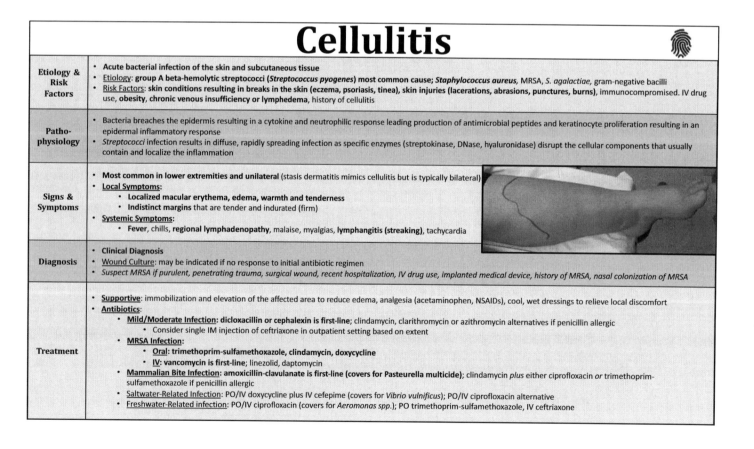

Erysipelas

Etiology & Risk Factors	• Variant of superficial cellulitis involving the superficial dermis layers and subcutaneous tissues (including lymphatics) • <u>Etiology</u>: group A beta-hemolytic streptococci (*Streptococcus pyogenes*) most common cause; *Staphylococcus aureus*, MRSA • <u>Risk Factors</u>: **skin breaks (surgical incisions, insect bites, stasis ulcerations, , eczema, tinea, venous stasis are most common), saphenous vein harvesting for bypass surgery, chronic venous insufficiency or lymphedema,** lymphatic obstruction, immunocompromised, obesity, IV drug abuse, poorly controlled diabetes, liver disease
Patho-physiology	• Bacteria breaches the epidermis resulting in a cytokine and neutrophilic response leading production of antimicrobial peptides and keratinocyte proliferation resulting in an epidermal inflammatory response

Signs & Symptoms	• **Most common in lower extremities or face**
	• <u>Local Symptoms</u>:
	  • **Intensely erythematous, shiny, raised, indurated, tender plaques**
	  • **Sharply demarcated borders**
	• <u>Systemic Symptoms</u>:
	  • **Fever**, chills, malaise, headache, tachycardia, nausea/vomiting
	  • *More commonly present with systemic symptoms than cellulitis*

Diagnosis	• **Clinical Diagnosis**

Treatment	• <u>Supportive</u>: immobilization and elevation of the affected area to reduce edema, analgesia (acetaminophen, NSAIDs), cool, wet dressings to relieve local discomfort
	• <u>Antibiotics</u>:
	  • <u>Mild/Moderate Infection</u>:
	    • <u>Oral</u>: **penicillin V is first-line**; cephalexin, amoxicillin-clavulanate are alternatives; clindamycin or erythromycin if penicillin allergic
	    • <u>IV</u>: cefazolin, ceftriaxone or levofloxacin
	  • <u>MRSA Infection</u>:
	    • <u>Oral</u>: **trimethoprim-sulfamethoxazole, clindamycin, doxycycline**
	    • <u>IV</u>: **vancomycin is first-line**; linezolid, daptomycin

Key Words & Most Common	• Variant of superficial cellulitis involving superficial dermis layers, subcutaneous tissues and lymphatics • *Streptococcus pyogenes* is most common cause • Most common on lower extremities or face • **Intensely erythematous, shiny, raised, indurated, tender plaques with sharply demarcated borders** • Penicillin V is first-line; TMP-SMX or clindamycin indicated if MRSA suspected

Intensely erythematous, raised, indurated plaques of the face

Lymphangitis

Etiology & Risk Factors	• **Acute inflammation or infection of peripheral deep dermal/subdermal lymphatic channels** • <u>Etiology</u>: *Streptococcal* infection most common; *Staphylococcal*, *Pasteurella*, anthrax, herpes simplex virus, lymphogranuloma venereum, rickettsia, sporotrichosis, malignancy • <u>Risk Factors</u>: **skin infection (cellulitis) spread to lymphatic vessels, injury or trauma to skin,** immunocompromised, diabetes mellitus, **lymphedema**
Patho-physiology	• Inoculation of skin flora through superficial abrasion, wound or coexisting infection (cellulitis) results in infection spreading to lymphatic channels

Signs & Symptoms	• <u>Local Symptoms</u>:
	  • **Erythematous, irregular, warm, tender streaking extends proximally from a peripheral lesion toward regional lymph nodes**
	  • **Enlarged and tender regional lymph nodes (lymphadenitis)**
	• <u>Systemic Symptoms</u>:
	  • **Fever**, chills, malaise, headache, tachycardia, nausea/vomiting

Diagnosis	• **Clinical Diagnosis**

Treatment	• <u>Supportive</u>: immobilization and elevation of the affected area to reduce edema, analgesia (acetaminophen, NSAIDs), cool, wet dressings to relieve local discomfort
	• <u>Antibiotics</u>: treat like cellulitis
	  • <u>Mild/Moderate Infection</u>: **dicloxacillin or cephalexin is first-line**; clindamycin, clarithromycin or azithromycin alternatives if penicillin allergic
	    • Consider single IM injection of ceftriaxone in outpatient setting based on extent
	  • <u>MRSA Infection</u>:
	    • <u>Oral</u>: **trimethoprim-sulfamethoxazole, clindamycin, doxycycline**
	    • <u>IV</u>: **vancomycin is first-line**; linezolid, daptomycin
	  • <u>Mammalian Bite Infection</u>: amoxicillin-clavulanate is first-line (covers for *Pasteurella multicide*); clindamycin *plus* either ciprofloxacin *or* trimethoprim-sulfamethoxazole if penicillin allergic
	  • <u>Saltwater-Related Infection</u>: PO/IV doxycycline plus IV cefepime (covers for *Vibrio vulnificus*); PO/IV ciprofloxacin alternative
	  • <u>Freshwater-Related infection</u>: PO/IV ciprofloxacin (covers for *Aeromonas spp.*); PO trimethoprim-sulfamethoxazole, IV ceftriaxone

Key Words & Most Common	• Acute inflammation/infection of lymphatic channels • Streptococcal infection most common • skin infection (cellulitis) spread to lymphatic vessels most common cause • Streaking erythema extending proximally from cellulitis toward regional lymph nodes • Treat like cellulitis

Erythematous streaking

Furuncle and Carbuncle

Etiology & Risk Factors	• Localized collection of pus surrounded by inflamed tissue, usually secondary to bacterial infection • Etiology: *Staphylococcus aureus* (including MRSA) is most common; *Streptococcus* • Risk Factors: poor hygiene, trauma to skin (cuts, scrapes, insect bites), obesity, poor nutrition, occupational exposures (dirt, oil, chemicals), immunocompromised, diabetes mellitus, hot and humid climates, occlusion or abnormal follicular anatomy (comedones in acne)
Patho-physiology	• Furuncles: deep skin abscesses involving a hair follicle and surrounding tissue (in contrast to folliculitis which is superficial) • Carbuncles: clusters of furuncles that are subcutaneously interconnected, causing deeper suppuration and scarring from multiple hair follicles

Signs & Symptoms	• Most common on the nape of the neck, breasts, face, back, axillae, groin and buttocks
	• Local Symptoms:
	  • Erythematous, tender nodule or pustule with surrounding induration
	  • Fluctuance (abscess); may discharge sanguineous pus
	• Systemic Symptoms: more common with carbuncles
	  • Regional lymphadenopathy, fever, fatigue, malaise

Diagnosis	• Clinical Diagnosis • Bacterial Culture and Sensitivities: helpful to identify organism and guide antibiotic therapy

Treatment	• Supportive: warm, moist compresses with dry covering and/or warm saline soaks if spontaneously draining
	• Incision and Drainage: mainstay of treatment
	  • Local anesthetic (1% lidocaine)
	  • #11 blade is used to make an incision into the cavity with peripheral manual pressure to express the purulent material
	  • Sterile hemostat may be used to break up any loculations followed by repeat peripheral manual pressure
	  • Cavity packing with iodoform strips or gauze to assist with further drainage
	• Antibiotics: indicated for lesions >5mm or <5mm not resolving with I&D, multiple lesions, cellulitis, immunocompromised, fever
	  • Oral: trimethoprim-sulfamethoxazole, clindamycin, or doxycycline; MRSA coverage
	  • IV: vancomycin is first-line; linezolid, daptomycin
	• Recurrence: bathe with a benzoyl peroxide wash or antibacterial soap; decolonization of the nares (application of mupirocin twice daily to the inner nares for 2-4 weeks)

Key Words & Most Common	• Furuncles: deep skin abscesses involving a hair follicle and surrounding tissue (in contrast to folliculitis which is superficial) • Carbuncles: clusters of furuncles that are subcutaneously interconnected, causing deeper suppuration and scarring from multiple hair follicles • *S. aureus* (MRSA) most common cause • Erythematous, tender nodule/pustule with surrounding induration +/- fluctuance • I&D is first-line treatment +/- antibiotics (TMP-SMX, clindamycin or doxycycline)

Erythematous pustule

Impetigo

Etiology & Risk Factors	• Highly contagious, superficial, vesiculopustular skin infection with crusts (nonbullous) or vesicles (bullous) • Etiology: *Staphylococcus aureus* and/or *Streptococcus pyogenes* most common, MRSA • Risk Factors: age (2-6 years old most common), trauma to skin (cuts, scrapes, insect bites, eczema), poor hygiene, low socioeconomic status, warm and humid climate, high risk exposures (daycare or school settings)
Patho-physiology	• Bacteria enter through a break in the skin and multiply to cause infection; bacteria produce toxins that cause the characteristic symptoms • *S. aureus* is the most common cause of nonbullous impetigo and all cases of bullous impetigo; bullae are formed due to the exfoliative toxin produced by staphylococci

Signs & Symptoms	• Nonbullous Impetigo: most common type
	  • Clusters of vesicles or pustules that rupture and develop a "honey-colored, golden crust" (exudate from the lesion base) over the lesions
	  • Smaller lesions may coalesce into larger crusted plaques
	  • Usually occur at signs of superficial skin trauma (insect bites) of the face, arms, ankles
	• Bullous Impetigo: bullae form as a result of staphylococci toxin
	  • Vesicles enlarge rapidly to form bullae that rupture to form larger bases resulting in "honey-colored varnish"
	• Ecthyma:
	  • Small, shallow, punched-out, pyodermic ulcers the develop thick, brown/black crusts and surrounding erythema

Diagnosis	• Clinical Diagnosis • Gram Stain and Wound Culture: indicated if recurrent or no response to empiric therapy

Treatment	• Supportive: gentle cleansing with soap and water several times a day to remove crusts prior to topical treatment; maintain adequate hygiene, avoid high risk exposures
	• Topical Antibiotics: indicated for localized, uncomplicated nonbullous impetigo
	  • Mupirocin 2% ointment (TID for 5-10 days) is first-line topical antibiotic; retapamulin ointment or ozenoxacin cream are alternatives
	• Oral Antibiotics: indicated if immunocompromised, extensive or resistant impetigo lesions or ecthyma
	  • Dicloxacillin or cephalexin are first-line oral antibiotics; clindamycin or erythromycin if penicillin allergic
	  • Trimethoprim-sulfamethoxazole, clindamycin, or doxycycline indicated if resistant or MRSA identified on culture
	• Complications: cellulitis, acute glomerulonephritis (streptococci), lymphangitis, furunculosis, and hypo/hyperpigmentation

Key Words & Most Common	• Superficial vesiculopustular skin infection with crusts (nonbullous) or vesicles (bullous) • S. aureus and/or S. pyogenes most common • Nonbullous: clusters of vesicles that rupture to form a "honey-colored, golden crust" • Bullous: vesicles enlarge rapidly and form larger bases • Topical mupirocin + proper hygiene is first-line treatment

Clusters of vesicles with crust

Tinea Capitis

Scalp Ringworm	**Tinea Capitis**	

Etiology & Risk Factors	• Dermatophyte infection of the scalp • <u>Etiology</u>: *Trichophyton tonsurans* is the most common cause; *Microsporum canis, M. audouinii* or other *Trichophyton* spp. • <u>Risk Factors</u>: **age (3-7 years old most common), male, close exposure (sharing combs, hair trimmers, hats, pillows)**, ethnicity (African American), hot and humid climate, **immunocompromised**, prolonged corticosteroid use, anemia
Patho-physiology	• Descending fungal growth and invasion into the stratum corneum and keratin (hair); infected hair eventually becomes brittle and is exposed to breakage leading to hair loss

Signs & Symptoms	• <u>General Presentation</u>:
	  • **Erythematous papules that increase in size is most common initial symptom**
	  • Patchy alopecia that may be normal at the center with an irritated, erythematous, or inflamed border
	• <u>Black Dot Tinea Capitis</u>: **classic presentation; patches of alopecia with multiple black dots due to infection and fracture of the hair shafts**
	• <u>Scaly Patch Tinea Capitis</u>: single or multiple scaly patches with alopecia; erythema and pruritus may be present
	• <u>Kerion</u>: severe infection leading to inflammatory plaque formation with pustules and crusting; may progress to scarring alopecia
	• <u>Favus</u>: boggy inflammatory type presenting with boggy, oozing nodules, abscesses or crusting (composed of dried scalp secretion, fungi, and skin and inflammatory cells)

Diagnosis	• <u>Clinical Diagnosis</u> • <u>Potassium Hydroxide (KOH) Wet Mount</u>: most common initial test; identifies fungal element inside (endothrix) or outside (ectothrix) the hair shaft to help guide treatment • <u>Wood Light Examination</u>: blue-green fluorescence indicates *Microsporum* infection; no fluorescence indicates *Trichophyton* infection • <u>Fungal Culture</u>: definitive diagnosis

Treatment	• <u>Supportive</u>: avoid sharing hats, trimmers, combs, pillows; disinfecting of combs and hair trimmers
	• <u>Oral Antifungals</u>:
	  • <u>Griseofulvin</u>: **first-line treatment**; treatment course is 6-12 weeks and taken with food (fatty foods aid in absorption)
	    • *No labs required prior to griseofulvin treatment; if repeat courses or if therapy continued beyond 8 weeks then obtain CBC and LFTs*
	  • <u>Terbinafine</u>: **alternative first-line treatment**; treatment course is 2-4 weeks and can be taken without regard to meals
	    • *Labs (CBC and LFTs) are required prior to initiating treatment*
	  • Fluconazole or Itraconazole are second-line treatments
	<u>Adjunctive Treatment</u>: selenium sulfide 1 or 2.5%, ciclopirox 1%, or ketoconazole 2% shampoo twice weekly (decreases shedding of fungal spores)

Key Words & Most Common	• Dermatophyte infection of scalp, most commonly caused by *Trichophyton tonsurans* • 3-7 years old, male, close exposures (sharing hats, combs, pillows) most common • Scaly, pruritic, patchy alopecia • Clinical diagnosis +/- KOH prep • Griseofulvin is first-line; longer treatment but doesn't require initial CBC/LFTs • Terbinafine is alternative first-line; shorter treatment but requires initial CBC/LFTs

---

Tinea Barbae

Barber's Itch	**Tinea Barbae**	

Etiology & Risk Factors	• **Dermatophyte infection of the beard area** • <u>Etiology</u>: ***Trichophyton mentagrophytes* or *Trichophyton verrucosum* are the most common causes** • <u>Risk Factors</u>: **male, poor hygiene, sharing trimmers or razors, trauma to skin (shaving, ingrown hairs, acne)**, occupational exposure (use of protective gear [firefighters, welders, healthcare workers]), close exposure to infected individual, immunocompromised, **contact with infected pets or animals**
Patho-physiology	• Invasion of the hair shaft by the fungus, leading to inflammation and destruction of the hair follicle
Signs & Symptoms	• **Superficial annular lesions of the beard area** • **Erythematous, boggy, tender, weeping nodule or plaque with pustules of the beard area** • Loss of hair or brittle hair that is easily plucked present at beard area
Diagnosis	• <u>Clinical Diagnosis</u> • <u>Potassium Hydroxide (KOH) Wet Mount</u>: identifies the fungal element (hyphae) on plucked beard hairs • <u>Fungal Culture</u>: definitive diagnosis

Treatment	• <u>Supportive</u>: maintain adequate hygiene, avoid sharing contaminated items
	• <u>Oral Antifungals</u>: mainstay of treatment
	  • <u>Griseofulvin</u>: **first-line treatment**
	  • <u>Terbinafine</u>: **alternative first-line treatment**
	• <u>Oral Corticosteroids</u>: may be indicated if lesions are severely inflamed to reduce symptoms and chance of scarring
	  • Prednisone 40mg; tapering over 2 weeks

Key Words & Most Common	• Dermatophyte infection of beard area • *Trichophyton mentagrophytes* or *Trichophyton verrucosum* most common • Male, sharing trimmers/razors, trauma to skin, occupational exposure, contact with infected pets/animals • Erythematous, boggy, tender, weeping nodule or plaque with pustules of the beard area • Griseofulvin is first-line treatment

Athlete's Foot	# Tinea Pedis	

Etiology & Risk Factors	• **Dermatophyte infection of the feet** • Etiology: ***Trichophyton rubrum* (chronic hyperkeratotic) is most common cause**, *T. mentagrophytes* var. *interdigitale* (acute ulcerative), *Epidermophyton floccosum* • Risk Factors: **prolonged wearing of occlusive footwear, high-risk exposure (barefoot exposure to locker room floors, gyms, swimming pool decks)**, hot and humid climate, excessive sweating, prolonged exposure to water
Patho-physiology	• Fungus releases enzymes (keratinases) that invade the keratin layer of skin resulting in skin breakdown and infection; dermatophyte cell wall also contains immunosuppressive molecules (mannans) that suppresses the normal local immune response
Signs & Symptoms	• **Interdigital Tinea Pedis: most common type; pruritic, erythematous erosions or scales between the toes; may have painful fissures;** 3rd/4th interdigital space most common • **Hyperkeratotic Tinea Pedis: diffuse, hyperkeratotic rash of the soles, lateral and medial sides of the feet**; follows a "moccasin distribution" of hyperkeratosis • Vesiculobullous Tinea Pedis: pruritic or painful vesicles or bullous eruptions with underlying erythema (inflammatory type); often affects the medial foot • Ulcerative Tinea Pedis: interdigital erosions or ulcers (uncommon; usually associated with secondary bacterial infection)
Diagnosis	• **Clinical Diagnosis** • **Potassium Hydroxide (KOH) Wet Mount**: most common initial test on skin scraping sample; identifies segmented hyphae • Fungal Culture: definitive diagnosis

Treatment	• Supportive: wearing sandals in high-risk exposure areas; moisture reduction (cotton socks, drying agents), frequent cleaning of floors to help prevent reinfection
	• **Topical Antifungals: first-line treatment**
	  • **Terbinafine 1%, clotrimazole 1%, ketoconazole 1% for 2-4 weeks** and continued for 7-10 days after resolution
	• **Oral Antifungals**: reserved for cases refractory to topical treatment
	  • **Itraconazole** for 4 weeks
	  • Terbinafine for 2-6 weeks

Key Words & Most Common	• Dermatophyte infection of the feet; *Trichophyton rubrum* most common cause • Interdigital Tinea Pedis: pruritic, erythematous erosions or scales between the toes • Hyperkeratotic Tinea Pedis: diffuse, hyperkeratotic rash of the soles, lateral and medial sides of the feet • Clinical diagnosis +/- KOH prep of skin scrapings • Topical antifungals (terbinafine, clotrimazole, ketoconazole) → oral antifungals (itraconazole, terbinafine)

Fissure

Erythematous erosions/scales between toes

Jock Itch	# Tinea Cruris	

Etiology & Risk Factors	• **Dermatophyte infection of the groin** • Etiology: ***Trichophyton rubrum* most common**; *Trichophyton mentagrophytes*, *Epidermophyton floccosum* • Risk Factors: **males** (apposition of scrotum and thigh), moist environments, **excessive sweating**, hot and humid climate, **restrictive clothing, poor hygiene, obesity (constant apposition of skinfolds)**, immunocompromised, diabetes mellitus
Patho-physiology	• Fungus releases enzymes (keratinases) that invade the keratin layer of skin resulting in skin breakdown and infection; dermatophyte cell wall also contains immunosuppressive molecules (mannans) that suppresses the normal local immune response • Tinea pedis or onychomycosis may be source of infection
Signs & Symptoms	• **Intensely pruritic, annular patches or plaques of the groin** • **Diffuse erythema of the crural folds extending to the adjacent proximal medial thigh** • **Sharply demarcated, raised, erythematous borders** • **Often spares the scrotum** (scrotum is often involved in candidal intertrigo or lichen simplex chronicus)
Diagnosis	• **Clinical Diagnosis** • **Potassium Hydroxide (KOH) Wet Mount**: most common initial test on skin scraping sample; identifies segmented hyphae • Fungal Culture: definitive diagnosis

Treatment	• Supportive: adequate hygiene, avoid restrictive clothing; moisture reduction (cotton underpants, drying agents)
	• **Topical Antifungals: first-line treatment**
	  • **Terbinafine, clotrimazole, miconazole or ketoconazole for 10-14 days** and continued for 2-3 days after resolution
	• **Oral Antifungals**: reserved for cases refractory to topical treatment
	  • **Itraconazole** for 4 weeks
	  • Terbinafine for 2-6 weeks

Key Words & Most Common	• Dermatophyte infection of the groin; Trichophyton rubrum most common • Males, excessive sweating, restrictive clothing, poor hygiene, obesity are greatest risk factors • Annular, erythematous, pruritic plaque of proximal medial thigh involving the crural folds and sparing the scrotum • Sharply demarcated, raised borders • Clinical diagnosis +/- KOH prep • Topical antifungals (terbinafine, clotrimazole, miconazole, ketoconazole) → oral antifungals (itraconazole, terbinafine)

Erythema of crural fold

Penis/ Scrotum

Medial thigh

Tinea Corporis

Body Ringworm

Erythematous annular patch with raised scaly borders

Etiology & Risk Factors	• **Dermatophyte infection of the face, trunk, and/or extremities** • Etiology: ***Trichophyton rubrum* is most common cause**; *Trichophyton mentagrophytes*, *Microsporum canis* • Risk Factors: **direct skin contact to infected person, contact sports (wrestling)**, sharing personal items (towels, razors, clothing), moist environments, **excessive sweating**, hot and humid climate, **restrictive clothing, poor hygiene, obesity**, immunocompromised, diabetes mellitus, **contact with infected pets or animals**
Patho-physiology	• Fungus releases enzymes (keratinases) that invade the keratin layer of skin resulting in skin breakdown and infection; dermatophyte cell wall also contains immunosuppressive molecules (mannans) that suppresses the normal local immune response • Tinea pedis or onychomycosis may be source of infection
Signs & Symptoms	• **Pruritic, erythematous, annular patches and plaques** • **Well-defined, raised, scaly borders** • **Borders expands outwardly with a central clearing**
Diagnosis	• **Clinical Diagnosis** • Potassium Hydroxide (KOH) Wet Mount: most common initial test on skin scraping sample; identifies segmented hyphae • Fungal Culture: definitive diagnosis

Treatment	• Supportive: adequate hygiene, avoid restrictive clothing; moisture reduction (cotton, linen, wool clothing, drying agents)
	• **Topical Antifungals: first-line treatment**
	   • **Terbinafine, clotrimazole, miconazole or ketoconazole** for 2-4 weeks and continued for 7-10 days after resolution
	• Oral Antifungals: reserved for cases refractory to topical treatment
	   • **Itraconazole** for 2-3 weeks
	   • **Terbinafine** for 2-3 weeks

Key Words & Most Common	• Dermatophyte infection of the groin; *Trichophyton rubrum* most common • Direct skin contact to infected person, contact sports (wrestling), excessive sweating, poor hygiene, contact with infected pets/animals greatest risk factors • Pruritic, erythematous, annular patches and plaques with well-defined, raised scaly borders that expand outwardly with a central clearing • Clinical diagnosis +/- KOH prep • Topical antifungals (terbinafine, clotrimazole, miconazole, ketoconazole) → oral antifungals (itraconazole, terbinafine)

Intertrigo

Etiology & Risk Factors	• **Superficial inflammatory skin condition of the intertriginous areas precipitated by moisture, warmth, friction, poor ventilation or maceration** • Etiology: fungal (***Candida* spp. most common**); gram-positive and gram-negative bacteria, other fungi and viruses • Risk Factors: **warm, moist environments (skin folds, excessive sweating, incontinence, obesity**), friction, immunocompromised (**diabetes mellitus**), **restrictive clothing**, corticosteroid use, hot and humid environment
Patho-physiology	• Friction between two adjacent skin surfaces causes inflammation of the epidermis; sweat and moisture accumulate in these areas leading to maceration of the stratum corneum and epidermis which accommodates bacterial or fungal (yeast) infection

Signs & Symptoms	• **Most common locations are inframammary, infrapannicular**, interdigital, **axillary**, infragluteal, and **genitocrural folds**
	• **Pruritus, burning, and pain in the skin folds and flexural surfaces**
	• Physical Exam:
	   • **Erythematous, "beefy red", macerated patch or plaques on both sides of the skin fold**
	   • **Satellite papules and pustules are pathognomic for *Candida* infection**

Diagnosis	• Clinical Diagnosis • Potassium Hydroxide (KOH) Wet Mount: most common initial test on skin scraping sample; identifies budding yeast with or without pseudohyphae (*Candida*) • Skin Culture: definitive diagnosis
Treatment	• Supportive: **weight loss**, adequate hygiene, avoid restrictive clothing; moisture reduction (cotton, linen, wool clothing, drying agents, antiperspirants) • **Topical Antifungals: first-line treatment** • **Clotrimazole, miconazole or ketoconazole** (nystatin if only *Candida* suspected) daily until rash resolves • Oral Antifungals: **fluconazole**; indicated if refractory to topical treatment or severe infection • Topical Corticosteroids: hydrocortisone; adjunctive treatment for severe inflammation (low-dose should be used to avoid skin thinning of macerated epidermis)
Key Words & Most Common	• Skin condition precipitated by moisture, warmth, friction • *Candida* spp. most common cause • Most common beneath the breast, the panniculus, and axilla • Erythematous, "beefy red" macerated rash of the skin folds with pruritus and burning • Satellite lesions pathognomonic for candida • Clinical diagnosis + KOH prep • Weight loss + topical antifungals (clotrimazole, miconazole) +/- oral antifungals (fluconazole)

Scabies

Etiology & Risk Factors	• Highly contagious infestation of the skin with the mite *Sarcoptes scabiei* • Etiology: mite infestation by *Sarcoptes scabiei* • Risk Factors: **crowded living conditions (dorms, schools, homeless shelters, military barracks, nursing homes, prisons)**, immunocompromised, sexual activity, **close exposure (sharing bedding, towels, or clothing)**; *no clear association with poor hygiene*
Patho-physiology	• Female mite burrows within the stratum corneum of the host and lays eggs, feed and defecate which precipitate a skin hypersensitivity reaction • Mites live within burrowed tunnels of the stratum corneum

Signs & Symptoms	• **Most common areas include finger web spaces, wrists**, elbows, areolae, navel region, penile shaft
	• **Intense pruritus especially at night**
	• Physical Exam:
	  • **Multiple, small erythematous papules**
	  • **Linear burrows (thin, wavy, slightly scaly lines that are several millimeters long) are pathognomonic**

Diagnosis	• **Clinical Diagnosis** • Microscopic Examination of Burrow Scrapings: visualization of mites, ova or fecal pellets on microscopy confirms diagnosis

Treatment	• General Care: all personal items (bed linens, towels, clothes) should be washed in hot water and dried on high heat or bagged and sealed for minimum 72 hours
	• Topical Scabicides: *close contacts should also be treated simultaneously*
	  • **Topical Permethrin 5%: first-line treatment**; apply from neck down and leave on for 8-12 hours before bathing; may reapply after 1-2 weeks if incomplete effect
	  • Topical Lindane: effective treatment but **typically avoided due to toxicity** (neurotoxicity, seizures); do not use after bath/shower (increased absorption through pores)
	  • Precipitated Sulfur 6-10% in Petroleum Jelly: indicated for pregnant women or infants <2 years old
	• Oral Scabicides:
	  • **Oral Ivermectin**: indicated for extensive or refractory cases

Key Words & Most Common	• Highly contagious skin infestations by *Sarcoptes scabiei* • Close exposures, crowded living conditions greatest risk factors • Most common on finger web spaces and volar wrists • Intense pruritus at night • Multiple erythematous papules + linear burrows • Topical permethrin 5% is first-line **Erythematous papules of finger web spaces**

Pediculosis Pubis

Pubic Lice or "Crabs"

Etiology & Risk Factors	• **Parasitic infestation of the pubic hair** • Etiology: **louse species *Phthirus pubis*** • Risk Factors: **sexual activity, multiple sexual partners, age (most common in adolescents and young adults)**, close contact exposure (sharing bed, clothing), **poor hygiene**, living in crowded or unsanitary conditions, **unkept or excessive body hair**
Patho-physiology	• Transmission: sexually transmitted or fomite transmitted (sharing towels, bedding, clothing) • Pruritus is secondary to immune-mediated hypersensitivity reaction to pubic louse bites

Signs & Symptoms	• **Pruritus of the pubic or perianal area**
	  • May spread to thighs, trunk, and facial hair (beard, mustache, eyelashes)
	• Physical Exam:
	  • **Excoriations** and regional lymphadenopathy
	  • Maculae Cerulae: pale, bluish gray skin macules (secondary to anticoagulant activity of louse saliva while feeding); rare finding

Diagnosis	• **Clinical Diagnosis** • Microscopic Examination: **visualized nits** on microscopy of hair shafts or tape sample (sticky tape to pick up adult lice) • Wood Light Examination: greenish-yellow fluorescence of the nits

Treatment	• General Care: all personal items (bed linens, towels, clothes) should be washed in hot water and dried on high heat or bagged and sealed for minimum 72 hours, adequate hygiene, trimming of body hair
	• Topical Pediculicides: *close contacts and sexual partners should also be treated simultaneously*
	  • **Topical Permethrin 1%: first-line treatment**; apply to affected area once per week for 2 weeks
	  • Topical Pyrethrin: apply to affected areas and wash off after 10 min
	  • Topical Lindane: effective treatment but **typically avoided due to toxicity** (neurotoxicity, seizures); do not use after bath/shower (increased absorption through pores)
	  • Petroleum Jelly: indicated for eyelash lice; apply 3–4 times a day for 7-10 days
	  • Fluorescein Drops: 10-20%: indicated for eyelash lice
	• Oral Pediculicides:
	  • **Oral Ivermectin**: indicated for extensive or refractory cases

Key Words & Most Common	• Louse infestation of pubic hair by *Phthirus pubis* • Pruritus of pubic or perianal area • Wash personal items in hot water, adequate hygiene, trimming of body hair • Topical permethrin 1% is first-line treatment • Petroleum jelly or fluoresceine drops indicated for eyelash lice • Oral ivermectin in extensive or refractory cases

Pediculosis Capitis

	Head Lice

Etiology & Risk Factors	• **Parasitic infestation of the scalp** • Etiology: louse species *Pediculus humanus* var. *capitis* • Risk Factors: **female, age (most common in children 5-11 years old), long hair**, close contact exposure (sharing bed, clothing, combs, brushes), **poor hygiene**, crowded living conditions, **children attending school or daycare**
Patho-physiology	• Transmission: person-to-person (direct contact, static electricity, wind); fomites (hats, headsets, clothing, bedding, combs, brushes) • Lice crawl onto the scalp and hair shafts and feed on blood and lay eggs (nits) which attach to hair shafts close to scalp and eventually hatch into nymphs which then grow into adult lice within 1-2 weeks; pruritus and skin inflammation are secondary to lice bites and saliva exposure

Signs & Symptoms	• **Intense pruritus of the scalp** (especially occipital area)
	• **Papular urticaria near lice bites**
	• Physical Exam:
	   • **Scalp excoriations and posterior cervical adenopathy**
	   • **Visualization of crawling nymphs or adult lice**
	   • Visualization of nits (grayish-white, oval-shaped egg capsules fixed to the base of hair shaft) alone does not confirm infestation

Diagnosis	• **Clinical Diagnosis**

Treatment	• General Care: all personal items (bed linens, towels, clothes) should be washed in hot water and dried on high heat or bagged and sealed for minimum 72 hours, adequate personal hygiene, trimming of hair; use of fine tooth comb to remove the nits
	• Topical Pediculicides:
	   • **Topical Permethrin 1%: first-line treatment**; apply to affected area once per week for 2 weeks
	   • **Topical Malathion 0.5%: alternative first-line medication**; causes paralysis of arthropods
	   • Topical Lindane: effective treatment but **typically avoided due to toxicity** (neurotoxicity, seizures); do not use after bath/shower (increased absorption through pores)
	   • Petroleum Jelly: may be used to suffocate lice
	   • Other: benzyl alcohol, Spinosad 0.9% topical, topical ivermectin
	• Oral Pediculicides:
	   • **Oral Ivermectin**: indicated for extensive or refractory cases

Key Words & Most Common	• Louse infestation of scalp by *Pediculus humanus* var. *capitis* • Intense pruritus of scalp + popular urticaria near lice bites • Visualization of crawling nymphs, adult lice, nits • Wash personal items in hot water, adequate hygiene, trimming of hair • Topical permethrin 1% is first-line treatment; topical malathion is alternative first-line • Oral ivermectin in extensive or refractory cases

Head louse — Nit (louse egg)

Pediculosis Corporis

	Body Lice

Etiology & Risk Factors	• **Parasitic infestation of the clothing or bedding that feed on the body** • Etiology: louse species *Pediculus humanus* var. *corporis* • Risk Factors: **poor personal hygiene is greatest risk factor, homelessness, crowded living conditions**(homeless shelters, prisons, crowded unsanitary conditions), **poverty or low socioeconomic status**, close contact exposure (sharing bed, clothing, towels)
Patho-physiology	• Transmission: person-to-person (direct contact, static electricity, wind); fomites (clothing, bedding, towels) • *Body lice are main vectors of Rickettsia prowazekii (epidemic typhus), Bartonella quintana (trench fever) and Borellia recurrentis (relapsing fever)* • Lice crawl onto the body and feed on blood and lay eggs (nits) on clothing or bedding that eventually hatch into nymphs which then mature into adult lice within 1-2 weeks • Body lice do not live on the skin and move to the skin to feed; pruritus and skin inflammation are secondary to lice bites and saliva exposure

Signs & Symptoms	• **Intense pruritus**
	• **Papular urticaria near lice bites**
	• Physical Exam:
	   • **Small, erythematous puncta (caused by bites), usually associated with linear excoriations, urticaria, or superficial bacterial infection**
	   • Visualization of nits (grayish-white, oval-shaped egg capsules) on clothing or bedding (**usually at the seams**)

Diagnosis	• **Clinical Diagnosis**

Treatment	• General Care:
	   • **Improvement of personal hygiene is first-line**
	   • **Launder all personal items (bed linens, towels, clothes)** should be washed in hot water and dried on high heat or bagged and sealed for minimum 72 hours or replaced based on extent of infestation
	• Topical Pediculicides: use is not required for the eradication of body lice infestation but often utilized if body lice or nits are found on body hair
	   • **Topical Permethrin 1%: first-line treatment**; apply to affected area once per week for 2 weeks
	   • Other: 5% benzyl alcohol lotion, 0.5% ivermectin lotion, 0.5% malathion lotion, 0.9% Spinosad topical suspension, and 1% lindane shampoo
	      • *Topical lindane usually avoided due to toxicity (neurotoxicity, seizures); do not use after bath/shower (increased absorption through pores)*
	• Oral Scabicides:
	   • **Oral Ivermectin**: indicated for extensive or refractory cases

Key Words & Most Common	• Louse infestation by *Pediculus humanus* var. *corporis* • *Lice live on clothing/bedding and migrate to body to feed* • Intense pruritus + popular urticaria near lice bites • Wash personal items in hot water + adequate personal hygiene is first-line treatment • Topical permethrin 1% may be indicated • Oral ivermectin in extensive or refractory cases

Molluscum Contagiosum

"Water Warts"	
Etiology & Risk Factors	• Self-limited, benign skin condition • <u>Etiology</u>: **Molluscum Contagiosum Virus (member of the *poxvirus* family)** • <u>Risk Factors</u>: **age (most common 0-12 years old)**, close contact exposure, participation in certain sports (wrestling, gymnastics), crowded environments, **immunocompromised**
Patho-physiology	• <u>Transmission</u>: **direct skin-to-skin (sexual activity, wrestling) contact** or indirect (towels, clothes, toys, razors) contact; sharing swimming pools, bath water possible • Virus enters the body through direct skin-to-skin contact or contact with contaminated objects and then infects epidermal skin cells, leading to the formation of characteristic lesions that contain the virus and can spread to other areas of the body through self-inoculation or close contact

Signs & Symptoms	• **Single or cluster of raised, flesh-colored to pearly-white, waxy papules**
	  • **Dome-shaped with central umbilication**
	  • **Usually 2-5mm in diameter**
	  • Usually **non-painful and non-pruritic** (may become inflamed if scratched or friction from clothing)
	  • Contains virus-filled white caseous "curd like" material that can be manually expressed
	• Lesions most common on the face, trunk, and extremities (children) or pubis, penis, or vulva (adults) but can affect any part of the body; palms and soles of feet are spared

Diagnosis	• **Clinical Diagnosis** • <u>Biopsy</u>: confirms diagnosis; shows enlarged keratinocytes with an abundant cytoplasm containing viral inclusions (Henderson-Paterson bodies)

Treatment	• <u>Supportive</u>: **no treatment necessary; self-limited condition and usually resolves spontaneously within 6-18 months**
	  • Treatment may be indicated in immunocompromised patients, **to preserve cosmesis or prevent autoinoculation**
	  • Hygiene is key to reduce spread
	• <u>Physical Removal</u>: **curettage or cryotherapy (liquid nitrogen, dry ice) are first-line for removal**; laser therapy (carbon dioxide or pulsed dye laser), electrocautery
	• <u>Topical Irritants</u>: trichloroacetic acid, cantharidin, tretinoin, podophyllotoxin, potassium hydroxide, salicylic acid; induces an inflammatory reaction to accelerate recovery
	• <u>Oral Antivirals</u>: cidofovir (DNA polymerase inhibitor) may be indicated in immunocompromised patients

Key Words & Most Common	• Self-limited, benign skin condition caused by Molluscum Contagiosum Virus (member of the *poxvirus* family) • Raised, flesh-colored to pearly-white dome-shaped papules with central umbilication • Non-painful and non-pruritic • Supportive treatment (most spontaneously resolve in months) • Curettage or cryotherapy are first-line for removal (indicated to preserve cosmesis or prevent autoinoculation)

Common, Flat, Plantar Warts

Etiology & Risk Factors	• **Common, benign, epidermal lesions** • <u>Etiology</u>: **human papillomavirus (HPV) infection** • <u>Risk Factors</u>: direct contact to virus, **skin-to-skin contact (sexual activity, contact sports)**, immunocompromised, damage or broken skin, poor personal hygiene
Patho-physiology	• <u>Transmission</u>: direct or indirect contact, autoinoculation; disruption of the normal epithelial barrier (trauma or maceration) increase the likelihood of developing a wart • Viral infection occurs with break or cut in the superficial, keratinized skin layer causing excessive proliferation and retention of the stratum corneum leading to lesion formation

Signs & Symptoms	• <u>Verruca Vulgaris (Common Wart)</u>:
	  • **Sharply demarcated, rough, round or irregular, firm hyperkeratotic papules**; may have pedunculated, "cauliflower-like" projection
	  • **Light gray, yellow, brown, or grayish-black nodule with reddish-brown punctations (thrombosed capillaries)**
	  • Usually 2-10 mm in diameter
	  • **Most common on areas subject to trauma (fingers or toes, elbows, knees**, face), but may occur anywhere
	• <u>Verruca Plana (Flat Wart)</u>:
	  • **Numerous, small, smooth, flat-topped, yellow-brown or flesh-colored papules**
	  • Usually 1-7mm in diameter; may develop dozens to hundreds of lesions
	  • Usually found on the face, hands, shins or along scratch marks
	• <u>Verruca Plantaris (Plantar Wart)</u>:
	  • **Sharply demarcated, rough, round or irregular, firm hyperkeratotic papule found on the sole of the foot**; flattened by pressure, surrounded by cornified epithelium
	  • **Light gray, yellow, brown, or grayish-black nodule with reddish-brown punctations (thrombosed capillaries)**
	  • May be tender and can make walking and standing uncomfortable

Diagnosis	• **Clinical Diagnosis** • <u>Biopsy</u>: confirms diagnosis; demonstrates koilocytotic squamous cells with hyperplastic hyperkeratosis

Treatment	• <u>Supportive</u>: **no treatment necessary; self-limited condition and usually resolves spontaneously within 2 years**
	  • Treatment indicated for warts that are cosmetically unacceptable, in locations that interfere with function or are painful
	• <u>Topical Irritants</u>: work by eliciting an immune response to HPV
	  • **Salicylic acid**, trichloroacetic acid, 5-fluorouracil, podophyllum resin, tretinoin, cantharidin
	  • Topical imiquimod induces skin cells to locally produce antiviral cytokines
	• <u>Physical Removal</u>: **cryotherapy**, laser, electrocautery, curettage, excision
	• <u>Intralesional Injections</u>: used for refractory lesions or lesions in sensitive areas; injection with immunotherapy (*Candida*), bleomycin, interferon alfa to induce antiviral effects

Key Words & Most Common	• Common Wart: rough, round, firm hyperkeratotic papule with reddish0brown punctations • Flat Wart: numerous, small, flat-topped, yellow-brown or flesh-colored papules • Plantar Wart: rough, round, firm hyperkeratotic papule on sole of foot, flattened by pressure • Supportive → salicylic acid → cryotherapy

Condyloma Acuminata

Genital Warts

Etiology & Risk Factors	• Skin-colored, fleshy papules in the anogenital region • Etiology: human papillomavirus (HPV) infection (type 6 and 11 most common) • Risk Factors: sexual activity (unprotected sex or having multiple sexual partners), immunocompromised, age (young adults are most commonly affected), lack of vaccination
Patho-physiology	• Virus enters body through skin or mucous membranes and primarily infects the nucleus of differentiated squamous epithelial cells; human papillomavirus (HPV) contains an oncogene that produces proteins responsible for promoting cell growth and facilitating viral replication • As the number of infected host cells increases, the skin layers thicken, resulting in the formation of warts at a macroscopic level due to acanthosis

Signs & Symptoms	• Warts appear after 1-6 month incubation period
	• Small, raised, soft, skin-colored, fleshy papules of the anogenital region
	  • May enlarge or become pedunculated ("cauliflower-like"), have rough surface, and/or appear in clusters
	    • Most common under foreskin, on coronal sulcus, or penile shaft of men; may occur around the anus or in the rectum in men who have sex with men
	    • Most common on vulva, vaginal wall, cervix, and perineum of women
	• Usually asymptomatic; may cause pruritus, bleeding, burning or general discomfort

Diagnosis	• Clinical Diagnosis • Acetic Acid Test: 5% solution of acetic acid applied to lesion causes lesions to whiten • Polymerase Chain Reaction (PCR): confirms diagnosis • HPV Serologies: confirms diagnosis • Colposcopy/Anoscopy: direct visualization of lesion • Biopsy: koilocytes (large keratinocytes with abundant cytoplasm and small nuclei) and papillomatosis

Treatment	• Supportive: most cases will experience spontaneous resolution; relapses are frequent and often require multiple retreatments
	  • Treatment indicated for warts that are cosmetically unacceptable, in locations that interfere with function or are painful
	• Physical Removal:
	  • Cryotherapy (Liquid Nitrogen): first-line treatment to remove lesions; 3-5 applications weekly for 6-10 weeks
	  • Electrocauterization, laser ablation or surgical excision are alternatives
	• Topical Management: considered second-line
	  • Antimitotics: podophyllotoxin, podophyllin, 5-fluorouracil; podophyllotoxin cannot be used for anogenital warts
	  • Caustics: trichloroacetic acid
	  • Interferon Inducers: imiquimod; lower rates of recurrence compared to podophyllotoxin
	  • Sinecatechins: alternative topical treatment with unknown mechanism
	• Prevention: recommended at age 11-12 years old males and females, previously unvaccinated or not adequately vaccinated patients through 26 years old
	  • 9-Valent HPV Vaccine (Gardasil-9): protects against HPV type 6, 11, 16, 18, 31, 33, 45, 52, 58
	  • Quadrivalent HPV Vaccine (Gardasil): protects against HPV type 6, 11, 16, 18

Seborrheic Keratosis

Etiology & Risk Factors	• Common, benign, superficial epidermal skin tumor • Etiology: benign proliferation of immature keratinocytes • Risk Factors: age (>40 years old most common), family history, prolonged sun exposure, fair skin, hormonal changes (pregnancy or undergoing hormonal treatment)
Patho-physiology	• Benign clonal expansion of immature epidermal keratinocytes
Signs & Symptoms	• Well-demarcated, round or oval shaped, velvety wart-like lesions with a "greasy" or "stuck-on" appearance • Flesh-colored, brown, or black lesions • May have a verrucous, velvety, waxy, scaling, or crusted surface • Most common on the trunk or temples • Vary in size and grow slowly
Diagnosis	• Clinical Diagnosis • Biopsy: confirms diagnosis; demonstrates proliferation of keratinocytes with keratin-filled cysts

Treatment	• Supportive: no treatment necessary; benign condition with no premalignant potential
	• Physical Removal: indicated to preserve cosmesis or for lesions that are consistently irritated and cause discomfort
	  • Cryotherapy: first-line for removal; liquid nitrogen or CO_2 rapidly freezes/thaws the targeted cells, resulting in cell death; may cause hypopigmentation
	  • Curettage, electrodessication, laser ablation therapy
	• Topical Management: considered second-line
	  • Tazarotene, imiquimod cream, alpha-hydroxy acids, urea ointment, vitamin D analogs (tacalcitol, calcipotriol)

Key Words & Most Common	• Common, benign, superficial epidermal skin tumor • Elderly patient with fair skin and prolonged sun exposure most common • Well-demarcated, round/oval, velvety, wart-like lesion with "stuck-on" appearance • Supportive → cryotherapy if bothersome or cosmetically unappealing

Actinic Keratosis

Etiology & Risk Factors	• Premalignant cutaneous lesions characterized by changes in skin cells (keratinocytes) that may progress to squamous cell carcinoma • Etiology: develop as a result of the **damaging effects of ultraviolet (UV) radiation to the skin most commonly from sunlight exposure** • Risk Factors: **increased age, excessive or chronic sun exposure, males, fair skin**, geographic location (closer to the equator), immunosuppression
Patho-physiology	• UV radiation exposure from the sun results in epidermal keratinocyte changes including cell growth and differentiation and results in inflammation and immunosuppression causing intraepidermal proliferation of dysplastic keratinocytes
Signs & Symptoms	• **Dry, rough macules or papules** • **Rough, gritty "sandpaper-like" feel of the scale** • May have **transparent or yellow scaling** • **Flesh-colored, erythematous or hyperkeratotic (hyperpigmented)** • **Thickened and hypertrophic; may form a cutaneous horn (skin projection)** • **Most common on sun-exposed areas** (balding scalp, face, lateral neck, distal upper or lower extremities)
Diagnosis	• **Clinical Diagnosis** • Shave or Punch Biopsy: confirms diagnosis; may be performed to distinguish from squamous cell carcinoma • Demonstrates **atypical epidermal keratinocytes** limited to the lower third of the epidermis

Treatment	• Supportive: **sun-protective measures (limit sun exposure, use of sunscreen, protective clothing)**
	• Lesion-Directed Therapy: indicated for localized or limited extent; targets individual lesions
	  • Physical Removal: **cryotherapy is most common**; dermabrasion, electrodessication, curettage
	• Field-Directed Therapy: indicated for multiple, widespread, and subclinical lesions
	  • Dermabrasion, laser, chemical peels, photodynamic therapy
	  • **Topical 5-fluorouracil (5-FU) or imiquimod cream are first-line treatments**
	  • Topical diclofenac sodium, tirbanibulin are alternatives

Key Words & Most Common	• Premalignant skin lesions that has possibility to progress to squamous cell carcinoma • Most common as a result of prolonged sunlight exposure • Dry, rough, gritty, "sandpaper-like" macules or papules with scale • Biopsy confirms diagnosis and distinguishes from squamous cell carcinoma • Sun-protective measures → cryotherapy

Squamous Cell Carcinoma

Etiology & Risk Factors	• **Malignant tumor of epidermal keratinocytes that invades the dermis** • **Bowen's Disease: squamous cell carcinoma in situ (has not invaded dermis)** • Etiology: **ultraviolet (UV) solar radiation is the most common cause**, chemical exposure, **severe burn scar, chronic ulcerations**, human papillomavirus (HPV) • Risk Factors: **increased age, excessive or chronic sun exposure, males, fair skin, preexisting actinic keratosis**, geographic location (closer to the equator), immunosuppression
Patho-physiology	• Exposure to UV solar radiation results in mutation and damage of squamous cell DNA (specifically the p53 protein) which disrupts the normal cell function and leads to uncontrolled cell growth and the formation of malignant tumors
Signs & Symptoms	• *Commonly arises from preexisting actinic keratosis* • **Slow-growing, flesh-colored to erythematous, elevated, thickened lesion** • May be flat, nodular or plaque-like • **Adherent white scale or crust** • **May present as a non-healing ulceration or erosion on sun-exposed area of the skin** • **Most common on sun exposed areas** (balding scalp, lips, face, neck, distal upper or lower extremities)
Diagnosis	• Biopsy: **essential for diagnosis** • Demonstrates irregular and atypical keratinocytes and malignant cells of the epidermis and invasion of the dermis

Treatment	• Surgery: **primary means of treatment**
	  • **Surgical Excision with Clear Margins: most common treatment**
	  • **Mohs Micrographic Surgery**: treatment of choice for lesions of head and neck, immunosuppressed patients, recurrent or aggressive cases, or depth ≥2mm of depth
	• Local Destruction: indicated for small, low-risk lesions
	  • Electrodesiccation and Curettage: indicated for small, well-defined, superficial lesions not on cosmetically sensitive areas
	  • Cryotherapy: indicated for low-risk, in situ lesions
	  • Topical Chemotherapy: imiquimod or 5-fluorouracil indicated for low-risk, in situ lesions
	• Supportive: **sun-protective measures (limit sun exposure, use of sunscreen, protective clothing)**

Key Words & Most Common	• Malignant tumor of epidermal keratinocytes caused by UV solar radiation • Age, chronic sun exposure, male, fair skin most common risk factors • Can arise from actinic keratosis • Slow-growing, flesh-colored, elevated, thickened lesions with adherent scale/crust • Non-healing ulceration on sun-exposed area of body • Biopsy • Surgery (surgical excision vs Mohs) is treatment of choice

Kaposi Sarcoma

Etiology & Risk Factors	• **Multicentric vascular tumor associated with human herpesvirus type 8 infection** • <u>Etiology</u>: **human herpesvirus type 8 (HHV-8) infection** • <u>Risk Factors</u>: **immunocompromised (HIV with CD4 count <100/mm³ or post-transplant most common)**, advanced age, male, **Eastern European and Mediterranean descent**
Patho-physiology	• HHV-8 infects the endothelial cells lining blood vessels, leading to the formation of abnormal blood vessels and proliferation of spindle-shaped tumor cells • The virus promotes inflammatory cytokine and growth factors release, further contributing to tumor growth and angiogenesis
Signs & Symptoms	• **Asymptomatic (painless, nonpruritic) purple, pink, red macules that may coalesce into blue/violet to black plaques and nodules** • Nodules may fungate or penetrate soft tissue, invading the underlying bone • Regional lymphadenopathy may be present
Diagnosis	• <u>Biopsy</u>: **confirms diagnosis via punch biopsy** • Demonstrates spindle-shaped cell proliferation with leukocytic infiltration and neovascularization in the dermis
Treatment	• <u>Superficial Lesions</u>: **surgical excision**, cryotherapy or electrocoagulation, intralesional chemotherapy (<u>vinblastine</u> or interferon alfa) • <u>Multiple or Diffuse Lesions and Lymph Node Involvement</u>: 10-20 Gy of radiation therapy and chemotherapy • <u>AIDS-Associated Disease</u>: **highly active antiretroviral therapy (HAART) demonstrates marked response (may lead to regression or complete resolution)**
Key Words & Most Common	• Vascular tumor associated with HHV-8 infection • Most common in HIV and/or elderly male of Eastern European or Mediterranean descent • Asymptomatic purple macule that coalesces into blue/violet/black plaques and nodules • Biopsy: spindle-shaped cell proliferation and neovascularization in the dermis • Surgical excision → radiation and chemotherapy • HAART if associated with HIV

Melanoma

Etiology & Risk Factors	• **Tumor developed by the malignant transformation of melanocytes most commonly affecting the skin** • <u>Etiology</u>: combination of genetic and environmental factors • <u>Risk Factors</u>: **ultraviolet (UV) radiation exposure is greatest risk factor (sun exposure with blistering sunburns, tanning bed use)**, **advanced age**, male, family history, personal characteristics (**fair skin**, light-colored eyes), **dysplastic nevi (atypical moles)**, immunosuppression, low socioeconomic status, xeroderma pigmentosum
Patho-physiology	• Ultraviolet (UV) radiation exposure over the course of a lifetime leads to accumulated DNA damage and mutations in genes involved in cell cycle regulation, DNA repair, and cell signaling pathways which disrupt the normal control preventative mechanisms that inhibit excessive cell proliferation and promotes malignant cell spread

Signs & Symptoms	• <u>Superficial Spreading Melanoma</u>: **most common type (70%)**
	  • **Asymptomatic plaque with irregular, raised, indurated, and tan or brown areas; average about 2cm in diameter**
	  • May have areas of red, white, black or blue spots or protuberant nodules
	• <u>Nodular Melanoma</u>: second most common type (15-30%)
	  • Dark gray or black protuberant plaque or papule
	• <u>Lentigo Maligna Melanoma</u>: most common on face
	  • Asymptomatic, flat, tan/brown, irregularly shaped flat lesion (macule or patch) with darker-colored spots irregularly distributed on the surface
	• <u>Acral-Lentiginous Melanoma</u>: **most common type among darker-skinned individuals; most common on palmar, plantar, and subungual skin**
	• <u>Desmoplastic</u>: most aggressive type; Infiltrative growth pattern and dense fibrous stroma
	  • Flesh-colored or pink nodule (mimics scar tissue development which makes for challenging diagnosis
	• <u>Hutchinson Sign</u>: hyperpigmentation extending across the lunula to the proximal nail fold

Diagnosis	• **"ABCDE"**: used to determine high-risk nevi • **A**symmetry (asymmetric appearance), **B**orders (irregular borders), **C**olor (unusual or significantly darker nevi), **D**iameter (>6mm), **E**volution (new or changing mole) • <u>Biopsy</u>: **full-thickness, wide excisional biopsy indicated for most lesions** (unless sensitive or cosmetic areas)

Treatment	• <u>Complete Wide Surgical Excision and Sentinel Lymph Node Biopsy</u>: **definitive treatment for early-stage melanoma**; elective lymph node dissection
	  • 1cm lateral tumor-free margin indicated for lesions <2mm thick
	  • 2cm lateral tumor-free margin indicated for lesions >2mm thick
	• <u>Adjuvant Therapy</u>: indicated for high-risk, advanced cases or lesions in sensitive areas
	  • Interferon alfa, immune therapy (nivolumab, ipilimumab)
	• Immunotherapy (pembrolizumab, nivolumab, ipilimumab), targeted therapy (vemurafenib, dabrafenib), and radiation therapy indicated for metastatic or unresectable lesions

Key Words & Most Common	• UV radiation is greatest risk factor • <u>Superficial Spreading Type</u>: asymptomatic plaque with irregular, raised, indurated, tan/brown area • <u>Nodular</u>: dark gray or black protuberant plaque/papule • <u>Acral-Lentiginous</u>: most common among darker-skinned individuals; most common on palmar, plantar, subungual skin • Complete wide surgical excision +/- sentinel lymph node biopsy

Basal Cell Carcinoma

Etiology & Risk Factors	• Superficial, slow-growing lesions that derives from keratinocytes near the basal layer of the epidermis; most common type of skin cancer • Etiology: combination of genetic and environmental factors • Risk Factors: ultraviolet (UV) radiation exposure is greatest risk factor (sun exposure with blistering sunburns, tanning bed use), advanced age, male, family history, personal characteristics (fair skin, light-colored eyes), immunosuppression, exposure to arsenic, genetic syndromes (xeroderma pigmentosum, Gorlin syndrome)
Patho-physiology	• Ultraviolet (UV) radiation exposure over the course of a lifetime leads to accumulated DNA damage and mutations in genes involved in cell cycle regulation, DNA repair, and cell signaling pathways which disrupt the normal control preventative mechanisms that inhibit excessive cell proliferation and promotes malignant cell spread
Signs & Symptoms	• Small, firm, shiny papules or nodules with a pearly, shiny, raised, rolled border with prominent engorged vessels (telangiectasias) on the surface and a central ulceration • Recurrent crusting or bleeding; "wound that never fully heals" • Most common on face, nose, neck or trunk
Diagnosis	• Biopsy: shave, punch or excisional biopsy indicated for most lesions • Demonstrates clusters or nests of basaloid cells, with a palisade arrangement of the nuclei at the periphery of the clusters
Treatment	• Mohs Microscopically Controlled Surgery: provides the best long-term cure rate of any treatment modality; gold standard due to high cure rate and tissue-sparing benefit • Indicated for facial or neck involvement, high-risk or difficult cases, recurrent or incompletely treated cancers, large cancers • Electrodessication and Curettage: most commonly indicated for non-facial lesions; small, superficial lesions without aggressive features and lesions with low recurrence risk • Surgical Excision: indicated for large, deep, or aggressive lesions • Radiation Therapy: indicated for lesions that cannot be surgically removed due to location or if the patient is not a suitable surgical candidate • Topical Medications: imiquimod or 5-fluorouracil (5-FU); indicated for superficial lesions or in patients that are not surgical candidates • Photodynamic Therapy (PDT): alternative treatment that involves applying a photosensitizing agent to the lesion followed by exposure to a specific light source
Key Words & Most Common	• Slow-growing lesion derived from keratinocytes near the basal layer • UV radiation exposure is greatest risk factor • Small, firm, shiny papule/nodule with pearly, shiny, rolled border with telangiectasias and central ulceration • Recurrent bleeding • Most common on sun-exposed areas • Biopsy • Mohs microscopically controlled surgery is preferred treatment • Electrodessication and curettage most commonly used for non-facial or small lesions

Perioral Dermatitis

Etiology & Risk Factors	• Benign skin eruption of the perioral area; may involve the periocular and paranasal skin • Etiology: combination of genetic, hormonal, and environmental factors • Risk Factors: topical corticosteroid use, use of fluoride-containing toothpaste, frequent use of chewing gum, female, age (20-45 years old most common), frequently licking lips, certain cosmetic products, hormonal changes (pregnancy, menstruation, oral contraceptives), environmental factors (exposure to extreme heat, cold, wind, excessive humidity)
Patho-physiology	• Disruption of the skin barrier leads to increased permeability and susceptibility to irritants leading to perifollicular and perivascular inflammation • Abnormal immune response and alterations in the skin's microflora may contribute to the development and persistence
Signs & Symptoms	• Grouped erythematous papulopustular lesions that primarily affect the perioral area • May involve the periorbital or paranasal skin • Pruritus or burning is common; worse when exposed to irritant • Vermillion borders of the lips are typically spared
Diagnosis	• Clinical Diagnosis • Culture: consider if bacterial etiology suspected • Potassium Hydroxide (KOH) Wet Mount: consider if *Candida* is suspected etiology (intensely pruritic rash with satellite lesions)

Treatment	• Discontinue Irritant: discontinue topical corticosteroids or offending skin care product (cosmetics, lotions, etc.)
	   • *Slow weaning may be required if medium-high potency corticosteroid to avoid significant rebound flaring*
	• Topical Management:
	   • Topical metronidazole, clindamycin, or erythromycin are first-line medical therapy; antibiotics are helpful for their anti-inflammatory properties
	   • Topical sulfur preparations and azelaic acid gel
	• Oral Management:
	   • Tetracycline, doxycycline or minocycline may be indicated if extensive or refractory to conservative or topical treatment

Key Words & Most Common	• Benign skin eruption of perioral area most commonly caused by topical corticosteroid use or cosmetics • Grouped erythematous papulopustular lesions • Vermillion border is spared • Discontinue irritant → topical metronidazole, clindamycin or erythromycin → oral tetracyclines

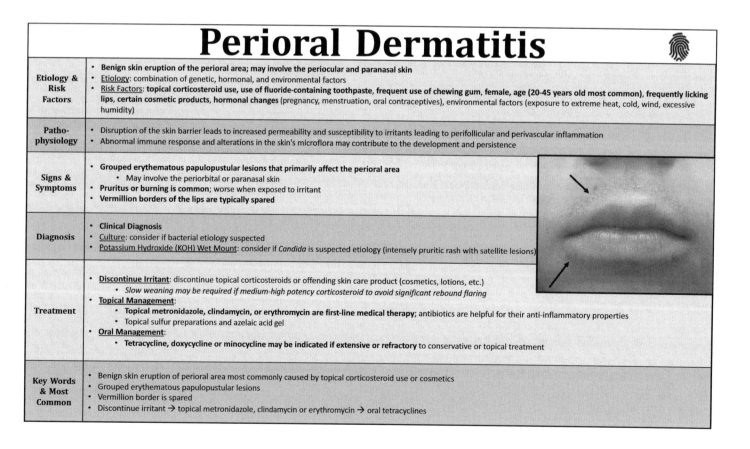

Contact Dermatitis

Etiology & Risk Factors	• Inflammation of the skin caused by direct contact with irritants (irritant contact dermatitis) or allergens (allergic contact dermatitis)
	• Etiology: **irritants or allergens**
	  • Irritant: **chemical agents** (acids or alkalis, solvents, cleaners, creams), **soaps** (abrasives, detergents, alcohols), **physical agents** (friction, abrasions, occlusions), **environmental factors** (photosensitivity, heat, low humidity), **chronic moisture** (body fluids, prolonged water exposure, urine, saliva)
	  • Allergic: **poison ivy is most common cause, nickel**, chemicals (fragrances, glues, dyes), chemicals (cleaners, acids), other metals
	• Risk Factors: **females** (more likely to wear jewelry, cosmetics, fragrances), **extremes of age** (infants, elderly), **light complexion** (red hair, fair skin),

Patho-physiology	• Irritant: nonspecific, **immediate**, inflammatory reaction secondary to exposure to toxic substances contacting the skin • Allergic: type IV, T-cell–mediated, **delayed-type** hypersensitivity reaction to an environmental allergen

Signs & Symptoms	• **Irritant**: symptoms appear immediately after exposure
	  • **More painful than pruritic**
	  • Generalized erythema, scaling, edema or erosions, crusting, blistering
	• **Allergic**: symptoms are delayed by hours to days after exposure
	  • **More pruritic than painful**
	  • Erythematous papules or vesicles, scaling, edema or erosions, crusting, blistering
	  • **Often occurs in a pattern or distribution that suggests a specific exposure** (linear pattern with exposure to poison ivy, circumferential pattern with nickel wristwatch, geometric shape)

Diagnosis	• **Clinical Diagnosis** • <u>Patch Testing</u>: standard contact allergens are applied to the upper back with adhesive and contain small amounts of allergen; allergen removed after 48 hours and patches are monitored for degree of erythema, size of the reaction, swelling, and vesiculation/crusting to identify specific allergy

Treatment	• <u>**Discontinue and Avoid Offending Agent**</u>: most important first-step in management
	• <u>**Supportive**</u>: cool compresses, cool saline washes or cool baths, emollients, calamine lotion, aloe vera
	• <u>**Topical Management**</u>:
	  • **Topical corticosteroids (triamcinolone or betamethasone) are first-line for medical management**
	  • Topical antihistamines (diphenhydramine)
	  • Topical calcineurin inhibitors (tacrolimus or pimecrolimus) are alternatives
	  • Drying agents (aluminum acetate) may be used if weeping or oozing
	• <u>**Oral Management**</u>:
	  • **Oral corticosteroids (prednisone) indicated for severe or extensive reactions; often required for 7-21 days**
	  • Oral antihistamines (diphenhydramine or hydroxyzine)

Diaper Rash

Irritant Contact Dermatitis

Etiology & Risk Factors	• Type of irritant contact dermatitis characterized by an inflammatory reaction of the skin exposed to a diaper (perineum, buttocks, genitalia, upper thighs, lower abdomen)
	• Etiology: inflammation or infection
	  • Inflammation (reaction due to increased moisture, prolonged contact with urine or feces, or other irritants like fragrances or detergents)
	  • Fungal (*Candida albicans*) or bacterial (*S. aureus* or *S. pyogenes*) infection
	• Risk Factors: **newborns or young infants** (skin immaturity), infrequency of diaper changes, **diet** (changes in intestinal microbiota and stool pH; breastfeeding is protective)

Patho-physiology	• Increased moisture, prolonged exposure to irritants (urine, feces, diaper fragrances or detergents) leads to increased friction and maceration • Breakdown of urinary urea may increase fecal enzyme activity resulting in further damage to the skin

Signs & Symptoms	• <u>Irritant Contact Dermatitis</u>:
	  • **Erythematous papules present around the perineum, buttocks, upper thighs, genitalia and suprapubic area**
	  • **May develop maceration or superficial erosions in severe cases**
	  • Often spares the skin folds (unless superimposed *Candida* infection present)
	• <u>*Candida* Dermatitis</u>: may be superimposed
	  • **Erythematous, edematous and scaly plaques**
	  • **Presence of satellite pustules or papules (most characteristic feature)**
	  • **Often involves the skin folds**
	  • Erosions and ulceration may occur in severe cases
	• *S. aureus* Infection: range of signs from small papules and pustules to large, blisters of bullous impetigo
	• *S. pyogenes* Infection: "fiery-red" erythema and maceration involving the skin folds

Diagnosis	• **Clinical Diagnosis** • <u>Potassium Hydroxide (KOH) Wet Mount</u>: consider if *Candida* is suspected etiology (intensely pruritic rash with satellite lesions) • <u>Culture</u>: consider if bacterial etiology suspected

Treatment	• <u>**Supportive**</u>: general skin care is first-line treatment
	  • **Good hygiene (keep affected area clean and dry), frequent diaper changes**, use of disposable diapers, periods of rest without a diaper, use of appropriate baby wipes (without fragrances, detergents, essential oils, etc.)
	  • **Barrier ointments (petroleum jelly, zinc oxide) may be used for treatment and to prevent further breakdown**
	• <u>Low-Potency Corticosteroids</u>: hydrocortisone 0.5% indicated if dermatitis does not improve in 2-3 days of implementing supportive measures
	• <u>Topical Antifungals</u>: nystatin is first-line for *Candida* dermatitis; Clotrimazole, miconazole, or ketoconazole may be used if no response in 1-3 days of nystatin use
	• <u>Antibiotics</u>: topical or oral antibiotics may be indicated for bacterial infection

Key Words & Most Common	• Irritant dermatitis of the diaper area; usually inflammatory reaction but may have superimposed *Candida* infection • Erythematous papules +/- maceration or erosions (satellite lesions and skin fold involvement if *Candida* dermatitis present) • General skin care → low-potency corticosteroids → topical antifungals (nystatin → -azoles if *Candida* dermatitis present)

Toxicodendron Dermatitis

Etiology & Risk Factors	• Type of allergic contact dermatitis caused by plants of the *Toxicodendron* genus including poison ivy, poison oak, and poison sumac
	• <u>Etiology</u>: **skin exposure to urushiol** (oil found in *Toxicodendron* plants), producing a type IV hypersensitivity reaction
	   • <u>Poison Ivy</u>: appears on a vine with almond-shaped leaves in groups of three; leaves change from green to red in the fall; most common in eastern US
	   • <u>Poison Oak</u>: shrub with lobed leaves in groups of three that resemble true oak leaves; most common in western US
	   • <u>Poison Sumac</u>: tree or tall shrub with red stems and feather-like leaf arrangement comprised of oval-shaped leaves; most common in swampy areas of southeastern US
	• <u>Risk Factors</u>: **exposure through occupation or activity (forestry work, landscaping, gardening, hiking, camping, hunting)**, increased sensitivity to urushiol

Patho-physiology	• Urushiol is the oil compound found in Toxicodendron plants primary that incites the release of local cytokines and inflammatory mediators • Oil compound is lipophilic resulting in rapid absorption and is subsequently picked up by Langerhans cells in the epidermis (makes washing of the compound ineffective)

Signs & Symptoms	• **Intensely pruritic, well-demarcated, erythematous papular or vesicular rash**
	   • **Associated burning or stinging**
	   • **Linear distribution** is common
	• **Most common on distal extremities** (ankles, shins; wrists, forearms)

Diagnosis	• **Clinical Diagnosis** • <u>Patch Testing</u>: may help identify patients with severe urushiol sensitivity

Treatment	• <u>Supportive</u>: first-line as dermatitis is usually self-limited, resolving within a couple of weeks
	   • **Immediate irrigation with soap and water**, decontamination of clothing after exposure
	   • Cool, moist compresses, oatmeal baths, calamine lotion, topical astringents
	• <u>High-Potency Topical Corticosteroids</u>: **clobetasol propionate 0.05% or triamcinolone 0.1%;** indicated for focal involvement
	• <u>Oral Corticosteroids</u>: **prednisone;** 7-21 day taper indicated for severe or extensive involvement; longer course required to prevent rebound dermatitis
	• <u>Oral and Topical Antihistamines</u>: generally not indicated as ineffective outside of the sedative effects (biochemical process is not due to histamine release)

Key Words & Most Common	• Allergic contact dermatitis secondary to exposure to poison ivy, poison oak, poison sumac • Outdoor occupations or activities greatest risk factors (landscaping, gardening, hiking, camping, hunting) • Pruritic, erythematous papules or vesicles in a linear distribution • Supportive → topical corticosteroids → oral corticosteroids

Hand and Foot Dermatitis
Acute Palmoplantar Eczema / Dyshidrotic Dermatitis

Etiology & Risk Factors	• **Dermatitis affecting the hands and/or feet** • <u>Etiology</u>: contact dermatitis (allergic or irritant) or atopic dermatitis • <u>Risk Factors</u>: **age (most common <40 years old), environmental factors (exposure to hot and humid conditions, excessive sweating, or frequent hand washing), skin barrier dysfunction, allergic or hypersensitivity reactions**, family history, stress and emotional factors (influences immune response)
Patho-physiology	• Edema accumulates between epidermal keratinocytes (spongiosis) resulting in rupture of cells and leading to the formation of microvesicles • Microvesicles may persist longer and become visible as the thicker stratum corneum of the hands and feet prevents rupture

Signs & Symptoms	• **Erythema, scaling, thickening of skin of soles, palms and fingers (lateral digits)**
	   • **May progress to tense, pruritic vesicles** that can desquamate (rupture) and lead to erosions and crusting
	• <u>Pompholyx</u>: severe form of dyshidrotic dermatitis
	   • Coalescence of vesicles that form larger bullae

Diagnosis	• **Clinical Diagnosis**

Treatment	• <u>Discontinue and Avoid Offending Agent</u>: **most important first-step in management**
	   • Avoid frequent or prolonged contact with water, soaps and detergents
	• <u>Supportive</u>: cool compresses, cool saline washes or cool baths, emollients, calamine lotion, aloe vera
	• <u>Topical Management</u>:
	   • **Topical corticosteroids (triamcinolone or betamethasone) are first-line for medical management**
	   • Topical antihistamines (diphenhydramine) may alleviate pruritus
	   • Drying agents (aluminum acetate) may be used if weeping or oozing
	• <u>Phototherapy</u>: narrowband ultraviolet B (UVB) or with soak ultraviolet A (patients soak hands and/or feet in psoralen solution before exposure to UVA) may be indicated for frequent episodes not controlled with corticosteroids

Key Words & Most Common	• Dermatitis of the hands/feet • Most common due to excessive sweating, frequent hand washing or prolonged exposure to water (washing dishes) • Erythema, scaling, thickening → tense, pruritic vesicles → rupture • Discontinue and avoid prolonged contact with water → supportive measures → topical corticosteroids → phototherapy

Lichen Planus

Etiology & Risk Factors	• Acute or chronic inflammatory disorder of the skin and mucous membranes • Etiology: **idiopathic; T-cell-mediated autoimmune disease** • Risk Factors: **hepatitis C infection**, certain medications (NSAIDs, ACEI, beta-blockers, sulfonylureas, thiazides, antimalarial), **dental restorations using mercury, copper, or gold**
Patho-physiology	• Not fully understood; T cell-mediated autoimmune reaction against basal epithelial keratinocytes in specific persons with a genetic predisposition
Signs & Symptoms	• **6 P's: pruritic, violaceous (purple), polygonal, flat-topped (planar) papules or plaques** • 2-4mm in size and may have fine scale, **irregular/angular borders** • Symmetric distribution **most commonly affecting the flexor aspects of the extremities, wrists, ankles**, legs, trunk, glans penis, and **oral** and vaginal mucosae • Lesions may coalesce or become hyperpigmented, atrophic, and/or hyperkeratotic over time • **Koebner's Phenomenon: new lesions appear at sites of minor skin injury (such as a superficial scratch or abrasion)** • **Wickham Striae: reticulated, lacy, bluish white, linear lesions of the oral mucosa is hallmark of oral lichen planus** • Nail bed scarring, discoloration, longitudinal ridging and thinning may occur
Diagnosis	• **Clinical Diagnosis** • Biopsy: confirms diagnosis; demonstrates irregular stratum corneum and granulosum, alteration or loss of rete ridges resulting in a sawtooth pattern; lymphocytes infiltration • Direct Immunofluorescence: helpful to differentiate between lichen planus and lupus erythematosus • *Consider hepatitis B and C testing if lichen planus diagnosis is made*
Treatment	• **Topical Corticosteroids: first-line treatment**; high-dose (clobetasol, fluocinonide) used on thicker lesions of extremities, low-dose (hydrocortisone) on face, groin, axilla • Occlusive dressings (polyethylene wrapping or flurandrenolide tape) may increase potency • **Oral Corticosteroids: prednisone (20mg for 2-6 weeks with taper); indicated for severe cases** • Intralesional Corticosteroid Injection: triamcinolone acetonide; indicated for hyperkeratotic plaques, scalp lesions, or persistent/resistance lesions • Oral Retinoids: acitretin (30 mg QD for 8 weeks); indicated for otherwise recalcitrant cases • Phototherapy: psoralen plus ultraviolet A (PUVA) or narrowband ultraviolet B (NBUVB) are alternatives; indicated for recalcitrant cases or generalized eruptions • Viscous Lidocaine: indicated to reduce symptoms in oral lichen planus
Key Words & Most Common	• T-cell mediated autoimmune disease of skin and mucous membranes • 6 P's: pruritic, violaceous (purple), polygonal, flat-topped (planar) papules or plaques of the extremities, wrists, ankles • Koebner's Phenomenon: new lesions at site of skin trauma • Wickham Striae: fine white lines of oral mucosa • Topical corticosteroids are first-line

Wickham Striae

Lichen Simplex Chronicus

Neurodermatitis

Etiology & Risk Factors	• **Thickened and leathery (lichenified) skin secondary to repeated skin rubbing and/or scratching of the skin ("itch-scratch" cycle)** • Etiology: **repetitive rubbing and/or scratching**, mechanical skin trauma • Risk Factors: **underlying skin conditions** (eczema, psoriasis, allergic dermatitis) **resulting in frequent scratching, psychological factors** (emotional stress, anxiety, depression), **skin trauma or injury** (burns, insect bites, surgical scars), **environmental factors** (irritants, allergens, harsh chemical)
Patho-physiology	• Frequent scratching or rubbing leads to altered sensory processing, resulting in an "itch-scratch" cycle; continued scratching causes further damage to the skin barrier, perpetuating the inflammatory response
Signs & Symptoms	• **Single or multiple pruritic, well-demarcated, hyperpigmented, plaques that are dry, scaling, and rough** • **Exaggerated skin lines** • **Thickened, leathery (lichenified) appearance** • Irregular, oval, or angular shapes • **Most common on easy-to-reach areas such as the scalp, arms, legs, neck, upper trunk, and genitals**
Diagnosis	• **Clinical Diagnosis**
Treatment	• **Avoid Rubbing/Scratching the Lesions**: first-line recommendation to decrease the "itch-scratch" cycle • **Treat or Remove Underlying Etiology**: address eczema, psoriasis, allergic dermatitis, radiculopathy, ill-fitting footwear, etc. • **Supportive**: oral H1-blocking antihistamines (diphenhydramine), emollients, and topical capsaicin cream may reduce pruritic symptoms • **High-Potency Topical Corticosteroids**: clobetasol; indicated as second-line treatment; patient may wrap lesion in plastic wrap overnight to increase potency • Intralesional Corticosteroid Injection: triamcinolone acetonide; indicated for small, resistance lesions
Key Words & Most Common	• Initiated by repetitive rubbing or scratching of the skin • Pruritic, well-demarcated, hyperpigmented plaques with thickened, leathery appearance • Avoid rubbing/scratching + address underlying etiology → diphenhydramine, emollients → high-potency topical corticosteroids

Atopic Dermatitis (Eczema)

Etiology & Risk Factors	• Chronic, relapsing, inflammatory skin disorder • <u>Etiology</u>: multiple genetic and environmental factors; **disruption and abnormalities of the epidermis and the immune system lead to symptomology** • <u>Risk Factors</u>: **atopy (eczema + allergic rhinitis + asthma), family history, food sensitivities** (eggs, milk, peanuts, soy, wheat), **environmental exposures** (heat or cold, dryness, perspiration, allergens), **contact irritants** (wool, nickel, harsh soaps/detergents, rough or synthetic fibers), immunocompromised
Patho-physiology	• Loss-of-function mutation of the filaggrin gene leads to disruption of the skin barrier • Allergens and irritants are then able to penetrate the epidermis, triggering an immune response and promoting inflammation
Signs & Symptoms	• **Intense pruritus is hallmark feature** • **Ill-defined, erythematous, thickened, scaly patches or plaques** • Lesions may become eroded (dry and lichenified) secondary to scratching • **Most common on the face, scalp, neck, extremity extensor surfaces in infants** (crawling and rubbing skin) • **Most common on neck and flexor creases (antecubital and popliteal folds) in children/adults** • <u>Nummular Eczema</u>: sharply defined, discoid ("coin-shaped") lesions most common on dorsum of hands and feet and extensor surfaces (knees and elbows)
Diagnosis	• **Clinical Diagnosis** • <u>Immunoglobulin E (IgE) Antibodies</u>: elevated test can help confirm atopic diathesis • <u>Testing for Type I Allergens</u>: prick, scratch, and intracutaneous testing may help confirm diagnosis
Treatment	• <u>**Supportive**</u>: avoidance of triggers or irritants, moisturizers **(especially ceramide-containing products applied after shower/bath),** oral probiotics, gentle skincare routine (avoid fragrances and hot water), wet wrap therapy (applying moisturizers or topical medications and covering with wet bandages to enhance the absorption), elimination diet, stress reduction, keep fingernails short (avoid excoriation from scratching) • <u>**Topical Corticosteroids**</u>: **mainstay of therapy; low- to mid-potency corticosteroids indicated to control skin inflammation**; prolonged use may cause skin atrophy • <u>Topical Calcineurin Inhibitors</u>: tacrolimus, pimecromilus; alternatives to corticosteroids that do not cause skin atrophy; indicated for sensitive areas (axilla, groin, face) • <u>Topical Crisaborole</u>: topical phosphodiesterase-4 inhibitor may be considered in refractory cases • <u>Oral Antihistamines</u>: hydroxyzine, diphenhydramine, loratadine, cetirizine indicated to alleviate pruritus via sedating properties • <u>Phototherapy</u>: psoralen plus ultraviolet A (PUVA) or narrowband ultraviolet B (NBUVB) are alternatives; indicated for recalcitrant cases or generalized eruptions • <u>Systemic Immunosuppressants</u>: cyclosporine, mycophenolate, methotrexate, azathioprine indicated for widespread, recalcitrant, disabling cases that fail other therapies • <u>Systemic Biological Agents</u>: dupilumab; human monoclonal IgG4 antibody indicated for moderate to severe cases that fail other therapies
Key Words & Most Common	• Part of atopic triad (eczema + allergic rhinitis + asthma) • Intensely pruritic, erythematous, thickened, scaly patches/plaques of neck and flexor creases • Supportive → topical corticosteroids

Pityriasis Rosea

Etiology & Risk Factors	• **Acute self-limiting papulosquamous disorder** • <u>Etiology</u>: **unknown; may be associated with viral infections (human herpesviruses 6 and 7)**, bacterial infection (*Streptococcus*), or spirochete infection • <u>Risk Factors</u>: **age (10-35 years old most common), recent immunization** (Bacillus Calmette-Guerin (BCG), influenza, diphtheria, hepatitis B, and *Pneumococcus*), seasonal (most common in spring and fall), **family history**, emotional stress and immune system dysregulation
Patho-physiology	• Viral infection leads to an increased immune response and subsequent release of inflammatory cytokines (T-cell mediated immunity), resulting in the characteristic skin rash and associated symptoms.

Signs & Symptoms	• <u>Herald Patch</u>: **large (2-10cm), solitary, salmon-colored macule on the trunk or proximal limb followed by general exanthem 7-14 days later**
	• <u>General Exanthem</u>: **general eruption of small (0.5-2cm), round/oval, salmon- or fawn-colored papules and plaques with a scaly, slightly raised border (collarette)**
	   • **Centripetal distribution, scaling in a Christmas-tree pattern (along skin cleavage lines)**
	   • Lesions are confined to the trunk and proximal extremities (face, palms, soles are usually spared)
	   • *Lesions may resemble ringworm (tinea corporis)*

Diagnosis	• **Clinical Diagnosis** • <u>Syphilis Testing</u>: RPR ordered to rule out secondary syphilis • Indicated with palm or sole involvement, lack of a preceding herald patch is not seen, or unusual distribution
Treatment	• <u>**Supportive**</u>: **mainstay of therapy;** most cases spontaneously resolve within 6-12 weeks • Education, reassurance, exposure to natural sunlight, oatmeal baths, moisturizers or emollients • <u>Antipruritic Therapy</u>: oral or topical corticosteroids, oral or topical antihistamines • <u>Antivirals</u>: acyclovir may alleviate symptoms in patients who present early and have widespread disease but are not routinely used
Key Words & Most Common	• Acute, self-limiting, papulosquamous disorder • May be associated with HHV 6 and 7 • <u>Herald Patch</u>: large, solitary, salmon-colored macule of trunk • <u>General Exanthem</u>: general eruption of small, round/oval, salmon/fawn-colored papules and plaques following skin cleavage lines (Christmas-tree pattern) • Supportive treatment

Psoriasis

Etiology & Risk Factors	• Chronic hyperproliferation of epidermal keratinocytes and epidermal and dermal inflammation; may also affect joints and eyes • Etiology: unknown; immune stimulation of epidermal keratinocytes has been implicated • Risk Factors: **age (bimodal distribution of 15-20 years old and 55-60 years old), genetic factors (HLA-C gene), family history,** immune system dysfunction, other autoimmune conditions, **environmental factors** (cold weather), **lifestyle factors** (smoking, excessive alcohol consumption, obesity, sedentary lifestyle) • Precipitating Factors: **skin trauma (Koebner phenomenon),** sunburn, infection, medications (beta-blockers, ACEI, NSAIDs, steroids), emotional stress, alcohol, smoking, obesity
Patho-physiology	• Infiltration of the skin by activated T cells which causes keratin hyperplasia, hyperproliferation of cells within the stratum basale and stratum spinosum, and cytokine release • Dysregulation of keratinocyte turnover results in the formation of thick plaques and hyposecretion of lipids by the epidermal cells leading to flaky and scaly skin

Signs & Symptoms	• **Plaque:** most common type (90%)
	   • **Raised, well-defined, erythematous plaques with thick silvery-white scales**
	   • Most common on extensor surfaces of extremities (knees, elbows), **scalp, nape of the neck** or lumbosacral region
	   • **Auspitz Sign:** punctate (pinpoint) bleeding seen with removal of the plaque or scale
	   • Koebner's Phenomenon: new lesions precipitated at sites of skin trauma
	• **Guttate:** small, erythematous and scaly "raindrop-shaped" papules with fine scales mainly over the trunk and back; **most commonly appears after** *Streptococcal* infection
	• **Pustular:** small, non-infectious pus-filled lesions with surrounding erythema; generalized type associated with hypocalcemia
	• **Erythrodermic:** generalized, wide-spread, inflammation and erythema involving >90% of the body; associated with severe itching, swelling, and pain
	• **Inverse:** smooth (lacks scale), erythematous, sharply demarcated patches affecting intertriginous areas (groin, axilla, intergluteal and inframammary region)
	• **Nail:** pitting, stippling, fraying, **yellow-brown discoloration (oil spot sign),** and thickening of the nails, may have separation of the nail plate (onycholysis)

Diagnosis	• **Clinical Diagnosis**

Treatment	• **Topical Management:**
	   • **Topical Corticosteroids: first-line treatment;** potency depends on severity and extent of disease
	   • **Topical Vitamin D₃ Analogs:** calcipotriene, calcitriol; induces normal keratinocyte proliferation and differentiation; often used in conjunction with corticosteroids
	   • Topical Calcineurin Inhibitors: tacrolimus, pimecromilus; alternatives to corticosteroids that do not cause skin atrophy; indicated for sensitive areas (axilla, groin, face)
	   • Topical Retinoids: tazarotene; vitamin A analog that is used as adjunct to corticosteroids
	   • Other: emollients, salicylic acid, coal tar, anthralin
	• **Phototherapy:** psoralen plus ultraviolet A (PUVA) or narrowband ultraviolet B (NBUVB) are alternatives; indicated for recalcitrant cases or generalized eruptions
	• **Immunosuppressants:**
	   • **Methotrexate:** effective treatment that is reserved for severe, disabling psoriasis; works by interfering with the rapid proliferation of epidermal cells
	   • Cyclosporine: alternative for severe cases
	   • Mycophenolate: alternative to severe cases that do not respond to methotrexate or cyclosporine
	• Systemic Retinoids: isotretinoin, acitretin; effective treatment for severe and recalcitrant cases of psoriasis; generally reserved for pustular or erythrodermic psoriasis
	• Immunomodulatory Biologic Agents: TNF inhibitors, etanercept, adalimumab, infliximab; manufactured proteins interrupt the immune process and are indicated for moderate to severe cases of psoriasis

Tinea Versicolor
Pityriasis Versicolor

Etiology & Risk Factors	• **Benign, superficial fungal infection of the skin** • Etiology: **overgrowth of the yeast** *Malassezia furfur* (part of normal skin flora) • Risk Factors: **warm and humid environments** (tropical climates), **age (adolescents and young adults most common due to the increase of sebum production), excessive sweating, oily skin,** immunosuppression (corticosteroid use, pregnancy, malnutrition, diabetes, etc.), application of oily lotions and creams
Patho-physiology	• Excessive oil or sebum production creates a lipid-rich environment that allows *M. furfur* to grow • Hypopigmentation is secondary to tyrosinase inhibition caused by *M. furfur* production of azelaic acid
Signs & Symptoms	• Asymptomatic • **Multiple tan, brown, salmon or pink-colored, hyper or hypopigmented, well-demarcated round macules with a fine scale** • **Lesions coalesce into patches** • Most common on trunk, neck, abdomen, and proximal extremities • **Affected area does not tan with sun exposure** (diagnosis in summer is more common)
Diagnosis	• **Clinical Diagnosis** • **Potassium Hydroxide (KOH) Wet Mount: identifies hyphae and clusters of yeast cells** ("spaghetti and meatballs") • Woods Lamp: reveals golden-white or coppery-orange fluorescence

Treatment	• **Topical Antifungals: first-line therapy;** selenium sulfide shampoo 2.5%, topical ketoconazole 2%, daily bathing with **zinc pyrithione soap 2% or sulfur-salicylic shampoo 2%**
	• **Oral Antifungals:** itraconazole or fluconazole weekly for 2-4 weeks; indicated in widespread, severe, recalcitrant or recurrent cases
	   • Fluconazole is delivered to the skin via perspiration therefore patients must be educated not to shower for several hours after taking medication
	• Prevention: recurrence is common as *M. furfur* is a commensal fungal inhabitant of the normal skin flora
	   • Adequate hygiene, regular use of zinc pyrithione soap, and/or once-monthly topical antifungal therapy lowers recurrence rate

Key Words & Most Common	• Benign fungal infection of the skin caused by overgrowth of Malassezia furfur • Warm/humid climates, excessive sweating, oily skin, adolescents are greatest risk factors • Multiple tan hyper/hypopigmented, round macules with fine scale that coalesce into patches • Most common on trunk, neck, abdomen • Affected area does not tan with sun exposure • KOH prep reveals hyphae and budding cells • Topical antifungals (topical ketoconazole or selenium sulfide shampoo) → oral antifungals (fluconazole)

	Cradle Cap	**Infantile Seborrheic Dermatitis** 🖐
Etiology & Risk Factors		• Common, self-limiting, non-inflammatory scaling skin condition affecting neonates and infants • Etiology: not fully understood • Risk Factors: **age (most common in neonates and infants; peaks at 3 months old)**, family history, excessive oil production, maternal hormonal influences
Patho-physiology		• Secondary influence of maternal circulating hormones results in increased sebaceous gland activity which results in excessive sebum production, creating a lipid-rich environment that allows excess *M. furfur* to grow • Overproduction of sebum causes the dead corneocytes (scale) to remain adherent to the scalp instead of undergoing normal desquamation
Signs & Symptoms		• **Asymptomatic** (non-painful, non-pruritic) • **Greasy, non-inflammatory plaques with overlying yellowish scale** • **Most common on the vertex and frontal regions of the scalp**
Diagnosis		• **Clinical Diagnosis**

Treatment		• Observation: benign, self-limiting condition that often resolves spontaneously by one year of age
		• Conservative: removal of the scale
		  • Apply emollient (white petrolatum, mineral oil, baby oil, olive oil) to the scalp and allow to sit for 15 minutes (possibly overnight) which will soften the scale
		  • Gentle removal of the scale with a soft brush or fine-tooth comb
		  • Wash scalp with gentle baby shampoo
		  • After scale is removed, scalp should be washed daily with baby shampoo to prevent recurrence
		• Topical Management: topical ketoconazole or low-potency topical corticosteroids may be considered in extensive or persistent cases

Key Words & Most Common		• Common condition affecting neonates and infants • Peaks at 3 months old • Greasy, non-inflammatory plaques with overlying yellowish scale • Most common on vertex and forehead • Observation → manual removal with emollient + removal with comb + wash with baby shampoo

	Adult Seborrheic Dermatitis 🖐	
Etiology & Risk Factors		• **Common inflammatory skin condition presenting with a papulosquamous morphology in areas with sebaceous gland prevalence** • Etiology: not fully understood • Risk Factors: **age (most common 30-70 years old), male**, increased sebaceous gland activity, **immunodeficiency (HIV), neurological/psychiatric conditions (Parkinson disease, stroke, Alzheimer dementia)**, certain medications (dopamine antagonists, lithium, immunosuppressants), **emotional stress, seasonal (fall and winter)**
Patho-physiology		• Disruption of the skin's normal microbiota causes sebaceous gland overactivity, causing excessive sebum production which creates a lipid-rich environment and allows excess *M. furfur* to grow • Overproduction of sebum causes the dead corneocytes (scale) to remain adherent to the scalp instead of undergoing normal desquamation
Signs & Symptoms		• **Occurs on areas rich in sebaceous glands (scalp, face, eyelids, beard, mustache, nasolabial folds, postauricular area, chest, groin)** • **Erythematous papules and plaques with a fine, white scale, and a yellowish, greasy crust** • **Dry flakes or greasy diffuse scalp scale (dandruff)** • **May be associated with variable burning and pruritus**
Diagnosis		• **Clinical Diagnosis**
Treatment		• Topical Antifungals: first-line therapy; selenium sulfide shampoo, topical ketoconazole, zinc pyrithione soap or sulfur-salicylic shampoo 2% (keratolytic shampoos) • Topical Corticosteroids: low-dose preparations (0.01% fluocinolone acetonide, 1% hydrocortisone, 0.025% triamcinolone); effective short-term treatment • Topical Calcineurin Inhibitors: tacrolimus, pimecromilus; alternatives to corticosteroids that do not cause skin atrophy; indicated for sensitive areas (axilla, groin, face) • **Oral Antifungals: itraconazole or fluconazole; indicated in widespread, severe, recalcitrant or recurrent cases**
Key Words & Most Common		• Common inflammatory skin condition • Most common in elderly males with Parkinson disease or HIV • Most common on scalp or face (rich in sebaceous glands) • Erythematous papules/plaques with a fine scale and yellow, greasy crust +/- burning/pruritus • Dandruff • Topical antifungals → topical corticosteroids

Hypersensitivity Reactions

Type I Reaction	<ul><li>**Immediate (<1 hour after exposure) hypersensitivity**</li><li>IgE mediated (antigen binds to IgE that is bound to tissue mast cells and blood basophils, triggering release of mediators such as histamine</li><li>Mediators result in vasodilation, increased capillary permeability, mucus hypersecretion, smooth muscle spasm, and tissue infiltration with eosinophils, type 2 helper T cells, and other inflammatory cells</li><li>Examples:<ul><li>**Allergic Rhinitis**: triggered by allergens (pollen, dust mites, pet dander) leading to symptoms including sneezing, itching, nasal congestion, and watery eyes</li><li>**Asthma**: triggered by allergens (pollen, mold spores, pet dander) can cause bronchial inflammation and airway constriction</li><li>**Anaphylaxis**: severe, life-threatening reaction occurring as a response to various triggers, including insect stings (bees, wasps), foods (peanuts, shellfish), medications (penicillin), or latex. It manifests rapidly and involves symptoms like difficulty breathing, swelling of the throat or tongue, urticaria, dizziness, and hypotension</li><li>**Allergic Conjunctivitis**: exposure to allergens (pollen or animal dander) results in conjunctival inflammation leading to redness, itching, tearing, and swollen eyelids</li><li>**Atopic Dermatitis (Eczema)**: exposure to allergens or irritants triggers an immune response, resulting in a chronic inflammatory skin condition</li></ul></li></ul>
Type II Reaction	<ul><li>**Antibody-dependent cytotoxic hypersensitivity**</li><li>Activation of IgG and IgM antibodies against specific antigens on cells or tissues that can bind to target cells, resulting in cell destruction through complement activation, antibody-dependent cell-mediated cytotoxicity (ADCC), and phagocytosis</li><li>Examples:<ul><li>**Hemolytic Transfusion Reaction**: incompatibility between the blood types of the donor and recipient can lead to the activation of complement proteins and the destruction of transfused red blood cells</li><li>**Hemolytic Disease of the Newborn (HDN)**: incompatibility between the blood types of a pregnant woman and her fetus (most commonly due to Rh factor incompatibility) result in the production of maternal antibodies that attack and destroy fetal red blood cells</li><li>**Autoimmune Hemolytic Anemia**: immune system antibodies target and destroys the body's own red blood cells by complement activation or by phagocytes</li><li>**Goodpasture Syndrome**: autoimmune disorder characterized by the production of autoantibodies against the basement membrane of the lungs and kidneys</li><li>**Drug-Induced Hemolytic Anemia**: certain medications (antibiotics and NSAIDs), can induce the production of antibodies that bind to red blood cells, leading to their destruction and subsequent anemia.</li></ul></li></ul>

Hypersensitivity Reactions

Type III Reaction	<ul><li>**Immune antibody-antigen complex-mediated hypersensitivity**</li><li>Immune complexes are formed through antigen and antibody (usually IgG or IgM) binding that is then deposited into tissues and activates the complement system; these immune complexes may trigger and inflammatory response which damages tissue</li><li>Examples:<ul><li>**Systemic Lupus Erythematosus (SLE)**: autoantibodies (particularly anti-nuclear antibodies), form immune complexes with self-antigens that are deposited in joint, skin, kidney and vascular tissue</li><li>**Serum Sickness**: hypersensitivity reaction occurring in response to the administration of certain medications in which immune complexes are formed between the drugs and antibodies, leading to their deposition in tissues and the activation of complement</li><li>**Post-Streptococcal Glomerulonephritis**: immune complexes composed of streptococcal antigens and antibodies are deposited in the glomeruli of the kidneys triggering an inflammatory response that results in glomerular damage Reactive Arthritis: inflammatory condition occurring in response to a GI or GU infection secondary to immune complex deposition in the affected joints</li></ul></li></ul>
Type IV Reaction	<ul><li>**Delayed (24-72 hours after exposure), cell-mediated hypersensitivity**</li><li>T cells mediated reaction in which sensitized T cells recognize specific antigens and release cytokines, leading to further recruitment of inflammatory cells</li><li>Examples:<ul><li>**Allergic Contact Dermatitis**: skin condition occurring when skin comes into contact with an allergen or irritant substance. The immune response is T cell mediated (specifically CD4+ and CD8+ T cells), which recognize the allergen or irritant as foreign, leading to local inflammation.</li><li>**Tuberculin Skin Test (Mantoux Test)**: this test is used to screen for tuberculosis (TB) infection. It involves injecting a purified protein derivative (PPD) of *Mycobacterium tuberculosis* into the skin. In patients with positive prior exposure to TB, a delayed-type hypersensitivity reaction occurs within 48-72 hours, resulting in erythema and induration at the injection site.</li><li>**Poison Ivy Dermatitis**: hypersensitivity reaction caused by exposure to urushiol (oily resin found in poison ivy, poison oak, and poison sumac plants) producing a T cell mediated immune response leading to the development of a rash, blisters, and intense itching.</li><li>**Autoimmune Diseases**: Some autoimmune diseases, such as rheumatoid arthritis and multiple sclerosis, involve a type IV hypersensitivity reaction. In these conditions, autoreactive T cells recognize self-antigens as foreign and mount an immune response against them, leading to chronic inflammation and tissue damage.</li></ul></li></ul>

Exanthematous Drug Eruption 🔎

Etiology & Risk Factors	• Inappropriate or exaggerated, hypersensitive immune response to systemic drugs • <u>Etiology</u>: **systemic drug administration** • **Penicillins, sulfonamides, NSAIDs, chemotherapy, anesthetics [lidocaine, propofol], contrast medium, monoclonal antibodies, vaccines are most common causes** • <u>Risk Factors</u>: family history, **previous drug hypersensitivity**, history of allergies or atopy, concurrent medications (drug-drug interactions), **underlying medical condition** (immunocompromised, autoimmune disorder), **increased duration and dosage of drug exposure**
Patho-physiology	• Type IV (delayed) cell-mediated hypersensitivity reaction • T cells mediated reaction in which sensitized T cells recognize specific antigens and release cytokines, leading to further recruitment of inflammatory cells
Signs & Symptoms	• **Delayed eruption** occurring 5-14 days after initiating offending medication or 24-72 hours after exposure in previously sensitized individuals • **Generalized distribution of morbilliform or maculopapular lesions that coalesce to form plaques** • **Primarily affect trunk and proximal extremities** • May be accompanied by **low-grade fever, arthralgias and generalized pruritus**
Diagnosis	• **Clinical Diagnosis** • <u>Skin Testing</u>: prick or scratch tests, intradermal tests or patch tests; helps identify immediate type I hypersensitivity reactions • <u>Labs</u>: complete blood count (CBC) may show eosinophilia, elevated levels of serum tryptase may indicate anaphylaxis, specific IgE testing to detect IgE antibodies against specific drugs and can help confirm type I hypersensitivity reactions • <u>Drug Provocation Testing</u>: indicated in certain cases where the diagnosis is uncertain or when tolerance to a suspected drug is required; involves administering the drug under controlled conditions while closely monitoring for any adverse reactions

Treatment	• <u>**Discontinue Offending Medication**</u>: **mainstay of treatment**; most cutaneous reactions are self-limited once the offending drug is discontinued
	• <u>**Symptomatic and Supportive Treatment**</u>:
	   • <u>**Oral Antihistamines**</u>: first-generation (**diphenhydramine**, hydroxyzine) or second-generation (cetirizine, loratadine, fexofenadine) indicated for pruritus
	   • <u>NSAIDs</u>: ibuprofen indicated for arthralgias
	   • <u>**Oral Corticosteroids**</u>: prednisone indicated for severe cutaneous reactions
	• <u>Rapid Desensitization Therapy</u>: may be indicated if IgE-mediated hypersensitivity with no essential or alternative treatment to produce temporary tolerance

Key Words & Most Common	• Hypersensitive immune response to systemic drugs (penicillins, sulfonamides and NSAIDs most common) • Delayed eruption • Generalized distribution of morbilliform or maculopapular lesions that coalesce to form plaques • Primarily affect trunk and proximal extremities • Discontinue offending medication → oral antihistamines +/- oral corticosteroids

Angioedema 🔎

Etiology & Risk Factors	• **Paroxysmal, localized swelling of dermal or submucosal layers of skin or mucosa**
	• <u>Etiology</u>: may be mast-cell (histamine) or bradykinin mediated
	   • <u>**Mast-Cell (Histamine) Mediated**</u>: **allergic reaction**; IgE-mediated type I hypersensitivity reaction
	   • <u>**Bradykinin Mediated**</u>: **angiotensin converting enzyme inhibitor (ACEI)-induced** or hereditary (secondary to C1 esterase inhibitor deficiency)
	     • Highest incidence with ACEI-induced angioedema occurs in first month but **can occur at any time**
	• <u>Risk Factors</u>: **exposures to certain foods (nuts, shellfish), acute use medications (antibiotics, NSAIDs, contrast agents) or insect stings, chronic use medications (ACEI)**, certain genetic conditions (hereditary angioedema), family history, comorbid autoimmune condition (SLE), environmental factors (exposure to heat or cold, stress, or trauma)

Patho-physiology	• <u>Mast-Cell (Histamine) Mediated</u>: IgE-mediated type I hypersensitivity reaction secondary to mast-cells and basophil activation • <u>Bradykinin Mediated</u>: ACEI-associated secondary to decreased bradykinin degradation; hereditary secondary to C1 esterase inhibitor deficiency causing bradykinin production • Excessive bradykinin and histamine increases vascular permeability leading to edema

Signs & Symptoms	• **Non-pitting edema of the mucosal tissue of the face, lips, and/or tongue is most common presentation**
	   • May involve hands, feet, and genitalia
	• <u>**Mast-Cell (Histamine) Mediated**</u>: develops over minutes to hours; accompanied by other allergic reaction symptoms
	   • <u>Upper Airway Edema</u>: **stridor, respiratory distress**, bronchospasm
	   • <u>Cutaneous Edema</u>: **generalized pruritus, urticaria**, flushing
	   • <u>Gastrointestinal Edema</u>: **nausea/vomiting, colicky abdominal pain**, diarrhea
	• <u>Bradykinin Mediated</u>: develops over hours to days; not accompanied by allergic reaction symptoms

Diagnosis	• **Clinical Diagnosis** • <u>**C1 and C4 Esterase Inhibitor Levels**</u>: decreased levels confirms diagnosis of hereditary angioedema

Treatment	• <u>Airway Management</u>: **securing airways is the highest priority**; endotracheal intubation
	   • Prepare for difficult airway if edema is severe; fiberoptics, ENT/anesthesia assistance, surgical airway, OR transfer
	• <u>**Mast-Cell (Histamine) Mediated**</u>:
	   • <u>**Antihistamines**</u>: IV/IM diphenhydramine
	   • <u>**Corticosteroids**</u>: IV/IM methylprednisolone or PO prednisone
	   • <u>**Epinephrine**</u>: 0.3mg IM given immediately if angioedema unless the mechanism is obviously bradykinin-mediated
	• <u>Bradykinin Mediated</u>: epinephrine, corticosteroids, and antihistamines have not been shown to be effective
	   • <u>ACEI-Induced</u>: discontinue ACEI (most cases resolve after 24-48 hours), consider tranexamic acid, fresh frozen plasma, icatibant, ecallantide
	   • <u>Hereditary</u>: C1 inhibitor concentrate, ecallantide (kallikrein inhibitor which is required for bradykinin generation), icatibant (bradykinin antagonist)

Urticaria

Etiology & Risk Factors	• **Edema of the superficial layers of the skin secondary to histamine-release** • Etiology: **type I IgE-mediated hypersensitivity reaction** • Risk Factors: **exposures to certain foods (nuts, shellfish) or food additives (artificial dyes or sweeteners or flavor enhancers [MSG]), medications (antibiotics, NSAIDs, contrast agents), insect stings,** environmental factors (pet dander, pollen, exposure to heat or cold), comorbid autoimmune conditions, emotional stress, intense exercise
Patho-physiology	• Exposure to an allergen causes a release of histamine and other inflammatory mediators from mast cells in the skin; histamine causes dilation and increased blood vessel permeability leading to characteristic urticarial lesions • Other inflammatory substances, such as leukotrienes and prostaglandin from mast cells and basophils in the skin, further contribute to the inflammatory response
Signs & Symptoms	• **Sudden onset of intensely pruritic, migratory, circumscribed, blanchable, raised, erythematous plaques with central pallor** • **Most common on pressure-prone areas (waistline, axilla, groin)** but can affect any part of the skin • Lesions may coalesce • **Lesions are transient** (remains for <24 hours without any residual ecchymosis or pigmentation)
Diagnosis	• Clinical Diagnosis • Skin Testing: prick or scratch tests, intradermal tests or patch tests; helps identify immediate type I hypersensitivity reactions; indicated in recurrent, or persistent cases • Consider laboratory testing to determine underlying etiology if chronic
Treatment	• **Antihistamines:** first-generation (**diphenhydramine**, hydroxyzine) or second-generation (cetirizine, loratadine, fexofenadine) • Second-generation often preferred due to less anticholinergic side effects, minimally sedating and less drug-drug interactions • **Corticosteroids: IV/IM methylprednisolone or PO prednisone** indicated for severe, recurrent, or persistent cases • **Epinephrine:** 0.3mg IM given immediately if angioedema or respiratory compromise present
Key Words & Most Common	• Type I IgE-mediated hypersensitive reaction due to histamine release • Foods, food additives, medications, inset stings, environmental exposures most common cause • Pruritic, blanchable, raised plaques with central pallor • Antihistamines → corticosteroids → epinephrine

Stasis Dermatitis

Etiology & Risk Factors	• **Inflammatory skin change associated with chronic edema** • Etiology: **chronic edema due to chronic venous insufficiency** (deep vein thrombosis, varicose veins, superficial thrombophlebitis), **right heart failure, or lymphedema** • Risk Factors: **history of chronic venous insufficiency, advanced age, obesity, prolonged standing or sitting, pregnancy,** history of injury, trauma or surgery, family history, diabetes, history of smoking, sedentary lifestyle, undergoing radiation therapy
Patho-physiology	• Impaired venous circulation in the lower extremities leads to venous hypertension and increased capillary pressure that compromises microvascular endothelial integrity resulting in fibrin leakage and epithelial barrier function disruption eventually leading to local inflammation

Signs & Symptoms	• **Generalized pain, pruritus, and erythema of the lower extremities (most commonly on the shins)**
	• **Most common bilaterally** and worse after prolonged standing or sitting and improves with ambulation and lower extremity elevation
	• Pain described as a burning, fatigue, aching, throbbing, cramping, heaviness
	• Physical Exam:
	  • **Eczematous, erythematous rash with excoriations, weeping erosions, scaling, and lichenification with dry, tight, hairless skin**
	  • Purpura Jaune D'ocre: **yellow-brown, purplish discoloration due hemosiderin deposits in the dermis**
	  • Lipodermatosclerosis: sclerosis of subcutaneous fat
	  • Atrophie Blanche: white, scar-like, hypopigmented patches surrounded by telangiectasias and punctate red dots that occurs after a venous ulcer heals
	  • **Venous Stasis Ulcers: shallow, irregularly-shaped painful sores most common on the medial malleolus**

Diagnosis	• **Clinical Diagnosis** • Venous Doppler Ultrasound: may be indicated depending on underlying etiology

Treatment	• **Treat Underlying Etiology: treating the underlying venous insufficiency is the mainstay of treatment**
	• **Supportive: leg elevation, compression therapy,** exercise, weight management, avoid prolonged periods of standing or sitting
	• General Hygiene Measures: gentle skin cleansing, petroleum-based emollients
	• Topical Corticosteroids: triamcinolone acetonide 0.1%; indicated for noneroded stasis dermatitis
	• Venous Stasis Ulcers:
	  • Compression Bandaging Systems and Bland Dressings: elastic bandages, zinc oxide paste, or hydrocolloid dressings
	  • Topical Antibiotics: mupirocin or silver sulfadiazine; indicated for partial or full-thickness ulcers
	  • Oral Antibiotics: cephalosporins, dicloxacillin; indicated for superimposed cellulitis

Key Words & Most Common	• Inflammatory skin secondary to chronic venous insufficiency • Generalized pain, pruritus, erythema of bilateral lower extremities (shins) with excoriations, weeping erosions, scaling plaques • Venous Stasis Ulcers: shallow, irregularly-shaped painful sores most common on the medial malleolus • Treat underlying etiology • Leg elevation, compression therapy, exercise, weight management

Vitiligo

Etiology & Risk Factors	• **Loss of skin melanocytes that results in areas of skin depigmentation** • <u>Etiology</u>: not fully understood; combination of genetic, autoimmune, and environmental factors • <u>Risk Factors</u>: **family history, comorbid autoimmune conditions (thyroid disorders, alopecia areata, and type 1 diabetes), certain environmental factors (stress, sunburn, chemical exposure, or traumatic skin injury)**, ethnicity (more noticeable in patients with darker skin tones), immune system disorders
Patho-physiology	• Not fully understood; cytotoxic, autoimmune, oxidant-antioxidant mechanism destruction of melanocytes leading to skin depigmentation has been theorized
Signs & Symptoms	• **Irregular, sharply-demarcated, discrete white (hypopigmented or depigmented) macules and patches** • **Most common on the the face, digits, dorsum of the hands, flexor wrists**, elbows, lower extremities, axilla, inguinal and anogenital area, umbilicus, and nipples • Hair in vitiliginous areas is usually white
Diagnosis	• **Clinical Diagnosis** • <u>Woods Lamp</u>: lesions are accentuated with a chalk-white appearance of the hypopigmented or depigmented skin • <u>Biopsy</u>: rarely performed; demonstrates absence of melanocytes and complete epidermal pigmentation loss
Treatment	• <u>Protection from Sunlight</u>: clothing or sunscreen required to protect skin as depigmented area is very prone to sunburn • <u>Cosmetic Concealment</u>: small or scattered lesions can be camouflaged with makeup • <u>Topical Corticosteroids</u>: **first-line medication**; prolonged use may cause skin atrophy • <u>Topical Calcineurin Inhibitors</u>: tacrolimus, pimecromilus; alternatives to corticosteroids that do not cause skin atrophy; indicated for sensitive areas (axilla, groin, face) • <u>Topical Vitamin D$_3$ Analogs</u>: calcipotriene, calcitriol • <u>Phototherapy</u>: **narrowband UVB is often the preferred initial treatment for widespread vitiligo** • <u>Other</u>: laser therapy, autologous micrografting, suction blister grafting, and tattooing are alternatives
Key Words & Most Common	• Autoimmune destruction of melanocytes leading to skin depigmentation • Irregular, sharply-demarcated, depigmented macules or patches • Most common on face, hands and wrists and skin folds • Protect from sunlight + cosmetic concealment • Topical corticosteroids or phototherapy

Melasma

Etiology & Risk Factors	• Hypermelanosis (hyperpigmentation) of sun-exposed areas of the skin • <u>Etiology</u>: not fully understood; combination of hormonal, environmental, and genetic factors • <u>Risk Factors</u>: **females, hormonal changes (pregnancy or oral contraceptive use), certain skin tones (darker complexion)**, ethnicity (Asian, Hispanic, or Middle Eastern descent most common), **prolonged sun exposure**, family history, certain cosmetics, topical hormone replacement therapies, exposure to phytotoxic drugs, history of thyroid disease
Patho-physiology	• Exposure to UV radiation induces production of melanocyte stimulating hormone, corticotropin, interleukin 1 and endothelin 1, which contributes to increased melanin production by intraepidermal melanocytes; subsequent dermal inflammation and fibroblast activation results in increased melanogenesis
Signs & Symptoms	• **Symmetrically distributed hyperpigmented macules** • **Most common on sun-exposed areas** (cheeks, upper lip, chin, forehead, neck)
Diagnosis	• **Clinical Diagnosis** • <u>Woods Lamp</u>: determines pattern of pigment disposition; epidermal pigmentation becomes accentuated • <u>Biopsy</u>: rarely performed; demonstrates increased melanin deposition in dermal and epidermal layers

Treatment	• <u>Sun Protection</u>: avoidance of sun exposure, wear protective clothing and hats, use of tinted sunscreen (contains zinc oxide or titanium dioxide) with an SPF of 30 or higher
	• <u>Triple Topical Therapy</u>: **hydroquinone 2-4% + tretinoin 0.05-1% + low-potency corticosteroid** (fluocinolone acetonide 0.01%; triamcinolone 0.1%; hydrocortisone 1%)
	   • <u>Hydroquinone</u>: depigmentation by inhibiting the enzymatic oxidation of tyrosine(DOPA which inhibits melanocyte metabolic processes
	   • <u>Tretinoin</u>: promotes keratinocyte turnover exfoliates skin that contains epidermal pigment
	   • <u>Corticosteroid</u>: inhibits synthesis and secretion of melanin
	   • <u>Hydroquinone 3-4%</u>: may be used as monotherapy if triple topical therapy is not available
	• <u>Azelaic Acid 15 or 20%</u>: tyrosinase inhibitor that reduces melanin production that **may be used during pregnancy** (hydroquinone and tretinoin are unsafe during pregnancy)
	• Chemical peels (with glycolic acid or 30 to 50% trichloroacetic acid) or laser therapy indicated for severe or dermal melasma

Key Words & Most Common	• Hyperpigmentation of sun-exposed areas of the skin • Female, hormone change (pregnancy or OCP use), prolonged sun exposure are greatest risk factors • Symmetrically distributed hyperpigmented macules on sun-exposed areas (cheeks most common) • Sun protection • Hydroquinone + tretinoin + corticosteroids • Azelaic acid if pregnant

Pressure Injury

| | Decubitus Ulcer | |

Etiology & Risk Factors	• Areas of necrosis and ulceration where soft tissues are compressed between bony prominences and an external surfaces • Etiology: constant or prolonged pressure exerted on the skin • Risk Factors: **age (>65 years old most common)**, **decreased mobility** (prolonged hospital stay, **bedrest**, spinal cord injury, sedation, weakness, cognitive impairment), **exposure to irritants** (urinary or fecal incontinence), **impaired wound healing** (diabetes, malnutrition, venous insufficiency, peripheral artery disease), impaired sensation
Patho-physiology	• Compression of soft tissues causes microvascular occlusion resulting in tissue ischemia, hypoxia, and impairs delivery of nutrients • Friction and shear forces from clothing or bedding initiates skin ulceration by causing local erosion and disrupts the epidermis and superficial dermis protection • Moisture (perspiration, incontinence) results in tissue breakdown and maceration which exacerbates pressure injuries

Signs & Symptoms	• Most common on bony prominences (**sacrum**, ischial tuberosities, trochanters, malleoli, calcaneus)
	• **Stage I**: superficial skin involvement
	  • **Intact skin with nonblanchable erythema**
	  • Erythema does not dissipate after pressure is relieved
	• **Stage II**: partial-thickness skin involvement; **extends into the dermis**
	  • **Shallow loss of epidermis (erosion or blister) with a pink to red base** (no slough or necrotic tissue is present)
	  • May have ulceration (defect beyond the level of the epidermis)
	  • **Subcutaneous tissue is not exposed**
	• **Stage III**: full-thickness skin involvement; **extends into the subcutaneous layer**
	  • **Crater-like wound without underlying muscle or bone exposure**; may extend down to (but not include) the underlying fascia
	• **Stage IV**: full thickness skin involvement; **extends beyond the fascia into the muscle, tendon, or bone**
	  • Extensive destruction and tissue necrosis

Diagnosis	• **Clinical Diagnosis** • Bone Biopsy and Culture or MRI with Gadolinium Contrast: may be indicated to evaluate for osteomyelitis
Treatment	• **Pressure Reduction**: **frequent repositioning (every 2 hours) of the patient**, **protective devices** (pillows, foam wedges, heel protectors, soft seat cushions), support surfaces • **Friction Reduction**: application of barrier protectants (petroleum jelly) • **Urinary and Fecal Diversion**: frequent replacement of absorbent products; urinary catheter or rectal tube may be required in severe cases • **Cleaning**: pressure-wash irrigation with normal saline • **Debridement**: necessary to remove necrotic tissue; includes mechanical (pressure irrigation, wet-to-dry dressings, hydrotherapy), surgical, autolytic (synthetic occlusive [hydrocolloid] or semi-occlusive [transparent film] dressings), biosurgery (maggot therapy used for selective debridement of necrotic tissue as maggots only eat dead tissue) • **Dressings**: transparent film for stage I; hydrocolloids or hydrogels, alginates, polyurethane foam for stage II; copolymer starch or hydrogel for stage III-IV • Infection Control: topical antimicrobials (silver sulfadiazine, bacitracin, mupirocin etc.) used sparingly (impairs visualization of wound), oral or IV antibiotics may be required • **Nutritional Support**: oral, nasogastric, or parenteral supplementation indicated in patients with nutritional deficiency (albumin<3.5 g/dL or weight <80% of ideal) • Adjunctive Therapy: negative-pressure therapy (vacuum-assisted closure), topical recombinant growth factors, electrical stimulation therapy, therapeutic ultrasonography • **Surgery**: surgical closure indicated for large defects with exposure of musculoskeletal structures or skin grafts for large, shallow defects

Inhalation Injury

Etiology & Risk Factors	• Pulmonary exposure to smoke and/or the toxic products of combustion or chemicals leading to airway tissue injury and metabolic effects • Etiology: **exposure to direct heat or smoke, gases, vapors, or fumes** • Risk Factors: **exposure to direct heat** (fires or explosions, steam), **occupational exposures** (manufacturing, mining, chemical plants, construction, painting, or chemical cleaning processes), **exposure to structural collapse** (dust, smoke, or debris)
Patho-physiology	• Exposure to heat or toxic products causes damage to the airways (nasal passages, posterior oropharynx, larynx, trachea, bronchi) or parenchymal damage (alveoli) • Damage to airway tissue causes increased mucus production, edema, denudation of epithelium, and mucosal ulceration and hemorrhage leading to further airflow obstruction

Signs & Symptoms	• Burning sensation in nose or throat
	• **Productive cough**
	• **Dyspnea, wheezing, dysphagia, odynophagia**
	• Physical Exam:
	  • **Burns of the face and neck**, voice hoarseness, **loss of facial and intranasal hair, carbonaceous material or soot in the mouth or nose (black sputum)**
	  • Accessory muscle usage, **tachypnea**, cyanosis, **stridor**, and rhonchi/rales/**wheezing**

Diagnosis	• Chest Imaging: serial CXR (often negative early) or chest computed tomography (CT) scan • Pulse Oximetry: may be falsely elevated if carbon monoxide exposure • Labs: CBC, electrolytes, **arterial blood gas (ABG), carboxyhemoglobin level (evaluates for carbon monoxide poisoning)** • Cardiac Monitoring: electrocardiogram (ECG) and telemetry to monitor for arrhythmias • **Bronchoscopy and Direct Laryngoscopy**: visualizes upper airways and trachea to determine extent of edema, tissue damage, and soot in the airways
Treatment	• **Oxygen**: 100% oxygen provided by face mask initially for all patients • **Maintain Airway**: most important management; have low threshold for intubation or tracheostomy if necessary • **Intubation**: indicated for respiratory distress, altered mental status, full thickness burns to face/perioral region, circumferential neck burn, major burns (40-60% TBSA) • **Bronchodilators**: beta-2-adrenergic agonists (**albuterol** and salbutamol) indicated in bronchospasm or obstruction secondary to airway reactivity
Key Words & Most Common	• Pulmonary exposure to heat, smoke, gases, vapors or fumes • Productive cough, wheezing, dyspnea, dysphagia • Burns to face and neck, loss of nasal hair, soot in mouth/nose • Chest imaging + pulse oximetry + ABG + carboxyhemoglobin + ECG → bronchoscopy/direct laryngoscopy • Supplemental oxygen + maintain airway +/- bronchodilators

Burns

Etiology & Risk Factors	• Injuries of skin or other tissue caused by thermal, radiation, chemical, or electrical contact
	• Etiology: **thermal, radiation, chemical, or electrical contact**
	  • **Thermal**: contact with any external heat source (flame, hot liquid, hot solid object, or steam)
	  • **Radiation**: prolonged exposure to solar ultraviolet radiation (prolonged sun exposure, tanning bed)
	  • **Chemical**: strong acids (certain cleaning products), strong alkalis (lye, cement), phenols, phosphorus, and certain petroleum products (gasoline, paint thinner)
	  • **Electrical**: heat generation and electroporation of cell membranes associated with massive electron current
	    • **Electrical burns cause extensive deep tissue damage to electrically conductive tissues (muscles, nerves, blood vessels) with minimal cutaneous injury**
	• Risk Factors: age (children and elderly at higher risk due to mobility limitations), **certain occupations** (firefighters, industrial workers, chefs), **substance abuse, physical or cognitive disabilities**, low socioeconomic status (lack of safe cooking facilities or heating sources)

Patho-physiology	• Heat causes protein denaturation and coagulative necrosis resulting in poor vessel constriction and poorly perfused tissue which promotes bacterial invasion, external fluid loss, and impaired thermoregulation

Signs & Symptoms	• **Superficial (First-Degree)**: burn limited to the epidermis
	  • Erythematous, painful,, dry appearing skin that blanches markedly and **does not blister**
	• **Partial-Thickness (Second-Degree)**: burn involving part of the dermis and can be superficial (involving the superficial dermis) or deep (involving the deeper dermis)
	  • **Superficial**: erythematous, blistering, moist skin that blanches with pressure (intact capillary refill); is **very painful/tender**; bases of vesicles and bullae are pink
	  • **Deep**: erythematous, white, or mottled, blistering, dry skin that does not blanch (absent capillary refill); **less painful/tender; decreased 2-point discrimination**
	• **Full-Thickness (Third-Degree)**: burns extend through the entire dermis and into the underlying subcutaneous tissue
	  • **Waxy, white, brown-leathery or black-charred, dry skin that does not blister and doe not blanch** with pressure; usually **painless**

Burns

Diagnosis	• **Clinical Diagnosis** • **Burn Size Calculation: rule of 9's:** (adult) or Lund-Browder chart (children) are used to determine extent of burn • **Rule of 9's only counts second- and third-degree burns and excludes areas of first-degree burns in the calculation** • Workup: includes CBC (hemoglobin and hematocrit), CMP (electrolytes [hyperkalemia], kidney and liver function), albumin, phosphate, creatine kinase, ionized calcium, ECG, UA (myoglobin), CXR; consider carboxyhemoglobin and serum lactate (for carbon monoxide and cyanide poising in smoke inhalation patients)

Treatment	• Initial Care: **maintain airway**, address tetanus status, remove clothing and jewelry
	• **Cooling**: submerge/irrigate with room temperature or cool tap water or saline to prevent progression of burning and to reduce pain; hypothermia treated
	• **Cleaning**: mild soap and water or antimicrobial wash (chlorhexidine); large blisters are debrided, small blisters or blisters involving the palms/soles are left intact
	• **Comfort**: analgesia with opioids, NSAIDs, acetaminophen; splints may be applied to reduce tension and improve ergonomics
	• **Covering**: wound covered with layered dressing with topical antimicrobial or emollient, nonadherent gauze, dry gauze, and elastic bandage
	• **Topical Emollients**: petrolatum; indicated for superficial first-degree burns
	• **Topical Antimicrobials**: indicated for partial-thickness (second-degree) or full-thickness (third-degree) burns
	  • **Bacitracin Zinc, Polymyxin B Sulfate, Neomycin, or Mupirocin**: antibiotic indicated for **superficial** partial-thickness (second-degree) burns
	  • **Silver Sulfadiazine**: antimicrobial with anti-inflammatory properties indicated for **deep** partial-thickness (second-degree) burns or full-thickness (third-degree) burns
	    • *Silver sulfadiazine inhibits keratinocytes thus impeding epithelialization and therefore should be discontinued when epithelialization is seen*
	  • Mafenide acetate: carbonic anhydrase inhibitor; alternative to silver sulfadiazine
	• **Fluid Resuscitation**: IV fluids **(ringer's lactate is fluid of choice)** given to patients in shock or with partial and full thickness burns > 10% TBSA
	  • **Parkland Formula**: used to estimate fluid volume needs in first 24 hours and determines the rate of IV fluid administration
	    • **4mL/kg × % TBSA of burns (not including superficial burns)**
	    • **Half of fluid given over first 8 hours with remainder given over the next 16 hours**
	  • Maintain urine output at 0.5 mL/kg/hour in adults and 1.0 mL/kg/hour in children (< 30 kg)
	• **Nutritional Support**: indicated for patients with burns > 20% TBSA or preexisting undernutrition; support with feeding tube necessary if oral nutrition is not attainable
	• **Antibiotics:**
	  • Prophylactic systemic antibiotics are not recommended
	  • Empiric antibiotic treatment for infection during the first 5 days should target staphylococci and streptococci
	  • Empiric antibiotic treatment for infection after the first 5 days should target gram-positive and gram-negative bacteria
	• **Surgery: indicated for burns not expected to heal within 2 weeks** (most deep partial-thickness burns and all full-thickness burns)
	  • Escharotomy followed by skin grafting with partial-thickness autografts (the patient's skin) preferred; allografts (cadaver skin) or xenografts (porcine skin) if TBSA >40%
	• Physical and Occupational Therapy: indicated to minimize scarring and contractures especially of areas with high skin tension and frequent movement (face, hands)

Classification of Burns

Degree	Burn Thickness	Depth	Appearance	Sensation	Capillary Refill	Prognosis
First	Superficial	Epidermis	• Erythematous • Dry • **No blister formation**	**Painful**	**Intact** (blanches with pressure)	Heals without scarring in 5-10 days
Second	**Superficial Partial-Thickness**	Superficial dermis (papillary)	• Erythematous (red to pink) • Moist • **Blister formation**	**Painful** (most painful of all burns)	**Intact** (blanches with pressure)	Heals without scarring in 2-4 weeks
Second	**Deep Partial-Thickness**	Deep dermis (reticular)	• Erythematous (red, yellow, pale white) • Dry • **Blister formation**	**Mildly painful** Pain with pressure Decreased 2-point discrimination	**Absent**	Heals with scarring in 3-8 weeks
Third	**Full Thickness**	Subcutaneous structures	• Waxy, white, leathery • Dry	**Painless**	Absent	Heals by contracture in >8 weeks with scar formation
Fourth	**Full Thickness**	Subcutaneous structures, muscle, bone	• Black, charred • Dry • Eschar formation	**Painless**	Absent	Requires surgical debridement and tissue reconstruction

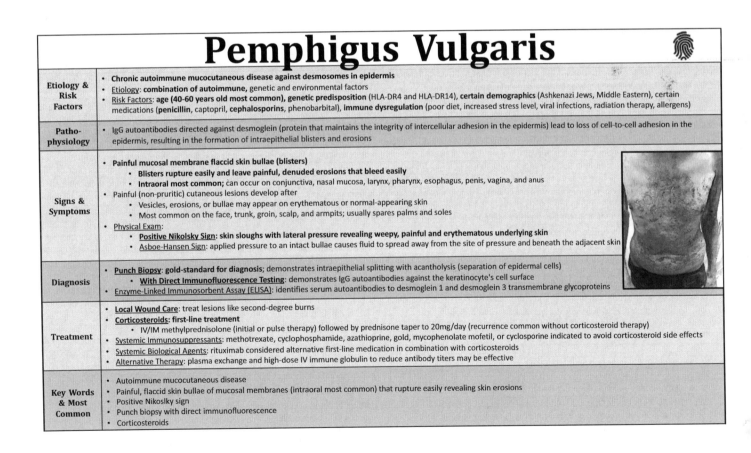

Head and Neck – 9%
- 4.5% anterior head/neck
- 4.5% posterior head/neck

Trunk
- 18% anterior trunk
- 18% posterior trunk

Genitalia = 1%
- 1% genitalia or perineum

Upper Limbs = 9% each limb
- 4.5% anterior left arm/hand
- 4.5% anterior right arm/hand
- 4.5% posterior left arm/hand
- 4.5% posterior right arm/hand

Lower Limbs = 18% each limb
- 9% anterior left leg/foot
- 9% anterior right leg/foot
- 9% posterior left leg/foot
- 9% posterior right leg/foot

Rule of 9's

Pemphigus Vulgaris

Etiology & Risk Factors	• **Chronic autoimmune mucocutaneous disease against desmosomes in epidermis** • Etiology: **combination of autoimmune,** genetic and environmental factors • Risk Factors: **age (40-60 years old most common), genetic predisposition** (HLA-DR4 and HLA-DR14), **certain demographics** (Ashkenazi Jews, Middle Eastern), certain medications (**penicillin,** captopril, **cephalosporins,** phenobarbital), **immune dysregulation** (poor diet, increased stress level, viral infections, radiation therapy, allergens)
Pathophysiology	• IgG autoantibodies directed against desmoglein (protein that maintains the integrity of intercellular adhesion in the epidermis) lead to loss of cell-to-cell adhesion in the epidermis, resulting in the formation of intraepithelial blisters and erosions

Signs & Symptoms	• **Painful mucosal membrane flaccid skin bullae (blisters)**
	  • **Blisters rupture easily and leave painful, denuded erosions that bleed easily**
	  • **Intraoral most common;** can occur on conjunctiva, nasal mucosa, larynx, pharynx, esophagus, penis, vagina, and anus
	• Painful (non-pruritic) cutaneous lesions develop after
	  • Vesicles, erosions, or bullae may appear on erythematous or normal-appearing skin
	  • Most common on the face, trunk, groin, scalp, and armpits; usually spares palms and soles
	• Physical Exam:
	  • **Positive Nikolsky Sign: skin sloughs with lateral pressure revealing weepy, painful and erythematous underlying skin**
	  • Asboe-Hansen Sign: applied pressure to an intact bullae causes fluid to spread away from the site of pressure and beneath the adjacent skin

Diagnosis	• **Punch Biopsy: gold-standard for diagnosis;** demonstrates intraepithelial splitting with acantholysis (separation of epidermal cells) • **With Direct Immunofluorescence Testing:** demonstrates IgG autoantibodies against the keratinocyte's cell surface • Enzyme-Linked Immunosorbent Assay (ELISA): identifies serum autoantibodies to desmoglein 1 and desmoglein 3 transmembrane glycoproteins
Treatment	• **Local Wound Care:** treat lesions like second-degree burns • **Corticosteroids: first-line treatment** • IV/IM methylprednisolone (initial or pulse therapy) followed by prednisone taper to 20mg/day (recurrence common without corticosteroid therapy) • Systemic Immunosuppressants: methotrexate, cyclophosphamide, azathioprine, gold, mycophenolate mofetil, or cyclosporine indicated to avoid corticosteroid side effects • Systemic Biological Agents: rituximab considered alternative first-line medication in combination with corticosteroids • Alternative Therapy: plasma exchange and high-dose IV immune globulin to reduce antibody titers may be effective
Key Words & Most Common	• Autoimmune mucocutaneous disease • Painful, flaccid skin bullae of mucosal membranes (intraoral most common) that rupture easily revealing skin erosions • Positive Nikoslky sign • Punch biopsy with direct immunofluorescence • Corticosteroids

Bullous Pemphigoid

Etiology & Risk Factors	• Chronic, autoimmune, subepidermal skin disorder resulting in generalized, bullous lesions in elderly patients • <u>Etiology</u>: combination of **autoimmune**, genetic and environmental factors • <u>Risk Factors</u>: **elderly age (60-80 years old most common)**, comorbid autoimmune condition, certain medications (diuretics [furosemide], antibiotics [penicillins, cephalosporins], and anti-inflammatories [NSAIDs, sulfasalazine]), **certain disorders** (Parkinson disease, diabetes, rheumatoid arthritis, ulcerative colitis, **multiple sclerosis**)
Patho-physiology	• Autoantibodies against specific skin components (particularly hemidesmosomal proteins) arranged at the dermal-epidermal junction leading to an inflammatory response • Immune cell recruitment and inflammatory mediator release result in separation of the epidermis and underlying dermis resulting in **subepidermal blistering**

Signs & Symptoms	• Prodrome of moderate-to-severe pruritus with or without urticarial popular lesions
	• Large (1-4cm), tense bullae develop over subsequent weeks to months
	  • Typically contain clear fluid and persist for several days before leaving erosions and crusts
	  • Most common on the axilla, flexor surface of the forearms, groin, trunk, and abdomen
	• <u>Physical Exam</u>:
	  • **Negative Nikolsky Sign: no skin sloughing with lateral pressure**

Diagnosis	• <u>Biopsy</u>: **gold-standard for diagnosis**; demonstrates subepidermal split with a superficial perivascular inflammatory infiltrate and numerous eosinophils • <u>With Direct Immunofluorescence Testing</u>: deposition of C3 and IgG in a linear homogeneous pattern at the basement membrane zone • <u>Enzyme-Linked Immunosorbent Assay (ELISA)</u>: identifies autoantibodies against BP180 and BP230

Treatment	• <u>Antihistamines</u>: diphenhydramine; indicated for pruritus
	• <u>Topical Corticosteroids</u>: clobetasol indicated in localized disease (<20% TBSA involvement in an elderly patient)
	  • May be combined with nicotinamide plus tetracycline, minocycline, or doxycycline for increased effectiveness
	• <u>Systemic Corticosteroids</u>: **mainstay of treatment**
	  • Oral prednisone tapered over weeks to months
	• <u>Systemic Immunosuppressants</u>: methotrexate, cyclophosphamide, azathioprine, gold, mycophenolate mofetil, or cyclosporine indicated to avoid corticosteroid side effects

Key Words & Most Common	• Chronic, autoimmune skin disorder resulting in bullous lesions in elderly • Prodrome of pruritus followed by tense bullae development • Negative Nikoslky sign • Biopsy with direct immunofluorescence testing is gold-standard • Antihistamines + topical corticosteroids → systemic corticosteroids

Acanthosis Nigricans

Etiology & Risk Factors	• Hyperpigmented cutaneous manifestation of an underlying condition
	• <u>Etiology</u>:
	  • <u>Insulin Resistance</u>: **most common cause**; diabetes mellitus, obesity, metabolic syndrome
	  • <u>Hormone Disorders</u>: **polycystic ovarian syndrome (PCOS)**, acromegaly, hypothyroidism
	  • <u>Certain Medications</u>: **oral contraceptives**, corticosteroids, nicotinic acid, estrogen, growth hormone therapy and certain antiretrovirals
	  • <u>Family History</u>: genetic predisposition
	  • <u>Malignancy</u>: gastrointestinal adenocarcinoma and genitourinary cancers such as prostate, breast, and ovary

Patho-physiology	• Insulin resistance results in increased circulating insulin that activates insulin-like growth factor-1 (IGF-1) receptors leading to keratocyte and melanocyte proliferation in the epidermis which results in characteristic hyperpigmented skin lesions
Signs & Symptoms	• **Asymptomatic darkening and thickening of the skin** • **Poorly defined, velvety, hyperpigmented macules and patches and progress to palpable plaques** • **Most common on skin folds (posterior neck**, forehead, groin, navel, axillae)
Diagnosis	• Clinical Diagnosis • <u>Biopsy</u>: confirms diagnosis; hyperkeratosis, leukocyte infiltration, epidermal folding, and melanocyte proliferation may be seen • <u>Labs</u>: lab testing to determine underlying etiology (hemoglobin A1c, fasting glucose, fasting insulin, glucose tolerance test etc.)

Treatment	• <u>Lifestyle Modification</u>: weight reduction, exercise, proper diet
	• <u>Treat Underlying Etiology</u>: blood glucose management, discontinue offending medication, lipid lowering medications (niacin, statin therapy)
	• <u>Keratolytics</u>:
	  • <u>Topical Retinoids</u>: **tretinoin** promotes epidermal cell turnover and exfoliation (reduces hyperkeratosis and hyperpigmentation)
	  • <u>Topical Vitamin D Analogs</u>: **calcipotriol (calcipotriene)** decrease keratinocyte proliferation

Key Words & Most Common	• Insulin resistance (diabetes, obesity, metabolic syndrome) or PCOS most common causes • Asymptomatic darkening and thickening of skin • Velvety, hyperpigmented macules on skin folds (posterior neck most common) • Lifestyle modification + treat underlying etiology

Hidradenitis Suppurativa

Acne Inversus

Etiology & Risk Factors	• Chronic inflammatory skin condition of intertriginous areas and other apocrine gland rich areas • <u>Etiology</u>: **chronic inflammation** as a result of multiple genetic, environmental, hormonal and behavioral influences • <u>Risk Factors</u>: **age (most common after puberty), female, obesity**, smoking, poor diet, fluctuations in hormone levels (menstruation, PCOS), history of acne, comorbid autoimmune conditions, environmental factors (stress, excessive heat, perspiration)
Patho-physiology	• Defective hair follicle becomes occluded and ruptures resulting in release of keratin and bacteria into the surrounding dermis resulting in inflammation and formation of abscesses, sinus tracts and scarring
Signs & Symptoms	• **Deep-seated, inflamed, painful nodules, sinus tracts, abscesses, and fibrotic hypertrophic scarring** • **Most commonly affects intertriginous areas and other apocrine gland rich areas (axillary most common**, groin, perianal, perineal, and inframammary locations)

Diagnosis	• **Clinical Diagnosis**
	• <u>Hurley Staging System</u>: utilized to further classify the case to guide treatment
	   • Hurley Stage I: abscess formation without tracts or scars
	   • Hurley Stage II: recurrent abscesses with sinus tracts and scarring; may be single or separate lesions
	   • Hurley Stage III: diffuse involvement with multiple interconnected sinus tracts, and abscesses across an entire area

Treatment	• <u>Lifestyle Modification</u>: proper diet (avoidance of high glycemic foods), **smoking cessation, weight reduction**, local skin hygiene (antiperspirants, benzoyl peroxide wash), avoid tight-fitting and synthetic clothing (polyester) • <u>**Topical Clindamycin 1%**</u>: **first-line treatment** • <u>**Oral Antibiotics**</u>: **tetracycline, doxycycline**, minocycline, erythromycin; clindamycin + rifampin in severe cases • <u>**Intralesional Corticosteroid Injection**</u>: triamcinolone acetonide injected once per month to decrease local inflammation • <u>Antiandrogen Therapy</u>: oral estrogen or combination oral contraceptives, spironolactone, finasteride, or combinations may be indicated in severe recurrent cases in females • <u>Debridement</u>: punch Debridement (excision with a punch instrument followed by digital debridement and curettage or scrubbing) indicated for small lesions, sinus tracts should be unroofed and debrided • <u>Incision and Drainage</u>: indicated for large, painful abscesses • <u>Surgery</u>: wide excision of the lesions, tracts, and scars of the entire affected area indicated for severe and recurrent cases
Key Words & Most Common	• Chronic inflammatory skin condition most commonly affecting axilla • Post-puberty, female, obesity most common risk factors • Deep, painful, inflamed nodules that progress to sinus tract development and scarring • Lifestyle modifications → topical clindamycin + oral antibiotics

Lipoma

Etiology & Risk Factors	• **Benign subcutaneous tumors composed of adipocytes (fat cells)** • <u>Etiology</u>: **mature adipose tissue** • <u>Risk Factors</u>: age (40-60 years old most common), male, family history, certain metabolic disorders (familial multiple lipomatosis and Gardner syndrome)
Patho-physiology	• Not fully understood, may involve genetic mutations that cause alterations in the genes responsible for adipocyte proliferation, accumulation, growth and differentiation • The growth of lipomas is typically slow, and they are encapsulated, non-invasive, and do not spread to surrounding tissues.

Signs & Symptoms	• **Soft, solitary, painless, subcutaneous nodules**
	   • Range in size from 1-10+ cm
	   • **Easily mobile**
	   • Not associated with epidermal change
	• **Most common on the trunk, neck, forearms, and proximal extremities**

Diagnosis	• **Clinical Diagnosis** • <u>Biopsy</u>: indicated for pain, rapid enlargement, fixation to underlying tissues, or location in deep tissues, the thigh, or retroperitoneal space
Treatment	• <u>**Observation**</u>: **no treatment required as tumor is benign** • <u>**Surgical Excision**</u>: indicated for cosmetic reasons or if rapidly enlarging tumor; complete surgical excision of the capsule is recommended to prevent recurrence
Key Words & Most Common	• Benign subcutaneous tumor composed of adipocytes • Soft, painless, subcutaneous nodule that is easily mobile • Most common on trunk, neck, forearms, proximal extremities • Observation • Surgical excision to preserve cosmesis

Epidermoid Cysts

Etiology & Risk Factors	• **Benign, encapsulated, subepidermal nodules filled with fibrous and keratin material** • Sebaceous cysts is a misnomer because epidermoid cysts do not originate from sebaceous glands • <u>Etiology</u>: **sporadic accumulation of keratin** • <u>Risk Factors</u>: **age (20-40 years old most common), male**, family history, **trauma to skin** (cuts, punctures, surgical incisions), hormonal changes (puberty, pregnancy, menopause)
Patho-physiology	• Epidermoid cysts are lined with stratified squamous epithelium that leads to an accumulation of keratin within the subepidermal layer or dermis leading to plugging of the follicular orifice

Signs & Symptoms	• Most common on the face, neck, chest, upper back, scrotum, and genitals
	• **Flesh-colored, non-fluctuant, compressible cyst or nodule**
	   • **Central punctum (dark comedone)**
	• **Ruptured cysts will have tenderness to palpation, erythema, and swelling**
	   • **Foul-smelling yellowish cheese-like material discharged**

Diagnosis	• **Clinical Diagnosis** • <u>Biopsy</u>: rarely performed; demonstrates epithelial-lined cyst filled with laminated keratin located within the dermis
Treatment	• <u>Observation</u>: no treatment required as may spontaneously resolve • <u>Surgical Excision</u>: **complete excision of the cyst with the cyst wall intact is most effective treatment**; indicated for cosmetic reasons or if recurrent
Key Words & Most Common	• Encapsulated, subepidermal nodules filled with fibrous/keratin material • Flesh-colored, compressible cyst or nodule with central punctum • Ruptured cyst will be painful, red, and swollen • Foul-smelling yellowish cheese-like material discharged • Observation → surgical excision

Pyoderma Gangrenosum

Etiology & Risk Factors	• **Chronic, progressive, neutrophilic, ulcerative skin condition**; *not infectious nor gangrenous as the name implies* • <u>Etiology</u>: **unknown**; may be mediated by an abnormal immune response • <u>Risk Factors</u>: **age (25-55 years old most common), certain inflammatory disorders (inflammatory bowel disease [Crohn disease, ulcerative colitis], rheumatoid arthritis,** solid tumors or hematologic malignancies), trauma, family history, certain medications (oral contraceptives, antibiotics [especially sulfonamides], anti-inflammatories)
Patho-physiology	• Not fully understood; may involve genetic mutations, neutrophil dysfunction, and immune/inflammatory dysregulation • Abnormal immune response causes in an exaggerated inflammatory reaction in the skin and soft tissues, leads to destruction of the skin and surrounding tissue and results in the characteristic ulcers and necrosis
Signs & Symptoms	• **Inflamed erythematous papule, pustule, or nodule initially** (may resemble furuncle or insect bite) • **Progresses to painful, necrotic ulcer with a swollen base and a raised, dusky to violaceous border** • May have **undermined borders** (loss of underlying support tissue at the border) • **Most common on the lower extremities or trunk** (especially buttocks and perineum) • May have fever and malaise • Lesions may heal with a **cribriform scar** • May have an exaggerated response to a minor skin injury (pathergy)
Diagnosis	• **Clinical Diagnosis of exclusion** • <u>Biopsy</u>: utilized to rule out other ulcerative skin lesions; demonstrates neutrophil infiltration of the dermis and may have necrotic dermal vessels

Treatment	• <u>Treat Underlying Systemic Disease</u>: management of underlying disorder may slow progression and manage symptoms
	• <u>**Wound Care**</u>: daily wound cleansing and application of occlusive dressings for less exudative lesions and absorptive dressings for highly exudative lesions
	   • Debridement must be performed carefully due to risk of pathergy
	• <u>**Topical High-Potency Corticosteroids**</u>: clobetasol, fluocinolone; indicated for superficial and early lesions
	• <u>Topical Calcineurin Inhibitors</u>: tacrolimus; indicated for superficial and early lesions
	• <u>**Oral Corticosteroids**</u>: **prednisone (60-80mg per day) is first-line for severe manifestations or rapid, deep or refractory cases**
	• <u>Immunosuppressive Therapy</u>:
	   • <u>Oral Calcineurin Inhibitors</u>: **cyclosporine** indicated for rapidly progressive disease
	   • <u>TNF-Alpha Inhibitors</u>: infliximab, adalimumab, etanercept are effective in patients with concomitant inflammatory bowel disease
	• <u>Other</u>: canakinumab (IL-1 beta monoclonal antibody) and tocilizumab (anti-IL-6 monoclonal antibody)

Key Words & Most Common	• Chronic, progressive, ulcerative skin condition of unknown origin • Associated with inflammatory disorders (inflammatory bowel disease most common) • Inflamed, erythematous papule or pustule → painful, necrotic ulcer with raised, purple/violet border • Clinical diagnosis of exclusion • Treat underlying disease + wound care → topical vs oral corticosteroids → immunosuppressive therapy

Keloids

Etiology & Risk Factors	• **Benign overgrowth of fibroblastic tissue arising from an injury site** • <u>Etiology</u>: **scarring secondary to skin trauma** (surgery, piercings, acne, tattooing, insect bites, burns, lacerations, abrasions, vaccinations) • <u>Risk Factors</u>: **darker-skinned individuals** (African, Asian, Hispanic descent), **age** (10 and 30 years old most common), **female**, **hormonal influences** (puberty, pregnancy, hormonal therapy)
Patho-physiology	• Prolonged fibroblastic phase of wound healing leads to overproduction of collagen and cytokines • Collagen synthesis in keloids is 20x greater than that of healthy skin and 3x greater than a standard hypertrophic scar

Signs & Symptoms	• **Firm, rubbery nodules that project above the underlying skin**
	  • **Erythematous, flesh-colored, or hyperpigmented**
	  • **May grow pedunculate** or broadly into a plaque
	  • May have associated **pruritus**, pain, or burning
	• Lesions develop 1-3 months after skin trauma (may occur up to a year later)
	• Most commonly occurs on the upper body (deltoid, pre-sternal chest, upper back, face and earlobes)

Diagnosis	• Clinical Diagnosis
Treatment	• <u>**Intralesional Corticosteroid Injections**</u>: **first-line treatment**; triamcinolone acetonide injections once per month suppress inflammation and reduce collagen synthesis • <u>**Cryotherapy**</u>: **second-line treatment**; freeze-thaw cycles of 10-20 seconds to achieve scar tissue necrosis • <u>**Laser Therapy**</u>: **second-line treatment**; utilized to induce flattening and regression of keloids • Other: topical imiquimod, intralesional Botox, intralesional bleomycin, intralesional 5-fluorouracil, silicone gel sheet application
Key Words & Most Common	• Benign overgrowth of fibroblastic tissue secondary to skin trauma • Most common in darker-skinned individuals • Flesh-colored, firm, rubbery nodules projecting above injury site • Intralesional corticosteroid injections → laser therapy or cryotherapy

Dermatitis Herpetiformis

Etiology & Risk Factors	• **Chronic, pruritic, autoimmune skin disorder** • <u>Etiology</u>: **immune system reaction to gluten** • <u>Risk Factors</u>: **history of Celiac disease (gluten sensitive enteropathy) is greatest risk factor**, age (young adults most common), male, family history, ethnicity (northern European descent)
Patho-physiology	• IgA dominant autoimmune response to transglutaminase molecules results in IgA immune complex deposition in the dermal papillary that attracts neutrophils and produces an inflammatory reaction
Signs & Symptoms	• **Intensely pruritic, erythematous, grouped papules and vesicles** • Vesicles often rupture quickly secondary to itching (pruritus) • **Most common on extensor surfaces of the elbows, forearms, knees, buttocks, sacrum and occiput** • May have symptoms associated with gluten sensitive enteropathy (bloating, diarrhea and other gastrointestinal complaints)
Diagnosis	• **Clinical Diagnosis** • <u>**Serologic Testing for Celiac Disease**</u>: IgA anti-tissue transglutaminase antibody, IgA anti-epidermal transglutaminase antibody, and IgA anti-endomysial antibody • <u>**Biopsy and Direct Immunofluorescence**</u>: **definitive diagnosis**; demonstrates granular IgA deposition in the dermal papillary tips
Treatment	• <u>**Dapsone**</u>: **first-line treatment for acute phase; dramatically relieves symptoms** • <u>**Sulfonamides**</u>: sulfapyridine and sulfasalazine are alternatives for patients are unable to tolerate dapsone • <u>**Gluten-Free Diet**</u>: **mainstay of long-term management**
Key Words & Most Common	• Chronic, autoimmune skin disorder associated with Celiac disease • Intensely pruritic, erythematous papules and vesicles on the extensor surfaces (elbows, forearms, knees) • Clinical diagnosis + serologic testing for celiac disease → biopsy and direct immunofluorescence • Dapsone for acute phase treatment • Gluten-free diet for long-term management

Pyogenic Granuloma

Lobular capillary hemangioma	

Etiology & Risk Factors	• Benign vascular tumor that arises in tissue of the skin and/or mucous membranes • <u>Etiology</u>: not fully understood • <u>Risk Factors</u>: **age (most common in young adults), female, history of trauma, hormonal influences (increased incidence in pregnancy)**, certain medications (retinoids, antivirals [indinavir], chemotherapy/immunosuppressives)
Patho-physiology	• Injury or irritation triggers an exaggerated, inflammatory response leading to release of growth factors and cytokines which promotes small blood vessel formation (angiogenesis) and proliferation of fibroblasts and inflammatory cells which accumulate in the tissue

Signs & Symptoms	• **Small, solitary, red nodule or papule**
	  • **Friable and bleeds easily**
	  • Does not blanch with pressure
	  • **Base of the lesion may be pedunculated** and surrounded by a collarette of epidermis
	• Most common on arms, hands, fingers, back and legs **(higher incidence of oral mucosal or gingival involvement in pregnancy)**
	• May rapidly grow over weeks to months before stabilizing in size

Diagnosis	• **Clinical Diagnosis** • <u>Biopsy</u>: confirms diagnosis and rules out malignancy; demonstrates highly vascular granulation tissue with proliferation of capillary vessels within a loose fibrous stroma
Treatment	• <u>**Complete Surgical Excision:** preferred treatment</u> indicated for lesions on non-cosmetic areas; lower rates of recurrence • <u>**Shave Excision or Curettage followed by Electrocautery:** indicated for lesions on cosmetic areas</u> • <u>Non-Surgical Modalities</u>: cryotherapy, electrocautery or chemical cautery with silver nitrate, laser therapy • <u>Intralesional Injections</u>: corticosteroids or sclerosants (ethanolamine oleate, sodium tetradecyl sulfate, polidocanol) may have some efficacy • <u>Topical Therapy</u>: generally ineffective
Key Words & Most Common	• Benign vascular tumor • Small, solitary red nodule that is friable and bleeds easily • Base may be pedunculated • Complete surgical excision is preferred treatment for non-cosmetic areas • Shave excision or curettage followed by electrocautery for cosmetic areas

Erythema Nodosum

Etiology & Risk Factors	• **Acute, nodular septal panniculitis** (inflammation of adipose layer below the skin)
	• <u>Etiology</u>: not fully understood; may be related to an immunologic reaction as associated with other infectious or inflammatory disorders
	• <u>Risk Factors</u>: age (20-40 years old most common), female, history of infection, medication use, inflammatory disorder or exposure to estrogen
	  • <u>Infection</u>: **bacterial (Streptococcal infection is most common**, Yersinia, Salmonella, Mycoplasma, **Tuberculosis)**, viral (**EBV**, hepatitis B), fungal (**Coccidioidomycosis)**
	  • <u>Medications</u>: sulfonamides, penicillins, iodides, bromides, **oral contraceptives**
	  • <u>Inflammatory Disorders</u>: **inflammatory bowel disease** (Crohns disease, ulcerative colitis), **sarcoidosis**
	  • <u>Estrogen Exposure</u>: **oral contraceptives**, pregnancy

Patho-physiology	• Delayed type IV hypersensitivity reaction to an antigen that leads to inflammation of the subcutaneous fat tissue and infiltration of neutrophils into the affected areas

Signs & Symptoms	• **Prodrome of nonspecific fever, malaise, arthralgia** for 3-6 days
	• **Sudden onset of erythematous, tender, firm, subcutaneous nodules or plaques**
	  • **Most common in the pretibial region** (extensor surfaces of the legs) and usually bilateral; may occur on other parts of the body
	  • May evolve into bruise-like areas over several weeks

Diagnosis	• **Clinical Diagnosis** • *Consider testing to determine underlying etiology*
Treatment	• <u>**Supportive:** lesions are generally self-limited and resolve spontaneously within several weeks</u> • Bed rest or work restrictions, elevation, cool compresses, and analgesia (NSAIDs) • <u>Treat Underlying Etiology</u>: if identified • <u>Systemic Corticosteroids</u>: indicated if persistent condition and underlying etiology is not due to infection
Key Words & Most Common	• Nodular panniculitis (inflammation of fat layer) • May be related to infection, medication use, IBD, sarcoidosis, oral contraceptives, pregnancy • Prodrome of nonspecific fever, malaise, arthralgia → sudden onset of red/pink, tender, firm, subcutaneous nodule in the pretibial region • Supportive treatment + treat underlying etiology

Cherry Hemangioma

Etiology & Risk Factors	• Acquired vascular proliferation of the skin • Etiology: abnormal mature capillary proliferation • Risk Factors: age (middle-aged adults and elderly most common), family history (mutations in *GNAQ* and *GNA11* genes), hormonal factors, UV exposure
Patho-physiology	• Abnormal proliferation and dilation of small blood vessels close to the skin's surface
Signs & Symptoms	• Small (1-5mm), well-demarcated, dome-shaped, bright red papules with a pale halo • Usually multiple lesions • Most common on the trunk or proximal extremities
Diagnosis	• Clinical Diagnosis

Treatment	• Supportive: asymptomatic condition that generally requires no treatment
	• Removal of Lesion: indicated for cosmetically unappealing lesions or lesions subject to bleeding
	   • Electrocautery: indicated for small lesions
	   • Shave Excision with Electrocauterization of the Base: indicated for larger lesions
	   • Cryotherapy: indicated for larger lesions
	   • CO_2 Laser Therapy: indicated for superficial lesions

Key Words & Most Common	• Acquired mature capillary proliferation most common in elderly • Small, dome-shaped, bright red papule • Most common on trunk or proximal extremities • No treatment necessary if asymptomatic • Excision if cosmetically unappealing or bleeding

Lacerations

Etiology & Risk Factors	• Tears in soft tissue of the body • Etiology: trauma (accidents, falls, sharp objects, blunt force), surgical procedures, animal bites, self-inflicted injuries • Risk Factors: age (more common in young adults), occupation (construction workers, firefighters, workplaces with sharp objects, machinery), high-impact activity (football, hockey, martial arts, biking), substance abuse, chronic medical conditions
Patho-physiology	• Inflammatory Phase: activation of platelets and formation of a blood clot in response to bleeding; inflammatory cells (neutrophiles and macrophages) migrate to injury site to clear debris and prevent infection • Proliferative Phase: migration and proliferation of fibroblasts which produce collagen and other extracellular matrix components allow new blood vessels to form which supply oxygen and nutrients to healing tissue • Remodeling Phase: newly formed collagen fibers reorganize and align along lines of tension to provide strength and stability to the healing wound
Signs & Symptoms	• Visible break or tear in the skin • Localized pain, swelling, bleeding • May have impaired sensation
Diagnosis	• Clinical Diagnosis • *Must assess neurovascular function and sensation and evaluate for contamination of the wound or foreign bodies present*

Treatment	• Wound Preparation:
	   • Debridement: most important step to decrease risk of infection; high pressure irrigation with sterile saline or tap water; *avoid betadine/chlorhexadine in wound*
	   • Hemostasis: holding direct pressure, chemical cautery (silver nitrate), electrocautery, tourniquets methods may be used to control bleeding
	   • Exploration: remove any debris, foreign bodies, or hair (may use topical antibiotic ointment or petroleum jelly to smooth hair out of field), assess neurovascular status, assess for tendon injury
	• Anesthesia: may be topical or injected
	   • Topical: preparations with lidocaine or prilocaine or combination; onset is 20-30 minutes to 2 hours
	   • Injected: lidocaine 1-2% with or without epinephrine is most common (*avoid epinephrine preparations for lacerations of fingers, toes, genitalia, nose or ears*)
	      • Consider nerve blocks to avoid tissue distortion for cosmetic areas such as vermillion border; digital block for finger lacerations
	• Suturing: techniques vary based on wound size and location
	   • Simple Interrupted: allows to alignment adjustment and carries less potential for wound edema or impaired circulation
	   • Running Subcuticular: useful for long, linear wounds but carries risk of dehiscence if suture is disrupted
	   • Horizontal Mattress: useful for high-tension wounds as suture spreads tension over larger area
	   • Vertical Mattress: useful for wound eversion to close both superficial and deep layers when deep sutures are contraindicated or unable to be performed
	• Steri-Strips and Skin Glue: indicated for superficial lacerations on low-tension areas that are well approximated
	• Aftercare:
	   • Antibiotics: indicated for contaminated wounds, animal bites, neglected wounds, immunocompromised, retained foreign body, decreased perfusion
	   • Wound Care: keep area clean and covered, antibiotic ointment generally not indicated; topical vitamin E cream and avoidance of sun exposure to reduce scarring

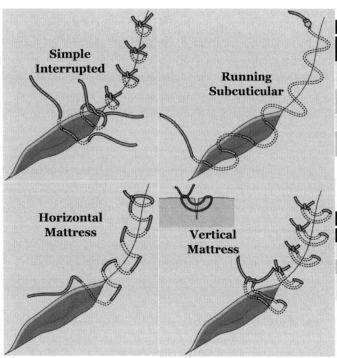

Simple Interrupted

Running Subcuticular

Horizontal Mattress

Vertical Mattress

Absorbable Sutures			
Suture Type	Days of Tensile Strength	Complete Absorption	Description
Chromic Gut	7-21 days	90 days	Chromium treated to decrease tissue reactivity
PDS (Polydioxone)	14 days	180-240 days	Monofilament synthetic absorbable suture
Vicryl	21 days	90 days	Synthetic
Vicryl Rapid	10 days	42 days	Synthetic with radiation treatment for increased absorption

Favor absorbable sutures for lacerations on the face (especially children), lip, mucosa, or genitals

Non-Absorbable Sutures			
Suture Type	Tensile Strength	Body Reactivity	Description
Nylon	High	Low	Monofilament
Silk	Low	High	Multifilament
Prolene (Polypropylene)	Moderate	Low	Monofilament

Favor non-absorbable sutures for lacerations of the body, extremities, or scalp (staples)

References

1. File:Acne vulgaris on a very oily skin.jpg. (2023, February 14). *Wikimedia Commons*. Retrieved 14:02, April 28, 2023 from https://commons.wikimedia.org/w/index.php?title=File:Acne_vulgaris_on_a_very_oily_skin.jpg&oldid=732416775.
2. File:Rosacea.jpg. (2022, June 27). *Wikimedia Commons*. Retrieved 14:00, April 28, 2023 from https://commons.wikimedia.org/w/index.php?title=File:Rosacea.jpg&oldid=668920223.
3. File:Folliculitis2.jpg. (2021, January 15). *Wikimedia Commons*. Retrieved 13:54, April 28, 2023 from https://commons.wikimedia.org/w/index.php?title=File:Folliculitis2.jpg&oldid=525999721.
4. File:Erythema Multiforme EM 01 ajustement niveaux auto.jpg. (2020, October 28). *Wikimedia Commons*. Retrieved 13:50, April 28, 2023 from https://commons.wikimedia.org/w/index.php?title=File:Erythema_Multiforme_EM_01_ajustement_niveaux_auto.jpg&oldid=505433520.
5. File:Stevens-johnson-syndrome.jpg. (2021, July 2). *Wikimedia Commons*. Retrieved 17:00, May 1, 2023 from https://commons.wikimedia.org/w/index.php?title=File:Stevens-johnson-syndrome.jpg&oldid=572862575.
6. File:Alopecia areata 1.jpg. (2020, September 27). *Wikimedia Commons*. Retrieved 17:01, May 1, 2023 from https://commons.wikimedia.org/w/index.php?title=File:Alopecia_areata_1.jpg&oldid=473586251.
7. File:Alopecia.jpg. (2022, November 8). *Wikimedia Commons*. Retrieved 17:53, May 1, 2023 from https://commons.wikimedia.org/w/index.php?title=File:Alopecia.jpg&oldid=703773361.
8. File:Onychomycosis due to Trichophyton rubrum, right and left great toe PHIL 579 lores.jpg. (2022, August 16). *Wikimedia Commons*. Retrieved 19:43, May 1, 2023 from https://commons.wikimedia.org/w/index.php?title=File:Onychomycosis_due_to_Trichophyton_rubrum,_right_and_left_great_toe_PHIL_579_lores.jpg&oldid=682794542.
9. File:Right index finger paronychia cellulitis.jpg. (2023, February 10). *Wikimedia Commons*. Retrieved 20:50, May 1, 2023 from https://commons.wikimedia.org/w/index.php?title=File:Right_index_finger_paronychia_cellulitis.jpg&oldid=731519969.
10. File:Toe (5).JPG. (2020, September 13). *Wikimedia Commons*. Retrieved 23:22, May 1, 2023 from https://commons.wikimedia.org/w/index.php?title=File:Toe_(5).JPG&oldid=458323598.
11. "My Brown Recluse bite in 07" by K2sleddogs is licensed under CC BY-SA 2.0.
12. File:SWS Bite.JPG. (2021, September 13). *Wikimedia Commons*. Retrieved 15:55, May 3, 2023 from https://commons.wikimedia.org/w/index.php?title=File:SWS_Bite.JPG&oldid=590884928.
13. File:Wasp bite (366189894).jpg. (2022, January 28). *Wikimedia Commons*. Retrieved 16:33, May 3, 2023 from https://commons.wikimedia.org/w/index.php?title=File:Wasp_bite_(366189894).jpg&oldid=625333787.
14. File:Slapped cheek Erythema Infectiosum.png. (2022, March 16). *Wikimedia Commons*. Retrieved 18:04, May 3, 2023 from https://commons.wikimedia.org/w/index.php?title=File:Slapped_cheek_Erythema_Infectiosum.png&oldid=639366013.
15. File:Morbillivirus measles infection.jpg. (2022, May 14). *Wikimedia Commons*. Retrieved 20:12, May 3, 2023 from https://commons.wikimedia.org/w/index.php?title=File:Morbillivirus_measles_infection.jpg&oldid=656039846.
16. File:Koplik spots, measles 6111 lores.jpg. (2020, November 1). *Wikimedia Commons*. Retrieved 20:12, May 3, 2023 from https://commons.wikimedia.org/w/index.php?title=File:Koplik_spots,_measles_6111_lores.jpg&oldid=508858717.
17. File:Hand Foot Mouth Disease.png. (2020, October 3). *Wikimedia Commons*. Retrieved 22:07, May 3, 2023 from https://commons.wikimedia.org/w/index.php?title=File:Hand_Foot_Mouth_Disease.png&oldid=479750247.
18. File:Hand foot and mouth disease on child feet.jpg. (2020, September 5). *Wikimedia Commons*. Retrieved 22:08, May 3, 2023 from https://commons.wikimedia.org/w/index.php?title=File:Hand_foot_and_mouth_disease_on_child_feet.jpg&oldid=448668064.
19. File:Herpangina2016.jpg. (2022, July 5). *Wikimedia Commons*. Retrieved 22:48, May 3, 2023 from https://commons.wikimedia.org/w/index.php?title=File:Herpangina2016.jpg&oldid=671557273.
20. File:Cellulitis leg (44699140442).jpg. (2023, April 22). *Wikimedia Commons*. Retrieved 13:56, May 4, 2023 from https://commons.wikimedia.org/w/index.php?title=File:Cellulitis_leg_(44699140442).jpg&oldid=753306667.
21. File:Facial erysipelas.jpg. (2020, October 6). *Wikimedia Commons*. Retrieved 18:10, May 4, 2023 from https://commons.wikimedia.org/w/index.php?title=File:Facial_erysipelas.jpg&oldid=482619180.
22. File:Lymphangitis after bed bug bites.jpg. (2022, December 15). *Wikimedia Commons*. Retrieved 18:36, May 4, 2023 from https://commons.wikimedia.org/w/index.php?title=File:Lymphangitis_after_bed_bug_bites.jpg&oldid=715257007.
23. File:Furoncle.jpg. (2022, May 13). *Wikimedia Commons*. Retrieved 19:22, May 4, 2023 from https://commons.wikimedia.org/w/index.php?title=File:Furoncle.jpg&oldid=655830350.
24. File:Impetigo2020.jpg. (2020, September 25). *Wikimedia Commons*. Retrieved 21:10, May 4, 2023 from https://commons.wikimedia.org/w/index.php?title=File:Impetigo2020.jpg&oldid=470793440.
25. File:Teigne tondante enfant.jpg. (2023, February 9). *Wikimedia Commons*. Retrieved 21:44, May 4, 2023 from https://commons.wikimedia.org/w/index.php?title=File:Teigne_tondante_enfant.jpg&oldid=731124543.

References

26. File:Tinea barbae 4807 lores.jpg. (2023, February 7). *Wikimedia Commons*. Retrieved 22:49, May 4, 2023 from https://commons.wikimedia.org/w/index.php?title=File:Tinea_barbae_4807_lores.jpg&oldid=730765211.
27. File:Tinea pedis interdigitalis.jpg. (2023, January 26). *Wikimedia Commons*. Retrieved 23:31, May 4, 2023 from https://commons.wikimedia.org/w/index.php?title=File:Tinea_pedis_interdigitalis.jpg&oldid=727977420.
28. File:Jock itch in groin.jpg. (2022, November 27). *Wikimedia Commons*. Retrieved 03:16, May 6, 2023 from https://commons.wikimedia.org/w/index.php?title=File:Jock_itch_in_groin.jpg&oldid=709948167.
29. File:Ringworm on the arm, or tinea corporis due to Trichophyton mentagrophytes PHIL 2938 lores.jpg. (2017, March 10). *Wikimedia Commons*. Retrieved 03:30, May 6, 2023 from https://commons.wikimedia.org/w/index.php?title=File:Ringworm_on_the_arm,_or_tinea_corporis_due_to_Trichophyton_mentagrophytes_PHIL_2938_lores.jpg&oldid=236614457.
30. File:Scabies hand and fingers 1.jpg. (2023, February 9). *Wikimedia Commons*. Retrieved 02:05, May 8, 2023 from https://commons.wikimedia.org/w/index.php?title=File:Scabies_hand_and_fingers_1.jpg&oldid=731129309.
31. File:SOA-Pediculosis-pubis.jpg. (2021, November 12). *Wikimedia Commons*. Retrieved 02:50, May 8, 2023 from https://commons.wikimedia.org/w/index.php?title=File:SOA-Pediculosis-pubis.jpg&oldid=606751617.
32. Head lice.jpg. (2023, February 12). *Wikimedia Commons*. Retrieved 18:25, August 17, 2023 from https://commons.wikimedia.org/w/index.php?title=File:Head_lice.jpg&oldid=731916640.
33. File:Molluscum bumps.jpg. (2020, June 21). *Wikimedia Commons*. Retrieved 14:27, May 17, 2023 from https://commons.wikimedia.org/w/index.php?title=File:Molluscum_bumps.jpg&oldid=428016328.
34. File:Dornwarzen.jpg. (2021, October 20). *Wikimedia Commons*. Retrieved 02:47, May 18, 2023 from https://commons.wikimedia.org/w/index.php?title=File:Dornwarzen.jpg&oldid=600720693.
35. File:SOA-Condylomata-acuminata-around-anus.jpg. (2023, January 13). *Wikimedia Commons*. Retrieved 17:55, May 18, 2023 from https://commons.wikimedia.org/w/index.php?title=File:SOA-Condylomata-acuminata-around-anus.jpg&oldid=724881042.
36. File:Seborrheic keratosis on human back.jpg. (2020, October 21). *Wikimedia Commons*. Retrieved 19:09, May 18, 2023 from https://commons.wikimedia.org/w/index.php?title=File:Seborrheic_keratosis_on_human_back.jpg&oldid=496824251.
37. File:Actinic keratosis of the scalp.jpg. (2020, September 19). *Wikimedia Commons*. Retrieved 03:06, May 19, 2023 from https://commons.wikimedia.org/w/index.php?title=File:Actinic_keratosis_of_the_scalp.jpg&oldid=464706147.
38. File:Squamous Cell Carcinoma, Right Upper Cheek.png. (2023, February 13). *Wikimedia Commons*. Retrieved 14:22, May 19, 2023 from https://commons.wikimedia.org/w/index.php?title=File:Squamous_Cell_Carcinoma,_Right_Upper_Cheek.png&oldid=732190259.
39. File:Kaposi's Sarcoma.jpg. (2021, November 7). *Wikimedia Commons*. Retrieved 03:14, May 20, 2023 from https://commons.wikimedia.org/w/index.php?title=File:Kaposi%27s_Sarcoma.jpg&oldid=605903262.
40. File:Basal cell carcinoma3.JPG. (2022, September 20). *Wikimedia Commons*. Retrieved 03:13, May 25, 2023 from https://commons.wikimedia.org/w/index.php?title=File:Basal_cell_carcinoma3.JPG&oldid=690035490.
41. File:Lip licker's dermatitis.jpg. (2023, March 26). *Wikimedia Commons*. Retrieved 02:23, May 28, 2023 from https://commons.wikimedia.org/w/index.php?title=File:Lip_licker%27s_dermatitis.jpg&oldid=744060789.
42. File:Dermite de contact.jpg. (2022, June 10). *Wikimedia Commons*. Retrieved 14:28, May 29, 2023 from https://commons.wikimedia.org/w/index.php?title=File:Dermite_de_contact.jpg&oldid=663585771.
43. File:Irritant diaper dermatitis.jpg. (2022, November 19). *Wikimedia Commons*. Retrieved 13:58, May 30, 2023 from https://commons.wikimedia.org/w/index.php?title=File:Irritant_diaper_dermatitis.jpg&oldid=707990070.
44. File:Urushiol induced contact dermatitis.jpg. (2022, November 1). *Wikimedia Commons*. Retrieved 14:44, May 30, 2023 from https://commons.wikimedia.org/w/index.php?title=File:Urushiol_induced_contact_dermatitis.jpg&oldid=701294464.
45. File:Pompholyx-Hand.jpg. (2023, May 8). *Wikimedia Commons*. Retrieved 03:26, May 31, 2023 from https://commons.wikimedia.org/w/index.php?title=File:Pompholyx-Hand.jpg&oldid=760804031.
46. File:Lichen planus.jpg. (2023, February 7). *Wikimedia Commons*. Retrieved 15:58, June 4, 2023 from https://commons.wikimedia.org/w/index.php?title=File:Lichen_planus.jpg&oldid=730677857.
47. File:Lichen simplex chronicus 1.jpg. (2021, January 13). *Wikimedia Commons*. Retrieved 16:50, June 4, 2023 from https://commons.wikimedia.org/w/index.php?title=File:Lichen_simplex_chronicus_1.jpg&oldid=525820402.
48. File:Dermatitis atopica 04.JPG. (2020, October 19). *Wikimedia Commons*. Retrieved 18:13, June 4, 2023 from https://commons.wikimedia.org/w/index.php?title=File:Dermatitis_atopica_04.JPG&oldid=494690141.
49. File:Pityriasisrosa.png. (2020, October 23). *Wikimedia Commons*. Retrieved 20:05, June 4, 2023 from https://commons.wikimedia.org/w/index.php?title=File:Pityriasisrosa.png&oldid=498409830.
50. File:Psoriasis on elbow.jpg. (2020, September 15). *Wikimedia Commons*. Retrieved 14:47, June 5, 2023 from https://commons.wikimedia.org/w/index.php?title=File:Psoriasis_on_elbow.jpg&oldid=460589806.
51. File:Tinea versicolor1.jpg. (2021, November 1). *Wikimedia Commons*. Retrieved 16:45, June 5, 2023 from https://commons.wikimedia.org/w/index.php?title=File:Tinea_versicolor1.jpg&oldid=604836245.

References

52. File:Baby With Cradle Cap.jpg. (2020, October 15). *Wikimedia Commons*. Retrieved 18:18, June 5, 2023 from https://commons.wikimedia.org/w/index.php?title=File:Baby_With_Cradle_Cap.jpg&oldid=490627662.
53. File:Seborrhoeic dermatitis highres.jpg. (2020, October 17). *Wikimedia Commons*. Retrieved 19:24, June 5, 2023 from https://commons.wikimedia.org/w/index.php?title=File:Seborrhoeic_dermatitis_highres.jpg&oldid=492826749.
54. File:Angioedema of the face.jpg. (2020, September 22). *Wikimedia Commons*. Retrieved 13:56, June 7, 2023 from https://commons.wikimedia.org/w/index.php?title=File:Angioedema_of_the_face.jpg&oldid=467773045.
55. File:Angioedema2013.JPG. (2020, September 23). *Wikimedia Commons*. Retrieved 13:57, June 7, 2023 from https://commons.wikimedia.org/w/index.php?title=File:Angioedema2013.JPG&oldid=468376919.
56. File:Rash.jpg. (2023, February 12). *Wikimedia Commons*. Retrieved 15:30, June 7, 2023 from https://commons.wikimedia.org/w/index.php?title=File:Rash.jpg&oldid=732087910.
57. File:Stasis dermatitis (Gravitational eczema).jpg. (2022, July 25). *Wikimedia Commons*. Retrieved 16:42, June 7, 2023 from https://commons.wikimedia.org/w/index.php?title=File:Stasis_dermatitis_(Gravitational_eczema).jpg&oldid=677643515.
58. File:Vitiligo and Poliosis.jpg. (2021, March 1). *Wikimedia Commons*. Retrieved 15:55, June 7, 2023 from https://commons.wikimedia.org/w/index.php?title=File:Vitiligo_and_Poliosis.jpg&oldid=537785007.
59. File:Melasmablemish.jpg. (2020, October 22). *Wikimedia Commons*. Retrieved 20:42, June 7, 2023 from https://commons.wikimedia.org/w/index.php?title=File:Melasmablemish.jpg&oldid=497636201.
60. File:Wallace rule of nines-en.svg. (2022, December 7). *Wikimedia Commons*. Retrieved 21:19, June 7, 2023 from https://commons.wikimedia.org/w/index.php?title=File:Wallace_rule_of_nines-en.svg&oldid=713080206.
61. File:Decubitus 01.JPG. (2020, October 28). *Wikimedia Commons*. Retrieved 13:23, June 10, 2023 from https://commons.wikimedia.org/w/index.php?title=File:Decubitus_01.JPG&oldid=505264341.
62. File:Pemphgoid vulgaris.jpg. (2020, October 27). *Wikimedia Commons*. Retrieved 18:52, June 11, 2023 from https://commons.wikimedia.org/w/index.php?title=File:Pemphgoid_vulgaris.jpg&oldid=504191669.
63. File:Bullous pemphigoid new image.jpg. (2020, September 16). *Wikimedia Commons*. Retrieved 20:18, June 11, 2023 from https://commons.wikimedia.org/w/index.php?title=File:Bullous_pemphigoid_new_image.jpg&oldid=461411024.
64. File:Acanthosis nigricans.jpg. (2023, February 12). *Wikimedia Commons*. Retrieved 21:51, June 11, 2023 from https://commons.wikimedia.org/w/index.php?title=File:Acanthosis_nigricans.jpg&oldid=732034176.
65. File:Hidradenitis suppurativa (stage II) in axilla.jpg. (2020, September 19). *Wikimedia Commons*. Retrieved 16:45, June 13, 2023 from https://commons.wikimedia.org/w/index.php?title=File:Hidradenitis_suppurativa_(stage_II)_in_axilla.jpg&oldid=464638644.
66. File:Lipoma 02.jpg. (2020, October 2). *Wikimedia Commons*. Retrieved 18:34, June 13, 2023 from https://commons.wikimedia.org/w/index.php?title=File:Lipoma_02.jpg&oldid=478443914.
67. File:Sebaceous cyst01.jpg. (2022, November 28). *Wikimedia Commons*. Retrieved 21:31, June 13, 2023 from https://commons.wikimedia.org/w/index.php?title=File:Sebaceous_cyst01.jpg&oldid=710375309.
68. File:Crohnie Pyoderma gangrenosum.jpg. (2022, September 18). *Wikimedia Commons*. Retrieved 15:55, June 14, 2023 from https://commons.wikimedia.org/w/index.php?title=File:Crohnie_Pyoderma_gangrenosum.jpg&oldid=689450000.
69. File:Keloid.jpg. (2020, September 24). *Wikimedia Commons*. Retrieved 17:38, June 14, 2023 from https://commons.wikimedia.org/w/index.php?title=File:Keloid.jpg&oldid=469585928.
70. File:Dermatitis Herpetiforme 4.jpg. (2020, October 15). *Wikimedia Commons*. Retrieved 19:51, June 14, 2023 from https://commons.wikimedia.org/w/index.php?title=File:Dermatitis_Herpetiforme_4.jpg&oldid=490092328.
71. File:Pyogenic granuloma on a finger-1.jpg. (2020, September 19). *Wikimedia Commons*. Retrieved 22:44, June 14, 2023 from https://commons.wikimedia.org/w/index.php?title=File:Pyogenic_granuloma_on_a_finger-1.jpg&oldid=465104126.
72. File:ENlegs.JPG. (2020, September 23). *Wikimedia Commons*. Retrieved 23:38, June 14, 2023 from https://commons.wikimedia.org/w/index.php?title=File:ENlegs.JPG&oldid=468421008.
73. File:Cherry angioma.jpg. (2020, November 11). *Wikimedia Commons*. Retrieved 14:39, June 15, 2023 from https://commons.wikimedia.org/w/index.php?title=File:Cherry_angioma.jpg&oldid=512003499.
74. File:Simple interrupted suture.svg. (2021, September 22). *Wikimedia Commons*. Retrieved 15:45, June 15, 2023 from https://commons.wikimedia.org/w/index.php?title=File:Simple_interrupted_suture.svg&oldid=592853956.
75. File:Subcuticular suture.svg. (2021, June 23). *Wikimedia Commons*. Retrieved 15:45, June 15, 2023 from https://commons.wikimedia.org/w/index.php?title=File:Subcuticular_suture.svg&oldid=570869210.
76. File:Vertical mattress suture.svg. (2022, June 13). *Wikimedia Commons*. Retrieved 15:45, June 15, 2023 from https://commons.wikimedia.org/w/index.php?title=File:Vertical_mattress_suture.svg&oldid=664220404.
77. File:Continous-Horizontal mattress suture.svg. (2022, July 2). *Wikimedia Commons*. Retrieved 15:46, June 15, 2023 from https://commons.wikimedia.org/w/index.php?title=File:Continous-Horizontal_mattress_suture.svg&oldid=670512420.
78. File:Pilonidal abscess.jpg. (2021, October 25). *Wikimedia Commons*. Retrieved 13:59, June 19, 2023 from https://commons.wikimedia.org/w/index.php?title=File:Pilonidal_abscess.jpg&oldid=601867940.

Chapter 13

Infectious Disease

ANTIBIOTIC CHART

ANTIBIOTIC CHART	MRSA	MSSA	Streptococci	E. coli	Proteus mirabilis	Klebsiella spp.	Pseudomonas	ESCAPPM	Neisseria gonorrhoeae	Neisseria meningitidis	Anaerobes	Atypicals
Natural Penicillins			Penicillin G									
Penicillinase-Resistant PCN		Nafcillin/Dicloxacillin										
Aminopenicillin			Ampicillin/Amoxicillin						Amp/Amox			
Aminopenicillins with Beta-Lactamase Inhibitors		Amoxicillin-Clavulanate / Ampicillin-Sulbactam									Amox-Clav / Amp-Sulb	
1st Gen Cephalosporin		Cefazolin, Cephalexin										
2nd Gen Cephalosporin		Cephotetan, Cefoxitin									Cephotetan / Cefoxitin	
3rd Gen Cephalosporin		Ceftriaxone							Ceftriaxone			
4th Gen Cephalosporin		Ceftazidime										
Anti-Pseudomonal PCN		Piperacillin + Tazobactam							Piperacillin + Tazobactam			
Carbapenems		Ertapenem / Imipenem, Meropenem							Ertapenem			
Quinolones	Cipro		Ciprofloxacin / Levofloxacin / Moxifloxacin						Moxifloxacin			Levo
Tetracyclines		Doxycycline							Doxycycline			Doxy
Macrolides		Azithromycin							Azithromycin			Azithro
Clindamycin	Clindamycin										Clinda	
Aminoglycosides				Gentamicin/Tobramycin/Amikacin								
Metronidazole											Metro	
Trimethoprim-Sulfamethoxazole		Trimethoprim-Sulfamethoxazole					TMP/SMX		TMP/SMX			

Column groups: **Gram Positive Cocci** (MRSA, MSSA, Streptococci); **Gram Negative Bacilli** (E. coli, Proteus mirabilis, Klebsiella spp., Pseudomonas, ESCAPPM); **Gram Negative Cocci** (Neisseria gonorrhoeae, Neisseria meningitidis); Anaerobes; Atypicals

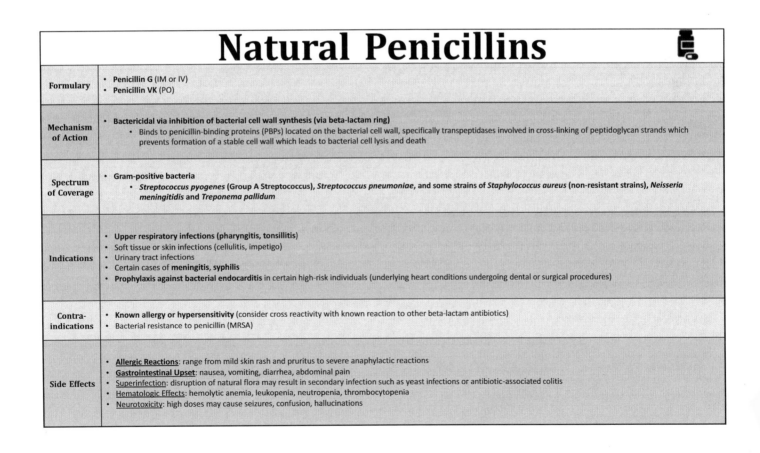

Natural Penicillins

Formulary	• **Penicillin G** (IM or IV) • **Penicillin VK** (PO)
Mechanism of Action	• **Bactericidal via inhibition of bacterial cell wall synthesis (via beta-lactam ring)** • Binds to penicillin-binding proteins (PBPs) located on the bacterial cell wall, specifically transpeptidases involved in cross-linking of peptidoglycan strands which prevents formation of a stable cell wall which leads to bacterial cell lysis and death
Spectrum of Coverage	• **Gram-positive bacteria** • *Streptococcus pyogenes* (Group A Streptococcus), *Streptococcus pneumoniae*, and some strains of *Staphylococcus aureus* (non-resistant strains), *Neisseria meningitidis* and *Treponema pallidum*
Indications	• **Upper respiratory infections (pharyngitis, tonsillitis)** • Soft tissue or skin infections (cellulitis, impetigo) • Urinary tract infections • Certain cases of **meningitis, syphilis** • **Prophylaxis against bacterial endocarditis** in certain high-risk individuals (underlying heart conditions undergoing dental or surgical procedures)
Contra-indications	• **Known allergy or hypersensitivity** (consider cross reactivity with known reaction to other beta-lactam antibiotics) • Bacterial resistance to penicillin (MRSA)
Side Effects	• <u>Allergic Reactions</u>: range from mild skin rash and pruritus to severe anaphylactic reactions • <u>Gastrointestinal Upset</u>: nausea, vomiting, diarrhea, abdominal pain • <u>Superinfection</u>: disruption of natural flora may result in secondary infection such as yeast infections or antibiotic-associated colitis • <u>Hematologic Effects</u>: hemolytic anemia, leukopenia, neutropenia, thrombocytopenia • <u>Neurotoxicity</u>: high doses may cause seizures, confusion, hallucinations

Penicillinase-Resistant Penicillin

Formulary	• Oxacillin (IV, IM) • Nafcillin (IV) • Dicloxacillin (PO)
Mechanism of Action	• **Bactericidal via inhibition of bacterial cell wall synthesis (via beta-lactam ring)** • Binds to penicillin-binding proteins (PBPs) located on the bacterial cell wall, specifically transpeptidases involved in cross-linking of peptidoglycan strands which prevents formation of a stable cell wall which leads to bacterial cell lysis and death • **Resistant to the enzymatic degradation by penicillinase or beta-lactamase enzymes produced by certain bacteria**

Spectrum of Coverage	• **Gram-positive bacteria**
	  • **Methicillin-susceptible** *Staphylococcus aureus* (MSSA), *Streptococcus pyogenes* (group A streptococcus), and *Streptococcus pneumonia*
	• **Gram-negative bacteria**
	  • Limited activity

Indications	• Skin and soft tissue infections • Bone and joint infections • Respiratory tract infections
Contra-indications	• **Known allergy or hypersensitivity** (consider cross reactivity with known reaction to other beta-lactam antibiotics) • Severe liver disease (potential risk of hepatotoxicity) • Bacterial resistance to penicillin (MRSA)
Side Effects	• <u>Allergic Reactions</u>: range from mild skin rash and pruritus to severe anaphylactic reactions • <u>Gastrointestinal Upset</u>: nausea, vomiting, diarrhea, abdominal pain • <u>Superinfection</u>: disruption of natural flora may result in secondary infection such as yeast infections or antibiotic-associated colitis • <u>Hematologic Effects</u>: hemolytic anemia, leukopenia, neutropenia, thrombocytopenia • <u>Neurotoxicity</u>: high doses may cause seizures, confusion, hallucinations

Aminopenicillins

Formulary	• Amoxicillin (PO) • Ampicillin (IV)
Mechanism of Action	• **Bactericidal via inhibition of bacterial cell wall synthesis (via beta-lactam ring)** • Binds to penicillin-binding proteins (PBPs) located on the bacterial cell wall, specifically transpeptidases involved in cross-linking of peptidoglycan strands which prevents formation of a stable cell wall which leads to bacterial cell lysis and death

Spectrum of Coverage	• **Gram-positive bacteria**
	  • *Streptococcus pneumonia, Streptococcus pyogenes* (group A *Streptococcus*), ***Streptococcus agalactiae*** (group B *Streptococcus*), ***Enterococcus faecalis***, some strains of *Staphylococcus aureus* (non-beta-lactamase producing)
	• **Gram-negative bacteria**
	  • *Haemophilus influenzae, Escherichia coli, Proteus mirabilis, Salmonella spp., Shigella spp.*

Indications	• **Respiratory tract infections** (otitis media, sinusitis, bronchitis, community-acquired pneumonia) • **Urinary tract infections** • **Skin and soft tissue infections** (cellulitis, impetigo, erysipelas) • **Dental infections** (dental abscesses and infections associated with tooth extraction) • Gastrointestinal infections • **Prophylaxis against bacterial endocarditis** in certain high-risk individuals (underlying heart conditions undergoing dental or surgical procedures)
Contra-indications	• **Known allergy or hypersensitivity** (consider cross reactivity with known reaction to other beta-lactam antibiotics) • **Infectious mononucleosis** (produces rash) • Severe liver disease (potential risk of hepatotoxicity) • Renal insufficiency (dose adjustment may be required) • Bacterial resistance to penicillin (MRSA)
Side Effects	• <u>Allergic Reactions</u>: range from mild skin rash and pruritus to severe anaphylactic reactions • <u>Gastrointestinal Upset</u>: nausea, vomiting, diarrhea, abdominal pain • <u>Superinfection</u>: disruption of natural flora may result in secondary infection such as yeast infections or antibiotic-associated colitis • <u>Hematologic Effects</u>: hemolytic anemia, leukopenia, neutropenia, thrombocytopenia • <u>Neurotoxicity</u>: high doses may cause seizures, confusion, hallucinations

Aminopenicillins with Beta-Lactamase Inhibitors

Formulary	• **Amoxicillin-clavulanate** (PO) • **Ampicillin-sulbactam** (IV)
Mechanism of Action	• **Bactericidal via inhibition of bacterial cell wall synthesis (via beta-lactam ring)** • Binds to penicillin-binding proteins (PBPs) located on the bacterial cell wall, specifically transpeptidases involved in cross-linking of peptidoglycan strands which prevents formation of a stable cell wall which leads to bacterial cell lysis and death • **Beta-lactamase inhibitors (clavulanate) have the ability to irreversibly bind to beta-lactamase enzymes** (enzymes that can inactivate beta-lactam antibiotics by breaking the beta-lactam ring, rendering them ineffective) **to prevent the inactivation of the primary antibiotic**

Spectrum of Coverage	• **Gram-positive bacteria**
	  • ***Streptococcus pneumonia, Streptococcus pyogenes*** (group A *Streptococcus*), ***Streptococcus agalactiae*** (group B *Streptococcus*), ***Enterococcus faecalis***, some strains of *Staphylococcus aureus* (non-beta-lactamase producing)
	• **Gram-negative bacteria**
	  • ***Haemophilus influenzae, Escherichia coli, Proteus mirabilis, Moraxella catarrhalis***, *Salmonella spp., Shigella spp.*
	• **Anaerobes**
	  • *Bacteroides fragilis* and other *Bacteroides spp.*

Indications	• **Respiratory tract infections (otitis media, sinusitis, bronchitis, community-acquired pneumonia)** • **Urinary tract infections** • **Skin and soft tissue infections** (cellulitis, impetigo, erysipelas) • **Dental infections** (dental abscesses and infections associated with tooth extraction) • **Gastrointestinal infections** • **Prophylaxis against bacterial endocarditis** in certain high-risk individuals (underlying heart conditions undergoing dental or surgical procedures)
Contra-indications	• **Known allergy or hypersensitivity** (consider cross reactivity with known reaction to other beta-lactam antibiotics) • **Infectious mononucleosis** (produces rash) • Severe liver disease (potential risk of hepatotoxicity) • Renal insufficiency (dose adjustment may be required) • Bacterial resistance to penicillin (MRSA)
Side Effects	• <u>Allergic Reactions</u>: range from mild skin rash and pruritus to severe anaphylactic reactions • <u>Gastrointestinal Upset</u>: nausea, vomiting, diarrhea, abdominal pain • <u>Superinfection</u>: disruption of natural flora may result in secondary infection such as yeast infections or antibiotic-associated colitis • <u>Hematologic Effects</u>: hemolytic anemia, leukopenia, neutropenia, thrombocytopenia • <u>Neurotoxicity</u>: high doses may cause seizures, confusion, hallucinations

Anti-Pseudomonal Penicillins

Formulary	• **Piperacillin-tazobactam** • **Ticarcillin-clavulanate** • Carbenicillin
Mechanism of Action	• **Bactericidal via inhibition of bacterial cell wall synthesis (via beta-lactam ring)** • Binds to penicillin-binding proteins (PBPs) located on the bacterial cell wall, specifically transpeptidases involved in cross-linking of peptidoglycan strands which prevents formation of a stable cell wall which leads to bacterial cell lysis and death • Anti-pseudomonal beta-lactamase inhibitor (tazobactam or clavulanate) irreversibly binds to the beta-lactamase enzymes produced by *Pseudomonas aeruginosa*, preventing the enzymes from inactivating the penicillin component and allowing the penicillin to exert its antimicrobial effect

Spectrum of Coverage	• **Gram-positive bacteria**
	  • ***Streptococcus pneumonia, Streptococcus pyogenes*** (group A *Streptococcus*), ***Streptococcus agalactiae*** (group B *Streptococcus*), ***Enterococcus faecalis***, some strains of *Staphylococcus aureus* (non-beta-lactamase producing)
	• **Gram-negative bacteria**
	  • ***Haemophilus influenzae, Escherichia coli, Proteus mirabilis, Moraxella catarrhalis***, *Klebsiella pneumoniae*
	• **Pseudomonas**
	  • *Pseudomonas aeruginosa*

Indications	• **Severe infections, especially those caused by *Pseudomonas aeruginosa*** • **Hospital-acquired pneumonia** • **Complicated urinary tract infections** • **Intra-abdominal infections (peritonitis or abscesses)**
Contra-indications	• **Known allergy or hypersensitivity** (consider cross reactivity with known reaction to other beta-lactam antibiotics) • Bacterial resistance to penicillin
Side Effects	• <u>Allergic Reactions</u>: range from mild skin rash and pruritus to severe anaphylactic reactions • <u>Gastrointestinal Upset</u>: nausea, vomiting, diarrhea, abdominal pain • <u>Superinfection</u>: disruption of natural flora may result in secondary infection such as yeast infections or antibiotic-associated colitis • <u>Hematologic Effects</u>: hemolytic anemia, leukopenia, neutropenia, thrombocytopenia • <u>Neurotoxicity</u>: high doses may cause seizures, confusion, hallucinations

Cephalosporins

	First-Generation	Second-Generation	Third-Generation	Fourth-Generation	Fifth Generation
Formulary	• Cephalexin (PO) • Cefazolin (IV) • Cefadroxil (PO)	• Cefaclor (PO) • Cefuroxime (IM, IV, PO) • Cefoxitin (IV) • Cefotetan (IM, IV)	• Ceftriaxone (IM, IV) • Ceftazidime (IM, IV) • Cefotaxime (IM, IV) • Cefixime (PO)	• Cefepime (IV)	• Ceftaroline (IV)
Gram Negative Coverage	• *Escherichia coli, Proteus mirabilis, Klebsiella pneumoniae, Haemophilus influenzae*	• Added coverage against *Bacteroides fragilis*	• Added coverage against *Serratia spp.* and enteric organisms • Improved CNS penetration	• Added coverage against *Pseudomonas aeruginosa*	• MRSA and gram negatives (excluding Pseudomonas or anaerobes)
Gram Positive Coverage	• *Increasing level of gram-negative activity and decreasing level of gram-positive activity with increasing generation* • *Streptococcus pneumonia, Streptococcus pyogenes* (group A *Streptococcus*), *Streptococcus agalactiae* (group B *Streptococcus*), *Enterococcus faecalis*, some strains of *Staphylococcus aureus* (non-beta-lactamase producing)				
Mechanism of Action	• **Bactericidal via inhibition of bacterial cell wall synthesis (via beta-lactam ring)** • Binds to penicillin-binding proteins (PBPs) located on the bacterial cell wall, specifically transpeptidases involved in cross-linking of peptidoglycan strands which prevents formation of a stable cell wall which leads to bacterial cell lysis and death • **Intrinsically effective against beta-lactamase producing bacteria**				
Indications	• **Skin and soft tissue infections Surgical prophylaxis** • **Upper and lower respiratory tract infections** • **Urinary tract infections**	• **Abdominal infections** • **Pelvic inflammatory disease**	• **Meningitis (ceftriaxone)** • **Lyme disease**	• *Pseudomonas aeruginosa* **infection**	• **MRSA infection**
Contra-indications	• **Known allergy or hypersensitivity** (consider cross reactivity with known reaction to other beta-lactam antibiotics) • Renal insufficiency (dose adjustment may be required) • Bacterial resistance				
Side Effects	• <u>Allergic Reactions</u>: range from mild skin rash and pruritus to severe anaphylactic reactions • *5-15% cross reactivity with penicillins (should not be used in any patient with anaphylactic reaction to penicillins)* • <u>Gastrointestinal Upset</u>: nausea, vomiting, diarrhea, abdominal pain • <u>Superinfection</u>: disruption of natural flora may result in secondary infection such as yeast infections or antibiotic-associated colitis • <u>Hematologic Effects</u>: leukopenia, neutropenia, thrombocytopenia; **hypoprothrombinemia due to vitamin K-dependent clotting factors with cefotetan and cefoxitin**				

Carbapenems

Formulary	• Imipenem-cilastatin (IV) • Meropenem (IV) • Ertapenem (IM, IV)
Mechanism of Action	• **Synthetic beta-lactam antibiotic** • **Bactericidal via inhibition of bacterial cell wall synthesis (via beta-lactam ring)** • Binds to penicillin-binding proteins (PBPs) located on the bacterial cell wall, specifically transpeptidases involved in cross-linking of peptidoglycan strands which prevents formation of a stable cell wall which leads to bacterial cell lysis and death • Addition of cilastatin reduces deactivation of antibiotic by the proximal renal tubule

Spectrum of Coverage	• **Broad spectrum of activity against both gram-positive and gram-negative bacteria, including many multidrug-resistant strains**
	• **Gram-positive bacteria**
	  • Methicillin-sensitive Staphylococcus aureus (MSSA), Streptococcus pneumoniae, and Enterococcus faecalis
	• **Gram-negative bacteria**
	  • *Escherichia coli, Klebsiella pneumoniae, Proteus mirabilis*, non-lactose fermenting bacteria such as *Pseudomonas aeruginosa*
	• **Anaerobic bacteria**
	  • *Bacteroides fragilis, Clostridium* spp., and *Prevotella* spp.
	• Not effective against MRSA, bacteria without peptidoglycan cell walls (*Mycoplasma* spp.), some *Pseudomonas* spp.

Indications	• **Considered a "last resort" antibiotic**; use is restricted due to the risk of promoting antibiotic resistance • **Empirical treatment of severe infections** (complicated intra-abdominal infections, hospital-acquired pneumonia, or complicated urinary tract infections) • **Multidrug-resistant bacterial infections** • **Polymicrobial infections** (intra-abdominal infections, diabetic foot infections, or necrotizing soft tissue infections) • **Bone and joint infections**
Contra-indications	• **Known allergy or hypersensitivity** (consider cross reactivity with known reaction to other beta-lactam antibiotics) • **History of seizures or central nervous system disorders** (may lower the seizure threshold)
Side Effects	• <u>Allergic Reactions</u>: range from mild skin rash and pruritus to severe anaphylactic reactions • *Patients with a known hypersensitivity to beta-lactam antibiotics (penicillins or cephalosporins) may be at an increased risk* • <u>Gastrointestinal Upset</u>: nausea, vomiting, diarrhea, abdominal pain • <u>Central Nervous System Effects</u>: risk of seizures, myoclonus and altered mental status (particularly in patients with a history of epilepsy, impaired renal function or receiving high doses of carbapenems) • <u>Superinfection</u>: disruption of natural flora may result in secondary infection such as yeast infections or antibiotic-associated colitis • <u>Laboratory abnormalities</u>: abnormal liver function tests, increased serum creatinine levels, or hematological abnormalities (eosinophilia, neutropenia)

Monobactam

Formulary	• Aztreonam (IV)
Mechanism of Action	• **Bactericidal via inhibition of bacterial cell wall synthesis** • Specifically binds to penicillin-binding proteins 3 (PBP3), which is predominantly found in Gram-negative bacteria • PBP3 is located on the bacterial cell wall, which inhibits transpeptidase activity and prevents formation of a stable cell wall which leads to bacterial cell lysis and death • **Minimal cross-reactivity with other beta-lactam antibiotics**
Spectrum of Coverage	• **Primarily gram-negative aerobes (*Enterobacteriaceae* and *Pseudomonas aeruginosa*)** • **Minimal coverage against gram positive organisms and anaerobes**
Indications	• *Infections caused by susceptible susceptible gram-negative bacteria, particularly when other antibiotics may be ineffective or contraindicated* • **Complicated urinary tract infections** (*Escherichia coli, Klebsiella pneumoniae,* and *Pseudomonas aeruginosa*) • **Intra-abdominal infections** • **Lower respiratory tract infections** (pneumonia, bronchitis) • **Skin and soft tissue infections**
Contra-indications	• **Known allergy or hypersensitivity** (consider cross reactivity with known reaction to other beta-lactam antibiotics)
Side Effects	• *Generally well tolerated, minimal cross reactivity with other beta-lactam antibiotics* • <u>Allergic Reactions</u>: range from mild skin rash and pruritus to severe anaphylactic reactions • <u>Gastrointestinal Upset</u>: nausea, vomiting, diarrhea, abdominal pain • <u>Local Reactions</u>: pain, redness, or swelling at the injection site (phlebitis)

Polymyxin

Formulary	• **Polymyxin B** • **Polymyxin E** (colistin) • *Topical, ophthalmic, otic; IM or IV*
Mechanism of Action	• Binds to the lipopolysaccharide component of the outer membrane of gram-negative bacteria leading to permeability of the outer membrane of gram-negative organisms resulting in leaking of cellular contents and cell death
Spectrum of Coverage	• **Gram-negative bacteria** • Multidrug-resistant strains such as *Pseudomonas aeruginosa, Acinetobacter baumannii*, and *Klebsiella pneumoniae* • **Gram-positive bacteria and anaerobes** • Limited activity and are generally not effective
Indications	• Topical treatment for infections of the eye, ear, and skin • *May be part of triple therapy with neomycin and bacitracin*
Contra-indications	• **Known allergy or hypersensitivity**
Side Effects	• <u>Topical</u>: • **Allergic contact dermatitis** • <u>IM/IV</u>: • **Nephrotoxicity** • **Neurotoxicity** (neurological effects such as numbness or tingling) • <u>Allergic Reactions</u>: range from mild skin rash and pruritus to severe anaphylactic reactions • Respiratory depression, muscle weakness

Vancomycin

Formulary	• Oral • IV
Mechanism of Action	• **Glycopeptide antibiotic that works by inhibiting bacterial cell wall synthesis through phospholipid and peptidoglycan inhibition** • Specifically targets and binds to the D-alanyl-D-alanine portion of the peptidoglycan precursors, preventing their incorporation into the growing cell wall, leading to bacterial cell death

Spectrum of Coverage	• **Gram-positive bacteria**
	  • Particularly those that are resistant to other antibiotics such as **methicillin-resistant *Staphylococcus aureus* (MRSA) and methicillin-resistant *Staphylococcus epidermidis* (MRSE) infections**
	  • *Streptococcus pneumoniae, Streptococcus pyogenes, Enterococcus faecalis*, and ***Clostridium difficile*** (oral formulary only)

Indications	• <u>Oral</u>: ***Clostridium difficile* colitis** • <u>IV</u>: methicillin-resistant *Staphylococcus aureus* (MRSA) and methicillin-resistant *Staphylococcus epidermidis* (MRSE) infections
Contra-indications	• **Known allergy or hypersensitivity**
Side Effects	• <u>Gastrointestinal Upset</u>: nausea, vomiting, diarrhea, abdominal pain • <u>Red Man Syndrome</u>: **flushing, rash, pruritus secondary to histamine release during rapid IV infusion** • **Prevented or minimized by slowing infusion rate** (slow infusion over 1-2 hours) **and antihistamine administration** • <u>Local Reactions</u>: pain, redness, or swelling at the injection site (phlebitis) • <u>Ototoxicity</u>: tinnitus or hearing loss • <u>Nephrotoxicity</u>: particularly with high doses or prolonged therapy or if given with other antibiotics with similar side effects (aminoglycosides)

Tetracyclines

Formulary	• **Doxycycline (oral, IM, IV)** • Tetracycline (oral) • Minocycline (oral)
Mechanism of Action	• **Inhibition of bacterial protein synthesis by binding to the bacterial ribosomes (specifically the 30S subunit)**, which prevents the attachment of aminoacyl-tRNA molecules to the mRNA-ribosome complex • **Bacteriostatic**
Spectrum of Coverage	• **Broad spectrum of activity against both gram-positive and gram-negative bacteria** • **Atypical bacteria such as *Chlamydia* spp., *Mycoplasma pneumoniae*, and *Rickettsia* spp.**
Indications	• **Sexually transmitted infections** (Chlamydia spp., pelvic inflammatory disease, lymphogranuloma venereum) • **Respiratory tract infections** (*Chlamydia pneumophila* pneumonia, *Mycoplasma pneumoniae* pneumonia) • Urinary tract infections • **Tick-borne illnesses (Lyme disease, Rocky Mountain spotted fever)** • Acne or rosacea (tetracycline or minocycline) • <u>Other</u>: Vibrio cholerae, Q fever, bubonic plague, cat scratch fever
Contra-indications	• **Known allergy or hypersensitivity** • **Infants and children (<8 years old for more than 21 days) and pregnant women due to potential for tooth discoloration and inhibited bone growth**
Side Effects	• <u>Gastrointestinal Upset</u>: nausea, vomiting, diarrhea, abdominal pain • <u>Phototoxicity</u>: increased sensitivity to sunlight • <u>Hepatotoxicity</u>: especially in pregnancy • <u>Deposition in Calcified Tissue</u>: **deposition may cause teeth discoloration and inhibit bone growth with prolonged use in children** • <u>Nephrotoxicity</u>: tetracycline and minocycline preparations • <u>Vestibular Dysfunction</u>: hearing loss, tinnitus with tetracycline preparations • <u>Impaired Absorption</u>: for optimal absorption, the medication should be taken 2-3 hours before or after consuming any supplements or drugs with magnesium, zinc, calcium, aluminum, iron, or sodium bicarbonate

Macrolides

Formulary	• **Azithromycin** (oral, IV, ophthalmic) • **Clarithromycin** (oral, IV) • **Erythromycin** (oral, IM, IV, topical, ophthalmic)
Mechanism of Action	• **Inhibition of bacterial protein synthesis by binding to the 50S subunit of the bacterial ribosome** which inhibits bacterial growth and replication • Bacteriostatic at low doses, bactericidal at high doses

Spectrum of Coverage	• **Gram-positive bacteria**
	  • Broad spectrum; *Streptococcus pneumoniae*, *Staphylococcus aureus* (including some methicillin-resistant strains), and *Streptococcus pyogenes*
	• **Gram-negative bacteria**
	  • *Neisseria meningitidis*
	• **Atypical organisms**
	  • *Mycoplasma pneumoniae*, *Legionella pneumophila*, and *Chlamydia* spp.

Indications	• **Upper respiratory infections** (Streptococcal pharyngitis, sinusitis, bronchitis, community acquired pneumonia) • Azithromycin has best coverage for atypicals (*Mycoplasma, Chlamydia, Legionella*) and exhibits anti inflammatory properties within the lung • **Sexually transmitted infections** (*Chlamydia*) • **Acne vulgaris** (topical erythromycin) • **Bacterial conjunctivitis** (erythromycin ophthalmic ointment) • **Peptic ulcers caused by *Helicobacter pylori*** (clarithromycin)
Contra-indications	• **Known allergy or hypersensitivity** • **Liver dysfunction** (carries risk of hepatotoxicity) • **Niacin or statin therapy** (increases muscle toxicity)
Side Effects	• <u>**Gastrointestinal Upset**</u>: nausea, vomiting, diarrhea, abdominal pain • <u>**QT Interval Prolongation**</u>: especially when used in high doses or in combination with other drugs that can also prolong the QT interval • <u>**Ototoxicity**</u>: may cause deafness (usually reversible) • <u>**Cytochrome P-450 Inhibition**</u>: many drug-drug interactions; may increase levels of warfarin, digoxin, theophylline, carbamazepine, statins

Bacitracin

Formulary	• **Topical** • **Ophthalmic** • **IM**
Mechanism of Action	• Bactericidal antibiotic that **inhibits bacterial cell wall synthesis** through interference of the dephosphorylation of the lipid carrier that transports the peptidoglycan precursors across the cell membrane, leading to the inhibition of peptidoglycan synthesis and bacterial cell wall formation
Spectrum of Coverage	• **Narrow spectrum** • **Gram-positive bacteria only** • *Staphylococcus aureus*, *Staphylococcus epidermidis*, *Streptococcal pyogenes* and some strains of *Streptococcus pneumoniae*
Indications	• **Skin and wound infections** (topical preparation for minor skin injuries, abrasions, lacerations, burns) • May be part of triple therapy ointment with neomycin and polymyxin B • Superficial ocular infections (topical ophthalmic preparation)
Contra-indications	• **Known allergy or hypersensitivity** • **Extensive or deep wounds or mucous membrane involvement**
Side Effects	• <u>**Allergic Contact Dermatitis**</u>: erythema, pruritus, rash • <u>Nephrotoxicity</u>: with IM form

Clindamycin

Formulary	• Oral • Oral solution • Topical • Vaginal • IM or IV
Mechanism of Action	• Bacteriostatic antibiotic that **inhibits bacterial protein synthesis by binding to the 50S subunit of the bacterial ribosome** which prevents the addition of amino acids to the growing peptide chain, thereby interfering with bacterial protein production

Spectrum of Coverage	• **Gram-positive bacteria**
	    • ***Staphylococcus aureus* (including methicillin-resistant strains)**, *Streptococcus pyogenes*, *Streptococcus pneumoniae*
	• Gram-negative bacteria
	    • Minimal coverage
	• Anaerobes
	    • *Bacteroides fragilis*

Indications	• **Skin and soft tissue infections** (cellulitis, abscesses, infected wounds) • **Gynecologic infections** (bacterial vaginosis, pelvic inflammatory disease) • **Bone and joint infections** • **Intra-abdominal infections** (anaerobic infection) • **Aspiration pneumonia** • **Acne vulgaris** (topical preparations)
Contra-indications	• **Known allergy or hypersensitivity** • **History of antibiotic-associated colitis (*Clostridium difficile*)**
Side Effects	• <u>Allergic Reactions</u>: range from mild skin rash and pruritus to severe anaphylactic reactions • <u>Gastrointestinal Upset</u>: **most common adverse reaction**; nausea, vomiting, diarrhea, abdominal pain • *<u>Clostridium difficile</u>* <u>Colitis</u>: altered GI flora + C. difficile resistance to clindamycin leads to overgrowth and pseudomembranous colitis • <u>IV</u>: thrombophlebitis, metallic taste • <u>Topical</u>: allergic contact dermatitis • <u>Vaginal</u>: vaginal candidiasis, pruritus, vaginitis

Chloramphenicol

Formulary	• Oral • Ophthalmic • IV
Mechanism of Action	• Bacteriostatic antibiotic that **inhibits bacterial protein synthesis by binding to the 50S subunit of the bacterial ribosome** which prevents the addition of amino acids to the growing peptide chain, thereby interfering with bacterial protein production
Spectrum of Coverage	• **Broad spectrum of activity** • **Good coverage against gram-positive and gram-negative bacteria, anaerobes and other** (*Rickettsia rickettsii*)
Indications	• **Rocky Mountain spotted fever (*Rickettsia rickettsii*) during pregnancy** • **Severe anaerobic infections** (reserved due to high incidence of toxicity)
Contra-indications	• **Known allergy or hypersensitivity** • **History of bone marrow suppression**
Side Effects	• <u>Bone Marrow Suppression</u>: which may lead to anemia (**aplastic**, reversible, hemolytic), leukopenia, leukemia, and thrombocytopenia • <u>Allergic Reactions</u>: range from mild skin rash and pruritus to severe anaphylactic reactions • <u>Gastrointestinal Upset</u>: nausea, vomiting, diarrhea, abdominal pain • <u>Gray Baby Syndrome</u>: secondary to abnormal mitochondrial activity in neonates leads to gray skin, cyanosis, abdominal distention, hypotension • <u>Cytochrome P-450 Inhibition</u>: many drug-drug interactions; may increase levels of warfarin, phenytoin, chlorpropamide, digoxin, theophylline, carbamazepine, statins

Aminoglycosides

Formulary	• **Gentamicin** (oral, topical, ophthalmic, otic, IM, IV) • **Tobramycin** (ophthalmic, IM, IV) • **Neomycin** (oral, topical) • **Streptomycin** (IM, IV)
Mechanism of Action	• Bactericidal antibiotic that **inhibits bacterial protein synthesis by irreversibly binding to the 30S subunit of the bacterial ribosome** which disrupts the formation of the initiation complex and causes misreading of the genetic code leading to the production of faulty proteins and bacterial cell death

Spectrum of Coverage	• **Gram-negative aerobic bacilli**
	   • *Enterobacteriaceae* (such as *Escherichia coli* and *Klebsiella pneumoniae*), *Pseudomonas aeruginosa,* and other bacteria (*Acinetobacter* spp.)
	• **Limited activity against gram-positive bacteria**
	   • **Synergistic effect when combined with beta-lactam antibiotic or vancomycin**

Indications	• <u>Gentamicin</u>: hospital-acquired pneumonia, gram-negative bacteremia, genitourinary infections, septic shock, neonatal meningitis (used with ampicillin) • <u>Tobramycin</u>: increased activity against *Pseudomonas* • <u>Neomycin</u>: skin and wound infections (topical preparation for minor skin injuries, abrasions, lacerations, burns) • <u>Streptomycin</u>: *Tuberculosis, Yersinia* infections
Contra-indications	• **Known allergy or hypersensitivity** • **Renal insufficiency**
Side Effects	• <u>Nephrotoxicity</u>: acute tubular necrosis • <u>Ototoxicity</u>: vestibular and cochlear impairment; especially with use with other ototoxic medications (cisplatin, furosemide, bumetanide, high-dose NSAIDs) • <u>Neuromuscular Paralysis</u>: increased muscular weakness seen in patients with myasthenia gravis • <u>Allergic Reactions</u>: range from mild skin rash and pruritus to severe anaphylactic reactions • <u>Gastrointestinal Upset</u>: **most common adverse reaction**; nausea, vomiting, diarrhea, abdominal pain • <u>IV</u>: thrombophlebitis • <u>Topical</u>: allergic contact dermatitis • <u>Vaginal</u>: vaginal candidiasis, pruritus, vaginitis

Linezolid

Formulary	• Oral • IV
Mechanism of Action	• Oxazolidinone antibiotic that **inhibits bacterial protein synthesis by specifically targeting the 23S rRNA of the 50S subunit of the bacterial ribosome** which prevents the formation of the initiation complex and blocks the production of bacterial proteins resulting in impaired bacterial growth • **Bacteriostatic against *Staphylococcus* and *Enterococci*** • **Bactericidal against *Streptococcus* and *Clostridium perfringens***

Spectrum of Coverage	• **Gram-positive bacteria**
	   • Methicillin-resistant *Staphylococcus aureus* (MRSA), vancomycin-resistant *Enterococcus* (VRE), *Streptococcus pneumoniae*, and other streptococcal species
	• Gram-negative bacteria
	   • Minimal coverage
	• **Atypicals**
	   • *Mycoplasma, Chlamydia, Legionella*

Indications	• **Complicated skin and soft tissue infections** • **Nosocomial and community-acquired pneumonia** • **Infections caused by multi-drug resistant organisms** (MRSA and VRE)
Contra-indications	• **Known allergy or hypersensitivity** • **Current or recent (within 2 weeks of discontinuing) any monoamine oxidase inhibitors (MAOIs) due to the risk of serotonin syndrome**
Side Effects	• <u>Allergic Reactions</u>: range from mild skin rash and pruritus to severe anaphylactic reactions • <u>Gastrointestinal Upset</u>: **most common adverse reaction**; nausea, vomiting, diarrhea, abdominal pain • <u>Myelosuppression</u>: thrombocytopenia, anemia, and leukopenia (especially with treatment duration >2 weeks) • <u>Neurologic</u>: may cause irreversible nerve damage (peripheral neuropathy) • <u>Serotonin Syndrome</u>: risk of serotonin syndrome if used in combination with monoamine oxidase inhibitors (MAOIs) or selective serotonin reuptake inhibitors (SSRIs) and serotonin-norepinephrine reuptake inhibitors (SNRIs)

Metronidazole

Formulary	• Oral • Topical • Vaginal • IV
Mechanism of Action	• Nitroimidazole antibiotic that exerts its antimicrobial activity through **disruption of the DNA helical structure and inhibition of DNA synthesis** in susceptible microorganisms • Medication is selectively taken up by anaerobic bacteria and protozoa, where it undergoes reduction and forms toxic metabolites that damage the microbial DNA, leading to cell death

Spectrum of Coverage	• **Anaerobic bacteria**
	  • *Bacteroides fragilis, Clostridium difficile, Gardnerella vaginalis,* some *Fusobacterium* spp.
	• **Protozoa**
	  • *Entamoeba histolytica, Giardia lamblia, Trichomonas vaginalis., Helicobacter pylori*

Indications	• Intra-abdominal infections • Gynecologic infections (vaginitis, vaginosis, pelvic inflammatory disease) • Gastrointestinal infections (pseudomembranous colitis, parasitic diarrhea [giardiasis, amoebiasis], peptic ulcers caused by *H. pylori*)
Contra-indications	• **Known allergy or hypersensitivity** • History of blood dyscrasias or central nervous system disorders
Side Effects	• <u>**Disulfiram-Like Reaction: if used with alcohol (acetaldehyde accumulation)**</u> • <u>**Allergic Reactions**</u>: range from mild skin rash and pruritus to severe anaphylactic reactions • <u>**Gastrointestinal Upset**</u>: nausea, vomiting, diarrhea, abdominal pain, metallic taste in mouth • <u>Neurotoxicity:</u> may cause peripheral neuropathy, headache, encephalopathy, dizziness

Daptomycin

Formulary	• IV
Mechanism of Action	• Cyclic lipopeptide antibiotic that exerts its function by disrupting bacterial cell membrane function by binding to the bacterial cell membrane causing depolarization and rapid loss of membrane potential • Rapid loss of membrane potential leads to the inhibition of protein, DNA, and RNA synthesis, ultimately resulting in bacterial cell death

Spectrum of Coverage	• **Gram-positive bacteria**
	  • **Methicillin-resistant** *Staphylococcus aureus* (MRSA), **vancomycin-resistant** *Enterococcus* (VRE), and *Streptococcus* spp.
	• Gram-negative bacteria
	  • Ineffective

Indications	• **Complicated skin and soft tissue infections** (caused by multi-drug resistant gram-positive bacteria) • **Bacteremia** • **Infective endocarditis**
Contra-indications	• **Known allergy or hypersensitivity** • **Pneumonia treatment** (inactivated by pulmonary surfactant and is not effective in the lung tissues) • **Statin therapy** (increases muscle toxicity risk)
Side Effects	• <u>**Myopathy**</u>: muscle toxicity secondary to increases in creatine phosphokinase (CPK) and risk of rhabdomyolysis • <u>**Allergic Reactions**</u>: range from mild skin rash and pruritus to severe anaphylactic reactions • <u>**Gastrointestinal Upset**</u>: nausea, vomiting, diarrhea, abdominal pain • <u>**Other**</u>: arthralgias, headache, eosinophilic pneumonia

Trimethoprim-Sulfamethoxazole

Formulary	• Oral IV
Mechanism of Action	• <u>Trimethoprim</u>: inhibits bacterial dihydrofolate reductase • <u>Sulfamethoxazole</u>: inhibits bacterial dihydropteroate synthetase • Together, they inhibit two sequential steps in the synthesis of folic acid (**folic acid antagonism**), an essential component for bacterial growth and replication

Spectrum of Coverage	• **Gram-positive bacteria**
	   • *Staphylococcus aureus* (second best oral medication for MRSA after linezolid), *Streptococcus pneumoniae*
	   • **Not active against group A *Streptococcus***
	• **Gram-negative bacteria**
	   • *Escherichia coli*, *Klebsiella* spp., and *Enterobacter* spp.
	• **Opportunistic bacteria**
	   • *Pneumocystis jirovecii* (formerly known as *Pneumocystis carinii*)

Indications	• **Skin and soft tissue infections (including MRSA)** • **Urinary tract infections** • **Respiratory tract infections** (acute exacerbations of chronic bronchitis) • *Pneumocystis pneumonia* (PCP) in immunocompromised individuals • Traveler's diarrhea
Contra-indications	• **Known allergy or hypersensitivity (sulfa component)** • **Pregnancy, nursing mothers and neonates <6 weeks old** • Severe liver or kidney dysfunction • Folate deficiency
Side Effects	• <u>**Allergic Reactions**</u>: range from mild skin rash and pruritus to severe anaphylactic reactions • May include severe allergic reactions (such as **Stevens-Johnson syndrome** or toxic epidermal necrolysis) • <u>**Gastrointestinal Upset**</u>: nausea, vomiting, diarrhea, abdominal pain, loss of appetite • <u>**Hematologic Abnormalities**</u>: hemolytic anemia (with G6PD deficiency), folic acid inhibition, hyperkalemia • <u>Other</u>: fatigue, dizziness, tinnitus

Nitrofurantoin

Formulary	• Oral
Mechanism of Action	• Bactericidal medication that exerts its effects by damaging bacterial DNA, RNA, protein and various enzymes involved in bacterial cell wall synthesis • Interference with bacterial metabolism which disrupts essential cellular processes, leading to bacterial cell death • Excreted in the urine where the active metabolites can address multiple bacterial sites

Spectrum of Coverage	• **Gram positive bacteria**
	   • **Staphylococcus saprophyticus**
	   • **Limited activity against gram-positives**
	• **Gram-negative**
	   • *Escherichia coli, Klebsiella species, Enterobacter* spp.
	   • Less effective against other gram-negatives
	   • Not effective against *Proteus* or *Pseudomonas* spp.

Indications	• **Urinary tract infections** (including cystitis and asymptomatic bacteriuria) • **Safe in pregnancy** (except at term between 38-42 weeks' gestation or during active labor)
Contra-indications	• **Known allergy or hypersensitivity (sulfa component)** • **Caution or avoided in patients with renal impairment** (creatinine clearance <60mL/min) due to the risk of drug accumulation and potential for toxicity • **Pregnant women at term** between 38-42 week's gestation or during active labor (risk of hemolytic anemia secondary to immature erythrocyte enzyme systems)
Side Effects	• <u>**Allergic Reactions**</u>: range from mild skin rash and pruritus to severe anaphylactic reactions • <u>**Gastrointestinal Upset**</u>: nausea, vomiting, diarrhea, abdominal pain, hepatotoxicity, loss of appetite • <u>**Pulmonary Toxicity**</u>: hypersensitivity pneumonitis, chronic pulmonary fibrosis (especially if >65 years old) • <u>Neurotoxicity</u>: peripheral neuropathy, headache

Fluoroquinolones

	Second-Generation Increased activity against aerobic gram-negative bacteria		Third-Generation Increased activity against gram-positive and atypical bacteria	
	Ciprofloxacin	**Ofloxacin**	**Levofloxacin**	**Moxifloxacin**
Formulary	• Oral, ophthalmic, IV	• Oral, ophthalmic, IV	• Oral, ophthalmic, IV	• Oral, ophthalmic, IV
Spectrum of Coverage	• *Best Gram-negative coverage* • **Pseudomonas, enteric organisms** • *Salmonella* spp., *Campylobacter* spp., *Shigella* spp., *Clostridium difficile* and certain strains of *Escherichia coli*), *Neisseria* spp. *Haemophilus influenzae*	• **Enhanced coverage against gram-positive bacteria** • Additional coverage against *Staphylococcus* spp. and *Streptococcus* spp.	• Enhanced coverage against gram-positive bacteria • Additional coverage against *Streptococcus pneumoniae*	• Best gram-positive, atypical, and anaerobe coverage of the fluoroquinolones
Mechanism of Action	• **Inhibition of bacterial enzymes (DNA gyrase and topoisomerase IV)** which are essential for DNA replication, repair, and transcription and result in DNA fragmentation • DNA Gyrase Inhibition: removes excess positive supercoiling in the DNA helix (primary target for gram-negative bacteria) • Topoisomerase IV Inhibition: inhibits cell division by inhibition topoisomerase IV which is necessary to separate bacterial DNA			
Indications	• **Urinary tract infections (prostatitis, pyelonephritis,** complicated cases) • **Gastrointestinal infections** (infectious diarrhea, Typhoid, intra-abdominal) • **Skin and soft tissue infections** • **Bone and joint infections** • **Meningitis prophylaxis** • **Sexually transmitted infections**	• Same as ciprofloxacin + **acute exacerbation of chronic bronchitis, community acquired pneumonia**	• **Respiratory tract infections (community acquired pneumonia, sinusitis)**	• **Intra-abdominal infections** • **Respiratory tract infections** • **Ocular infections** • **Skin and soft tissue infections**
Contra-indications	• **Known allergy or hypersensitivity** • **High-impact athletes due to risk of tendon rupture** • Children and pregnant women due to potential adverse effects on bone and cartilage development			
Side Effects	• <u>Allergic Reactions</u>: range from mild skin rash and pruritus to severe anaphylactic reactions • <u>Gastrointestinal Upset</u>: nausea, vomiting, diarrhea, abdominal pain • <u>Neurological Dysfunction</u>: headache, memory impairment, agitation, peripheral neuropathy, myasthenia gravis exacerbation, dizziness, confusion, hallucinations • <u>Arthropathy</u>: may be associated with tendinitis or tendon rupture in adults • <u>Other</u>: renal or hepatic dysfunction, QT interval prolongation, risk of hyperglycemia or hypoglycemia, aortic aneurysm			

Rheumatic Fever

Etiology & Risk Factors	• **Nonsuppurative, acute, autoimmune inflammatory, multi-systemic complication of group A streptococcal infection** • <u>Etiology</u>: **group A streptococcal pharyngitis infection** (specifically *Streptococcus pyogenes*) • <u>Risk Factors</u>: **age (5-15 years old most common), inadequately treated streptococcal infection,** genetic predisposition, low-socioeconomic status
Patho-physiology	• Autoimmune response triggered by a prior infection with Group A Streptococcus bacteria which contain antigens that resemble proteins found in various tissues of the body, particularly the heart, joints, and central nervous system • The immune system inappropriately targets these tissues, leading to inflammation and tissue damage (carditis, arthritis, neurological involvement)

Signs & Symptoms	• <u>Migratory Polyarthritis</u>: **most common symptom**
	   • Arthritis appears in one or more joints, resolves, then appears again in another joint
	   • **Medium/large joints most commonly affected** (knees, ankles, elbows and wrist most common, hips, shoulders, and feet may be affected)
	   • **Erythematous, warm, painful joints with effusion**
	• <u>Carditis</u>:
	   • **High fever, chest pain**
	   • **Pancarditis** (involves the endocardium, myocardium, and pericardium) **with valvulitis** (especially aortic and mitral valves)
	   • **Pericardial rub, murmurs, cardiac enlargement, or heart failure**
	     • <u>Mitral Regurgitation</u>: apical pansystolic blowing murmur radiating to the axilla
	     • <u>Aortic Regurgitation</u>: soft diastolic blowing murmur at the left sternal border
	• <u>Sydenham's Chorea</u>: insidious onset (1-8 months after initial infection)
	   • Sudden, irregular involuntary, jerky movements beginning with the hands then becomes generalized, involving the feet and face
	   • May be preceded by inappropriate laughing or crying
	• <u>Cutaneous Features</u>:
	   • <u>Erythema Marginatum</u>: serpiginous, flat or slightly raised, nonscarring, erythematous, painless macules with sharply demarcated borders of the trunk and proximal extremities (spares the face)
	   • <u>Subcutaneous Nodules</u>: firm, painless nodules; most common on the extensor surfaces of large joints (knees, elbows, wrists), scalp, spinal column
	• <u>Other</u>: abdominal pain, fever, anorexia, malaise, facial tics/grimaces, epistaxis

Diagnosis	• <u>Modified Jones Criteria</u>: 2 major or 1 major + 2 minor
	   • <u>Major Criteria</u>: carditis, migratory polyarthritis, Sydenham's chorea, erythema marginatum, subcutaneous nodules
	   • <u>Minor Criteria</u>: fever, arthralgia, history of rheumatic fever, prolonged PR interval, elevated ESR/CRP
	   • <u>Supporting Evidence of Recent Group A Streptococcal Infection</u>: positive throat culture, positive rapid GAS test or elevated streptococcal antibody titers

Treatment	• <u>Antibiotics</u>: **penicillin G is antibiotic of choice**; oral penicillin V or amoxicillin for 10 days; erythromycin if penicillin allergic • <u>Aspirin</u>: indicated for arthralgia and mild carditis (high-dose aspirin for 2-4 weeks followed by taper over following 4 weeks) • <u>Corticosteroids</u>: prednisone for 2-4 weeks followed by taper indicated for moderate to severe carditis • <u>Haloperidol</u>: consider for cases of chorea

Erythema Marginatum

Scarlet Fever

Etiology & Risk Factors	• Diffuse, blanching, papular skin eruption occurring as a result of group A *Streptococcus* infection • Etiology: group A *Streptococcus* infection (*Streptococcus pyogenes*) • Risk Factors: age (**5-15 years old most common**; uncommon before age 3), previous streptococcal pharyngitis infection, crowded environment (schools, daycare centers, households with multiple people), poor hygiene, immunocompromised, lack of immunity (no previous exposures), seasonal (fall and winter most common)
Patho-physiology	• Group A *Streptococcus* bacteria produces a toxin (erythrogenic toxin) which causes dilation and increased permeability of blood vessels leading to a local inflammatory response which produces the characteristic red, flushed appearance of the skin

Signs & Symptoms	• Prodrome: fever, chills, sore throat, headache, abdominal pain followed by rash 1-2 days later
	• Enanthem: mucosal membrane involvement
	   • **Tonsillar/pharyngeal erythema with exudate**
	   • Exudate of tongue followed by erythema (**"strawberry tongue"**)
	   • Petechial lesions of soft palate
	• Exanthem: cutaneous rash
	   • **Begins 1-2 days after prodrome**
	   • **Multiple small (1-2mm), finely punctate, erythematous papules with a sandpaper texture that blanch with pressure**
	   • **Starts on neck, axillae, groin then spreads to trunk and extremities**
	   • May have flushed face with circumoral pallor
	   • Pastia Lines: linear petechial lesions on pressure points of the axillary, antecubital, abdominal or inguinal areas

Diagnosis	• **Clinical Diagnosis** • **Rapid Antigen Test: best initial test**; high specificity, low sensitivity • **Throat Culture: gold-standard**; confirmatory test; should be obtained if antigen test negative

Treatment	• Antibiotics: indicated to reduce risk of rheumatic fever and nephritis
	   • **Penicillin G or V; Amoxicillin: first-line and treatment of choice**
	   • Macrolides: **azithromycin indicated if penicillin-allergic**
	   • Cephalosporins: cephalexin, cefdinir alternatives if refractory to penicillins or macrolides and no anaphylactic allergy to penicillins
	• *Children may return to school/daycare 24 hours after initiation of antibiotics*

Key Words & Most Common	• Diffuse skin eruption that occurs as a result of group a Streptococcus infection (*Streptococcus pyogenes*) • Prodrome of fever, sore throat, abdominal pain, headache → small, erythematous papules with sandpaper texture that blanc with pressure • Starts on neck, axillae → spreads to trunk/extremities • Clinical diagnosis + GAS antigen or throat culture to confirm • Penicillin/Amoxicillin first-line → azithromycin if penicillin allergic

"Sandpaper-Like" erythematous rash

Septic Arthritis

Etiology & Risk Factors	• Inflammation of a joint secondary to infectious etiology (bacteria most common) that constitutes an orthopedic emergency • **Knee is most common joint affected in adults and older children. Hip is most common joint affected in younger children;** sternoclavicular and sacroiliac joint in IVDU • Etiology: **direct penetration** (surgery, trauma, bites), infection extension (osteomyelitis, adjacent abscess), hematogenous spread • Risk Factors: **advanced age, immunosuppression, prosthetic joint implant, trauma,** chronic arthropathy (gout, RA, OA), **diabetes,** sickle cell disease,

Patho-physiology	• Bacterial inoculation of the synovium lead to joint destruction mediated by inflammatory cytokines and proteases • Neutrophiles then migrate to joint, phagocytose the organism resulting in lysosomal enzyme release which damages the cartilage, synovium, and ligaments	**Organisms** • *Staphylococcus aureus*: most common organism; MRSA seen with IVDU • *Staphylococcus epidermis*: prosthetic joint implant • *Streptococcal* spp: 2nd most common organism; more common in young kids/neonates • *Neisseria gonorrhoeae*: sexually active young adults • *Pseudomonas* spp: immunocompromised; trauma/puncture wounds; IVDU • *Salmonella*: sickle cell disease

Signs & Symptoms	• Constitutional Symptoms: **fever,** chills, malaise/fatigue, diaphoresis, myalgias, tachycardia • Local Symptoms: **swollen, warm, erythematous, painful joint; limited ROM** with active and passive movement,

Diagnosis	• **Arthrocentesis with Synovial Fluid Analysis: most useful and accurate test**; culture, Gram stain, crystals analysis, white blood cell count with differential
	   • **WBC >50,000** (90% neutrophil predominance); WBC>1,100 considered positive in prosthetic joints
	• **Elevated ESR and CRP** (nonspecific)
	• Blood cultures
	   • If Neisseria suspected, cultures from the cervix, rectum, and/or throat.
	• X-Ray: nonspecific; joint space widening, soft tissue bulging, or subchondral bony change

Treatment	• Antibiotics: empiric treatment followed by guided therapy based on culture results • Empiric: **Vancomycin (preferred)** or Nafcillin or Oxacillin **PLUS** 3rd **generation cephalosporin** (cefepime or ceftazidime or **cefotaxime; ceftriaxone**) • Surgery: open surgical debridement vs arthroscopic irrigation
Key Words & Most Common	• Knee most common in adults/older children; hip most common in young children • S.. Aureus most common organism; S. epidermis most common with prosthetic joint • Fever + warm/swollen/erythematous joint • Synovial fluid analysis (WBC>50k); elevated ESR/CRP • Antibiotics (Vanco + cephalosporin) +/- surgical drainage or irrigation

Urethritis

Etiology & Risk Factors	• Lower urinary tract infection causing inflammation of the urethra
	• Etiology:
	  • ***Chlamydia trachomatis*: most common cause**; 5-8 day incubation period
	  • ***Neisseria gonorrhea***: abrupt onset; 3-4 day incubation period
	  • Other Infectious: *Trichomonas vaginalis, Ureaplasma urealyticum, Mycoplasma genitalium*, Herpes Simplex virus, *Treponema pallidum, Candida*
	  • Other Non-Infectious: trauma, irritation (friction from clothing or sex, physical activity such as biking, soaps, detergents, lotions)
	• Risk Factors: male, age (young adults most common), **unprotected sexual intercourse, multiple sexual partners**

Patho-physiology	• Bacterial infection of the lower urinary tract causes inflammation of the urethra; most commonly transmitted via unprotected sexual intercourse

Signs & Symptoms	• **Commonly asymptomatic**
	• **Urethral discharge**
	  • ***Chlamydia trachomatis***: tends to be more mucoid or thin/watery discharge; 5-8 day incubation period
	  • ***Neisseria gonorrhea***: purulent or mucopurulent discharge; 3-4 day incubation period
	• **Dysuria**
	• **Penile or vaginal pruritus**

Diagnosis	• **Clinical Diagnosis**
	• **Nucleic Acid Amplification Test: most sensitive and specific test**; first-catch urine or urethral swab
	• **Gram Stain Test**: >2 WBC/hpf on gram stain
	  • ***Chlamydia trachomatis***: no organisms generally seen on Gram stain (organism is a small, gram-negative obligate intracellular parasitic bacteria)
	  • ***Neisseria gonorrhea*: gram-negative diplococci** bacteria on Gram stain
	• Urinalysis: suspect with positive leukocyte esterase or >10 WBCs/hpf (pyuria) on microscopy
	  • Suspect *Chlamydia* in a young, sexually active female patient with pyuria and no bacteriuria

Treatment	• Coinfection of *Gonorrhea* and *Chlamydia* is common; empiric treatment of <u>both</u> is recommended if one entity suspected and/or test results are not available
	• ***Chlamydia trachomatis*: doxycycline 100mg BID for 7 days**
	  • Azithromycin 1g oral (single dose) if pregnant
	• ***Neisseria gonorrhea*: ceftriaxone 500mg IM**; (1g if weight >150kg)
	  • Gentamicin 240mg IM + Azithromycin 2g oral (single dose) if ceftriaxone contraindicated (anaphylaxis to penicillins or cephalosporin allergy)

Key Words & Most Common	• *Chlamydia trachomatis* is most common cause; *Neisseria gonorrhea* is second most common cause • Asymptomatic → urethral discharge + dysuria in sexually active patient • NAAT is most sensitive and specific test • Empiric treatment with doxycycline 100mg BID for 7 days (*Chlamydia*) and ceftriaxone 500mg IM (*Gonorrhea*)

Lymphogranuloma Venereum

Etiology & Risk Factors	• Ulcerative sexually transmitted infection of the genital area • Etiology: **serovars L1, L2, and L3 of *Chlamydia trachomatis*** • Risk Factors: **unprotected sexual contact, multiple sexual partners, high-risk sexual behavior** (unprotected anal intercourse, rough sexual activity that may cause tissue damage, engaging in sex work), men who have sex with men (MSM), tropical and sub-tropical climates
Patho-physiology	• After sexual transmission, the bacterium infects the epithelial cells of the genital or rectal mucosa and invades the regional lymph nodes through the lymphatic system leading to lymphadenopathy, lymphatic obstruction, and subsequent granulomatous inflammation

Signs & Symptoms	• **1st Stage**: approximately 3 day incubation period
	  • Small, painless genital ulcer at site of inoculation that often heals quickly
	• **2nd Stage**: begins after about 2-4 weeks
	  • **Painful inguinal and/or femoral lymphadenopathy** that may enlarge forming large, tender, fluctuant masses or abscesses (**buboes**)
	  • Buboes may adhere to deeper tissues, causing the overlying skin to become inflamed
	• **3rd Stage**:
	  • Lesions heal with scarring; untreated infection may lead to lymphatic obstruction
	  • *Individuals who engage in receptive anal sex may develop proctocolitis (rectal discharge, constipation, anal pain, tenesmus)*

Diagnosis	• **Clinical Diagnosis** • Antibody Detection: antibodies to chlamydial endotoxin or genotyping using a polymerase chain reaction-based NAAT
Treatment	• **Doxycycline: 100mg BID for 21 days is treatment of choice** • **Erythromycin**: 500mg QID for 21 days is preferred treatment for pregnant and lactating females • Azithromycin: 1g weekly for 3 weeks is an alternative for pregnant women • Treat Sexual Partner: doxycycline 100mg BID for 7 days or azithromycin 1g single dose • Nodal Aspiration: may be indicated for symptomatic relief of fluctuant or pus-filled buboes; I&D is not recommended as it can delay the healing process
Key Words & Most Common	• Ulcerative STI of the genital area caused by Chlamydia trachomatis L1, L2 and L3 • 1st Stage: small, painless ulcer • 2nd Stage: painful inguinal lymphadenopathy + fluctuant masses (buboes) • 3rd Stage: healing with scarring + proctocolitis • Doxycycline is treatment of choice

Chancroid

Etiology & Risk Factors	• **Rare sexually transmitted infection of the genital skin or mucous membranes causing genital ulcers, lymphadenopathy and bubo formation** • <u>Etiology</u>: *Haemophilus ducreyi*; gram-negative fastidious coccobacillus • <u>Risk Factors</u>: male, age (young adults most common), **unprotected sexual intercourse**, multiple sexual partners, immunocompromised, certain areas (Asia, Africa, Caribbean)
Patho-physiology	• Break in the skin allows bacterial transmission through sexual contact; bacteria invades the epithelial cells of the genital mucosa, leading to the formation of painful ulcers • The bacteria release various virulence factors, including enzymes and toxins, contributing to tissue damage and inflammation
Signs & Symptoms	• 3-7 day incubation period • **Small, painful papules occur at the inoculation site** • **Papules rapidly break down into shallow, soft, painful ulcers with ragged, undermined edges and an erythematous border** • **Painful inguinal lymphadenopathy**; may form a bubo (enlarged and tender group of regional lymph nodes)
Diagnosis	• **Clinical Diagnosis** • <u>Polymerase Chain Reaction (PCR)</u>: may be used for indeterminant cases • <u>Serologic Testing</u>: syphilis, HIV and HSV testing to rule out other causes of genital ulcers

Treatment	• <u>Aspiration or Incision and Drainage</u>: may be indicated for symptomatic relief of large/painful bubos
	• **Antibiotics**:
	   • **Azithromycin 1g oral as a single dose**
	   • **Ceftriaxone 250mg IM as a single dose**
	   • Erythromycin 500mg three times daily for 1 week
	   • Ciprofloxacin 500mg twice daily for 3 days

Key Words & Most Common	• Sexually transmitted infection caused by *Haemophilus ducreyi* • Genital ulcers with ragged, erythematous borders • Painful inguinal lymphadenopathy • Clinical diagnosis • Azithromycin 1g oral or ceftriaxone 250mg IM

Trichomoniasis

Etiology & Risk Factors	• Sexually transmitted infection caused by a flagellated protozoan that may infect the male or female genital tract • <u>Etiology</u>: *Trichomonas vaginalis*; a flagellated protozoan • <u>Risk Factors</u>: history of STIs, **multiple or new sex partners or a partner who does not use a condom**, contact with infected sexual partner, IV drug abuse,	
Patho-physiology	• *Trichomonas vaginalis* is a flagellated protozoan that resides urogenital tract lumen and releases cytotoxic proteins that disrupt the epithelial lining; may increase vaginal pH	
	Women	**Men**

Signs & Symptoms	• **Copious, yellow/green, frothy, malodourous vaginal discharge**
	• **Soreness of vulva or perineum**
	• Dyspareunia, dysuria, urinary frequency
	• <u>Physical Exam</u>:
	   • **Copious yellow/green, frothy malodourous vaginal discharge**, vulvovaginal erythema, **cervical petechiae** ("strawberry cervix")
		• **Mostly asymptomatic**
		• **Urethritis**; epididymitis and prostatitis are rare complications
		• <u>Physical Exam</u>:
		   • Often benign; may have moisture at urethral meatus

Diagnosis	• <u>Microscopic Examination</u>: saline wet mount of vaginal secretions demonstrates **trichomonads (motile protozoan with flagella), numerous neutrophils, vaginal pH >4.5** • <u>Nucleic Acid Amplification Test (NAAT)</u>: more sensitive than microscopic examination or culture for diagnosis • <u>Urine or Urethral Swab Culture</u>: only validated test for detecting *T. vaginalis* in men	

Treatment	• <u>Sexual Education</u>: encourage safe-sex behavior with barrier contraceptives
	• <u>Antibiotics</u>: exposed sexual partners must be treated
	   • **Metronidazole: treatment of choice**; oral 500mg BID for 7 days (women) or 2g one time dose (men or pregnant women)
	   • <u>Tinidazole</u>: 2g one time dose is an alternative
	   • *Topical medications have high failure rates and should not be used*
	• NAAT test of cure recommended for all women treated within three months of treatment	

Key Words & Most Common	• *Trichomonas vaginalis* is a flagellated, sexually transmitted protozoan
	• <u>Women</u>: copious, yellow/green, frothy vaginal discharge +/- cervical petechiae ("strawberry cervix")
	• <u>Men</u>: mostly asymptomatic; may develop urethritis
	• Microscopic exam with saline wet mount shows motile flagellated protozoan
	• NAAT is more sensitive; urine/urethral swab culture for men
	• Oral metronidazole is treatment of choice
	   • 500mg BID for 1 days for women
	   • 2g one time dose for men or pregnant women	

Syphilis

Etiology & Risk Factors	• Systemic, bacterial infection characterized by 3 sequential symptomatic stages separated by asymptomatic latent periods • <u>Etiology</u>: *Treponema pallidum*; a spirochetal (spiral-shaped) bacterium • <u>Risk Factors</u>: males, **men who have sex with men (MSM), unprotected sexual activity, high-risk sexual behavior**, substance abuse, low socioeconomic status • <u>Transmission</u>: **sexual contact (vaginal, anal, oral)**, skin-to-skin (open wound/sore), blood transfer (blood transfusion or needle sharing), transplacental vertical transmission
Patho-physiology	• Bacteria enters the body through direct contact of a mucocutaneous lesions and can disseminate through the bloodstream to various organs; the immune response to the infection leads to the characteristic manifestations of syphilis

Signs & Symptoms	• <u>Primary Syphilis</u>: appears 10-90 days after exposure
	  • **Chancre**: erythematous papules that progresses to a painless ulcer with indurated edges, develops at or near the inoculation site and resolves without treatment within 3-4 weeks
	  • **Regional Lymphadenopathy**: nontender, rubbery lymphadenopathy near chancre
	• <u>Secondary Syphilis</u>: appears 2-8 weeks after chancre resolves
	  • **Systemic Symptoms**: fever, lymphadenopathy, anorexia, fatigue, arthritis, headache (meningitis), hearing loss (otitis), nausea, vestibular symptoms (labyrinthitis), visual disturbances (uveitis, retinitis), bone pain (periostitis)
	  • **Syphilitic Dermatitis**: diffuse, symmetric, maculopapular lesions that commonly involve the palms and soles
	  • **Condyloma Lata**: highly contagious, hypertrophic, flattened, pinkish-gray papules involving mucous membranes and moist areas (groin, perineum, inframammary)
	• <u>Tertiary Syphilis</u>: may occur years to decades after initial infection
	  • **Gumma**: noncancerous soft, destructive, inflammatory granulomatous masses on skin, bones, and/or internal organs
	  • **Cardiovascular**: aneurysmal dilation of ascending aorta, aortic regurgitation, coronary artery narrowing
	  • **Neurosyphilis**: several forms
	    • **Meningovascular**: headache, neck stiffness, dizziness, blurred vision, behavioral abnormalities, memory loss, inability to concentrate, insomnia
	    • **Parenchymatous: mimics mental disorder or dementia**; irritability, memory deterioration, impaired judgment, headaches, insomnia, fatigue, lethargy
	    • **Tabes Dorsalis**: demyelination of dorsal columns; stabbing back and leg pain with loss of vibratory sense, proprioception, and reflexes
	    • **Argyll-Robertson Pupil**: pupils that constrict with accommodation for near vision but do not respond to light

Diagnosis	• <u>Serologic Non-Treponemal Reaginic Tests (screening)</u>: rapid plasma reagin (RPR) or Venereal Disease Research Laboratory (VDRL) testing utilized for screening • <u>Serologic Treponemal Tests (confirmatory)</u>: fluorescent treponemal antibody absorption (FTA-ABS) or microhemagglutination assay for antibodies to *T. pallidum* • <u>Darkfield Microscopy</u>: most sensitive and specific test for primary syphilis; allows for direct visualization of spirochetes in chancre exudate or lymph node aspirate sample

Treatment	• <u>Benzathine Penicillin G</u>: **treatment of choice for all stages**
	  • **Early (primary, secondary or early latent)**: 2.4 million units IM given as a single dose; *doxycycline BID for 14 days is alternative if penicillin allergic*
	  • **Late (tertiary or late latent)**: 2.4 million units IM once weekly for 3 weeks
	  • **Neurosyphilis: IV penicillin G**; 3-4 million units every 4 hours for 10-14 days
	• <u>Jarisch-Herxheimer Reaction</u>: acute, self-limiting febrile reaction occurring within the first 24 hours after receiving treatment for spirochetal infection
	  • Fever, chills, rigors, headaches, myalgias, diaphoresis, anxiety, or a temporary exacerbation of the syphilitic lesions

Toxic Shock Syndrome

Etiology & Risk Factors	• Acute onset illness caused by exotoxins produced by *Staphylococcus aureus* or *Streptococcus pyogenes* • <u>Etiology</u>: **toxigenic strain of *Staphylococcus aureus* or Group A Strep (*Streptococcus pyogenes*) is most common cause** • <u>Risk Factors</u>: **use of high absorbency tampons is most common**; soft tissue infections and abscess, burns, post-surgical infection, **retained foreign body (nasal packing, tampon)**, dialysis catheters, intrauterine device (IUD)
Patho-physiology	• Exotoxin-producing *S. aureus* produce superantigens which activates T-cells and causes hyperactivation of cytokines and inflammatory mediators (IL-2, IL-1, TNF) • This over-activation of inflammatory cells causes **capillary leakage**, circulatory collapse, and multi-organ failure

Signs & Symptoms	• **Trio of fever, rash and hypotension**
	• **Fever**: rapid onset fever (>102.2°F)
	• **Rash**: diffuse, blanching, erythroderma (diffusely erythematous macular rash); may resemble a sunburn
	  • **Desquamation of skin (full-thickness peeling) occurs 3-7 days later; involves palms and soles**
	  • May have mucosal involvement with hyperemia of vaginal, oropharyngeal, or conjunctival mucosa
	• **Hypotension**: systolic BP less than 90 mmHg
	• **Multisystem Organ Failure**: renal impairment (elevated BUN/creatinine), coagulopathy, liver impairment (elevated AST/ALT/bilirubin), acute respiratory distress (hypoxemia, diffuse pulmonary infiltrates), soft tissue necrosis, muscular (elevated creatine phosphokinase), CNS (altered mental status, focal neurologic deficits)
	• May have prodrome of fever and chills, nausea and vomiting, myalgias, headache, pharyngitis that progresses

Diagnosis	• **Clinical Diagnosis** • <u>Labs</u>: CBC (may show leukocytosis or leukopenia), CMP, creatine kinase (CK), coagulation studies • **Culture: blood cultures and culture of suspected source (nasal sinus, vagina) should be obtained**

Treatment	• **Local Treatment**: decontamination of infection source; irrigation of surgical incision, debridement of devitalized tissue, irrigation of colonized sites (nasal sinus, vagina), removal of retained foreign body (tampon, nasal packing)
	• **Supportive**: fluid and electrolyte replacement (due to systemic capillary leakage); circulatory, ventilation, and hemodialysis support
	• **Antibiotics**: **clindamycin is preferred antibiotic as it suppresses toxin synthesis**; pending culture results
	  • <u>Group A *Streptococcus*</u>: clindamycin + beta lactam
	  • <u>Methicillin-Susceptible *S. aureus* (MSSA)</u>: clindamycin + oxacillin or nafcillin
	  • <u>Methicillin-Resistant *S. aureus* (MRSA)</u>: vancomycin + clindamycin or linezolid

Key Words & Most Common	• Toxigenic S. aureus or GAS is most common cause; associated with high-absorbency tampon use, wound/burn infection, or retained foreign body (nasal packing, tampon, IUD) • Fever, rash (diffuse, blanching erythroderma with peeling), hypotension • Clinical diagnosis + labs to identify organ involvement + culture • Decontamination + fluid/electrolyte replacement + antibiotics (clindamycin preferred)

Tetanus

Etiology & Risk Factors	• Infection characterized by a state of generalized hypertonia and muscle spasms • Etiology: *Clostridium tetani*; spores found in soil, dust and animal feces • May enter the human body through **puncture wounds, crush injuries**, laceration, skin breaks, insect bites or inoculation with an infected syringe • Risk Factors: **incomplete or absent immunization, deep puncture wounds, poor wound care**, rural environment, intravenous drug use, chronic wounds (diabetic ulcers)
Patho-physiology	• The bacterium *Clostridium tetani* releases a neurotoxin called tetanospasmin which irreversibly binds to motor neurons in the nervous system, inhibiting the release of inhibitory neurotransmitters (GABA and glycine) leading to uncontrolled and sustained muscle contractions

Signs & Symptoms	• Incubation period of 2-50 days (5-10 days most common)
	• **Generalized Tetanus: most common form**
	  • **Pain and tingling at the inoculation site**, headache, restlessness, fatigue, hyperirritability followed by drooling, sore throat
	  • **Trismus** (spasm of the masticator muscle group; **"lockjaw") is the most common presenting symptom**
	  • **Muscle spasms exacerbated by minor stimuli** (lights, movement or sudden noise)
	  • **Risus sardonicus** (fixed smile and elevated eyebrows)
	  • **Opisthotonus** (generalized rigidity of the body with arched back and neck)
	  • Apnea secondary to prolonged muscle spasms of respiratory muscles (respiratory failure is most common cause of death)
	  • **Hypersympathetic state** (tachycardia, diaphoresis, hyperpyrexia, hyperreflexia, hypertension, fever)
	• **Neonatal**: often fatal
	  • **Inadequately cleansed umbilical stump in neonates born of inadequately immunized mothers**
	  • Rigidity, spasms, and poor feeding presenting within first 2 weeks of life
	• **Localized**: spasticity of muscles near the entry wound but no trismus; uncommon variant
	• **Cephalic**: form of localized tetanus that affects the cranial nerves (VII most commonly affected); follows injuries to head or otitis media

Diagnosis	• **Clinical Diagnosis**
Treatment	• Respiratory Support: if needed • Wound Care: thorough irrigation and debridement of wound to control source of toxin production • **Management of Muscle Spasms: benzodiazepines (diazepam) can help control seizures, counter muscle rigidity, and induce sedation**; intrathecal baclofen, dantrolene • **Management of Autonomic Dysfunction**: morphine for analgesia and cardiovascular dysfunction; beta blockers (esmolol) for hypertension and tachycardia • **Antibiotics: metronidazole**, doxycycline or penicillin G • **Antitoxin and Toxoid: tetanus immune globulin injected directly into wound and intramuscular**; 3,000-6,000 units IM with adequate mL to wound • **Prophylaxis**: unimmunized adults receive Tdap initially, then Td 4 weeks and 6-12 months later, and Td every 10 years thereafter • Td given for major/dirty wounds if last booster was received >5 years ago • **Prevention**: DTaP (5 doses at 2, 4, 6, 15-18 months and 4-6 years old); **Tdap during *every* pregnancy, preferably at 27 to 36 weeks gestation**

Botulism

Etiology & Risk Factors	• **Diffuse, flaccid paralysis caused by botulinum neurotoxin (BoNT)** • Etiology: *Clostridium botulinum*; anaerobic, gram-positive, spore-forming bacilli • Risk Factors: **home-canned foods, are the most common sources of ingested toxin, ingestion of honey contaminated with spores is most common cause of infantile botulism**, substance abuse (IV drug use), contaminated wound
Patho-physiology	• *Clostridium botulinum* toxin inhibits the release of acetylcholine (neurotransmitter responsible for muscle contraction) at the neuromuscular junction, impairing nerve signal transmission, leading to muscle weakness and flaccid paralysis

Signs & Symptoms	• **Foodborne**: abrupt onset 6-18 hours after ingestion
	  • **Prodromal GI Symptoms**: nausea, vomiting, diarrhea, abdominal pain
	  • **8 D's: Dry mouth, Dysphagia, Dilated, fixed pupils, Dysarthria, Dysphonia, Diplopia, Decreased muscle strength (flaccid paralysis), Decreased deep tendon reflexes**
	  • **Neurological Symptoms**: bilateral and symmetric, start with the cranial nerves and progresses to descending weakness or paralysis
	• **Infantile**: most common form
	  • **Constipation is most common initial symptom followed by neuromuscular paralysis** (begins with cranial nerves and progresses to peripheral and respiratory paralysis)
	  • **Cranial Nerve Deficits**: ptosis, extraocular muscle palsies, lethargy, weak cry, feeding difficulty, decreased gag reflex, pooling of oral secretions, hypotonia ("floppy baby syndrome"), expressionless face
	• Wound: neurological symptoms without prodromal GI symptoms

Diagnosis	• **Clinical Diagnosis** • Toxin Assay: confirms diagnosis by finding *C. botulinum* toxin in serum, wound or stool

Treatment	• **Foodborne/Infantile**:
	  • Supportive: respiratory support (nasogastric intubation preferred)
	  • **Heptavalent Equine-Derived Botulinum Antitoxin: may slow or halt further progression indicated for children >1 years old or adults**
	  • **Human-Derived Botulism Immune Globulin: indicated for infantile botulism**
	  • Antibiotics: contraindicated because they may lyse *C. botulinum* in the gut and increase toxin availability
	• Wound:
	  • Antitoxin + antibiotics (penicillin G is first line) + wound debridement

Key Words & Most Common	• Diffuse, flaccid paralysis caused by *Clostridium botulinum* toxin • Prodromal GI symptoms + flaccid paralysis, dysphagia, dilated pupils, neurological deficits • Constipation → neuromuscular paralysis + CN deficits + hypotonia ("floppy baby syndrome") • Equine-derived botulinum antitoxin if >1 years old • Human-derived botulism immune globulin if <1 year old • No antibiotics in foodborne or infantile cases

Gas Gangrene	**Clostridial Soft-Tissue Infections**	
Etiology & Risk Factors	• **Cellulitis, myositis, and clostridial myonecrosis** (life-threatening muscle infection) • <u>Etiology</u>: ***Clostridium perfringens* is most common cause** • <u>Risk Factors</u>: **trauma** (deep penetrating or crush injuries), **postoperative state** (recent GI or biliary surgery), diabetes, immunocompromised state, vascular disease, substance abuse (IV drug use)	
Patho-physiology	• Severe crushing or penetrating trauma devitalizes tissue and creates an anaerobic condition where Clostridium bacteria can enter and multiply • Clostridium perfringens produces several toxins (alpha-toxin [lecithinase], theta-toxin [perfringolysin O]), and other tissue-damaging enzymes which cause direct damage to the muscle tissue, disrupt the cell membranes, promote tissue necrosis, and lead to the release of additional toxins and bacteria	

Signs & Symptoms	• <u>Cellulitis</u>: localized infection in a superficial wound
	  • Infections spreads along fascial planes with crepitation and abundant gas bubbling
	  • **Bullae present with foul-smelling, serous, brown ("blood-tinged") exudate**
	• <u>Myositis</u>: suppurative infection of muscle without necrosis
	  • **Most commonly associated with IV drug use**
	  • **Edema, pain, and gas within the tissues**
	  • Spreads rapidly and may progress to myonecrosis
	• <u>Myonecrosis</u>: gas gangrene
	  • **Severe pain and tensely edematous**
	  • **Pale wound that progresses to a bronze or red color and progresses to blackish-green discoloration**
	  • **Crepitus (gas) in tissues on palpation**
	  • Patient appears toxic (fever, hypotension, tachycardia, pallor)	

Diagnosis	• **Clinical Diagnosis** • <u>Imaging</u>: **x-rays may show local gas production**; CT and MRI delineate the extent of gas and necrosis • <u>Labs</u>: **culture** or smear of exudates (demonstrates **gram-positive bacilli with few** few polymorphonuclear neutrophils [PMNs]); blood cultures	

Treatment	• <u>Surgical Debridement</u>: rapid and aggressive intervention is required
	  • May require fasciotomy
	• <u>Antibiotics</u>: initiated immediately
	  • **IV penicillin G + IV clindamycin indicated (clindamycin alone is inadequate)**; metronidazole + clindamycin indicated if penicillin allergic
	• <u>Hyperbaric Oxygen Therapy</u>: may be helpful in extensive myonecrosis as a supplement to antibiotics and surgical debridement	

Key Words & Most Common	• Most commonly caused by *Clostridium perfringens* after trauma or surgery • Severe pain and edema + pale wound progressing to bronze/red then black/green + crepitus (gas) in the tissues • Gas evident on x-ray • Surgical debridement + antibiotics (IV penicillin G + clindamycin)	

Rabies

Etiology & Risk Factors	• **Viral encephalitis transmitted by the saliva of infected bats and certain other infected mammals** • Etiology: ***Rhabdoviridae* family of viruses** • <u>Risk Factors</u>: **exposure to infected mammal (bats are most common, raccoons, skunks, foxes, or dogs in developing countries)**, occupational exposure (park ranger, veterinarian, animal handler), lack of access to rabies vaccination programs and inadequate animal control measures
Patho-physiology	• After a bite or scratch from an infected animal, the virus enters the body and replicates in the muscle tissue near the site of entry; the virus then spreads via acetylcholine receptor cellular uptake along peripheral nerve pathways, eventually reaching the central nervous system and causing inflammation of the brain (encephalitis)

Signs & Symptoms	• <u>Prodrome</u>:
	  • **Pain or paresthesia develops at the site of the bite**
	  • Nonspecific flu-like symptoms (fever, headache, and malaise)
	• <u>Encephalitic Form</u>: most common form; "furious" rabies
	  • <u>Encephalitis</u>: restlessness, **hyperexcitability**, confusion, **agitation**, **bizarre behavior**, hallucinations, insomnia, paresthesias, paralysis, autonomic dysfunction
	  • <u>Hydrophobia</u>: **painful spasms of laryngeal and pharyngeal muscles in response to drinking, seeing, or hearing water**
	  • <u>Aerophobia</u>: **spasms of larynx, pharynx or diaphragm in response to air or changes in temperature**
	  • <u>Hypersalivation</u>: **excessive salivation ("foaming at the mouth") with thick sputum**
	• <u>Paralytic Form</u>: "dumb" rabies
	  • **Ascending paralysis** and quadriplegia, altered mental status, **weakness**
	  • **Respiratory muscle paralysis**

Diagnosis	• <u>Skin Biopsy with Fluorescent Antibody Testing</u>: **biopsy specimen of skin from the nape of the neck is the diagnostic test of choice** • <u>Polymerase Chain Reaction (PCR)</u>: performed on cerebrospinal fluid (CSF), saliva, or tissue • <u>Autopsy</u>: immunochemical staining demonstrate virion deposits in the nerve cytoplasm; **Negri bodies** visualized on light microscopy

Treatment	• <u>Wound Care</u>: appropriate wound care has been shown to be almost 100% effective if initiated within three hours of inoculation
	  • Scrub wound and surrounding area with soap and water (20% soap solution, povidone iodine, and/or alcohol solutions) + pressure wash irrigation
	• <u>Supportive</u>: no effective management once symptoms occur as patients rarely survive (death within 3-10 days)
	  • <u>Sedation</u>: ketamine and midazolam given for comfort care
	• <u>Prophylaxis</u>:
	  • <u>Pre-Exposure Prophylaxis</u>: human diploid cell rabies vaccine (HDCV) indicated for high-risk individuals (veterinarians, animal handlers, spelunkers [cave explorer], travelers to endemic areas)
	  • <u>Post-Exposure Prophylaxis</u>:
	    • <u>Rabies Vaccine</u>: given on days 0, 3, 7, and 14; additional 5th dose on day 28 for immunocompromised
	    • <u>Rabies Immune Globulin</u>: half given IM, half infiltrated around the wound for passive immunization

Anthrax

Etiology & Risk Factors	• Etiology: *Bacillus anthracis*; an encapsulated, spore-forming, gram-variable bacilli • Risk Factors: **exposure to infected animals (naturally found in livestock such as cattle, horses, goats, sheep) or animal products (wool, animal hide or hair)**, occupational exposure (farmers, veterinarians), travel to endemic areas (Africa, Asia, and the Middle East)
Patho-physiology	• Bacillus anthracis spores enter the body through inhalation, ingestion, or skin contact where they germinate inside macrophages, migrate to regional lymph nodes and release toxins that cause tissue damage and inflammation; the toxins produced by the bacteria interfere with the immune response and can lead to severe systemic effects

Signs & Symptoms	• **Cutaneous**: forms 1-10 days after exposure
	  • **Painless, pruritic, brawny, erythematous papule at inoculation site that forms a central ulceration and followed by a painless, black eschar**
	  • Vesiculation and induration are present
	  • **Local lymphadenopathy**, malaise, myalgia, headache, fever, nausea, and vomiting
	• **Gastrointestinal**: contracted through ingestion of meat contaminated with spores
	  • Fever, nausea, vomiting, abdominal pain, bloody diarrhea
	• **Oropharyngeal**:
	  • Voise hoarseness, sore throat, fever, dysphagia
	  • Edematous lesions with central necrosis on the tonsils, posterior pharynx, or hard palate
	  • Marked soft-tissue swelling of the neck with cervical lymphadenopathy
	• **Inhalation**: rapidly fatal
	  • Flu-like symptoms followed by worsening fever, dyspnea, hypoxia, severe respiratory distress
	  • Severe hemorrhagic necrotizing lymphadenitis that spreads to mediastinum

Diagnosis	• **Clinical Diagnosis** • **Gram Stain and Culture**: demonstrates encapsulated, gram-positive bacilli • Direct Fluorescent Antibody (DFA) Test and Polymerase Chain Reaction (PCR) Assay: aids in diagnosis • **CXR or Chest CT**: widened mediastinum (hemorrhagic lymphadenitis), infiltrates, pleural effusion, hyperdense mediastinal lymphadenopathy

Treatment	• **Antibiotics**:
	  • **Cutaneous**: fluoroquinolones are first-line **(ciprofloxacin,** levofloxacin, moxifloxacin) for 7-10 days; doxycycline is alternative
	  • **Inhalation**: antibiotic therapy to include ≥2 antibiotics with bactericidal activity and ≥1 should be a protein synthesis inhibitor to block toxin production
	    • **Bactericidal Activity**: **fluoroquinolone (ciprofloxacin,** levofloxacin, moxifloxacin) or carbapenem or vancomycin or penicillin G (to penicillin-susceptible strains)
	    • **Protein Synthesis Inhibitor**: linezolid, clindamycin, rifampin, chloramphenicol; doxycycline is an alternative
	• Pleural Fluid Drainage: supportive care and mechanical ventilation may be indicated for inhalation anthrax; possible continuous pleural fluid drainage by chest tube
	• *Contact CDC Emergency Hotline for all suspected bioterrorism cases*

Diphtheria

Etiology & Risk Factors	• **Acute upper respiratory or cutaneous infection caused by *Corynebacterium diphtheriae*** • Etiology: *Corynebacterium diphtheriae*; gram-positive bacillus • Risk Factors: **inadequate vaccination or lack of immunization**, living in overcrowded or unsanitary conditions, poor hygiene practices, immunocompromised, travel history from endemic regions (South-East Asia, Africa), low socioeconomic status • Transmission: respiratory droplets, nasopharyngeal secretions, contact with infected skin lesions
Patho-physiology	• *Corynebacterium diphtheriae* colonizes the respiratory tract and release a potent exotoxin (diphtheria toxin) which inhibits protein synthesis and damages host tissue resulting in formation of a grayish pseudomembrane in the respiratory tract; affects various organs, particularly the heart, nervous system, and respiratory system

Signs & Symptoms	• **Pharyngeal Infection**:
	  • **Nonspecific Flu-Like Symptoms**: mild sore throat, dysphagia, low-grade fever, tachycardia, **cervical lymphadenopathy**, nausea, vomiting, headache
	  • **Pseudo membrane**: white, glossy exudate that progresses to a gray, tough, fibrinous, and adherent membrane on the pharynx that is friable and bleeds if scraped
	  • **Local Edema**: visibly swollen neck ("bull neck"), voice hoarseness, stridor, dyspnea, dysphagia
	• **Cutaneous Infection**:
	  • Ulcerating skin lesions covered with a gray membrane that do not spread or invade the surrounding tissues
	• **Complications**:
	  • Myocarditis: usually presents 1-2 weeks after upper respiratory symptoms; arrhythmias, heart failure,
	  • Neurotoxicity: toxin causes a demyelinating polyneuropathy that affects cranial and peripheral nerves

Diagnosis	• **Clinical Diagnosis** • Gram Stain: reveals club-shaped, nonencapsulated, nonmotile bacilli found in clusters • Culture: special culture media (Loffler medium or Tindale media) required; black colony with halos seen on Tindale media, metachromatic granules seen on a Loffler medium • ECG: required to assess for myocarditis; consider cardiac enzymes

Treatment	• **Diphtheria Antitoxin (DAT)**: most important to reduce sequelae and improve recovery time
	  • Neutralizes the unbound diphtheria toxin in the blood
	• Antibiotics: required to eradicate the organism and prevent spread
	  • Erythromycin or procaine penicillin G; vancomycin or linezolid if resistance detected
	• **Prophylaxis**:
	  • Diphtheria booster + erythromycin or IM benzathine penicillin G
	• **Prevention**:
	  • DTaP: 5 doses at 2, 4, 6, 15-18 months and 4-6 years old
	  • Tdap: given at 11-12 years old and to pregnant women during *every* pregnancy (preferably at 27 to 36 weeks gestation)

Cholera

Etiology & Risk Factors	• Gastrointestinal infection due to ***Vibrio cholerae*** • Etiology: ***Vibrio cholerae***; a gram-negative, enterotoxin-producing bacteria • Risk Factors: patients with blood type O are more likely to have severe disease, residing in or travel to endemic areas (Asia, Africa, and Central/South America); poor sanitary conditions, regions afflicted by natural disasters and/or humanitarian crises • Transmission: **fecal-oral route** through contaminated food/water (**seafood/shellfish**); humans are only known host; can live freely in fresh/salt water
Patho-physiology	• Small intestine is colonized by bacterium that produces enterotoxins causing increase in cell cAMP leading to hypersecretion of isotonic electrolytes by the mucosa into the gut lumen causing intense secretory diarrhea
Signs & Symptoms	• Onset 24-72 hours after exposure • **Abrupt onset of copious, watery diarrhea (white/gray stool with flecks of mucous "rice water stool"**; may have "fishy odor"), **vomiting,** abdominal cramping • May develop **severe dehydration** (tachycardia, dry mucous membranes, decreased urine output, weakness, muscle cramps) **from fluid and electrolyte loss** • Fluid loss can be as high as 1L/hr • *Fatality rate as high as 70% without treatment due to dehydration, arrythmia (electrolyte abnormalities), paralytic ileus*
Diagnosis	• **Clinical Diagnosis** • Stool Culture: on TCBS medium; confirms diagnosis • Polymerase Chain Reaction (PCR): detects specific antigens or genetic material in stool sample • Labs: indicated to evaluate hypovolemia/electrolyte abnormalities (CBC, CMP); may show hyponatremia, hypokalemia, hypoglycemia, hemoconcentration

Treatment	• Fluid Replacement: mainstay of therapy
	   • **Oral Hydration: preferred method of rehydration**(oral glucose-electrolyte solution, bouillon, broths)
	   • **IV Hydration:** reserved for intractable vomiting, hypovolemia, severe dehydration
	• Antibiotics: antibiotics have been shown to decrease the severity and duration of disease
	   • **Doxycycline is first-line;** azithromycin or ciprofloxacin are alternatives
	• Proper Hygiene: wash hands with warm soap and water, avoiding contaminated foods/water, using clean filtered or bottled water
	• *Antiemetics and antidiarrheals are found to have little benefit*

Key Words & Most Common	• Contaminated food/water source (seafood/shellfish) • Abrupt onset of watery diarrhea; white/gray flecks of mucous "rice water" stool • Severe dehydration • Clinical diagnosis • Oral hydration vs IV hydration • Doxycycline is first line antibiotic

Plague

Etiology & Risk Factors	• Etiology: ***Yersinia pestis***; a gram-negative bacillus • Risk Factors: **residing in or travel to endemic areas** (Africa; the Democratic Republic of Congo and Madagascar, Peru), **close contact with infected animals (rats, mice, squirrels, prairie dogs),** poor sanitation and hygiene practices • Transmission: rodent-to-human by the bite of an infected **rat flea vector**; human-to-human transmission occurs by inhaling droplets from patients with pulmonary infection
Patho-physiology	• After entering the body, *Y. pestis* disseminates through the lymphatic system and enters the bloodstream, leading to systemic infection • The bacterium's ability to evade the immune response and multiply rapidly within host tissues contributes to the development of severe symptoms

Signs & Symptoms	• **Bubonic Plague: most common form**
	   • **Abrupt onset of fever and chills,** restlessness, delirium, confusion, incoordination
	   • Primary cutaneous lesion (pustule, ulcer, **eschar**) may develop at the site of the flea bite
	   • **Acute, enlarged, warm, painful lymph nodes near site of inoculation (buboes);** axillary or inguinal lymph nodes are most common; femoral and cervical possible
	• **Pneumonic Plague: most lethal form**; most patients with pneumonic plague die within 48 hours of symptom onset if left untreated
	   • Abrupt onset of high fever and chills, tachycardia, chest pain, headache
	   • **Productive cough with pink or bright red and foamy sputum** ("red death"), tachypnea, dyspnea
	• Septicemic Plague: subsequent, advanced illness that may be fatal
	   • Disseminated Intravascular Coagulopathy (DIC): extensive purpura
	   • Gangrene: necrosis of tissue involving distal extremities, nose, penis ("black death")

Diagnosis	• Stain and Culture: stained smears of peripheral blood, sputum, or needle aspiration of a lymph node bubo • **Demonstrates bipolar-staining, ovoid, gram-negative organisms with a "safety pin" appearance** • Polymerase Chain Reaction (PCR): confirms diagnosis

Treatment	• Isolation: strict respiratory isolation and droplet precautions
	• **Antibiotics:**
	   • **Streptomycin or gentamicin is first-line treatment**
	   • **Doxycycline is second-line**

Key Words & Most Common	• *Yersinia pestis*; transmitted through rat flea bite • Bubonic: eschar near flea bite followed by acutely warm and painful lymph node (buboes) • Pneumonic: productive cough with pink or bright red and foamy sputum • Septicemic: DIC and gangrene • Stain demonstrates bipolar-staining, gram-negative organisms with a "safety pin" appearance • Streptomycin or gentamicin is first-line

Campylobacter Enteritis

Etiology & Risk Factors	• Most common cause of bacterial enteritis in the US; commonly affects children and young adults • <u>Etiology</u>: ***Campylobacter jejuni***; a motile, gram-negative, non-spore-forming bacteria • <u>Risk Factors</u>: consumption of **raw/unpasteurized milk, undercooked poultry, and contaminated water**; contact with animal feces (puppies) • <u>Transmission</u>: **fecal-oral route**
Patho-physiology	• ***C. jejuni*** **is strongly associated with subsequent development of Guillain-Barré syndrome (GBS)** secondary to a cross-reaction between *C. jejuni* antibodies and human gangliosides; autoantibodies may react with peripheral nerves causing demyelination and ascending paralysis • Bacterial invasion of intestinal epithelium causes inflammatory lesions and mucosal damage leading to bloody and mucous-like diarrhea
Signs & Symptoms	• Onset is 1-3 days after exposure with symptoms lasting 5-7 days • Prodrome phase of fever, rigors, body aches, dizziness • **Diarrhea (initially watery progressing to bloody or mucous-like), fever, abdominal pain, nausea, vomiting** • **Periumbilical pain (may mimic appendicitis)**
Diagnosis	• <u>Stool Culture</u>: **confirms diagnosis**; gram-stain may reveal "S or comma shaped organism" • <u>Rapid Molecular or Antigen Test</u>: detects specific antigens in stool sample • <u>Enzyme-linked Immunosorbent Assays (ELISA) or Polymerase Chain Reaction (PCR)</u>: detects the genetic material in stool samples; not commonly used • <u>Ultrasound or CT</u>: utilized to rule out acute appendicitis if warranted

Treatment	• <u>Fluid Replacement</u>: mainstay of therapy
	  • <u>Oral Hydration</u>: **preferred method of rehydration**(oral glucose-electrolyte solution, bouillon, broths)
	  • <u>IV Hydration</u>: reserved for intractable vomiting, hypovolemia, severe dehydration
	• <u>Antibiotics</u>: indicated for severe cases, elderly, immunocompromised, or diabetics
	  • **Azithromycin is first-line;** ciprofloxacin may be used but growing resistance
	• <u>Antidiarrheals</u>: avoided in invasive diarrheas
	• <u>Prevention</u>: proper hygiene habits, safe food processing, treated water consumption

Key Words & Most Common	• Most common source is raw milk or undercooked poultry • Watery diarrhea that may become bloody or mucous-like • Stool culture • Oral rehydration • Azithromycin for severe cases

Salmonellosis

Etiology & Risk Factors	• Foodborne disease caused by *Salmonella enteriditis;* most common cause of foodborne illness in US • Etiology: ***Salmonella enteriditis***; a gram-negative bacilli • <u>Transmission</u>: **fecal-oral route** • <u>Risk Factors</u>: **consumption of contaminated water or foods** (poultry, eggs, peanut butter, unwashed produce), contact with reptiles (**turtles**)
Patho-physiology	• Bacteria is ingested and invades epithelium wall of intestine through transferring of bacterial proteins or M cells (epithelial cells serving as antigen-present cells in gut mucosa or lymphoid tissue) or direct penetration of gut mucosa • Pathogen may become systemic through lymphatic and bloodstream infiltration; may colonize in gallbladder of chronic carriers
Signs & Symptoms	• Onset is 8-72 hours after exposure • <u>Initial Symptoms</u>: may be gradual; **abdominal pain, fever, constipation and headache** • <u>Subsequent Symptoms</u>: **diarrhea** (may be "pea soup" green or bloody), **"step-ladder" fever** (rises one day, falls the next), cough, anorexia, malaise • *Constipation may be predominant over diarrhea in some cases due to Payer patch hypertrophy* • <u>Physical Exam</u>: **bradycardia relative to fever; Rose spots** (pink/salmon-colored macular rash of trunk and extremities), **hepatosplenomegaly**, dehydration, delirium
Diagnosis	• <u>Blood, Urine and Stool Cultures</u>: **best way to detect**; order with antibiotic susceptibility due to increasing drug resistance • <u>Bone Marrow Culture</u>: gold standard; highly invasive and expensive so rarely ordered • <u>Enzyme-Linked Immunosorbent Assays (ELISA) or Polymerase Chain Reaction (PCR)</u>: expensive and not commonly used

Treatment	• <u>Fluid Replacement</u>: mainstay of therapy
	  • <u>Oral Hydration</u>: **preferred method of rehydration**(oral glucose-electrolyte solution, bouillon, broths)
	  • <u>IV Hydration</u>: reserved for intractable vomiting, hypovolemia, severe dehydration
	• <u>Antibiotics</u>: guided treatment based on culture susceptibility
	  • **Ciprofloxacin is first-line**
	  • **Azithromycin or ceftriaxone are alternatives**
	• <u>Prevention</u>: proper hygiene habits, safe food processing, treated water consumption

Key Words & Most Common	• Most common source is contaminated water; contact with contaminated eggs, poultry, turtles; travel to endemic area • Abdominal pain, fever, constipation, headache progressing to diarrhea, cough, general symptoms • Bradycardia relative to fever, Rose spots, hepatosplenomegaly • Blood, urine and stool cultures; bone marrow culture is gold standard • Fluid replacement • Ciprofloxacin is first-line; azithromycin or ceftriaxone

Shigellosis

Etiology & Risk Factors	• Bacterial diarrhea caused by the anaerobic gram-negative bacilli *Shigella* spp. • <u>Etiology</u>: ***Shigella sonnei* (most common in US)**, *flexneri, boydii,* and *dysenteriae* (produces most toxin) • <u>Risk Factors</u>: consumption of **contaminated water/food**, immunocompromised, age (elderly, children <5yo), overcrowded areas with inadequate sanitization (**daycare**) • <u>Transmission</u>: **fecal-oral route**; humans are only natural reservoirs; can be spready by flies; *requires very small inoculum to cause disease*
Patho-physiology	• Bacteria is ingested and then multiplies in the small intestine before entering colon. Shigella bacterium invades colonic mucosa and produces a "Shiga" enterotoxin which is cytotoxic, neurotoxic and enterotoxic; intestinal mucosal cells may slough off causing bloody diarrhea • Shiga toxin can have systemic effects causing vasculitis which manifests as hemolytic uremic syndrome
Signs & Symptoms	• Onset is 1-4 days after exposure • **Generalized crampy abdominal pain, fever, tenesmus** (urgency to defecate) • **Explosive watery diarrhea (progresses to bloody or mucous-like)** • <u>Severe Symptoms</u>: delirium, anuria, encephalopathy, seizures (febrile seizures may be more common in young children) • <u>Physical Exam</u>: fever, tachycardia, hypotension, evidence of dehydration, distended abdomen, hyperactive bowel sounds, lower abdominal tenderness
Diagnosis	• <u>Labs</u>: shows **marked leukocytosis** • <u>Stool Culture</u>: confirms diagnosis; stool analysis may show fecal leukocytes and blood • <u>Polymerase Chain Reaction (PCR)</u>: detects specific antigens or genetic material in stool sample • <u>Sigmoidoscopy</u>: diffuse erythema with small punctate ulcerations

Treatment	• <u>Fluid Replacement</u>: mainstay of therapy
	  • **Oral Hydration: preferred method of rehydration**(oral glucose-electrolyte solution, bouillon, broths)
	  • **IV Hydration**: reserved for intractable vomiting, hypovolemia, severe dehydration
	• <u>Antibiotics</u>: guided treatment based on culture susceptibility
	  • **Ciprofloxacin is first-line**
	  • **Azithromycin (first-line for pediatrics) or ceftriaxone are alternatives**
	• <u>Antidiarrheals</u>: should be avoided as retained toxins can worsen or prolong illness
	• <u>Prevention</u>: proper hygiene habits, safe food processing, treated water consumption

Key Words & Most Common	• Most common source is contaminated water; contact with contaminated eggs, poultry, turtles; travel to endemic area • Crampy abdominal pain, fever, tenesmus • Explosive watery diarrhea (bloody or mucous-like) • Stool cultures; CBC shows marked leukocytosis • Fluid replacement • Ciprofloxacin is first-line; azithromycin or ceftriaxone

Listeriosis

Etiology & Risk Factors	• <u>Etiology</u>: ***Listeria monocytogenes***; gram-positive, beta-hemolytic, facultative anaerobic, endotoxin-producing bacilli that is non-spore forming • <u>Risk Factors</u>: **immunocompromised**, neonates, elderly, **pregnant women** (*Listeria* can cross placental barrier), certain medical conditions (diabetes, malignancy, liver and kidney disease), **consumption of contaminated food (unpasteurized dairy products, melons, soft cheese, undercooked meats, and ready-to-eat deli meats and hot dogs)**
Patho-physiology	• The bacteria invades and replicate within host cells, allowing it to evade immune defenses and spread throughout the body leading to severe systemic infection, inflammation, tissue damage, and potentially life-threatening complications • Bacterium grows at refrigerator temperatures and produces biofilms to survive harsh environments by utilizing surface and host proteins

Signs & Symptoms	• <u>Listerial Febrile Illness</u>: self-limited; most common presentation
	  • **General Flu-Like Symptoms: fever, diarrhea**, headache, chills, **nausea, vomiting, abdominal pain**, myalgias
	  • **Pregnancy**: febrile illness associated with intrauterine infection, chorioamnionitis, premature labor, stillbirth, or neonatal infections
	    • *Infected pregnant women have a risk of miscarriage or stillbirth of approximately 20%*
	• <u>Listeriosis</u>: bacteremia and/or meningitis; most common in infants <2 months old, immunocompromised or elderly
	  • **Primary Bacteremia**: high fever without localizing symptoms and signs; endocarditis, peritonitis, osteomyelitis, septic arthritis, cholecystitis, pleuropneumonia possible
	  • **Meningitis**: fever, neck stiffness, altered consciousness, cranial nerve palsies, neurological deficits, cerebellar signs, and motor or sensory loss

Diagnosis	• **Culture: performed on blood, cerebral spinal fluid, or placental fluid** • Demonstrates gram-positive, facultative intracellular bacilli with colonies that are beta-hemolytic

Treatment	• <u>Supportive</u>: proper hand-washing technique, avoiding foods commonly contaminated (especially while pregnant)
	• <u>Antibiotics</u>:
	  • **IV ampicillin or penicillin G is initial treatment of choice**; trimethoprim-sulfamethoxazole is an alternative if the patient has a penicillin allergy
	  • **Gentamicin often added** based on synergy in vitro; utilized to cover for gram-negative etiologies of meningitis

Key Words & Most Common	• Infection caused by *Listeria monocytogenes* • Most commonly affects immunocompromised and pregnant women • Consumption of unpasteurized dairy, melons, soft cheeses, deli meat, hot dogs • General flu-like symptoms +/- bacteremia, meningitis • Febrile illness associated with risk of miscarriage or stillbirth in pregnant women • Culture of blood, CSF or placental fluid • IV ampicillin or penicillin G + gentamicin

474

Clostridium difficile

Etiology & Risk Factors	• Most common cause of antibiotic-associated colitis and infectious diarrhea in hospitalized patients • <u>Etiology</u>: *Clostridioides difficile* (formerly *Clostridium*); a spore-forming, toxin-producing, gram-positive anaerobic bacterium • <u>Risk Factors</u>: **recent antibiotic use (clindamycin,** cephalosporins, penicillin, fluoroquinolones), **advanced age,** recent hospitalization, resident at nursing home, use of PPI/H2 blockers, chemotherapy
Patho-physiology	• *C. diff* colonizes in large intestine; use of antibiotics then alter the microbial flora increasing susceptibility of infection and overgrowth of C. diff bacteria • Diarrhea and colitis secondary to clostridial glycosylation exotoxins and enterotoxins which leads to hypersecretion of fluid into intestinal lumen and develops characteristic pseudomembranes (yellow-white plaques), and watery, foul-smelling diarrhea
Signs & Symptoms	• Onset typically 5-10 days after starting antibiotic • **Foul-smelling, watery** diarrhea (may have mucous and occult blood), **abdominal cramping,** low-grade fever, nausea, vomiting, anorexia • <u>Fulminant Colitis</u>: severe diarrhea, diffuse abdominal pain/distension, hypovolemia that may lead to sepsis, toxic megacolon, or perforated bowel
Diagnosis	• *Consider testing patients with >3 loose stools within 24 hours + risk factors* • <u>Stool Assay</u>: tests for *C. difficile* **toxin (initial test of choice); glutamate dehydrogenase (GDH) antigen** and polymerase chain reaction (PCR) for toxin gene • <u>Labs</u>: **leukocytosis** and elevated WBC count • <u>Sigmoidoscopy</u>: confirms pseudomembrane presence; used for patients with high suspicion and negative toxin assay
Treatment	• <u>Discontinue Offending Antibiotic</u>: **first step in management if possible** • **Fluid Replacement:** • <u>Oral Hydration</u>: **preferred method of rehydration;** oral glucose-electrolyte solution, bouillon, broths • <u>IV Hydration</u>: reserved for hypovolemia or severe dehydration • <u>Antibiotics</u>: • **Oral vancomycin or oral fidaxomicin are first-line** • Metronidazole is an alternative • *Consider pulse-taper with oral vancomycin/fidaxomicin +/- metronidazole with recurrent cases* • <u>Fecal Transplant</u>: transplantation of microbiota using colonoscopy indicated for severe (3+) recurrence • <u>Prevention</u>: **proper hygiene, contact precautions;** hand washing with warm soap and water (spores resistant to alcohol-based hand sanitizer)
Key Words & Most Common	• Recent antibiotic use (clindamycin); common cause of infectious diarrhea in hospitalized patients • Foul-smelling, watery diarrhea • Stool Assay test for *C. diff* toxin • Discontinue antibiotic • Oral Vancomycin or oral Fidaxomicin • Contact precautions

Rotavirus Gastroenteritis

Etiology & Risk Factors	• Most common cause of viral gastroenteritis in worldwide; most common in unimmunized kids • <u>Etiology</u>: **rotavirus**; a double-stranded virus • <u>Transmission</u>: **fecal-oral route from contaminated hands or surface fomite contamination** (food/water contaminations less likely), seasonal (peak incidence in **later winter to early spring**; may occur at any time of year) • Common outbreaks seen in day dare facilities or elementary schools
Patho-physiology	• Viral replication occurs in mature enterocytes throughout small intestine lumen causing alteration in epithelial cells. This causes an osmotically active food bolus to rapidly transmit through large intestine and impairing water absorption thus causing the typical watery diarrhea
Signs & Symptoms	• Onset 24-72 hours after exposure • **Copious, watery diarrhea is predominant symptom, vomiting, fever** • May have general symptoms like fever, abdominal cramping, fatigue, malaise, headache, dehydration (tachycardia, dry mucous membranes, decreased urine output) • *Symptoms are more severe in infants and children*
Diagnosis	• **Clinical Diagnosis** • <u>Enzyme Immunoassays and Reverse Transcription Polymerase Chain Reaction (RT-PCR)</u>: may aid in detection but rarely used • <u>Labs</u>: CBC/CMP to evaluate hypovolemia/electrolyte abnormalities
Treatment	• **Fluid Replacement**: • <u>Oral Hydration</u>: **preferred** method of rehydration; oral glucose-electrolyte solution, bouillon, broths • <u>IV Hydration</u>: reserved for intractable vomiting, hypovolemia, severe dehydration • <u>Antiemetics</u>: **ondansetron** alleviates nausea to allow for proper oral hydration; avoid in children • <u>Antidiarrheals</u>: loperamide may offer symptomatic relief; avoid in children • <u>Prevention</u>: proper hygiene; wash hands with warm soap and water
Key Words & Most Common	• Fecal-oral transmission from contaminated hands or surface fomites • Copious, watery diarrhea, vomiting, fever • Clinical diagnosis • Oral hydration vs IV hydration • Ondansetron/loperamide for symptomatic relief; avoid in children

Norovirus Gastroenteritis

Etiology & Risk Factors	• Most common cause of viral gastroenteritis in US • <u>Etiology</u>: norovirus; a nonenveloped, positive-sense, single-stranded virus • <u>Risk Factors</u>: **crowded living spaces** (common outbreaks seen on **cruise ships**, schools, military barracks, **restaurants, healthcare facilities), seasonal** (peak incidence in **winter**; may occur at any time of year), consumption of high-risk foods (**raw foods**, particularly fruits and vegetables, oysters, fish/sushi) • <u>Transmission</u>: **fecal-oral route from contaminated food/water or surface fomite contamination** • Very low inoculum to cause infection (highly contagious)
Patho-physiology	• Norovirus invades, infects and replicates in immune cells including macrophages, dendritic cells, and B cells; may directly invade enterocytes lining the gut lumen • Virus may interact with host's gut flora to enhance infection and replication

Signs & Symptoms	• Onset 12-72 hours after exposure (24 hours average); may be abrupt onset
	• <u>General Symptoms</u>: fever, malaise, headache, anorexia
	• <u>Gastrointestinal Symptoms</u>:
	   • **Intense nausea and recurrent vomiting are predominant symptoms**
	   • Non-bloody diarrhea without mucous
	   • Abdominal cramping

Diagnosis	• **Clinical Diagnosis** • <u>Enzyme Immunoassays and Reverse Transcription Polymerase Chain Reaction (RT-PCR)</u>: may aid in detection but rarely used • <u>Labs</u>: CBC/CMP to evaluate hypovolemia/electrolyte abnormalities

Treatment	• **Fluid Replacement**:
	   • **Oral Hydration: preferred** method of rehydration; oral glucose-electrolyte solution, bouillon, broths
	   • **IV Hydration:** reserved for intractable vomiting, hypovolemia, severe dehydration
	• **Antiemetics: ondansetron** alleviates nausea to allow for proper oral rehydration
	• <u>Prevention</u>: proper hygiene; wash hands with warm soap and water; disinfect bathroom (*virus may aerosolize with vomiting, defecation, or when flushing toilet*)

Key Words & Most Common	• Fecal-oral transmission from contaminated food/water (raw fruits/vegetables, fish) • Abrupt onset of vomiting • Clinical diagnosis • Oral hydration vs IV hydration • Ondansetron for symptomatic relief

Enterohemorrhagic E. coli O157:H7

Etiology & Risk Factors	• <u>Etiology</u>: *Escherichia coli O157:H7;* a shiga-like toxin producing gram-negative bacteria • <u>Transmission</u>: fecal-oral route • <u>Risk Factors</u>: consumption of **raw/unpasteurized milk or apple cider, undercooked ground beef, and contaminated water or unwashed fruits/vegetables;** day care centers, petting zoos, age (most commonly affects children and elderly adults)
Patho-physiology	• Bacteria produce shiga-like verotoxins that cause direct damage to vascular endothelial cells and mucosal cells of the large intestinal wall • Intestinal mucosal cells may slough off causing bloody diarrhea • Shiga-like toxin can have systemic effects causing vasculitis which manifests as hemolytic uremic syndrome
Signs & Symptoms	• Onset is 4-9 days after exposure • **Acute onset of watery diarrhea progressing to grossly bloody diarrhea within 24 hours** • Abdominal pain, nausea, vomiting • Typically low-grade or no fever • <u>Hemolytic-Uremic Syndrome</u>: may have hypertension and evidence of fluid overload
Diagnosis	• <u>Labs</u>: most patients will have leukocytosis • Hemolytic-uremic syndrome may have sharp decrease in hematocrit and platelets, elevated creatinine • **Stool Culture: best way to detect** • <u>Stool Assay</u>: antigen stool test, enzyme-linked immunosorbent assays (ELISA) or polymerase chain reaction (PCR); not commonly used • *Evaluate for other causes of bloody diarrhea*

Treatment	• **Fluid Replacement**:
	   • **Oral Hydration: preferred** method of rehydration; oral glucose-electrolyte solution, bouillon, broths
	   • **IV Hydration:** reserved for intractable vomiting, hypovolemia, severe dehydration
	• <u>Antibiotics</u>: **should be avoided due to increase release of shiga-like toxins leading to hemolytic uremic syndrome**
	• <u>Antidiarrheals</u>: avoided in invasive diarrheas
	• <u>Prevention</u>: proper hygiene; wash hands with warm soap and water, safe food processing, treated water consumption

Key Words & Most Common	• Most common source is unpasteurized milk or apple cider, undercooked ground beef, contaminated water • Watery diarrhea that may become bloody • Stool culture • Oral rehydration • Avoid antibiotics due to increased chance of developing hemolytic uremic syndrome

Giardiasis

Etiology & Risk Factors	• Small intestine infection; most common cause of parasitic diarrhea worldwide • <u>Etiology</u>: ***Giardia lamblia (duodenalis)***; a flagellated intestinal protozoan parasite • <u>Risk Factors</u>: **consumption of contaminated water from remote streams or wells; wilderness travelers, international travelers, daycare workers**, poor sanitation • "Backpacker's diarrhea" or "beaver fever" • <u>Transmission</u>: fecal-oral; **contaminated water most common**; most common during summer months
Patho-physiology	• Infected animals excrete cysts into water; ingestion of cysts through consumption of contaminated water leads to infection • Cysts undergo excystation within the intestines which then release trophozoites that adhere to the intestinal epithelium. This disrupts the epithelial cell wall junctions and brush border enzymes leading to altered intestinal motility and permeability
Signs & Symptoms	• Onset is 1-14 days after exposure • **Most are asymptomatic**; *asymptomatic patients can still excrete infective cysts in stool* • **Watery, foul-smelling, pale diarrhea (no blood or mucous)** • **Abdominal cramping and distension, flatulence**, malaise, low-grade fever • Fat and sugar malabsorption can occur with chronic diarrhea
Diagnosis	• <u>Stool Antigen Assay</u>: uses enzyme-linked immunosorbent assays (ELISA); more sensitive than microscopy • <u>Stool Microscopy</u>: evaluation for ova and parasites; demonstrates motile trophozoites and cysts • <u>Labs</u>: normal WBCs, no eosinophilia

Treatment	• <u>Fluid Replacement</u>:
	   • **Oral Hydration: preferred method** for rehydration; oral glucose-electrolyte solution, bouillon, broths
	   • **IV Hydration:** reserved for hypovolemia or severe dehydration
	• <u>Antiparasitics</u>: **Metronidazole is first-line**; Tinidazole, Albendazole, Quinacrine are alternatives
	• <u>Prevention</u>: proper hygiene habits, safe food processing, treated water consumption

Key Words & Most Common	• Most common source is contaminated water from remote streams, lakes, or wells Most common among wilderness travelers, hikers or daycare workers • Watery, foul-smelling, pale diarrhea (no blood/mucous) • Stool antigen test • Fluid replacement • Metronidazole is first-line; albendazole, tinidazole are alternatives

Amebiasis

Etiology & Risk Factors	• Parasitic protozoan infection transmitted by ingestion of cysts from fecal contaminated food/water • <u>Etiology</u>: ***Entamoeba histolytica***; a motile protozoan • <u>Risk Factors</u>: **inadequate sanitation practices, contaminated food or water**, poor personal hygiene, **migrants from or travelers to endemic areas** (Central America, western South America, western and southern Africa, India), immunocompromised, living in crowded or institutional settings (refugee camps)
Patho-physiology	• Upon ingestion of contaminated food or water, the cysts of the parasite survive the acidic environment of the stomach and transform into trophozoites in the intestines where they feed on bacteria and tissue, reproduce and colonize the lumen and the mucosa of the large intestine. • The trophozoites can invade the intestinal lining, leading to inflammation, tissue damage, ulcer formation; trophozoites can spread to other organs, such as the liver

Signs & Symptoms	• **Mostly asymptomatic**
	• <u>Gastrointestinal Symptoms</u>: develop 1 to 3 weeks after ingestion of cysts
	   • **Intermittent diarrhea and constipation, flatulence, cramping abdominal pain**
	• <u>Amebic Dysentery</u>:
	   • Frequent semiliquid stools that often contain blood and mucous
	   • Abdominal pain, fever, weight loss
	• <u>Liver Abscess</u>: significantly more common in men
	   • Fever, chills, diaphoresis, nausea, vomiting, weakness, weight loss
	   • **RUQ pain (may radiate to right shoulder)**

Diagnosis	• <u>Stool Microscopy</u>: evaluation of ova and parasites; diagnosis supported by finding amebic trophozoites, cysts, or both in stool or tissues • <u>Enzyme Immunoassay (EIA)</u>: most widely used antigen test; sensitive and rapidly performed • <u>Stool Polymerase Chain Reaction (PCR)</u>: **diagnostic gold standard**; detects parasitic DNA in the stool • <u>Abdominal Imaging</u>: ultrasonography, CT, or MRI indicated to diagnose liver abscess; may require CT guided aspiration

Treatment	• <u>Fluid Replacement</u>:
	   • **Oral Hydration: preferred method of rehydration**(oral glucose-electrolyte solution, bouillon, broths)
	   • **IV Hydration:** reserved for intractable vomiting, hypovolemia, severe dehydration
	• <u>Amebicides</u>:
	   • **Metronidazole or tinidazole followed by paromomycin**, iodoquinol, or diloxanide furoate to eradicate residual cysts in the intestine
	   • *Asymptomatic cases should be treated with paromomycin, iodoquinol, or diloxanide furoate alone*

Key Words & Most Common	• Parasitic protozoan infection caused by Entamoeba histolytica contracted from contaminated food/water • Mostly asymptomatic → GI symptoms that range from mild to dysentery • Liver abscess (fever + RUQ pain) • Stool microscopy, EIA, PCR + abdominal imaging if concern for liver abscess • Metronidazole followed by paromomycin (to eradicate cysts)

Toxoplasmosis

Etiology & Risk Factors	• Infection caused by the parasite *Toxoplasma gondii* • <u>Etiology</u>: ***Toxoplasma gondii***; an obligate intracellular protozoan • <u>Transmission</u>: **foodborne** (ingestion of tissue cysts via undercooked/raw meat), **zoonotic (ingestion of oocysts via consumption of food and water contaminated with feline feces)**, vertical (Infected mother causes congenital infection through the placenta) • <u>Risk Factors</u>: exposure to contaminated soil, water, or food, **handling cat feces**, immunocompromised (AIDS/HIV when CD4 <100 cells/uL)
Patho-physiology	• Ingestion of the parasite through contaminated food, water, or contact with infected animals allows the parasite to invade host cells (particularly immune cells and muscle cells) and forms cysts, leading to a chronic infection

Signs & Symptoms	• <u>**Acute Toxoplasmosis**</u>: usually asymptomatic
	  • **May develop bilateral, nontender cervical or axillary lymphadenopathy**
	  • May develop flu-like symptoms (fever, malaise, myalgia, pharyngitis), hepatosplenomegaly (may mimic infectious mononucleosis)
	• <u>**Central Nervous System Toxoplasmosis**</u>: most common in immunocompromised (HIV/AIDs with CD4 <100 cells/uL)
	  • **Encephalitis**: headache, neurologic symptoms including focal neurologic deficits, fever, altered mental status
	• <u>**Congenital Toxoplasmosis**</u>: may be severe, particularly if acquired early in pregnancy
	  • Jaundice, rash, hepatosplenomegaly, and the classic tetrad of bilateral retinochoroiditis, cerebral calcifications, hydrocephalus, psychomotor retardation
	• <u>**Ocular Toxoplasmosis**</u>: usually results from congenital infection that is reactivated
	  • Ocular pain, blurred vision, floaters, decreased visual acuity or blindness
	• <u>**Disseminated Toxoplasmosis**</u>: occurs primarily in severely immunocompromised patients
	  • Pneumonitis, myocarditis, polymyositis, diffuse maculopapular rash, high fevers, chills, and prostration

Diagnosis	• <u>Serologic Testing</u>: most common diagnostic method; indirect fluorescent antibody (IFA) test or enzyme immunoassay (EIA) for anti-toxoplasma IgG and IgM • <u>Neuroimaging</u>: CT or MRI with contrast; demonstrates single or multiple rounded, ring-enhancing lesions • <u>Lumbar Puncture with CSF Analysis</u>: demonstrates lymphocytic pleocytosis and elevated protein
Treatment	• <u>**Immunocompetent**</u>: **pyrimethamine and sulfadiazine plus leucovorin** *(administer folinic acid if the treatment regimen includes leucovorin to prevent folic acid depletion)* • <u>**Immunocompromised**</u>: **trimethoprim-sulfamethoxazole is first-line**; pyrimethamine and leucovorin plus sulfadiazine or clindamycin or azithromycin • <u>**Pregnant**</u>: spiramycin
Key Words & Most Common	• Toxoplasma gondii infection most common in pregnant females handling cat feces or immunocompromised • Acute: bilateral, cervical lymphadenopathy + flu-like symptoms (may resemble mononucleosis) • CNS: encephalitis • Congenital: jaundice, rash, hepatosplenomegaly • Ocular: ocular pain, blurred vision, floaters • Serologic testing (IFA or EIA for anti-toxoplasma IgG and IgM) • pyrimethamine and sulfadiazine plus leucovorin (if immunocompetent); TMP-SMX (if immunocompromised)

Cat Scratch Disease

Etiology & Risk Factors	• Illness caused by bacterial infection caused by the scratch or bite from an infected cat or exposure to cat fleas • <u>Etiology</u>: *Bartonella henselae*; intracellular gram-negative bacilli • <u>Risk Factors</u>: age (children and young adults most common), **exposure to cats (especially kittens)**, immunocompromised, exposure to cat fleas
Patho-physiology	• Scratches or bites from infected cats allows the bacteria (*Bartonella henselae*) to enter the body where it multiplies within the regional lymph nodes near the inoculation site, leading to lymphadenopathy and granuloma formation; the immune response to the bacteria is responsible for the characteristic clinical manifestations
Signs & Symptoms	• **Erythematous, crusted, painless papule at the inoculation site** • **Regional lymphadenopathy**, fever, malaise, headache, and anorexia develop within 2 weeks • Lymphadenitis proximal to exposure
Diagnosis	• <u>Serologic Testing</u>: indirect fluorescence assay (IFA) or ELISA testing; *negative serologic tests do not rule out the diagnosis* • <u>Polymerase Chain Reaction (PCR) Testing</u>: performed on samples from lymph node aspirates • <u>Biopsy</u>: not routinely indicated; biopsy of skin lesions or lymph node demonstrates suppurative granulomatous changes

Treatment	• <u>**Supportive**</u>: warm compresses and analgesia (NSAIDs) indicated for immunocompetent patients (**usually self-limited disease**)
	• <u>**Antibiotics**</u>: indicated for moderate to severe cases or immunocompromised patients
	  • <u>**Moderate**</u>: **azithromycin is first-line**; doxycycline is an alternative
	  • <u>Severe</u>: rifampin, gentamycin, or ciprofloxacin

Key Words & Most Common	• Infection caused by Bartonella henselae secondary to a scratch/bite from an infected cat • Erythematous, crusted, painless papule at inoculation site • Regional lymphadenopathy • Serologic testing (IFA or ELISA) • Supportive treatment if immunocompetent • Azithromycin or doxycycline if immunocompromised or severe disease

Candidiasis

Etiology & Risk Factors	• **Opportunistic infection due to Candida** that may affect the oral cavity, vagina, penis, or other parts of the body • <u>Etiology</u>: *Candida albicans* is most common; a form of yeast that normally colonizes the oropharyngeal, esophageal, and gastrointestinal mucosa • <u>Risk Factors</u>: **recent antibiotic use, immunocompromised, diabetes**, hormonal changes, poor hygiene, certain medications (**corticosteroids**, immunosuppressants, oral contraceptives), **obesity**, sexual activity, restrictive clothing, warm and humid climate, infrequent diaper or undergarment changes in children and older patients
Patho-physiology	• Combination of disrupted normal microbial balance, a compromised immune response, or local tissue damage leading to opportunistic overgrowth of *Candida albicans* • An imbalance between the fungus and the body's immune defense allows the fungus to proliferate and invade tissues
Signs & Symptoms	• <u>**Esophagitis**</u>: substernal odynophagia, gastroesophageal reflux, epigastric pain, nausea/vomiting • <u>**Oropharyngeal (Thrush)**</u>: **friable, white plaques on oral mucous membranes** that may bleed when scraped • <u>**Intertrigo**</u>: **well-demarcated, pruritic, erythematous "beefy red" patches of intertriginous areas** (axillae, groin, gluteal folds, glans penis, inframammary) **with satellite lesions** • <u>**Vulvovaginal**</u>: **vulvar pruritus, burning, vaginal discharge (thick, white, "curd-like" discharge)** • <u>**Angular Cheilitis**</u>: cracks and tiny fissures at the corner of the mouth
Diagnosis	• **Clinical Diagnosis** • **Potassium Hydroxide (KOH) Wet Mount**: confirms diagnosis with identification of budding yeast and pseudohyphae
Treatment	• <u>**Esophagitis**</u>: oral fluconazole is first-line • <u>**Oropharyngeal (Thrush)**</u>: **nystatin oral suspension** (swish and swallow) or dissolving clotrimazole troche in mouth; oral fluconazole if refractory • <u>**Intertrigo**</u>: use of topical drying agents; topical antifungals (powdered miconazole or topical clotrimazole); oral fluconazole if refractory • <u>**Vulvovaginal**</u>: intravaginal miconazole, clotrimazole, tioconazole; oral fluconazole if severe or persistent • <u>**Angular Cheilitis**</u>: topical clotrimazole; oral fluconazole if severe or persistent
Key Words & Most Common	• Opportunistic infection caused by Candida albicans • Recent antibiotic use, immunocompromised, diabetes, corticosteroid use greatest risk factors • Signs and symptoms vary by affected region • Clinical diagnosis + KOH prep (budding yeast and pseudohyphae) • Topical antifungals vs oral fluconazole

Pneumocystis jirovecii Pneumonia

Etiology & Risk Factors	• **Common cause of pneumonia in immunosuppressed patients** • <u>Etiology</u>: *Pneumocystis jirovecii* (formerly known as *carinii*); an atypical yeast-like fungus • <u>Risk Factors</u>: **immunocompromised** (malignancy, cancer treatment, transplant recipients, HIV, immunosuppressive medication), malnutrition, chronic corticosteroid use • **Most common opportunistic infection associated with HIV, especially when CD4+ count < 200 cells/uL**
Patho-physiology	• Fungus is inhaled, attaches to alveolar epithelium and transitions from small trophic form to larger cystic form • Inflammation then leads to alveolar damage and further lung injury, impaired gas exchange, and possibly respiratory failure
Signs & Symptoms	• <u>**Classic Triad**</u>: **fever, nonproductive cough, progressive dyspnea** (starts with dyspnea on exertion and progresses to at-rest) • Hypoxemia, respiratory distress • <u>Physical exam</u>: 50% will have normal breath sounds; may have crackles, rhonchi, tachypnea/tachycardia
Diagnosis	• <u>Labs</u>: ↑**LDH**, ↑**beta-D-glucagon** (contained in fungi cellular wall), ↓**CD4+ count**, ABG if respiratory distress • <u>CXR</u>: **diffuse, bilateral, perihilar interstitial infiltrates**; normal CXR in 25% • <u>CT</u>: more sensitive and specific; shows ground glass infiltrative pattern • <u>Sputum Histopathology</u>: obtained through induced sputum or bronchoalveolar lavage • Methenamine silver stain, Wright-Giemsa stain, and modified monoclonal antibody stain may be used • <u>Lung Biopsy</u>: definitive diagnosis but rarely performed

Treatment	• <u>**Antibiotics**</u>:
	   • **Trimethoprim-sulfamethoxazole (TMP-SMX) is first line**; therapy for 21 days
	     • <u>Sulfa Allergy</u>: primaquine + clindamycin, atovaquone, trimethoprim + dapsone, or IV pentamidine
	• <u>**Corticosteroids**</u>: **prednisone indicated if HIV+ and severe respiratory compromise** (room air PaO$_2$<70mmHg *OR* A-a gradient>35mmHg *OR* hypoxic)
	• <u>Prophylaxis</u>: TMP-SMX once daily if CD4+ <200 cells/uL

Key Words & Most Common	• Most common in HIV+ patients with CD4+ <200 • Fever, nonproductive cough, progressive dyspnea • CXR: diffuse, bilateral, perihilar interstitial infiltrates • Trimethoprim-sulfamethoxazole (TMP-SMX) is first line; steroids if HIV+ and hypoxic

Histoplasmosis

Etiology & Risk Factors	• Pulmonary and hematogenous disease caused by *Histoplasma capsulatum*
	• <u>Etiology</u>: *Histoplasma capsulatum;* a dimorphic soil-based yeast
	   • Mold found in soil that contains bird or bat feces
	   • **Endemic to Ohio, Missouri, and Mississippi river valleys** and southeastern US
	• <u>Risk Factors</u>: **immunocompromised (AIDS with CD4+ ≤150 cells/uL)**; demolition of old buildings (inhabited by birds/bats), farmers, **cave explorers**, or cave excavators

Patho-physiology	• Disruption of soil containing the fungus causes spores to become airborne, inhaled by the host, and become lodged in the alveoli • Spore is engulfed by neutrophils and macrophages which then organize and form granulomas that fibrose and calcify

Signs & Symptoms	• <u>Asymptomatic</u>: **90% of cases**; usually self limited
	• <u>Symptomatic</u>: 1-4 weeks after exposure; **flu-like illness**
	   • Fever/chills, myalgias, headache, arthralgias, dyspnea, nonproductive cough (may have hemoptysis)
	• <u>Disseminated</u>: involves multiple organ systems & affects immunocompromised
	   • Hepatosplenomegaly, fever, weight loss, oropharyngeal mucosal or GI ulcers, bloody diarrhea, hematologic disturbance, pericarditis (mimics TB)

Diagnosis	• <u>Labs</u>: CBC (mild anemia); elevated alkaline phosphatase and elevated LDH in disseminated • <u>CXR</u>: may be normal in 40-70% of cases • Pneumonitis with **hilar/mediastinal lymphadenopathy**, focal pulmonary infiltrates (light exposure) or diffuse miliary pulmonary infiltrates (heavy exposure) • <u>Antigen Testing</u>: **serum or urine antigen testing is highly specific** • <u>Sputum Culture</u>: **most specific test**; poses serious risk to lab personnel (blood culture may be positive in disseminated)
Treatment	• <u>Asymptomatic</u>: **no treatment necessary**; resolves without treatment (pulmonary symptoms less than 1 month) • <u>Acute Primary</u>: **itraconazole is first line** if symptoms >1 month; treatment for 3 months • <u>Chronic Pulmonary</u>: **itraconazole** for 1 year • <u>Progressive Disseminated</u>: **amphotericin B** for 1 week followed by itraconazole for 1 year; untreated disseminated has >90% mortality rate
Key Words & Most Common	• Soil-based fungus found in soil containing bird or bat feces • Endemic to Ohio and Mississippi river valleys • Asymptomatic and self limiting in 90% of cases; flu-like illness if symptomatic • Serum or urine antigen testing; CXR may show hilar/mediastinal lymphadenopathy • Asymptomatic requires no treatment; Itraconazole if symptoms >1mo

Cryptococcosis

Etiology & Risk Factors	• Pulmonary or disseminated infection acquired by inhalation of soil contaminated with the encapsulated yeasts *Cryptococcus neoformans* or *C. gattii* • <u>Etiology</u>: ***Cryptococcus neoformans;*** encapsulated, budding, round yeast • **Fungus found in soil contaminated with bird droppings (especially pigeons)** • <u>Risk Factors</u>: **immunocompromised (AIDS [CD4+ <100 cells/uL]**, lymphoma, sarcoidosis, organ transplant, long-term corticosteroid use, diabetes)
Patho-physiology	• Disruption of soil containing the fungus causes spores to become airborne and inhaled by the host. • Spread of the disease is through hematogenous dissemination in immunosuppressed patients (frequently to brain and meninges)

Signs & Symptoms	• <u>Central Nervous System</u>: symptoms as a result of cerebral edema
	   • **Meningoencephalitis is most common clinical manifestation**; CNS symptoms as a result of cerebral edema
	   • Low-grade fever, **headache**, general malaise, **neck stiffness**, **photophobia**, nausea/vomiting, blurred vision, depression, agitation, confusion, altered mental status
	• <u>Respiratory</u>: nonspecific; cough, dyspnea, **pneumonia**
	• <u>Skin</u>: pustular, papular, nodular, or **ulcerated lesions** may be seen if disseminated

Diagnosis	• <u>Lumbar Puncture and Cerebrospinal Fluid Analysis</u>: ↑ or normal WBC, ↓glucose, ↑protein
	   • <u>Cryptococcal Antigen via latex agglutination or ELISA</u>: highly sensitive and specific
	   • <u>Cryptococcal Culture</u>: is 95-100% sensitive; takes 3-7 days
	   • <u>India Ink Stain</u>: **shows encapsulated yeast**
	• <u>CT Brain</u>: soap bubble lesions; may be normal
	• <u>CXR</u>: variable findings; may have infiltrates, mediastinal lymphadenopathy

Treatment	• <u>Pneumonia</u>:
	   • <u>AIDS-Associated</u>: **fluconazole for 6-12 months**
	   • <u>Not AIDS-Associated</u>: fluconazole or itraconazole for 6-12 months
	• <u>Meningoencephalitis</u>: amphotericin B + flucytosine for 4 weeks, **followed by oral fluconazole** for 8 weeks
	• *Therapy is discontinued when CD4+ count is >200 cells/uL and asymptomatic for 6 months*

Key Words & Most Common	• Pulmonary or disseminated infection caused by *Cryptococcus neoformans;* found in soil contaminated with pigeon droppings • Immunocompromised (AIDS patients with CD4+ count <100) • Meningoencephalitis is most common clinical manifestation • Diagnose with CSF analysis for antigen or identify encapsulated yeast on India ink stain • <u>Pulmonary</u>: Fluconazole • <u>Meningitis</u>: Amphotericin B + Flucytosine followed by oral fluconazole

Blastomycosis

Etiology & Risk Factors	• Pyogranulomatous fungal infection caused by inhaling spores of the dimorphic fungus *Blastomyces dermatitidis* • Etiology: *Blastomyces dermatitidis*; a dimorphic fungus • Fungus found in moist soil or decaying wood near **Mississippi & Ohio River valleys and Great Lakes** (also Northern Midwest, Upstate NY, & southern Canada) • Risk Factors: **more common in immunocompetent males,** occupational & recreational exposure **(outdoor activities near water);** immunocompromised
Patho-physiology	• Fungal colony disturbed during outdoor activity causing spores to become airborne and inhaled which are then phagocytized by mononuclear cells & killed by macrophages and neutrophils; in the lungs, the inhaled spores convert to larger invasive yeasts, forming broad-based buds and may disseminate hematogenous
Signs & Symptoms	• Up to 50% of cases will be asymptomatic; 3-6 week incubation period • General: flu-like symptoms (fever/chills, cough, myalgias, arthralgias, malaise), weight loss, night sweats • Pulmonary: **most common site of involvement;** acute or chronic pneumonia, diffuse pneumonitis, ARDS • Cutaneous: **most common extrapulmonary site;** verrucous (wart-like) lesions with irregular border, **subcutaneous nodules, well-demarcated ulcers** that bleed easily • Disseminated: bone involvement (osteomyelitis, paravertebral abscess, **lytic bone lesions),** central nervous system (meningitis, brain/epidural abscess) and genitourinary system (prostatitis, epididymitis)
Diagnosis	• CXR: alveolar infiltrates, mass lesion; lacks specificity • Vertebral X-Ray: well-circumscribed osteolytic lesion; may show lytic lesions at anterior vertebral body & destruction of disk space • Fungal Culture: sputum stained with fungal stain • Potassium Hydroxide (KOH) Wet Mount): sputum sample demonstrates **round yeast with thick double walls & broad-based budding;** may take 5-10 days • Antigen Testing: urine or serologic
Treatment	• Mild to Moderate: **itraconazole is first-line;** fluconazole for 6-12 months • Severe: **amphotericin B** if progressive, or CNS involvement
Key Words & Most Common	• Fungus found in moist soil/decaying wood near Mississippi & Ohio River valleys and Great Lakes • Immunocompetent male participating in outdoor activities near water • Flu-like symptoms; skin is most common extrapulmonary site • KOH shows round yeast with thick double walls & broad-based budding • Itraconazole if mild; Amphotericin B if severe

Aspergillosis

Etiology & Risk Factors	• Opportunistic infection affecting the lower respiratory tract and is caused by inhaling spores of the filamentous fungus *Aspergillus* • Etiology: *Aspergillus fumigatus;* a filamentous, monomorphic **fungus with septate hyphae that branch at 45° angles,** and affects the lungs, sinuses, and CNS • Fungus is most commonly found in garden and houseplant soils, decaying vegetation and compost • Risk Factors: **immunocompromised (AIDS, leukemia, organ transplant,** long-term corticosteroid use, diabetes), environmental or occupational exposure **(construction or farming industries),** smoking marijuana contaminated with fungus, chronic lung diseases (asthma, cystic fibrosis, COPD)		
Patho-physiology	• *Aspergillus* spores are inhaled and taken up by respiratory phagocytes that then germinate into hyphae due to increased body temperature within the lung • In immunocompetent patients, beta-D-glucan is secreted by phagocytes which activates neutrophils that kill the hyphae and prevent infection; inn immunocompromised patients, these defense mechanisms are impaired leading to infection		
	Allergic Bronchopulmonary Aspergillosis	**Aspergilloma**	**Acute Invasive Aspergillosis**
Signs & Symptoms	• **Type 1 hypersensitivity** to *A. fumigatus;* **most commonly affects patients with asthma or cystic fibrosis** • **Cough productive of brownish mucus plug** in sputum, hemoptysis, fever, malaise +/- allergic fungal sinusitis	• Affects those with preexisting pulmonary cavitary lung disease (TB, sarcoidosis); fungus colonizes the lesion **(fungal ball)** • May be asymptomatic and incidentally found on CXR; cough +/- hemoptysis if symptomatic	• Occurs in severely immunocompromised (leukemia, organ transplant, chemotherapy) • Fever, cough, dyspnea, **pleuritic chest pain, hemoptysis, invasive chronic sinusitis** (may develop necrotizing cutaneous lesions around sinus)
Diagnosis	• **Increased IgE** (2x increase from baseline), **eosinophilia;** positive skin test for *Aspergillus fumigatus* • CXR: central bronchiectasis, mucoid impaction, migratory pulmonary infiltrates (eosinophilic pneumonia)	• **Positive precipitin Ab test** • Biopsy: **septate hyphae that branch at 45° angles;** may be necrotic appearing • CXR/CT: **upper lobe "fungal ball" mass in preexisting cavity that changes position with patient; air crescent sign** (crescent of air outlining solid mass)	• Galactomannan level (cell wall component of *Aspergillus* release into blood); beta-D-glucan assay; sputum culture • CXR/CT: **halo sign** (nodules with surrounding ground glass opacities); cavitary lesions, wedge-shaped or pleural-based infiltrates
Treatment	• **Oral corticosteroids (3-6wks followed by taper) and chest physiotherapy is first-line;** add itraconazole if chronic	• **Oral itraconazole + surgical resection;** observation if asymptomatic	• **Voriconazole is drug of choice;** posaconazole or amphotericin B are alternatives
Key Words & Most Common	• Fungus found in gardens and decaying vegetation; affects immunocompromised • Allergic is type 1 hypersensitivity affecting asthma/cystic fibrosis; increased IgE and eosinophilia; treated with oral steroids • Aspergilloma affects preexisting pulmonary lung disease; "fungal ball" mass of upper lobe; air crescent sign; treated with itraconazole • Acute invasive: pleuritic chest pain & hemoptysis; halo sign (nodule with surrounding opacification); treated with voriconazole		

	Valley Fever	Coccidioidomycosis	

Etiology & Risk Factors	• Pulmonary or hematogenous spread disseminated disease caused by the fungi *Coccidioides immitis* and *C. posadasii* • Etiology: *Coccidioides immitis* or *C. posadasii* a dimorphic fungus • Fungus most commonly found in soil of arid/desert regions; endemic to southwestern US (New Mexico, Arizona, West Texas, Southern California) • Risk Factors: **immunocompromised (HIV)** 2nd & 3rd trimester **pregnancy**, advanced age, **certain ethnicities** (Filipino, African American, Native American, Hispanics, Asians), environmental exposure (hiking, outdoor recreation, **farming, construction work**); *about 30-60% of people that live in endemic area have been exposed during lifetime*
Patho-physiology	• Disruption of soil containing the fungus causes spores to become airborne and inhaled by the host where they convert to large spherules which may rupture and release thousands of endospores; local release of endospores causes host response and acute inflammation leading to fibrosis

Signs & Symptoms	• Primary Illness : 1-4 weeks after exposure; 60% are asymptomatic
	    • **Mild flu-like symptoms** that may resemble bronchitis/pneumonia (fever, cough, pleuritic chest pain, chills, sputum production, sore throat, hemoptysis)
	• Progressive Illness: 1-3 weeks after primary pulmonary disease presentation
	    • Fever, arthralgias (especially knee and ankles), anorexia, weight loss, and weakness.
	    • Erythema Nodosum: erythematous, painful, subcutaneous nodules most common on the lower extremities
	• Disseminated Illness: more common in the immunosuppressed and pregnant women
	    • CNS involvement (meningitis) in 50%; vertebral osteomyelitis; skin lesions; **joint involvement (knees)**, dramatic sweats, weight loss

Diagnosis	• Serologic Testing: enzyme immunoassay detects IgM and IgG antibodies (usually first test ordered); ↑ESR, eosinophilia • Fungal Culture: most definitive test • Microscopic Analysis: **thick-walled spherule containing endospores seen within samples of** sputum, pleural fluid, cerebrospinal fluid (CSF), exudate, or biopsied specimens • Polymerase Chain Reaction (PCR): highly sensitive and specific test; not widely available • CXR: unilateral infiltrates, miliary pneumonia, persistent cavitation • CSF: presence of complement-fixing antibodies is diagnostic; ↓glucose, lymphocytosis (ordered if meningitis suspected)
Treatment	• Asymptomatic or Mild: self-limited and requires no treatment • Mild to Moderate Nonmeningeal Extrapulmonary Involvement: **fluconazole or itraconazole** • Severe: **amphotericin B** • High dose fluconazole for meningitis
Key Words & Most Common	• Caused by fungus found in arid/desert regions of southwestern US • Primary Pulmonary (flu-like illness) followed by "Valley Fever" (triad of fever, arthralgias, and erythema nodosum); Dissemination may occur in immunocompromised • Labs: enzyme immunoassay to detect IgM & IgG; eosinophilia • Most cases self-limited; Fluconazole in moderate cases, Amphotericin B in severe cases

	Pneumocystis *Jirovecii* Pneumonia	Histoplasmosis	Cryptococcosis	Blastomycosis	Aspergillosis	Coccidioidomycosis
Etiology	• *Pneumocystis jirovecii*: atypical yeast-like fungus	• *Histoplasma capsulatum*: dimorphic soil-based yeast	• *Cryptococcus neoformans*: encapsulated yeast	• *Blastomyces dermatitidis*: dimorphic fungus	• *Aspergillus*: **fungus with septate hyphae that branch at 45° angles**	• *Coccidioides immitis*: dimorphic fungus
Risk Factors	• Most common opportunistic infection associated with HIV • **CD4+ count <200 cells/uL**	• Bird or **bat droppings** • OH, MO, and MS river valleys • **CD4+ ≤150 cells/uL**	• **Pigeon droppings** • CD4+ <100 cells/uL	• **Moist soil or decaying wood** • **MS & OH river valleys & Great Lakes**	• **Garden soil/compost**	• **Soil of arid/desert regions** • **Southwestern US**
Symptoms	• Classic Triad: **fever, nonproductive cough, progressive dyspnea**	• Acute: asymptomatic or flu-like illness • Disseminated: HSM, fever, oropharyngeal ulcers, bloody diarrhea	• Meningitis: MCC of fungal meningitis • **Pneumonia: cough, pleuritic pain, dyspnea**	• Flu-like symptoms • Skin is MC extrapulmonary site	• **Allergic**: hypersensitivity rxn in asthma and CF; cough with thick brown mucous plugs • **Aspergilloma**: colonizes preexisting cavitary lesion • **Invasive**: fever, cough, dyspnea, chest pain, hemoptysis	• Primary: flu-like illness • Valley Fever: fever, arthralgias, erythema nodosum • Disseminated: **meningitis**
Diagnosis	• Labs: ↑LDH, ↑beta-D-glucagon, ↓CD4+ count • CXR: diffuse, bilateral, perihilar interstitial infiltrates • CT: ground glass	• **Sputum cultures/antigen** • Urine antigen • Fungal blood cultures • CXR variable (**miliary infiltrates**)	• CSF: ↓glucose, ↑protein • **Cryptococcal Antigen** • **India Ink Stain** shows encapsulated yeast	• **Sputum/CSF/urine cultures budding yeast with thick double walls**	• **Allergic**: elevated IgE and eosinophilia • **Aspergilloma**: "fungal ball" with air crescent sign on CXR • **Invasive**: halo sign	• IgG and IgM antibodies • Histopathology with fungal culture
Treatment	• **Trimethoprim-sulfamethoxazole (TMP-SMX) is first line** • Steroids if HIV+ and hypoxic	• Acute: Itraconazole • Disseminated: Amphotericin B	• Pneumonia: **Fluconazole** • Meningoencephalitis: **Amphotericin B + Flucytosine**	• **Itraconazole is first line** • Amphotericin B if severe	• **Allergic**: corticosteroids • **Aspergilloma**: surgery + itraconazole • **Invasive**: voriconazole	• Mild: self limited • Moderate: Fluconazole • Severe: Amphotericin B

Tuberculosis

Etiology & Risk Factors	• Chronic, progressive multi-system disease caused by *Mycobacterium tuberculosis* and **spread through inhalation of airborne respiratory droplets** • Etiology: *Mycobacterium tuberculosis* • Risk Factors: close contact exposure to someone with TB, **crowded living conditions (homeless shelters, prisons)**, HIV (CD4+ <500 cell/uL, immunosuppression (steroid use, diabetes), **recent immigration from high-prevalence areas**, healthcare workers, malnutrition • Epidemiology: estimated that 1/4th of entire world population is infected; **most cases in Southeast Asia** (India, Indonesia), Africa, and the Western Pacific (China)
Patho-physiology	• *M. tuberculosis* is inhaled and deposit deep in lung (middle/lower lobe) and ingested by alveolar macrophages; infected macrophages can migrate to regional lymph nodes and enter the bloodstream; *M. tuberculosis* replicates inside which eventually kills host macrophage causing inflammatory mediators to go to area and creating a focal pneumonitis

Signs & Symptoms	• Primary: usually **asymptomatic**; may be rapidly progressive in immunocompromised
	 • Reactivation: **fever, night sweats**, malaise, fatigue, **weight loss**
	  • **Pulmonary**: cough with or without mucous production, hemoptysis, dyspnea, pleuritic chest pain
	  • **Extrapulmonary: painless lymphadenopathy (Scrofula), Pott's disease (TB osteomyelitis of vertebrae)**, pericarditis, adrenal insufficiency, meningitis, peritonitis
	 • Latent: asymptomatic, positive purified protein derivative (PPD), no CXR findings of active infection
		• Primary TB: initial infection (often self-limiting), primary progressive may be present in children in endemic areas; **contagious**
		 • Reactivation TB: **more common in immunocompromised patients**; cavitary lesions in upper lobe (secondary to ↑O_2 in lung apices); **contagious**
		 • Latent TB: **caseating granuloma formation** leads to central necrotic, acidic and ↓O_2 environment decreases *M. tuberculosis* growth and inhibits symptomatic infection; **not contagious**

Diagnosis	• **CXR: most common initial test**
	  • Primary: **middle or lower lobe consolidation**, hilar or mediastinal lymphadenopathy
	  • Reactivation: fibrocavitary lesions in **upper lobe**
	  • Latent: upper lobe/hilar nodules, fibrotic lesion, **Ghon's complex** (calcified caseating granuloma), **Ranke's complex** (healed Ghon's complex)
	  • Miliary TB: diffuse **millet-seed** (2-4mm) nodular lesions
	 • Sputum specimen: acid-fast bacilli, culture, nucleic acid amplification test

Treatment	• Active: 4-drug therapy (RIPE) **Rifampin + Isoniazid + Pyrazinamide + Ethambutol for 2 months**, followed by Isoniazid & Rifampin for 4 months • Latent: **Isoniazid + Pyridoxine (vitamin B6) for 9 months;** Consider treatment for newly positive PPD, close contact exposure to active TB, immunocompromised

Screening	• Purified Protein Derivative (PPD): transdermal administration & examined 48-72h after for transverse induration (erythema is not considered positive)
	  • Reaction considered POSITIVE in following situations
	   • ≥5mm: Immunosuppressed, HIV+, calcified granuloma or fibrotic changes on CXR, close contact exposure to active TB
	   • ≥10mm: Children <4yo, healthcare/prison employees, comorbid conditions (dialysis, diabetes, malignancy, IVDU), exposure to high prevalence area
	   • ≥15mm: No known risk factors
	 • Interferon Gamma Release Assay (QuantiFERON Gold Assay): blood test with no reader bias, no false positive with BCG vaccine, and improved specificity

Mycobacterium Avium Complex

Etiology & Risk Factors	• Nontuberculosis mycobacterial (NTM) species that almost exclusively affects immunocompromised patients • Etiology: *Mycobacterium avium* and *intracellulare*; nonmotile, non-spore-forming, gram-positive acid-fast bacillus • Risk Factors: **immunocompromised (HIV with CD4 ≤50 cell/uL**, organ transplant recipients, immunosuppressive therapy), advanced age, **underlying pulmonary disease** (bronchiectasis, COPD, cystic fibrosis), environmental exposure (water, soil, dust), occupational exposure (farmers, gardeners)
Patho-physiology	• Inhalation or ingestion of the bacteria, which then colonizes and invades macrophages within various tissues; the bacteria are able to resist killing by phagocytes, replicate within the host cells, and cause chronic granulomatous inflammation, leading to tissue damage and progression of the disease

Signs & Symptoms	• **Pulmonary**:
	  • Productive cough, fever, dyspnea, fatigue, night sweats, weight loss
	 • **Lymphadenitis**: more common in children (1-5 years old)
	  • Maxillary, submandibular and cervical lymphadenitis
	 • **Disseminated**: most commonly seen with HIV
	  • **Fever of unknown origin**, anemia, thrombocytopenia, diarrhea, diaphoresis, fatigue, dyspnea and abdominal pain

Diagnosis	• **Acid Fast Staining and Culture**: performed on sputum samples • CXR: fibronodular infiltrates that resemble Tuberculosis (cavitation usually thin-walled; pleural effusions are rare) • **Biopsy: confirms diagnosis in disseminated disease**; percutaneous fine-needle biopsy of liver or necrotic lymph nodes

Treatment	• **Antibiotics**:
	  • **Moderate Cases: clarithromycin or azithromycin plus rifampin plus ethambutol for 12-18 months**
	  • Severe or Progressive Cases: clarithromycin or azithromycin plus rifabutin plus ciprofloxacin plus clofazimine plus amikacin
	  • **Prophylaxis: clarithromycin or azithromycin required if CD4 count ≤100 cell/uL**
	 • **Surgery**:
	  • Surgical excision of infected lymph nodes is curative in most lymphadenitis cases

Key Words & Most Common	• Mycobacterium avium infection of immunocompromised patients (HIV with CD4 ≤50 cell/uL) • Nonspecific pulmonary symptoms • Lymphadenitis seen in children • Disseminated disease (fever) seen with HIV • Acid fast staining + culture • Clarithromycin or azithromycin plus rifampin plus ethambutol for 12-18 months

Leprosy

Etiology & Risk Factors	• Chronic granulomatous infection caused by *Mycobacterium leprae* and *Mycobacterium lepromatosis* • Etiology: *Mycobacterium leprae* and *Mycobacterium lepromatosis*; gram-positive, acid-fast bacilli; obligate intracellular organism • Risk Factors: **living in or travel to endemic areas particularly in tropical and subtropical areas (India, Brazil, Indonesia most common)**, close contact with infected person, immunocompromised (HIV/AIDS), genetic susceptibility, low socioeconomic status (poverty, overcrowded living conditions, lack of access to healthcare), **armadillo exposure**
Patho-physiology	• Bacteria primarily infect the skin and peripheral nerves, leading to a spectrum of clinical manifestations ranging from tuberculoid leprosy (characterized by a strong immune response) to lepromatous leprosy (characterized by a weak immune response) • The bacteria's affinity for peripheral nerve cells attacks Schwann cells resulting in nerve demyelination and loss of axonal conductance

Signs & Symptoms	• **Tuberculoid**: more common in immunocompetent patients
	  • **Non-pruritic, hypoesthetic (reduced sensation), centrally hypopigmented macules with sharp, raised borders**
	• **Lepromatous:**
	  • **Skin macules, papules, nodules, or plaques (lepromas) with poorly-defined borders** affecting many areas of the body
	    • **Lesions can be particularly disfiguring on the face**
	  • Loss of eyebrows and eyelashes
	  • **Peripheral neuropathy most prominent**
	• **Borderline:**
	  • Features of both tuberculoid and lepromatous leprosy are present

Diagnosis	• **Biopsy: with acid-fast bacillus smear**
	  • Tuberculoid: well-defined epithelioid non-caseating granulomas and few or absent acid-fast bacilli
	  • Lepromatous: macrophages with a vacuolar cytoplasm, plasma cells, lymphocytes, and numerous acid-fast bacilli

Treatment	• **Tuberculoid:**
	  • **Dapsone plus rifampin** for 6-12 months
	• **Lepromatous:**
	  • **Dapsone plus rifampin plus clofazimine** for 24 months

Key Words & Most Common	• Chronic granulomatous infection caused by *Mycobacterium leprae* and *Mycobacterium lepromatosis* • Endemic to tropical and subtropical areas (India, Brazil, Indonesia most common), armadillo exposure • Tuberculoid: non-pruritic, hypoesthetic (reduced sensation), hypopigmented macules • Lepromatous: skin macules, papules, nodules (lepromas) that may disfigure face; peripheral neuropathy • Biopsy • Dapsone + rifampin +/- clofazimine

Cytomegalovirus (CMV)

Etiology & Risk Factors	• Viral infection with a wide range of symptoms that primarily affects immunocompromised patients • Etiology: **cytomegalovirus; human herpesvirus 5** is a double-stranded DNA virus that lies dormant within the host • Risk Factors: **immunocompromised**, congenital transmission, close contact exposure (contact with bodily fluids, including saliva, urine, and blood), high-risk sexual activity, attending day-care as child (80% infected at day-care centers)
Patho-physiology	• After initial infection, CMV establishes latency within host myeloid cells, allowing it to evade immune surveillance • Replication and reactivation are contained primarily by cytotoxic T-cell immunity however may reactivate from latency during periods of immunosuppression

Signs & Symptoms	• **Primary Infection: mostly asymptomatic**
	  • Mononucleosis-Like Illness: **fever**, cough, myalgias/arthralgia, fatigue; *usually without sore throat or lymphadenopathy*
	• **Reactivation: most commonly seen in immunocompromised**
	  • **Esophagitis**: odynophagia, dysphagia, fever, nausea
	  • **Colitis: most common**; fever, anorexia, abdominal pain, diarrhea, bloody stool, weight loss, dehydration
	  • **Pneumonitis**: viral syndrome with cough
	  • **Retinitis**: most commonly seen in HIV when CD4 count is ≤50 cells/uL; changes in visual acuity, visual field cuts (scotoma, loss of central vision), floaters, photophobia
	  • **Neuritis: encephalitis** (impaired memory, motor deficits, CN palsies, ataxia, nystagmus), **polyradiculitis** (back pain, paresthesias, ascending paralysis, urinary retention)

Diagnosis	• **Polymerase Chain Reaction (PCR):** preferred method for viral detection • Serology: detects CMV-specific IgM and IgG antibodies • Viral Culture: cell culture from bodily fluids such as urine, saliva, or tissue • **Biopsy: gold standard; enlarged nuclei inclusion surrounded by a clear halo with cytoplasmic inclusions ("owl's eye" appearance)**

Treatment	• Supportive: self-limited in immunocompetent patient; does not require specific therapy other than symptomatic management
	• **Antivirals**: indicated for severe cases or infection in immunocompromised patient
	  • **Ganciclovir is first-line treatment of choice**
	  • Valganciclovir, foscarnet, cidofovir are alternatives

Key Words & Most Common	• Viral infection caused by the cytomegalovirus – human herpesvirus 5 • Primarily affects immunocompromised • Primary infection: asymptomatic or mononucleosis-like illness • Reactivation: esophagitis, colitis, pneumonitis, retinitis, neuritis • PCR; biopsy is gold standard ("owl's eye" appearance) • Ganciclovir is first-line

Cryptosporidiosis

Etiology & Risk Factors	• Most common cause of chronic diarrhea in HIV patients • Etiology: *Cryptosporidium hominis* and *Cryptosporidium parvum*; *an* obligate, intracellular coccidian protozoa that replicates within small-bowel epithelial cells • Risk Factors: **immunocompromised (HIV with CD4 <200 cells/uL)**, exposure to contaminated food/water, travel to endemic area (developing countries), occupational exposure (healthcare settings, childcare facilities, veterinarians, farmers), close contact with animals **(particularly cats and cattle)**
Patho-physiology	• Ingestion of the oocysts of the parasite allows invasion of the epithelial cells lining the small intestine; oocysts undergo replication and excystation that releases sporozoites; sporozoites settle within the walls of the small intestine where they produce thick- and thin-walled oocysts that are shed into the stool and persist in the environment • Sporozoites settling within the small intestinal wall leads to inflammation and damage to the intestinal lining, resulting in nutrient and water malabsorption
Signs & Symptoms	• Incubation period of about 1 week • **Abrupt onset of watery diarrhea** • Chronic diarrhea can occur in immunocompromised patients • **Abdominal cramping**, fever, nausea/vomiting, anorexia, malaise • **Dehydration, weight loss**
Diagnosis	• <u>Microscopic Examination of Stool</u>: mature oocyst is identified using modified acid-fast staining • <u>Polymerase Chain Reaction (PCR)</u>: molecular testing that can distinguish which species is present • <u>Enzyme Immunoassay</u>: testing for fecal *Cryptosporidium* antigen is more sensitive than microscopic examination for oocysts

Treatment	• <u>Supportive</u>: self-limited in immunocompetent patient; does not require specific therapy other than symptomatic management
	• <u>Antiparasitics</u>: indicated for immunocompromised or in severe or persistent infections
	  • <u>Nitazoxanide</u>: treatment for 14 days or longer has been effective in reducing symptoms in patients with CD4 counts >50 cells/uL
	  • <u>Paromomycin +/- Azithromycin</u>: may be initiated to decrease diarrhea and recalcitrant malabsorption of antimicrobial drugs
	• <u>Antiretroviral Therapy (ART)</u>: **recommended for all HIV+ patients**

Key Words & Most Common	• Most common cause of chronic diarrhea in HIV patients (CD4 <200 cells/uL) • Caused by *Cryptosporidium* spp. • Close contact with animals (cats and cattle) • Abrupt onset of watery diarrhea (chronic diarrhea possible in immunocompromised) → dehydration and weight loss • Abdominal cramping • Microscopy; PCR; EIA • Supportive if immunocompetent • Antiparasitics (nitazoxanide) + antiretroviral therapy if immunocompromised (HIV+)

Kaposi Sarcoma

Etiology & Risk Factors	• **Multicentric vascular tumor associated with human herpesvirus type 8 infection** • <u>Etiology</u>: human herpesvirus type 8 (HHV-8) infection • <u>Risk Factors</u>: **immunocompromised (HIV with CD4 count <100/mm³ or post-transplant most common)**, advanced age, male, **Eastern European and Mediterranean descent**
Patho-physiology	• HHV-8 infects the endothelial cells lining blood vessels, leading to the formation of abnormal blood vessels and proliferation of spindle-shaped tumor cells • The virus promotes inflammatory cytokine and growth factors release, further contributing to tumor growth and angiogenesis
Signs & Symptoms	• **Asymptomatic (painless, nonpruritic) purple, pink, red macules that may coalesce into blue/violet to black plaques and nodules** • Nodules may fungate or penetrate soft tissue, invading the underlying bone • Regional lymphadenopathy may be present
Diagnosis	• <u>Biopsy</u>: **confirms diagnosis via punch biopsy** • Demonstrates spindle-shaped cell proliferation with leukocytic infiltration and neovascularization in the dermis
Treatment	• <u>Superficial Lesions</u>: **surgical excision**, cryotherapy or electrocoagulation, intralesional chemotherapy (<u>vinblastine</u> or interferon alfa) • <u>Multiple or Diffuse Lesions and Lymph Node Involvement</u>: 10-20 Gy of radiation therapy and chemotherapy • <u>AIDS-Associated Disease</u>: **highly active antiretroviral therapy (HAART) demonstrates marked response (may lead to regression or complete resolution)**
Key Words & Most Common	• Vascular tumor associated with HHV-8 infection • Most common in HIV and/or elderly male of Eastern European or Mediterranean descent • Asymptomatic purple macule that coalesces into blue/violet/black plaques and nodules • Biopsy: spindle-shaped cell proliferation and neovascularization in the dermis • Surgical excision → radiation and chemotherapy • HAART if associated with HIV

Human Immunodeficiency Virus (HIV) ✺

Etiology & Risk Factors	• Infection resulting from retroviruses that destroy CD4+ lymphocytes and impair cell-mediated immunity, leading to an increased risk of certain infections and malignancies • <u>Etiology</u>: HIV-1 (most common) and HIV-2; an enveloped retrovirus that contains 2 copies of a single-stranded RNA genome • <u>Retroviruses</u>: enveloped RNA viruses that replicate via **reverse transcription** to produce DNA copies that integrate into the host cell's genome • <u>Risk Factors</u>: **substance abuse, unprotected sexual intercourse, men who have sex with men**, high-risk sexual behavior, the use of intravenous drugs, vertical transmission (birth or breastfeeding), receiving contaminated blood or blood products, low socioeconomic status
Patho-physiology	• HIV is a retrovirus that primarily targets CD4+ T cells of the immune system and binds to the CD4 receptor and co-receptors on the cellular surface and gain entry where the virus replicates and integrates its genetic material into the host DNA, gradually depleting CD4+ T cells and impairing immune function • Viral replication requires reverse transcriptase (an RNA-dependent DNA polymerase) copy HIV RNA to produce proviral DNA

Signs & Symptoms	• May be asymptomatic or cause nonspecific symptoms
	• <u>Acute Retroviral Syndrome</u>: begins within 1-4 weeks of infection; lasts 3-14 days
	  • **Flu-Like or Mononucleosis-Like Illness: fever, malaise, fatigue, myalgias, pharyngitis are most common symptoms**; mucocutaneous ulceration, generalized rash, headache, arthralgias, diarrhea, weight loss, sore throat, generalized lymphadenopathy, and septic meningitis
	• <u>Opportunistic Infection</u>:
	  • **Oral and esophageal candidiasis is most common opportunistic infection**
	  • CMV (proctitis, colitis), PCP pneumonia, cryptosporidiosis, fungal infections, unusually severe infections (herpes zoster, herpes simplex, vaginal candidiasis etc.)
	• <u>Acquired Immune Deficiency Syndrome (AIDS)</u>: defined as HIV infection with a CD4+ T lymphocyte count <200 cell/uL
	  • <u>AIDS Defining Illness</u>: serious opportunistic infections, certain cancers (Kaposi sarcoma, non-Hodgkin lymphoma), neurologic dysfunction, wasting syndrome

Diagnosis	• 4th <u>Generation Combination Antigen/Antibody Immunoassay (Screening)</u>: screening test to detect HIV-1 and HIV-2 antibodies and the p24 HIV antigen
	• <u>HIV RNA Level (Viral Load) Testing</u>: nucleic acid amplification assay or RT-PCR (sensitive to extremely low HIV RNA levels)
	  • Negative screening test + positive viral load = early infection; repeat testing should be performed in 1-2 weeks
	  • Positive screening test + positive viral load = early or established infection
	• <u>Monitoring</u>: HIV+ patients should be monitored to determine prognosis and treatment
	  • <u>CD4 Count</u>: product of WBC count + percentage of white blood cells that are lymphocytes + percentage of lymphocytes that are CD4+
	  • <u>HIV RNA Level (Viral Load) Testing</u>: reflects HIV replication rates

Treatment	• <u>Anti-Retroviral Therapy</u>: recommended for all HIV+ patients; goal to reduce the plasma HIV RNA level to an undetectable and restore the CD4 count to a normal level
	  • **Treatment typically involves a combination of at least 3 antiretroviral drugs from different classes, such as nucleoside reverse transcriptase inhibitors (NRTIs), non-nucleoside reverse transcriptase inhibitors (NNRTIs), protease inhibitors (PIs), and integrase strand transfer inhibitors (INSTI)**
	    • **2 NRTIs + NNRTI *OR* 2 NRTIs + PI *OR* 2 NRTIs + INSTI**
	  • **Typical first line regimens include combination reverse transcriptase inhibitor (NRTI) and an integrase strand transfer inhibitors (INSTI)**
	    • Tenofovir/emtricitabine (Truvada) **PLUS** raltegravir (Isentress)
	    • Tenofovir/emtricitabine (Truvada) **PLUS** dolutegravir (Tivicay)

HIV Opportunistic Infections

CD4 Count (cells/uL)	Disease/Organisms to Consider	Clinical Clues	Primary Prophylaxis	Secondary Prophylaxis
700-1,500	Normal			
>500	Community Acquired Organisms	• More likely to acquire bacterial pneumonia • More likely to HSV and herpes zoster reactivation		
200-500	Tuberculosis	• Hemoptysis • Night sweats • Weight loss	INH (if latent)	Rifampin
<200	Pneumocystis jiroveci	• Hypoxia induced by activity, interstitial infiltrates, ↑LDH	TMP-SMX	Dapsone, Atovaquone, Pentamidine
	Cryptosporidium	• Profuse, watery diarrhea		
	Candida	• Oral thrush, oral lesions	Fluconazole	Itraconazole
	Fungal Pneumonia	• Cavitary lesions or diffuse infiltrates on CXR	Itraconazole	Amphotericin B
<100	Toxoplasmosis	• Ring enhancing lesions on CT brain	TMP-SMX	Dapsone + Pyrimethamine + Folinic Acid
	Candidal, HSV or CMV Esophagitis	• Odynophagia, dysphagia		
	Cytomegalovirus	• Esophagitis, enteritis, encephalitis	Valganciclovir	Ganciclovir + Foscarnet
	Cryptococcus	• Headache, altered mental status, + India ink	Fluconazole	Amphotericin B
<50	Mycobacterium Avium Complex (MAC)	• Night sweats, weight loss, diarrhea, malaise	Azithromycin or Clarithromycin	Rifabutin
	Cytomegalovirus Retinitis	• Changes in visual acuity, visual field cuts, floaters, photophobia	Valganciclovir	Ganciclovir + Foscarnet

486

Rocky Mountain Spotted Fever ✳

Etiology & Risk Factors	• Acute, febrile, tick-borne illness • <u>Etiology</u>: *Rickettsia rickettsii*; gram-negative, coccobacillary, obligate intracellular bacteria with a predilection for vascular endothelial cells • <u>Risk Factors</u>: **tick exposure, geographical location** (southeastern and south-central United States most common), **seasonal** (March-September most common), **outdoor activities** (hiking, biking, camping, gardening), age (<15 years old most common) • <u>Vectors</u>: dog tick (*Dermacentor variabilis*) and the wood tick (*Dermacentor andersoni*),
Patho-physiology	• Following a tick bite, *Rickettsia rickettsii* bacteria enters the bloodstream and infects the endothelial cells that line blood vessels, leading to disseminated vascular inflammation, loss of barrier function and altered vascular permeability, triggering a cascade of immune responses, including the release of cytokines and activation of immune cells

Signs & Symptoms	• <u>**Non-Specific Symptoms**</u>: symptoms begin 2-14 days after inoculation from an infected tick
	  • Fever/chills, nausea/vomiting, abdominal pain, **myalgias (severe calf pain)**, headache, fatigue, conjunctivitis, lethargy
	• <u>Rash</u>: develops on day 1-6 of fever
	  • **Blanching, erythematous, macular rash**
	  • **Starts as faint pink then becomes darker, maculopapular, petechial rash**
	  • **First appears on the wrists, ankles**, palms, soles, then rapidly spreads to the neck, trunk, face, axillae, and buttocks
	  • <u>Rumpel-Leede Test</u>: development of petechiae at the site of blood pressure cuff and distally after compression
	• <u>Associated Symptoms</u>: arthralgias, periorbital and pedal edema, neurological symptoms (headache, restlessness, insomnia, delirium, coma)
	• <u>Complications</u>: vasculitis, myocarditis, interstitial pneumonitis, encephalitis

Diagnosis	• **Clinical Diagnosis** (treatment decision must be made before receiving results of confirmatory testing) • <u>Polymerase Chain Reaction (PCR)</u>: initial test of a biopsy specimen of the rash • <u>Serial Serologic Examinations</u>: indirect immunofluorescent antibody testing for IgM and IgG antibodies confirms diagnosis • <u>Other</u>: CBC (thrombocytopenia), CMP (hyponatremia), ECG (myocarditis), and lumbar puncture (cerebrospinal fluid pleocytosis [increased cell count])
Treatment	• <u>**Doxycycline**</u>: **first-line antibiotic indicated for all non-pregnant adults and children (including children <8 years old)**; 5-10 day course • <u>**Chloramphenicol**</u>: **second-line treatment; preferred treatment in pregnancy** • May cause aplastic anemia and grey baby syndrome with third trimester use; consider doxycycline in third trimester
Key Words & Most Common	• Acute tick-borne illness caused by Rickettsia rickettsii • Non-specific symptoms (fever, nausea, myalgias, abdominal pain, fatigue, headache) followed by rash • <u>Rash</u>: blanching, erythematous macular rash starts on wrist/ankles then spreads to trunk and extremities • Clinical diagnosis + PCR and serologies • Doxycycline is first-line antibiotic in all non-pregnant patients

Lyme Disease ✳

Etiology & Risk Factors	• Arthropod-borne disease spread by the deer tick • <u>Etiology</u>: *Borrelia burgdorferi*; a gram-negative spirochete • <u>Risk Factors</u>: **tick exposure, geographical location** (northeastern US most common [Maine to Virginia] and northern Midwest [Wisconsin, Minnesota, Michigan]), **seasonal** (May-August most common), **outdoor activities** (hiking, biking, camping, gardening), age (children and young adults most common) • <u>Transmission</u>: deer tick (*Ixodes scapularis*) in the nymphal phase
Patho-physiology	• The bacterium *Borrelia burgdorferi* is transmitted through the bite of infected deer tick and enters the skin and spreads to the lymphatic system or disseminates in the blood to infect various organ systems; the immune response to the infection leads to the characteristic symptoms affecting the skin, joints, heart, and nervous system.

Signs & Symptoms	• <u>**Early Localized**</u>: occurs between 3 days and 30 days after a tick bite
	  • **Erythema Migrans**: **erythematous, annular macule that expands and develops a central clearing (Bull's eye or target appearance)**; may have warmth or induration
	  • <u>Constitutional Symptoms</u>: fatigue, low grade fever, migrating arthralgia, lymphadenopathy, headache, nausea/vomiting, abdominal pain
	• <u>**Early Disseminated**</u>: occurs days or weeks after the appearance of the primary lesion
	  • <u>**Flu-Like Syndrome**</u>: fatigue, headache, fever, malaise, arthralgias, myalgias, lymphadenopathy
	  • <u>Cutaneous Abnormalities</u>: multiple annular lesions that spare the palm and soles
	  • <u>**Neurologic Abnormalities**</u>: cranial nerve palsies (CNVII [facial] palsy most common; can be bilateral), headache, meningoencephalitis, **peripheral neuropathy**
	  • <u>**Myocardial Abnormalities**</u>: atrioventricular block (1st-degree, Wenckebach, or 3rd-degree) is most common; myopericarditis, arrythmias, cardiomegaly
	• <u>**Late Disseminated**</u>: occurs months to years after initial infection
	  • **Arthritis**: intermittent, persistent asymmetric arthritis; large joints most commonly affected (knee most common)
	  • <u>**Chronic Neurologic Abnormalities**</u>: polyneuropathy, distal paresthesias, subtle cognitive changes or subacute encephalopathy with mood, memory, and sleep disorders

Diagnosis	• **Clinical Diagnosis** (especially in early localized disease)
	• <u>**Serologic Testing**</u>:
	  • <u>**Enzyme-Linked Immunosorbent Assay (ELISA)**</u>: initial quantitative screening test for serum antibodies
	  • <u>**Western Blot**</u>: confirmatory test indicated if ELISA test is positive or equivocal
	  • <u>Acute (IgM) and Convalescent (IgG) Antibody Titers</u>: indicated as an adjunct to patients with clinical symptoms suggestive of Lyme disease

Treatment	• <u>**Prophylaxis**</u>:
	  • <u>**Doxycycline**</u>: 200mg as a single dose may be given within 72 hours of tick removal if tick was present for at least 36 hours (no risk if tick was attached <24 hours)
	• <u>**Early Localized and Mild Early Disseminated**</u>:
	  • <u>**Doxycycline**</u>: **first-line antibiotic**; 100mg BID for 10 days; *acceptable for pediatric patients when used for 21 days or less*
	  • Amoxicillin: alternative antibiotic indicated in pregnant patients or those with contraindication to doxycycline; 500mg TID for 14 days
	• <u>**Late Disseminated or Severe Early Disseminated**</u>:
	  • <u>**IV Ceftriaxone**</u>: indicated for cases with neurological (meningitis) or myocardial abnormalities
	• <u>Jarisch-Herxheimer Reaction</u>: acute, self-limiting febrile reaction occurring within the first 24 hours after receiving treatment for spirochetal infection
	  • Fever, chills, rigors, headaches, myalgias, diaphoresis, anxiety, or a temporary exacerbation of the syphilitic lesions

Enterobiasis (Pinworms)

Etiology & Risk Factors	• **Intestinal nematode infection** • Etiology: ***Enterobius vermicularis***; most common cause of helminthic infection in the US • Risk Factors: **age (5-10 years old most common), close contact exposure**, crowded living conditions (**schools, daycares**, prisons), poor hygiene, thumb sucking in child
Patho-physiology	• Ingested pinworm eggs hatch in the small intestine and the larvae migrate to the large intestine; the female worms then migrate to the anal area at night to lay their eggs, causing intense itching and leading to the transmission of the infection • Transmission: **fecal-oral, autoinoculation** (thumb sucking in child) **or hand-mouth contact with contaminated fomites** (clothing, bedding, furniture, rugs, toys, toilet seats)

Signs & Symptoms	• **Perianal pruritus**
	   • **Worse at night** (females migrate at night to lay eggs)
	   • May develop excoriations due to scratching
	• Abdominal pain, nausea and vomiting may be present in severe cases

Diagnosis	• Direct Visualization: may be seen in the perianal region 1 or 2 hours after a child goes to bed at night or in the morning • Cellophane Tape Test: samples are obtained in the early morning by applying strip of cellophane tape the perianal skinfolds and then visualized under a microscope • **Oval-shaped ova with a thin shell that contains a curled-up larva**

Treatment	• Supportive: hand washing, trimming fingernails, redirection when child is thumb sucking, taking bath early in morning (reduces egg contamination)
	• Anthelmintics:
	   • **Albendazole, mebendazole or pyrantel** (pyrantel is most cost-effective and available over the counter)
	   • *Treatment of entire household may reduce risk of reinfection*

Key Words & Most Common	• Intestinal nematode infection by Enterobius vermicularis • Children attending daycare most at risk • Intense nocturnal perianal pruritus • Cellophane tape test to visualized eggs • Albendazole, mebendazole or pyrantel

Ascariasis

Etiology & Risk Factors	• Parasitic roundworm infection of the intestine • Etiology: ***Ascaris lumbriocoides***; most common helminth infection worldwide • Risk Factors: age (children most common), **poor sanitation and hygiene practices**, living in crowded or unsanitary conditions, **consuming contaminated food or water**, consuming undercooked vegetables or fruits contaminated with pig feces
Patho-physiology	• Ingestion of the infective eggs which hatch in the intestine and release larvae that penetrate the intestinal wall and migrate through the bloodstream and reach the lungs, where they are coughed up and swallowed, returning to the intestine to mature into adult worms • Adult worms may cause obstruction of the intestine, impair nutrient absorption, and elicit an immune response leading to inflammation and tissue damage
Signs & Symptoms	• Minor Infection: asymptomatic • **Moderate infection: gastrointestinal distress (cramping abdominal pain, nausea, vomiting, anorexia, diarrhea)**, malaise, weakness, impaired cognitive / physical development, malnutrition • **Severe Infection: intestinal obstruction** (small bowel obstruction, volvulus, appendicitis, intussusception); **biliary and pancreatic duct obstruction** (cholecystitis, cholangitis, pancreatitis) • **Löeffler Syndrome**: occurs as larvae pass through the lung • Non-productive cough, chest pain, wheezing, dyspnea, hemoptysis, fever
Diagnosis	• Microscopic Examination of Stool: evaluate for ova and parasites within stool • Direct Visualization: adult worm may be seen in the stool or coming out of the rectum; may be coughed up or passed in the urine • Abdominal Imaging: US and CT scans may be used to identify worms in the biliary duct and gallbladder • Löeffler Syndrome: marked eosinophilia and diffuse pulmonary infiltrates on CXR
Treatment	• Anthelmintics: • **Albendazole, mebendazole or ivermectin** • Surgical or Endoscopic Extraction: indicated for obstructive complications • Löeffler Syndrome: corticosteroids and/or corticosteroids
Key Words & Most Common	• Intestinal infection with *Ascaris lumbriocoides* • GI distress → intestinal obstruction • Löeffler Syndrome: nonspecific respiratory symptoms + marked eosinophilia and diffuse pulmonary infiltrates on CXR • Stool ova and parasites to diagnosis • Albendazole, mebendazole or ivermectin

Trichinosis

Etiology & Risk Factors	• Parasitic roundworm infection of the intestine • Etiology: *Trichinella spiralis* or related *Trichinella* species; consumption of raw or undercooked meat (especially pigs, wild boar, or bear) • Risk Factors: **consumption of raw/undercooked meat** or meat from animals raised in uncontrolled or unhygienic environments, poor food handling and preparation practices
Patho-physiology	• After ingestion, the larvae invade the small intestine and mature into adult worms and reproduce; the newly formed larvae then penetrate the intestinal wall and encapsulate in striated muscle tissue and/or migrate through the blood stream to various tissues causing an inflammatory response

Signs & Symptoms	• **Enteral Phase**: week 1
	  • **Gastrointestinal Symptoms**: nausea, vomiting, diarrhea, abdominal cramps, dyspepsia
	• **Parenteral Phase**: week 1-2
	  • **General**: headache, persistent fever
	  • **Myositis**: myalgia, swelling, weakness; muscles of respiration, speech, mastication, and swallowing may be painful
	  • **Ophthalmic**: facial or periorbital edema, retinal hemorrhages, subconjunctival hemorrhages and petechiae
	• Severe Infections: involve multiple organ systems
	  • Cardiac: **myocarditis** (secondary to eosinophilia), heart failure, arrhythmia
	  • Neurologic: encephalitis, meningitis, visual or auditory disorders, seizures
	  • Pulmonary: pneumonitis, pleurisy

Diagnosis	• **Clinical Diagnosis (periorbital edema + myositis + eosinophilia)** • Enzyme Immunoassay (EIA): using *T. spiralis* excretory-secretory (ES) antigen • Labs: **eosinophilia is hallmark finding; increased muscle enzymes** (elevated creatine kinase [CK] and lactic dehydrogenase [LDH] due to muscle involvement)

Treatment	• **Anthelmintics**: early administration prevents muscular invasion and disease progression
	  • **Albendazole or mebendazole**
	  • **Pyrantel indicated for pregnant women and children**
	• Corticosteroids: prednisone; indicated in severe cases with CNS, cardiac, or pulmonary involvement

Key Words & Most Common	• Parasitic roundworm infection caused by Trichinella spiralis • Raw or undercooked meat (pork, wild boar, bear) • GI symptoms --> myositis + periorbital/facial edema • Myocarditis, encephalitis, meningitis, pneumonitis may be seen in severe cases • Clinical diagnosis + eosinophilia + elevated muscle enzymes • Albendazole or mebendazole +/- prednisone

Hookworm
Ancylostomiasis

Etiology & Risk Factors	• **Nematode parasite infection causing ancylostomiasis**
	• Etiology:
	  • *Ancylostoma duodenale* occurs in the Middle East, North Africa, and southern Europe
	  • *Necator americanus* occurs in North and South America, Australia, Central Africa, South Pacific, India
	  • *Ancylostoma ceylanicum* occurs in India and Southeast Asia
	• Risk Factors: **poor hygiene and sanitation, walking barefoot** (direct exposure to contaminated soil allows larvae to penetrate skin), **occupational exposure to contaminated soil** (farming, mining, construction), crowded living conditions with poor sanitation

Patho-physiology	• Contact of skin to human fecal contaminated soil allow larvae of hookworm species to penetrate the skin and migrate through the bloodstream to the pulmonary capillaries; larvae are then carried to the mouth via the mucociliary escalator and swallowed, reaching the small intestine where they mature into adult worms • Adult worms attach to the intestinal wall and feed on blood, causing chronic intestinal inflammation and resulting in symptoms such as abdominal pain, diarrhea, and anemia

Signs & Symptoms	• **Cutaneous Larvae Migrans**:
	  • **Pruritic erythematous serpiginous, 1-5 cm skin lesions** (occurs as larvae becomes unable to penetrate the deep layers of the skin)
	  • Most common on feet and ankles (direct contact to contaminated soil)
	• **Pulmonary Stage**: usually asymptomatic
	  • Mild cough, pharyngitis, sneezing, bronchitis
	  • Löeffler Syndrome: eosinophilic pneumonia characterized by low-grade fever, productive cough, wheezing
	• **Gastrointestinal Stage**: nonspecific abdominal symptoms
	  • Abdominal pain and distension (mid-epigastric) worse postprandial, nausea, vomiting, diarrhea; occasional GI bleeding (melena)
	• **Chronic Nutritional Impairment**: occurs due to direct parasite consumption of blood or blood leakage from the parasite attachment site within the GI tract
	  • Iron deficiency anemia, hypoalbuminemia, occasional geophagia (infected patients crave soil and ingest dirt)
	  • Chronic fatigue, pallor, dyspnea, weakness, tachycardia, lassitude, and peripheral edema

Diagnosis	• *Occasionally clinical diagnosis* • **Microscopic Examination of Stool**: egg concentration or Kato-Katz techniques; serial exams necessary to detect • Examination for ova and parasites within stool; demonstrates thin-shelled ova detected in fresh stool • Labs: CBC (eosinophilia), iron deficiency anemia (hypochromic microcytic anemia), positive stool guaiac **Cutaneous Larvae Migrans**

Treatment	• **Supportive**: adequate dietary iron intake, iron supplementation, multivitamins
	• **Anthelmintics**:
	  • **Intestinal Infection**: albendazole, mebendazole or pyrantel (ivermectin ineffective)
	  • **Cutaneous Larvae Migrans**: albendazole or ivermectin

Malaria

Etiology & Risk Factors	• Mosquito-borne parasitic infection caused by *Plasmodium* spp. and transmitted via the *Anopheles* mosquito • Etiology: *Plasmodium* spp. (*P. falciparum* is most severe; *P. vivax, P. ovale, P. malariae, P. knowlesi*) and transmitted via the *Anopheles* mosquito • Risk Factors: **living in or traveling to endemic area**, mosquito exposure, lack of immunity, immunocompromised, poor living conditions, occupational exposure (forestry workers, miners, and military personnel), recreational activity exposure (camping, hiking), lack of preventative measures; *sickle cell and thalassemia traits are protective* • Distribution: endemic to Africa, India, Southeast Asia, North and South Korea, Mexico, Central America, Haiti, the Dominican Republic, South America (including northern parts of Argentina), the Middle East (Turkey, Syria, Iran, Iraq), and Central Asia
Patho-physiology	• An infected female *Anopheles* mosquito bites a human, sporozoites are released into the bloodstream which then invade hepatocytes and rapidly divide to form merozoites that infect red blood cells; within erythrocytes, *Plasmodia* consume hemoglobin and develop into trophozoites which disrupt erythrocyte cell membrane integrity, leading to capillary endothelial adherence and cell lysis

Signs & Symptoms	• **Abrupt fever, chills and rigors are hallmark**
	  • Fever is then followed by headache, fatigue, malaise, gastrointestinal distress, polyuria, upper respiratory symptoms, myalgias
	  • Fever then subsides after 2-6 hours; diaphoresis and extreme fatigue occurs
	• Hepatomegaly and **splenomegaly**
	• Severe cases may have jaundice, confusion, seizures, and dark urine
	• **P. falciparum Infection**: most severe disease because of its microvascular effects; fatal if untreated
	  • **Cerebral malaria** (altered mental status, delirium, seizures, coma)
	  • Acute respiratory distress syndrome (ARDS), diarrhea, icterus, epigastric tenderness, retinal hemorrhages, and severe thrombocytopenia may also occur
	  • **Renal insufficiency** (secondary to volume depletion, vascular obstruction by parasitized erythrocytes, or immune complex deposition)
	  • Blackwater Fever: severe intravascular hemolysis resulting in anemia with hemoglobinuria (dark urine) and renal failure;

Diagnosis	• Occasionally, clinical diagnosis (fever + travel)
	• **Light Microscopy of Blood: thin and thick smears**
	  • Thin blood smears stained with Wright-Giemsa stain allow assessment of parasite morphology within red blood cells (RBCs)
	  • Thick blood smears are more difficult to prepare as the RBCs are lysed before staining
	• **Rapid Diagnostic Tests**: antigen or antibody testing; comparable sensitivity to microscopy
	• Labs: leukopenia, **hemolytic anemia**, thrombocytopenia

Treatment	• **Uncomplicated *P. falciparum* Infection**: artemether/lumefantrine is first-line
	  • Alternatives include atovaquone/proguanil or quinine sulfate + doxycycline, tetracycline or clindamycin
	  • **Chloroquine or hydroxychloroquine are additional alternatives**
	• **Chloroquine Resistant *P. falciparum* Infection**: artemether/lumefantrine or atovaquone/proguanil plus primaquine or tafenoquine
	• Uncomplicated *P. vivax* or *P. ovale* Infection: chloroquine or hydroxychloroquine plus primaquine or tafenoquine
	• Severe or Life-Threatening Infection: **IV artesunate or IV quinidine**
	• Prophylaxis: atovaquone-proguanil, doxycycline, and mefloquine

Zika Virus

Etiology & Risk Factors	• **Mosquito-borne flavivirus transmitted by the *Aedes* mosquito** • Etiology: Zika virus transmitted by the bite of the female *Aedes aegypti* and *Aedes albopictus* mosquitoes • Risk Factors: **residing in or travel to endemic area (more common in Central and South America, the Caribbean and the Pacific)**, having unprotect sexual intercourse
Patho-physiology	• The virus enters the body and targets various tissues and cells, including immune cells and neural progenitor cells • Transmission: person-to-person contact (**sexual contact**), blood transfusion, organ transplant, and **perinatally (maternal-fetal vertical transmission)** can also transmit infection • The virus can cross the placental barrier during pregnancy and may infect fetal tissues, leading to potential developmental abnormalities

Signs & Symptoms	• **Most are asymptomatic**
	• Fever, maculopapular rash, conjunctivitis, arthralgias (especially small joints of hands/feet), myalgias, retro-orbital pain, headache
	• Complications:
	  • Guillain-Barré Syndrome: rapidly progressive, self-limited inflammatory polyneuropathy
	  • **Congenital Zika Syndrome: microcephaly** (impaired brain development and small head size), intracranial cerebral malformation, ocular lesions, congenital contractures

Diagnosis	• **Nucleic Acid Amplification Test (NAAT) with Reverse Transcriptase-Polymerase Chain Reaction (RT-PCR) Testing**: detects viral RNA in serum or urine • Serologic Testing: **enzyme-linked immunosorbent assay (ELISA) for IgM**; plaque reduction neutralization test [PRNT] is confirmatory test for Zika virus antibodies
Treatment	• **Supportive**: adequate hydration, rest, **acetaminophen** for fever and arthralgias • **Avoid aspirin and other NSAIDs** until dengue fever can be ruled out due to risk of hemorrhage) • Pregnancy: consider fetal ultrasound every 3-4 weeks to monitor fetal anatomy and growth
Key Words & Most Common	• Mosquito-borne flavivirus transmitted by the female *Aedes aegypti* and *Aedes albopictus* mosquitoes • Can be transmitted through sexual contact or vertical transmission (maternal-fetal) • Most cases are asymptomatic • Congenital Zika syndrome results in microcephaly, decreased brain tissue, eye damage, congenital contractures, and hypertonia • NAAT with RT-PCR or serologic testing • Supportive care

Chicken Pox

Etiology & Risk Factors	• **Acute, primary infection caused by varicella-zoster virus** • <u>Etiology</u>: **varicella-zoster virus** (human herpesvirus type 3) • <u>Risk Factors</u>: age (**children are most common**), lack of immunity (never had chickenpox or received the varicella vaccine), close contact exposure, immunocompromised
Patho-physiology	• <u>Transmission</u>: mucosal (nasopharyngeal) inoculation via infected airborne droplets or aerosolized particles or direct contact with the virus (exposure to open skin lesions) • Highly contagious virus; enters the body through the respiratory tract and then replicates in the respiratory epithelium and spreads to the regional lymph nodes

Signs & Symptoms	• <u>Prodrome</u>: occurs 24-36 hours prior to rash development
	  • **Mild headache, moderate fever, pharyngitis and malaise**
	  • Macular eruption with a rapidly fading flush; usually starts on head or scalp
	• <u>Evolution</u>:
	  • **Intensely-pruritic, erythematous papules with teardrop vesicles on an erythematous base (pathognomonic)**
	  • **Lesions develop in crops** (various stages of development throughout body)
	  • **Lesions then become pustular and crust over**

Diagnosis	• **Clinical Diagnosis** • <u>Polymerase Chain Reaction (PCR)</u>: used to confirm diagnosis • <u>Viral Culture</u>: performed on fluid from ruptured vesicles • <u>Tzanck Smear</u>: performed with Wright-Giemsa or toluidine blue stain; shows multinucleated giant cells • <u>Serologic Testing</u>: IgM antibodies to varicella-zoster virus (VZV)

Treatment	• <u>**Supportive**</u>: symptomatic treatment
	  • **Cool, wet compresses, systemic antihistamines, colloidal oatmeal baths, trimming of fingernails** (prevents secondary bacterial infection from scratching)
	• <u>Antivirals</u>: may reduce severity and duration of symptoms if initiated within 72 hours
	  • Oral acyclovir, valacyclovir, famciclovir considered for patients >12 years old, history of eczema, chronic lung disease, receiving long-term salicylates or corticosteroids
	  • Oral acyclovir or valacyclovir may be considered in pregnant patients
	  • IV acyclovir indicated for immunocompromised children or adults
	• *Patient is contagious from 48 hours prior to onset of rash until all lesions have crusted over*

Key Words & Most Common	• Acute primary infection caused by varicella-zoster virus • Most common in children • Prodrome of headache, fever, malaise → macular eruption → pruritic papules with vesicles on erythematous base → lesions become pustular and crust over • Clinical diagnosis • Supportive treatment • Antivirals indicated in certain cases (immunocompromised, pregnancy)

Herpes Zoster (Shingles)

Etiology & Risk Factors	• **Viral syndrome that occurs when the varicella-zoster virus reactivates from its latent state in a posterior dorsal root ganglion** • <u>Etiology</u>: **varicella-zoster virus** (human herpesvirus type 3) • <u>Risk Factors</u>: **advancing age (>50 years old most common)**, immunocompromised (HIV/AIDS, chemotherapy, organ transplant recipient), **physical, emotional or immunologic stress**, certain medical conditions (malignancy or autoimmune diseases)
Patho-physiology	• After recovery from chickenpox, the virus remains dormant in the posterior dorsal root ganglia; virus reactivation occurs secondary to declining immunity and age-related changes in the immune system, and travels along the sensory nerve fibers to the skin, resulting in the characteristic painful rash and blisters

Signs & Symptoms	• <u>Prodrome</u>: headache, malaise, photophobia, **sensory changes (pain, pruritus, burning, paresthesia to dermatome 2-3 days prior to rash development)**
	• <u>Rash Development</u>: lasts 10-14 days
	  • Painful maculopapular rash progressing to vesicles on an erythematous base; may coalesce to bullae
	  • **Follows a dermatomal distribution (does not cross the midline)**
	  • **Most commonly affects chest or face**; may affect cervical, trigeminal, facial, or lumbosacral nerves
	• <u>Herpes Zoster Oticus (Ramsay-Hunt Syndrome)</u>: reactivation of virus in geniculate ganglion of the facial nerve (CNVII)
	  • Ipsilateral facial paralysis, ear pain, vertigo, **vesicles on the external auditory canal and/or auricle**
	  • Loss of taste on the anterior 2/3rd of the tongue
	• <u>Herpes Zoster Ophthalmicus</u>: sight-threatening disorder
	  • Occurs with reactivation of the virus involving the ophthalmic division of the trigeminal nerve (CNV)
	  • Conjunctivitis, uveitis, episcleritis, keratitis; vesicles on side or tip of the nose (Hutchinson sign)
	• <u>Post-Herpetic Neuralgia</u>: persistent pain or sensory symptoms that last >90 days after onset
	  • Persistent, burning, sharp pain or sensory changes (allodynia)

Diagnosis	• **Clinical Diagnosis** • <u>Polymerase Chain Reaction (PCR)</u>: used to confirm diagnosis • <u>Viral Culture</u>: performed on fluid from ruptured vesicles • <u>Tzanck Smear</u>: performed with Wright-Giemsa or toluidine blue stain; shows multinucleated giant cells • <u>Slit-Lamp Examination</u>: indicated if concern of herpes zoster ophthalmicus; demonstrates dendritic (branching) uptake of fluorescein if keratoconjunctivitis present
Treatment	• <u>Supportive</u>: cool, wet compresses, **analgesia** (topical lidocaine, nerve blocks, acetaminophen, NSAIDs, opioids) • <u>Antivirals</u>: decreases the severity and duration of the acute eruption and reduces risk of complications including post-herpetic neuralgia • **Valacyclovir or famciclovir are preferred** due to increased bioavailability and dosing requirements; acyclovir is alternative • <u>Corticosteroids</u>: consider methylprednisolone and/or prednisone in severe cases or herpes zoster oticus/ophthalmic cases (blunts inflammatory response) • <u>Post-Herpetic Neuralgia</u>: **gabapentin or pregabalin is initial treatment**; topical capsaicin or lidocaine; tricyclic antidepressants or opioids in severe cases • <u>Post-Exposure Prophylaxis</u>: varicella zoster immune globulin indicated for immunocompromised, patients on immunosuppressive therapy or neonates • <u>Prevention</u>: recombinant zoster vaccine is recommended for immunocompetent adults ≥ 50 years (2 doses given 2-6 months apart)

Human Papillomavirus (HPV)

Etiology & Risk Factors	• Skin-colored, fleshy papules in the anogenital region • Etiology: human papillomavirus (HPV) infection (type 6 and 11 most common) • Risk Factors: **sexual activity (unprotected sex or having multiple sexual partners)**, immunocompromised, age (young adults are most commonly affected), lack of vaccination
Patho-physiology	• Virus enters body through skin or mucous membranes and primarily infects the nucleus of differentiated squamous epithelial cells; human papillomavirus (HPV) contains an oncogene that produces proteins responsible for promoting cell growth and facilitating viral replication • As the number of infected host cells increases, the skin layers thicken, resulting in the formation of warts at a macroscopic level due to acanthosis

Signs & Symptoms	• Incubation period of 1-6 months
	• Small, raised, soft, skin-colored, fleshy papules of the anogenital region
	   • May **enlarge or become pedunculated ("cauliflower-like")**, have rough surface, and/or appear in clusters
	   • **Most common under foreskin, on coronal sulcus, or penile shaft of men;** may occur around the anus or in the rectum in men who have sex with men
	   • **Most common on vulva, vaginal wall, cervix, and perineum of women**
	   • **Usually asymptomatic;** may cause pruritus, bleeding, burning or general discomfort

Diagnosis	• **Clinical Diagnosis** • **Acetic Acid Test: 5% solution of acetic acid applied to lesion causes lesions to whiten** • Polymerase Chain Reaction (PCR): confirms diagnosis • HPV Serologies: confirms diagnosis • Colposcopy/Anoscopy: direct visualization of lesion • Biopsy: koilocytes (large keratinocytes with abundant cytoplasm and small nuclei) and papillomatosis

Treatment	• **Supportive: most cases will experience spontaneous resolution;** relapses are frequent and often require multiple retreatments
	   • Treatment indicated for warts that are cosmetically unacceptable, in locations that interfere with function or are painful
	• **Physical Removal:**
	   • **Cryotherapy (Liquid Nitrogen): first-line treatment to remove lesions;** 3-5 applications weekly for 6-10 weeks
	   • Electrocauterization, laser ablation or surgical excision are alternatives
	• Topical Management: considered second-line
	   • Antimitotics: podophyllotoxin, podophyllin, 5-fluorouracil; podophyllotoxin cannot be used for anogenital warts
	   • Caustics: trichloroacetic acid
	   • Interferon Inducers: imiquimod; lower rates of recurrence compared to podophyllotoxin
	   • Sinecatechins: alternative topical treatment with unknown mechanism
	• Prevention: recommended at age 11-12 years old males and females, previously unvaccinated or not adequately vaccinated patients through 26 years old
	   • 9-Valent HPV Vaccine (Gardasil-9): protects against HPV type 6, 11, 16, 18, 31, 33, 45, 52, 58
	   • Quadrivalent HPV Vaccine (Gardasil): protects against HPV type 6, 11, 16, 18

Influenza

Etiology & Risk Factors	• Viral illness affecting the upper and lower respiratory tract • Etiology: **influenza viruses** (classified as type A or B) • Risk Factors: age (<2 or >65 years old), chronic medical comorbidities, immunocompromised, pregnancy, obesity, seasonal (fall/winter months in temperate climates) • Complications: primary viral pneumonia, secondary bacterial pneumonia, acute respiratory distress syndrome, meningitis, myocarditis, death • Transmission: droplet transmission occurs within 3-6ft radius; viral shedding lasts about 5days (24-48hr prior to symptom onset); *n95 or surgical mask reduces transmission*
Patho-physiology	• Acute viral illness targeting upper and lower respiratory tract; immune reaction and interferon response cause viral symptom syndrome as a result of viral infection • Influenza A can have multiple subtypes based on combination of hemagglutinin (H) and neuraminidase (N) protein expression on viral surface (i.e. H1N1, H3N2, etc.) • Hemagglutinin binds to respiratory tract epithelial cells allowing infection to progress; neuraminidase breaks bond holding virus together allowing transmission
Signs & Symptoms	• *Influenza A is associated with a more severe disease course* • **Sudden onset fever/chills, headache,** nonproductive cough, fatigue, pharyngitis • **Myalgias (particularly lower back and legs)** • Acute symptoms generally subside after 2-3 days; fever may persist for 5 days
Diagnosis	• **Clinical Diagnosis** • Rapid Influenza Nasal Swab or Viral Culture: specific but variable sensitivity • Reverse Transcriptase-Polymerase Chain Reaction (RT-PCR): sensitive and specific; used in hospital or ER setting • CXR: may be ordered to rule out primary viral or secondary bacterial pneumonia

Treatment	• **Supportive: symptomatic treatment** with acetaminophen/NSAIDs as needed (avoid aspirin if <18 due to risk of Reye syndrome); adequate hydration; rest
	• Antivirals: recommended for hospitalized or high-risk patients; **all antivirals are most effective if initiated within 48 hours of symptoms**
	   • Neuraminidase Inhibitors: **Oseltamivir (Tamiflu)** slow spread by interfering viral release from infected cells
	   • Endonuclease Inhibitor: **Baloxavir (Xofluza)** block viral RNA transcription to interfere with viral replication
	   • Adamantanes: Amantadine & Rimantadine are no longer indicated due to 99% resistance
	• Prevention: **annual influenza vaccination;** pre/post-exposure prophylactic antivirals

Key Words & Most Common	• Seasonal virus characterized by abrupt onset of fever/chills, headache, myalgias of lower back and legs • Diagnosed clinically; rapid influenza may be used in office but lacks sensitivity; RT-PCR more sensitive but usually only used in inpatient/ER setting • Supportive symptomatic treatment is mainstay • Antivirals may be initiated if <48 hours since onset of symptoms • Prevention with annual vaccination

Measles (Rubeola)

Etiology & Risk Factors	• Highly contagious RNA virus that primarily affects the respiratory system • Etiology: **measles virus, part of the Paramyxovirus family** • Risk Factors: **lack of immunization, international travel to areas with outbreaks, exposure to international terminal at airports or interaction with foreign visitors** (U.S. tourist attractions), crowded areas (schools, dorms, military barracks, daycare centers, public transportation), immunocompromised
Patho-physiology	• Transmission: respiratory droplets; **7-14 day incubation period** • Virus enters the respiratory tract (nasopharynx) and infects the mucous membranes, then spreads throughout the body via the bloodstream, causing a systemic infection; viral replication initially occurs in immune cells of the lymphatic system and may also infect and damage the respiratory epithelium and skin, leading to characteristic rashes

Signs & Symptoms	• **Prodrome:**
	  • **Fever, coryza, cough and conjunctivitis** followed by Koplik spots
	• **Koplik Spots: pathognomonic enanthem**
	  • **Small 1-3mm pale white papules with erythematous base on the buccal mucosa**; precedes rash by about 24-48 hours
	  • **Most commonly on oral mucosa opposite the 1st and 2nd upper molars;** may be extensive
	  • Spots resemble "grains of white sand surrounded by red base"
	• Generalized Exanthem: appears 3-5 days after symptom onset; 1-2 days after Koplik spots appear
	  • **Morbilliform (maculopapular), erythematous rash beginning on face at the hairline and behind the ears**
	  • **Descending rash spreads to trunk and extremities (including palms and soles) as the lesions fade on the face**
	  • Rash usually lasts 3-5 days and may fade rapidly, leaving a darkened, coppery-brown discoloration followed by desquamation
	
	Morbilliform Rash

Diagnosis	• **Clinical Diagnosis** • **Viral Detection via Polymerase Chain Reaction (PCR): preferred testing method to confirm diagnosis** • Measles IgM Serology: frequent false positives; no longer recommended

Treatment	• **Supportive: mainstay of treatment;** self-limited disease
	  • **Analgesia/antipyretics (acetaminophen and/or NSAIDs)**
	  • Oral hydration
	• **Vitamin A Supplementation:** reduces morbidity and mortality
	  • Dose is once per day for 2 days
	    • >1 Year: 200,000 international units (IU)
	    • 6-11 Months: 100,000 IU
	    • <6 Months: 50,000 IU
	• Prevention: live-attenuated virus vaccine containing measles, mumps, and rubella
	  • First dose recommended at 12-15 months; second dose recommended at 4-6 years old
	
	Koplik Spots

Viral Parotitis

Etiology & Risk Factors	• Acute inflammation of the parotid gland • Etiology: **paramyxovirus (mumps) is most common;** influenza, parainfluenza, coxsackie • Risk Factors: **age (<15 years old most common),** immunosuppression, **unimmunized or partially immunized (MMR),** congregate settings (college campus/dorms)
Patho-physiology	• Virus enters upper respiratory tract through nose or mouth; following exposure, virus spreads to parotid gland causing local inflammation
Signs & Symptoms	• **Prodrome of fever, headache, arthralgias/myalgias, malaise** • **Unilateral or bilateral parotid gland pain and swelling** • May have pain with chewing • **Unilateral orchitis** (20-30% of male patients)
Diagnosis	• **Clinical Diagnosis** • **Mumps immunoglobulin (IgM and IgG) or Polymerase Chain Reaction (PCR): confirms diagnosis;** may require reporting to local health department • **Testicular Ultrasound:** if concern for orchitis
Treatment	• **Supportive: mainstay of treatment;** rest, hydration, analgesia (NSAIDs), soft diet • Testicular Support: scrotal sling or supportive, non-restrictive underwear to minimize tension, ice packs
Key Words & Most Common	• Acute inflammation of parotid gland • Paramyxovirus (mumps) most common; influenza • Unimmunized/partially immunized against MMR • Prodrome of fever, headache, body/muscle aches • Unilateral/bilateral parotid gland pain and swelling • Orchitis • Clinical diagnosis + Mumps immunoglobulin or PCR to confirm diagnosis • Testicular ultrasound as indicated • Supportive care Unilateral parotid gland swelling

Rubella

Etiology & Risk Factors	• Mild viral illness also known as **German Measles** • <u>Etiology</u>: **Rubella virus**; genus Rubivirus within the *Matonaviridae* family • <u>Risk Factors</u>: **age (5-9 years old most common), unimmunized or partially immunized (MMR),** crowded living conditions (**daycare centers** or households with multiple children), seasonal (**late winter and early spring most common**), immunocompromised
Patho-physiology	• The virus enters the body through respiratory droplets and spreads to various organs, including the lymph nodes, skin, and joints • The virus primarily infects and replicates within cells of the respiratory epithelium, lymph nodes, and other organs

Signs & Symptoms	• Incubation period of 14-21 days
	• <u>Prodrome</u>:
	  • Low-grade fever, cough, anorexia, malaise, conjunctivitis
	• <u>Exanthem</u>:
	  • **Erythematous (pink or light-red), nonconfluent, maculopapular rash beginning on the face and neck and quickly spreading to the trunk and extremities**
	  • Rash coalesces on face as it reaches extremities and may become more scarlatiniform (pinpoint) with a reddish flush
	  • **Rash lasts 3-5 days**
	• <u>**Forchheimer Spots**</u>: petechiae on the soft palate
	• <u>**Lymphadenopathy**</u>: suboccipital, **postauricular**, posterior cervical

Diagnosis	• **Clinical Diagnosis** • <u>Polymerase Chain Reaction (PCR)</u>: testing of throat, nasal, or urine specimens • <u>Serum Rubella IgM Antibody Testing</u>: **confirms diagnosis**; testing necessary for pregnant women and neonates and patients with signs of encephalitis

Treatment	• <u>**Supportive**</u>: **mainstay of treatment; self-limiting illness**
	  • Rest, adequate hydration, antipyretics (acetaminophen, ibuprofen)
	• <u>Proper Hygiene</u>: adequate handwashing to prevent spread of infection
	• <u>Prevention</u>: live-attenuated virus vaccine containing measles, mumps, and rubella
	  • First dose recommended at 12-15 months; second dose recommended at 4-6 years old

Key Words & Most Common	• Most common among unimmunized children • Prodrome of mild constitutional symptoms • Erythematous maculopapular rash of face and neck spreading to trunk/extremities • Postauricular lymphadenopathy • Clinical diagnosis → PCR or IgM Ab testing to confirm • Supportive

Erythema Infectiosum

Etiology & Risk Factors	• Viral infection also known as **fifth disease** • <u>Etiology</u>: **parvovirus B19** • <u>Risk Factors</u>: seasonal (**most common in spring**), age (**most common among children 5-7 years old**), high risk exposures (**daycare or school settings**)
Patho-physiology	• <u>Transmission</u>: respiratory droplets; **4-14 day incubation period** • Parvovirus B19 infects and destroys reticulocytes resulting in a transient suppression of erythropoiesis (**leading to aplastic crisis in patients with sickle cell disease**) • Transplacental transmission possible in pregnant females without immunity; can result in stillbirth or severe fetal anemia with widespread edema (hydrops fetalis)
Signs & Symptoms	• **Nonspecific flu-like symptoms** (low-grade fever, malaise, coryza, pharyngitis) **initially** • **Erythematous malar rash appears over the cheeks ("slapped-cheek" appearance) and circumoral pallor for 2-4 days** • **Symmetric, reticular or lacy, maculopapular rash appears on the extremities (especially upper) and/or trunk**; usually spares the palms and soles usually lasting for 5-10 days • Rash may recur for several weeks, exacerbated by sunlight, exercise, heat, fever and/or emotional stress • **Arthralgias** may be present in older children and adults
Diagnosis	• **Clinical Diagnosis** • <u>Serologies</u>: Parvovirus B19 specific IgM-antibody confirms diagnosis

Treatment	• <u>**Supportive**</u>: **mainstay of treatment**; self-limited disease
	  • **Analgesia/antipyretics (acetaminophen and/or NSAIDs)**
	  • Oral hydration
	• <u>IV Immunoglobulin</u>: indicated for immunocompromised children
	• <u>Pregnancy</u>: regular fetal monitoring and close follow-up with obstetrician

Key Words & Most Common	• AKA fifth disease • Viral infection caused by parvovirus B19 • Most common in spring and in children • 4-14 day incubation period • Nonspecific flu-like symptoms → erythematous malar rash over cheeks → reticular/lacy maculopapular rash of extremities and trunk • Clinical diagnosis • Supportive treatment

Erythematous malar rash with a "slapped-cheek" appearance

Roseola Infantum

Etiology & Risk Factors	• Common disease of childhood; also known as **sixth disease** • Etiology: **human herpesvirus-6 (HHV-6) is most common**; human herpesvirus 7 (HHV-7) possible • Risk Factors: **age (<2 years old most common)**, crowded living conditions (**daycare centers** or households with multiple children), seasonal (fall and spring most common), immunocompromised • Transmission: saliva via respiratory droplets
Patho-physiology	• The virus enters the body through respiratory secretions and infects lymphocytes, including T-cells and B-cells • The virus then spreads to multiple organs, leading to the characteristic symptoms of high fever followed by a rash

Signs & Symptoms	• Incubation period of 5-15 days
	• Prodrome:
	  • **Abrupt onset of high fever (may exceed 104°F) lasting 3-5 days without localizing signs or symptoms**
	  • Child generally appears well and alert; *febrile seizures possible*
	  • **Fever often resolves prior to onset of the rash**
	  • Cervical and posterior auricular lymphadenopathy often develops
	• Exanthem:
	  • **Erythematous (rose/pink colored), blanching, macular or maculopapular rash that begins on the trunk and neck and spreads to the face**
	    • *Only viral exanthem that starts on the trunk*
	  • **Lasts a few hours up to 2 days**
	• Uvulopalatoglossal Spots (Nagayama Spots): erythematous papules found on the soft palate and uvula
	• Erythematous tympanic membranes

Diagnosis	• **Clinical Diagnosis**
Treatment	• **Supportive: mainstay of treatment; self-limiting illness** • Rest, adequate hydration, antipyretics (acetaminophen, ibuprofen) • Proper Hygiene: adequate handwashing to prevent spread of infection
Key Words & Most Common	• Common disease of childhood caused by HHV-6 • 3-5 day prodrome of high fever → defervescence → macular rash that begins on trunk lasting for 1-2 days • Clinical diagnosis • Supportive treatment

Epstein-Barr Virus (Infectious Mononucleosis)

Etiology & Risk Factors	• Herpesvirus that infects 50% of children before 5 years old and 90% of adults • Etiology: **Epstein Barr Virus (EBV)**; a double-stranded DNA virus that infects B lymphocyte cells • Risk Factors: **contact with saliva of an infected individual (kissing, sharing utensils), age (most common in adolescents and young adults)**, immunocompromised
Patho-physiology	• **EBV primarily infects B lymphocytes**, leading to the expansion of infected B cells and their dissemination throughout the body; the virus enters the host cells through binding to CD21 receptors on B cells, initiating a complex interplay between viral and host factors • EBV establishes a latent infection in B cells, where the viral genome persists, allowing reactivation and production of infectious viral particles

Signs & Symptoms	• Tetrad: fever, pharyngitis, lymphadenopathy, fatigue
	  • **Fever**: typically peaks in the afternoon or early evening
	  • **Pharyngitis**: severe, painful, **exudative**; may have petechiae on the hard palate
	  • **Lymphadenopathy**: usually symmetric and involves anterior and posterior cervical chains; **posterior cervical chain is most common**
	  • **Fatigue: maximal during the first 2-3 weeks; may** persist for several months
	• Other: may be associated with **splenomegaly**, hepatomegaly, **fatigue**, headache, general malaise
	• Morbilliform Rash: may develop if patient on amoxicillin or ampicillin

Diagnosis	• Heterophile Antibody Test: measured using various agglutination card (monospot) tests; 87% sensitive and and 91% specific • **EBV-Specific Antibody Testing: highly sensitive and specific**; can determine if primary infection, reactivation, or latent infection • Tests for EBV viral capsid antigen (VCA), VCA-IgG antibody, EBV nuclear antigen (EBNA-IgG), EBV early antigen and VCA-IgM antibody • Splenic Ultrasound: consider with splenomegaly for return-to-play protocol

Treatment	• **Supportive: self-limited illness**; adequate rest, analgesia (acetaminophen, NSAIDs), oral rehydration, avoid overly strenuous exercise
	  • *Fatigue may last for months*
	• **Avoiding Contact Sports: avoid trauma, heavy lifting or contact sports for at least 4 weeks to reduce risk of splenic rupture**
	  • *Consider splenic ultrasound for return-to-play protocol*
	• Corticosteroids: indicated for complications such as airway obstruction, severe thrombocytopenia, and hemolytic anemia

Key Words & Most Common	• Transmission through contact with saliva ("kissing disease") • EBV primarily infects B lymphocytes • Tetrad of fever, pharyngitis, lymphadenopathy, fatigue • Morbilliform rash if given penicillin • Heterophile antibody vs EBV specific antibody test • Supportive care • Avoid contact sports due to risk of splenic rupture

Exudative Pharyngitis

EBV Specific Antibody Interpretation				
Interpretation	VCA-IgM	EA-IgG	VCA-IgG	EBNA-IgG
No Infection	−	−	−	−
Early Phase Infection	+	−	−	−
Acute Primary Infection	+	+ or −	+	−
Past Infection	−	+ or −	+	+
Reactivation of Latent Infection	+ or −	+	+	+

Herpes Simplex Virus 1

Etiology & Risk Factors	• Virus that causes recurrent infection affecting the skin, mouth, lips, eyes, and genitals • <u>Etiology</u>: **human herpesviruses types 1** • <u>Risk Factors</u>: **direct oral-to-oral contact (kissing or sharing utensils, drinks, or lip balm)**, childhood exposure (contact with infected family members), immunocompromised
Patho-physiology	• HSV-1 and HSV-2 can both cause oral or genital infection; HSV-1 typically causes gingivostomatitis, herpes labialis, and herpes keratitis • Virus infects epithelial cells, where it replicates and causes local tissue damage and then enters sensory neurons and establishes latency in the sensory ganglia, leading to recurrent outbreaks of oral herpes lesions triggered by various factors, such as stress or immune system compromise

Signs & Symptoms	• <u>**Acute Herpetic Gingivostomatitis**</u>: caused by primary infection of HSV; most common in children
	   • Intraoral and gingival vesicles that rupture and form ulcers
	• <u>**Herpes Labialis (Cold Sores)**</u>: reactivation of latent viral infection
	   • Prodromal symptoms of pruritus, burning, paresthesia, pain
	   • Within 24 hours, grouped vesicles on an erythematous base and ulceration develop on the vermilion border of the lip
	• <u>**Herpes Simplex Keratitis**</u>: infection of the corneal epithelium
	   • Ocular pain, tearing, photophobia, and corneal ulcers with a branching dendritic pattern (seen on fluorescein stain)
	• <u>**Herpetic Whitlow**</u>: inoculation of HSV through the skin; common in dentists and health care workers
	   • Edematous, painful, erythematous lesion of the finger

Diagnosis	• **Clinical Diagnosis** • <u>Polymerase Chain Reaction (PCR)</u>: used to confirm diagnosis • <u>Viral Culture</u>: performed on fluid from ruptured vesicles • <u>Tzanck Smear</u>: performed with Wright-Giemsa or toluidine blue stain; shows multinucleated giant cells • <u>Serologic Testing</u>: gold standard for diagnosis

Treatment	• <u>**Acute Herpetic Gingivostomatitis**</u>:
	   • <u>Supportive</u>: symptomatic relief with topical anesthetics (benzocaine, viscous lidocaine)
	   • <u>Antivirals</u>: acyclovir, valacyclovir indicated in severe cases
	• <u>**Herpes Labialis (Cold Sores)**</u>:
	   • <u>**Antivirals**</u>: **valacyclovir 2g BID for 1 day**; famciclovir 1500mg as single dose is alternative
	• <u>**Herpes Simplex Keratitis**</u>: referral to ophthalmologist is indicated
	   • <u>Topical Antivirals</u>: trifluridine
	• <u>**Herpetic Whitlow**</u>:
	   • <u>Supportive</u>: keep lesions covered to reduce spread; resolves within 2-3 weeks without treatment

Herpes Labialis

Herpes Simplex Virus 2

Etiology & Risk Factors	• Virus that causes recurrent infection affecting genitals • <u>Etiology</u>: **human herpesviruses types 2** • <u>Risk Factors</u>: **unprotected sexual activity** (particularly vaginal or anal intercourse), having multiple sexual partners, high-risk sexual behavior, immunocompromised
Patho-physiology	• Virus infects epithelial cells, where it replicates and causes local tissue damage and then enters sensory neurons and establishes latency in the sensory nerve ganglia; reactivation can occur intermittently leading to recurrent outbreaks of painful, genital lesions • HSV-2 is primarily transmitted through sexual contact and can also be transmitted from mother to infant during childbirth
Signs & Symptoms	• **Prodromal symptoms of pruritus, burning, paresthesia, pain** • Within 24 hours, **grouped vesicles on an erythematous base and painful, shallow ulceration develop on the genitals** • Inguinal lymphadenopathy is common
Diagnosis	• **Clinical Diagnosis** • <u>Polymerase Chain Reaction (PCR)</u>: used to confirm diagnosis • <u>Viral Culture</u>: performed on fluid from ruptured vesicles • <u>Tzanck Smear</u>: performed with Wright-Giemsa or toluidine blue stain; shows multinucleated giant cells • <u>Serologic Testing</u>: gold standard for diagnosis

Treatment	• <u>**Initial Episode**</u>:
	   • <u>**Valacyclovir**</u>: 1g BID for 7-10 days
	   • <u>**Acyclovir**</u>: 400mg TID for 7-10 days
	   • <u>**Famciclovir**</u>: 250mg TID for 7-10 days
	• <u>**Recurrence**</u>:
	   • <u>**Valacyclovir**</u>: 500mg BID for 3 days or 1g QD for 5 days
	   • <u>**Acyclovir**</u>: 400mg TID for 5 days or 800mg BID for 5 days
	   • <u>**Famciclovir**</u>: 125mg BID for 5 days
	• <u>**Suppressive Therapy**</u>:
	   • <u>**Valacyclovir**</u>: 1g daily
	   • <u>**Acyclovir**</u>: 400mg BID daily
	   • <u>**Famciclovir**</u>: 250mg BID daily

Genital herpes on the vulva

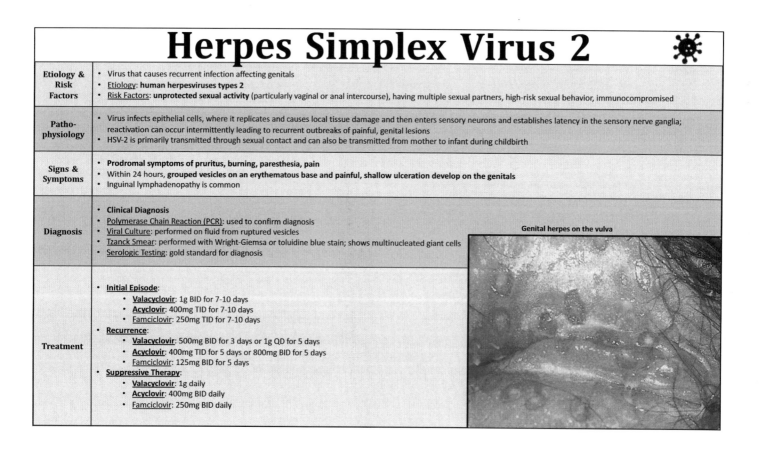

Parainfluenza Virus

Etiology & Risk Factors	• Common respiratory illness that causes inflammation of the upper and lower airways particularly the larynx and subglottic airway; also known as laryngotracheitis • <u>Etiologies</u>: **Parainfluenza virus is most common cause** • <u>Risk Factors</u>: age (6 months to 3 years old most common; peaks at 2 years old), seasonal (most common during fall and winter)
Patho-physiology	• Infection causes edema of the larynx, trachea, and bronchi as a result of white blood cell infiltration leading to subglottic airway obstruction. • Airway obstruction leads to labored breathing and the characteristic turbulent airflow (stridor)
Signs & Symptoms	• **Croup** • **Upper airway infection symptoms for 1-3 days followed by a harsh, spasmodic, "seal-like barking" cough and inspiratory stridor most commonly occurring at night** • Total duration of illness is 4-7 days; most severe on days 3-4 • May have low grade fever, voice hoarseness, dyspnea • Child may awaken at night with tachypnea, retractions, and/or respiratory distress • **NO drooling or dysphagia** • Severe cases may have hypoxia and cyanosis
Diagnosis	• **Clinical diagnosis** (obstructive conditions such as epiglottitis, bacterial tracheitis, and airway foreign body should be ruled out) • <u>AP Neck X-Ray</u>: may show subglottic airway stenosis (**steeple sign**) but is rarely performed
Treatment	• <u>Supportive</u>: **cool mist humidifier**, antipyretics, hydration • <u>Steroids</u>: **first line treatment; Dexamethasone PO/IM** provides significant relief and associated with faster resolution and decreased relapse • <u>Nebulized Epinephrine</u>: provides symptomatic relief through vasoconstriction; reserved for moderate to severe cases; patient should be observed for 3-4 hours after • <u>Intubation</u>: rarely required; ½ size smaller tube should be used due to airway edema • Do NOT give albuterol as may worsen airway edema (vasodilation)
Key Words & Most Common	• Common respiratory illness resulting in upper/lower airway inflammation • Most common in 6mo-3yo (peaks at 2yo) • URI symptoms for 1-3 days followed by harsh, "seal-like barking" cough and inspiratory stridor; worse at night • Clinical diagnosis; steeple sign on AP neck x-ray • Supportive with cool mist humidifier; Dexamethasone is first-line for symptomatic relief

Respiratory Syncytial Virus (RSV)

Etiology & Risk Factors	• Common lower respiratory viral infection typically occurring in young patients • <u>Etiology</u>: respiratory syncytial virus (RSV) • <u>Risk Factors</u>: **age (most common in infants <2 years old; peak incidence 2-6 months old), premature infants** (<36weeks of gestation), parental smoking, crowded environment **(day care)** • Patients with congenital heart disease and chronic lung diseases, younger age (<3mo) & immunodeficiency are at risk for severe disease
Patho-physiology	• Virus infects airway epithelial cells which induce an inflammatory response and cause mucociliary dysfunction and accumulation of cellular debris • Cytokine release causes airway edema which progresses to decreased lung compliance and air trapping
Signs & Symptoms	• **Upper respiratory infection symptoms (low grade fever, cough, rhinorrhea) for 24–72 hours** • Progresses to symptoms of **respiratory distress** (apnea, wheezing, tachypnea, retractions, nasal flaring) • **Dehydration** as a result of vomiting and decreased oral intake (tachypnea interferes with feeding) • Severe disease may have apnea/tachypnea, cyanosis/hypoxemia, respiratory failure, lethargy
Diagnosis	• **Clinical Diagnosis** • <u>**Polymerase Chain Reaction (PCR) or Rapid Antigen**</u>: **may aid in confirming diagnosis** • <u>**Pulse Oximeter**</u>: best predictor of disease course in children; further testing not required if normal spO_2 • <u>CXR</u>: not routinely necessary; nonspecific findings (hyperinflation, hilar markings); consider if diagnosis is unclear or severe symptoms
Treatment	• <u>Supportive</u>: mainstay of treatment; **aggressive hydration (oral and/or IV), humidified oxygen**, nebulized saline, cool mist humidifier, suction of secretions • <u>Supplemental Oxygen</u>: goal spO_2>90% with high flow nasal canula • <u>Endotracheal Intubation</u>: reserved for severe cases with apnea, hypoxemia, or unable to clear secretions • <u>Bronchodilators</u>: generally not effective and may aggravate symptoms • <u>Corticosteroids</u>: dexamethasone; reserved for severe cases
Key Words & Most Common	• Acute, viral, lower respiratory infection typically occurring in young patients <2yo with peak incidence in 2-6-month-olds • URI symptoms for 24-72 hours that progress to respiratory distress; MC complication is dehydration • Clinical diagnosis, pulse oximeter should be monitored • Supportive treatment with aggressive hydration and supplemental oxygen with goal spO2 >90%

Hand-Foot-and-Mouth Disease ✹

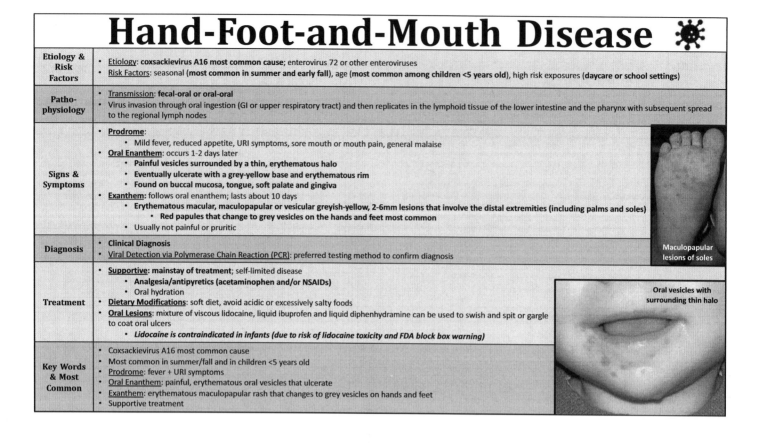

Etiology & Risk Factors	• Etiology: **coxsackievirus A16 most common cause**; enterovirus 72 or other enteroviruses • Risk Factors: seasonal **(most common in summer and early fall)**, age **(most common among children <5 years old)**, high risk exposures **(daycare or school settings)**
Patho-physiology	• Transmission: **fecal-oral or oral-oral** • Virus invasion through oral ingestion (GI or upper respiratory tract) and then replicates in the lymphoid tissue of the lower intestine and the pharynx with subsequent spread to the regional lymph nodes

Signs & Symptoms	• **Prodrome:**
	  • Mild fever, reduced appetite, URI symptoms, sore mouth or mouth pain, general malaise
	• **Oral Enanthem:** occurs 1-2 days later
	  • **Painful vesicles surrounded by a thin, erythematous halo**
	  • **Eventually ulcerate with a grey-yellow base and erythematous rim**
	  • **Found on buccal mucosa, tongue, soft palate and gingiva**
	• **Exanthem:** follows oral enanthem; lasts about 10 days
	  • **Erythematous macular, maculopapular or vesicular greyish-yellow, 2-6mm lesions that involve the distal extremities (including palms and soles)**
	    • **Red papules that change to grey vesicles on the hands and feet most common**
	  • Usually not painful or pruritic

Diagnosis	• **Clinical Diagnosis** • Viral Detection via Polymerase Chain Reaction (PCR): preferred testing method to confirm diagnosis

Treatment	• **Supportive: mainstay of treatment**; self-limited disease
	  • **Analgesia/antipyretics (acetaminophen and/or NSAIDs)**
	  • Oral hydration
	• **Dietary Modifications:** soft diet, avoid acidic or excessively salty foods
	• **Oral Lesions:** mixture of viscous lidocaine, liquid ibuprofen and liquid diphenhydramine can be used to swish and spit or gargle to coat oral ulcers
	  • ***Lidocaine is contraindicated in infants (due to risk of lidocaine toxicity and FDA block box warning)***

Key Words & Most Common	• Coxsackievirus A16 most common cause • Most common in summer/fall and in children <5 years old • Prodrome: fever + URI symptoms • Oral Enanthem: painful, erythematous oral vesicles that ulcerate • Exanthem: erythematous maculopapular rash that changes to grey vesicles on hands and feet • Supportive treatment

Maculopapular lesions of soles

Oral vesicles with surrounding thin halo

References

1. Antibiotics coverage diagram.jpg. (2020, September 16). *Wikimedia Commons*. Retrieved 21:02, August 17, 2023 from https://commons.wikimedia.org/w/index.php?title=File:Antibiotics_coverage_diagram.jpg&oldid=461160643.
2. Leg with erythema marginatum Wellcome L0061869.jpg. (2020, September 7). *Wikimedia Commons*. Retrieved 20:17, August 17, 2023 from https://commons.wikimedia.org/w/index.php?title=File:Leg_with_erythema_marginatum_Wellcome_L0061869.jpg&oldid=450778383.
3. Scarlet fever 2.jpg. (2022, April 25). *Wikimedia Commons*. Retrieved 20:22, August 17, 2023 from https://commons.wikimedia.org/w/index.php?title=File:Scarlet_fever_2.jpg&oldid=651836410.
4. Chancroid lesion haemophilus ducreyi PHIL 3728 lores.jpg. (2023, February 16). *Wikimedia Commons*. Retrieved 20:27, August 17, 2023 from https://commons.wikimedia.org/w/index.php?title=File:Chancroid_lesion_haemophilus_ducreyi_PHIL_3728_lores.jpg&oldid=733171728.
5. Anthrax 2033.png. (2020, September 16). *Wikimedia Commons*. Retrieved 20:29, August 17, 2023 from https://commons.wikimedia.org/w/index.php?title=File:Anthrax_PHIL_2033.png&oldid=461471416.
6. Rocky mountain spotted fever.jpg. (2019, May 8). *Wikimedia Commons*. Retrieved 20:33, August 17, 2023 from https://commons.wikimedia.org/w/index.php?title=File:Rocky_mountain_spotted_fever.jpg&oldid=349236177.
7. Erythema migrans - erythematous rash in Lyme disease - PHIL 9875.jpg. (2022, August 9). *Wikimedia Commons*. Retrieved 20:31, August 17, 2023 from https://commons.wikimedia.org/w/index.php?title=File:Erythema_migrans_-_erythematous_rash_in_Lyme_disease_-_PHIL_9875.jpg&oldid=681183153.
8. Threadworm.jpg. (2020, September 13). *Wikimedia Commons*. Retrieved 20:37, August 17, 2023 from https://commons.wikimedia.org/w/index.php?title=File:Threadworm.jpg&oldid=458269518.
9. Cutaneous-larva-migrans-foot.jpg. (2023, June 9). *Wikimedia Commons*. Retrieved 20:39, August 17, 2023 from https://commons.wikimedia.org/w/index.php?title=File:Cutaneous-larva-migrans-foot.jpg&oldid=772861935.
10. Chickenpox leg.JPG. (2020, September 28). *Wikimedia Commons*. Retrieved 20:40, August 17, 2023 from https://commons.wikimedia.org/w/index.php?title=File:Chickenpox_leg.JPG&oldid=473945284.
11. Shingles on the chest.jpg. (2020, September 30). *Wikimedia Commons*. Retrieved 20:42, August 17, 2023 from https://commons.wikimedia.org/w/index.php?title=File:Shingles_on_the_chest.jpg&oldid=476526303.
12. File:Morbillivirus measles infection.jpg. (2022, May 14). *Wikimedia Commons*. Retrieved 20:12, May 3, 2023 from https://commons.wikimedia.org/w/index.php?title=File:Morbillivirus_measles_infection.jpg&oldid=656039846.
13. File:Koplik spots, measles 6111 lores.jpg. (2020, November 1). *Wikimedia Commons*. Retrieved 20:12, May 3, 2023 from https://commons.wikimedia.org/w/index.php?title=File:Koplik_spots,_measles_6111_lores.jpg&oldid=508858717.
14. Parotiditis (Parotitis; Mumps).JPG. (2020, October 10). *Wikimedia Commons*. Retrieved 20:47, August 17, 2023 from https://commons.wikimedia.org/w/index.php?title=File:Parotiditis_(Parotitis;_Mumps).JPG&oldid=485515925.
15. Rash of rubella on back (crop).JPG. (2020, August 27). *Wikimedia Commons*. Retrieved 20:48, August 17, 2023 from https://commons.wikimedia.org/w/index.php?title=File:Rash_of_rubella_on_back_(crop).JPG&oldid=444125689.
16. File:Slapped cheek Erythema Infectiosum.png. (2022, March 16). *Wikimedia Commons*. Retrieved 18:04, May 3, 2023 from https://commons.wikimedia.org/w/index.php?title=File:Slapped_cheek_Erythema_Infectiosum.png&oldid=639366013.
17. Sestamalattia (2).JPG. (2020, September 24). *Wikimedia Commons*. Retrieved 20:50, August 17, 2023 from https://commons.wikimedia.org/w/index.php?title=File:Sestamalattia_(2).JPG&oldid=470276226.
18. Herpes labialis - opryszczka wargowa.jpg. (2021, November 7). *Wikimedia Commons*. Retrieved 20:52, August 17, 2023 from https://commons.wikimedia.org/w/index.php?title=File:Herpes_labialis_-_opryszczka_wargowa.jpg&oldid=605906333.
19. SOA-Herpes-genitalis-female.jpg. (2020, October 9). *Wikimedia Commons*. Retrieved 20:54, August 17, 2023 from https://commons.wikimedia.org/w/index.php?title=File:SOA-Herpes-genitalis-female.jpg&oldid=484907508.
20. Mononucleosis.JPG. (2020, October 28). *Wikimedia Commons*. Retrieved 20:55, August 17, 2023 from https://commons.wikimedia.org/w/index.php?title=File:Mononucleosis.JPG&oldid=504599461.
21. File:Hand Foot Mouth Disease.png. (2020, October 3). *Wikimedia Commons*. Retrieved 22:07, May 3, 2023 from https://commons.wikimedia.org/w/index.php?title=File:Hand_Foot_Mouth_Disease.png&oldid=479750247.
22. File:Hand foot and mouth disease on child feet.jpg. (2020, September 5). *Wikimedia Commons*. Retrieved 22:08, May 3, 2023 from https://commons.wikimedia.org/w/index.php?title=File:Hand_foot_and_mouth_disease_on_child_feet.jpg&oldid=448668064.

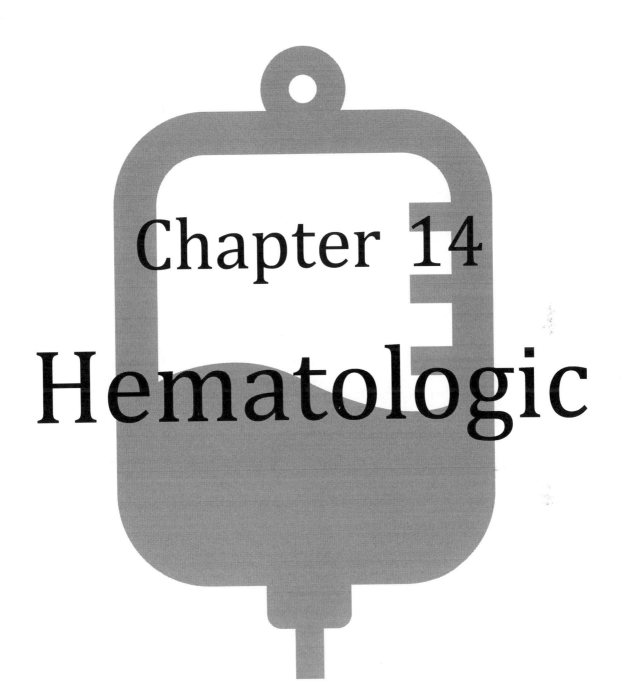

Chapter 14
Hematologic

	Hematologic Finding	Characteristics	Conditions
	Rouleaux Formation	• Red blood cells (RBCs) stack together like a "**stack of coins**" due to increased plasma proteins (such as fibrinogen or immunoglobulins) • Increased density of RBCs cause the stacks to settle resulting in **increased erythrocyte sedimentation rate (ESR)**	• **Multiple myeloma** • General inflammation • Acute or chronic infections

	Auto-Agglutination	• **Clumping of RBCs** due to the presence of IgM autoantibodies that coat the RBC surface leading to increased RBC destruction by macrophages
		• Cold IgM antibody agglutinins are reactive at colder temperatures
		• Can be distinguished from rouleaux formation by performing a saline dilution test (the clumping is disrupted in autoagglutination)
			• **Cold agglutinin autoimmune hemolytic anemia**
			  • Mycoplasma pneumoniae,
			  • Epstein-Barr Virus (EBV)
			• Cryoglobulinemia
			• Antigen-Antibody reaction if incorrect blood match
			• Certain infections

	Howell-Jolly Bodies	• Small, dense, basophilic, round remnants of nuclear material (inclusions) seen in RBCs
		• Typically removed by the spleen
			• **Splenic dysfunction**
			  • Autosplenectomy (sickle cell disease)
			  • Post splenectomy
			• Severe hemolytic anemia
			• Megaloblastic anemia

	Hemolytic Cells	• **Bite Cells (Degmacytes)**: type of hemolytic cell characterized by the presence of a "bite" or "pit" taken out of the RBC membrane • Caused by macrophages removing denatured hemoglobin precipitates from the RBC surface	• **G6PD deficiency** • Hemoglobinopathy (Thalassemia)
		• **Schistocytes**: fragmented RBCs resulting from mechanical damage and shearing forces within the circulation	• Microangiopathic hemolytic anemia • Thrombotic microangiopathies (thrombotic thrombocytopenic purpura, hemolytic-uremic syndrome, disseminated intravascular coagulation)
		• **Keratocytes**: irregularly shaped RBCs with two or more spicules protruding from the cell membrane • Also known as "**helmet cells**" due to the characteristic shape	• Fragmentation hemolysis, (microangiopathic hemolytic anemias [thrombotic thrombocytopenic purpura, hemolytic-uremic syndrome, disseminated intravascular coagulation]) • **Mechanical injury to RBCs (prosthetic heart valves)** • Liver disease

	Hematologic Finding	Characteristics	Conditions
	Basophilic Stippling	• Presence of fine, dark blue granules (RNA remnants) seen in RBCs, indicating impaired erythropoiesis • Similar to reticulocytes but basophilic stippling is evenly distributed	• Sideroblastic anemia • Heavy metal poisoning (lead, arsenic) • Hemoglobinopathies (Thalassemia) • Myelodysplasia • Chronic alcohol abuse
	Echinocytes	• "Burr Cells" • RBCs with numerous short, evenly spaced projections due to abnormal cell membrane • Resemble thorny projections	• **Uremia** • Liver disease • Pyruvate kinase deficiency • Hypophosphatemia
	Acanthocytes	• "Spur Cells" • Irregularly spiky or thorny projections on the RBC membrane	• Liver disease (alcoholic cirrhosis) • Abetalipoproteinemia • Post splenectomy • Autoimmune hemolytic anemia • Severe vitamin E deficiency
	Codocytes	• "Target Cells" • Hypochromic RBCs with a central bullseye appearance due to excess cell membrane compared to hemoglobin content	• Liver disease • Hemoglobinopathies (sickle cell, Thalassemia, severe iron deficiency anemia) • Asplenia
	Spherocytes	• Small, dense, spherical RBCs lacking central pallor	• **Hereditary spherocytosis** • **Autoimmune hemolytic anemia**
	Hyper-segmented Neutrophils	• Neutrophils with more than 5 lobes in their nucleus	• Megaloblastic anemias such as **vitamin B12 or folate deficiency** (due to impaired DNA synthesis)

Approach to Microcytic Anemia

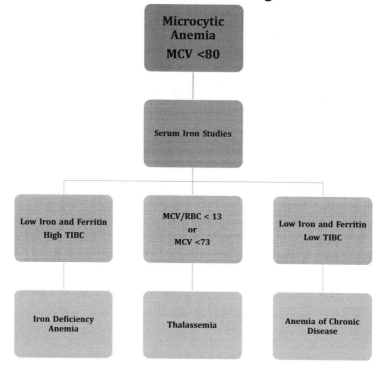

Microcytic Anemia MCV <80

Serum Iron Studies

- Low Iron and Ferritin High TIBC → **Iron Deficiency Anemia**
- MCV/RBC < 13 or MCV <73 → **Thalassemia**
- Low Iron and Ferritin Low TIBC → **Anemia of Chronic Disease**

Approach to Normocytic Anemia

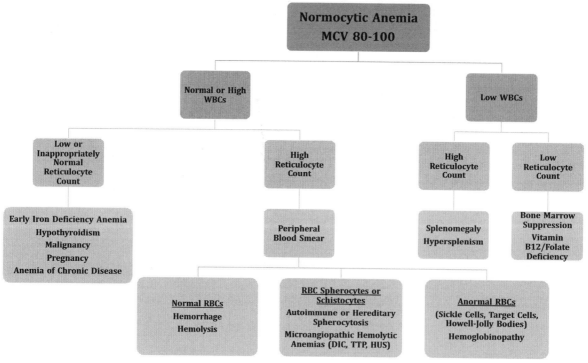

Normocytic Anemia MCV 80-100

Normal or High WBCs

- Low or Inappropriately Normal Reticulocyte Count
  - Early Iron Deficiency Anemia
  - Hypothyroidism
  - Malignancy
  - Pregnancy
  - Anemia of Chronic Disease
- High Reticulocyte Count
  - Peripheral Blood Smear
    - Normal RBCs
      - Hemorrhage
      - Hemolysis
    - RBC Spherocytes or Schistocytes
      - Autoimmune or Hereditary Spherocytosis
      - Microangiopathic Hemolytic Anemias (DIC, TTP, HUS)
    - Anormal RBCs (Sickle Cells, Target Cells, Howell-Jolly Bodies)
      - Hemoglobinopathy

Low WBCs

- High Reticulocyte Count
  - Splenomegaly
  - Hypersplenism
- Low Reticulocyte Count
  - Bone Marrow Suppression
  - Vitamin B12/Folate Deficiency

Approach to Macrocytic Anemia

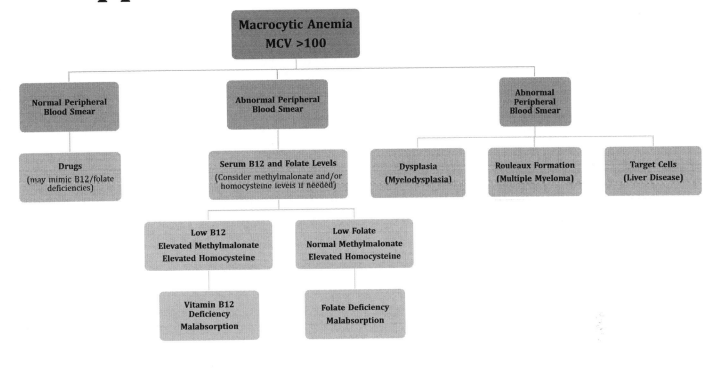

Iron Deficiency Anemia

Etiology & Risk Factors	• Insufficient amount of iron available to produce adequate number of red blood cells and reduced production of hemoglobin results in decreased oxygen-carrying capacity
	• Etiology: decreased iron availability through blood loss, decreased intake or absorption, increased requirements
	  • Blood Loss: **most common cause**; excessive menstruation, GI blood loss (ulcers, gastritis, **colon cancer**), parasitic hookworms
	  • **Decreased Iron Availability**: low dietary intake (**vegan diet**), increased systemic requirements for iron (pregnancy, lactation), decreased iron absorption (Celiac disease, bariatric surgery, *H. pylori*)
	• Risk Factors: age (**elderly** more at risk for chronic blood loss, **infants** more at risk due to dietary intake or depleted stores), **chronic kidney disease** (reduced erythropoietin production which stimulates RBC production)

Patho-physiology	• Iron Absorption: iron is primarily absorbed in the duodenum and upper jejunum; heme iron (meat) is more readily absorbed than nonheme iron (nonheme iron absorption is influenced by various factors such as food components [milk products, vegetable fiber], certain antibiotics, and ascorbic acid) • Iron Transport and Usage: iron from the intestinal mucosal cells is transferred to transferrin (iron-transport protein synthesized in the liver) which transports iron to various cells, including erythroblasts, placental cells, and liver cells, for heme synthesis. • Iron Storage and Recycling: iron not utilized for erythropoiesis is stored in ferritin and hemosiderin; ferritin (the primary storage form) is a soluble and active fraction found in the liver, bone marrow, spleen, and serum. It can release stored iron as needed.
Signs & Symptoms	• Classic Anemia Symptoms: **fatigue**, exercise intolerance, shortness of breath, **weakness**, dizziness, **pallor** • **Neurologic Dysfunction: difficulty concentrating**, irritability, **poor school performance**, cognitive disturbances, **restless leg syndrome** • **Pica**: abnormal craving to eat nonfood substances (**ice [pagophagia]**, dirt, paint, starch, chalk, ashes) • Severe Deficiency: **glossitis** (smooth tongue), **cheilosis** (inflammation of corners of mouth), and **koilonychia** (concave spooning of the nails)

Diagnosis	• **Complete Blood Count (CBC)**:
	  • Low hemoglobin; **microcytic hypochromic anemia**
	  • Increased red cell distribution width, anisocytosis, **low reticulocyte count**
	• Iron Studies: serum iron, iron-binding capacity, transferrin, serum ferritin
	  • **Increased iron-binding capacity**
	  • **Decreased transferrin saturation**
	  • **Decreased serum ferritin**
	  • **Decreased serum iron**
	• **Bone Marrow Examination**: bone marrow stores of iron is definitive diagnosis; rarely performed
	• *Consider evaluation to determine underlying etiology (endoscopy/colonoscopy for GI bleed)*

Treatment	• **Oral Iron Supplementation: ferrous sulfate**, ferrous gluconate, ferrous fumarate once per day or every other day
	  • **Increased Absorption**: take on an empty stomach 30 minutes before a meal with ascorbic acid (vitamin C) as an oral supplement or glass of orange juice
	• Parenteral Iron: ferrous sucrose; rapid therapeutic response
	  • Indicated for those that cannot tolerate oral iron or for patients that require immediate repletion (severe anemia, elective surgery, third trimester of pregnancy)

Alpha Thalassemia

Etiology & Risk Factors	• Alpha-globin gene deletion resulting in reduced or absent production of alpha-globin chains • <u>Etiology</u>: **mutations or deletions of the Hb genes**, resulting in underproduction or absence of alpha or beta chains • **Alpha Thalassemia**: caused by deletions or mutations of alpha-globin genes on chromosome 16 • <u>Risk Factors</u>: **family history (autosomal recessive** [both the parents must be affected with or carriers for the disease to transfer it to the next generation]), certain ethnicities (Mediterranean, Middle Eastern, Southeast Asian, and African descent), consanguinity (marriages between close relatives)
Patho-physiology	• Deficiency or absence of one or more of the globin chains that make up hemoglobin leading to ineffective erythropoiesis (formation of red blood cells) and abnormal red blood cell morphology, resulting in chronic anemia and other complications • <u>Alpha-Thalassemia</u>: normally four alpha genes (two on each pair of chromosomes); deletion of alpha genes results in decreased production of alpha-polypeptide chains

Signs & Symptoms	• <u>**Defect in a Single Allele**</u>:
	  • Asymptomatic; "silent carrier"
	• <u>**Defect in Two Alleles**</u>:
	  • Asymptomatic with mild to moderate microcytic anemia; carrier of alpha-thalassemia trait
	• <u>**Defect in Three Alleles**</u>:
	  • **Symptomatic at birth (neonatal jaundice**, hemolytic anemia, **hepatosplenomegaly**, respiratory distress)
	  • **Frontal bossing**, maxilla overgrowth (increased bone marrow hematopoiesis)
	• <u>**Defect in Four Alleles**</u>:
	  • <u>**Hemoglobin Bart Syndrome**</u>: **hydrops fetalis** (excessive fluid accumulation in the fetus) **resulting in severe fetal anemia and tissue hypoxia**; lethal condition in utero (hemoglobin lacks alpha chains and is unable to transport oxygen)

Diagnosis	• <u>**Complete Blood Count (CBC)**</u>: **low hemoglobin and low MCV, increased RBC count**
	  • <u>**Mentzer Index**</u>: **index of less than 13** indicates thalassemia (mean corpuscular volume divided by red cell count)
	• <u>**Peripheral Blood Smear**</u>: **microcytic, hypochromic, hemolytic anemia (schistocytes**, tear drop cells, **increased reticulocyte count**)
	  • **Heinz bodies**, Target cells, basophilic stippling
	• <u>**Hemoglobin Electrophoresis**</u>: **presence of HbH (beta chain tetramer)**
	• <u>Recombinant DNA Gene Mapping</u>: standard for prenatal diagnosis and genetic counseling

Treatment	• <u>**Mild Thalassemia**</u>: Hb 6-10 g/dL
	  • No treatment necessary; **episodic blood transfusion may be required** after surgery, infection or following childbirth to reduce complications
	• <u>**Moderate to Severe Thalassemia**</u>: Hb <5-6 g/dL
	  • <u>**Frequent Blood Transfusions**</u>: regular blood transfusions (every few weeks) with a goal of maintaining Hb at 9-10 mg/dl
	  • <u>**Chelation Therapy**</u>: iron chelators (deferasirox, **deferoxamine**, deferiprone) are given to remove extra iron from the body due to chronic blood transfusions
	  • <u>Stem Cell Transplant</u>: bone marrow transplant is potential option in limited cases (child born with severe thalassemia)
	  • <u>Splenectomy</u>: stops RBC destruction and therefore limits the number of required blood transfusions and controls the spread of extramedullary hematopoiesis

Beta Thalassemia

Etiology & Risk Factors	• Beta-globin gene deletion resulting in reduced or absent production of beta-globin chains • <u>Etiology</u>: **mutations or deletions of the Hb genes**, resulting in underproduction or absence of beta chains • **Beta Thalassemia**: caused by a point mutation or small insertions/deletions in the beta-globin gene, located on chromosome 11 • <u>Risk Factors</u>: **family history (autosomal recessive** [both the parents must be affected with or carriers for the disease to transfer it to the next generation]), certain ethnicities (Mediterranean **[Greek, Italian]**, Middle Eastern, Southeast Asian, and African descent), consanguinity (marriages between close relatives)
Patho-physiology	• Deficiency or absence of one or more of the globin chains that make up hemoglobin leading to ineffective erythropoiesis (formation of red blood cells) and abnormal red blood cell morphology, resulting in chronic anemia and other complications • <u>Beta-Thalassemia</u>: decreased production of beta-polypeptide chains due to mutations or deletions in the beta globin gene results in impaired production of hemoglobin (Hb)

Signs & Symptoms	• <u>**Beta Thalassemia Minor (or Train)**</u>: most common type; heterozygous form where only one gene is defective
	  • Asymptomatic; may have mild-moderate microcytic anemia
	• <u>**Beta Thalassemia Intermedia**</u>: mild homozygous form
	  • Variable clinical picture between thalassemia minor/major; microcytic anemia, hepatosplenomegaly, bone hyperactivity
	• <u>**Beta Thalassemia Major (Cooley's Anemia)**</u>: both beta genes are mutated; *symptoms often occur after 6 months old*
	  • <u>**Severe Anemia**</u>: pallor, dyspnea, mental delays, dyspnea, irritability; jaundice, hepatosplenomegaly (hemolytic)
	  • <u>**Extramedullary Hematopoiesis**</u>: **bone hyperactivity**, abnormal/delayed skeletal development, extramedullary expansion (frontal bossing, osteoporosis, abnormal ribs)
	  • <u>**Endocrine Abnormalities**</u>: secondary to iron overload; hypogonadism, hypothyroidism, diabetes, stunted grown

Diagnosis	• <u>**Complete Blood Count (CBC)**</u>: **low hemoglobin and low MCV, increased RBC count**
	  • <u>**Mentzer Index**</u>: **index of less than 13** indicates thalassemia (mean corpuscular volume divided by red cell count)
	• <u>**Peripheral Blood Smear**</u>: **microcytic, hypochromic, hemolytic anemia (schistocytes**, tear drop cells, **increased reticulocyte count**)
	  • **Heinz bodies**, Target cells, basophilic stippling
	• <u>**Hemoglobin Electrophoresis**</u>: decrease in or absence of hemoglobin A (HbA) and an increase in hemoglobin F (HbF) and/or hemoglobin A2 (HbA2) levels
	• <u>Recombinant DNA Gene Mapping</u>: standard for prenatal diagnosis and genetic counseling

Treatment	• <u>**Mild Thalassemia**</u>: Hb 6-10 g/dL
	  • No treatment necessary; **episodic blood transfusion may be required** after surgery, infection or following childbirth to reduce complications
	• <u>**Moderate to Severe Thalassemia**</u>: Hb <5-6 g/dL
	  • <u>**Frequent Blood Transfusions**</u>: regular blood transfusions (every few weeks) with a goal of maintaining Hb at 9-10 mg/dl
	  • <u>**Chelation Therapy**</u>: iron chelators (deferasirox, **deferoxamine**, deferiprone) are given to remove extra iron from the body due to chronic blood transfusions
	  • <u>Stem Cell Transplant</u>: bone marrow transplant is potential option in limited cases (child born with severe thalassemia)
	  • <u>Splenectomy</u>: stops RBC destruction and therefore limits the number of required blood transfusions and controls the spread of extramedullary hematopoiesis

Vitamin B12 (Cobalamin) Deficiency 🛝

Etiology & Risk Factors	• Water-soluble vitamin that is a cofactor for synthesis of DNA, fatty acids, and myelin
	• <u>Sources</u>: **animal products**; red meat, eggs, dairy products, seafood/shellfish
	• <u>Etiology</u>: **decreased absorption is most common cause**; decreased intake
	   • <u>Decreased Absorption</u>: **pernicious anemia is most common cause** (lack of intrinsic factors due to parietal cell antibodies leading to malabsorption and gastric atrophy), **Crohn disease** (affects terminal ileum), pancreatic insufficiency, gastric bypass surgery, gastritis, Celiac disease, alcoholism, certain medications (**oral contraceptive pills**, H2 blockers/PPIs [decreased acidity decreases absorption], metformin, anticonvulsants), parasites
	   • <u>Decreased Intake</u>: **vegetarian or vegan diet**
	• <u>Risk Factors</u>: **inadequate dietary intake, vegetarian or vegan diet**, gastrointestinal disorders resulting in chronic diarrhea, advanced age, liver disorders, dialysis, alcoholism, gastric bypass surgery

	• Vitamin B12 is involved with nucleic acid metabolism, methyl transfer, and myelin synthesis; necessary for multiple metabolic pathways, neurologic and hematologic function • Vitamin B12 is bound to intrinsic factor (protein secreted by gastric parietal cells); B12 intrinsic factor complex is absorbed by the terminal ileum and stored in liver
Patho-physiology	• <u>Hematologic</u>: **anemia symptoms; fatigue, pallor**, exercise intolerance • <u>Gastrointestinal</u>: **diarrhea, malabsorption**, hepatomegaly/splenomegaly, weight loss • <u>Neurologic</u>: **symmetrical peripheral neuropathy is most common initial symptom**; ataxia, weakness • <u>Dorsal Column Demyelination</u>: impaired vibratory and proprioception senses, hypotonia
Signs & Symptoms	• <u>CBC with Peripheral Smear</u>: **macrocytic anemia (Increased MCV)** • **Megaloblastic Anemia**: hyper-segmented neutrophils, high RDW, low reticulocyte count; leukopenia/thrombocytopenia if severe • <u>Serum B12</u>: **decreased** • <u>Methylmalonic Acid</u>: **elevated methylmalonic acid distinguishes B12 from folate deficiency** (MMA is normal in folate deficiency) • LDH and bilirubin may be elevated; **elevated homocysteine**

Diagnosis	• <u>Nutritious Diet</u>: **consumption of foods high in riboflavin**; eggs, milk, cheese, liver, fortified cereal product
	• <u>Vitamin B12 Supplementation</u>: dosing based on severity of deficiency
	   • <u>Intramuscular Injection</u>: weekly cyanocobalamin injection then tapered; indicated for symptomatic anemia or neurologic symptoms
	   • *Pernicious anemia patients need lifelong IM B12 injections*

Treatment	• Water-soluble vitamin found in animal products; red meat, eggs, dairy • Risks include pernicious anemia, inadequate diet, veganism, OCP pills, malabsorption/diarrhea, alcoholism • Anemia symptoms (fatigue, pallor); malabsorption, diarrhea • Symmetrical peripheral neuropathy is most common initial symptom • CBC with peripheral smear: macrocytic anemia • Nutritious Diet + Vitamin B12 Supplementation (IM injections if symptomatic or pernicious anemia patient)

Folate Deficiency 🛝

Etiology & Risk Factors	• Water-soluble vitamin that is crucial for various physiological processes including DNA synthesis, red blood cell formation, and cell division; also known as vitamin B9
	• <u>Sources</u>: **animal products** (red meat, eggs, organ meats [**liver**]) raw green leafy vegetables, fruits, fortified cereal products
	• <u>Etiology</u>: **inadequate intake is most common cause**
	   • <u>Inadequate Intake</u>: **most common cause, alcoholism, undernutrition**
	   • <u>Increased Requirements</u>: pregnancy or lactation, infancy, malignancy, hemolytic anemias
	   • <u>Impaired Absorption</u>: Celiac disease, chronic diarrhea, inflammatory bowel disease, anticonvulsant medications
	   • <u>Inadequate Utilization</u>: folate antagonists (metformin, **methotrexate**, triamterene, **trimethoprim**), antiseizure drugs, congenital/acquired enzyme deficiency, alcoholism
	   • <u>Increased Excretion</u>: dialysis

Patho-physiology	• Folate is necessary for the synthesis of thymidine, a component of DNA, and its deficiency results in ineffective DNA replication and impaired cell division, leading to the impaired production of red blood cells and the formation of large, immature red blood cells (megaloblastic anemia)
Signs & Symptoms	• Similar symptoms to vitamin b12 deficiency without neurologic abnormalities • <u>Hematologic</u>: **anemia symptoms; fatigue, pallor**, exercise intolerance • <u>Epithelial</u>: **glossitis** (smooth tongue), **cheilosis** (inflammation of corners of mouth), aphthous ulcers
Diagnosis	• <u>CBC with Peripheral Smear</u>: **macrocytic anemia (increased MCV)** • **Megaloblastic Anemia**: hyper-segmented neutrophils, high RDW, low reticulocyte count; leukopenia/thrombocytopenia if severe • <u>Serum Folate</u>: **decreased** • <u>Methylmalonic Acid</u>: **normal methylmalonic acid distinguishes folate from B12 deficiency** (MMA is elevated in B12 deficiency) • LDH and bilirubin may be elevated; **elevated homocysteine**
Treatment	• <u>Oral Folate Supplementation</u>: • Folate 400 to 1000 mcg orally once a day • *CAUTION: In patients with megaloblastic anemia, vitamin B12 deficiency must be ruled out prior to folate supplementation; if vitamin B12 deficiency is present, folate supplementation may treat the anemia but will possible exacerbate the neurological deficits*

Anemia of Chronic Disease

Etiology & Risk Factors	• Anemia secondary to decreased red blood cell (RBC) production in the setting of chronic disease • <u>Etiology</u>: **chronic inflammatory disorders; chronic infection is most common** (HIV/AIDS, tuberculosis, hepatitis), **autoimmune disease** (rheumatoid arthritis, systemic lupus erythematosus, inflammatory bowel disease), chronic kidney disease, heart failure, malignancy, trauma, post-surgery
Patho-physiology	• <u>Hemophagocytosis</u>: increased hemophagocytosis by macrophages lead to shortened lifespan of red blood cells • <u>Impaired Erythropoiesis</u>: decreases in erythropoietin production and bone marrow response; inflammatory cytokines suppress production and lifespan of red blood cells • <u>Impaired Iron Metabolism</u>: increase in hepcidin blocks release of iron from macrophages and inhibits iron absorption and recycling which leads to iron sequestration.
Signs & Symptoms	• Symptoms of the underlying disorder (infection, inflammation, malignancy) • <u>**Classic Anemia Symptoms**</u>: fatigue, weakness, pallor, shortness of breath, reduced exercise tolerance, tachycardia, dizziness or lightheadedness, cognitive impairment

Diagnosis	• <u>**CBC with Peripheral Smear**</u>: hemoglobin usually not <8mg/dL
	    • **Mild normocytic normochromic anemia**
	    • Decreased reticulocyte count, normal to increased RDW
	• <u>**Iron Studies**</u>: serum iron, iron-binding capacity, transferrin, serum ferritin
	    • **Normal to decreased iron-binding capacity**
	    • **Normal to decreased transferrin saturation**
	    • **Normal to increased serum ferritin**
	    • **Decreased serum iron**
	• **Erythropoietin Level: low in setting of chronic kidney disease**

Treatment	• <u>**Treat Underlying Disorder**</u>: various approaches, including anti-inflammatory medications, immunosuppressants, disease-specific treatments, or lifestyle modifications • <u>**Blood Transfusions**</u>: indicated in severe cases where the hemoglobin levels are significantly low and symptoms are severe • <u>**Erythropoiesis-Stimulating Agents (ESAs)**</u>: **erythropoietin-alpha** indicated in severe anemia or cases associated with chronic kidney disease or malignancy • Stimulates the production of red blood cells
Key Words & Most Common	• Anemia secondary to chronic inflammatory disorders (chronic infection, autoimmune) • Classic anemia symptoms • <u>CBC</u>: normal to low hemoglobin; mild normocytic, normochromic anemia • <u>Iron Studies</u>: ↔ to ↓ iron-binding capacity, ↔ to ↓ transferrin saturation, ↔ to ↑ serum ferritin • Treat underlying disorder → erythropoietin-alpha if severe anemia associated with CKD or malignancy

Sideroblastic Anemia

Etiology & Risk Factors	• **Anemia that results from abnormal utilization of iron during erythropoiesis**
	• <u>Etiology</u>: congenital or acquired
	    • <u>**Congenital**</u>: mutations in genes that are involved in heme synthesis, iron-sulfur cluster biogenesis, or mitochondrial metabolism
	    • <u>**Acquired**</u>: **associated with myelodysplastic syndrome**, medications (antibiotics, hormones, isoniazid, linezolid, copper-chelating agents, chemotherapy), toxins (**lead toxicity**, alcohol), copper deficiency (may be from excessive zinc ingestion) or chronic malignancy

Patho-physiology	• Impaired heme synthesis that results due to the abnormal production of iron-containing molecules called sideroblasts • Defect in the utilization or incorporation of iron into the heme molecule within RBC precursors leads to iron accumulation in mitochondria and ineffective erythropoiesis
Signs & Symptoms	• <u>**Classic Anemia Symptoms**</u>: **fatigue, weakness, pallor**, shortness of breath, reduced exercise tolerance, tachycardia, dizziness or lightheadedness, cognitive impairment • May have cold intolerance or neurological symptoms (paresthesias, difficulty with coordination and balance)

Diagnosis	• <u>**Complete Blood Count (CBC) with Peripheral Smear**</u>: moderate to severe anemia (Hgb 4-10mg/dL)
	    • **Microcytic (low MCV) anemia**
	    • **Decreased mean corpuscular hemoglobin and increased red blood cell distribution width**
	• <u>**Peripheral Blood Smear**</u>: RBC dimorphism or basophilic stippling (accumulation of ribosomal RNA in periphery)
	• <u>**Iron Studies**</u>: serum iron, iron-binding capacity, transferrin, serum ferritin
	    • Normal or increased serum iron
	    • Normal or decreased iron binding capacity
	    • Increased serum ferritin level
	• <u>**Bone Marrow Biopsy**</u>: definitive diagnosis; utilized to identify the presence of ringed sideroblasts, assess cellularity, and rule out other potential causes of anemia
	    • <u>**Ringed Sideroblasts**</u>: iron staining reveals the iron-engorged perinuclear mitochondria in developing RBCs
	• <u>Genetic Testing</u>: performed to identify specific gene mutations associated with the condition (ALAS2, SLC25A38, or ABCB7 genes)
	• <u>Serum Lead Level</u>: indicated if sideroblastic anemia present with unknown cause

Treatment	• <u>**Treat Underlying Etiology**</u>: elimination of toxin (alcohol cessation, identifying lead exposure source) or medication (discontinuing zinc supplementation), treat underlying condition, lifestyle changes
	• <u>**Vitamin/Mineral Supplementation:**</u> indicated in specific cases
	    • <u>**Vitamin B6 (Pyridoxine) Supplementation**</u>: vitamin B6 can improve heme production and alleviate anemia in individuals with specific gene mutations
	    • Copper Supplementation: copper necessary for enzymatic function involved in iron utilization and heme synthesis
	• <u>Iron Chelation or Phlebotomy Therapy</u>: may be indicated in certain cases associated with iron overload to help remove excess iron from the body
	• <u>Blood Transfusions</u>: indicated in severe cases where the hemoglobin levels are significantly low and symptoms are severe

Aplastic Anemia

Etiology & Risk Factors	• **Hematopoietic stem cell disorder resulting in a loss of blood cell precursors, bone marrow hypoplasia, and cytopenias of 2+ cell lines (RBCs, WBCs, and/or platelets)**
	• Etiology: **most cases are idiopathic**; may be caused by infection, medications, or other conditions
	   • Chemicals: benzene, inorganic arsenic
	   • Medications: chemotherapy, antibiotics (**chloramphenicol, sulfa drugs**), NSAIDs, **antiepileptics (carbamazepine**, phenytoin), acetazolamide, penicillamine, quinine
	   • Infection: seronegative viral hepatitis, **parvovirus B19** in patients with baseline hemolytic anemias (sickle cell, G6PD deficiency), Epstein-Barr virus

Patho-physiology	• Two interrelated mechanisms: extrinsic immune-mediated suppression of hematopoietic stem cells and intrinsic abnormality of marrow progenitors • In the immune-mediated pathway, damaged hematopoietic stem cells mature into self-reactive T-helper cells that release cytokines (interferon-gamma and tumor necrosis factor) leading to the suppression and destruction of other hematopoietic stem cells • The intrinsic abnormality pathway involves inherent defects in stem cells, resulting in their inability to differentiate and proliferate, leading to clonal evolution into hematologic neoplasms or premature exhaustion of hematopoietic stem cells

Signs & Symptoms	• Pancytopenia:
	   • **Thrombocytopenia: mucocutaneous bleeding** (epistaxis, bleeding gums, petechia, purpura), easy bruising, menorrhagia
	   • **Anemia: fatigue, weakness, pallor**, shortness of breath, reduced exercise tolerance, tachycardia, dizziness or lightheadedness, cognitive impairment
	   • Neutropenia: frequent or recurrent infections, sudden onset fever
	• *Absence of splenomegaly (presence suggests alternative diagnosis)*

Diagnosis	• **Complete Blood Count (CBC) with Peripheral Smear:** demonstrates pancytopenia
	   • **Reticulopodia:** <1% or <40,000/microL
	   • **Neutropenia:** <500/microL
	   • **Thrombocytopenia:** <20,000/microL
	• **Bone Marrow Biopsy: essential to confirm diagnosis**
	   • **Bone marrow hypocellularity** (affecting all three cell lineages; red blood cells, white blood cells, platelets)
	   • **Fatty infiltration or fibrosis** (indicating the replacement of normal hematopoietic cells by non-functional adipose tissue or scar tissue)
	   • Normal or abnormal cell morphology (dysplasia)

Treatment	• **Supportive: initial treatment;** identify and remove underlying etiology (if possible)
	   • Antibiotics: infectious prophylaxis with broad-spectrum antibiotics
	   • Blood Transfusions: indicated for hemoglobin <7mg/dL or platelets <10,000
	• **Allogeneic Hematopoietic Stem Cell Transplant (HCT): treatment of choice for young patients (<50 years old) in good health with severe aplastic anemia**
	• **Immunosuppressive Therapy:** indicated for older patients (>50 years old), younger patients without a matched donor or patients unfit for transplant
	   • Anti-thymocyte globulin (ATG), cyclosporine, eltrombopag

Autoimmune Hemolytic Anemia

Etiology & Risk Factors	• Decompensated acquired hemolysis secondary to the **autoantibody production that react with red blood cells (RBCs)**
	• Etiology: warm agglutin or cold agglutin
	   • **Warm Agglutin: idiopathic is most common;** underlying autoimmune disorder (systemic lupus erythematosus [SLE]), lymphoproliferative disorders (chronic lymphocytic leukemia, lymphoma), viral infection, **medications (methyldopa, levodopa, penicillin, cephalosporins, quinidine)**
	   • **Cold Agglutin:** idiopathic, infection (***Mycoplasma pneumoniae,* Epstein-Barr virus,** HIV), lymphoproliferative disorders (chronic lymphocytic leukemia, lymphoma)

Patho-physiology	• **Warm Agglutin:** production of **immunoglobulin G (IgG) autoantibodies** that bind to surface proteins on red blood cells at body temperature leading to the destruction of red blood cells by splenic macrophages through extravascular hemolysis • **Cold Agglutin:** production of **immunoglobulin M (IgM) autoantibodies** that agglutinate and cause the destruction of red blood cells at temperatures below normal body temperature; cold agglutinins primarily target red blood cells in the peripheral circulation, leading to cold-induced, complement-mediated RBC lysis

Signs & Symptoms	• **Warm Agglutin:** symptoms due to anemia
	   • Classic anemia symptoms; fatigue, weakness, pallor, dyspnea, reduced exercise tolerance, tachycardia, dizziness or lightheadedness, cognitive impairment
	   • Fever, chest pain, syncope, or liver or heart failure may occur in severe cases
	   • Mild splenomegaly
	• **Cold Agglutin:** symptoms due to hemolysis
	   • Hemoglobinuria, jaundice, splenomegaly
	   • **Acrocyanoses (numbness or mottling of fingers, toes, nose, ears), Raynaud phenomenon, cold-associated occlusive changes**

Diagnosis	• **Complete Blood Count (CBC) with Peripheral Smear:** decreased hemoglobin
	   • Smear demonstrates **microspherocytes and a high reticulocyte count with few or no schistocytes (indicates extravascular hemolysis)**
	• **Labs:** hemolysis (increased LDH, elevated indirect bilirubin, decreased haptoglobin)
	• **Direct Antiglobulin (Direct Coombs) Test:** reveals antibody-coated RBCs
	   • **Warm Agglutin:** IgG and C3 present
	   • **Cold Agglutin:** only C3 is present (IgG is usually absent)

Treatment	• **Blood Transfusions: most important treatment;** indicated in severe cases where the hemoglobin levels are significantly low and symptoms are severe
	• **Warm Agglutin:**
	   • **Drug Induced:** discontinue offending medication (if possible)
	   • **Idiopathic: corticosteroids are first-line,** rituximab (anti-CD20) is second-line, folic acid, and/or splenectomy
	     • Immunosuppressive Therapy: cyclosporine, cyclophosphamide, azathioprine; indicated if no response with splenectomy or corticosteroids
	• **Cold Agglutin:**
	• **Avoidance of Cold: mainstay of treatment**
	• Rituximab: second-line treatment
	• **Plasmapheresis:** effective temporary treatment in severe cases

Hereditary Spherocytosis

Etiology & Risk Factors	• **Autosomal dominant disease** characterized by hemolysis of spheroidal RBCs and anemia • <u>Etiology</u>: genetic mutations in the genes encoding proteins involved in the red blood cell membrane leading to the formation of spherical-shaped red blood cells. • <u>Risk Factors</u>: **family history, Northern Europeans**
Patho-physiology	• Deficiency in the red blood cell membrane (particularly in proteins such as spectrin, ankyrin, and band 3) results in a loss of structural integrity, causing the red blood cells to become spherical and fragile; the altered shape and decreased flexibility of these cells lead to their premature destruction by the spleen (hemolysis)

Signs & Symptoms	• Usually mild anemia symptoms
	• <u>**Recurrent Episodes of Hemolysis**</u>: hallmark
	  • <u>**Hemolytic Anemia**</u>: chronic anemia leading to fatigue, weakness, and pallor
	  • <u>**Jaundice**</u>: yellowing of the skin and eyes.
	  • <u>**Splenomegaly**</u>: LUQ abdominal pain and fullness
	• <u>**Cholelithiasis**</u>: pigmented stones (calcium bilirubinate) is common

Diagnosis	• <u>**Complete Blood Count (CBC) with Peripheral Smear**</u>: decreased hemoglobin
	  • **Increased mean corpuscular hemoglobin concentration (MCHC)**
	  • **Presence of spherocytes (small, dense, spherical red blood cells lacking central pallor)** on the peripheral blood smear
	  • **Increased reticulocyte count** indicating increased red blood cell production in response to hemolysis
	• <u>**Eosin-5-Maleimide (EMA) Binding Test**</u>: most accurate test; measures the binding capacity of EMA (a fluorescent dye), to RBCs; reduced binding indicates the presence of abnormal RBC membrane proteins
	• <u>**Osmotic Fragility Test**</u>: increased osmotic fragility of red blood cells due to increased membrane permeability, causing them to lyse in hypotonic solutions
	• <u>**Direct Antiglobulin (Direct Coombs) Test**</u>: **negative test** distinguishes from autoimmune hemolytic anemia

Treatment	• <u>**Folate Supplementation**</u>: non-curative; may aid in sustaining RBC production and DNA synthesis due to the increase in erythropoietic activity compensating for hemolysis • <u>**Splenectomy**</u>: **curative treatment** as the spleen is the principal organ where erythrocyte destruction takes place • Indicated in patients with severe hemolysis or complications such as biliary colic or persistent aplastic crisis
Key Words & Most Common	• Autosomal dominant disease • Recurrent episodes of hemolysis (anemia, jaundice, splenomegaly) +/- cholelithiasis • <u>CBC</u>: decreased hemoglobin, increased MCHC • <u>Peripheral Smear</u>: presence of spherocytes (small, dense, spherical red blood cells lacking central pallor), increased reticulocyte count • <u>EMA Binding Test</u>: most accurate test • <u>Direct Coombs Test</u>: negative test differentiates between autoimmune hemolytic anemia • Splenectomy is curative treatment

Sickle Cell Disease

Etiology & Risk Factors	• Inherited autosomal recessive disorder that affects the beta-globin gene leading to abnormal hemoglobin and rigid, sickle-shaped red blood cells • <u>Etiology</u>: **genetic mutation in the hemoglobin gene (HBB gene)** leading to abnormal hemoglobin (hemoglobin S [HbS]) • <u>Risk Factors</u>: **family history**, certain ethnicities (**African most common** [affects 1 in 600], South Asian, Middle Eastern, Mediterranean descent)
Patho-physiology	• Point mutation on the beta-globin gene leading to production of abnormal hemoglobin (HbS) which causes red blood cells to become rigid and assume a sickle shape, increasing the chance of cells to "clump" together which leads to the obstruction of small blood vessels, reduced blood flow, and tissue damage • The shortened lifespan of the sickle cells leads to chronic anemia, as the bone marrow is unable to meet the demand for new red blood cells

Signs & Symptoms	• *Highly variable with wide range of complications*
	• <u>**Hemolytic Anemia**</u>: fatigue, weakness, **pallor, jaundice**, pigmented gallstones
	• <u>**Dactylitis**</u>: pain and swelling in both hands and feet is most common initial symptom; may start as early as six months of age
	• <u>**Vaso-Occlusive Crisis**</u>: **most common presentation**; may be triggered by hypoxia, cold weather, infection, dehydration, alcohol use, pregnancy
	  • <u>**Severe Bone Pain**</u>: **worst in long bones, the hands and feet, back, and joints**; hip or shoulder pain secondary to **avascular necrosis** of bone (femoral or humeral head)
	  • <u>**Acute Chest Syndrome**</u>: sudden onset of fever, cough, tachypnea, hypoxia, dyspnea
	  • <u>**Abdominal Pain**</u>: may be secondary to hepatic vein thrombosis; with or without vomiting
	• <u>**Infections**</u>: **at risk for infections with encapsulated organisms** (*S. pneumoniae, H. influenzae, N. meningitidis*, GBS, *Klebsiella, Salmonella*) due to **functional asplenia**
	  • <u>**Osteomyelitis**</u>: *Salmonella* spp. is most common organism
	  • <u>**Aplastic Crisis**</u>: associated with parvovirus B19 infections
	• <u>**Splenic Sequestration**</u>: potentially catastrophic complication; characterized by an acute decrease in hemoglobin resulting in severe abdominal pain and circulatory collapse
	• <u>**Complications**</u>: increased risk for CVA/stroke, pulmonary hypertension, pulmonary embolism, proliferative retinopathy, priapism, cholelithiasis,

Diagnosis	• <u>**Complete Blood Count (CBC) with Peripheral Smear**</u>: **best initial test**
	  • <u>**CBC**</u>: assess for significant anemia (usually baseline 8-10g/dL), decreased hematocrit, increased reticulocyte count
	  • <u>**Peripheral Smear**</u>: Target cells, **sickled erythrocytes** (crescent-shaped, often with elongated or pointed ends), **Howell-Jolly bodies** (indicates functional asplenia),
	  <u>**Hemoglobin Electrophoresis**</u>: gold standard test; separates different types of hemoglobin based on electrical charge; increased amount of HbS and a decrease or absence of normal HbA
	• <u>**DNA Genetic Testing**</u>: confirms diagnosis by identifying the specific mutation in the HBB gene

Treatment	• <u>**Antibiotics**</u>: broad-spectrum antibiotics indicated for suspected serious bacterial infections or acute chest syndrome • <u>**Analgesia**</u>: liberal administration of analgesics including opioids (**IV morphine**) is recommended for managing painful crises; NSAIDs used with cautiously with renal disease • <u>**Intravenous Hydration**</u>: **maintaining normal intravascular volume is a mainstay of therapy** to reverse and prevent sickling • <u>**Oxygen**</u>: administered if needed to prevent or treat hypoxia • <u>**Blood Transfusion**</u>: indicated for acute splenic sequestration, aplastic crises, cardiopulmonary symptoms, preoperative use, priapism, life-threatening events, pregnancy • Chronic transfusion therapy is used to prevent recurrent cerebral thrombosis, aiming to maintain the Hb S percentage less than 30% • <u>**Hydroxyurea**</u>: **mainstay of treatment to reduce frequency and severity of pain episodes**; increased production of HbF and reduces RBC sickling • <u>**Allogeneic Hematopoietic Stem Cell Transplant (HCT)**</u>: only curative treatment for advanced disease complications

Thrombotic Thrombocytopenic Purpura (TTP) 🩸

Etiology & Risk Factors	• Microangiopathic hemolytic anemia characterized by fever, hemolytic anemia, thrombocytopenia, and renal and neurologic dysfunction • Etiology: congenital or acquired deficiency of **ADAMTS13** (a plasma enzyme responsible for breaking down von Willebrand factor [vWF] in the bloodstream) • Congenital: hereditary (Upshaw-Schulman syndrome) • Acquired: **concomitant autoimmune condition (SLE)**, malignancy, bone marrow transplantation, certain medications (**clopidogrel**, immunosuppressives, estrogen-containing birth control, quinidine), pregnancy, HIV • Risk Factors: female, African-American descent, pregnancy
Patho-physiology	• Severe deficiency or dysfunction of ADAMTS13 (an enzyme responsible for cleaving von Willebrand factor [vWF] multimers) leads to accumulation of large vWF monomers which promote platelet aggregation and thrombus formation • Resultant microvascular occlusion leads to tissue ischemia, organ dysfunction, and thrombocytopenia due to excessive platelet consumption
Signs & Symptoms	• Pentad: **FAT RN** (Fever, Anemia, Thrombocytopenia, Renal, Neurologic symptoms); rarely are all 5 present • **Fever**: rare sign/symptom • **Anemia**: microangiopathic hemolytic anemia; weakness, fatigue, pallor, jaundice, and dark urine • **Thrombocytopenia**: bruising, petechiae, or **mucosal bleeding (epistaxis, bleeding gums, menorrhagia)** • **Renal Pathology**: uncommon • **Neurologic Abnormalities**: headache, visual changes, altered mental status, seizure CVA, coma
Diagnosis	• PLASMIC Score: <5 features effectively rules out TTP • **(1)** Platelets <30 x 10⁹/L **(2)** Hemolysis with reticulocyte count >2.5%, indirect bilirubin >2mg/dL, or low haptoglobin **(3)** MCV <90fL **(4)** INR <1.5 **(5)** Creatinine <2mg/dL **(6)** No Current Cancer • Complete Blood Count (CBC) with Platelets and Peripheral Blood Smear: best initial test; thrombocytopenia and anemia • Thrombocytopenia and anemia • **Hemolysis**: fragmented red blood cells, **schistocytes** (helmet cells; triangular RBCs, distorted-appearing RBCs), elevated reticulocyte count, increased serum LDH and bilirubin, decreased haptoglobin • Coagulation Studies: normal PT and PTT; helps distinguish TTP and HUS from DIC • Direct Antiglobulin (Direct Coombs) Test: negative test • ADAMTS13 Activity and Autoantibody Testing: decreased ADAMTS13 level (<10%) with the presence of antibody against ADAMTS13
Treatment	• **Plasmapheresis**: initial treatment of choice; >85% of patients recover completely • Plasma exchange removes antibodies against ADAMTS13 and repletes ADAMTS13 • **Corticosteroids**: high-dose corticosteroid therapy is continued with plasma exchange and subsequently tapered off based on clinical response • **Rituximab**: anti-CD20 monoclonal antibody used to help treat TTP refractory to plasma exchange • Other: splenectomy, cyclosporine, cyclophosphamide, vincristine • Platelet Transfusions: contraindicated as may potentiate thrombi formation or renal failure; only used for life-threatening bleeding or intracranial hemorrhage

Hemolytic Uremic Syndrome (HUS) 🩸

Etiology & Risk Factors	• **Thrombotic microangiopathy characterized by thrombocytopenia, microangiopathic hemolytic anemia, and renal dysfunction** • Etiology: two variants termed typical and atypical HUS • **Typical**: caused by Shiga-like toxin (verotoxin) produced by **enterohemorrhagic** *Escherichia coli* **(O157: H7)** and Shiga toxin by *Shigella dysenteriae* • **Atypical**: bacteria (*Streptococcus pneumoniae, Mycoplasma pneumoniae, C. difficile*, HIV, histoplasmosis, coxsackievirus, H1N1 Influenza A), medication/drugs (cyclosporine, cisplatin, cocaine, quinine), or immune processes capable of endothelial damage • Risk Factors: **age** (primarily affects children under ten years old; **<5 years old most common**), **recent history of gastroenteritis** (*Escherichia coli*), geographics (rural communities, seasonal (summer and fall most common)
Patho-physiology	• Enterohemorrhagic strains of *Escherichia coli* (O157:H7) produce Shiga toxins which damage the lining of blood vessels, leading to the formation of blood clots in small blood vessels (microthrombi) throughout the body which obstruct the flow of blood and result in red blood cell destruction, platelet activation, and kidney damage
Signs & Symptoms	• Prodromal Gastroenteritis: occurs 5-10 days prior • **Fever, abdominal pain, nausea, vomiting, bloody diarrhea** • Anemia: microangiopathic hemolytic anemia; weakness, fatigue, pallor, jaundice, and dark urine • Thrombocytopenia: may have small ecchymosis and mucosal bleeding; petechiae and purpura are uncommon • Acute Renal Failure: oliguria/anuria, hematuria, dark urine
Diagnosis	• Complete Blood Count (CBC) with Platelets and Peripheral Blood Smear: best initial test; thrombocytopenia and anemia • Thrombocytopenia and anemia • **Hemolysis**: fragmented red blood cells, **schistocytes** (helmet cells; triangular RBCs, distorted-appearing RBCs), elevated reticulocyte count, increased serum LDH and bilirubin, decreased haptoglobin • Metabolic Panel: **elevated BUN and creatinine** (often more pronounced than TTP), uremia, hyponatremia and hyperkalemia (renal failure) • Urinalysis: hematuria and proteinuria • Coagulation Studies: normal PT and PTT; helps distinguish TTP and HUS from DIC • Direct Antiglobulin (Direct Coombs) Test: negative test • ADAMTS13 Activity and Autoantibody Testing: normal activity; differentiates TTP and HUS • Stool Testing: *Shiga* toxin enzyme-linked immunosorbent assay (ELISA) or specific culture media for *E. coli* O157:H7 helps identify specific etiology
Treatment	• Supportive Care: initial management choice • Rehydration and electrolyte replacement, discontinue nephrotoxic medications • Hemodialysis: typically reserved for symptomatic uremia, azotemia (BUN >80 mg/dL), fluid overload or electrolyte abnormalities refractory to medical therapy • Plasmapheresis: indicated if anuria or neurologic sequela • AVOID Antibiotics: may lead to worsening lysis of bacteria and further Shiga toxin release • AVOID Anti-Motility Agents: leads to prolonged gut exposure to toxins and increased risk of toxic megacolon

Disseminated Intravascular Coagulation (DIC) 💉

Etiology & Risk Factors	• Widespread and inappropriate activation of the coagulation and fibrinolytic systems that may lead to microvascular and macrovascular clotting and impaired blood flow
	• Etiology:
	  • **Infection: gram-negative sepsis is most common cause**
	  • **Obstetric Complications: abruptio placentae,** pre-eclampsia, amniotic fluid embolism, septic abortion, HELLP Syndrome
	  • **Malignancy:** mucin-secreting pancreatic cancer, prostate cancer, acute myelogenous leukemia
	  • **Tissue Injury and Trauma:** head trauma, burns, frostbite, gunshot wounds, ARDS, aortic aneurysms, liver disease

Patho-physiology	• Inappropriate activation of the coagulation cascade leads to uncontrolled fibrin production and formation of small blood clots (**microthrombi**) within the blood vessels • Clots consume clotting factors (V, VIII, fibrinogen) and platelets, leading to the depletion of these essential components and subsequent **thrombocytopenia** (manifested as **diffuse bleeding** from skin, respiratory and GI tract), and the release of pro-inflammatory substances that damage blood vessels and impair organ function
Signs & Symptoms	• **Bleeding:** persisting bleeding from skin puncture sites (IV, drains, or arterial punctures), bruising at sites of parenteral injections, serious gastrointestinal bleeds • **Thrombosis:** symptoms of venous thrombosis and/or symptoms of pulmonary embolism may be present; gangrene, multi-organ failure
Diagnosis	• **Complete Blood Count (CBC) with Platelets and Peripheral Blood Smear: thrombocytopenia** present in 98% of cases; **low or dropping platelets** (may need to trend) • Peripheral Blood Smear: fragmented RBCs, schistocytes • **Coagulation Studies: prolonged PT and PTT;** PT (not INR) is used for monitoring • **Fibrinogen: decreased** fibrinogen levels (from consumption) • Fibrin Degradation Products (FDP): elevated level • **D-Dimer: elevated** level; *FDP and d-dimer may increase sensitivity and specificity*
Treatment	• **Treat Underlying Etiology:** mainstay of treatment • Broad-spectrum antibiotic treatment of suspected gram-negative sepsis, evacuation of the uterus in abruptio placentae, blood volume repletion etc. • **Platelet Transfusion:** indicated in severe bleeds to correct thrombocytopenia in cases of rapidly declining platelet count or platelet count <10,000-20,000/microL • **Fresh Frozen Plasma:** indicated in severe bleeds to increase levels of other clotting factors and natural anticoagulants (antithrombin, proteins C, S, and Z) • **Cryoprecipitate:** indicated in severe bleeds to replace fibrinogen (and factor VIII) if the fibrinogen level is rapidly declining or is <100mg/dL • Heparin: may be used in the treatment of slowly evolving DIC with venous thrombosis or pulmonary embolism
Key Words & Most Common	• Inappropriate activation of coagulation and fibrinolytic systems leading to clotting and impaired blood flow • Causes include infection, obstetric complications, malignancy, and tissue injury/trauma • Results in uncontrolled fibrin production and formation of microthrombi in blood vessels • Symptoms include bleeding, thrombosis, thrombocytopenia, and organ damage/failure • Thrombocytopenia + prolonged PT/PTT + decreased fibrinogen + elevated d-dimer • Treatment involves addressing the underlying cause → platelet transfusion, fresh frozen plasma, cryoprecipitate in severe cases

Immune Thrombocytopenic Purpura (ITP) 💉

Etiology & Risk Factors	• **Acquired, immune-mediated disease characterized by a thrombocytopenia, purpura, and hemorrhagic episodes caused by antiplatelet autoantibodies**
	• Etiology: may be primary or secondary; exact cause not fully understood, may be combination of genetic predisposition, immune dysregulation, and environmental triggers.
	  • Primary: **idiopathic; most common after viral infection**
	  • Secondary: immune-mediated; associated with underlying disorders such as infection (HIV), autoimmune disorders (SLE, autoimmune hepatitis and thyroid disease), malignancy (adenocarcinoma and lymphoma)
	• Risk Factors: **concomitant autoimmune disorders,** history of viral infection, certain medications (anticonvulsants, NSAIDs), certain vaccinations (MMR), family history

Patho-physiology	• Destruction of platelets by antiplatelet autoantibodies which bind to platelet surface antigens leading to their premature destruction by macrophages in the spleen and liver • Decreased platelet count results in a reduced ability to form blood clots and leads to symptoms such as easy bruising, petechiae, and mucosal bleeding
Signs & Symptoms	• **Often asymptomatic** • **Bleeding:** secondary to thrombocytopenia; bruising, petechiae, purpura, ecchymosis or **mucosal bleeding (epistaxis, gingival bleeding, menorrhagia)** • Severe Bleeding: intracranial hemorrhage, gastrointestinal (GI) bleeding and hematuria are less common • ***Not associated with splenomegaly***
Diagnosis	• **Complete Blood Count (CBC) with Platelets and Peripheral Blood Smear: isolated thrombocytopenia** (otherwise normal CBC and peripheral blood smear) • **Coagulation Studies:** normal PT, PTT • Bone Marrow Biopsy: not required for diagnosis; reserved for elderly patients or if patients fail to respond to standard therapy • **Normal or increased numbers of megakaryocytes** (large-sized platelets) in an otherwise normal bone marrow sample
Treatment	• **Corticosteroids: first-line therapy;** prednisone (14 days) or dexamethasone (4 days) indicated for newly diagnosed ITP with bleeding and a platelet count <30,000/mcL • **IV Immunoglobulin (IVIG): second-line therapy** or if treatment if rapid rise in platelet counts is required (tooth extractions, childbirth, surgery, or other invasive procedures) • Thrombopoietin Receptor Agonists (TPO-RA): romiplostim, eltrombopag, avatrombopag; may be used before invasive procedures or in steroid-refractory cases (should not be used for childbirth) • **Rituximab:** anti-CD20 monoclonal antibody used in steroid-refractory cases • **Splenectomy:** reserved for patients with severe or persistent thrombocytopenia (<15,000/mcL) and bleeding risk cannot be controlled with medical therapy • Shown to achieve complete remission in about 2/3rd of patients who fail initial corticosteroid therapy
Key Words & Most Common	• Thrombocytopenia caused by antiplatelet autoantibodies • Often asymptomatic • Bruising, petechiae, purpura, ecchymosis or mucosal bleeding; not associated with splenomegaly • Isolated thrombocytopenia with normal CBC/blood smear/coagulation studies • Corticosteroids → IVIG → rituximab or splenectomy

Hemophilia

Etiology & Risk Factors	• X-linked recessive hereditary bleeding disorders • <u>Etiology</u>: **mutations, deletions, or inversions affecting either clotting factor VIII (hemophilia A) or IX (hemophilia B)** • <u>Risk Factors</u>: **family history**; consanguinity (marriages between close relatives)
Patho-physiology	• Deficiency or dysfunction of clotting factor VIII (hemophilia A) or clotting factor IX (hemophilia B) leading to impaired blood clotting and a prolonged bleeding time • The defective clotting factor hinders the formation of fibrin, a key component of blood clots, resulting in the inability to control bleeding effectively

Signs & Symptoms	• <u>**Hemarthrosis**</u>: **most common bleeding sign/symptom**
	  • **Bleeding into weight-bearing joints** leading to joint destruction and chronic synovitis and arthropathy
	  • **Ankles most common in kids**
	  • **Knees, elbow, ankles most common in adults**
	• <u>**Hematomas**</u>: bleeding into soft tissues or muscle
	  • Neck (airway compromise), limbs (compartment syndrome), eye (retro-orbital hematoma), spine (epidural hematoma), retroperitoneum (iliopsoas bleeds)
	• <u>**Mucocutaneous Bleeding**</u>: spontaneous bleeding from oropharynx, GI or urinary tract, epistaxis, hemoptysis
	• <u>**CNS Bleeding**</u>: **intracranial hemorrhage is most common cause of hemorrhagic death**; subdural hematomas can occur spontaneously or with minimal trauma
	• <u>**Hematuria**</u>: common, usually not serious
	• <u>Excessive Bleeding</u>: during trauma, surgery or incisional procedure (surgery or dental extraction)
	• *Hemophilias less commonly present with purpura or petechiae (normal platelet function)*

Diagnosis	• <u>**Complete Blood Count (CBC) with Platelets**</u>: **normal platelet level** • <u>**Coagulation Studies**</u>: **prolonged PTT; normal PT** • <u>**Factor VIII and IX Assay**</u>: determines the type and severity of the hemophilia; low factor VIII seen in hemophilia A, low factor IX seen in hemophilia B

Treatment	• <u>**Replacement of Deficient Factor**</u>: **first-line therapy**; levels transiently raised to 25-100% of normal depending on severity
	  • <u>**Factor VIII Infusion**</u>: **indicated in hemophilia A**
	  • <u>**Factor IX Infusion**</u>: **indicated in hemophilia B**
	• <u>Desmopressin</u>: may temporarily raise factor VIII and vWF levels in hemophilia A prior to minor procedures to prevent bleeding
	  • *Ineffective in hemophilia B*

Key Words & Most Common	• X-linked recessive bleeding disorder affecting clotting factor VIII (hemophilia A) or IX (hemophilia B) • Hemarthrosis (ankles most common in kids; knees most common in adults), hematomas, mucocutaneous bleeding, hematuria, intracranial bleeding • Normal platelets, normal PT, prolonged PTT • Replacement of deficient factors is first-line therapy

Von Willebrand Disease (vWD)

Etiology & Risk Factors	• **Autosomal dominant** bleeding disorder resulting in ineffective platelet adhesion
	• <u>Etiology</u>: **qualitative or quantitative deficiency of the pro-von Willebrand factor**
	  • <u>Type 1 (Most Common)</u>: quantitative deficiency of VWF; concentration and activity are both reduced proportionally.
	  • <u>Type 2</u>: qualitative impairment in synthesis and function of VWF
	  • <u>Type 3</u>: rare autosomal recessive disorder in which homozygotes have no detectable VWF
	• <u>Risk Factors</u>: **family history**, Caucasian descent, female

Patho-physiology	• Von Willebrand factor (VWF) is a glycoprotein that promotes platelet adhesion by by binding with a receptor on the platelet surface membrane (glycoprotein Ib/IX) with collagen, thus connecting the platelets to the vessel wall; acts as carrier protein for factor VIII extending its half-life

Signs & Symptoms	• <u>**Bleeding**</u>: **bruising or mucosal bleeding (epistaxis, gingival bleeding, menorrhagia)**
	  • Prolonged bleeding from minor cuts that may stop and start over hours
	  • Increased bleeding after surgical procedures (tooth extraction, tonsillectomy)
	• *VWD less commonly present with purpura or petechiae (normal platelet function)*

Diagnosis	• <u>**Complete Blood Count (CBC) with Platelets**</u>: **normal platelet level** • <u>**Coagulation Studies**</u>: **slightly prolonged PTT; normal PT** • <u>**Von Willebrand Factor Antigen**</u>: protein levels are tested for a quantitative defect; **decreased antigen levels seen in type I VWD** • <u>**Von Willebrand Factor Activity**</u>: qualitative analysis for von Willebrand factor physiological function; **decreased activity levels (<30IU) seen in type II VWD** • <u>**Factor VIII Activity**</u>: decreased von Willebrand factor leads to increased degradation of factor VIII • *Type 3 VWD have no detectable VWF and a marked deficiency of factor VIII.*

Treatment	• <u>**Desmopressin**</u>: **indicated for type I and most type II VWD cases**
	  • Analog of vasopressin (antidiuretic hormone) stimulates release of VWF into the plasma and may increase factor VIII levels
	  • Given 15-30 minutes prior to minor procedures (tooth extraction, minor surgery)
	• <u>**Von Willebrand Factor Replacement**</u>: indicated for type 3 or severe type 1 or type 2 variants with minimal desmopressin response
	  • Given when undergoing invasive or extensive procedures
	  • Replacement of VWF by infusion of human-derived factor VIII concentrates, purified VWF concentrates or recombinant VWF

Key Words & Most Common	• Autosomal dominant bleeding disorder caused by a qualitative or quantitative VWF deficiency • Bleeding: bruising or mucosal bleeding; less commonly presents with purpura or petechiae (normal platelet function) • Normal platelet level, normal PT, slightly prolonged PTT • VWF Antigen = quantitative defect; VWF activity = qualitative defect • Desmopressin indicated in type I and most type II • VWF Replacement indicated in type 3 or severe type 1 or 2 variants

Factor V Leiden Mutation

Etiology & Risk Factors	• Autosomal dominant genetic mutation of factor V which causes hypercoagulability (thrombophilia) and increases the risk of thrombosis • <u>Etiology</u>: **point mutation of factor V** • <u>Risk Factors</u>: **family history**, certain ethnicities (Caucasian or European descent); female, pregnancy, obesity, smoking, and prolonged immobility increase risk of clotting
Patho-physiology	• Genetic alteration in the factor V gene that leads to an abnormal form of the F5 protein involved in the blood clotting process • The mutation makes factor V resistant to inactivation by protein C (a natural anticoagulant) leading to an increased tendency of blood clot formation (hypercoagulability)

Signs & Symptoms	• <u>**Hypercoagulability**</u>: **increased risk of spontaneous venous thromboembolism (VTE)**
	   • Increased incidence of deep vein thrombosis (DVT), pulmonary embolism (PE), portal or hepatic vein thrombosis
	   • Increased incidence of cerebral vein thrombosis (especially with combination oral contraceptives)
	   • Increased risk of miscarriage and VTE during pregnancy (controversial)

Diagnosis	• <u>**Functional Activated Protein C (APC) Resistance Assay**</u>: does not become prolonged; if positive, confirm with genetic or DNA mutation analysis • <u>Genetic Testing</u>: indicated for those with a family history of factor V Leiden or positive positive functional assay for APC resistance to confirm diagnosis • <u>**DNA Mutation Analysis**</u>: polymerase chain reaction methods can detect factor V Leiden mutation • <u>Coagulation Studies</u>: normal PT/PTT
Treatment	• <u>**Anticoagulation**</u>: **parenteral heparin or low molecular weight heparin (LMWH) followed by oral warfarin** • Indicated for for venous thrombosis or prophylaxis for patients at increased thromboembolic risk (immobilization, severe injury, surgery) • <u>Direct Oral Anticoagulant (DOAC) Inhibitors</u>: thrombin inhibitor (dabigatran) or factor Xa inhibitor (rivaroxaban, apixaban) may be used in place of warfarin; *not yet certain*
Key Words & Most Common	• Autosomal dominant genetic mutation of factor V • Hypercoagulability → spontaneous VTE (DVT or PE) • Functional APC resistance assay → genetic or DNA mutation analysis • Anticoagulation (heparin or LMWH → warfarin)

Protein C or S Deficiency

Etiology & Risk Factors	• **Protein C and protein S are vitamin K-dependent anticoagulant glycoproteins that stimulate fibrinolysis and inactivate factors V and VIII**; synthesized in the liver
	• <u>Etiology</u>: deficiencies secondary to inherited or acquired causes
	   • <u>Inherited Deficiencies</u>: **autosomal dominant genetic mutations;** lead to reduced or dysfunctional protein C or S
	   • <u>Acquired Deficiencies</u>: severe liver disease, vitamin K deficiency, certain medications (warfarin), or certain medical conditions (DIC or thrombotic microangiopathies)
	• <u>Risk Factors</u>: **family history**, liver disease, vitamin K deficiency, warfarin use; female, pregnancy, obesity, smoking, prolonged immobility increase risk of clotting

Patho-physiology	• Protein C inhibits the activity of clotting factors; protein S enhances the anticoagulant function of protein C • Deficiency in either protein C or protein S results in impaired regulation of blood clotting, leading to an increased risk of abnormal blood clot formation (hypercoagulability)
Signs & Symptoms	• <u>**Hypercoagulability**</u>: **increased risk of spontaneous venous thromboembolism (VTE)** • Increased incidence of deep vein thrombosis (DVT), pulmonary embolism (PE) • <u>**Warfarin-Induced Skin Necrosis**</u>: possible in patients with an underlying hereditary protein C deficiency • <u>Neonatal Purpura Fulminans</u>: severe neonatal type of (DIC); manifests as ecchymoses and extensive venous and arterial thromboses on the first day of life
Diagnosis	• <u>**Functional Protein C and S Assay**</u>: preferred assay in the clinical setting to assess the protein activity • <u>Genetic Testing</u>: not routinely performed
Treatment	• <u>**Anticoagulation**</u>: **parenteral heparin or low molecular weight heparin (LMWH) followed by oral warfarin** • *Risk of warfarin causing thrombotic skin infarction in protein C deficiency* • <u>Protein C Concentrate</u>: indicated for acute thrombosis or neonatal purpura fulminans cases • <u>Fresh Frozen Plasma Transfusion</u>: indicated to replace protein S during a thrombotic emergency • <u>Direct Oral Anticoagulant (DOAC) Inhibitors</u>: thrombin inhibitor (dabigatran) or factor Xa inhibitor (rivaroxaban, apixaban) may be used in place of warfarin; *not yet certain*
Key Words & Most Common	• Vitamin K-dependent anticoagulant proteins that may lead to hypercoagulability • Increased risk of spontaneous venous thromboembolism (VTE) • Warfarin-induced skin necrosis • Neonatal purpura fulminans • Functional protein C and S assay • Anticoagulation

Antithrombin III Deficiency

Etiology & Risk Factors	• Decreased levels of antithrombin III lead to hypercoagulable state
	• <u>Etiology</u>: may be inherited or acquired
	   • <u>Inherited</u>: most common cause; **autosomal dominant genetic mutation** affecting the production or function of antithrombin
	   • <u>Acquired</u>: liver disease, nephrotic syndrome, DIC, certain medications (heparin), certain conditions that increase the consumption of antithrombin (severe infections, major surgery)
	• <u>Risk Factors</u>: **family history**, liver disease, nephrotic syndrome, certain medications (oral contraceptives)

Patho-physiology	• Antithrombin protein inhibits coagulation by neutralizing thrombin (factors IIa, IXa, and Xa) activity • Deficiency disrupts the normal balance between clot formation and clot dissolution, leading to an increased risk of blood clot formation (hypercoagulability)
Signs & Symptoms	• <u>**Hypercoagulability**</u>: **increased risk of spontaneous venous thromboembolism (VTE)** • Increased incidence of deep vein thrombosis (DVT), pulmonary embolism (PE)
Diagnosis	• <u>Antithrombin III Assay</u>: involves quantification of the capacity of plasma to inhibit <u>thrombin</u> in the presence of <u>heparin</u>
Treatment	• <u>**Warfarin**</u>: used for prophylaxis against venous thromboembolism • <u>Direct Oral Anticoagulant (DOAC) Inhibitors</u>: thrombin inhibitor (dabigatran) or factor Xa inhibitor (rivaroxaban, apixaban) may be used in place of warfarin; *not yet certain*
Key Words & Most Common	• Decreased level of antithrombin lead to hypercoagulable state • Increased risk of spontaneous venous thromboembolism (VTE) • Antithrombin assay • Anticoagulation therapy

Heparin-Induced Thrombocytopenia (HIT)

Etiology & Risk Factors	• Thrombocytopenia acquired within the first 5-10 days after initiating heparin therapy • <u>Etiology</u>: **unfractionated heparin** or LMWH (**10x more common in unfractionated**) • <u>Risk Factors</u>: **heparin exposure** (prolonged heparin therapy [>5 days], high-dose heparin, previous exposure to heparin within the past 3 months)
Patho-physiology	• Pathologic activation/consumption of platelets secondary to autoantibodies against heparin-platelet complex (hapten of heparin + platelet factor 4) leading to platelet aggregation, thrombus formation and subsequent thrombocytopenia; activated platelets release microparticles that contribute to the prothrombotic state

Signs & Symptoms	• <u>4 T's</u>: **T**hrombocytopenia, **T**iming, **T**hrombosis, no o**T**her causes
	   • **Thrombocytopenia**: bruising, petechiae, or **mucosal bleeding (epistaxis, bleeding gums, menorrhagia)**
	   • **Timing**: occurs **5-10 days** after initiating heparin therapy
	   • **Thrombosis**: **increased risk of spontaneous venous thromboembolism (VTE), gangrene, organ infarction and skin necrosis**
	     • Increased incidence of DVT/PE, limb arterial occlusion, CVA, MI

Diagnosis	• **Complete Blood Count (CBC) with Platelets**: **thrombocytopenia (low platelet level)** • **Platelet Activation Assays**: serotonin release assay **(gold standard)** or heparin-induced platelet activation assay • <u>Enzyme-Linked Immunosorbent Assay (ELISA)</u>: evaluate for antibodies against platelet factor 4 (PF4)

Treatment	• **Discontinuation of All Heparin Products**: immediate discontinuation is most important
	• **Initiate Non-Heparin Anticoagulants:**
	   • **Direct Thrombin Inhibitor: lepirudin, argatroban**
	   • <u>Direct Xa Inhibitor</u>: fondaparinux, danaparoid
	   • <u>Direct Oral Anticoagulants</u>: apixaban, edoxaban, rivaroxaban, dabigatran
	• *Do not give platelets (may precipitate thrombosis)*
	• *Avoid warfarin until platelets >100K-150K*

Key Words & Most Common	• Thrombocytopenia secondary to unfractionated heparin • **T**hrombocytopenia + **T**iming + **T**hrombosis + no o**T**her causes • Serotonin release assay is gold standard • Discontinue all heparin products → initiate non-heparin anticoagulants

Hemochromatosis

Etiology & Risk Factors	• **Genetic disorder characterized by excessive iron (Fe) deposition in parenchymal cells of heart, liver, pancreas and endocrine organs resulting in tissue damage** • <u>Etiology</u>: **mutations of the C282Y HFE (human homeostatic iron regulator) genotype is most common**; autosomal recessive pattern • <u>Risk Factors</u>: **Northern European descent (most common in people of Celtic ancestry)**; chronic liver disease, excessive iron supplementation, repeated blood transfusions, certain conditions causing increased iron absorption or accumulation (thalassemia or chronic alcoholism)
Patho-physiology	• Genetic mutations in the HFE protein cause decreased hepcidin levels, disrupting the normal regulation of iron absorption in the intestine which increases the intestinal absorption of iron; this causes excessive iron accumulation in parenchymal cells of the heart, liver pancreas and endocrine organs resulting in tissue damage and dysfunction
Signs & Symptoms	• *Symptoms relate to the organs with the largest iron deposits* • <u>Liver</u>: fatigue, weakness, abdominal pain, **cirrhosis**, hepatomegaly • <u>Pancreas</u>: **diabetes** (due to iron deposition in pancreas causing beta cell damage) • <u>Heart</u>: **restrictive or dilated cardiomyopathy**, arrhythmias, heart blocks, heart failure • <u>Reproductive</u>: **hypogonadism, erectile dysfunction**, testicular atrophy • <u>Musculoskeletal</u>: arthralgias, arthritis, synovitis • <u>Cutaneous</u>: **metallic or bronze skin** (due to iron deposition); also known as "bronze diabetes"

Diagnosis	• <u>Iron Studies</u>: initial test of choice
	  • **Elevated serum ferritin is most simple and direct initial test** (>300ng/mL in males and postmenopausal women; >150ng/mL in premenopausal women)
	  • Elevated transferrin saturation (>45-50% suggestive of iron overload)
	  • Elevated serum iron (usually >300 mg/dL)
	• <u>Genetic Testing</u>: testing for the *HFE* gene mutations indicated if iron studies are abnormal
	• <u>Liver Testing</u>: indicated to test for fibrosis and cirrhosis
	  • Liver function studies (elevated ALT/AST)
	  • MRI with noncontrast MR elastography (noninvasive alternative for estimating hepatic iron content and fibrosis)
	  • **Liver biopsy is most accurate test** (shows increased hemosiderin in liver parenchyma with Prussian blue staining)

Treatment	• <u>Phlebotomy</u>: **mainstay of treatment**; indicated for symptomatic patients, elevated serum ferritin levels or elevated transferrin saturation • Performed weekly or biweekly until serum ferritin levels reach 50-100 ng/mL • <u>Chelation Therapy</u>: iron chelators (deferasirox, **deferoxamine**, deferiprone) indicated for patients unable to undergo phlebotomy • <u>Lifestyle Modifications</u>: avoid iron supplementation (not necessary to restrict iron-containing foods [red meat, liver]), avoid vitamin C supplementation, avoid alcohol
Key Words & Most Common	• Genetic disorder characterized by excessive iron deposition in tissue caused by HFE mutation • Diabetes, restrictive/dilated cardiomyopathy, cirrhosis, metallic or bronze skin, hypogonadism, ED • Elevated serum ferritin → elevated transferrin saturation and serum iron → genetic testing → liver testing • Phlebotomy is mainstay of treatment

Polycythemia Vera

Etiology & Risk Factors	• **Acquired myeloproliferative disorder characterized by an increased production of normal red cells, white cells and platelets** • <u>Etiology</u>: **mutation in the Janus kinase-2 (JAK2) gene** • <u>Risk Factors</u>: **male, age (>60 years old most common)**, family history, prior history of blood disorders
Patho-physiology	• Overproduction of red blood cells, white blood cells, and platelets caused by a mutation in the JAK2 gene which leads to the activation of the JAK-STAT signaling pathway • The abnormal signaling pathway promotes uncontrolled proliferation and survival of blood cells in the bone marrow, resulting in an increased number of mature and functional blood cells in circulation

Signs & Symptoms	• Symptoms related to hyperviscosity and thrombosis (impaired oxygenation); may often be asymptomatic
	• <u>Hyperviscosity</u>: headache, dizziness, tinnitus, blurry vision, lightheadedness, fatigue, weakness, insomnia, claudication, early satiety
	  • **Aquagenic Pruritus**: pruritus after a hot bath or shower (due to a histamine surge from mast cell and basophil degranulation)
	• <u>Thrombosis</u>: symptoms at the affected site
	  • Neurologic deficits (stroke or TIA), leg pain or swelling (DVT), dyspnea (PE), unilateral vision loss (retinal vascular occlusion)
	• <u>Erythromelalgia</u>: burning/throbbing pain in the hands and feet with erythema or pallor
	• <u>Other</u>: **hepatosplenomegaly**, facial plethora (flushed face) may be present

Diagnosis	• <u>Complete Blood Count (CBC)</u>:
	  • **Elevated Hemoglobin**: >16.5g/dL in men or >16.0g/dL in women
	  • **Elevated Hematocrit (Hct)**: >49% in men or >48% in women
	  • **Increased RBC Mass**: >25% above mean normal predicted
	• <u>Bone Marrow Biopsy</u>: hypercellularity; prominent erythroid, granulocytic, and megakaryocytic proliferation
	• <u>Genetic Testing</u>: testing for JAK2 gene mutation
	• <u>Serum Erythropoietin Level</u>: **decreased** level below the reference range

Treatment	• <u>Phlebotomy</u>: **mainstay of treatment**
	  • Goal of treatment is hematocrit < 45% in men and < 42% in women
	• <u>Aspirin</u>: indicated for symptomatic treatment; alleviates symptoms of microvascular events (erythromelalgia)
	  • *Does not reduce the incidence of macrovascular events*
	• <u>Myelosuppressive Therapy</u>: interferon alfa or ruxolitinib is preferred
	  • <u>Interferon Alfa</u>: specifically targets the affected cell and not normal stem cells
	  • <u>Ruxolitinib</u>: nonspecific JAK inhibitor
	  • *Alkylating agents such as chlorambucil and hydroxyurea can increase the incidence of acute leukemia and solid tumors and are no longer recommended*
	• <u>Antihistamines</u>: indicated for pruritus

Myelodysplastic Syndrome

Etiology & Risk Factors	• **Acquired clonal pre-leukemic disorder of hematopoietic stem cells**, leading to hypercellular marrow, abnormal cell morphology, and **pancytopenia** • Etiology: idiopathic; may involve a combination of genetic, environmental, and immune dysregulation factors • Risk Factors: **advanced age (>65 years old most common)**, radiation exposure, chemical exposure (benzene, pesticides, industrial chemicals, mercury, lead), previous chemotherapy (hydroxyurea), smoking, certain genetic factors
Patho-physiology	• Mutations of hematopoietic stem cells results in ineffective and dysplastic hematopoiesis as bone marrow becomes crowded with abnormal and dysfunctional cells leading to cytopenia in one or more lineages; abnormal bone marrow cells may have a higher risk of transformation into acute myeloid leukemia (AML) in some cases

Signs & Symptoms	• May be asymptomatic
	• **Symptoms reflect the most affected cell line**
	  • **Thrombocytopenia: mucocutaneous bleeding** (epistaxis, bleeding gums, petechia, purpura), easy bruising, menorrhagia
	  • **Anemia: fatigue, weakness, pallor**, shortness of breath, reduced exercise tolerance, tachycardia, dizziness or lightheadedness, cognitive impairment
	  • **Neutropenia**: frequent or recurrent infections, sudden onset fever

Diagnosis	• **Complete Blood Count (CBC) with Platelets and Peripheral Blood Smear**: decreased numbers of one or more cell lines (red cells, platelets or neutrophils)
	  • Thrombocytopenia: platelets may be larger in size and lack granules
	  • Anemia: marked normocytic or macrocytic anemia
	  • Neutropenia: commonly with abnormal neutrophil morphology (hypogranular and hyposegmented neutrophils)
	  • Peripheral Blood Smear: may contain myeloblasts
	• **Bone Marrow Biopsy: required for diagnosis**; may be normal or hypercellular
	  • **Dysplastic bone marrow is hallmark** (abnormal morphology and maturation of various cell lineages, including erythrocytes, granulocytes, and megakaryocytes)
	  • Increased blasts (but <20%)

Treatment	• **Supportive Care**: may require chronic blood and platelet transfusions • **Erythrocyte-Stimulating Agents (ESA): erythropoietin**; may be used in low-risk patients with mild pancytopenia • Thalidomide Derivatives: lenalidomide; may be indicated in patients with symptomatic anemia with deletion 5q syndrome • Pyrimidine Analogues: azacitidine and decitabine; may allow differentiation of blasts into mature cells and induce remission • **Allogenic Hematopoietic Stem Cell Transplantation: only effective curative treatment**; indicated in younger, medically fit patients
Key Words & Most Common	• Acquired disorder of hematopoietic stem cells leading to pancytopenia • Advanced age, chemical and radiation exposure greatest risk factors • Symptoms of thrombocytopenia, anemia, neutropenia • CBC shows decreased numbers of 1+ cell lines → bone marrow biopsy shows dysplastic bone marrow • Allogenic stem cell transplant only effective cure

Multiple Myeloma

Etiology & Risk Factors	• **Clonal plasma cell proliferation disorder that produces ineffective monoclonal antibodies (especially IgG and IgA) that invade and destroy bone tissue** • Etiology: not fully understood; may be related to chromosomal and genetic factors and radiation or chemical exposure • Risk Factors: **males, age (>65 years old most common), African-American descent**, family history, radiation exposure, exposure to certain chemicals (**benzene** and herbicides)
Patho-physiology	• Abnormal plasma cells accumulate in the bone marrow, interrupt the normal cell production and form tumors; the malignant plasma cells produce excessive amounts of abnormal antibodies, which can lead to bone damage, kidney dysfunction, and suppressed immune function

Signs & Symptoms	• **Bone Involvement: most common sign/symptom**; caused by plasma cell proliferation in bone marrow
	  • **Bone Pain: most commonly involves back, ribs**, extremities; worse with movement
	  • **Pathologic Fractures**: due to osteolytic lesions and osteopenia
	• **Renal Impairment**: due to light-chain protein deposition in kidneys
	  • **Elevated BUN and creatinine**, hypercalcemia, vulnerability to nephrotoxic agents
	• **Hematologic**: due to plasma cell infiltration in marrow
	  • **Anemia Symptoms**: fatigue, weakness pallor, weight loss, hepatosplenomegaly
	• Neurologic: spinal cord compression due to vertebral fracture or collapse; paresthesias, peripheral neuropathy, radiculopathy
	• **Infection**: most common cause of death; due to leukopenia and ineffective antibody production

Diagnosis	• **Complete Blood Count (CBC) with Peripheral Blood Smear**: normocytic-normochromic anemia • **Rouleaux Formation**: RBCs with a "stack of coins" appearance due to increased plasma protein • Labs: basic metabolic panel (**elevated BUN and creatinine**), elevated LDH, elevated beta-2 microglobulin, and elevated serum uric acid level; hypercalcemia • **Serum Protein Electrophoresis**: identifies **monoclonal (M-protein) spike (IgG most common; IgA)** • Urine Protein Electrophoresis: Bence-Jones proteins (large, waxy, laminated casts due to free monoclonal light-chain proteins) • Skeletal Survey: x-rays of skull, long bones, spine, pelvis, and ribs; demonstrate **"punched-out" lytic lesions** or diffuse osteoporosis • **Bone Marrow Biopsy: definitive diagnosis**; demonstrates sheets or clusters of plasma cells (**plasmacytosis**)

Treatment	• Autologous Stem Cell Transplanation: preferred therapy for stable patients who have adequate cardiac, hepatic, pulmonary, and renal function
	• Allogeneic Stem Cell Transplantation: performed after nonmyeloablative chemotherapy (low-dose cyclophosphamide and fludarabine) or low-dose radiation therapy
	  • *Experimental therapy that may produce myeloma-free survival of 5-10 years in some patients*
	• Chemotherapy: may temporarily alleviate symptoms
	  • Immunomodulatory drugs (thalidomide, lenalidomide, pomalidomide), proteasome inhibitors (bortezomib, carfilzomib, ixazomib), targeted therapy (monoclonal antibodies; daratumumab or elotuzumab)
	• Treat Underlying Complications: anemia, hypercalcemia, hyperuricemia, infection

Acute Lymphocytic Leukemia (ALL) 🝆

Etiology & Risk Factors	• Malignancy of B or T lymphoblasts characterized by uncontrolled proliferation of abnormal, immature lymphocytes • Etiology: not fully understood; combination of genetic and environmental factors • Risk Factors: **males, age (2-5 years old most common)**, certain genetic syndromes (**Down syndrome**), exposure to ionizing radiation, chemical exposures (benzene, pesticides)
Patho-physiology	• Dysregulation of signaling pathways, genetic alterations, impaired immune responses contribute to changes in hematopoietic stem cell DNA that leads to the disruption of normal cell development and maturation and promotes uncontrolled growth • Blasts (abnormal immature lymphocytes), accumulate in the bone marrow and suppress the production of normal blood cells, resulting in bone marrow failure

Signs & Symptoms	• **Pancytopenia**: nonspecific symptoms that reflect the most affected cell line
	  • **Thrombocytopenia**: mucocutaneous bleeding (epistaxis, bleeding gums, petechia, purpura), easy bruising, menorrhagia
	  • **Anemia**: fatigue, weakness, pallor, shortness of breath, reduced exercise tolerance, tachycardia, dizziness or lightheadedness, cognitive impairment
	  • **Neutropenia**: frequent or recurrent infections, sudden onset fever
	• **Organ Infiltration by Leukemic Cells**:
	  • **Liver Infiltration: hepatosplenomegaly**, abdominal pain/distention, anorexia
	  • **Lymph Node Infiltration**: lymphadenopathy
	  • **Bone Marrow and Periosteal Infiltration**: bone and joint pain (bone marrow and periosteal infiltration)
	  • **CNS and Meningeal Infiltration**: cranial nerve palsies, headache, visual or auditory symptoms, altered mental status, and transient ischemic attack/stroke

Diagnosis	• **Complete Blood Count (CBC) with Platelets and Peripheral Blood Smear**:
	  • **Pancytopenia**: thrombocytopenia, anemia, neutropenia (WBC 5,000-100,000)
	  • **Peripheral Smear: blast cells** may approach 90% of WBC count
	• **Bone Marrow Biopsy: definitive diagnosis; hypercellular with >20% blast cells** (typically 25-95%)

Treatment	• **Combination Chemotherapy: highly responsive (remission achieved in >85% of cases); 4 phases**
	  • Induction Chemotherapy: corticosteroids (dexamethasone, prednisone), anthracycline (daunorubicin, doxorubicin, idarubicin), vincristine to achieve remission
	  • Post-Remission Consolidation: combination of chemotherapy medication to prevent leukemic regrowth
	  • Interim Maintenance and Intensification: less intense combination of chemotherapy
	  • Maintenance Therapy: regimens include monthly vincristine, weekly methotrexate, daily mercaptopurine, and 5 days/month corticosteroid
	• **CNS Prophylaxis and Treatment: intrathecal methotrexate**, cytarabine, hydrocortisone used in combination or as monotherapy

Key Words & Most Common	• Malignancy of B or T lymphoblasts • Most common in children ages 2-5 years old and males • Pancytopenia + organ infiltration symptoms • Blast cells >20% on bone marrow biopsy • Combination chemotherapy

Chronic Lymphocytic Leukemia (CLL) 🝆

Etiology & Risk Factors	• **Chronic lymphoproliferative disorder characterized by monoclonal B cell proliferation** • Etiology: not fully understood; combination of genetic and environmental factors • Risk Factors: **males, advanced age (70 years old average age of diagnosis)**, family history, exposure to certain chemicals (**benzene**, herbicides), radiation exposure, smoking, certain ethnicities (Caucasians, Jews of Eastern European descent)
Patho-physiology	• Malignant transformation of CD5+ B cells; starts with monoclonal B-cell lymphocytosis and progresses as genetic abnormalities accumulate leading to CLL • CLL characterized by accumulation of abnormal lymphocytes in bone marrow, lymph nodes, and lymphoid tissues, resulting in organ enlargement and systemic symptoms

Signs & Symptoms	• **Often asymptomatic at time of presentation**
	• **Nonspecific Symptoms**: fatigue, weakness, anorexia, weight loss, fever, and/or **night sweats**
	• Physical Exam:
	  • **Lymphadenopathy: cervical, supraclavicular, and axillary lymph nodes most commonly involved**; lymph nodes are firm, non-tender, round, and freely mobile
	  • Splenomegaly and hepatomegaly are less common

Diagnosis	• **Complete Blood Count (CBC) with Platelets and Peripheral Blood Smear**:
	  • **Lymphocytosis: absolute peripheral lymphocytosis of >5000/mcL**
	  • **Peripheral Smear**: small, well-differentiated, normal-appearing lymphocytes with **"smudge cells"** (fragile cells that are disrupted during preparation of glass slide)
	• Peripheral Blood Flow Cytometry: confirms clonality in circulating B cells; lymphocytes express CD5 (B cell maturity), CD19, CD20, CD23, and kappa or lambda light chains
	• Other: hypogammaglobulinemia, elevated lactate dehydrogenase (LDH), elevated uric acid, elevated liver enzymes, and hypercalcemia
	• Bone Marrow Biopsy: not required for diagnosis; demonstrates >30% lymphocytes

Treatment	• **Observation**: indicated in indolent, asymptomatic patients; treatment held until patient becomes symptomatic or progressive lymphocytosis occurs • **Chemotherapy**: various chemotherapy regimens including **fludarabine**, cyclophosphamide, and rituximab; indicated in symptomatic or progressive cases • Targeted Therapy: ibrutinib and venetoclax; agents that specifically target the B-cell receptor signaling pathway • Immunotherapy: monoclonal antibodies (rituximab, obinutuzumab, ofatumumab) may be used to enhance the immune response and transiently palliate symptoms • Allogenic Stem Cell Transplantation: treatment considered in younger, medically fit patients
Key Words & Most Common	• Chronic lymphoproliferative disorder • Most common in males of advanced age • Often asymptomatic → nonspecific symptoms (fatigue, anorexia, weight loss) • Lymphadenopathy (cervical, supraclavicular, axillary) is most common finding • Absolute lymphocytosis of >5000/mcL • Peripheral smear shows "smudge cells" • Observation → chemotherapy

Acute Myeloid Leukemia (AML) 🩸

Etiology & Risk Factors	• Hematopoietic neoplasm characterized by **clonal proliferation of immature "blast cells" in the peripheral blood and bone marrow** resulting in ineffective erythropoiesis and bone marrow failure; **most common acute leukemia in adults** • <u>Etiology</u>: not fully understood; combination of genetic and environmental factors • <u>Risk Factors</u>: **history of myelodysplastic syndrome is most common risk factor, advanced age (68 years old average age of diagnosis)**, certain genetic syndromes (**Down syndrome**), radiation exposure, chemical exposure (benzene, pesticides/herbicides), smoking, previous treatment with chemotherapy
Patho-physiology	• Hematopoietic neoplasm characterized by the uncontrolled growth and accumulation of immature myeloid cells (blasts) resulting from genetic mutations that disrupt the normal processes of cell differentiation, proliferation, and apoptosis • Accumulation of these leukemic blasts (immature white blood cells cells) interferes with the production of normal blood cells, leading to pancytopenia

Signs & Symptoms	• <u>Pancytopenia</u>: nonspecific symptoms that reflect the most affected cell line
	  • <u>Thrombocytopenia</u>: **mucocutaneous bleeding** (epistaxis, bleeding gums, petechia, purpura), easy bruising, menorrhagia
	  • <u>Anemia</u>: **fatigue, weakness, pallor**, shortness of breath, reduced exercise tolerance, tachycardia, dizziness or lightheadedness, cognitive impairment
	  • <u>Neutropenia</u>: frequent or recurrent infections, sudden onset fever
	• <u>Organ Infiltration by Leukemic Cells</u>: **less common in AML than ALL**
	  • <u>Liver Infiltration</u>: hepatosplenomegaly, abdominal pain/distention, anorexia
	  • <u>Lymph Node Infiltration</u>: lymphadenopathy
	  • <u>Bone Marrow and Periosteal Infiltration</u>: bone and joint pain (bone marrow and periosteal infiltration)
	  • <u>CNS and Meningeal Infiltration</u>: cranial nerve palsies, headache, visual or auditory symptoms, altered mental status, and transient ischemic attack/stroke

Diagnosis	• <u>Complete Blood Count (CBC) with Platelets and Peripheral Blood Smear</u>: **best initial test**
	  • <u>Pancytopenia</u>: thrombocytopenia, normocytic normochromic anemia, neutropenia, decreased reticulocyte count
	  • <u>Peripheral Smear</u>: circulating myeloblasts may approach 90% of WBC count
	• <u>Bone Marrow Biopsy</u>: **definitive diagnosis; hypercellular with >20%** (typically 25-95%) **myeloblast cells** (immature cells with prominent nucleoli)
	• <u>Histochemical Studies</u>: staining for **myeloperoxidase** (positive in cells of myeloid origin)
	  • Crystallization of myeloperoxidase-rich granules results in formation of <u>**Auer rods**</u> **(linear pink/red rod-like granular inclusions in the cytoplasm of blast cells)**
	• <u>Other</u>: hyperuricemia, hyperphosphatemia, hyperkalemia, hypocalcemia, elevated LDH

Treatment	• <u>Combination Chemotherapy</u>: induction and consolidation indicated in medically fit patients • **Cytarabine and daunorubicin** • <u>All-*Trans* Retinoic Acid (Tretinoin)</u>: added to promyelocytic leukemia cases to correct DIC • <u>Allogenic Hematopoietic Stem Cell Transplantation</u>: **only effective curative treatment**; indicated in younger, medically fit patients

Chronic Myeloid Leukemia (CML) 🩸

Etiology & Risk Factors	• Myeloproliferative neoplasm characterized by **uncontrolled proliferation of mature and immature granulocytes** • <u>Etiology</u>: not fully understood • <u>Risk Factors</u>: **advanced age (64 years old average age of diagnosis)**, presence of the Philadelphia chromosome, exposure to high levels of radiation (medical treatments or nuclear accidents), certain genetic conditions (Down syndrome)
Patho-physiology	• Genetic abnormality known as the **Philadelphia chromosome** (Ph chromosome) which results from a reciprocal translocation between chromosomes 9 and 22 • BCR-ABL fusion gene produces a constitutively active tyrosine kinase that drives the uncontrolled growth and proliferation of myeloid cells, leading to the accumulation of mature and immature myeloid cells in the bone marrow and peripheral blood • <u>Chronic Phase</u>: asymptomatic, indolent period lasting 5-6 years; may be detected incidentally on routine CBC • <u>Accelerated Phase</u>: neutrophil differentiation becomes more impaired and leukocyte count unable to be controlled resulting in worsening anemia, progressive thrombocytopenia, worsening splenomegaly, increasing basophils, and increasing marrow or blood blasts • <u>Blastic Crisis</u>: acute leukemia with accumulation of blasts in extramedullary sites (bone, central nervous system, lymph nodes, skin/soft tissues)

Signs & Symptoms	• Often asymptomatic early in course
	• <u>Non-Specific Symptoms</u>: **fatigue, weakness**, anorexia, **weight loss**, malaise, night sweats, abdominal fullness (splenomegaly), gouty arthritis
	  • <u>Splenomegaly</u>: **most common finding**
	  • <u>Aquagenic Pruritus</u>: pruritus after a hot bath or shower (due to a histamine surge from mast cell and basophil degranulation)

Diagnosis	• <u>Complete Blood Count (CBC) with Platelets and Peripheral Blood Smear</u>: best initial test
	  • <u>CBC</u>: marked leukocytosis with granulocytic cells (neutrophilia, **basophilia**, eosinophilia); **may be 200,000-1,000,000/mcL in symptomatic patients**
	  • <u>Platelets</u>: normal or moderately increased; thrombocytopenia present in accelerated phase
	  • <u>Peripheral Smear</u>: immature granulocytes, absolute eosinophilia and basophilia
	• <u>Bone Marrow Biopsy</u>: granulocytic hyperplasia, blasts (chronic = <5%; accelerated 5-30%; blastic crisis >20%)
	• <u>Genetic Testing</u>: **Philadelphia chromosome; cytogenetic analysis, fluorescent *in situ* hybridization (FISH), and/or reverse transcriptase-polymerase chain reaction (RT-PCR)**

Treatment	• <u>Tyrosine Kinase Inhibitors</u>: **imatinib**, nilotinib, dasatinib; **initial treatment of choice**
	  • Inhibit the *BCR-ABL* oncogene on the Philadelphia chromosome
	  • Effective in achieving complete hematologic and cytogenetic remissions and prolong survival in cases of Philadelphia chromosome positive CML
	• <u>Hematopoietic Stem Cell Transplantation</u>: **only effective curative treatment**; indicated in younger, medically fit patients

Key Words & Most Common	• Myeloproliferative disorder with uncontrolled proliferation of granulocytes • Presence of Philadelphia chromosome • Non-specific symptoms + splenomegaly + aquagenic pruritus • Marked leukocytosis with granulocytic cells • Tyrosine kinase inhibitors (imatinib) are initial treatment of choice • Hematopoietic stem cell transplant in select patients

Hodgkin Lymphoma

Etiology & Risk Factors	• Localized or disseminated malignant proliferation of B-cells of the lymphoreticular system • <u>Etiology</u>: not fully understood; combination of genetic and environmental factors • <u>Risk Factors</u>: age **(most common 15-40 years old and >55 years old)**; males, immunosuppression, **Epstein-Barr virus infection**, family history
Patho-physiology	• Type of cancer originating in the lymphatic system involving abnormal growth and proliferation of large, malignant cells derived from B-lymphocytes (Reed-Sternberg cells) • These cells interact with surrounding immune cells and cytokines, creating a microenvironment that contributes to the characteristic inflammatory response

Signs & Symptoms	• <u>**Painless Cervical Lymphadenopathy**</u>**: most common presentation**
	   • **Pain in lymph nodes occurs with alcohol consumption within minutes** (paraneoplastic symptom)
	• <u>Systemic "B" Symptoms</u>: may signify involvement of internal lymph nodes (mediastinal or retroperitoneal), viscera (liver), or bone marrow
	   • **Fever, night sweats, loss of appetite resulting in unintentional weight loss (> 10% of body weight in previous 6 months)**
	   • **Splenomegaly**; hepatomegaly is unusual
	   • <u>**Pel-Ebstein Fever**</u>: cyclical fever lasting for a few days alternating with a few days to several weeks of normal to below-normal temperatures
	   • Cachexia in advanced disease

Diagnosis	• <u>**Excisional Whole Lymph Node Biopsy**</u>**: definitive diagnosis; demonstrates Reed-Sternberg cells** • <u>**Reed-Sternberg Cells**</u>**: large, binucleated cells** with an "owl eye appearance", and nucleoli inclusions • <u>Labs</u>: workup includes complete blood count (CBC), complete metabolic panel (CMP), erythrocyte sedimentation rate (ESR), Hepatitis B virus, hepatitis C virus, LDH, HIV • <u>Imaging</u>: staging of disease with combined chest x-ray, CT chest/abdomen/pelvis, and PET/CT scans
Treatment	• <u>**Limited Stage Disease**</u>**: limited chemotherapy regimen** (doxorubicin, bleomycin, vinblastine, and dacarbazine) **with or without radiation therapy** • <u>**Advanced Stage**</u>**: combination chemotherapy regiment** (bleomycin, etoposide, doxorubicin, cyclophosphamide, vincristine, procarbazine, and prednisone) • <u>Hematopoietic Stem Cell Transplantation</u>: considered for patients with aggressive or recurrent disease
Key Words & Most Common	• Malignant proliferation of B-cells in lymphoreticular system • Bimodal distribution (15-40 years old and >55 years old) • Associated with Epstein-Barr virus infection • Painless cervical lymphadenopathy • <u>"B" Symptoms</u>: fever, night sweats, weight loss, splenomegaly • Excisional lymph node biopsy demonstrates Reed-Sternberg cells (large, binucleated cells) • Chemotherapy

Non-Hodgkin Lymphoma

Etiology & Risk Factors	• **Malignant monoclonal proliferation of lymphoid cells in lymphoreticular sites (lymph nodes bone marrow and spleen)** • <u>Etiology</u>: not fully understood; combination of genetic and environmental factors • <u>Risk Factors</u>: **age (>60 years old most common)**, immunosuppression, **certain infections (HIV, HCV, EBV, HHV-8, *H. pylori*)**, family history, chemical exposure (pesticides, solvents, herbicides), radiation exposure, **certain autoimmune disorders** (RA, SLE, Sjögren's syndrome, Hashimoto thyroiditis), obesity
Patho-physiology	• Malignancy arising from either from B cells (most common), T cells, or natural killer cells due to chromosomal translocation or mutation/deletion • Malignant monoclonal proliferation of abnormal lymphocytes leads to the formation of tumor masses in lymph nodes, spleen, bone marrow, and other lymphoid tissues • <u>Diffuse Large B-cell Lymphoma (DLBCL)</u>: most common subtype; characterized by aggressive, rapidly growing B-cell lymphomas arising in various parts of the body • <u>Follicular Lymphoma</u>: second most common subtype; characterized by slow-growing B-cell lymphomas that typically form small clusters of cells called follicles • <u>Mantle Cell Lymphoma</u>: rare subtype arising from B-cells in the mantle zone of lymph nodes • <u>Marginal Zone Lymphoma</u>: subtype involving B-cells that develop from the marginal zone of lymphoid tissues • <u>3 Subtypes</u>: extranodal marginal zone lymphoma (MALT lymphoma), nodal marginal zone lymphoma, and splenic marginal zone lymphoma • <u>Burkitt Lymphoma</u>: rapidly growing subtype arising from B-cells and is associated with genetic changes; associated with EBV • <u>T-Cell Lymphomas</u>: subtypes involving malignant transformation of T-cells

Signs & Symptoms	• <u>**Local**</u>**: painless peripheral lymphadenopathy is most common presenting symptom**
	   • Cervical, axillary, inguinal, and femoral most common location
	   • Waxing and waning episodes of lymphadenopathy
	• <u>**Extranodal Involvement**</u>:
	   • <u>**Gastrointestinal Tract**</u>**: most common extranodal site**; epigastric pain, anorexia, weight loss, nausea/vomiting, GI bleeding, early satiety
	   • <u>Cutaneous</u>: slightly raised, erythematous nodules of scalp or legs; hypersensitivity reactions to insect bites, generalized fatigue, pruritus
	   • <u>Central Nervous System</u>: headache, lethargy, focal neurologic deficits, seizures, paralysis, spinal cord compression, lymphomatous meningitis
	• <u>**Systemic "B" Symptoms**</u>: may signify involvement of internal lymph
	   • **Fever, night sweats, loss of appetite resulting in unintentional weight loss**

Diagnosis	• <u>**Excisional Whole Lymph Node Biopsy**</u>**: gold standard for diagnosis; required for classification of NHL** • <u>Imaging</u>: staging of disease with combined chest x-ray, CT chest/abdomen/pelvis, and PET/CT scans
Treatment	• <u>**Limited Stage Disease**</u>**: observation in asymptomatic cases**; external beam radiation therapy, combination chemotherapy with or without radiation therapy • <u>**Advanced Stage**</u>**: combination chemotherapy regiment** • <u>R-CHOP</u>: <u>R</u>ituximab plus <u>C</u>yclophosphamide, <u>H</u>ydroxydaunorubicin (doxorubicin), <u>O</u>ncovorin (vincristine), and <u>P</u>rednisone • <u>Hematopoietic Stem Cell Transplantation</u>: considered for patients with aggressive or recurrent disease

Works Cited

1. Rouleaux formation.jpg. (2020, October 8). *Wikimedia Commons*. Retrieved 16:28, July 9, 2023 from https://commons.wikimedia.org/w/index.php?title=File:Rouleaux_formation.jpg&oldid=484427634.
2. Red cell agglutination.jpg. (2020, August 28). *Wikimedia Commons*. Retrieved 16:35, July 9, 2023 from https://commons.wikimedia.org/w/index.php?title=File:Red_cell_agglutination.jpg&oldid=444491492.
3. Corps de Howell-Jolly-3.JPG. (2020, October 25). *Wikimedia Commons*. Retrieved 16:35, July 9, 2023 from https://commons.wikimedia.org/w/index.php?title=File:Corps_de_Howell-Jolly-3.JPG&oldid=500933243.
4. Cabot ring and basophilic stippling.jpg. (2022, October 30). *Wikimedia Commons*. Retrieved 20:21, July 9, 2023
   from https://commons.wikimedia.org/w/index.php?title=File:Cabot_ring_and_basophilic_stippling.jpg&oldid=700571170.
5. Crenated Red Cells.jpg. (2020, October 20). *Wikimedia Commons*. Retrieved 20:24, July 9, 2023 from https://commons.wikimedia.org/w/index.php?title=File:Crenated_Red_Cells.jpg&oldid=495108154.
6. Acanthocytes, Peripheral Blood (3884092551).jpg. (2023, July 4). *Wikimedia Commons*. Retrieved 20:28, July 9, 2023
   from https://commons.wikimedia.org/w/index.php?title=File:Acanthocytes,_Peripheral_Blood_(3884092551).jpg&oldid=780375199.
7. Target cells.jpg. (2020, October 30). *Wikimedia Commons*. Retrieved 20:29, July 9, 2023 from https://commons.wikimedia.org/w/index.php?title=File:Target_cells.jpg&oldid=507429690.
8. Sphérocytes-5.JPG. (2020, October 4). *Wikimedia Commons*. Retrieved 20:31, July 9, 2023 from https://commons.wikimedia.org/w/index.php?title=File:Sph%C3%A9rocytes-5.JPG&oldid=480374860.

F

G

H

Made in the USA
Middletown, DE
16 October 2023

40884220R00298